Organic Chemistry

[Volume 2]

AF659326

Anupa Saha
Anup Pathak

CELEBRATING 60 YEARS 1960-2020

Since BOOKS AND ALLIED 1960

[*Meant for Chemistry Hons./Major (CBCS) & Pharmacy students. Also useful to NET, SLET, GATE, IIT–JEE candidates*]

Organic Chemistry

[Volume 2]

Dr. Anupa Saha, M.Sc., Ph.D.
Assistant Professor, Chemistry Dept., Scottish Church College

Dr. Anup Pathak, M.Sc., Ph.D.
Associate Professor, Chemistry Dept., Bagnan College

BOOKS & ALLIED (P) LTD.

NO.1-E(1) "SHUBHAM PLAZA" (1st Floor)
83/1, BELIAGHATA MAIN ROAD, KOLKATA 700010 (INDIA)
Tel : (033)23740062, 8274085530
e-mail : booksandallied1960@gmail.com, booksmktng@gmail.com

Organic Chemistry

[Volume 2]

First Published : August 2013
Reprinted : 2015, 2017
Reprinted : 2021

Publisher : Ruba Sen
BOOKS & ALLIED (P) LTD.
8/1 Chintamoni Das Lane, Kolkata 700009

Typesetter : BOOKS & ALLIED (P) LTD.
8/1 Chintamoni Das Lane, Kolkata 700009

Printer : EUREKA
91/A, Baithakkhana Road, Kolkata 700009

Project Supervisor : Sukumar Patra

ISBN **978-81-87134-16-9**

***Price* : ₹ 675.00**

Preface to the First Edition

It has been almost two years since the publication of the First Volume of *Organic Chemistry*. The First Volume is in its 2nd Edition now and the praise heaped on us by students and scholars have more than made up for the hard labour required to prepare the book.

For quite some time now, we had been working on the Second Volume which includes reaction and mechanism based Chemistry on aromatic electrophilic and nucleophilic substitution, Carbonyl Compounds, Organonitrogen Compounds, Organometallic compounds and Spectroscopy comprising of UV, IR and ^{1}HNMR Spectroscopy with detailed text materials and a large number of solved problems. A close analysis of the books available in the market shows that no other text addresses the needs of students and scholars alike as this text. We have taken all measures to ensure the continuation of the high standard set by the First Volume. The focus, as before, has been to prepare a text that will not only provide suitable guidelines to students preparing for their examination but also arouse the intellectual curiosity of readers who wish to further pursue this fascinating branch of Organic Chemistry.

We, the authors, take moral responsibility of any shortcomings that this book might have while the credit for all its positive aspects go to all who inspired us in a million ways.

It will be impossible to acknowledge all people without whose help this book would not have seen the light of the day. Any omission in print is regretted, but we assure that their contributions and help will forever remain etched in our mind.

It would be injustice on our part to forget the contribution of some people, however, who have been an integral part of this book. We specially acknowledge the contributions made by Mr. Arunabha Sen, Managing Director of Books & Allied (P) Ltd., Mr. Sukumar Patra, Mr. Pradip Sen and Mr. Amit Kumar Ganguly of the publishing house. We also acknowledge our family members, friends, colleagues and elders who continuously inspired us to write the Second Volume. If students and scholars benefit from the book, we will consider it to be compensation enough for our hard work.

The 15th April, 2013

Authors

Contents

Chapter 1	**Spectroscopy**	**1–106**
	UV-VIS Spectroscopy	2-31
	IR spectroscopy	32-64
	NMR spectroscopy	65-106
Chapter 2	**Chemistry of Carbonyl Compounds**	**107–308**
	α,β-unsaturated carbonyl	308-322
	Quinones	322-332
	Enolates and enamines	332-346
	Tautomerism	346-372
	Carboxylic acids and their derivatives	373-453
	Alcohols and ethers	454-522
	Organometallic Compounds	523-587
Chapter 3	**Aromatic Electrophilic and Nucleophilic Substitution**	**589–673**
	Phenols	674-736
	Amines and diazonium compounds	737-824
	Nitroalkanes and alkylnitrites	825-838
	Aromatic nitro and nitroso compounds	838-857
	Alkyl nitrites and isonitriles	857-870
Chapter 4	**Aromatic Polynuclear Hydrocarbons**	**871–917**
	Naphthalene	871-888
	Anthracene	888-901
	Phenanthrene	901-917
	Index	**(i)-(viii)**

1 Spectroscopy

Spectroscopy

Spectroscopy is the method or means for calibration of energy of an excited system *i.e.*, a compound in excited state under the influence of an external energy by an instrument, in the form of light energy.

Classification : Spectroscopy can be divided into two broad heads:

(i) Emission Spectroscopy

(ii) Absorption Spectroscopy

(i) Emission Spectroscopy : An emission spectrum is obtained by spectroscopic analysis of some light source such as a flame or of an electric arc. This phenomenon is preliminarily caused by excitation of an atom by thermal or electrical means. The absorbed energy causes the electrons in ground state to be promoted to a higher energy level. The life time of such excited electrons is metastable *i.e.*, very short, and they return to some lower energy state, and as it happens, the absorbed energy is released as "light", the measurement of which demonstrates the **emission spectroscopy**.

Examples : **Fluorescent light** and **colours obtained in a flame during flame test** when inorganic salts are heated directly in to the flame are the examples of **emission spectra**.

Phosphorescence : In some cases the electrons promoted to a higher energy level due to excitation, are some what more stable than the metastable state and return to the lower energy level at a very slower rate even though the source of energy is removed. For such cases, the radiation occurs for a longer period and the phenomenon is termed as "**Phosphorescence**".

Example : Some barium salts show radiation for a much longer time, thus glow even in darkness: $Ba_3(PO_4)_2$.

(ii) Absorption Spectroscopy : An absorption spectrum is obtained by placing a substance between the spectrometer and the source of light that provides electromagnetic radiation in the frequency range being studied. The spectrometer analyses the transmitted energy relative to incident energy for given frequency and produces **absorption spectra**.

Absorption spectroscopy may be divided into **six** major heads:

(a) Ultraviolet-Visible (UV-VIS)

(b) Infra Red (IR)

(c) Nuclear Magnetic Resonance (NMR)

(d) Mass Spectroscopy

(e) Raman Spectroscopy

(f) Electron Spin Resonance (ESR)

Description of spectrometers

1. A source of radiation of appropriate frequency (a UV lamp or IR lamp or a radio frequency transmitter etc.)
2. A sample holder to permit efficient irradiation of the sample.
3. A frequency analyser which separates out all the individual frequencies generated by the source.
4. A detector for measuring the intensity of radiation at each frequency allowing the measurement how much energy has been absorbed at each of these frequencies by the sample.
5. A recorder (either a pen-recorder) or a computerised data section for viewing the spectrum.

No single spectroscopic technique supplies enough information to deduce the structure of the molecule of any complexity but depending on the molecule, some methods are more helpful and amenable to analyse than others.

UV-VIS Spectroscopy

The UV-VIS spectroscopy falls under the category of "**Absorption Spectroscopy**". The absorption of ultraviolet or visible range of radiation by a molecule leads to transition among the energy of molecule and consequently shows spectra by these electronic transition in this range. For this reason, UV-VIS spectroscopy is often termed as "**Electronic spectroscopy**".

Method of expressing UV-VIS absorption

Electronic radiation (radio waves, ultraviolet, infrared, visible etc.) has properties of both of a wave and a particle. So, it is a wave occuring simultaneously in electric and magnetic fields and also a particle which consists of bunch of particles called "**quanta** or **photons**".

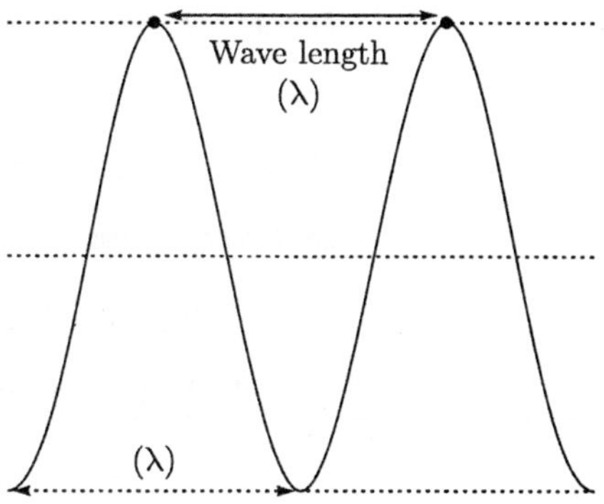

Fig. 1.1 :

Unit of a wave length is described in meter or millimeter (10^{-3} m) or micrometer (μm=10^{-6} m) or nanometer (nm=10^{-9}m). Radiation is also characterized by frequency (ν), which is number of complete cycles per second (cps).

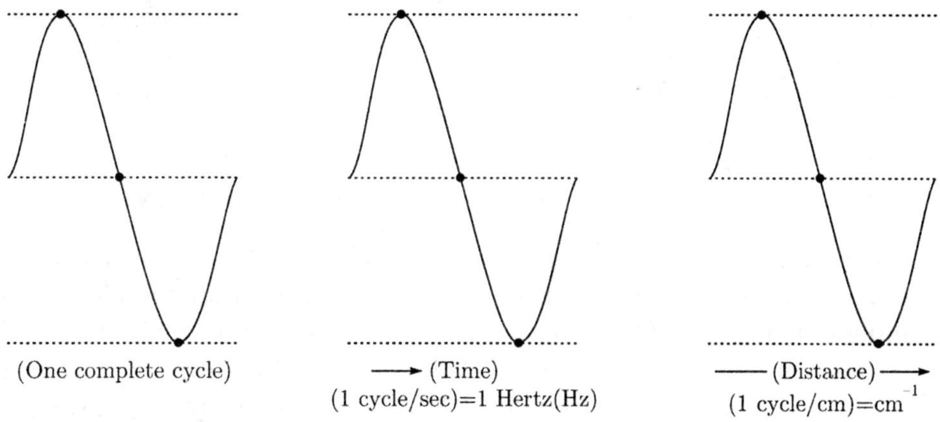

Fig. 1.2 :

$\nu=c/\lambda$ [ν=Frequency in Hz; c=Velocity of light = 3×10^{10} cm/sec;
λ=Wave length in cm]

and E=hν [Where h=Planck's constant; ν=Frequency in Hz]

therefore, $E=h\nu=h\ c/\lambda$

The higher frequency of radiation (or shorter the wavelength) the greater will be the energy and *vice versa.* So a photon of UV (Ultra violet) light (shorter wavelength, higher frequency) has more energy than a photon of visible light (longer wavelength, lower frequency).

Symbols used in ultra violet spectroscopy

Symbol	Designation/unit
ν	Frequency in Hertz (Hz) [cycles/sec]
λ	Wavelength
μm	Micrometer or micron $(\mu)=10^{-6}$ m
nm	Nanometer or milli micron $(m\mu)=10^{-9}$ m
Å	Angstrom, 10^{-1} nm
γ	Wave number, frequency in reciprocal cm (cm^{-1}), $1/\lambda$

Some terminologies

(a) **Chromophores** : Structural units which absorb radiation in the UV region and are responsible for imparting colour to a compound are known as "Chromophores". *e.g.*, C=C, C=O etc. When conjugation is present with these systems, the contributions of chromophores get largely increased to absorb at higher wavelength. These conjugated chromophores are called "**effective chromophores**". *e.g.*, Conjugated dienes and polyenes, α, β–unsaturated carbonyl compounds, arylazo compounds etc.

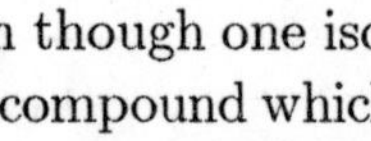, 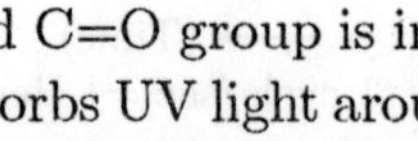, Ar—N=N—Ar

The term is retained within an extended interpretation to imply any functional group that absorbs electromagnetic radiation, whether or not a **colour** is thereby produced. Thus, C=O group is a chromophore in both ultraviolet and infrared terms, even though one isolated C=O group is insufficiently powerful to impart colour to a compound which absorbs UV light around 280 nm. Organic application of electronic spectroscopy is mainly concerned with conjugated chromophores, to a lower extent with those others that give rise to absorption above 200 nm and hardly at all with those below 200 nm.

Chromophores	Wavelength λ_{max} (nm)	Intensity ε_{max} (10^{-2} m^2 mol^{-1})
C=C	175	14000
C≡C	175	10000
	195	2000
C=O	223	18000
	160	5000
	185	15
	280	5000
RNO_2	200	5000
	274	15
Congjugated Systems		
R—C≡N	165	5
C=C—C=C	217	20000
C=C—C=O	220	10000
C=C—C≡C	315	30
	230	7500
Benzene	184, 204, 255	60000, 7400, 204

(a) **Auxochromes** : Groups which are not themselves chromophores, but when attached to a chromophores enhance the colour imparting properties, are known as "**auxochromes**". Exampls of auxochromes are as follows.

$$-\ddot{N}H_2,\ -\ddot{\underset{\cdot\cdot}{O}}H,\ -\ddot{\underset{\cdot\cdot}{X}}:,\ -\ddot{N}R_2,\ -\ddot{\underset{\cdot\cdot}{S}}R$$

(b) **Bathochromic Shift/Red shift** : Due to certain factors, if the energy of transition is decreased, so that the compound absorbs at a higher wavelength than normal one, the shift of λ_{max} is known as "Bathochromic shift or Red shift.

e.g., In alkali, *p*-nitrophenol shows a red shift in UV region.

(c) **Hypsochromic shift/Blue shift** : If the energy of transition is increased due to influence of certain factors, so that the compound absorbs at a lower wavelength than the normal λ_{max} value, the shift of wavelength is known as "Hypsochromic shift or Blue shift". *e.g.*, In acid, *p*-nitroaniline shows a strong blue shift as the lone pair on anilino nitrogen atom gets protonated in acid, so that the ground state is stabilized, and the $n \rightarrow \pi^*$ transition gets off, and the energy of transition is increased.

(d) **Hyperchromic effect** : Sometimes the presence of certain groups or by some external effects, the intensity of absorption (ε_{max}) increases. Such increase of intensity of absorption is known as **hyperchromic effect**. A hyperchromic shift of ε_{max} is observed when alkali is added to *p*-nitrophenol.

(e) **Hypochromic effect** : When presence of certain groups or by some external effects, the intensity of absorption (ε_{max}) decreases, and the effect is termed as **hypochromic effect.** A hypochromic effect is seen when N, N–dimethylaniline is treated with CH_3I to form quaternary ammonium salt, i.e., N, N, N–trimethylammonium iodide.

(f) **End Absorption** : Molecules containing O, N, S or halogens always show an absorption around or below 200-210 nm due to n $\rightarrow$ σ^* transition which increase in intensity toward shorter wavelength, though the particular compound may not show any absorption in the normal UV (>210 n.m.). Such absorption due to presence of heteroatoms in organic molecules or solvents, at one end of UV recording is known as "**End Absorption**". *e.g.*, MeOH shows n $\rightarrow$ σ^* transition: 183 nm (ε=150); Me_3N: at 227 nm (ε=900) which vanishes in aqueous solution due to protonation ($Me_3N: + H_2O \rightarrow Me_3NH^+$).

(g) **Vacuum ultraviolet** : The conventional electronic spectroscopic techniques can not be used below 200 nm, since oxygen (in the air) begins to absorb strongly there. To study the higher energy transitions below 200 nm, the entire path length must be evacuated, and for this reason, the region below 200 nm (100-200 nm) is usually referred to as **vacuum ultraviolet.** It has mainly been exploited in studying bond energies etc. and is **not usually very helpful in organic structural determination.**

Absorption of electromagnetic radiation by organic molecules

Organic molecules absorb radiation, in discrete packets of $\Delta E=h\nu$, which are called "Quanta of Energy".

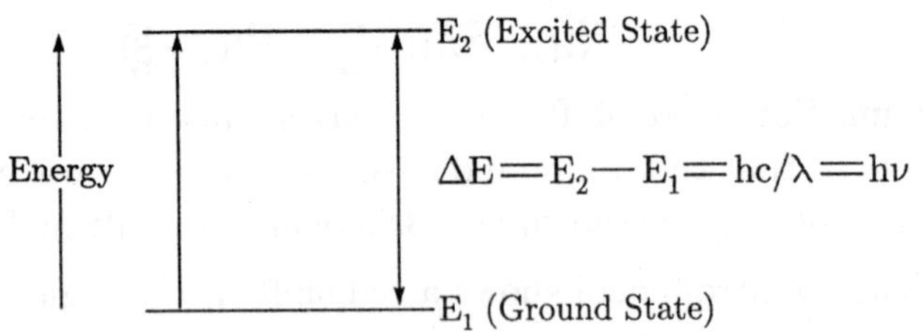

Fig. 1.3 :

ΔE for one gm mole of any molecule $=\frac{N_0hc}{\lambda}$ (N_0=Avogadro number) a molecule can only absorb a **particular frequency,** if there exists within the molecule an energy transition of magnitude $E=h\nu$.

The spectra of a compound, *i.e.* the response of a substance subjected to radiation of various wavelengths, are among the most important physical properties of an organic compound. Spectroscopy is therefore a powerful tool for structure determination of an organic molecule.

When we consider a molecule, it is found that, it is associated with several types of motion. The molecule as a whole **rotates, the bonds undergo vibrations** and even **the electrons move**. Each of these motions are quantized, *i.e.*, the molecules can exist only in distinct states which corresponds to discrete energy contents. The absorption occurs when the radiation supplies the right packet of energy to the compound under study. Each state is characterized by one or more quantum numbers and the energy difference between two such states. As ΔE is related to light frequency ν, spectroscopy is essentially a technical procedure by which the energy differences between the allowed states of a system are measured (Mapped and Recorded) by determining the frequencies of the corresponding light absorbed. The absorbed quanta of energy bring about different kinds of excitations in a molecule and each requires its own distinctive energy, ΔE. Each type of excitation motion corresponds to absorption of light in a different region of the electromagnetic spectrum. Ultraviolet and visible lights bring about movement of **valence shell electrons** typically from a filled molecular orbital (bonding and nonbonding) to an unfilled antibonding molecular orbital. This energy of transition from a bonding MO to an antibonding MO almost equals the bond energy, which is nearly 500 kJ/mol for organic molecules. The wavelength for this transition (bonding MO to antibonding MO) can be shown as follows:

$\lambda = N_0\ hc/\Delta E$, taking $\Delta E \approx 500$ kJ/mol, $\lambda = 250 \times 10^{-9}$ m = 250 nm. This falls in UV region. So an organic molecule will absorb UV radiation in the electronic level and the corresponding energy will promote one electron from occupied MO to an unoccupied MO. Generally transition occurs from HOMO to LUMO (highest occupied molecular orbital to lowest unoccupied molecular orbital) but other electronic transitions are also possible. There are some electronic transitions where ΔE for HOMO to LUMO is so small, that the energy is absorbed even in the visible region. For example, **benzil absorbs violet light and radiates yellow colour as complementary colour**.

Table

	Far UV	UV	Visible	IR
λ(nm)	50-150	200-400	400-800	2.5-15μ

When an organic molecule absorbs UV or visible light of a particular energy, as a **first approximation**, it is assumed that **only one electron** in lower level (generally form bonding or non bonding) is promoted to higher level (generally antibonding) and all other electrons remain **unaffected**.

Generally the absorption of light energy by organic molecules in UV or visible region involves promotion of electrons in the bonding σ or π and non bonding n orbitals from ground state to higher energy antibonding π^* or σ^* levels. The most probable ΔE of transition would appear to involve the promotion of one electron from **HOMO** to **LUMO** *i.e.*, to π^* or σ^* as the case may be and would be recognized as λ_{max} in the UV–VIS spectra. **As n -orbitals are nonbonding; they have no corresponding antibonding level associated with them.**

The possible transitions that can occur are:

$\sigma\rightarrow\sigma^*$,	$\sigma\rightarrow\pi^*$,	$\pi\rightarrow\pi^*$,	$\pi\rightarrow\sigma^*$,	$n\rightarrow\pi^*$,	&	$n\rightarrow\sigma^*$
$\Delta E \geq 712$ kJ		< 712 kJ		≈ 450 kJ		≤ 628 kJ
$\lambda_{max} \leq 150$ nm		170–190 nm		≈ 280 nm		185–200 nm

MO Diagram :

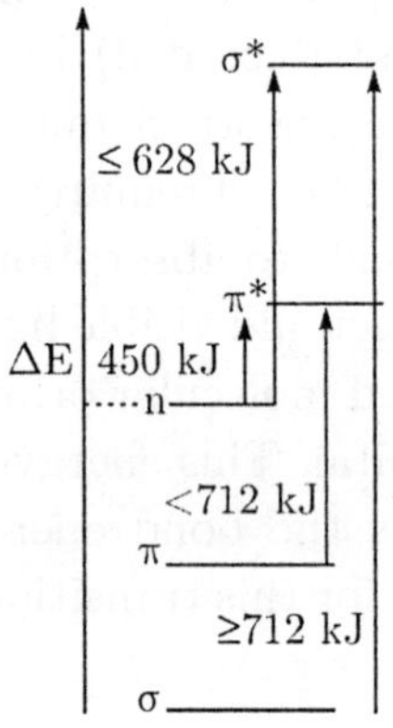

Fig. 1.4 :

From the energy difference data of bonding and antibonding MOs it is clear that normally the $n\rightarrow\pi^*$ transition if any present comes in the UV region. The other transitions like $\pi\rightarrow\pi^*$ and $n\rightarrow\sigma^*$ are very near to UV region. But due to certain reasons like resonance, hyperconjugation etc., the energy gaps diminish the λ_{max} values very much and allow entry into the UV periphery.

In summary, electronic transition in a molecule occurs when UV radiation is absorbed at its electronic level from an occupied MO to an unoccupied MO. The quantity of energy absorbed is E_2-E_1, where E_2 is the energy of the excited state and E_1 is the energy level of the ground state. So, $\Delta E=E_2-E_1=h\nu=hc/\lambda$.

This ΔE is also known as one quantum of energy, which is necessary for a "single electron transition".

Laws of Light Absorption (*Lambert and Beer's Law*) : Beer's law relates absorption to the concentration of the absorbing solution and Lambert's law relates total absorption to the optical path length. They are conveniently used as combined **Lambert–Beer's Law**.

If I_0 is the intensity of incident light passing through a cell and I is the intensity of light transmitted through the sample solution, then according to the combined law, $\log (I_0/I)=\varepsilon.c.l$ or $\varepsilon=A/c.l$

Where, **$\log (I_0/I)=A$**=absorbance of the solution formerly called optical density (O.D.) and ε is molar absorptivity, formerly known as molar extinction coefficient in l/mol/cm or $m^2mol^{-1}\times10^{-2}$ and l is path length of light through the sample in cm.

The molar absorptivity, ε, is a constant for a particular compound at a given wavelength and is most commonly expressed as ε_{max}, the molar absorptivity at an absorption band maximum. Since values for ε_{max} can be very large, an alternative convention is to quote its logarithm, $\log_{10} \varepsilon_{max}$.

The absorbance A defined as $\log I_0/I$ is recorded directly by all modern double-beam instruments.

If the molecular weight of a compound is unknown and consequently ε can not be calculated, a convenient expression used is A=a.c.l, where, 'a' is 'absorptivity', 'c' is 'concentration in g/l' and 'l' is the 'path length of the light through the sample in cm'.

Conventions : Absorption spectra in organic structure determination are most often plotted with increasing ε or log ε on the ordinate and the wavelength λ on the abscissa increasing from left to right. Some frequency units are often used on the abscissa i.e. 1/λ being plotted in similar fashion.

Meaning of $E_{1\,cm}^{x\%}$: $E_{1\,cm}^{x\%}$ means absorption $[\log_{10}(I_0/I)]$ of a x% solution in a cell with a 1cm path length. This is used in lieu of ε when the molecular weight is unknown or when a mixture is being examined.

The molar absorptivity ε is a constant for an organic compound at a given wavelength and is expressed as ε_{max}: the molar absorptivity at an absorption maximum. **ε is not dimensionless and the unit of ε is 10^{-2} m^2 mol^{-1}**. But conventionally unit is not expressed for ε. An alternative expression is to report its logarithm as $\log_{10} \varepsilon_{max}$.

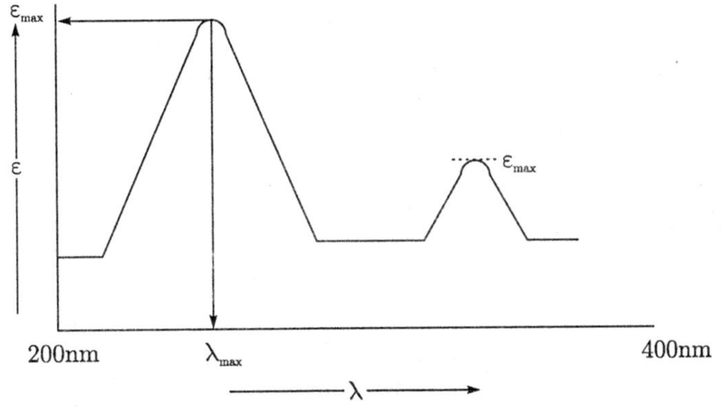

Fig. 1.5 :

UV absorption spectrum of any molecule shows a **broad band**, because there may exist more than one energy levels in rotational and vibrational energies. As a result, all the molecules either in the ground or excited states can not have a single value. So ΔE can not have a single value but, instead, can have many values very close to one another. The value of λ_{max} which are very close, often superimposes and as a result, a broad spectrum is seen. λ_{max} is calculated by choosing the electron transition from most populated energy level.

Conditions of UV absorption

(i) After absorption of UV radiation, the electron should be promoted to an unoccupied molecular orbital.

(ii) The energy difference between the excited state and ground state of electronic transition should be equal to 1(one) quantum of energy of the incident light so that $\Delta E = E_2 - E_1 = h\nu = hc/\lambda$.

(iii) **There are some restrictions regarding electronic transition.** These limitations can be evaluated from the solutions of "Group Theory". One of the limitations is due to different relative geometries of the orbitals. The probability of finding electron density along a nodal plane in an orbital is zero. So, regarding electron transition, the axis of unoccupied orbital in the excited state should not lie along the nodal plane of the ground state occupied orbital from which transition is taking place. If the axis of unoccupied orbital lies along the nodal plane of the occupied orbital, then no transition takes place from the occupied to unoccupied orbital. In other word, **no UV absorption takes place for this type of orbital orientation involved in transition and are designated as "Forbidden" transition.**

(iv) The electronic transition takes place by proper interaction with the oscillating magnetic field of radiation and a resultant change in the dipole moment occurs. The more the change in the magnitude of dipole moment, the more is the extent of absorption of UV radiation. So, we can say that the possibility of UV absorption by **symmetric molecules is quite low.**

Diagram of Elecronic Energy Levels

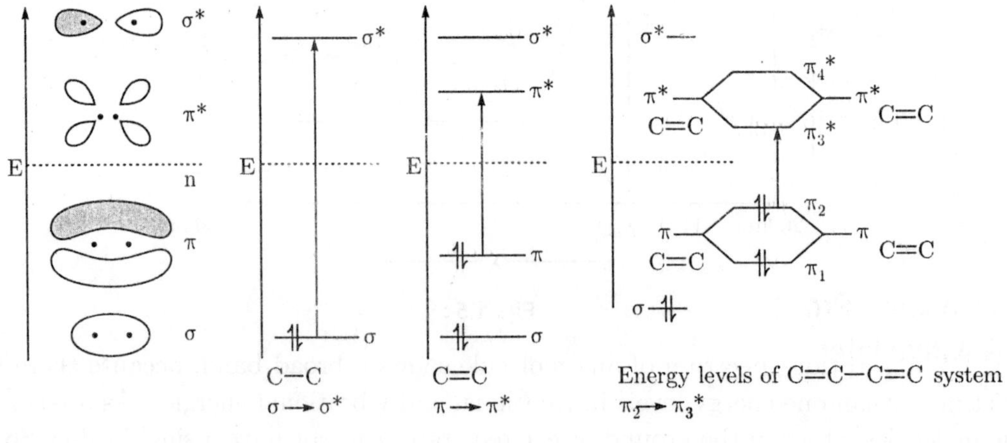

Fig. 1.6 : Relative Energies of orbitals most involved in electronic spectroscopy of organic molecules

Symmetry restrictions on the allowedness of electronic transitions

Even for the simple organic molecules, it is usually difficult to calculate the energies of the molecular orbitals that might be involved in electronic transitions, and hence in the absorption of ultraviolet or visible light; where this can be done, it is then necessary to decide which transitions are allowed and which are forbidden.

The allowedness of a transition is associated with the relationship between the geometries of the lower and higher energy molecular orbitals and the symmetry of the molecule as a whole, but the mathematics of group theory is an essential prerequisite to a full exposition of the restrictions that apply. A few qualitative generalisations may be stated which are indicators of symmetry rules that must be observed.

Symmetrical molecules (*i.e.*, molecules with a high degree of symmetry) have more restrictions on their electronic transitions than have less symmetrical molecules. As an example, benzene is highly symmetrical, having a large number of symmetry elements; many restrictions apply to the electronic transitions of the benzene molecule and therefore its electronic absorption spectrum is simple.

For a totally unsymmetrical molecule, the only symmetry operation that can be performed is the identity operation (which changes nothing). For such a molecule, no symmetry restrictions apply to the electronic transitions, so that transitions may be observed among all of its molecular orbitals except, of course, among filled orbitals; a complex electronic absorption spectrum will result.

Between these two extremes, lies the majority of organic compounds that absorb light in the ultraviolet visible region. For any of these compounds, to decide whether a transition between two given molecular orbitals is allowed or forbidden, and will give rise to **UV/visible** absorption, we must consider.

(a) The geometry of the ground state MO.

(b) The geometry of the excited state MO and

(c) The orientation of the electric dipole of the incident light that might induce the transition (when referred to the same coordinates).

Provided these three have an appropriate symmetry relationship, the transition will be allowed.

Transition Probability—Allowed and Forbidden Transitions; Relative Intensity of Absorption

The excitation of an electron may not always take place from bonding orbital or lone pair to an unoccupied antibonding or nonbonding orbital when a compound absorbs ultraviolet or visible light. The extinction coefficient, $\varepsilon_{max}=0.87\times10^{20}$ p.a. where p=*transition probability* with values from 0 to 1, and a=*Target area* of the absorbing system, *i.e.*, a chromophore. The value of ε_{max} is found to be around 10^5 when the chromophore has a length of the order 10Å or 10^{-7} cm. A chromophore with low transition probability will have $\varepsilon_{max} < 1000$. Thus there is a direct relationship between the area of the chromophore and the absorption intensity, ε_{max}. There are some other factors which also govern the transition probability. Depending upon the symmetry and the value of ε_{max}, the transitions may either be allowed or forbidden. The transitions with ε_{max} *more than* 10^4 *are* usually called allowed transitions. They generally arise due to $\pi \rightarrow \pi^*$ transition. In butadiene, the absorption at 217 nm (ε_{max}=21,000) is an allowed transition.

The forbidden transition is a result of the excitation of one electron from the lone pair present in the hetero atom to an antibonding π^* orbital. The $n \rightarrow \pi^*$ transition near

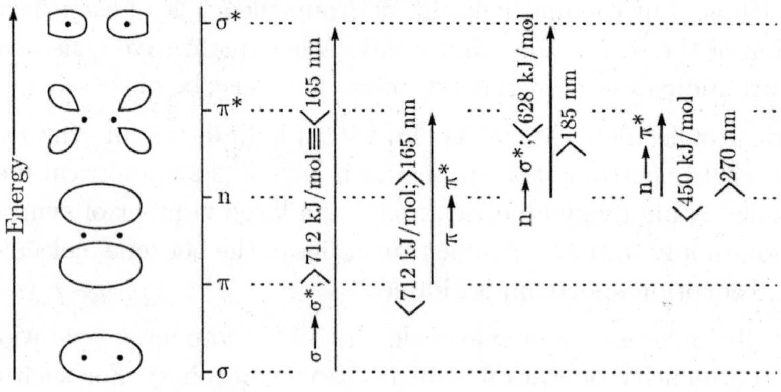

Fig. 1.7 : (MO Energy Diagram showing energy-wavelength relation for an electronic transition)

$$\Delta E_{HOMO \rightarrow LUMO\ (\sigma \rightarrow \sigma^*)} > \Delta E_{HOMO \rightarrow LUMO\ (\pi \rightarrow \pi^*)} > \Delta E_{HOMO \rightarrow LUMO\ (n \rightarrow \sigma^*)} > \Delta E_{HOMO \rightarrow LUMO\ (n \rightarrow \pi^*)}$$

300 nm in case of carbonyl compounds with ε_{max} between **10–100** is the result of forbidden transition. The ε_{max} for forbidden transitions are generally **below 10^4**. The allowedness of electronic transitions is related not only to the symmetries of lower and higher energy molecular orbitals but also with the symmetry of the molecule as a whole. Benzene is highly symmetrical and have more restrictions on the electronic transitions.

Designation of UV Absorption Bands

1. **$\sigma \rightarrow \sigma^*$ Transition :** A transition of an electron from a bonding sigma orbital to a higher energy antibonding sigma orbital is designated as $\sigma \rightarrow \sigma^*$ transition. For **alkanes**, the occupied and unoccupied molecular orbitals are σ C—H and σ C—C and σ* C—H and σ* C—C respectively. The value of $\Delta E_{\sigma \rightarrow \sigma^*}$ is so high that the UV radiation necessry to have a successful $\sigma \rightarrow \sigma^*$ transition has wave length around **150 nm or even less**. Aerial oxygen, nitrogen etc. can absorb wave length less than 200 nm, and so for UV radiation, wave length less than 200 nm is not applied generally. Sometimes vacuum UV radiation having wave length less than 200 nm is used to determine the bond energy of some molecules. *Alkanes are UV inactive or transparent to wave lengths of UV radiation more than 200 nm.*

2. **$n \rightarrow \sigma^*$ Transition :** This transition involves saturated centres with one hetero atom with unshared pair of electrons (n electrons), *i.e.*, saturated halides, alcohols,

ethers, amines etc. These compounds have probable electronic transitions like $\sigma \rightarrow \sigma^*$ and $n \rightarrow \sigma^*$. $n \rightarrow \sigma^*$ requires comparatively less energy than $\sigma \rightarrow \sigma^*$, but still is quite high and the wave length of UV radiation falls much below 200 nm. Water absorbs at 167 nm, MeOH at 174 nm, CH_3Cl at 169 nm and CH_3I at 258 nm. In saturated alkyl halides, the energy required for $n \rightarrow \sigma^*$ transition decreases with the increase in the size of the halogen atom. Hence, CH_3Cl atoms are comparatively difficult to excite than CH_3I atoms. $n \rightarrow \sigma^*$ transitions are sensitive to hydrogen bonding. Alcohols form hydrogen bonding through the non bonding electrons present on the oxygen atom with the solvent molecules, and thus energy (ΔE) required for the transition becomes more. *So the above stated compounds (alcohols, ethers, amines, halides etc.) are transparent to UV radiation and can be used as solvents for UV active molecules. It is to be noted that these compounds on the contrary are IR active and so can not be used as solvents in IR spectroscopy.*

3. **$\pi \rightarrow \pi^*$ transition (K–BAND)** : This transition is available in compounds with unsaturated centres, *e.g.*, simple alkenes, aromatic molecules etc. The possibility of electronic transitions are $\sigma \rightarrow \sigma^*$, and $\pi \rightarrow \pi^*$. $\pi \rightarrow \pi^*$ transition requires less energy than $\sigma \rightarrow \sigma^*$. For $\pi \rightarrow \pi^*$ electronic transition, an absorption band around 170-190 nm in *unconjugated alkenes* is found. Generally for $\pi \rightarrow \pi^*$ transition, the λ_{max} resides around **165 nm**. So the **unconjugated alkenes** are also **transparent** to **UV radiation**.

4. **$n \rightarrow \pi^*$ transition (R–BAND)** : In this transition, an electron of unshared electron pair on a heteroatom is excited to π^* antibonding orbital. This transition involves least amount of energy compared to all other transitions and therefore gives rise to an absorption band at longer wave lengths. In saturated aliphatic ketones, the $n \rightarrow \pi^*$ transition around 280 nm is the lowest energy transition. But this $n - \pi^*$ transition is forbidden by consideration thus the **intensity** of the **band** becomes **very low**, although λ_{max} is quite long due to less $\Delta E_{n \rightarrow \pi^*}$.

UV Spectra of Carbonyl Compounds

The electronic presentation of carbonyl group of an aldehyde or ketone is as follows.

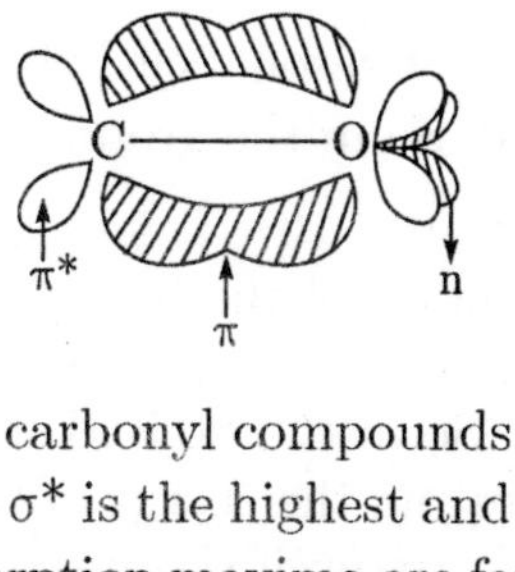

The electronic transitions for carbonyl compounds are $\sigma \rightarrow \sigma^*$, $n \rightarrow \sigma^*$, $\pi \rightarrow \pi^*$ and $n \rightarrow \sigma^*$. Among them, ΔE for $\sigma \rightarrow \sigma^*$ is the highest and consequently λ_{max} becomes very low. Under vacuum UV, three absorption maxima are found, λ_{max} ~ 165 nm ($\varepsilon \cong$ 18,000), λ_{max} ~ 185 nm ($\varepsilon \cong$ 5,000) and λ_{max} ~ 280 nm ($\varepsilon \cong$ 15).

π-Bond in case of carbonyl compounds is stronger than the π-bond present in alkenes. So we expect that ΔE for $\pi \rightarrow \pi^*$ transition for carbonyl compounds should be more than that for alkenes. ($\Delta E_{\pi \rightarrow \pi^*_{C=O}} > \Delta E_{\pi \rightarrow \pi^*_{C=C}}$). λ_{max} for $\pi \rightarrow \pi^*$ transition in case of **alkenes** is around 165 nm and so for $\pi \rightarrow \pi^*$ transition in case of *carbonyl compounds should be less than 165 nm.* The transition moment (change in dipole moment in the excited state due to electronic transition) is *more* for C=O compared to C=C. So $\varepsilon_{\pi \rightarrow \pi^*} > \varepsilon_{n \rightarrow \sigma^*}$. Again the geometry of π and π^* orbitals makes the electron promoted to the excited state in a very facile manner. So $\varepsilon_{\pi \rightarrow \pi^*}$ becomes *more than* $\varepsilon_{n \rightarrow \pi^*}$. λ_{max} at *185 nm* is due to $n \rightarrow \pi^*$ transition, λ_{max} with *poor* ε *at 280 nm* is due to $n \rightarrow \pi^*$ transition. $\Delta E_{n \rightarrow \pi^*}$ is *least* among all the transitions and consequently λ_{max} has got the highest value. The nodal plane of n orbital lies along the axis of p orbitals and so *$n \rightarrow \pi^*$ transition* is *symmetry forbidden* which is reflected in *very low value* of *molar absorptivity (ε).*

UV Absorption of Conjugated Systems

The molecules like conjugated polyene, conjugated carbonyl, aromatic compounds etc. which contain extended conjugation, absorb UV radiation at a wave length higher than 200 nm. The simplest member of conjugated diene is 1,3-butadiene (λ_{max} = 217 nm, ε_{max} = 20,000). The explanation for the longer λ_{max} of butadiene can be explained by both valence bond theory and molecular orbital theory.

1. **Valence bond theory (VBT)** : By valence bond theory, butadiene is a hybrid of following resonating structures.

   ψ = *wave function* of 1,3-butadiene and ϕ_I, ϕ_{II} and ϕ_{III} are the individual wave functions of resonating structures (I), (II) and (III) respectively. Now λ_{II} and λ_{III} tend to zero as they have negligible contribution in the ground state and λ_I so tends to one ($\lambda_I \rightarrow 1$). So at ground state the energy level of (I) is almost

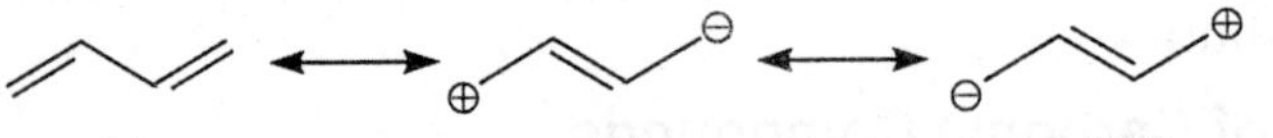

(I) (II) (III)

$$\psi = \phi_I \lambda_I + \phi_{II} \lambda_{II} + \phi_{III} \lambda_{III}$$

   equal to the energy level of resonance hybrid, or resonance energy (R.E) = $E_I - E_{(resonance\ hybrid)} \cong 0$. So in the ground state, resonance has practically no effect or negligible effect.

   Let us take the wave function of the hybrid be ψ', then $\psi' = \lambda_1' \phi_I' + \lambda_2' \phi_{II}' + \lambda_3' \phi_{III}'$. It is supposed that the dipole moment of excited state is greater than that in the ground state. So in the excited state, the contribution of structures (II) and (III) become more and the energy of the resonance hybrid is less than the energy of (I). In other words, the excited state configuration is stabilised by resonance.

   $\therefore$ Resonance Energy (R.E.) = $E_I' - E_{resonance\ hybrid} > 0$

In other words, resonance plays an important role regarding the stability of the molecule in the excited state and as a result, ΔE (energy needed for electron transition) gets *decreased* to a considerable amount and consequent λ_{max} becomes *longer*.

2. **Molecular orbital therory (M.O.T.)** : According to molecular orbital theory, 1,3-butadiene has four molecular orbitals.

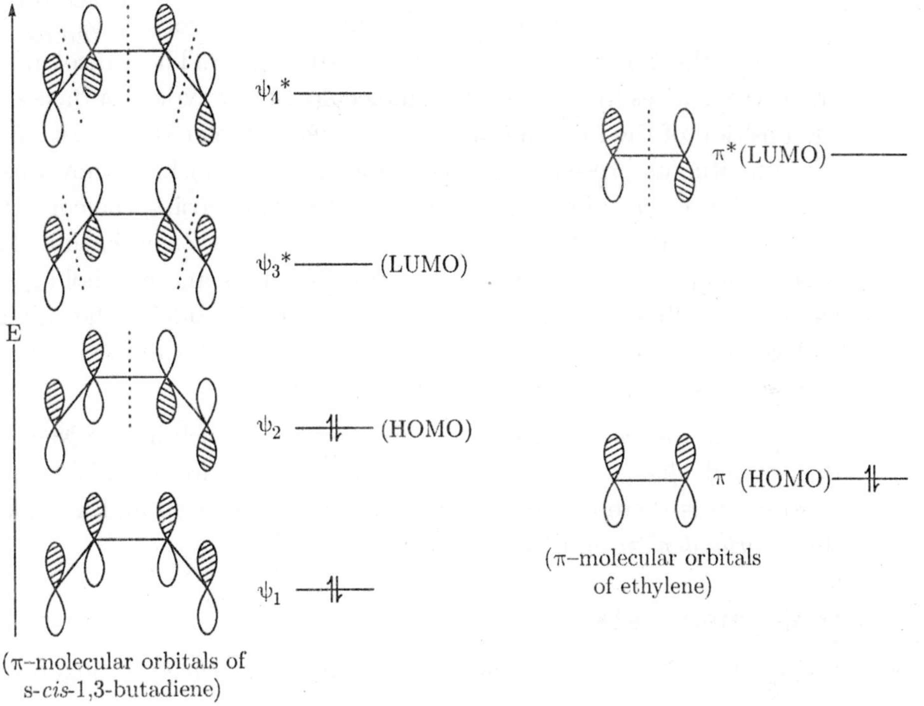

Fig. 1.8 :

In 1,3-butadiene, the energy of ψ_2 (HOMO) is ($\alpha + 0.618\beta$) and the energy of ψ_3* (LUMO) is (α–0.618β) (calculated from quantum mechanical calculations).

$\therefore \Delta E_{HOMO \rightarrow LUMO} = \alpha - 0.618\beta - (\alpha + 0.618\beta) = -1.236\beta$

The energy of HOMO (π) in ethylene is ($\alpha + \beta$) and the energy of LUMO (π^*) is $\alpha - \beta$.

$\therefore \Delta E_{HOMO \rightarrow LUMO} = \alpha - \beta - (\alpha + \beta) = -2\beta$

As the *value of β is always regative*, ΔE for electron transition from HOMO to LUMO is case of *1,3-butadiene* is *much less* than the corresponding $\Delta E_{HOMO \rightarrow LUMO}$ in case of *ethylene* which is reflected in *longer* λ_{max} for 1,3-butadiene. In case of butadiene, the delocalisation of π-electrons due to sidewise overlap of p orbitals is more effective than that present in ethylene which increases the λ_{max} of the former molecule. The extent of p–p conjugation depends on two factors.

(a) The extent of side wise overlap between the p orbitals *diminishes* if the p orbitals deviate from *parallel orientation.* As a result $\Delta E_{HOMO \rightarrow LUMO}$ *increases.*

(b) With increase in number of p orbitals, the extent of *lateral overlap increases* and consequently $\Delta E_{HOMO \rightarrow LUMO}$ *decreases.*

The characteristic progression in the electronic spectra of trienes to polyenes (*more than 20 double bonds in conjugation*) continuous upto *500-600 nm.* By this stage, the polyenes are strongly *yellow* in colour. The red colour of tomatoes and carrots arises from conjugated molecules of this type. For dienes and trienes, the position of the most intense band can be correlated in most instances with the substituents present, by some emperical relationships known as *Woodward Rules.* To use the rules, it is simply a matter of choosing the correct base value and summing the contributions made by each substituent feature. The rules are based emperically an analogous model compounds and will hold good for other compounds whose structures are close to these of models. The only general rule is that larger conjugation leads to higher intensity, the approximate relationship in many cases being $\varepsilon \propto$ (length of chromophore)^2.

Conjugated dienes therefore show absorption at much higher wave length than do isolated alkene groups, a typical value being around 217 nm. A stronger absorption is there due to "*allowed*" $\pi \rightarrow \pi^*$ transition and a weak absorption due "*forbidden*" $n \rightarrow \pi^*$ transition.

Cross-conjugated systems

Cross-conjugated systems are those which contain a "*branched*" conjugated systems.

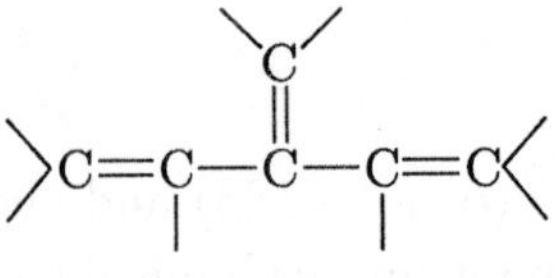

(*Triene*)

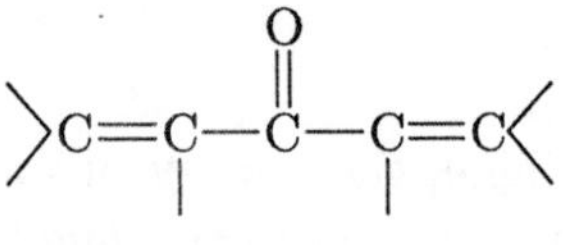

(*Dieneone*)

Two overlapping α, β–unsaturated chromophoric groups may be said to be present, each may give rise to transitions expected to have a reasonably high extinction coefficient. Both systems generally give rise to absorption, but because of the band nature of the spectra, only that system having absorption at longer wavelength and higher internsity is usually observed. In cross-conjugated systems, the position of absorption observed appears to be due to the most highly substituted simple conjugated system. An example is the following steroidal dienone.

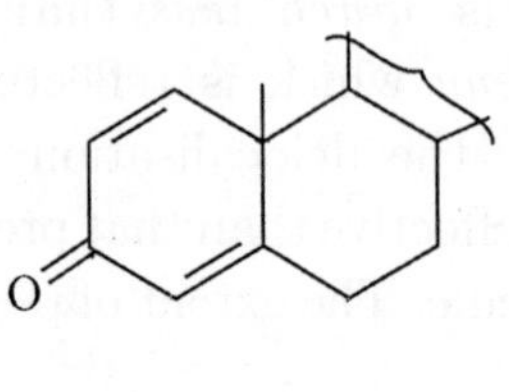

(λ_{max}=246 nm, ε_{max}=15,000)

Applications of electronic spectroscopy : conjugated polyeneynes and enynes

These compounds were discovered in plants, and electronic spectroscopy has been of paramount importance in structure elucidation. The number of possible permutations between triple and double bonds in polyeneynes is very large indeed, but two typical groupings are shown below.

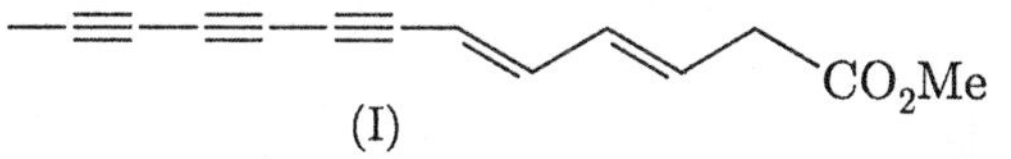

(I)

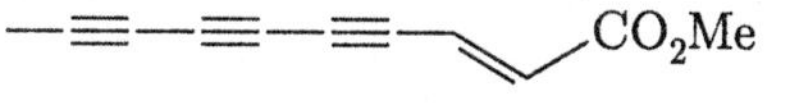

(II)

The intensity (ε) and λ_{max} values increase with increasing conjugation and substitution.

Applications of electronic spectroscopy—benzene and its substitution derivatives

The $\Delta E_{HOMO \rightarrow LUMO}$ transition for benzene is much more compared to a non aromatic system, having same number of π-electrons. When one electron is promoted from HOMO to the LUMO in benzene, the aromatic sextet gets disturbed and as a result aromatic stability is lost.

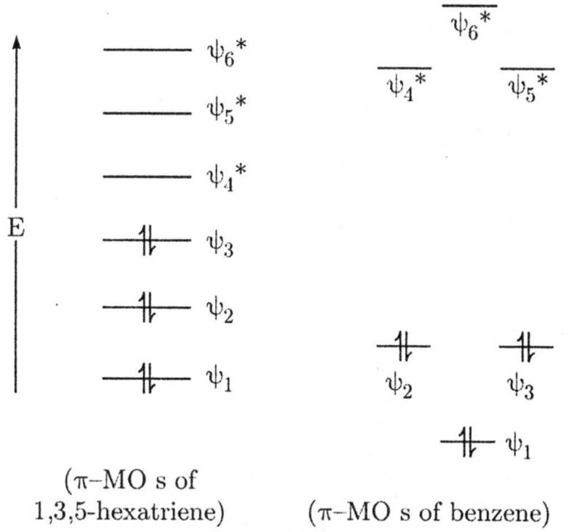

Fig. 1.9 :

In case of polycyclic aromatic compounds like naphthalene, anthracene etc., with the increase in the number of rings, the extent of conjugation increases and the extent of aromatic stability decreases. As a result, $\Delta E_{HOMO \rightarrow LUMO}$ decreases with increase in number of rings and λ_{max} *becomes longer.*

When any group or atom containing lone pair of electrons is attached to ethylenic double bond like $CH_2{=}CH{-}\ddot{A}$, the energy level of π-molecular orbitals get modified and can be shown as follows.

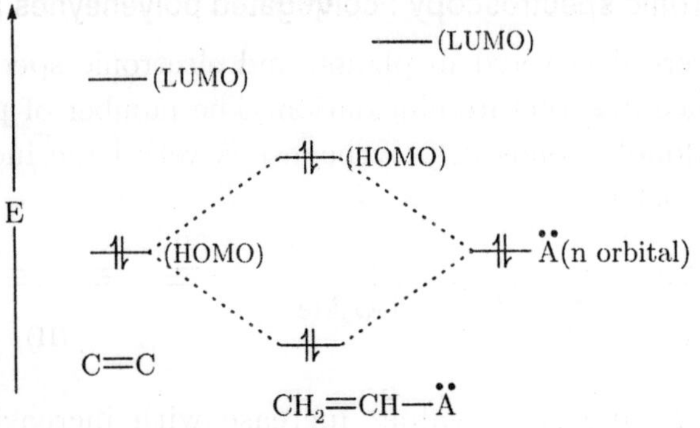

Fig. 1.10 :

Compared to $\Delta E_{HOMO \rightarrow LUMO}$ for ethylene, the $\Delta E_{HOMO \rightarrow LUMO}$ for $CH_2=CH-\ddot{A}$ molecule is *less.* The HOMO of $CH_2=CH-\ddot{A}$ has more similarity with non bonding orbital (n orbital) of isolated $\ddot{A}$ group.

When benzene ring contains similar substituents like $\ddot{A}$ with lone pair of electrons, the following π molecular orbitals are formed by lateral overlap of p–p interaction. In this case also HOMO of substituted benzene derivative bears a close similarity with non bonding orbital of $\ddot{A}$.

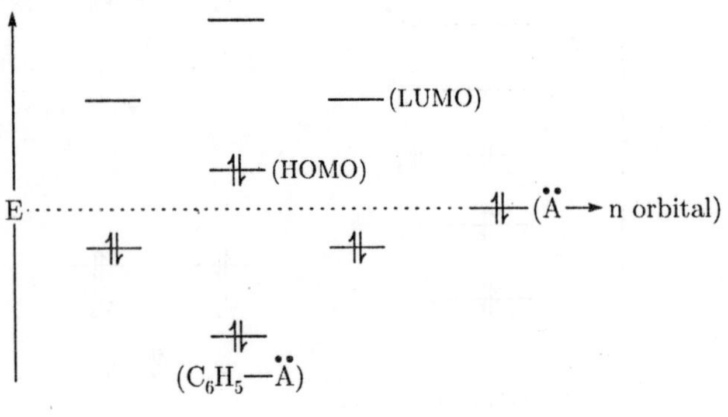

Fig. 1.11 :

Simple alkyl substituents shift the absorptions slightly to longer wave length, but do not destroy the fine structure, while substituents with nonbonded pair of electrons ($-\ddot{O}H$, $-\ddot{O}R$, $-\ddot{N}H_2$ etc) shift the absorption more substantially to longer wave length and severely diminish or wholly eliminate the fine structure.

Three points are to remember regarding substitution in the benzene ring.

1. The most "*influential*" combination of substituents is a –M(–R) group *para* to a + M(+R) group so that non bonding pair donation (by the + M(+R) group) is effectively complementary to the electron withdrawing –M(–R) group; the shift in λ_{max} is greater than the sum of the individual shifts.

   Examples : *p*-nitroaniline and *p*-nitrophenol.

2. Usually a –M(–R) group *ortho* or *meta* to a + M(+R) group produces merely a small shift from that of the isolated chromophores.
3. Altering the non bonding pair "availability" will alter the position of λ_{max}.

Applications of electronic spectrosocpy—α, β–unsaturated carbonyl compounds and other carbonyl compounds

1. **Saturated carbonyl compounds :** Carbonyl compounds show characteristic absorption due to non bonding electrons on oxygen atom. These *non bonding electrons* are *not tightly held* as π-electrons and are therefore excited to antibonding orbitals by lower energy UV radiation. Saturated aldehydes and ketones show three absorption bonds, two of which are absorved in the far UV region ($\pi \rightarrow \pi^*$, 150 nm; $n \rightarrow \sigma^*$, 190 nm). The third band ($n \rightarrow \pi^*$) occurs in near UV 270–300 nm, but as $n \rightarrow \pi^*$ is a forbidden transition ε_{max} is *very poor* ($\varepsilon_{max} < 30$), giving rise to low intensity of this band as typically in the case of acetone.

   Introduction of polar substituents, *e.g.*, a halogen on the α-carbon in the case of acyclic aliphatic ketone has no effect (for $n \rightarrow \pi^*$ transition). But in case of cyclic ketones, presence of such substituents *increases* λ_{max}, by 10-30 nm (when *axial*) and *lowers* by 4-10 nm (when *equatorial*) than the parent compound.

   Example : **2-chlorocyclohexanone may have either conformation.**

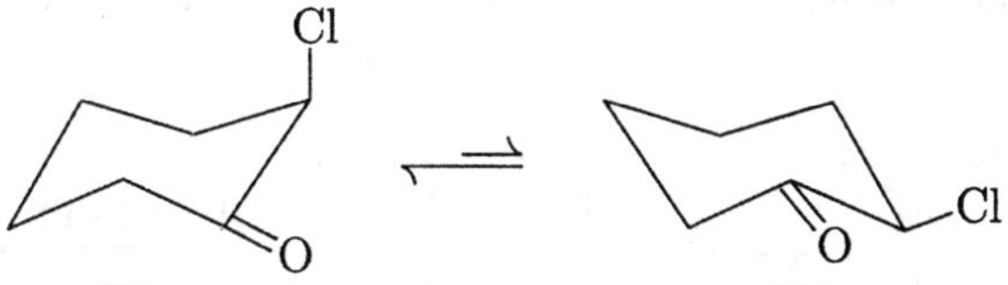

(I) (II)

(Parent cyclohexanone has λ_{max} 282 nm)

   2-chlorocyclohexanone *absorbs* at 293 nm (282 + 11 nm) corresponding to a shift of + 11 nm and indicates that the predominant conformer is (I), the axial conformer.

   When the carbonyl group is substituted by an auxochrome, e,g in acids, esters or amides, the π^* orbital is raised but the n-level of lone pair is left largely unaltered. So $\Delta E_{n \rightarrow \pi^*}$ becomes more and gets shifted to **200-220 nm range.** λ_{max} of CH_3CHO is 293 nm and ethyl acetate, acetic acid and acetamide show λ_{max} at 207, 204 and 220 nm respectively. The presence of a *weak band* at 275-295 nm gives a positive indication of ketone or aldehyde carbonyl group.

2. **α, β-unsaturated aldehydes and ketones :** Compounds in which *carbon-oxygen double bond* is *conjugated* with a *carbon-carbon double bond* (enones) have their absorptions at longer wave lengths due to a decrease in the energy difference between ground and excited states. Thus, both $\Delta E_{n \rightarrow \pi^*}$ and $\Delta E_{\pi \rightarrow \pi^*}$ become

less and occur at longer wave lengths. The excited state is relatively more stabilised by conjugation than the ground state, and, as a result, the magnitude of energy transition is decreased.

Examples :

(a) 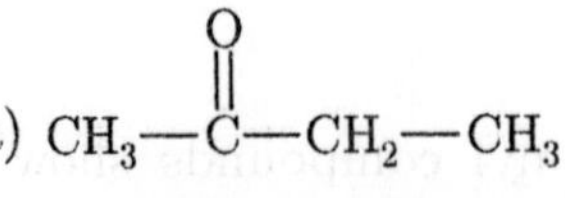 $n \rightarrow \pi^*$, λ_{max}=277nm

(2-Butanone) $\pi \rightarrow \pi^*$, λ_{max}=185nm

(b) 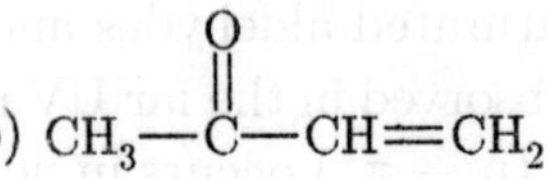 $n \rightarrow \pi^*$, λ_{max}=324nm, ε_{max}=24

(Methyl vinyl ketone) $\pi \rightarrow \pi^*$, λ_{max}=219nm, ε_{max}=10,000

(Intense band)

The enones can threfore be characterised by intense absorption band in the region 215-250 nm (ε_{max} 10,000–20,000) and a *weak* n → π* *band* at 310–330 nm. The change of solvent polarity effects the wave length of transition.

3. **Dicarbonyl compounds :** *Cyclic α-diketones* are *more stable* in their *enol-form* and so the absorption is related to an α, β-unsaturated carbonyl system.

(a) 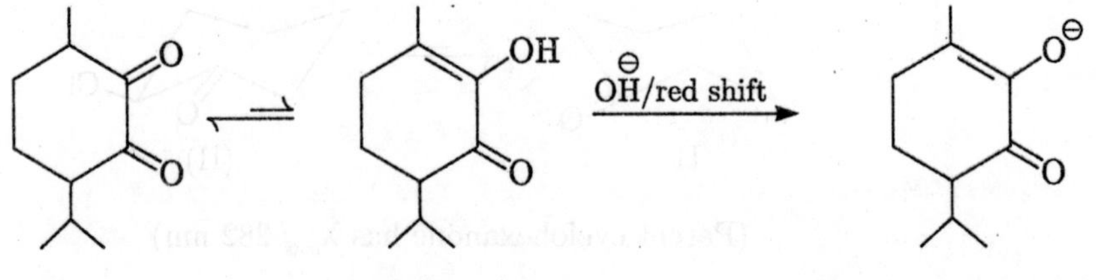

(α-diketone) λ_{max}(EtOH)=270nm (Stable enolate anion) λ_{max}(270+50)=320nm

(b) 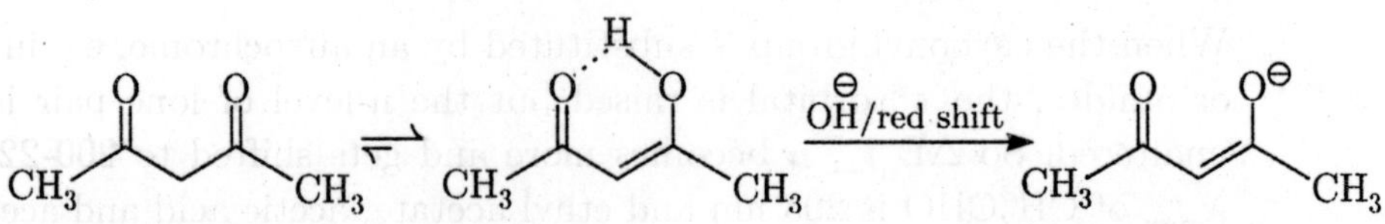

(Acetylacetone) (β-Diketone)

Isooctane λ_{max}=272nm, ε_{max}=12,000

H_2O λ_{max}=274nm, ε_{max}=2050

Isooctane λ_{max}=(272+20)nm =292nm

(c) 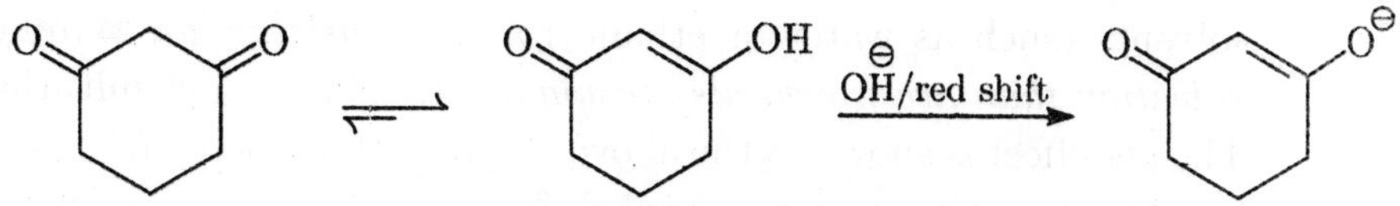

EtOH
λ_{max}=293nm
ε_{max}=22,000

(d) 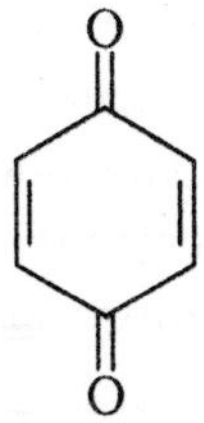

Hexane
λ_{max}=242nm, ε_{max}=24,000 ($\pi \rightarrow \pi^*$)
=281nm, ε_{max}=400
=434nm, ε_{max}=20 } ($n \rightarrow \pi^*$)

(*p*-Benzoquinone)
(vinylogous α-diketone)

Yellow colour of *p*-benzoquinone is due to weak ($n \rightarrow \pi^*$) transition in the visible region (434 nm).

Dependence of position of λ_{max}

1. **Effect of solvent :** The position and intensity of an absorption band may shift when the spectrum is recorded in different solvents. For changes to solvents of increased polarity, the normal pattern of shift are summarised as follows.
   (a) Conjugated dienes and aromatic hydrocarbons experience very little solvent effect.
   (b) **α, β-unsaturated carbonyl compounds** show *two* different shifts.
      (i) $\pi \rightarrow \pi^*$ band moves to longer wave length (red shift), while.
      (ii) The $n \rightarrow \pi^*$ band moves to shorter wave length (blue shift).

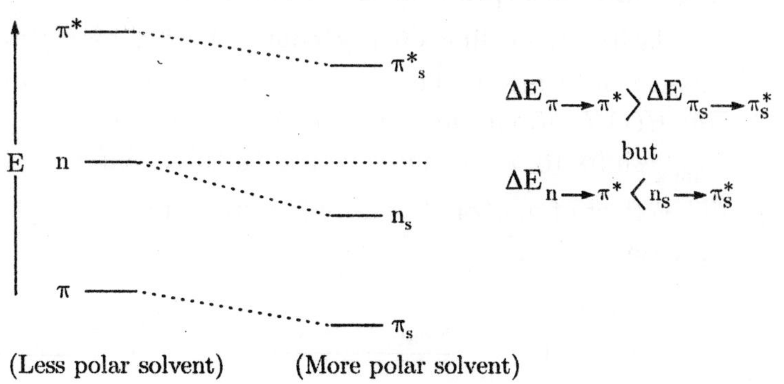

Fig. 1.12 :

Solvation by a polar solvent stabilises π–, π*– and n-orbitals; the stabilisation of non-bonding orbitals is particularly pronounced with hydrogen bonding solvents (such as water or ethanol) and *π^* orbitals are more stabilised by solvation than are π-orbitals presumably because π^* orbitals are more polar.* The net effect is shown in the above diagram. The energy of $\pi \rightarrow \pi^*$ transition becomes less with solvation (red shift) while the energy of $n \rightarrow \pi^*$ transition becomes greater (blue shift). For *α, β-unsaturated ketones* the maximum red shift of + 19 nm occurs in the $\pi \rightarrow \pi^*$ band on changing the solvent from hexane or cyclohexane to water.

Alternative explanation for the *stabilisation* of *π^*-orbital* by solvation is as follows. *π^*-orbital* is comparatively *away from the nucleus* compared to *bonding π-orbital* which resides comparatively nearer to the nucleus so the polar solvent molecules have greater solvating as well as stabilising effect with the π^*–orbital and make this antibonding orbital more stabilised than the corresponding bonding π–orbitals.

2. Effect of pH

(a) The compounds, which change their configuration on change of pH, also show change in λ_{max} to a considerable extent. When alkali is added to phenol, phenoxide anion is formed. The negative charge is generally accumulated on the oxygen atom and thereby the *energy of non bonded* MO *on oxygen atom increases.* The HOMO of phenoxide anion has a similarity with n-orbital of oxygen and due to negative charge on oxygen atom the energy of HOMO *increases.* As a result, $\Delta E_{HOMO \rightarrow LUMO}$ in *phenoxide anion decreases,* and we get a *longer* λ_{max} on addition of alkali to unionised phenols (red shift).

(b) When *acid* is added to *aniline, anilinium cation* ($C_6H_5\overset{\oplus}{N}H_3$) is produced where the non bonding electrons on nitrogen is used to form the cation. As the non bonding electrons are no longer available, non bonding orbitals also can not participate and in fact anilinium cation behaves as benzene molecule regarding absorption of UV radiation. The HOMO of aniline has close similarity (regarding energy content) with n-orbital of $-\ddot{N}H_2$ group, and upon acidification, the *energy level of HOMO changes* and now *resembles the HOMO of benzene molecule.* As a result, $\Delta E_{HOMO \rightarrow LUMO}$ *increases* and λ_{max} shifts to a *shorter* wave length (blue shift).

(c) The effect of *acid* on 2-or 4-hydroxypyridine is just the *reverse* what we find in case of phenol.

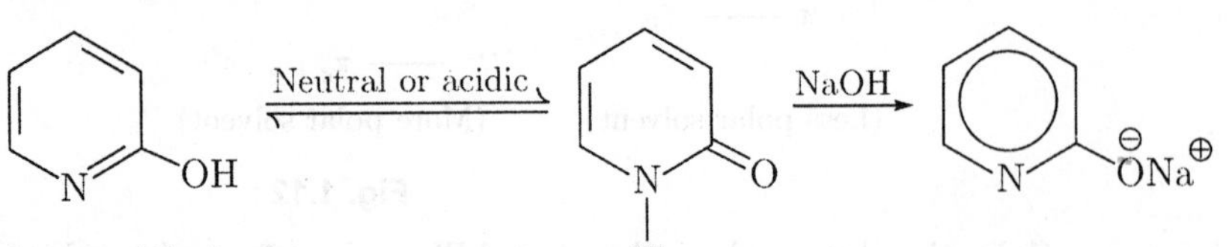

(2-hydroxypyridine)

(I) (II) (III)

In neutral or acidic solution, *2-hydroxypyridine* remains mainly as its *amide configuration* (II). (II) is *non aromatic* and can undergo extended conjugation. For this reason, $\Delta E_{HOMO \rightarrow LUMO}$ is *less* and λ_{max} shifts to *longer wave length.* When alkali is added to (I), (III) is formed which is *aromatic* and hence $\Delta E_{HOMO \rightarrow LUMO}$ becomes *high* and λ_{max} shifts to *shorter wave length.*

3. **Inductive effect :** The energy level of HOMO becomes higher when any group with (+I) effect is attached to the chromophore. The electron density on HOMO gets increased and the *energy levels* of other molecular orbitals also *increase.* As a result, $\Delta E_{HOMO \rightarrow LUMO}$ is *decreased slightly* and λ_{max} shifts to a *longer wave length.* The situation gets reversed with substituents containing (–I) effect.
4. **Steric effect :** The planar structure of a molecule gets disturbed if the structure experiences strain due to steric effects. The parallaly placed p-orbitals (essential condition to have effective sidewise overlap) are no longer parallel to one another and the *extent of p–p overlap* gets *decreased* to a considerable amount or even to a total loss. The result is higher value of $\Delta E_{HOMO \rightarrow LUMO}$ and λ_{max} shifts to a *shorter wave length.*

(a) 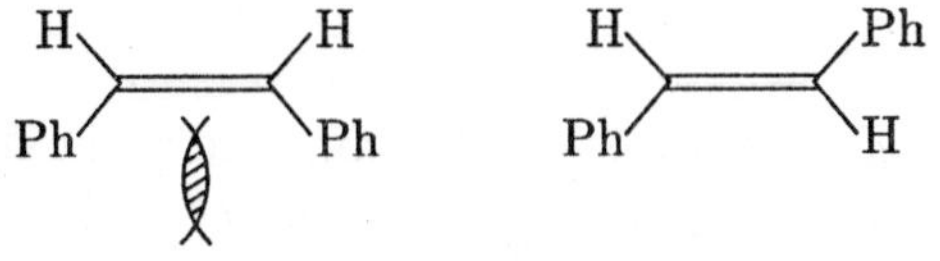

(*Cis*-stilbene) (*Trans*-stilbene)

In case of *cis*-stilbene, the two benzene rings can not be in the same plane with the olefinic double bond due to steric repulsion arising out of the bulk of two phenyl rings. On the other hand, no steric factor is present in the *trans*-isomer and effective p–p interaction is possible. As a result, $\Delta E_{HOMO \rightarrow LUMO}$ for *cis*-isomer becomes *more* than $\Delta E_{HOMO \rightarrow LUMO}$ for the *trans*-isomer and we get λ_{max} for *trans*-isomer longer compared to λ_{max} for *cis one.*

(b) **Biphenyls and binaphthyls :** Biphenyls are not completely planar (the angle between the two rings is about 45°) and in 2-substituted biphenyls, the rings are further out of coplanarity. The effect is manifested in decreased overlap between p orbitals in the 2-substituted biphenyls with shorter λ_{max} and intensity of ε_{max} also decreases.

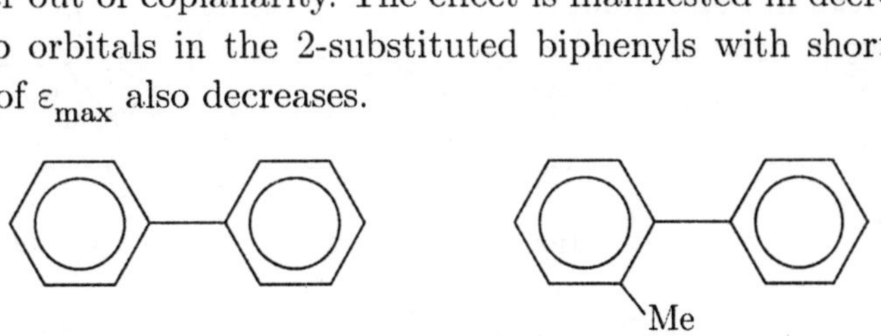

λ_{max}=250nm, ε_{max}=19,000 λ_{max}=237nm, ε_{max}=10,250

1,1′-Binaphthyls can not be coplanar (indeed are enantiomers) exhibit electronic absorption at a *shorter* λ_{max} than naphthalene itself.

(c) **Angular distortion, cross-conjugation and steric inhibition of resonance :**

(i) Woodward rules for conjugated dienes and carbonyl compounds give reliable results where there is no strain around the chromophore, *i.e.*, successful for acyclic and six-membered ring systems.

The following systems do not exhibit good electronic spectra.

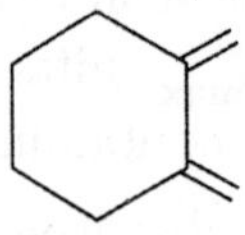
(I)

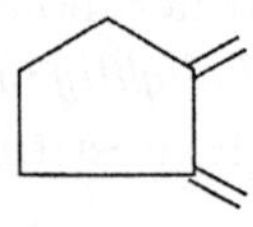
(II)

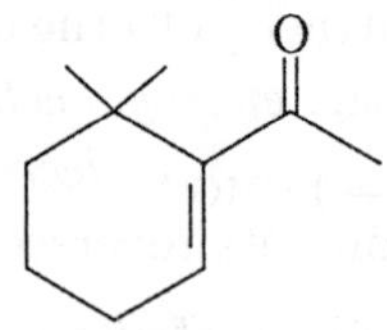
(III)

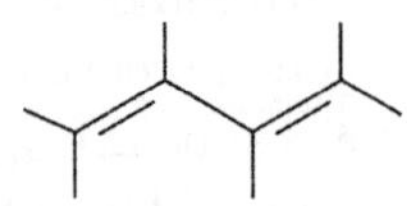
(IV)

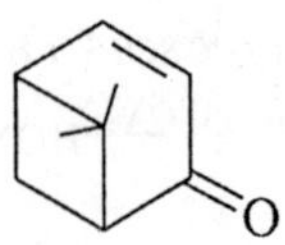
(V)

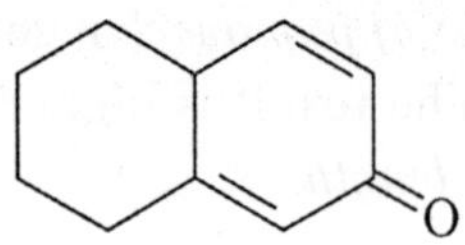
(VI)

All these compounds show steric inhibition of resonance and exhibit λ_{max} at shorter wave lengths and diminished ε_{max}. The same explanation can be cited for the following examples.

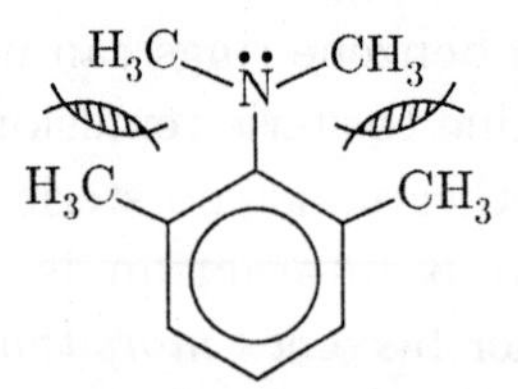
λ_{max}=194nm, ε_{max}=36,100

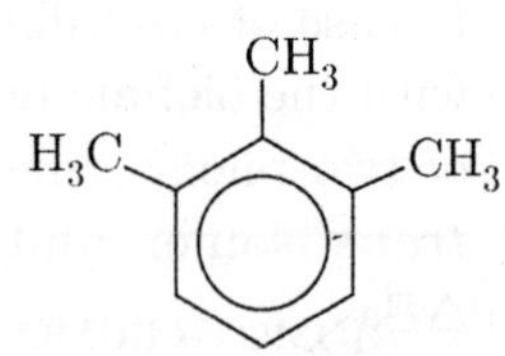
λ_{max}=195nm, ε_{max}=55,000

(b) In case of *homoannular dienes*, there is a *repulsion* between *two π bond pairs* which is *absent* in case of *heteroannular dienes.* So the energy level of ground

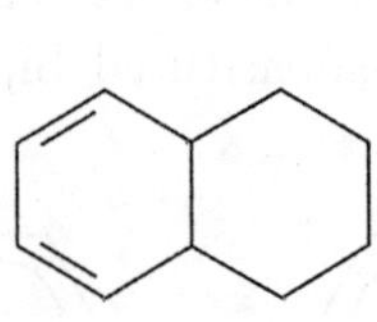
(Homoannular diene)

⇒

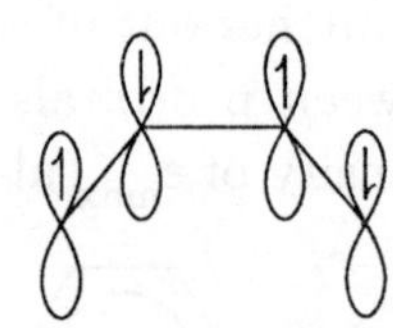
(*Cisoid* diene)

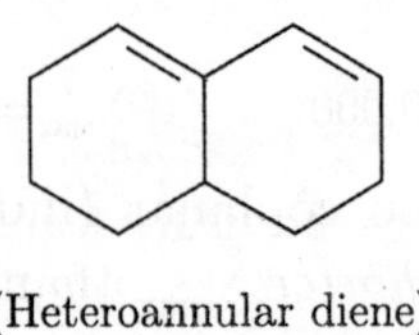
(Heteroannular diene)

⇒

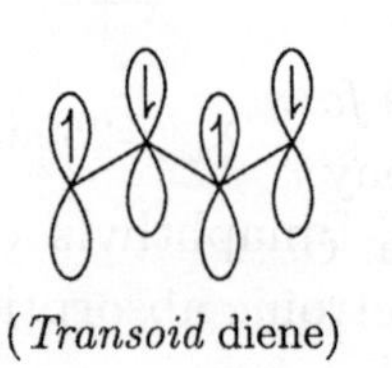
(*Transoid* diene)

state of homoannular dienes is more than the ground state energy content of heteroannular dienes. But in the excited state, the repulsion between the pairs of π bonds less in case of homoannular dienes and as a result they (homoannular dienes) absorb at a longer wave length. Alternatively, homoannular dienes have structural similarity with *cisoid* dienes and the effective p orbital overlap is more compared to that present in *transoid* dienes. As a result, homoannular dienes absorb at a longer wavelength.

5. Effect of exocyclic double bond :

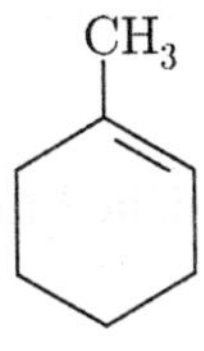

(*Endocyclic double bond*; more stable isomer as the double bond is more substituted.)

(I)

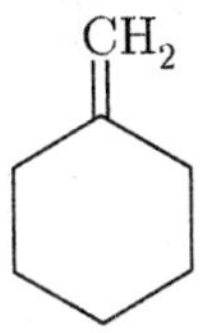

(*Exocyclic double bond*; less stable isomer as the double bond is less substituted.)

(II)

The isomer containing the exocyclic double bond (II) absorbs at a higher wave length (λ_{max} shifts to longer side by 5 nm; red shift) compared to the isomer containing endocyclic double bond.

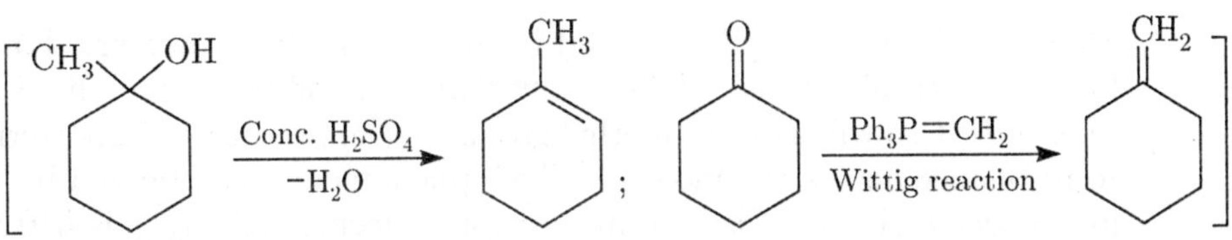

6. Effect of s-*cis* and s-*trans* (*cisoid* and *transoid*) conformations :

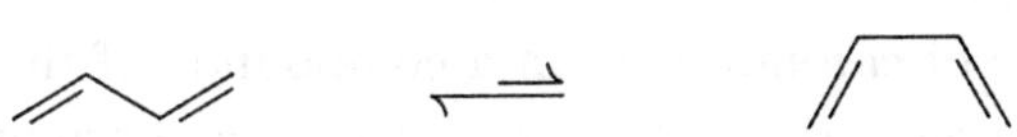

(s-*trans* 1,3-butadiene) (97.5%) (s-*cis*)–1,3-butadiene

λ_{max}=217nm

The acyclic dienes can rotate around single bond and hence exists *mostly* as s-*trans form.* In case of cyclic dienes, the s-*cis* form can not attain s-*trans* form as it may rupture the rigid ring structure and has some effect on the electronic spectra. *Cyclic dienes* absorbs at *lower wave lengths* with *diminished* ε (intensity) compared to their acyclic counterparts.

Mono- and polycylic dienes can be divided into two classes whether the double bonds are present in the same ring or in different rings.

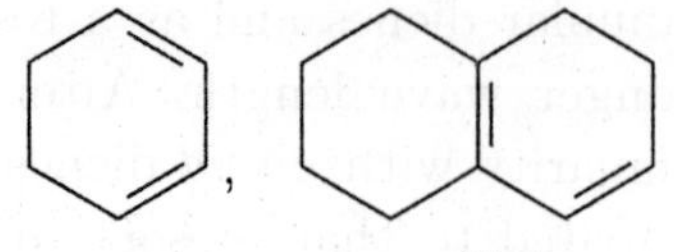

(I)

(*Homoannular diene*; where the two double bonds are present in the same ring– s-*cis* configuration.)

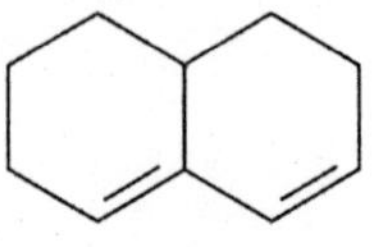

(II)

(*Heteroannular diene*; where the two double bonds are present in two different rings– s-*trans* configuration.)

(I) absorbs at a higher wave length but with diminished intensity (ε) compared to (II) which is a heteroannular diene.

7. 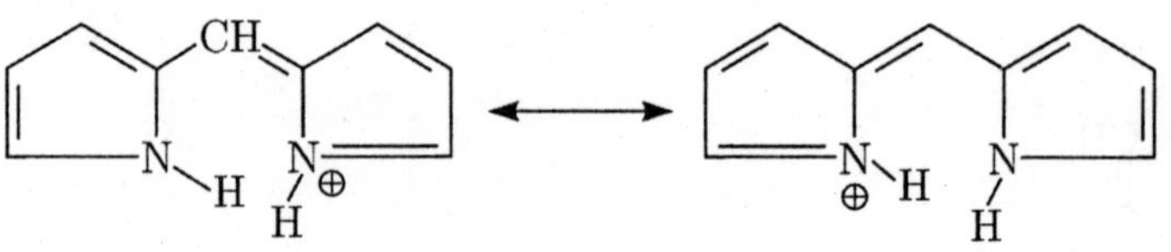

λ_{max}=470nm

(I)

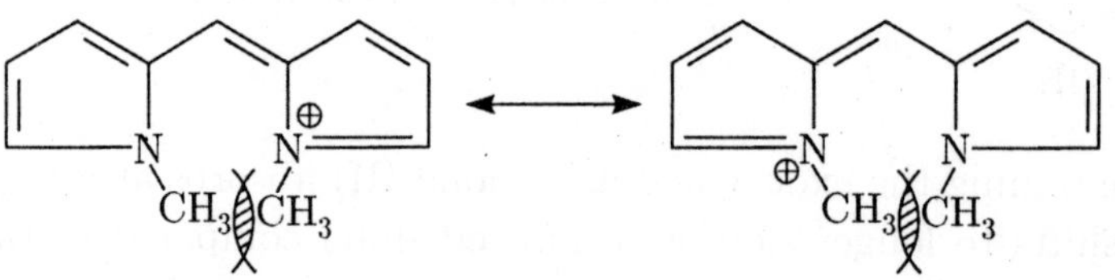

λ_{max}=510nm

(II)

Molecule (II) is primarily affected in the ground state by steric hindrance. ΔE for its electronic transition is *lower than* that of (I) where there is *no steric hindrance.* Crowding of two methyl groups in (II) produces severe steric hindrance to resonance across the molecule. This phenomenon is reflected in λ_{max} values; for molecule (I), λ_{max} is 470 nm but for molecule (II), λ_{max} is 510 nm.

Applications of UV Spectroscopy

1. **Presence of chromophore in a compound** : If the UV spectrum of an unknown molecule has resemblence with a known chromophore with an established UV spectrum, one may assume that the molecule may contain that chromophore. If an UV spectrum of an unknown compound bears close similarity with chromophores like benzene, polyalkylbenzene etc. it is highly probable that the molecule may contain those chromophores. Generally λ_{max} *increases* with *increase in number of alkyl groups* as substituent in the benzene ring and also ε_{max} increases accordingly. So any UV spectrum which has a close similarity with the UV spectrum of benzene, then we may say that the unknown molecule is a derivative of benzene.

2. **Determination of configuration** : The configuration of a conjugated diene or conjugated carbonyl compound can be determined from the corresponding λ_{max} values.

Example : The molecular formula of a compound is $C_6H_{10}O$. The number of double bonds present in it can be calculated by,

$$IHD = \frac{4\times6+2-(5\times2)-2-10}{2} = 2$$

IR spectra : Peak at 1680 cm^{-1} but *no peak* at ~2780 cm^{-1}. The compound may be a carbonyl compound (>C=O comes at ~1700cm $^{-1}$) and no aldehyde C—H is there (peak at ~ 2780 cm^{-1}) which is *absent.* The compound *does not respond* to *iodoform test*, so —C(=O)—CH_3 group is not present. In UV spectrum, one peak at *228 nm* with *high* ε_{max} and another at *314 nm* with low ε_{max} are found. First peak is due to $\pi \rightarrow \pi^*$ and the second peak is due to $n \rightarrow \pi^*$ transition. The compound contains two double bonds and one carbonyl group, so the skeleton of the molecule becomes:

C=C—C=O

and also the λ_{max} of the molecule comes *higher than 215 nm* confirms that the molecule is a *conjugated* one. The base value for α, β-unsaturated ketone is *215 nm* and this molecule absorbs at 228 nm (215 + 13 = 228 nm), so we may assume that one alkyl group is attached to *β-sp*^{2} carbon. So the emperical formula of the molecule becomes

R′—CH=CH—C(R)=O

but R′ is neither H nor CH_3. To satisfy the molecular formula, R′ should be CH_3 and R is CH_2CH_3.

∴ The *structure* of the molecule is CH_3CH=CH—C(CH_2CH_3)=O

As we apply Woodward's rule to the molecule, it must be the *trans-isomer* as Woodward's rule is *not obeyed* by *cis-isomer* due to steric reasons.

So the structure of the molecule is as follows.

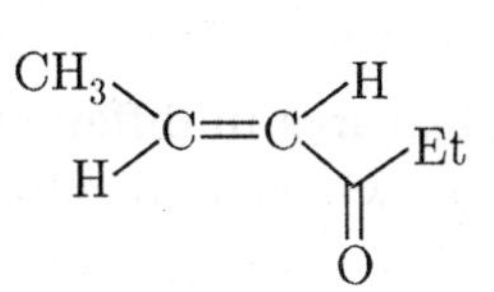

3. **Comparison and Determination of the structure of the compounds :**

(a) *p*-Toluidine absorbs at a longer λ_{max} *with a* high ε_{max} compared to those by benzylamine. So, from the UV spectra of the two compounds we can easily distinguish between them. If we add acid to both the compounds, the UV spectrum of benzylamine would not alter much, but the UV spectrum of *p*-toluidine changes considerably. In acid solution, *p*-toluidine shows both blue shift and hypochromic shift.

(b) *γ-Diketone* is *UV-inactive* whereas β-diketone is *UV active.* β-Diketone can enolise and the enol form behaves like a conjugated system and an intense peak (high ε_{max}) due to $\pi \rightarrow \pi^*$ transition at *270 nm* is found.

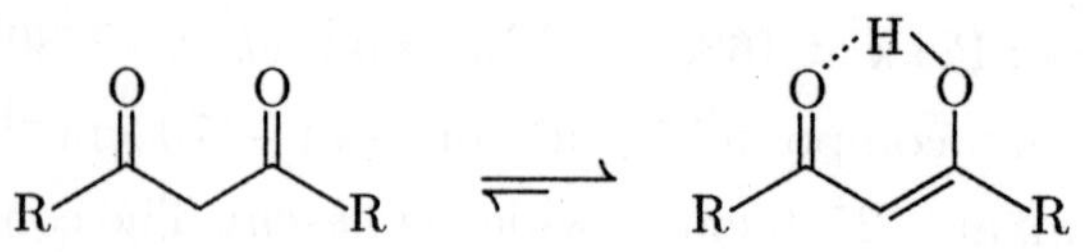

(β-Diketone) (Enol form)

(c)

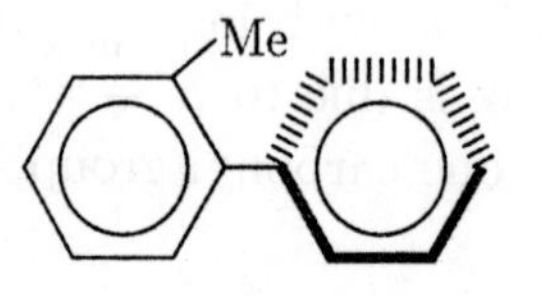

2-methylbiphenyl (I)
(Resonance is lost between the two rings due to the presence of ortho methyl group)
λ_{max}=237nm, ε_{max} ≅10,000

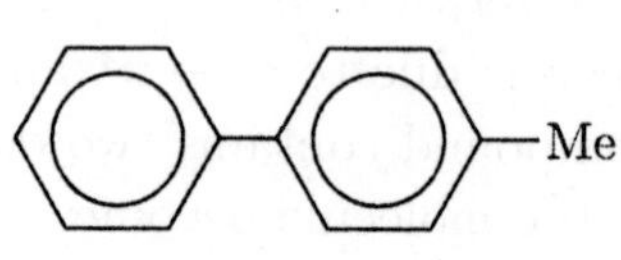

4-methylbiphenyl (II)
λ_{max}=255nm, ε_{max}=19,000

Due to steric effect (*ortho effect*), the two benzene rings in molecule (I) lose coplanarity and λ_{max} gets shorter with diminished ε_{max} compared to molecule (II) where no such steric inhibition of resonance is present.

4. **Detection of Intermediate in a reaction :** UV spectrum is helpful to detect π-complex during a reaction between benzene and an electrophile. At –72°C, benzene reacts with HCl to form $C_6H_6 \cdot HCl$. The UV spectrum of this compound shows close similarity with the UV spectrum of benzene itself. As the π-electronic structure remains intact in this addition compound, ($C_6H_6.HCl$) which is π-complex, the UV spectrum is not very different from the UV spectrum of benzene itself. But in the presence of $AlCl_3$ at –72°C, *benzene* forms an *addition compound* with *HCl* which shows an UV spectrum totally different from the UV spectrum of benzene. Here the π-electronic structure of benzene nucleus is changed and the complex is known as *σ-complex.*

5. **Study of structural features in different solvents :** Chloral hydrate shows λ_{max} at 290 nm in hexane, which is totally absent if the solvent is changed from hexane to water. This observation tells us that the structure of chloral ($Cl_3C—CHO \cdot H_2O$) in hexane changes to chloral hydrate $CCl_3CH(OH)_2$ in *aqueous solution.* Chloral hydrate is transparent to UV and so no λ_{max} appears around 290 nm.

Extent of Absorption

1. **Concentration of molecules which can absorb UV radiation :** When a molecule remains as tautomeric mixture in solution, the resultant UV spectrum is due to individual spectrum of both the tautomers. If one of the tautomers is UV inactive, then the spectrum we get is entirely due to the other tautomer which is UV active.

   From *Beer-Lambert's law* we find that Optical Density (O.D.) = ε.c.l, where *c is the concentration* of the compound under investigation. If the concentration of the UV active tautomer be C_a then optical density is proportional to C_a and also C_a is proportional to ε. In other words, if the *concentration* of *UV active tautomer increases*, ε_{max} also *increases* for that tautomer.

   Example :

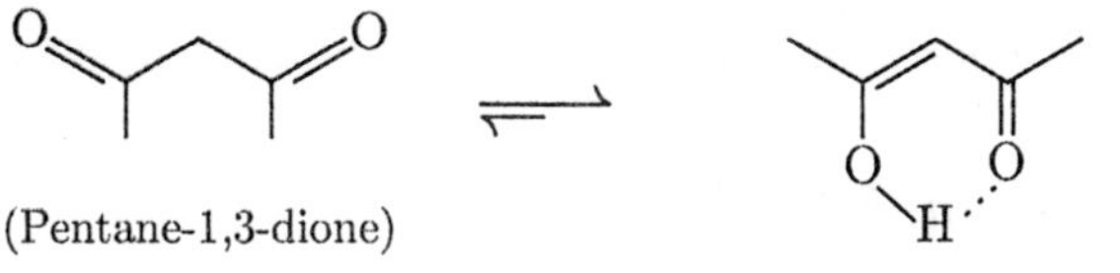

(Pentane-1,3-dione)

$\lambda_{max}^{H_2O}$=274nm; $\varepsilon_{max}^{H_2O}$=2000

The UV spectrum of pentane- 1,3-dione is entirely due to the enol form as this form resembles α, β-unsaturated carbonyl compound. λ_{max} is due to $\pi \rightarrow \pi^*$ electronic transition with $-\ddot{\underset{\cdot\cdot}{O}}H$ group as auxochrome. The *diketo form* is *UV inactive.* If the spectrum is taken in hexane instead of water, λ_{max} does not alter much (λ_{max} = 272 nm in hexane). But ε_{max} changes to a considerable extent ($\varepsilon_{max} \cong$ 12,000). *In hexane*, pentane–1,3-dione remain almost fully in its *enol form* (92%) and as the enol tautomer is only *UV active*, ε_{max} becomes large as the effective concentration of the compound (enol form) increases. On the other hand, in aqueous solution, the concentration of enol tautomer is much *less* ($\cong$ 15%).

$$\therefore \frac{H_2O}{\text{hexane}} = \frac{[C_{enol}]_{H_2O}}{[C_{enol}]_{hexane}} = \frac{1}{6}$$

Effective chromophore concentration

A compound may contain more than one UV active chromophore per molecule. Chromophores may interact with the UV radiation and with the increase in concentration of chromophores, the probability of interaction also increases. In other words, the UV absorption by any molecule increases with increase in the number of chromophores.

1,3,5-Trimethyl benzene and *2,2′,4,4′,6,6′-hexamethyl biphenyl* both have a common chromophore which is trimethyl benzene.

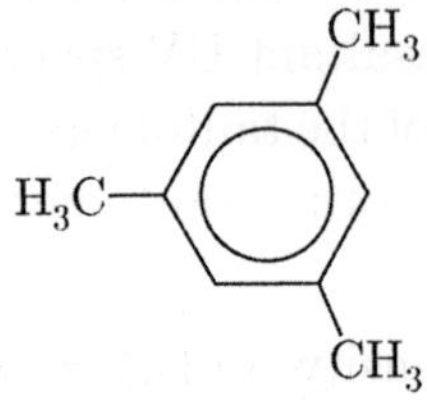

(1,3,5-Trimethyl benzene)(I)

λ_{max}=266nm, ε_{max}=20

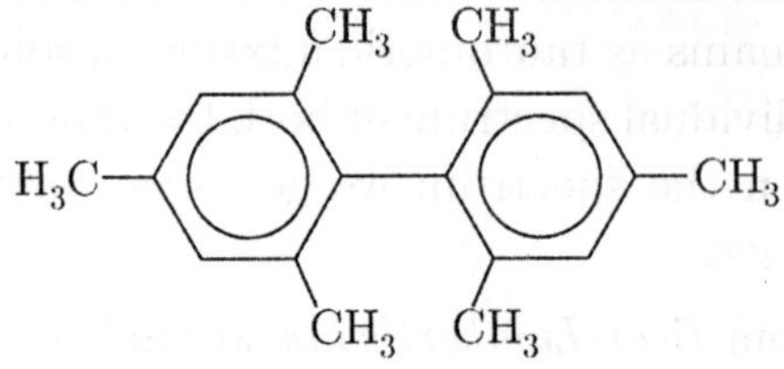

(2,2,4,4′,6,6′-Hexamethyl biphenyl)(II)

λ_{max}=266nm, ε_{max}=545

In molecule (II) the two benzene rings are almost at right angles to each other, and so there is practically no π-interaction between the two rings. Both the compounds show identical λ_{max} (266 nm); but in molecule (II), the number of effective chromophore is two. For this reason, the value of $\varepsilon(\varepsilon = 545)$ becomes more for molecule (II) compared to molecule (I) ($\varepsilon = 20$) where the number of effective chromphore is only *one.*

Magnitude of Transition Moment

A compound will absorb UV radiation more if the transition moment of the molecule is high; with increase in transition moment, the absorptivity (ε) also increases. ε of heteroannular diene is more compared to a homoannular diene. The magnitude of transition moment is different for homoannular and heteroannular dienes. It is assumed that, in the excited state (irradiated by UV radiation) the resonating structure of the diene which is *dipolar* contributes maximum to the resonance hybrid. Homoannular dienes have *cisoid* structures and the dipoles remain in comparatively shorter distance where the distance between the two poles in heteroannular dienes is longer, as the latter exist in transoid configuration. So we see that heteroannular dienes have higher dipole moment in the excited state and homoannular dienes have lower dipole moment in the excited state. This is reflected in the intensity of ε also. Heteroannular dienes have higher ε value over the homoannular ones. Naphthalene and azulene are two isomeric compounds. Resonance stabilises the ground state of naphthalene relative to its excited state as naphthalene is aromatic in nature. On the other hand, azulene is resonance stabilised in the excited state as this excited state of azulene is aromatic, which contains a dipolar structure. In other words, transition moment of azulene in its excited state is more than than its ground state. Increase in transition moment leads to better UV absorption and so $\Delta E_{HOMO \rightarrow LUMO}$ for azulene is less than $\Delta E_{HOMO \rightarrow LUMO}$ for naphthalene. For the same reason, fulvene (an isomer of benzene) is yellow (absorbs at higher λ_{max}) than *benzene* (*shorter* λ_{max}). Similarly, $C_6H_5CH = CHC_6H_5$ (λ_{max} = 319 nm) is colourless but $C_6H_5(CH = CH)_3C_6H_5$ (λ_{max} = 377 nm) and C_6H_5–$(CH{=}CH)_5C_6H_5$ (λ_{max} = 424 nm) are pale yellow and orange in colour respectively. In the latter two cases, the magnitude of transition moment is more than stilbene and their corresponding λ_{max} values shift to the *longer wave length* side.

UV spectroscopy and rate of reaction

The rate of following reaction is determined by UV spectral analysis.

$$CH_3CH_2NO_2 + \overset{\ominus}{O}H \rightleftharpoons CH_3\overset{\ominus}{C}HNO_2 + H_2O$$

(Nitroethane) (Nitroethane anion)

λ_{max}=240nm

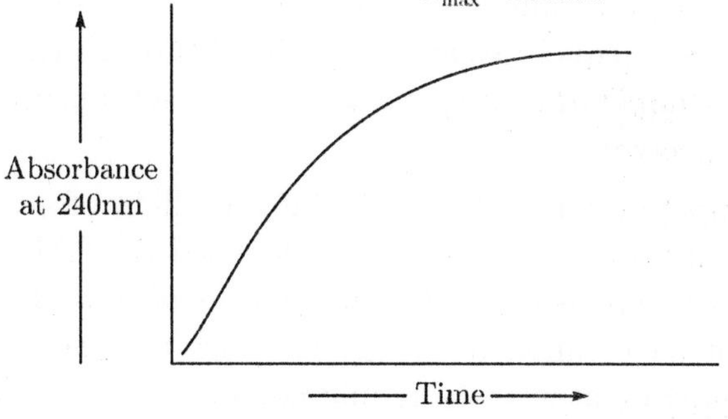

Fig. 1.13 :

Nitroethane is taken in the quartz cell of the spectrometer containing a basic solution and the rate of the reaction is monitored by rate of increase in absorbance at *240 nm.*

Determination of pK_a

The pK_a of a compound can be determined by UV spectroscopy provided either the acidic form or the basic form of the molecule under investigation is *UV active.* Phenolate anion absorbs at 287 nm (λ_{max}). If the absorbance at 287 nm is measured as a function of pH, the pK_a of phenol can be determined by determining the pH at which half the increase in absorbance takes place. At this pH, half of the phenol gets converted to phenolate anion and therefore, this pH represents the pK_a of the compound.

[*Henderson's equation* is $pH=pK_a+\log\frac{[salt]}{[acid]}$; at *half neutralisation point* [salt]=[acid] and hence pH becomes equal to pK_a.]

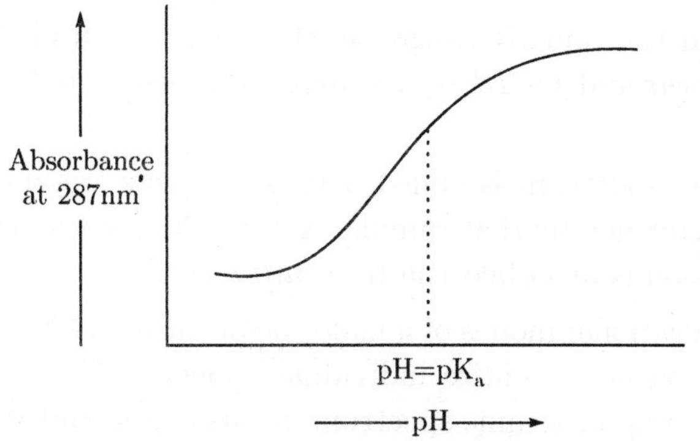

Fig. 1.14 :

Absorption Spectroscopy

Infrared Spectroscopy

Infrared spectroscopy is one of the most widely used tools for the detection of functional groups in pure compounds and in mixtures.

When infrared light [(2.5μ to 15μ) wave length or $4000 cm^{-1}$–$650 cm^{-1}$ ($\bar{\nu}$), (wave number)] is passed through a sample of an organic compound, some of the frequencies are absorbed, while other frequencies are transmitted through the sample without being absorbed. If we plot *transmittance (preferably)* or absorbance against *frequency*, the result is an infrared spectrum.

A particular compound will only absorb infrared light of a particular frequency, if there is an energy transition within the molecule, such that $\Delta E = h\nu$. The transitions involved in IR absorption are associated with *vibrational changes* within the molecule as IR radiation does not have sufficient energy to cause the excitation of an electron. It causes atoms or groups of atoms of organic compounds to vibrate faster about the covalent bond which connect them. The position of an infrared absorption band is specified in frequency units by its wave number ($\bar{\nu}$) in cm^{-1} or by its wave length. λ, measured in μm (*micrometre or micron*).

$$\bar{\nu} = \frac{1}{\lambda}\ (\lambda \text{ in cm}) \text{ or } \bar{\nu} = \frac{10{,}000}{\lambda}\ (\lambda \text{ in } \mu\text{m})$$

Different bonds (C—C, C=C, C≡C, C—O, C=O, O—H, N—H etc.) have different vibrational frequencies and we can detect the presence of these bonds in an organic molecule by identifying this characteristic frequency as an absorption band in the infrared spectrum.

The infrared region constitutes three parts.

1. Near infrared (>$4000 cm^{-1}$)
2. Mid infrared (4000-$650 cm^{-1}$, 15.4-2.5 μm) *(Important)*
3. Far infrared (<$650 cm^{-1}$)

Spectroscopy in the mid IR range (4000-$650 cm^{-1}$) is useful to study the organic compounds. Both *near* and *far IR region* are of *little use* as only few absorptions occur there.

Each dip in the spectrum is called a band or peak, represents absorption of IR radiation at that frequency by that sample. A *100% transmittance* means *no* absorption and if all the radiation is absorbed the *transmittance* is 0%.

Many of the vibrational modes of a molecule occur in (1400–$600 cm^{-1}$) depending on the complex vibration of the entire individual molecule. No two different compounds (excepting enantiomers) have same spectrum in this region and so this region is logically named as *fingerprint region* of the molecule.

Preparation of the sample

1. Sample (2-5mg) is ground together with the mulling agent (1-2 drops of Nujol, a high boiling fraction from petroleum) and IR spectrum is then taken. Nujol has its own band around 2920–2860 (C—H stretching) 1460 and 1380cm^{-1} (C—H bending of —CH_2— and —CH_3 respectively) and so no information can be gathered from this region.
2. Solid sample (1–3 mg) and KBr or KCl (100–200mg), ground together, dried at room temperature and made into a small disc under pressure. KBr *does not absorb IR* in 4000-650cm^{-1} and thus a complete spectrum of the solid sample is obtained.
3. For liquid samples, a small drop of liquid is placed on a sodium chloride pelette, another sodium chloride pelette is placed on the top of drop to get a thin film of the sample and the spectrum is then examined.

Molecular Vibrations

The idea of molecular vibration can be derived from classical mechanics. Two particles having masses m_1 and m_2 can be imagined connected by a bond which is a perfectly elastic spring. The two particles act as nuclei of two atoms and the elastic spring is the bonding orbital. When the particles are expanded or contracted from their normal positions, an opposing force is generated as the spring is ideally elastic in nature. The magnitude of force is proportional to expansion or contraction, and vibrational motion follows simple harmonic motion. If the normal equilibrium distance between the particles is r_0 and the changed distance is r, then the opposing force acting is,

$-f \propto (r_0-r)$ or $-f = k(r_0-r)$ where k is a *proportionality constant* and work done against this opposing force is as follows:

$$W = \text{Opposing force} \times \text{change in distance}$$
$$= k(r_0-r).\ (r_0-r)$$
$$= k(r_0-r)^2$$

In other words, vibration energy, $E_v=k(r_0-r)^2$. If the opposing force exceeds elastic limit, then there will be no harmonic oscillation and beyond breaking stress, the spring will break. This equation can also be applied to molecular vibration with a little correction. In case of spring, the change of E_v with r is continuous, but in case of molecular vibration we have to apply *quantum theory, i.e.*, the changing values of E_v are *discontinuous.* There are some definite values for E_v and for each value of E_v we get a *quantised vibrational energy level.* Each energy level can be designated by one *vibrational quantum number.* The different vibrational energy levels can be written as follows.

$$E_v = (v+\tfrac{1}{2})h\omega,\ v=0,1,2,3,\ ....$$

where v = *Vibrational quantum number*

and ω(Omega) = *Vibrational frequency*

The vibrational energy level for which v=0 is called *zero point energy level.* At *zero point energy level,* vibrational energy becomes,

$$E_0 = \frac{1}{2} h\omega \text{ (when v=0)}$$

From the equation it is evident that, for a spring where vibrational energy is continuous, a stable position for the molecule is possible where distance is r_0 when energy is zero. But for molecular vibrations, we never get a stable position as the minimum energy needed is $\frac{1}{2}h\omega$ where ω is the vibrational frequency.

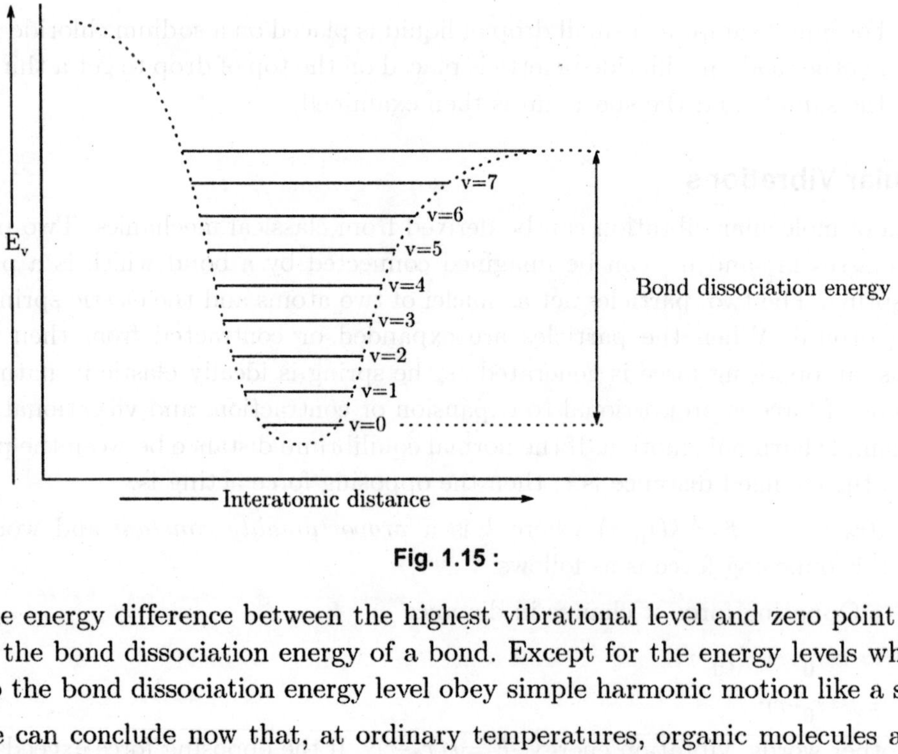

Fig. 1.15 :

The energy difference between the highest vibrational level and zero point energy level is the bond dissociation energy of a bond. Except for the energy levels which are close to the bond dissociation energy level obey simple harmonic motion like a spring.

We can conclude now that, at ordinary temperatures, organic molecules are in a constant state of vibration, where each bond has its characteristic stretching and bending frequencies and are capable of absorbing light at that frequency. As we have to apply more energy to stretch a spring rather to bend it, the stretching energy of a bond is more compared to its bending energy. In other words, *stretching absorptions of a bond appear at higher frequencies in the IR spectrum than the bending frequencies of the same bond.*

In general, molecular vibrations which leads to a *change in the dipole moment* of the molecule will give rise to absorption bands in the infrared. Otherwise they are said to be *IR inactive* and will show no absorption. For example, **the symmetrical stretching of the *C=C bond* in ethylene (a molecule with centre of symmetry) will not produce a change in the dipole moment of the molecule. This mode of vibration is therefore *IR inactive*.** This explains why symmetrical dichloroethylene (*trans* isomer) shows no C=C stretching but the *cis*-isomer shows this band.

Calculation of Vibrational Frequencies –The Hooke's Law and Force Constant

Hooke's law states that the frequency of vibration is directly proportional to the square root of the *force constant* of a bond. This force constant is characteristic of a bond with a definite value. Like other physical constants (m.p., b.p. etc.) it is another physical constant. The force constant may be linked to the *stiffness*, *i.e.*, strength of the bond. For the vibrations for which the molecule is *relatively flexible*, force constant is *less* and *vice versa.* Moreover, the frequency is inversely proportional to the square root of the reduced mass $\left(\frac{m_1.m_2}{(m_1+m_2)}\right)$ of the system. So according to Hooke's law,

$$\left.\begin{aligned} \nu &= \frac{1}{2\pi} \times \sqrt{\frac{k}{\frac{m_1.m_2}{(m_1+m_2)}}} \\ \text{and } \bar{\nu} &= \frac{1}{2\pi c} \times \sqrt{\frac{k}{\frac{m_1.m_2}{(m_1+m_2)}}} \end{aligned}\right\} \textit{(Hooke's law for diatomic molecule)}$$

where $\bar{\nu} = \frac{\nu}{c}$ and $\nu = \frac{1}{2\pi}\sqrt{\frac{k}{\mu}}$, μ=*reduced mass* $= \frac{m_1.m_2}{(m_1+m_2)}$

ν=frequency, $\bar{\nu}$ = wave number

k=force constant of the concerned bond (dyne cm^{-1}; g sec^{-2})

c=velocity of light (cm/sec)

m_1 and m_2=Masses of atoms

For an example, we can calculate the approximate frequency of C—H stretching vibration from the following data.

$k=500\ Nm^{-1}=5.0\times10^5 g\ sec^{-2}$ (since 1 Newton=10^3g.m.sec^{-2})

m_C=Mass of C atom = 20×10^{-24}g

m_H=Mass of hydrogen = 1.6×10^{-24}g

$$\nu = \frac{7}{2\times22}\left[\frac{5\times10^5 g.sec^{-2}}{\frac{(20\times10^{-24}g)\times(1.6\times10^{-24}g)}{(20+1.6)\times10^{-24}g}}\right]^{\frac{1}{2}} = 9.3\times10^{13}sec^{-1}$$

To express in wave number, the equation becomes

$$\bar{\nu} = \frac{\nu}{c} = \frac{9.3\times10^{13}\ sec^{-1}}{3.0\times10^8\ m\ sec^{-1}} = 3.1\times10^5\ m^{-1} = 3100\ cm^{-1}$$

The vibrational frequency of a bond is expected to increase when the bond strength increases and also when the reduced mass ($\mu = \frac{m_1.m_2}{m_1+m_2}$) of the system decreases.

Absorption Frequency

The frequency of radiation which is a simple multiple of vibrational frequency of that molecule gets absorbed and promotes the molecule from lower vibrational energy state to higher vibrational energy state. So in IR spectrum, the absorption maximum depends on the vibrational frequency. For highest absorption, the frequency of radiation becomes equal to the frequency of vibration.

Absorption of IR and Vibrational Transition

A bond must absorb *one quantum* of energy for transition from a lower vibrational energy level having vibrational quantum number v to a higher energy level having vibrational quantum number v+n.

$\therefore h\nu = E_{v+n} - E_v$

Now $E_v = (v+\frac{1}{2})h\omega$ where ω=frequency of vibration

$\therefore E_{v+n} - E_v = [v+n+\frac{1}{2}]h\omega - [v+\frac{1}{2}]h\omega = nh\omega$

$\therefore h\nu = nh\omega$ or $\nu = n\omega$

Therefore, a simple multiple of frequency of vibration will be the frequency of absorption of absorbed radiation. The probability of transition from one energy level to the *next energy level* is maximum. The probability of transition gets poor to the higher energy levels. In other words, when n=1, intensity of absorption is maximum; when n=2 intensity gets decreased (10% of first transition) and when n=3, the extent of absorption has *no practical use.* A bond absorb energy of one quantum per energy level from lowest or zero point energy level (v=0) and could be promoted to the highest energy level where the bond dissociates.

$\therefore$ *Bond dissociation energy* (B.D.E)=$\Sigma n\omega$

Conditions of IR absorption

1. The frequency of radiation should be that, when *1 quantum of energy* becomes equal to the difference in energy between the excited state vibrational level and ground state vibrational level of a molecule.

   $E_{excited} - E_{ground} = h\nu$

2. With vibration, the *dipole moment* of a molecule *should change, i.e.,* $\frac{d\mu}{dr} \neq 0$

3. For good absorption, the frequency of radiation should be simple multiple of frequency of vibration, *i.e.,*

   $\nu = n\omega$ and for *maximum absorption* $\nu = \omega$

Factors influencing vibrational frequency

1. **Mass of the atoms (Mass effect)** : If the masses of the atoms in a molecule increase, then reduced mass μ also increases. As a result, the magnitude of vibrational frequency decreases which is inversely proportional to the square root of reduced mass. The ratio of stretching frequencies of C—H and C—D (D=deuterium) bonds can be shown as follows.

$$\frac{\nu_{C-H}}{\nu_{C-D}} \cong \sqrt{\frac{\mu_{C-D}}{\mu_{C-H}}} = \sqrt{\frac{12\times2/(12+2)}{12\times1/(12+1)}} \cong \frac{\sqrt{2}}{1}$$

The force constant for both the frequencies is almost equal.

Similar conclusion can be drawn for O—H and O—D *stretching frequencies.*

The experimental result is in good agreement. The stretching absorption maxima for C—H and C—D are approximately 2900cm^{-1} and 2200cm^{-1} respectively.

The stretching frequency of any bond where hydrogen is present as one constituent has a high value of stretching frequency compared to other atoms, as hydrogen bears the lowest mass. For the same reason C—H and O—H stretching absorptions have high values compared to C—C and C—O stretching frequencies.

2. **Nature of vibration** : Stretching vibrational frequency of a bond is always higher than the bending frequency of the same bond. The molecule is relatively flexible towards bending (or *less stiff* towards bending) and so the force constant of bending is comparatively less compared to the stretching frequency counterpart. As a result,

$$\nu_{\text{stretching}} > \nu_{\text{bending}}$$

3. **Nature of bond**

(a) Bond length : The bond strength increases with decrease in bond length and *vice-versa.* The vibrational frequency increases with decrease in bond length. One can thus predict that C=C and C=O stretching frequencies will have higher values than C—C and C—O stretching frequencies.

(b) Bond multiplicity : Bond strength increases with increase in bond multiplicity. Double bond is stronger than a single bond and a triple bond is stronger than a double bond. So the stretching frequencies of the bonds follow the order—

$$\nu_{\text{triple bond}} > \nu_{\text{double bond}} > \nu_{\text{single bond}}$$

The *ratio of force constants* of C—C, C=C and C≡C is approximately 1:2:3. So, $\nu_{C-C} : \nu_{C=C} : \nu_{C\equiv C}$ is *approximately* $1:\sqrt{2}:\sqrt{3}$

	C≡C	C=C	C—C
	← Increasing bond strength —		
$\bar{\nu}$ in cm^{-1}	~ 2200	~ 1650	~ 1200

Sometimes, the nature of bond changes due to resonance which is manifested in the value of ν. Ketenes are more resonance stabilised than ketones and C=O stretching frequency of a ketene is higher than that of a ketone.

$$R_2C{=}C{=}\ddot{\underset{\cdot\cdot}{O}} \longleftrightarrow R_2\overset{\ominus}{\ddot{C}}{-}C{\equiv}\overset{\oplus}{O}:$$

(c) Dipolar nature of a bond : The stiffness of a bond increases when a dipole is generated in the molecule, as in that case, the molecule is held rigid by electrostatic attraction between the opposite charges. So,

$$\nu_{O-H_{str}} > \nu_{C-H_{str}} \text{ and } \nu_{C=O_{str}} > \nu_{C=C_{str}}$$

Regarding mass effect, the order should be reverse. Here electrostatic attraction between the atoms due to polarity difference takes a key role. But in the case of C—C, C—N, C—O etc. where the atoms are connected by single bonds, there is valence shell electron pair repulsion and as a result, the bond becomes weak, *i.e.*, bond strength becomes weakened.

$$\text{B.D.E}_{C-C} > \text{B.D.E}_{C-N} > \text{B.D.E}_{C-O} \quad (\text{B.D.E}=\textit{Bond dissociation energy})$$

With decrease in bond strength, force constant decreases and stretching frequency also decreases. Again atomic mass increases from carbon to oxygen for which also ν_{str} decreases and we get the following order.

$$\nu_{C-C_{str}} > \nu_{C-N_{str}} > \nu_{C-O_{str}}$$

(d) Percentage s-character : The bond strength decreases with increase in s-character and the bond also becomes *more stiff*. So,

$$\nu_{sp\,C-H_{str}} > \nu_{sp^2\,C-H_{str}} > \nu_{sp^3\,C-H_{str}}$$

The percentage s-character also depends on bond angle. With increase in bond angle, the extent of *s-character increases* and consequently ν *becomes higher*. In cyclobutanone, C—C=O bond angle is more than 120°. So the bonding orbital of C=O faces more s-character and the C=O bond becomes more *stiff*. On the other hand, the C—C=O bond angle in ditertiarybutyl ketone is less than 120° (due to steric repulsion between the two bulky tertiarybutyl groups) and the % s-character is less in C=O bond. As a result, C=O stretching frequency in cyclobutanone has a higher value compared to C=O stretching frequency in ditertiarybutyl ketone.

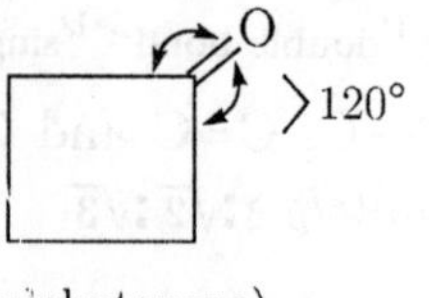

(Cyclobutanone)

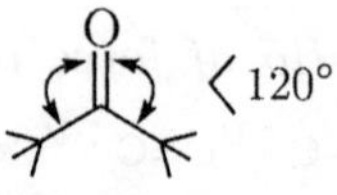

(Ditertiary butyl ketone)

Cyclopropane has higher C—H stretching frequency over C—H stretching frequency in *n*-propane. In cyclopropane, the bonding C—H orbital has more s-character and so C—H stretching absorbs at a higher frequency.

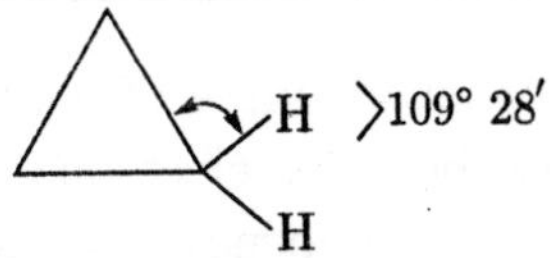

4. **Electronic effect** : Electronic effect includes inductive and resonance effects, together with occassional through space influence or field effect.

Conjugation lowers the frequency of $C{=}O_{str}$ and $C{=}C_{str}$ whether the conjugation is brought about by α, β unsaturation or by an aromatic ring.

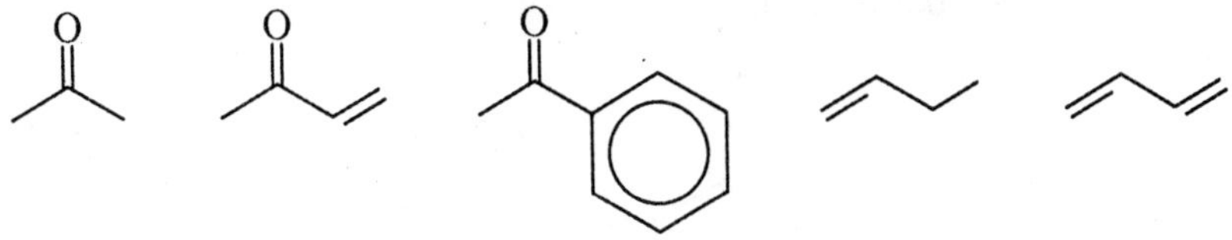

$\bar{\nu}_{C=O}$	(I)	(II)	(III)	(IV)	(V)
(cm^{-1})	1720	1700	1700	1650	1610

In (III), delocalisation of π-electrons between C=O and the ring increases the double bond character of the bond joining the C=O to the ring. This leads to a lower bond order in the C=O bond which is consequently weakened; the decrease in force constant lowers the stretching vibration frequency by 20-30 cm^{-1}.

One can also attribute such C=O frequency shifts to the mesomeric or resonance effect; any substituent that enhances the mesomeric shift will decrease the bond order of C=O bond and lead to lower C=O stretching frequency.

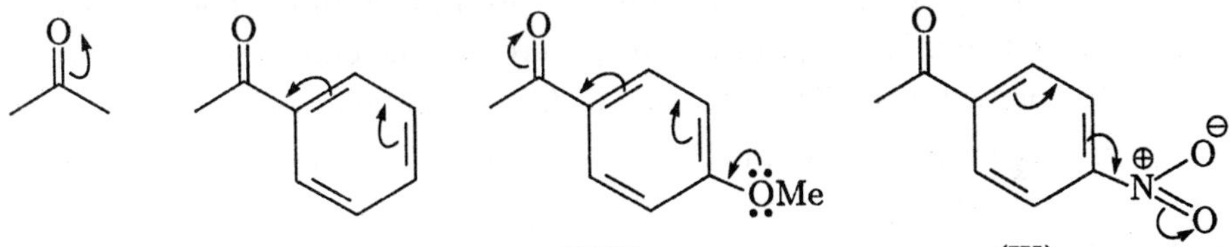

(VI) (VII) (VIII) (IX)

Conjugation with phenyl (VII) does so and a (+R) group such as *p*-OMe in (VIII) will lead to even lower frequencies. A *p*-NO_2 group (IX) (–R) will oppose these trends and lead to higher frequencies.

In amides, (XI) (+R) effect produces a lengthening (weakening) of the C=O bond, leading to lower frequency in the corresponding ketone, (X); the (–I) effect of Cl in acyl chlorides, (XII), is more influential than +R and here an opposite shift (to *higher frequency*) occurs.

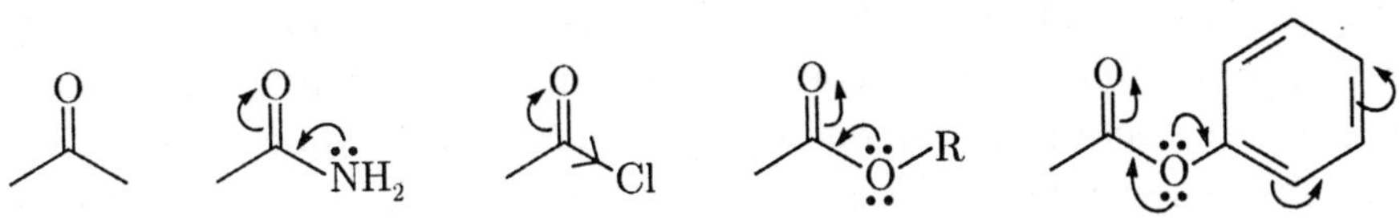

(X) (XI) (XII) (XIII) (XIV)

Esters represent another example of conflict between I and R effects. In alkyl esters (XIII), the non bonding electrons on oxygen increase (+R) conjugation, leading to lower the C=O frequency. The electronegativity of oxygen, (–I) operates in the opposite sense but (+R) is apparently dominant. In phenyl esters (XIV), the non bonding electrons are partly drawn into the ring, and their conjugation with C=O is consequently diminished. When this happens, the (–I) effect of oxygen becomes dominant and C=O moves to higher frequency.

Let us take the following series.

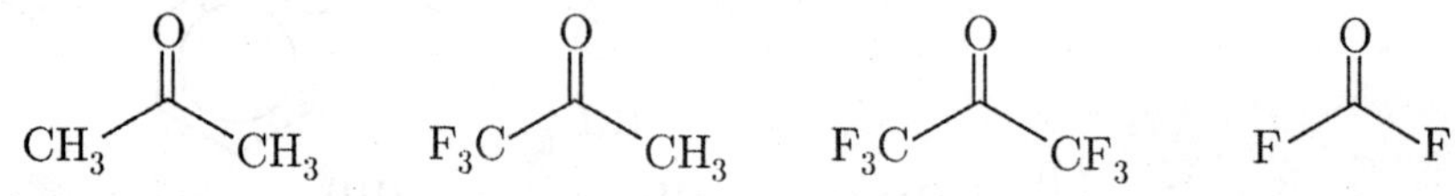

C=O str (cm^{-1})	1720	1769	1801	1928

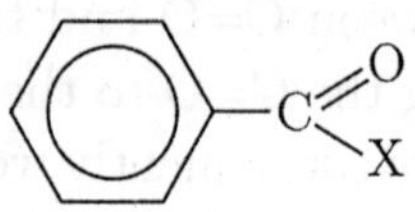

	X=Br	OPh	OMe	H	Me	NMe_2
C=O str (in cm^{-1})	1760	1750	1735	1714	1697	1660
	(–I)	(–I/+R)	(–I/+R)			(–I/+R)

Here also the double bond character in C=O is measured by both (–I) and (+R) effects. when X=Br, (–I) effect is prominent but when X=NMe_2, (+R) takes precedence. In the phenyl ester, there is some delocalisation of the electrons into the phenyl ring. The increase in C=O frequency of an ester as compared to a ketone suggests that, (–I) effect (of $\ddot{\underset{\cdot\cdot}{O}}$Me) is more important than (+M) effect.

Bond angles

In ketones, the highest C=O frequencies arise in the strained cyclobutanones, and we can explain this in terms of bond-angular strain; the *C—$\hat{C}$O—C bond angle* is reduced *below* the *normal 120°*, leading to *increased s-character* in the C=O bond. The C=O bond is shortened and therefore strengthened and so $\nu_{C=O}$ increases. If the bond angle is pushed outwards *above 120°*, the opposite effect operates and for this reason, ditertiary-butyl ketone has a very low $\bar{\nu}_{C=O}$ stretching frequency (1697cm^{-1}).

An alternative view involves no change in the C=O force constant but merely an increased rigidity in the C—CO—C bond system as ring size decreases; C=O stretching must in these circumstances couple more effectively with C—C stretching, leading to higher C=O stretching frequencies. Cycloalkanes also show such an effect, but a less simple relationship holds. Thus, in cycloalkenes (XV), $\bar{\nu}_{C=C}$ falls with increasing strain, but reaches a minimum in cyclobutene. In cyclobutene (XVI) stretching of C=C involves only bending of attached C—C bonds. In all the others (where internal angles are *not 90°*),

C=C stretching must involve some stretching of the adjacent C—C bonds which involves increasing the energy (*frequency*) of C=C stretching.

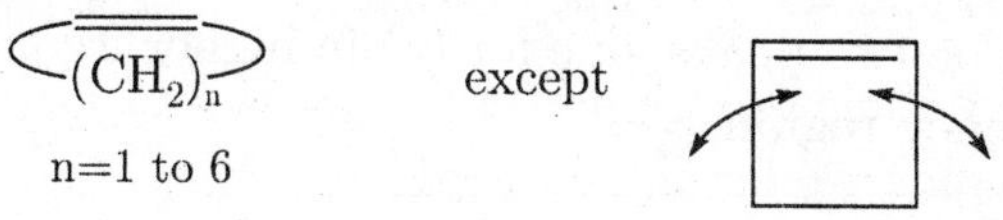

(XV) (XVI)

$\bar{\nu}_{C=C_{str}} \cong 1610\text{–}1650\ cm^{-1}$ 1566 cm^{-1}

C—H stretching vibrations move to higher frequency in the sequence alkane-alkene-alkyne. As the hybridisation goes from sp^3 to sp^2 to sp, the s-character of the C—H bond increases, bond lengths become shorter and frequencies arise. Cyclopropanes have high C—H stretching frequencies for the same reason (3070-3040cm^{-1}), the C—$\hat{C}$—C bond angle is substantially contracted below 109°28′ leading to increased s-character in the C—H bonds and thus to higher frequencies.

Field effects

Two groups often influence each other's vibrational frequencies by a through space interaction, which may be electrostatic and/or steric in nature. The best examples of this field effect are interactions between carbonyl groups and halogen atoms; for example, in the α-chloroketone derivatives of steroids, (XVIII), C=O stretching frequency is higher when chlorine is equatorial than when it is axial. Presumably the non bonding electrons of oxygen and chlorine undergo repulsion when they are close together in the molecule, this results in a change in the hybridisation state of oxygen and therefore a shift in C=O stretching frequency.

In *o*-chloro or hydroxybenzoic acid esters, this field effect shifts the C=O frequency in the rotational isomer (XVIII), and not in the isomer (XIX); both isomers are normally present, so that **two C=O stretching absorptions** are observed in the spectrum of this compound.

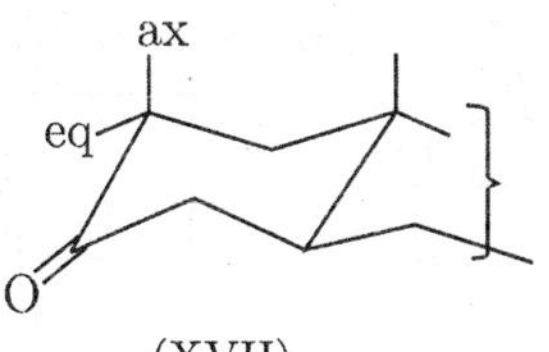

(XVII)

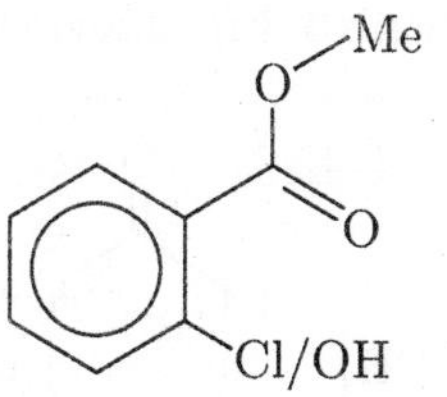

(XVIII)(a)

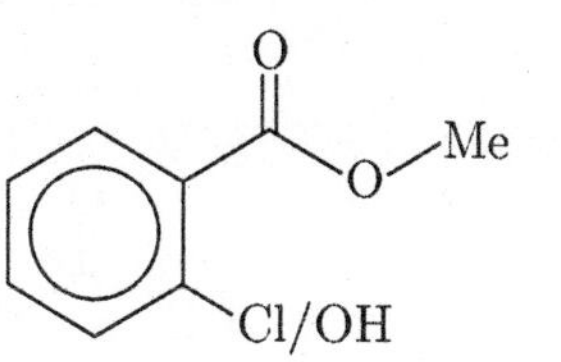

(XVIII)(b)

Two peaks are available for C=O stretching frequency a. one in normal region and b. the other in higher frequency region. In case (a), simple charges on oxygen and chlorine are close to each other in space. So, there is an electrostatic repulsion between the two (dipole-dipole interaction). So, in order to decrease the negative charge density on the oxygen atom (to minimise the repulsion), $>\overset{\oplus}{C}-\overset{\ominus}{O}$ will have less contribution than $>=O$. So C—O has more double bond character and $\bar{\nu}_{C=O}$ stretching shifts to higher frequency. But in (b), no such effect is operative and gives peak in normal frequency region. So there will be two peaks, one for (a) in higher frequency region and another for (b) in normal frequency region.

Effect of ring strain

Ring strain in cyclic compounds causes a comparatively large shift of C=O stretching to higher frequency. This provides a dependable test to distinguish clearly between 3–, 4– and 5– and also larger membered ring ketones. Six membered ring ketones show the normal frequency found for the open chain compounds. Two explanations have been advanced to explain this influence of strain on C=O stretching frequency. The C—$\hat{C}$O—C bond angle is reduced below the normal (~120° in acyclic and six-membered ring ketones) bond angle in strained rings. This leads to an increase in the s-character in the C=O bond, which is therefore, strengthened and consequently C=O stretching frequency is increased. The C=O stretching frequency displayed by the acyclic system like ditertiarybutyl ketone is very low (1698cm^{-1}), since now the opposite effect operates (increase in *p*-character), the C—$\hat{C}$O—C bond angle being pushed outwards above 120°.

In an alternate explanation, it has been suggested that C=O stretching is affected by the adjacent C—C stretching. When the ring is strained, the interaction with C—C bond stretching leads to an increase in the energy for C=O stretching and as a consequence, C=O stretching frequency increases.

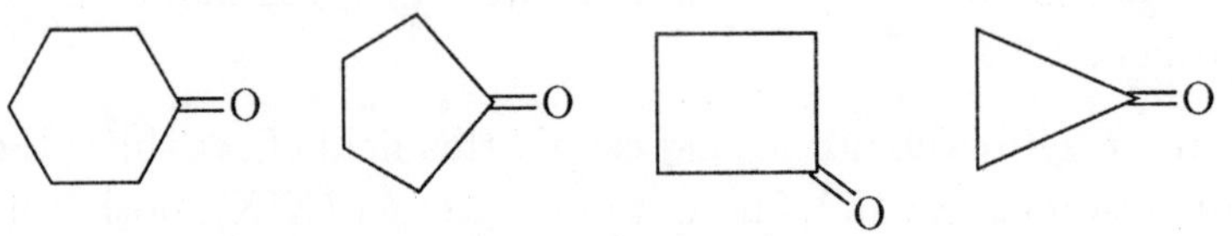

$\bar{\nu}_{C=O_{str}}$ (cm^{-1}) 1715 1740 1760 1780

——— Increasing s character ———→

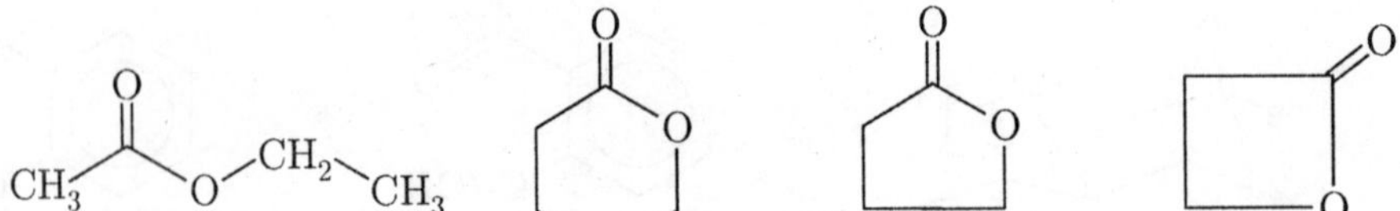

	(Ethyl acetate)	(δ-valerolactone)	(γ-butyrolactone)	(β-propiolactone)
$\bar{\nu}_{C=O_{str}}$ (cm^{-1})	1735	1735	1770	1800
	(no strain)	(no strain)	(moderate strain)	(high strain)

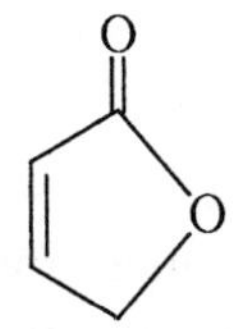 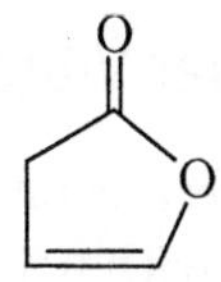

$\bar{\nu}_{C=O_{str}}$ (cm^{-1}) 1750 1800

So we see that, C=O stretching frequency depends on the position of the double bonds in the unsaturated lactones.

So *ring strain* in *lactones increases* the *C=O stretching frequency.*

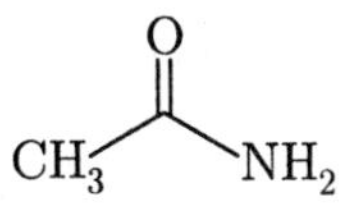 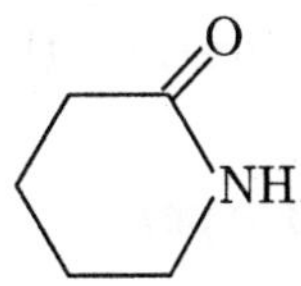 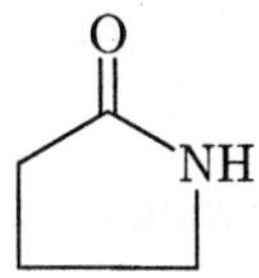 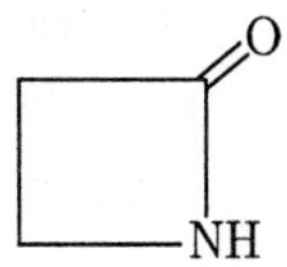

	(Acetamide)	(δ-Valerolactam)	(γ-Butyrolactam)	(β-Propiolactam)
$\bar{\nu}_{C=O_{str}}$ (cm^{-1})	1680	1670	1700	1745
	(no strain)	(no strain)	(moderate strain)	(high strain)

Ring strain in *lactams increases* the *C=O stretching frequency.*

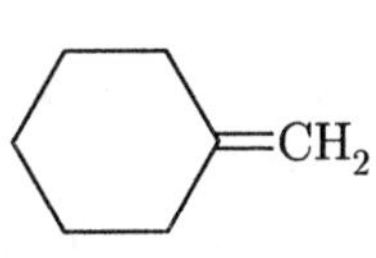 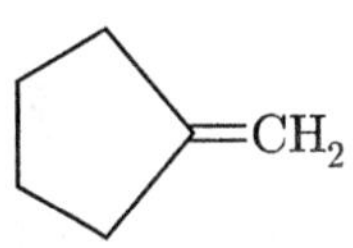 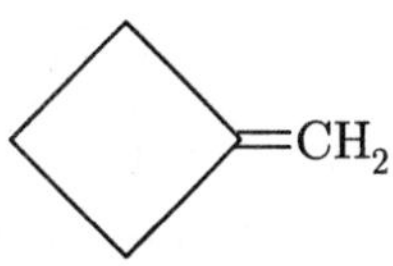 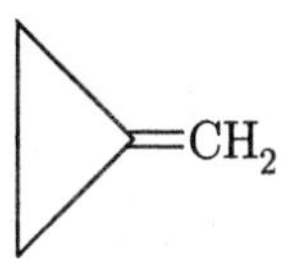

$\bar{\nu}_{C=C_{str}}$ (cm^{-1}) 1651 1657 1690 1750

The explanation is the same as stated earlier.

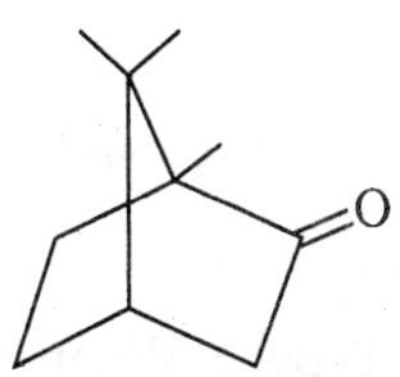 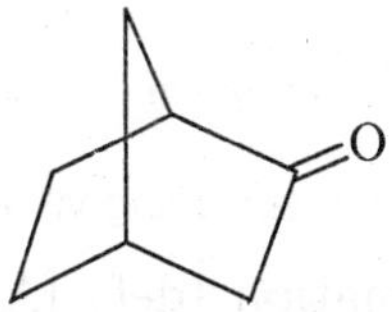 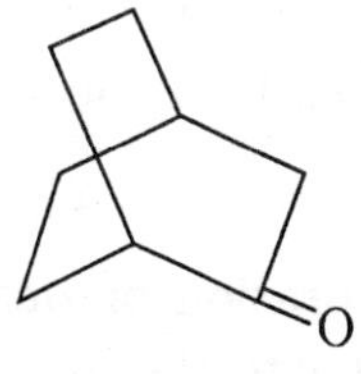 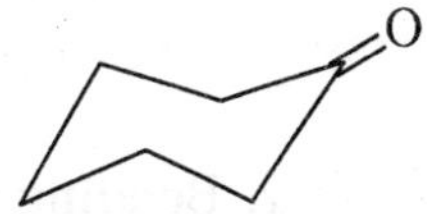

(Comphor)

$\bar{\nu}_{C=O_{str}}$ (cm^{-1}) 1740 1750 1731 1715

The bicyclic ketones show C=O stretching frequency for higher than expected for a cyclohexanone ring. In bicyclic systems, the cyclohexanone ring is present not as a chair, but in a boat conformation, which raises a strain in the bicyclic ketones. As a result, the force constant of C=O increases making C=O bond stiff and consequently they absorb at a higher frequency.

Modes of Molecular Vibration

Molecules with large assemblages of atoms possess many vibrational frequencies; for a *non-linear* molecule with n atoms, the number of vibrational modes is (3n–6); so methane theoretically possesses 9 and ethane has 18 modes of vibration. Does this lead to methane having 9 and not more than 9 absorption bands in the infrared? For *linear molecules*, the number of vibrational modes is (3n–5). Among these modes some vibrate along bond axis and some of them are perpendicular to the bond axis. According to the direction of vibration, they are divided into two categories.

1. **Stretching vibration** : Vibration along the bond-axis is known as stretching vibration. During stretching vibration, the bond length increases or decreases periodically.

   (a) ***For linear molecules (A–B type)***

A—B	A——B	A–B
(Average bond length)	(Expanded condition)	(Contracted condition)

   (b) ***For non-linear molecules (AB_2 system, e.g., $-NH_2$, $-NO_2$ etc.)*** : For *non-linear* (AB_2 type) molecules, stretching vibration may be divided into *two types* as follows.

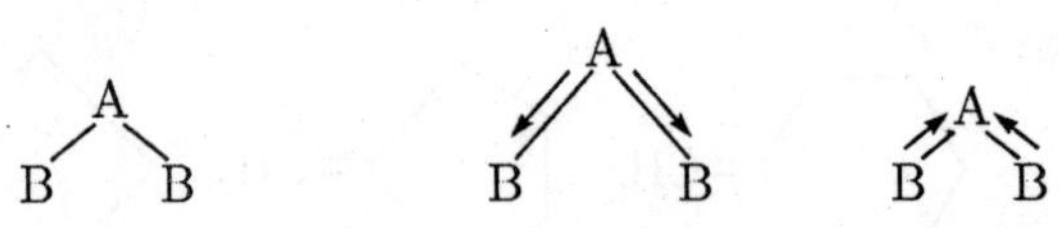

(Average bond length) (Expanded) (Contracted)

Symmetric streching vibrations

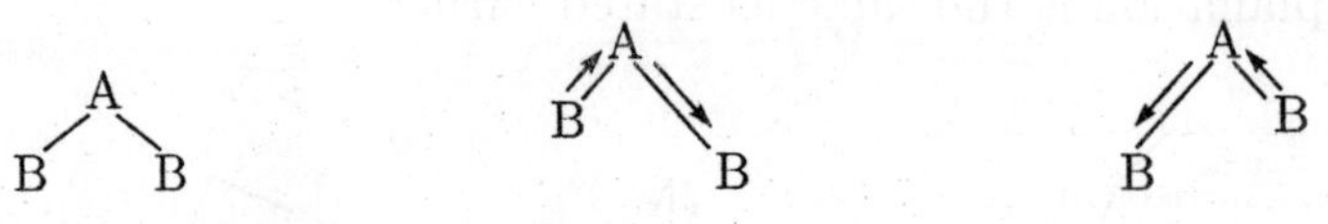

(Average bond length) (Contraction–Expansion) (Expansion–Contraction)

Asymmetric stretching vibrations

2. **Bending vibration or deformation (def) [AB_2 type]** : When vibration occurs *perpendicular* to the bond axis is known as bending vibration. The bond angle of a molecule increases or decreases periodically due to bonding vibration.

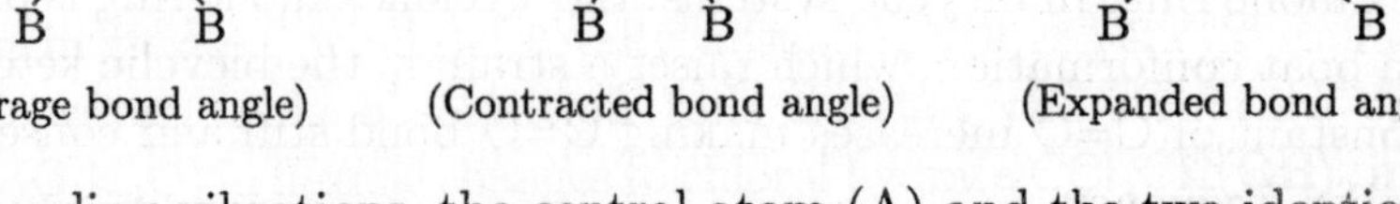

(Average bond angle) (Contracted bond angle) (Expanded bond angle)

In some bending vibrations, the central atom (A) and the two identical atoms connected to A (*i.e.*, *two* B atoms) lie in the same plane. Such type of bending vibration is known as *in plane bending vibrations.* But there are some bending vibrations where the two similar atoms attached to the central atom vibrate in a plane perpendicular to each other, and these types of bending vibrations are known as *out of plane bending vibrations.*

Examples :

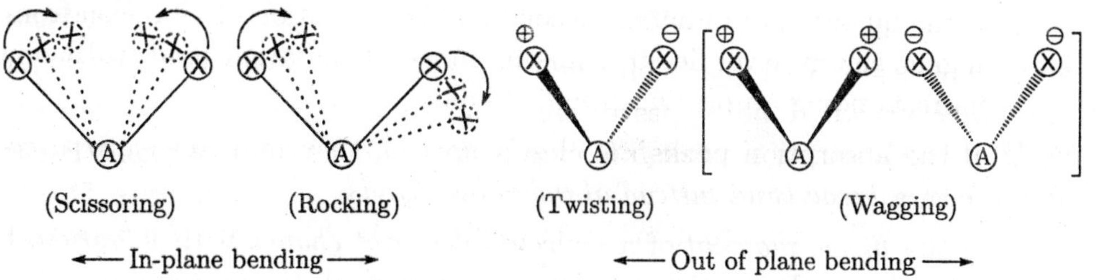

(The direction of arrows shows the direction of virbration)

Vibrational Coupling

An isolated C—H bond has only one stretching frequency but the stretching vibrations of C—H bonds in —CH_2– combine together to produce two coupled vibrations of different frequencies, the asymmetric $\bar{\nu}_{anti}$ and symmetric $\bar{\nu}_{sym}$. The C—H bonds in —CH_3 also give rise to symmetric and asymmetric vibrations. These vibrations (of —CH_3) are different from those of —CH_2– and can be seen in high resolution spectrum of the molecule.

Vibrational coupling takes place between two bonds vibrating with similar frequency, provided the bonds are reasonably closely situated in the molecule; the coupling vibrations may both be fundamental or a overtone where a fundamental vibration couples with some other vibration. The coupling of latter type is commonly called "**Fermi Resonance**" (named after the discoverer *Enrico Fermi*). Due to Fermi Resonance, the intensity of absorption increases and a very prominent band is found in the IR spectrum.

For polyatomic non-linear molecules, a number of absorption peaks are possible in IR spectrum and the reasons for the formation of those peaks are summarised below.

1. For *non-linear polyatomic molecules*, (3n–6) (n=number of atoms present in the molecule) different modes of stretching and bending vibrations are possible and for each different mode, one absorption peak appears.
2. Apart from fundamental tones of vibration ($\nu=\omega'$), overtones ($\nu=2\omega'$, $3\omega'$) are also possible. For both fundamental tones and overtones, absorption peaks are possible.
3. Due to vibrational coupling, combination band ($\nu=\nu_1+\nu_2$) and difference band ($\nu=\nu_1-\nu_2$) etc. are possible.
4. Some absorptions may get intensified due to Fermi Resonance, and can cite important absorption peaks.

In other words, we may conclude that, *the presence of absorption peaks does not confirm the presence of a particular functionality unambiguously, rather its absence confirms that, that particular functionality is not present in the molecule.*

There are some reasons for which the number of IR absorption peaks may get diminished.

1. If the quantum of radiation needed for the transition of vibration from lower to higher energy level lies beyond the range of radiation used in IR analysis, no corresponding absorption peak is found.
2. If the absorption peaks are closely spaced, they may get *superposed* and can form a *broad band instead of individual bands.*
3. If the *dipole moment* of a molecule *does not change* with *vibration*, then that vibration is IR inactive and no absorption peak can be absorved.

Some typical asymmetric and symmetric stretching frequencies for AB_2 type groups

Group	Asym (cm^{-1})	Sym (cm^{-1})
1. $—CH_2—$	3000	2900
2. $—NH_2$	3400	3300
3. $—NO_2$ ($—\overset{\oplus}{N}(=O)(—O^{\ominus})$)	1550	1400
4. $—SO_2—$ ($O=S=O$)	1350	1150
5. (salt of $—C(=O)OH$)	1600	1400

Vibrational coupling and carboxylic acid anhydrides

Carboxylic acid anhydrides give rise to two C=O stretching absorptions, $\bar{\nu}_{asym}$ and $\bar{\nu}_{sym}$ (around 1900–1800cm^{-1}, with a separation of about 65cm^{-1}); coupling occurs between

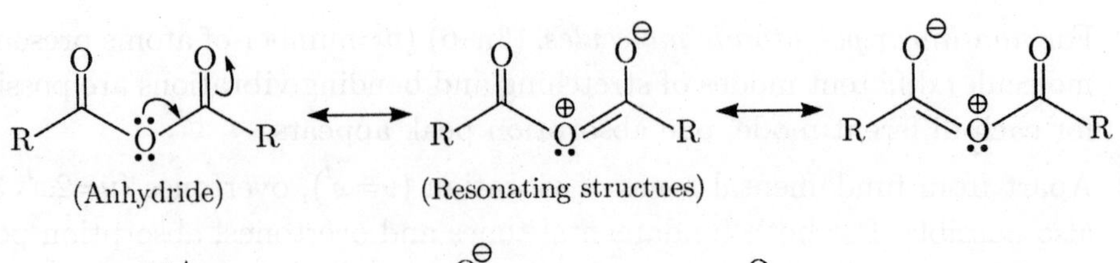

(Anhydride) (Resonating structuctes)

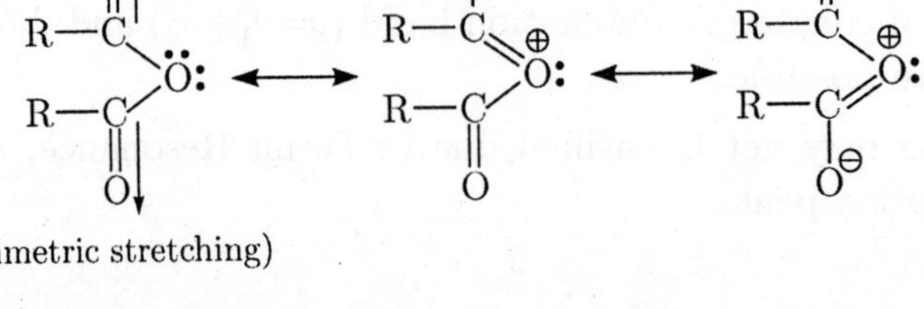

(Symmetric stretching)

two carboxyl groups, which are *indirectly* linked through —Ö—. The interaction is presumably encouraged because of the slight double bond character in the carboxyl-oxygen bonds brought about by resonance, since this will keep the system coplanar. The high frequency band in this case is the symmetric C=O stretching.

Amides

Amides show *two* absorption bands around 1700–1600cm^{-1} corresponding mainly to C=O *stretching* and N—H *bending* (def), but because of vibrational coupling, the original nature of the vibrations are modified. Two bands are not pure C=O stretching and N—H def, and are commonly referred to as amide (I) and amide (II) bands. Amide (I) may be as high as 80% C=O stretching in character but amide (II) is a strongly coupled interaction between N—H def and C—N stretching.

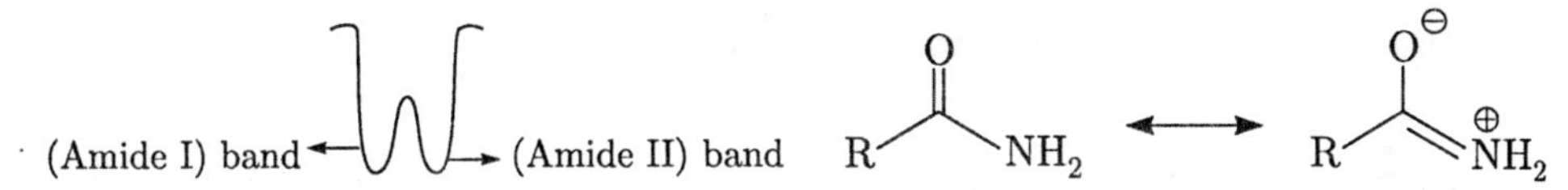

Higher is the energy of the orbital containing the lone pair, greater will be the extent of participation of lone pair of electrons in resonance. Nitrogen being less electronegative than oxygen, always contains higher energy orbital containing lone pair, and so mesomeric effect predominates over inductive effect in the case of amides.

Aldehydes

In aldehydes, C—H *stretching* usually appears as a doublet because of interaction between the C—H stretching fundamental and overtone of C—H def (*i.e.*, C—H bending frequency). If a sharp peak at 1900–1600cm^{-1} and a doublet at 2800–2700cm^{-1} () appears, that confirms the presence of 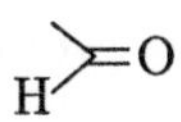 group.

Some common terms used in IR spectroscopy

Overtone Bands

Ovetone bonds appear at integral multiple of fundamental vibrations. For example, strong absorption at x cm^{-1} will also give rise to weaker absorption at 2x cm^{-1}.

Beat Bands

Two frequencies may interact to give beats which are combination or difference frequencies. For example, absorptions at x cm^{-1} and y cm^{-1} interact to produce two weaker BEAT frequencies at (x±y)cm^{-1}.

Vibrational coupling in some molecules

For —CH_2— group, the stretching frequency gives a doublet (W) one peak for symmetric stretching at lower frequency and another for asymmetric stretching at higher frequency. When the stretching frequency of two bonds are very close to each other, and the bonds are also close to each other, then coupling may take place in a molecule.

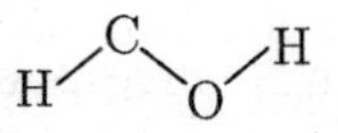

($\bar{\nu}$stretch are different for C—H and O—H bonds so no coupling is found)

or

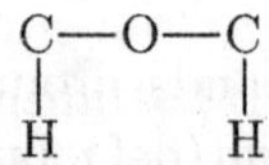

(no coupling as the C—H bonds are far apart)

R—NH_2 (primary amine) ⟹ 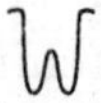 $\bar{\nu}_{strech}$ (3300–3500 cm^{-1}) (Two peaks)

R_2NH (secondary amine) ⟹ 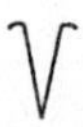 (one peak)

R_3N (tertiary amine) ⟹ no peak

Fermi resonance

When a fundamental vibration is coupling with a non fundamental vibration, then it is known as FERMI RESONANCE.

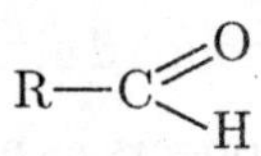

Overtone of C—H bending frequency and C—H stretching frequency couples with each other and a doublet (W) peak arises. If a sharp peak at (1900–1600 cm^{-1}) and a *doublet* at (2800–2700 cm^{-1}) arises, that confirms 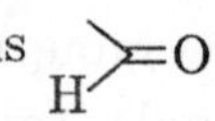 group is present.

Finger print region (900–1400 cm^{-1}) (F.P.R)

The region that contains a particularly large number of unassigned vibrations (and is most valuable in this respect) is roughly from 900–1400 cm^{-1} and this general area is called the **Finger print region**. No prominent stretching frequency is found in this region, most of them being instead bending frequencies.

If two diastereoisomers, who are different from each other in a very small aspect, especially only one centre is "R" for one and "S" for another (but they are *not enantiomers*), $\bar{\nu}_{\text{stretching frequency}}$ will be the same for two. But in the finger print region, the two compounds will give rise to different peaks.

F.P.R contains all types of bending vibrations (also some types of stretching vibration). It is rather complicated part of a spectrum, but *not impossible* to assign the vibrational peaks with the characteristic bands. However it is generally used for establishing the identity of a molecule. If F.P.R of two molecules are **indentical** in all respects; they are identical in stereochemistry, structures etc.

Characteristic and Diagnostic Stretching Frequencies of some Bonds

Analysis of IR spectra : The IR radiation used experimentally lies in the range 2.5 μ to 15 μ (wave length) or 4000 cm^{-1} to 650 cm^{-1} (wave number). Some characteristic stretching absorption peaks are found between 1500 to 4000 cm^{-1} which indicates the presence of some special functional groups. The stretching absorption of C—C, C—N, C—O etc. (σ-bonded) are found in the region 650 cm^{-1} to 1500 cm^{-1} and many bending absorption peaks are also found here. Sometimes the peaks get superposed and the individual characteristics are lost. This region is known as finger print region and except enantiomers no two molecules have similar finger print region.

The presence of some functional groups can be proved unambigously from IR spectra.

1. **O–H Bond and hydrogen bond regarding O–H$_{st}$** : If the IR spectrum shows a broad band as absorption peak in the region 3300 cm^{-1} to 3500 cm^{-1}, the molecule under investigation may contain O—H bond. The position of O—H stretching absorption maxima for phenols, alcohols, enols, carboxylic acids etc. come approximately around 3500 cm^{-1}. The above said molecules remain hydrogen bonded either in solid, liquid or in concentrated solution form. As a result, the charge density on the O—H dipole gets decreased compared to that present in unbonded or free O—H group and also the electrostatic attraction becomes less. In other words, the *stiffness of unbonded O—H bond is more.* Again the extent of stiffness is not equal for all O—H bonds present in the molecule. As a result, a number of closely spaced O—H stretching absorption maxima are possible and on superposition they give rise to **broad bands.**

   But in the gaseous state or in highly dilute solution, the molecules may get free from hydrogen bonding. The force constant of free O—H bond is more and a sharp absorption peak is found at a comparatively higher wave number (3650 cm^{-1}) where the stretching vibration is same for all the O—H bonds. For example, ethyl alcohol shows a broad band at 3500 cm^{-1} in liquid form. But when a solution of ethyl alcohol in carbon tetrachloride is diluted gradually, a new sharp peak at about 3600 cm^{-1} is found. In very dilute solution, the broad band (at 3500 cm^{-1}) may get vanished totally, and only the sharp peak (~3600 cm^{-1}) remains. The O—H stretching absorption band of phenols come at 3550 cm^{-1} as a broad band, which indicates that phenol molecules are also hydrogen bonded. But, 2,6–ditertiarybutylphenol shows absorption peak at about 3650 cm^{-1} as a **sharp band**. In first case, the phenol molecules are hydrogen bonded but in the second case, hydrogen bonding is inhibited due to the presence of steric repulsion exerted by bulky tertiarybutyl groups at the *o*-positions. For 2-tertiarybutyl phenol, two bands appear, one broad band at 3500 cm^{-1} and another, a sharp one at 3650 cm^{-1}. Some conformers of 2-tertiarybutylphenol are hydrogen-bonded (show broad spectrum at 3550 cm^{-1}) and some are free from hydrogen bonding (show sharp peak at 3650 cm^{-1}) and as a result, we get two absorption peaks.

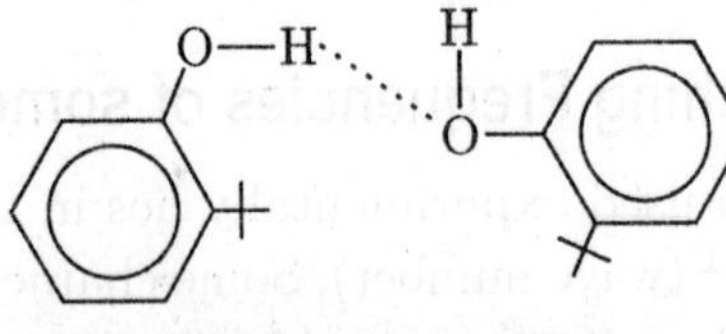

(Hydrogen bonded conformer of 2-tertiarybutylphenol)

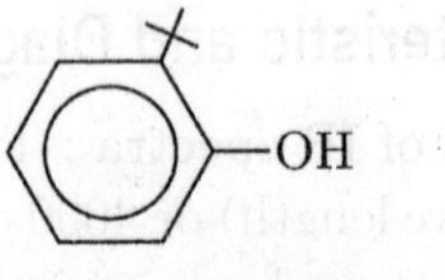

(2-tertiarybutylphenol free from H-bonding)

The molecules where O—H group is *internally* or *intramolecularly hydrogen bonded* give absorption peak of *broad nature* at about 3550 cm^{-1} and on dilution *no change* in the absorption band is observed. When the solution is sufficiently dilute, the molecules can be separated from one another which are *intermolecularly* hydrogen bonded but this technique does not help to separate the molecules which are *intramolecularly hydrogen* bonded free from hydrogen bonding. So this type of molecules show broad absorption band either in liquid, in concentrated solution or in dilute solution. For example, the IR spectrum of ethylene glycel shows a broad spectrum at about 3550 cm^{-1} which on sufficient dilution with carbon tetrachloride does not change its position or nature. (In highly dilute solution, ethylene glycel shows two absorption maxima at 32 cm^{-1} apart by high resolution technique.)

IR spectrum helps us to distinguish between the isomers, where one of them is capable of forming hydrogen bond and the other is not. Sometimes it is even possible to assign the conformation of one isomer.

***Examples* :**

1. **Separation of salicylaldehyde from *m*-or *p*-hydroxybenzaldehyde :** The IR spectra of pure salicylaldehyde and pure *m*- or *p*-hydroxybenzaldehyde are taken separately in carbon tetrachloride solution. Now, the IR spectrum of the mixture of salicylaldehyde and *p* or *m*-hydroxybenzaldehyde in carbon tetrachloride solvent is taken. Further dilution with carbon tetrachloride, the O—H band of *p*-hydroxy benzaldehyde (broad

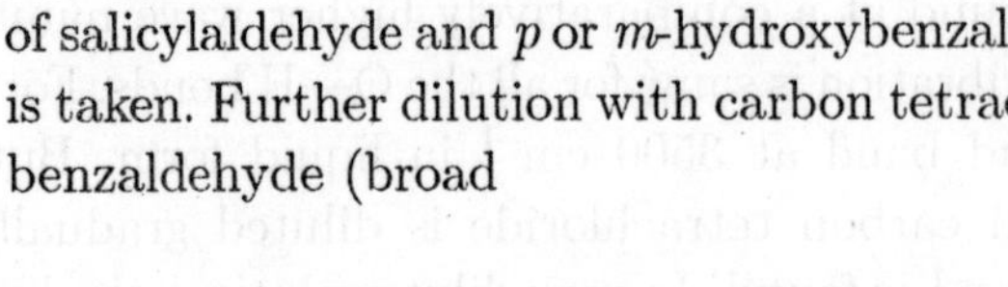

(*p*-hydroxybenzaldehyde)
(*intermolecularly* hydrogen bonded)

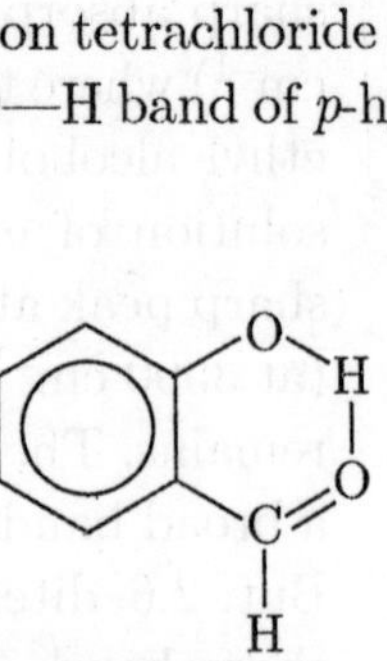

(Salicylaldehyde)
(*intramolecularly* hydrogen bonded)

at 3550 cm^{-1}) changed to a sharp peak for O—H stretching band at 3650 cm^{-1}. Salicylaldehyde does not change either its position or nature of O—H stretching band even on very high dilution. *p*-hydroxybenzaldehyde is intermolecularly hydrogen bonded under normal conditions which can be made free from hydrogen bonding on dilution but salicylaldehyde does not change its O—H stretching band position even on high dilution because it is intramolecularly hydrogen bonded.

2. ***Cis*-cyclohexane-1,3-diol can exist in two conformations which are shown as follows.**

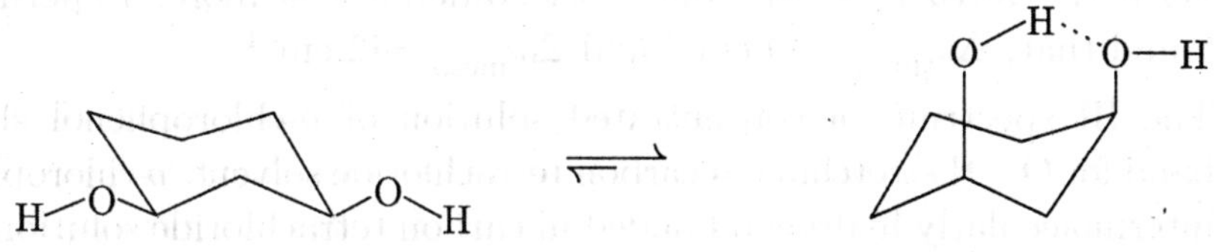

(*Diequatorial* conformer) *Cis*-cyclohexane-1,3-diol

(*Diaxial* conformer) (more stable conformer as a stable 6-membered chelate is formed on intramolecular *hydrogen bonding*)

The diequatorial conformer may undergo intermolecular hydrogen bond and so can be made free from it when diluted with carbon tetrachloride. But the diaxial conformer is intramolecularly hydrogen bonded and so does not change either its position or nature with dilution in the IR spectrum. This observation proves that *cis*- cyclohexane-1,3-diol mainly exists as a diaxial conformer.

3. **Separation of erythro- (*meso*-isomer) and *threo*- butane -2,3-diol (active isomer) by high resolution IR spectroscopy**

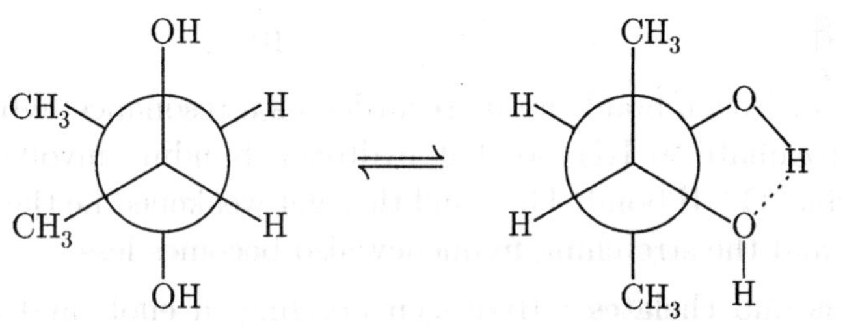

(*Threo*-isomer) (active) (I) (II)

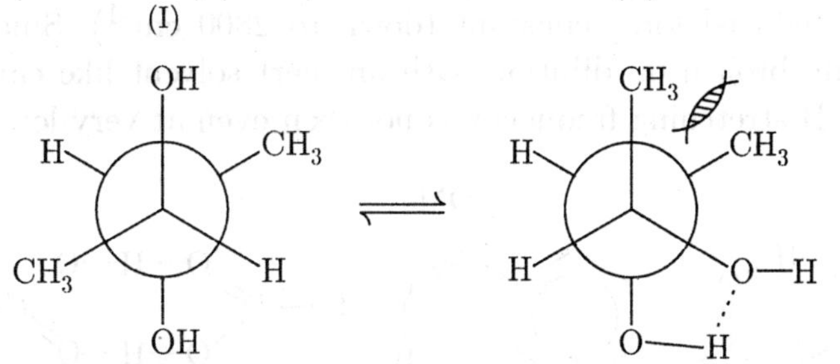

(*Meso*-isomer) (Inactive) (III) (IV)

If we compare (II) and (IV), we see that, (IV) contains are CH_3/CH_3 gauche butane interaction, which is absent in (II) and so conformation (II) is more stable and contains stronger hydrogen bonding. The force constant becomes less with increasing strength of hydrogen bonding and the difference in O—H stretching frequency between hydrogen bonded O—H and unbonded O—H stretching frequency becomes *more.* On dilution with carbon tetrachloride both (II) and (IV) show two absorption maxima for O—H stretching in high resolution IR. But the difference in absorption maxima is different for the two isomers. With the *threo* (active) isomer, the difference is more. Experimentally it is found that, $\Delta\nu_{threo} = 49\ cm^{-1}$ and $\Delta\nu_{meso} = 42\ cm^{-1}$.

4. The IR spectrum of concentrated solution of *o*-chlorophenol shows a broad band for O—H stretching in carbon tetrachloride solvent. *o*-chlorophenol remains intermolecularly hydrogen bonded in carbon tetrachloride solution and we get a broad band at 3550 cm^{-1}. On medium dilution with the same solvent and using high resolution IR, *three absorption maxima* are found instead of one peak. The peak corresponding to highest wave number is due to free O—H stretching, the second highest wave number corresponds to hydrogen bonded O—H stretching and the lowest wave number is due to O—H stretching which forms weak hydrogen bonding with chlorine atom. If we dilute the solution further, the O—H stretching corresponding to intermolecular hydrogen bonding vanishes and only two peaks then remain.

5. 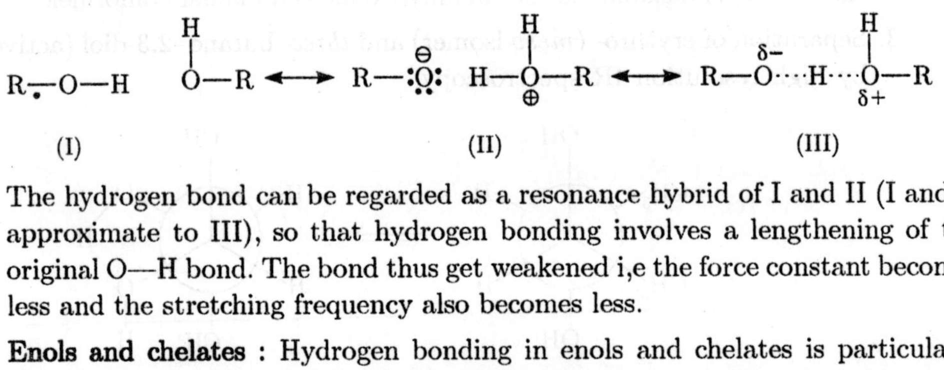

(I) (II) (III)

The hydrogen bond can be regarded as a resonance hybrid of I and II (I and II approximate to III), so that hydrogen bonding involves a lengthening of the original O—H bond. The bond thus get weakened i,e the force constant becomes less and the stretching frequency also becomes less.

6. **Enols and chelates** : Hydrogen bonding in enols and chelates is particularly strong and the observed O—H stretching frequencies may be very low due to the reduced force constant (down to 2800 cm^{-1}). Since these bonds are not easily broken on dilution with an inert solvent like carbon tetrachloride, free O—H stretching frequency is not seen even at very low concentration.

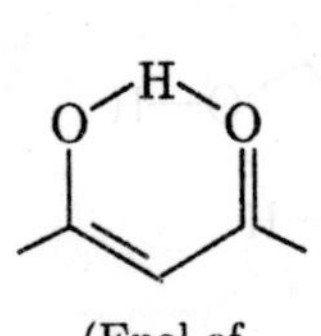

(Enol of acetylacetone)

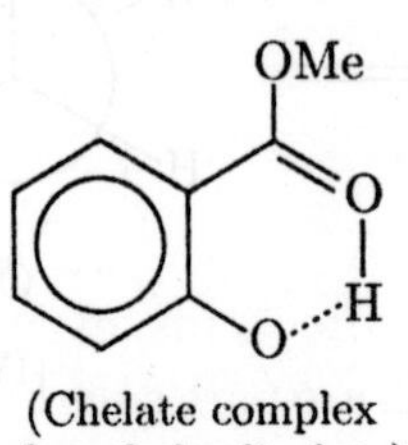

(Chelate complex of methyl salicylate)

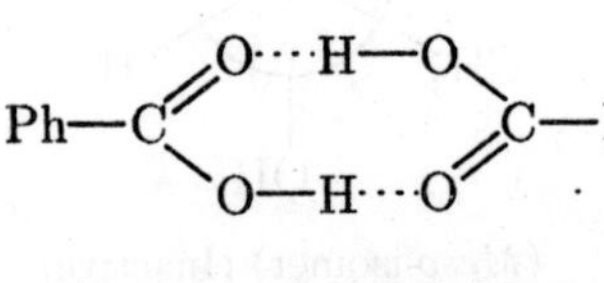

(Hydrogen bonded dimer of benzoic acid)

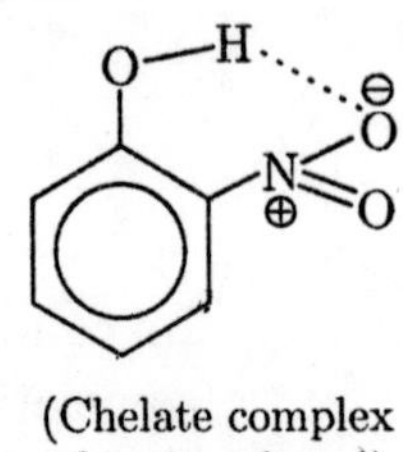

(Chelate complex of *o*-nitrophenol)

7. Alcohols and phenols in condensed phases, (bulk liquid or potassium bromide discs etc.) are strongly hydrogen bonded, usually in the form of a dynamic polymeric association, dimers, trimers and tetramers also exist and this leads to a wide envelope of absorptions and hence to broadening of the absorption band. In dilute solution, in inert solvents or in the vapour phase the proportion of the free molecules increases and these give rise to sharp 3650 cm^{-1} band.

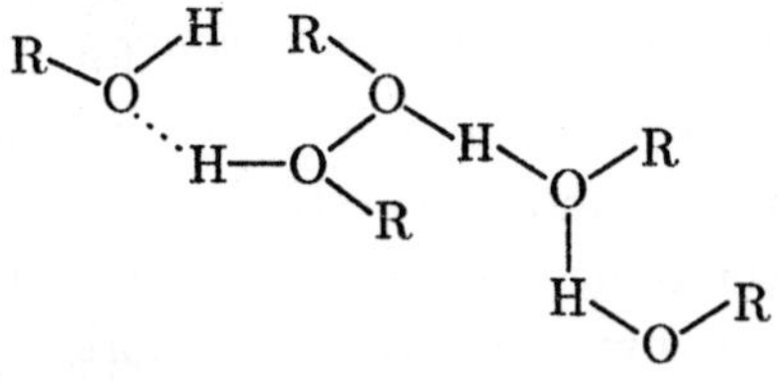

(Polymeric association of O–H groups)

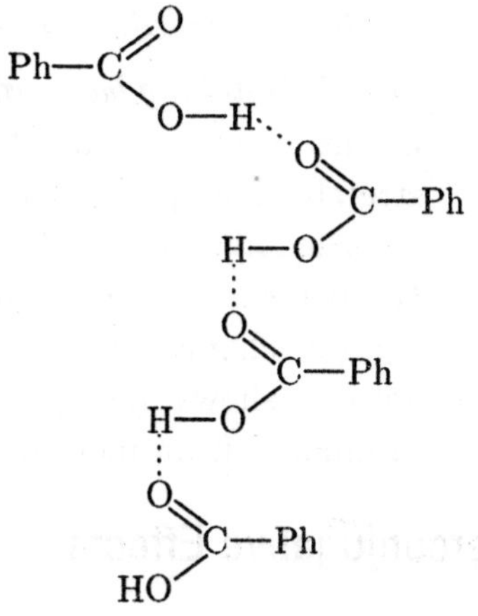

(Polymer of benzoic acid)

8. **Hydrogen bonding in carbonyl compounds** : In enols and chelates such as methyl salicylate, hydrogen bonding will influence not only the O—H vibration frequency but also the C=O vibration to which it hydrogen bonds. The key factor here is the basicity of the C=O group, the more basic it is, the stronger will be the hydrogen bond that it can form. The extreme case of protonation shows that C=O bond has increased single bond character and longer length; the same tendency occurs in hydrogen bonding leading to a lowering of vibration frequency.

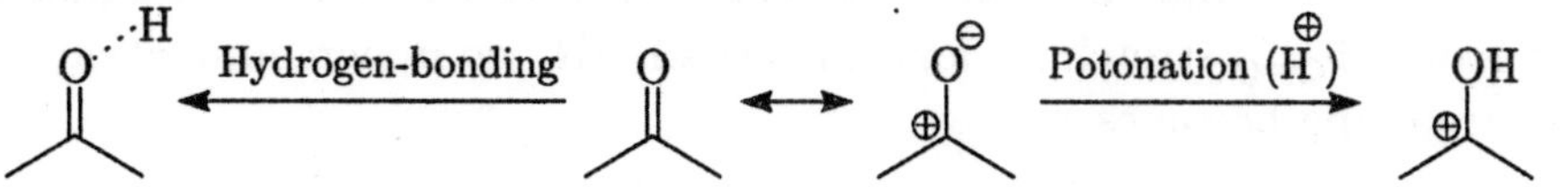

9. **Hydrogen bonding in carboxylic acids** : Carboxylic acids have an exceedingly broad band reaching from 2500 cm^{-1} to 3500 cm^{-1} is hydrogen bonded O—H stretching, for the carboxylic acid dimeric structure.

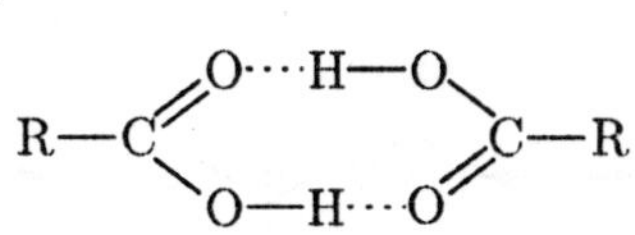

(Dimeric structure of carboxylic acid)

In condensed phases, all the carboxylic acids exists in this stable dimeric association in which the hydrogen bonds are particularly strong. The fine structure of the O—H stretching peak is usually attributed to vibrational coupling with overtones of lower frequencies. In very dilute solution in hexane, it is just possible to distinguish *free O—H* stretching, but this is extreme dilution. Even in carbon tetrachloride, some degree of hydrogen bonding to solvent arises and in extreme dilution in carbon tetrachloride, the free O—H stretching absorption is seen at lower frequency than in hexane. Polymeric association is also known as to occur in carboxylic acids, although dimeric association is the norm; *the proportion of monomer to dimer increases in solvents such as benzene and in dioxan there is no dimer formed since the acid prefers to be hydrogen bonded to the solvent.*

O—H stretching band and role of solvent : There may be a relation between the nature of solvent and the stretching band of O—H. The frequency of O—H stretching in phenols can be lowered by 40–100 cm^{-1} when the spectrum is recorded in benzene solution compared with carbon tetrachloride solution. When IR spectrum of a molecule is taken in solution, the position of absorption band can get changed under the influence of solvent. C=O stretching frequency of ketones shows absorption maximum at lower frequency as the electrical field originated from methanol stabilises the ketone.

Hyperconjugative Effects

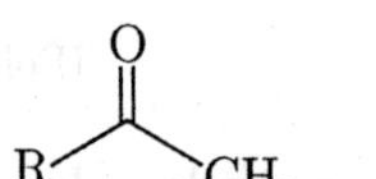
(I)

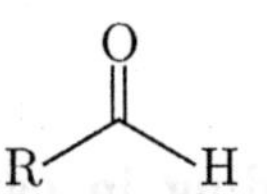
(II)

$\bar{\nu}_{C=O_{str}}$ is *less* $\bar{\nu}_{C=O_{str}}$ is *more*

In (I), hyperconjugation is possible, so contribution of C—O single bond increases, which makes $\bar{\nu}_{C=O}$ stretching *less.* In case of (II), *no* hyperconjugation is possible and $\bar{\nu}_{C=O}$ stretching becomes *more.*

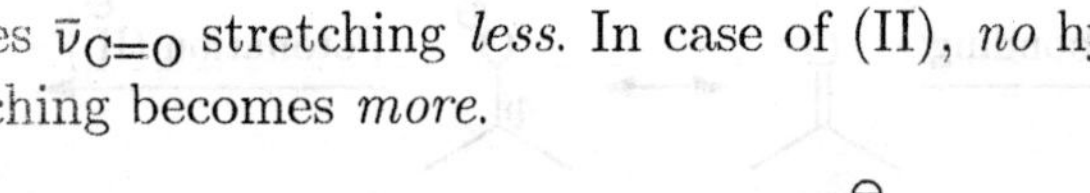
(III)

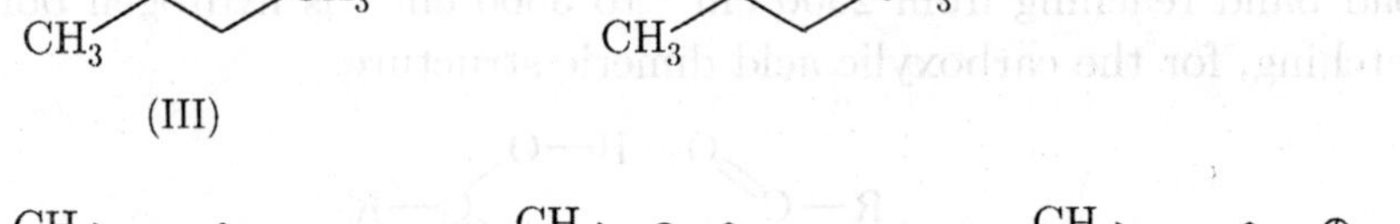
(IV)

In (IV), there are two resonating structures, where C—O bond has more single bond character (two of the resonating structures contain C—O single bond). But in

(III), there is only one such structure and so $\bar{\nu}_{C=O}$ *stretching* of (III) is *more* than $\bar{\nu}_{C=O}$ stretching of (IV).

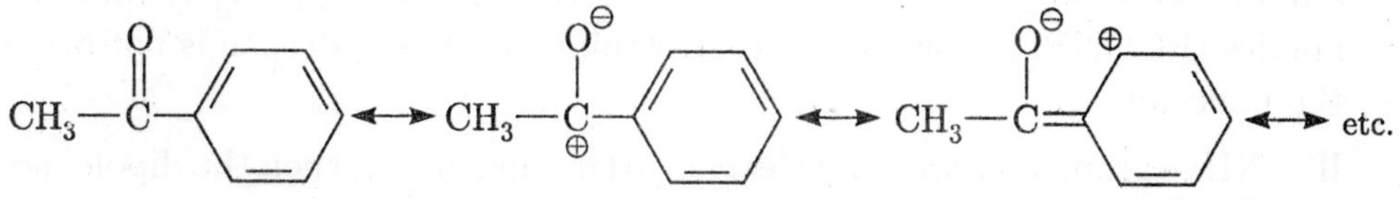

(V)

The molecule (V) has C=O bond with single bond character and thus, the value of C=O stretching frequency becomes less.

(X=F, Cl, Br, O, N, OH, OR, NH_2)

(VI) (VII)

(VII) is destabilised due to (–I) effect of X. So contribution of (VI) to the resonance hybrid is more where C=O double bond character is more. As a result, stretching frequency of C=O increases.

Individual Absorption Bands for Different Bonds

1. **N—H Bond** : The position of N—H stretching band is in between 3200 cm^{-1} to 3400 cm^{-1}. A broad band is formed mainly due to hydrogen bonding. Particularly all the —NH— containing compounds like primary and secondary amines, primary and secondary amides, amino acids, ammonium salts, all show N—H stretching band in this region. Apart from this stretching band, another peak at 1600 cm^{-1} is found due to N—H bending or deformation. Regarding N—H stretching band, it is close to O—H stretching band especially in amides and amines, and one may get confused. But nitrogen is less electronegative than oxygen, so the *stiffness* of O—H bond is *more* than N—H bond and a higher dipole is generated in O—H. So O—H stretching band is stronger than N—H stretching band. In dilute solution, O—H band shifts to a *sharp peak* at 3600 cm^{-1} but the hydrogen bond associated with, N—H group is usually weak and it never goes as high as free O—H around 3600 cm^{-1} in very dilute solution. The hydrogen bonded N—H stretching band is more sharp than the hydrogen bonded O—H stretching band, as the former is involved in weak hydrogen bonding. Primary amines and *amides* show **two** N—H stretching bands

(Symmetric stretching) (Asymmetric stretching)

due to symmetric and asymmetric stretching (3200 cm^{-1} and 3500 cm^{-1}), the **stronger band** is due to **asymmetric stretching**. Secondary amines and secondary amides show only one stretching band. Tertiary amines (R_3N) and tertiary amides ($RCONR_2$) show *no* N—H stretching band as hydrogen is not present in the molecule.

If —NH— group contains any electron attracting group, then the dipole moment of —NH— group increases and the stiffness of the bond also increases. As a result, N—H stretching band shifts to a higher frequency, like alcohols, in dilute solution.

The N—H stretching vibrations of amines are shifted to higher frequencies. But the shifts are not that dramatic as we find in case of alcohols, as the hydrogen bonds present in amines are weaker in nature compared to those present in alcohols. The shift is about 250 cm^{-1} for amines versus 300 cm^{-1} in case of alcohols.

2. **C—H Bond :** C—H stretching frequency depends on the state of hybridisation of carbon atom. The region where C—H absorbs to shown as follows.

   (a) $\bar{\nu}_{sp^3 \text{C-H}}$ *stretch* ~2850 cm^{-1}

   (b) $\bar{\nu}_{sp^2 \text{C-H}}$ *stretch* ~3000 cm^{-1}

   (c) $\bar{\nu}_{sp \text{ C-H}}$ *stretch* ~3300 cm^{-1}

   (d) Aldehyde C—H *stretch* ~2780 cm^{-1} ()

   —CH_3— and —CH_2— groups show symmetric and asymmetric C—H stretching and in many cases the IR spectra contain C—H stretching band with more than one peak, *i.e.*, they are found as multiplets. Apart from C—H stretching bands, bending of C—H band is also possible. *Two modes*—one *in-plane bending* and another *out of plane bending* is possible for which two bands near 4000 cm^{-1} and 900 cm^{-1} respectively are found. In some cases, particularly for out of plane bending overtone may be formed which is twice the frequency of vibration.

3. **C≡N Bond :** The IR spectrum of a nitrile shows C≡N stretching at around 2300 cm^{-1}. The intensity of absorption is quite strong, *i.e.*, the peak is a strong absorption peak. A strong dipole is generated in C≡N functionality during vibration and so we get a strong absorption band.

4. **C≡C Bond :** Terminal alkynes show C≡C stretching absorption peak at around 2200 cm^{-1} which is a weak band. For non terminal alkynes like R—C≡C—R′, the C≡C stretching band is not found at all. For this type of alkynes, the electron charge density is symmetrically arranged around the centre of the triple bond. As the molecule becomes symmetrical, no change in dipole moment is found with vibration, and the molecule becomes IR inactive. For terminal alkynes, change in dipole moment with vibration is very little and so a weak absorption band is found.

5. C=O Bond : The different C=O *stretching* absorption maxima are as follows.

	Molecule	$\bar{\nu}$ **(cm^{-1})**
1.	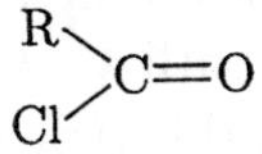	~1800 cm^{-1}
2.	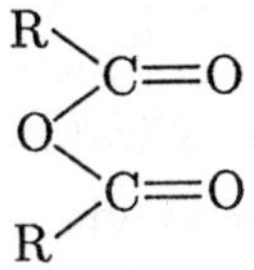	~1780-1840 cm^{-1} (Pure carbonyl stretching peak is *not* found due to the coupled vibration of $\bar{\nu}_{sym}$ and $\bar{\nu}_{asym}$ of C=O)
3.	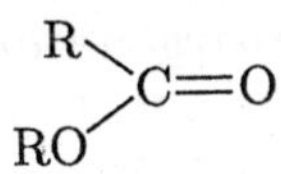	~1760 cm^{-1}
4.	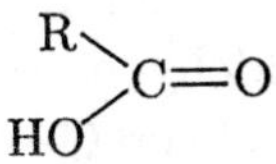	~1720 cm^{-1}
5.	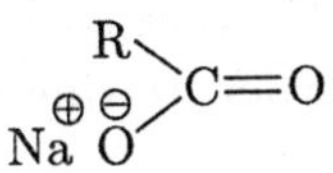	~1400-1500 cm^{-1} ($\bar{\nu}_{sym}$ and $\bar{\nu}_{asym}$)
6.	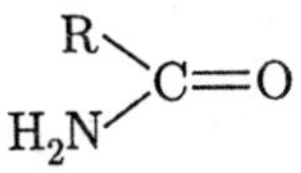	~1680 cm^{-1}
7.	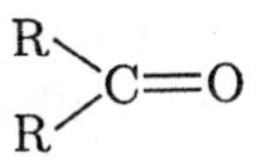	~1715 cm^{-1}
8.	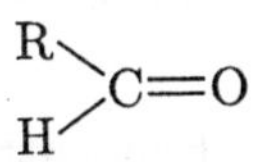	~1730 cm^{-1}

Acyl halides, acid anhydrides, esters, carboxylic acids and amides can be taken as resonance hybrid of the following structures.

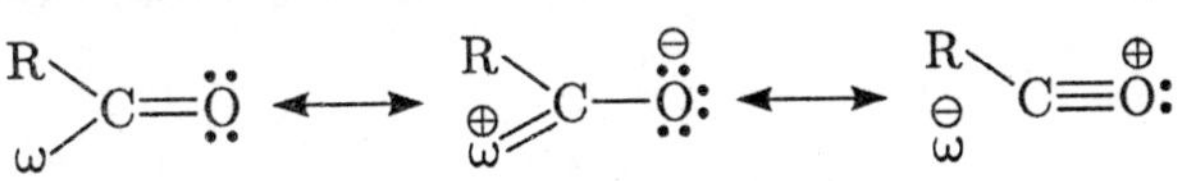

(I) (II) (III)

If ω is **electron withdrawing**, then extent of overlap increases between non bonding orbitals on oxygen carrying lone pairs of electrons and empty σ^* C—ω orbitals. As a result, C—O bond has partial triple bond like character and contribution of resonating structure (III) is more to the resonance hybrid. Moreover, ω being electron withdrawing, uses p orbital more to form C—ω bonding orbital and more s orbital is used to form C=O bonding orbital. So, the stiffness of C=O bond becomes more and vibrated at a higher frequency. When **ω is electron donating or less electron negative** the non bonding pair of electrons on w overlaps with p orbital of carbonyl carbon and C—O bond becomes more of single bond type. In other words, structure (II) contributes more to the resonance hybrid where the *stiffness* of C=O bond is *less* and band comes at a *lower frequency.* Carboxylic acids and amides can have intermolecular hydrogen bonding and C=O stretching frequency becomes less as the stiffness of the bond decreases. In amides, N—H bending vibration couples with C=O stretching vibration and the spectrum becomes complex. In general, this type of spectrum is called the "*amide band*". Anhydrides show vibrational coupling and due to symmetric and asymmetric stretching, the band becomes complex. In salts of carboxylic acids, the two oxygen atoms attain similar nature and two peaks are formed due to symmetric and asymmetric stretching. Carboxylate anions also contain carbon-oxygen bond intermediate between carbon-carbon double bond and carbon-carbon single bond. For this reason in *carboxylate anions,* C=O stretching absorbs at a lower frequency.

In aldehydes, the non-bonding lone pair of *electrons* on oxygen atom overlaps, with σ* C—H orbital. In other words, C=O bond in aldehydes is **stiffer** than C=O bond in ketones where this effect is not found. So aldehyde C—H stretching absorption occurs at a lower frequency than other C—H bonds. α, β-unsaturated carbonyl compounds can have following resonating structure due to extended conjugation.

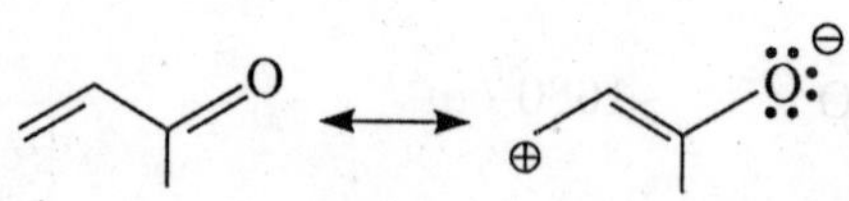

α, β-unsaturated carbonyl compounds have less double bond character and more single bond character for C=O bond. As a result, the stiffness *of* C=O bond becomes less and the absorption maximum shifts to lower frequency. $\bar{\nu}_{C=O}$ stretching of α, β-unsaturated ketone is 1680 cm^{-1}.

In esters like RCOOR′, if the R group is vinyl, then C=O bond attains partial single bond character due to resonance and the stiffness of the bond becomes less and the frequency shifts to the lower side. But if R′ is vinyl, then the vinyl group comes into resonance with the oxygen atom as follows.

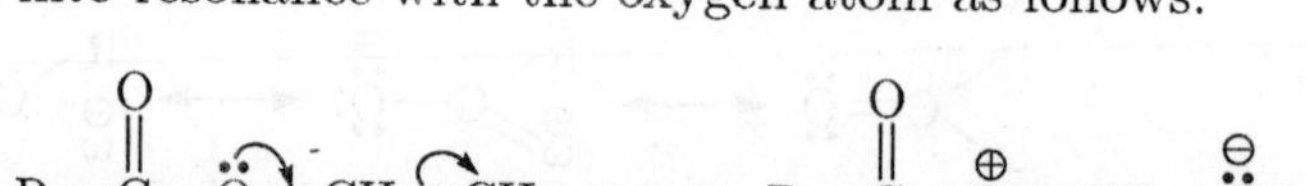

As a result, R′ becomes elecron withdrawing and the stiffness of C=O bond increases, and C=O stretching band absorbs at a higher frequency.

Compounds having the molecular formula A=C=O (ketens, isocyanates, carbon dioxide etc.) have C—O bond which has partial triple bond character due to resonance.

$$A{=}C{=}\ddot{O}: \longleftrightarrow \overset{\ominus}{\ddot{A}}{-}C{\equiv}\overset{\oplus}{O}:$$

Moreover, carbon atom is sp hybridised here and so the C=O bond contains more s orbital in carbonyl bonding orbital. For this reason, the stiffness of C=O bond becomes more and absorption maximum is found at a higher frequency. For CO_2 molecule, no change in dipole moment occurs due to symmetric stretching (as O=C=O is linear and symmetric) and this vibration is therefore IR **inactive.** CO_2 shows IR absorbance only due to **asymmetric stretching.**

The conformer of α-chloroketone, which contains C—Cl and C=O in eclipsed position has a stiffer C=O bond compared to other conformers.

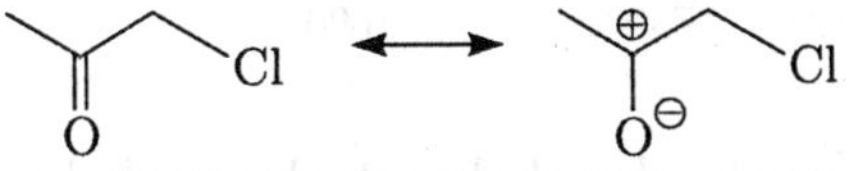

(I) (II)

Between the resonating structures (I) and (II); (II) has little contribution as it faces a strong dipole-dipole interaction and the resonance hybrid mainly consists of structure (I). For this reason the C=O stretching vibration of α-chloroketones occur at a higher frequency. If C—Cl and and C=O bonds remain in *anti* position, *e.g.*, in (III) and (IV), this effect becomes negligible and C=O stretching frequency absorbs at a normal region where C=O stretching of other ketones absorb.

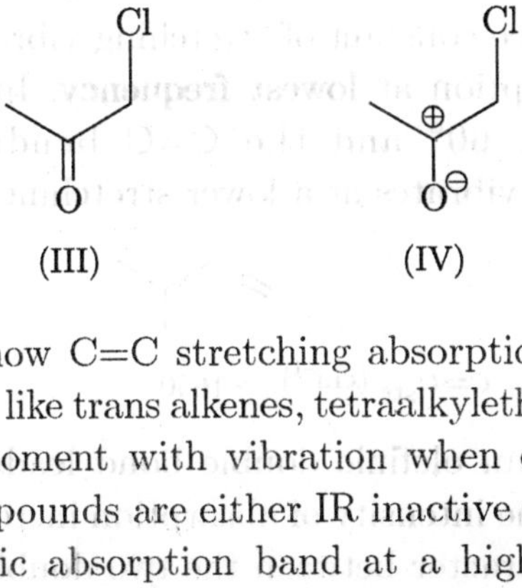

(III) (IV)

6. **C=C Bond** : Alkenes show C=C stretching absorption at around 1640 cm^{-1}. Centrosymmetric alkenes like trans alkenes, tetraalkylethylene etc. do not undergo any change in dipole moment with vibration when directed along the C=C bond axis. So these compounds are either IR inactive or show very weak band. Allenes show asymmetric absorption band at a higher frequency. Here, the central carbon atom is sp hybridised and so the bonding orbital contains more s character. As a result, the stiffness of C=C bond gets increased. Besides this, vibrational coupling also occurs which increases the frequency of asymmetric stretching.

   Conjugated polyenes show resonance which lowers the stiffness of C=C bond and the vibrational frequency shifts to lower side (~1620 cm^{-1}). For the same reason, benzenoids show further lowering in vibrational frequency.

   In cyclic unsaturated compounds, where the double bond is *exocyclic*, the value of C=C *stretching* frequency *increases* with *decrease in ring size.* The C—$\hat{C}$—C *bond angle* decreases as the ring becomes smaller. So C—C bonding orbital uses more p orbital and C=C bonding orbital uses more s character. As a result, stiffness of C=C bond increases and C=C stretching frequency thus shifts to higher frequency.

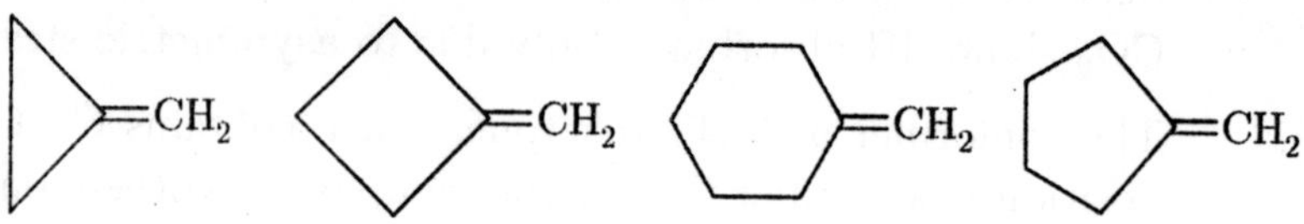

$\bar{\nu}_{C=C_{str}}$ (in cm^{-1}) 1750 1690 1657 1651

In case of endocyclic double bond, the angle between C=C and C—C becomes smaller than 120° for small ring compounds and for cyclobutene, it is 90°.

(Cyclobutene) (Cyclopropene)

In cyclobutene, only C—C bending vibration is found along with the stretching vibration of C=C. But, as the bond angle deviates from 90°, some stretching vibration with C—C is observed. The force constant for bending vibration is less than the force constant of stretching vibration. So cyclobutene shows C=C stretching absorption at **lowest frequency**. In case of cyclopropene, the bond angle is about 60° and the C=C bending orbital experiences more p character and vibrates at a lower stretching frequency.

$C=C_{str}$ (cm^{-1}) ~1650 ~1610

Conjugation of an olefinic double bond leads to lowering of C=C stretching frequency and the intensity of absorption increases. Resonance results in partial double bond character between the two double bonds, with decreased electron density and stiffness of the double bonds themselves. So conjugated polyenes vibrate at a lower C=C stretching frequency compared to isolated double bonds.

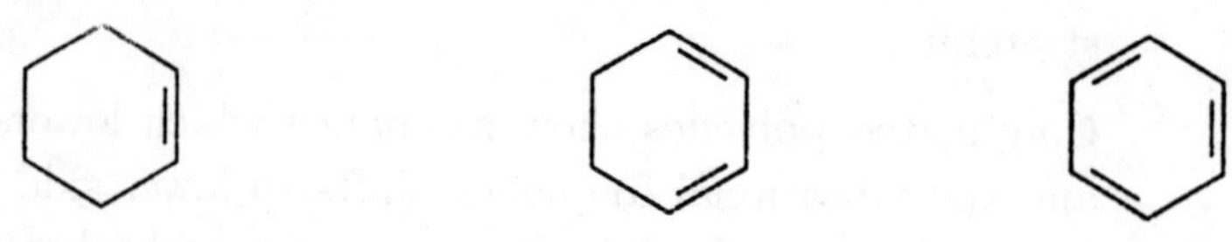

(Cyclohexene) (isolated double bond) (1,3-cyclohexadiene) (conjugated) (Benzene) (aromatic)

$\bar{\nu}_{C=C_{str}}$ (cm^{-1}) 1645 1620 1600

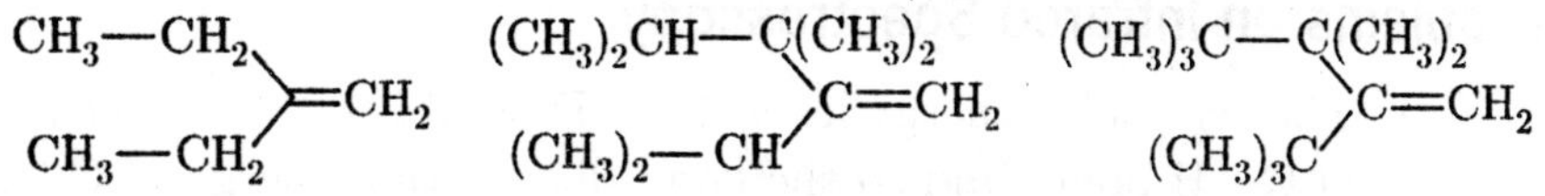

$\bar{\nu}_{C=C_{str}}$ (cm^{-1}) 1652 1639 1621

Spreading of the angle ($R'R{>}C{=}CH_2$) due to the size of R groups lowers C=C stretching of the vinylidene double bond in the compounds shown above.

Since alkenes and aromatic π bonds can behave as Lewis bases, it is not surprising that they can form hydrogen bonds to acidic hydrogens; the frequency of O—H stretching in phenols can be lowered by 40–100 cm^{-1} when the spectrum is recorded in benzene solution, compared with carbon tetrachloride solution.

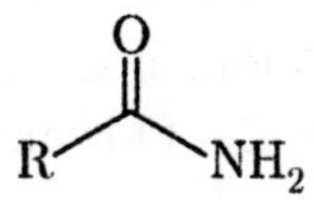

$\bar{\nu}_{C=O_{str}}$ (cm^{-1}) 1600–1650

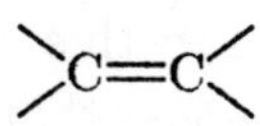

$\bar{\nu}_{C=C_{str}}$ (cm^{-1}) 1600–1650

These two stretching frequencies show identical value. But for C=C, **intensity of peak is lower** whereas for C=O, the **intensity of peak is higher**.

Problems on Infrared Spectroscopy

1. The zero point energy level of C—D bond is less than the zero point energy level of C—H bond, and so the bond dissociation energy of C—D is more than that of C—H bond. But although the zero point energy level of C—C is low, the corresponding C—C bond dissociation energy is less. Explain.

   Ans.: Generally if the zero point energy level of a particular bond is low, the bond dissociation energy of that bond becomes more. This is shown by C—D bond, of which the zero point energy level is lower than that of C—H bond, and so has a higher bond dissociation energy. But with C—C bond, which has low zero point energy level, has lower bond dissociation energy.

   Carbon atom with higher atomic weight than hydrogen has lower zero point energy level for C—C bond than C—H or C—D bond. But there is a valence shell electron pair repulsion between the valence shell pairs of two carbon atom and due to this electronic repulsion, bond dissociation energy of C—C bond becomes less than that C—H or C—D bond dissociation energy.

2. a. How many modes vibrations are possible for CO_2? b. There will be no symmetric stretching vibration for CO_2. Explain.

   Ans. : The structure of CO_2 is linear, *i.e.*, Ö=C=Ö. The number of modes of vibration possible for a linear molecule is (3n–5) where n is the number of atoms. So the number of modes of vibration theoretically possible for CO_2 molecule is (3×3–5)=4. But only three vibrational modes are possible.

   (a) Asymmetric stretching vibration.

   (b) Scissoring in plane bending vibration.

   (c) Rocking in plane bending vibration.

   CO_2 being a linear and planar molecule, the two oxygen atoms always lie in the same plane with the carbon atom, so out of plane bending vibration modes (twisting and wagging) are not possible. Symmetric stretching vibration mode is also not possible because CO_2 is a centrosymmetric molecule, and symmetric stretching vibration will not rise any change in dipole in the structure.

Expansion Contraction

   No change is dipole moment is observed in CO_2 with symmetric stretching.

3. H_2O molecule can have only three modes of vibration. Justify.

   Ans.: The number of modes of vibration possible for H_2O molecule is (3n–6) where n is the no. of atoms present in a molecule (=3) and H_2O is a nonlinear (angular) molecule.

So the number of modes of vibration = $3\times3-6 = 3$ are possible for water molecule which is angular. The modes are as follows.

(a) Asymmetric stretching vibration.

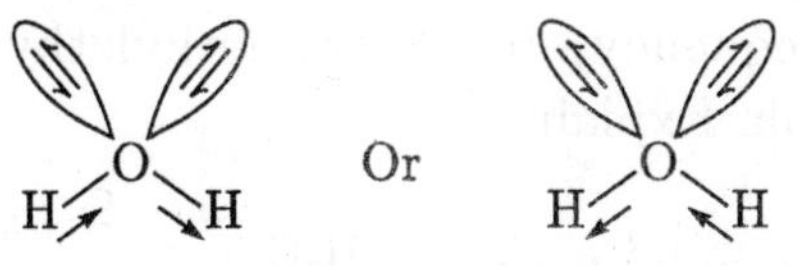

(b) Out of plane bending vibration (twisting)

(c) Out of plane bending vibration (wagging)

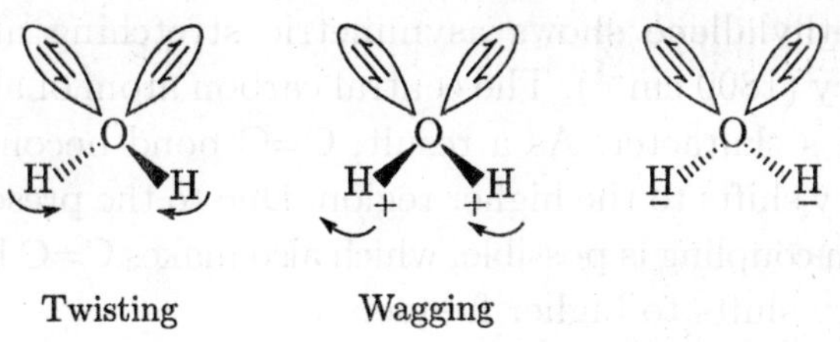

4. **Generally a compound gives broad band in IR in solution but a sharp band is observed in the gaseous state.**

Ans.: In solution, the electric field of one molecule of a compound can influence the electric field of another molecule and ΔE_{vib} becomes different and we get a broad spectrum for narrowly separated transitions. Again in liquid phase, one vibrational level is accompanied with a number of rotational energy levels and as a result the vibrational energy levels are not single valued. For this reason also, a broad spectrum is produced. Vibrational frequencies are different for different transitions theoretically but actually they are so close that we get a broad spectrum.

In gaseous phase, the molecules do not experience the effect of environment (field effect) as experienced in the solution phase (the electric field of one molecule is transmitted through medium to another molecule or in solid phase) and we get a sharp band.

5. What do you mean by force constant of vibration of a bond? What is its unit in C.G.S and S.I.?

Ans. : Force constant is defined as the opposing force generated due to vibrational motion of the atoms in a molecule and the magnitude of force constant is directly dependent to the stiffness of that motion. If the stiffness of a particular bond is more, the force constant is more and *vice versa.* The mode of motion to which the molecule is flexible has low value of force constant.

Unit of force constant (k) in C.G.S unit = 5.0×10^5 g$\times$sec^{-2}=dynes/cm and unit of force constant (k) in S.I unit 500 N$\times$m^{-1} (since 1 newton=10^3g.m.s^{-2})

$\bar{\nu}$ = Frequency of vibration = $\frac{1}{2\pi} \times \sqrt{\frac{k}{\mu}}$ where k = Force constant and μ = Reduced mass = $\frac{m_1 m_2}{m_1+m_2}$ for diatomic molecule.

6. Tetramethylallene shows its C=C stretching absorption peak at 1800 cm^{-1} (high vibrational frequency) but tetramethylethylene shows no C=C stretching absorption peak. Explain.

Ans. :

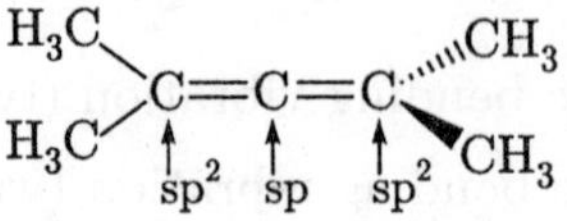

Tetramethylallene shows asymmetric stretching absorption band at a high frequency (1800 cm^{-1}). The central carbon atom of allene is sp hybridised which has 50% s character. As a result, C=C bond becomes stiff and the stretching frequency shifts to the higher region. Due to the presence of adjacent C=C bond vibration coupling is possible, which also makes C=C bond stiff and the stretching frequency shifts to higher frequency.

Tetramethylethylene is centrosymmetric, and there is no change in dipole moment due to vibration along the bond axis of C=C bond. As a result, tetramethylethylene becomes IR inactive. In other words $\frac{d\mu}{dr} = 0$. But the condition of a molecule to be IR active is that, with vibration, the dipole moment of a molecule should change i,e $d\mu/dr \neq 0$.

7. State the relative positions of C—H stretching absorption peaks of cyclopropane and *n*-propane.

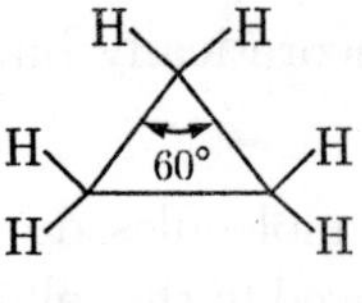

In cyclopropane, ∠HCH bond angle is much greater than the normal sp^3 bond angle 109°28′. With the increase in bond angle, the % s character increases in C—H bond and the stiffness of C—H bond thus increases. This stiffness of C—H bond shifts the stretching absorption peak to a high value of 3070–3040 cm^{-1}. In *n*-propane, unlike cyclopropane, no ring strain is present and rather propane is an acyclic molecule with ∠HCH bond angle nearly about 109°28′, and the stretching absorption peak appears at about 2850 cm^{-1}. Due to symmetric and asymmetric C—H stretching, C—H absorption (stretching) appears as a multiplet. Apart from it, due to in plane and out of plane bending vibrations, absorption peaks appears at 1400 cm^{-1} and 900 cm^{-1}.

The Proton Nuclear Magnetic Resonance (^{1}H–NMR) Spectroscopy

Nuclear magnetic resonance (NMR) is concerned with the magnetic properties of certain atomic nuclei, notably the nucleus of the hydrogen atom (the proton) and that of the carbon 13 (^{13}C) isotope of carbon. Studying a molecule by NMR spectroscopy enables us to record differences in the magnetic properties of the various magnetic nuclei present and to deduce what are the positions of these nuclei within the molecule. When we use hydrogen nucleus or proton for NMR spectroscopy, it is also called proton magnetic resonance (PMR) spectroscopy. PMR spectroscopy helps us to determine the position and number of hydrogen nucleus present in a molecule.

The ^{1}H–NMR Phenomenon

1. **The spinning nucleus :** The nucleus of the hydrogen atom, i,e the proton behaves as a tiny bar magnet, because it possesses both electric charge and mechanical spin as any spinning charged body generates a magnetic field.

2. **Precessional motion :** The subatomic particles like protons and neutrons spin around their own axis like a top. This rotation is known as the *spinning motion* of the nucleus. This is a common property of all subatomic particles. When a proton spins around its own axis, a magnetic field is generated *parallel to the rotational axis* i,e it behaves like a tiny bar magnet. Normally the direction of the magnetic field of this tiny bar magnet is oriented in every probable direction. But if an *external magnetic field is applied*, the proton adopts specific orientations with respect to the external magnetic field. Due to *quantum restrictions*, the proton adopts only two orientations either aligned to the field (the lower energy state) or opposed to the field (the higher energy state). These orientations are also described as *parallel* or *antiparallel* with the applied field. There are *two* preferred orientations come from the following quantum calculations. If S be the spin quantum number, then the number of orientations of the nucleus in the presence of external magnetic field is (2S+1). Only two orientations for a proton is possible as the spin quantum number of proton is $\pm$ ½. One orientation, aligned to the external magnetic field is of lower energy (parallel) and another, opposite to the external magnetic field is of higher energy (antiparallel).

   A spinning top, due to its spinning motion, performs a slow *Waltz-like* motion, in which the spinning axis of the top *moves slowly around the vertical.* This is called *precessional motion* and the top is said to be *precessing* around its vertical axis. As the proton is a spinning magnet, it will like the top *precess* around the *axis of an applied external magnetic field* and can have *two* orientations, one aligned to the field (low energy) and another opposed to the field (higher energy).

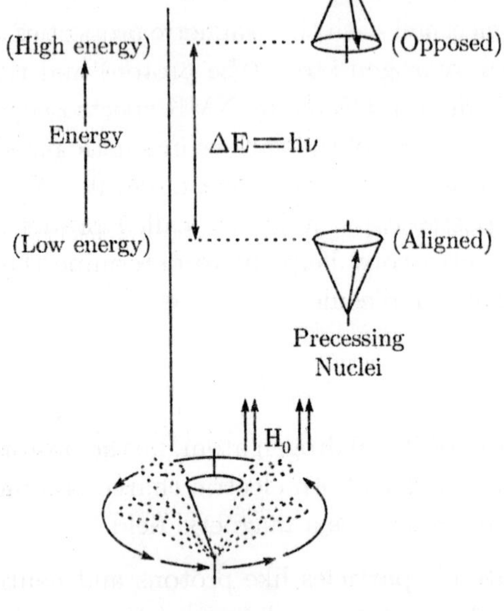

"Waltz like Motion of a Top"

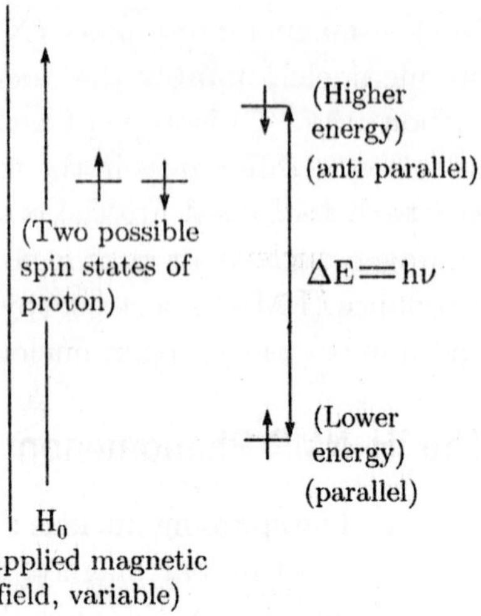

The number of spins in unit time, *i.e.*, the *spinning frequency* of a nucleus of a proton *does not change*, but the *precessional frequency* (number of precessions around the axis of the external magnetic field in unit time) *may change* and its magnitude depends on the strength of the applied external magnetic field. In fact, the precessional frequency, ν is directly proportional to H_0, the strength of external magnetic field. If the intensity of external magnetic field is 14,000 gauss, a proton precesses 60×10^6 times per second; *i.e.*, the precessional frequency is 60×10^6 Hertz, *i.e.*, 60 mega Hertz (MHz). If the external magnetic field is 23,000 gauss, ν is 100 MHz and if it is 117,000 gauss, then ν becomes 500 MHz. Precessional frequency also depends on the magnetic moment (μ) of the nucleus and ν increases with increase in magnetic momentum of a nucleus. The magnetic moment of a proton is higher than compared to those of other nuclei and this is the reason why proton is the most sensitive nucleus in NMR spectrosocpy. The use of D (deuterium) in NMR spectroscopy is of less worth as D has one third magnetic moment compared to that of proton.

Radiofrequency absorption : A proton with a particular precessional frequency can have two orientations regarding spinning in an external magnetic field—one parallel to the applied field with *lower* energy and another antiparallel to the applied field with *higher* energy. Under this condition, if the nucleus is irradiated with a radiowave having the same frequency as that of precessional frequency, the nucleus and the radiofrequency beam are called to be in *resonance* and a quantum of energy is absorbed by each proton to get promoted from the low energy state to high energy state. In other words transition of proton occurs from low energy to high energy state. This phenomenon is known as *nuclear magnetic resonance*, as resonance occurs between precessional frequency and radiowave frequency. When transition occurs from a high energy to low energy state, a *quantum* of energy is *radiated* or *emitted.* The transition of proton from higher to lower energy state may occur smoothly and *vice versa.* By this way the number of protons in the higher energy state becomes equal to the number of protons in the lower energy state; the former by emitting a quantum of radiation and the latter by absorbing a quantum of radiation. Under this condition, no further absorption of energy can occur and the observed resonance signal will fade out. Thus situation is referred as the *saturation* of the signal. In the recording of a normal NMR spectrum, the populations in the two spin states do not become equal because higher energy nuclei are constantly returning to the low energy spin state. We can calculate the ratio of protons in the two energy states by applying *Boltzmann Distribution Law.*

$\Delta E = N_0 . h. \nu$ (N_0 = Avogadro number
h = Planck's constant
ν = frequency of absorbed radiation
≡ precessional frequency)

With the increase in ΔE, the number of protons in low energy state increases. In this equation, ν is proportional to ΔE and ν can be increased by increasing the intensity of external magnetic field. Still, when H_0 is 117,000 gauss, which leads to precessional frequency ν to 500 MHz, then also *ΔE is too small* (about 10^{-4} kJ/mol). This means that the number of protons in low energy state is only 0.001% more than the protons present in high energy state. When recording NMR signals, we put the organic molecule under study in a strong magnetic field and the protons present in the molecule undergo precessional motion. The protons present in a particular compound can have same or different precessional frequencies. When we irradiate the molecule with radiowaves of different frequencies, those waves will be absorbed which are equal to the precessional frequencies of protons present in that molecule, and this absorption is manifested as NMR spectrum.

Theory of Nuclear Magnetic Resonance : The only nuclei that exhibit the NMR phenomenon are those for which the spin quantum number s is greater than zero; the spin quantum number s is associated with the mass number and the atomic number of the nuclei as follows.

Mass Number	Atomic Number	Spin quantum Number
Odd	Odd or even	$\frac{1}{2}, \frac{3}{2}, \frac{5}{2}, ...$
Even	Even	0
Even	Odd	1,2,3,4, ...

The nuclei of ^1H and ^{13}C have s= ½, whereas ^{12}C and ^{16}O have s=0 and so the latter nuclei are *non magnetic.* If ^{12}C and ^{16}O had been magnetic, the NMR spectra of organic molecules would have been much more complex. Other important magnetic nuclei for NMR are ^{11}B, ^{13}C, ^{14}N, ^{15}N, ^{17}O, ^{19}F and ^{31}P. ^2H(D) and ^{14}N have s=1.

Under the influence of an external magnetic field, a magnetic nucleus can take up different orientations with respect to that field, the number of possible orientations is given by (2S+1), so that for nuclei with spin ½(^{1}H, ^{13}C, ^{19}F etc.), only *two* orientations are allowed, D and ^{14}N have S=1 and so can take up *three* orientations. These nuclei do not simply possess magnetic dipoles but rather possess electric quadripoles.

In an applied magnetic field, magnetic nuclei like the proton *precess* at a frequency ν, which is proportional to the strength of the applied field. The exact frequency is given by,

$$\nu = \frac{\gamma . H_0}{2\pi}$$ [H_0=Applied magnetic field experienced by the proton

γ=Gyromagnetic ratio (or magnetogyric ratio)

$$= \frac{\text{nuclear magnetic momentum } (\mu)}{\text{nuclear angular momentum (I)}}$$]

For a proton μ=26753 and H_0=117,000 gauss ≡ 14.1 T(tesla) ν becomes 500 MHz.

Relaxation Process : A proton in the low energy state absorbs energy of radiofrequency radiation and gets promoted to the high energy state. Again the proton from the high energy state returns to the low energy state by emitting energy in the radiowave region. Generally, in the presence of radiowave irradiation, the rate of transition of proton from low to high energy state is more. If the rate of transition from high to low energy state becomes too low compared to the transition from low to high energy state, a situation may arise where the number of protons may be equal in the two energy levels and no further absorption of radiofrequency energy will be there. Even with large magnetic field (117,000 gauss or 14.1 T), the population of protons in low and high energy levels differs very small, only by 0.001%. As a result, the resonance signal will fade out (saturation of resonance signal). But in practice, this never happens and the population of the two spin states do not become equal because the higher energy nuclei constantly return to the lower energy spin state and keeps the lower level always more populated. Such process is known as *relaxation process.*

The relaxation process by which a proton returns from the high energy state to low energy state may be of *three* types.

1. The proton may radiate a radiowave of same frequency which it had absorbed for the transition from low energy state to high energy state. the *relaxation process* may follow two other *radiationless processes.*
2. ***Spin-lattice Relaxation*** : A higher energy nucleus can have its energy (relaxation) by transferring energy to some electromagnetic vector present in the surrounding environement, such as a nearby solvent molecule or the molecules themselves which undergo continuous vibrational and rotational changes thus associated with electrical and magnetical changes. These might be properly oriented and of the correct dimension to absorb ΔE. This relaxation process is known as spin-lattice relaxation where lattice implies the *entire framework* or *aggregate of neighbours.*

3. A second relaxation process involves transferring ΔE to a neighbouring nucleus, provided that the particular value of ΔE is common to both nuclei. This mutual exchange of spin-energy is termed as *spin-spin relaxation.* While one nucleus loses energy, the other nucleus gains energy so that no net change in the population of the two spin-states is involved.

   If the relaxation process is slow (half life approximately 1 sec), we get a definite value for the precessional frequency and as a result, a *sharp signal* is found in NMR signal. Generally non viscous liquids (solution of solids in non viscous solvents) have random molecular orientations and transfer of energy by spin-lattice relaxation is inefficient. In consequence, $t_{1/2}$ is large and non viscous systems give rise to *sharp signals.* On the other hand, if the relaxation process is rapid ($t_{1/2}$ is too short) we do not get a definite value for precessional frequency and the transfer of energy by spin-lattice interaction occurs with efficiency and a *broad signal* is found. *Viscous systems* have more interactions with protons leading to quick spin-lattice relaxation and they give generally *broad signals.* The proton attached to ^{14}N gives rise to a broad signal as quick spin-lattice relaxation occurs between proton and the nucleus of ^{14}N.

Chemical Shift : The precessional frequencies of all protons in a molecule in the same externally applied field (*e.g.*, ν=60 MHz, 1.4 T≡14,000 gauss) are not the same; the precise value for any one proton depends on a number of factors. As a result, the protons with different precessional frequencies absorb at different positions in an NMR spectrum to show different signals at different positions.

In reality, the protons present in a molecule reside in *different* chemical environments. The protons which have similar chemical environments, absorb radiowave of same frequency and show signal at the same position. Protons having different chemical environments show NMR signals at different positions of the spectrum. Because the *shift in frequency* depends on the *chemical environment*, this gives rise to the term *chemical shift.*

It is very difficult to get the absolute value of precessional frequency for proton or any other nucleus ($s \neq 0$) and it is also not needed essentially to analyse an NMR spectrum. In practice, the differences in frequencies are measured with respect to same reference group of nuclei. For protons and ^{13}C, the universally accepted reference is tetramethylsilane (Me_4Si) or TMS.

Reasons for taking tetramethylsilane (Me_4Si) or TMS as reference compound or internal standard :

1. TMS has *twelve* magnetically equivalent protons which give an intense *sharp* signal even at very low concentration (0.01–1.0%).

2. Since silicon is less electronegative than carbon, all the twelve hydrogens are in regions of high electron density and are as a result highly shielded. So its signal occurs in a spectrum where few other hydrogens absorb and seldom interferes with signals of other types of hydrogens.

3. TMS like other alkanes is *chemically inert.*

4. TMS is low boiling (27°C) so that it is easily removed by easy evaporation from a recoverable sample of valuable organic compound.
5. TMS is soluble in most organic solvents and can be added to sample solution (0.01–1.0%) as an *internal standard.* TMS is not *soluble* in water or in D_2O. So sodio salt of 3-(trimethylsilyl)-propanesulphonic acid, $Me_3SiCH_2CH_2CH_2SO_3^{\ominus}Na^{\oplus}$ is used as an internal standard instead of TMS.

Measurement of chemical shift and Units used in NMR spectroscopy : We always measure the differences in chemical shift position between the reference (TMS) and the signals from the compound being examined. By international convention, an NMR spectrum is always plotted with TMS on the right hand side, at low frequency and with high frequency on the left hand side. The region on the left hand side of the spectrum is known as downfield region (high frequency) and the region on the right hand side of the spectrum is called *upfield region (low frequency).* The molecule, the NMR spectrum of which is to be done is taken in $CDCl_3$ and irradiated with radiofrequencies like 60 MHz, 100 MHz, 500 MHz etc. Then the intensity of the magnetic field is increased slowly and the precessional frequencies of protons increase accordingly. When the precessional frequency of any proton becomes equal to the radiofrequency radiation, they come in resonance and the proton absorbs that radiowave. This absorption can be manifested on a NMR graph by a detector, as an NMR signal.

1. ***Delta Units (δ units)*** : Chemical shift positions are normally expressed in δ (delta) units, which are defined as proportional differences in *parts per million* (ppm), from an appropriate reference standard (TMS in case of ^{1}H-and ^{13}C NMRs).

$$\delta_X = \frac{H_X - H_R}{H_0} \times 10^6 \, ppm = \frac{\nu_X - \nu_R}{\nu_0} \times 10^6 \, ppm = \frac{\nu_X - \nu_{TMS}}{\nu_0} \times 10^6 \, ppm$$

(ν_{TMS}=0, taken as a standard)

Where δ_X=chemical shift in ppm, ν_X and ν_{TMS} are the frequencies in MHz of the signals for X and TMS, respectively, and ν_0 is the operating frequency of the instrument (in MHz).

Since δ unit is a proportionality, it is a dimensionless number. It is independent of field strength. A signal of δ value say 4.6 derived from a 60 MHz spectrum (1.4 T instrument) will be found at exactly the same value $\delta_{4.6}$ on a 100 MHz or an a 500 MHz (14.1 T) instrument.

2. ***Tau (τ) value*** : To correspond with the downfield values on the left and upfield on the right, a scale of units from 0 to 10, also running from left to right was proposed, so that δ=10–τ. It is an old convention.

Problems :

1. A benzyl alcohol sample shows the OH proton signal at 144 Hz higher frequency than TMS. Calculate the δ value of O—H proton signal, where the instrumental frequency is 60 MHz.

Answer : We know : $\delta = \frac{\text{Position of OH proton signal–Position of TMS peak}}{\text{Instrument frequency}} \times 10^6$

Here OH proton signal is higher by 144 Hz, hence we can write

$$\delta = \frac{144}{60 \times 10^6} \times 10^6 = 2.4$$

Hence $\delta_{OH\text{-}proton} = 2.4$

2. The signal for —CH_2— protons in pmr of benzyl alcohol ($C_6H_5CH_2OH$) appears at δ 4.6. Calculate the difference in frequency expressed in hertz, between this signal and TMS signal in a 300 MHz.

Answer : Difference in signal position $= \delta \times \frac{\text{frequency of the instrument in hertz}}{10^6}$

$$= \frac{4.6 \times 300 \times 10^6}{10^6} \text{ Hz}$$

$$= 1380 \text{ Hz}$$

Some values of δ in ppm (R=alkyl or H)

Type	ppm	Type	ppm	Type	ppm
1° alkyl	0.8–1.0	$R_2C\underline{H}F$	4.3–4.4	$RO\underline{H}$	0.5–0.5
2° alkyl	1.2–1.4	$RC\underline{H}Cl_2$	5.2–6.0		(*for enols* 11.0–16.0)
3° alkyl	1.4–1.8	$R_2C\underline{H}OR$	3.3–3.8	$ArO\underline{H}$	4.5
$R_2C{=}CRC\underline{H}R_2$	1.7–2.6	$R_2CHO\underline{H}$	3.4–3.8		(*H-bonded or*
$R{-}C{\equiv}C{-}C\underline{H}R_2$	2.0–2.2	$R_2C\underline{H}OCOR$	3.6–5.0		*chelated* 9.0–11.0)
$R_2C\underline{H}COOR$	2.0–2.2	$R_2C\underline{H}\overset{\oplus}{N}R_3$	3.3–3.5	$RCOO\underline{H}$	10.0–13.0
$R_2C\underline{H}CONR_2$	2.0–2.1	$R_2C\underline{H}NO_2$	4.3–4.6	$R_2N\underline{H}$	5.0–8.0
$R_2C\underline{H}COR$	2.1–2.5	$R{-}C{\equiv}C{-}\underline{H}$	1.8–1.9		(*broad signal*)
$R_2C\underline{H}NR_2$	2.1–2.9	$R_2C{=}C\underline{H}R$	4.6–5.0		
$ArC\underline{H}R_2$	2.3–2.9	$Ar\underline{H}$	7.0–8.0		
$R_2C\underline{H}Cl$	3.0–4.0	$RC\underline{H}O$	9.6–9.9		

The δ values given above may change if a strong electron withdrawing or electron-releasing group is present within the molecule.

Factors Influencing Chemical shift : The values of chemical shift and the position of NMR signal depends on the environment in which a proton under study resides.

1. ***Shielding or Deshielding by Sigma-bonded Electrons*** : In a magnetic field, the electrons around the proton are induced to circulate and in doing so, they generate a small secondary magnetic field which acts in opposition (*i.e.*, diamagnetically) to the applied field. The greater the electron density circulating around the proton, the greater is the induced *diamagnetic shielding effect* and the lower is the precessional frequency of the proton. Precessional frequency

must be increased to make it equal to the frequency of radiowave and the intensity of applied magnetic field should be increased. So, this type of protons absorb in *upfield region*, i,e *δ becomes less.* Electronic effects like +I and +R *effects increase sigma electron density* and ^1H *signal shifts upfield.*

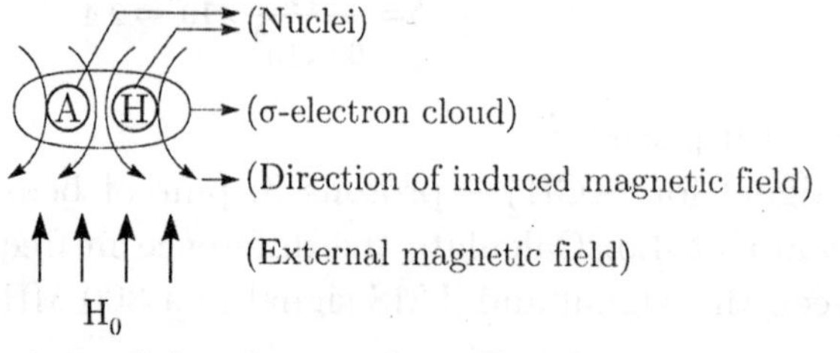

Silicon is more electropositive than carbon. For this reason, the electron density around the ^1H nucleus of methyl group increases in TMS and the proton of TMS absorbs maximum upfield compared to protons of other organic molecules. δ is taken zero as a standard for the methyl protons of TMS.

Deshielding effect is found if groups with –I or –R effect is present within the molecule. Electronegative groups such as fluorine in CH_3F withdraw electron density from the methyl group and this deshielding effect means that the methyl protons experience a greater net magnetic field, and, hence precess with higher frequencies. Cl in CH_3Cl is less electronegative than F, so the shift of ^1H of CH_3Cl occurs at a *less* downfield compared to shift of ^1H of CH_3F which is more downfield.

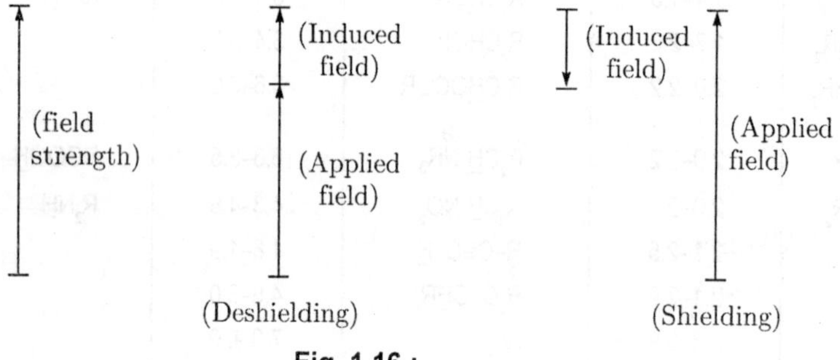

Fig. 1.16 :

The effect of charged species on chemical shift values is very marked. Protons adjacent to $\overset{\oplus}{N}$ (as in quaternary ammonium ion $R_4\overset{\oplus}{N}$) are very strongly deshielded (high δ values), while carbanionic centres, COO^-, O^- (all having +I effects) act as powerful shielding influences (low δ values).

van der Waals Deshielding : In a rigid molecule, it is possible for a proton to occupy a sterically hindered position, and in consequence, the electron cloud of the hindering group will *tend to repel*, by electrostatic repulsion, the electron cloud surrounding the proton. The proton will be deshielded and appear at higher δ values than would be predicted in the absence of the effect. This influence is small (usually less than 1 ppm) and is manifested in overcrowded molecules, such as highly substituted steroids and alkaloids.

One Example of Deshielding of Protons in the presence of groups containing –I effect.

1,1,2–Trichloroethane

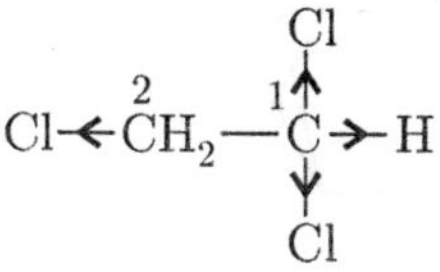

The protons of C–1 absorbs at a lower magnetic field strength with higher δ (δ=5.77 ppm) than the C–2 protons (δ=3.95 ppm). This is due to the reason that, two Cl atoms (–I effect) joined to C–1, making C–1 H more *deshielded* compared to C–2 protons where only one Cl atom is attached. The σ-electron density around the C–2 protons is higher.

2. **Effect of π-Orbital : Anisotropic Effects :** The δ values of protons attached to sp^3 carbons of an alkane is much *less* compared to δ values of protons attached to sp^2 carbon in alkenes. Only mere electronegativity difference between sp^3 and sp^2 hybrid orbitals cannot explain this vast difference in δ value. Again the δ value of protons attached to sp carbon is enough *upfield*, but the electronegativity of sp orbital is more than that of sp^2 orbital. Aldehydes and aromatic protons also have high δ values. This apparent anomalous behaviour of proton signal attached to π-bond is due to the complexity of the magnetic field generated by the circulation of π-electrons. The effect is complex and can lead to shifts to higher frequency (downfield or paramagnetic shifts), or to lower frequency (upfield or diamagnetic shifts). So the effects are paramagnetic in certain directions around the π-clouds and diamagnetic in ethers, so that these effects are described as ***anisotropic*** (non uniform) as opposed to ***isotropic*** (operating equally through space).

   (a) Alkenes : When an alkene group is so oriented that the plane of the double bond is at 90° to the direction of the applied field H_0, the induced circulation of the π-electrons generates a secondary magnetic field, which is *diamagnetic* around the carbon atoms but *paramagnetic* in the region of the alkene protons.

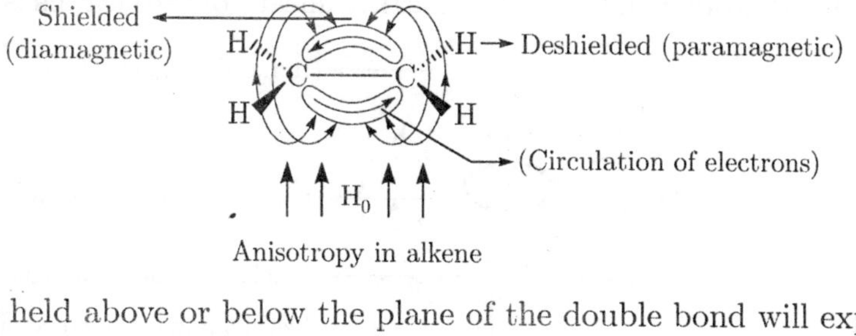

Anisotropy in alkene

Any group held above or below the plane of the double bond will experience a shielding effect, since in these areas, the induced field opposes H_0. In α-pinene, one of the geminal methyl groups is held in just such a shielded position, and comes to resonance at significantly lower δ than its twin. The third methyl group appears at higher δ, since it lies in the plane of the double bond and is thus deshielded.

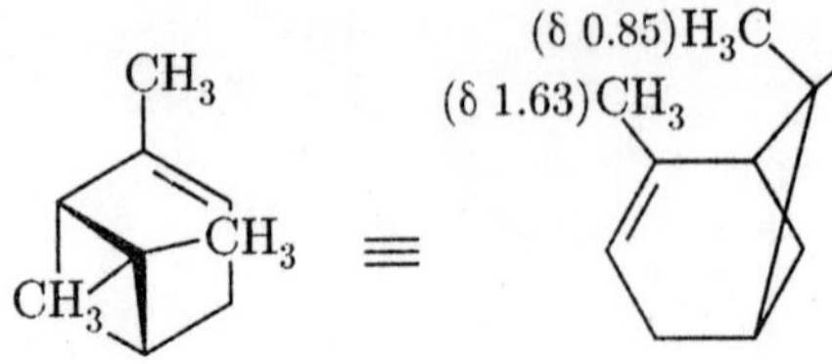

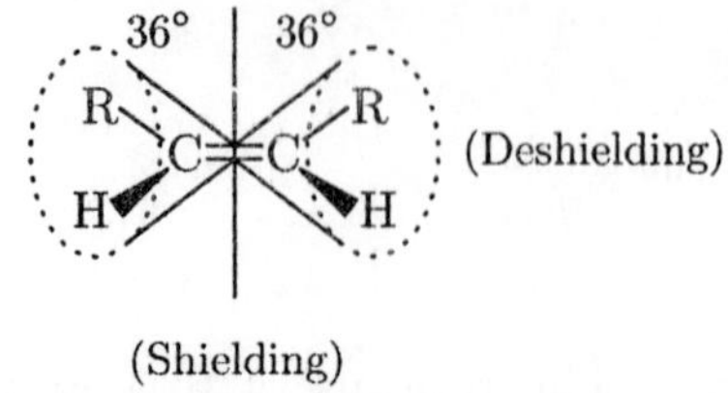

We can divide the space around a double bond into two categories. Deshielding occurs in the cone-shaped zones with higher δ values. Shielding is found outside the cones and protons in these zones are shielded with lower δ values.

(b) Carbonyl compounds : For the carbonyl group, a similar situation arises although the best representation of shielding and deshielding zones is slightly different from the alkene pattern.

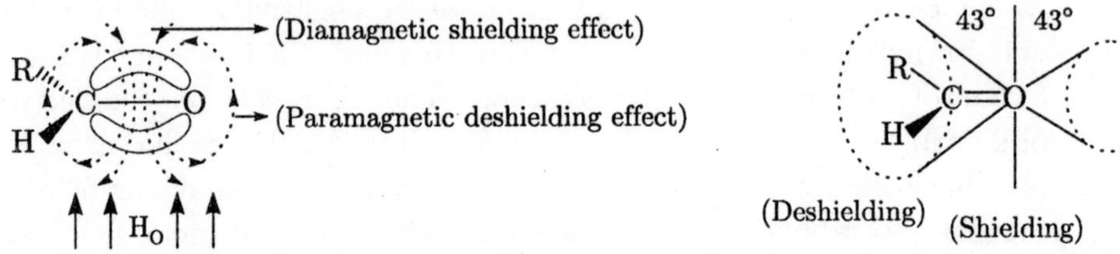

Anisotropy in carbonyl compounds

Two cone-shaped volumes, centred on the oxygen atom, lie parallel to the axis of the C=O bond, protons within these cones experience deshielding, so that *aldehydic protons* and the formyl protons of formyl esters appear at high δ values. Protons held above or below these cones will come to resonance at lower δ values.

(c) Alkynes : Whereas alkene and aldehydic protons appear at high δ values, alkyne protons appear around δ 1.5–3.5. Electron circulation around the triple bond occurs in such a way that the protons experience a *diamagnetic shielding effect*, when the axis of the alkyne group lies parallel to the direction of H_0, the external applied field. The cylindrical sheath of π-electrons is induced to circulate

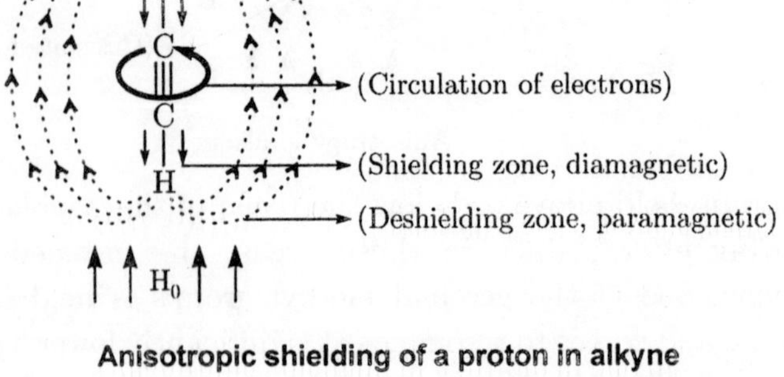

Anisotropic shielding of a proton in alkyne

around the axis, and the resultant annulus shaped magnetic field acts in a direction that opposes H_0 in the vicinity of the protons. These protons experience a shielding; therefore, acetylenic protons appear at lower δ values in the spectrum.

(d) Aromatic compounds : In the molecule of benzene and aromatic compounds, π-electrons are *delocalised cyclically* over the aromatic ring. These loops of electrons are induced to circulate in the presence of applied field H_0, producing a substantial electric current, called *ring current.* The magnetic field associated with this electric field has the geometry and direction as follows.

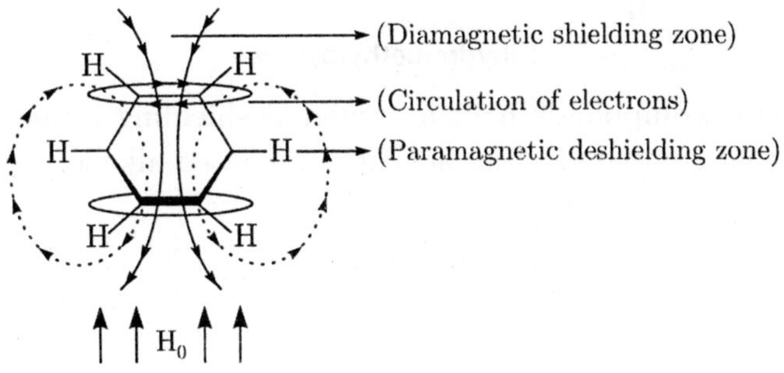

Anisotropic shielding and deshielding associated with the aromatic ring current. Protons attached to the ring fall under the paramagnetic deshielding zone, and such low field, absorption of aromatic protons (δ=6 to 9) is often used as a criterion for aromaticity for identification.

***Exceptions* :**

(a) Not all aromatic protons absorb at low magnetic field. For large ring aromatic compounds like [18] annulene, the internal H atom in the centre of the ring are highly shielded by the opposed induced field and absorbs at δ=–1.8 (much higher field) whereas the external protons are deshielded and show δ=8.9 as the phenyl protons. So *twelve* peripheral protons are deshielded and the six internal protons are highly shielded. (δ=–1.8), even upfield than TMS (δ=0).

(a)

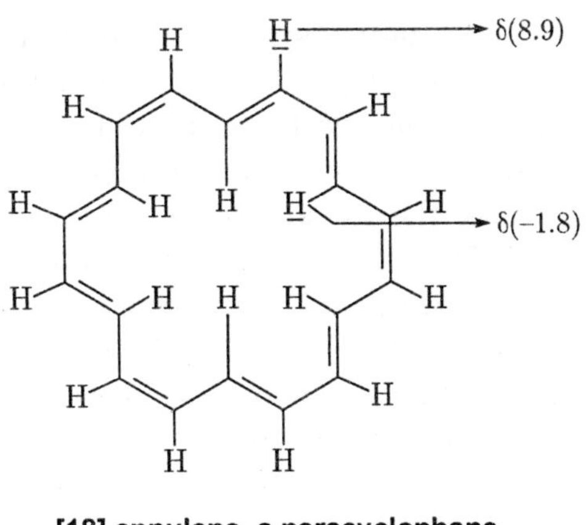

[18] annulene, a paracyclophane

(b)

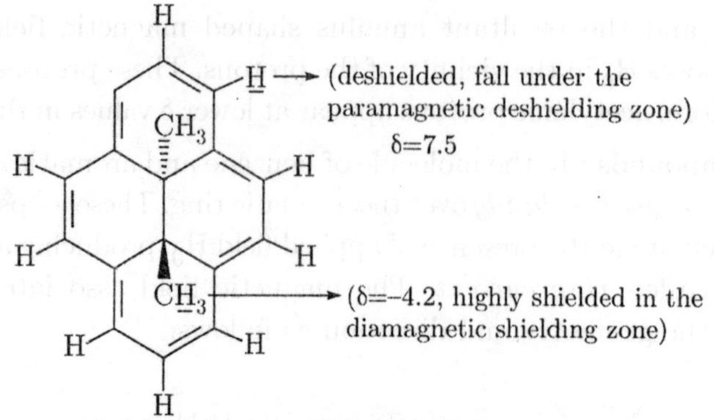

Dihydromethylpyrene

Aromatic compounds have a greater deshielding influence of the ring current than that compared to an acyclic conjugated alkene.

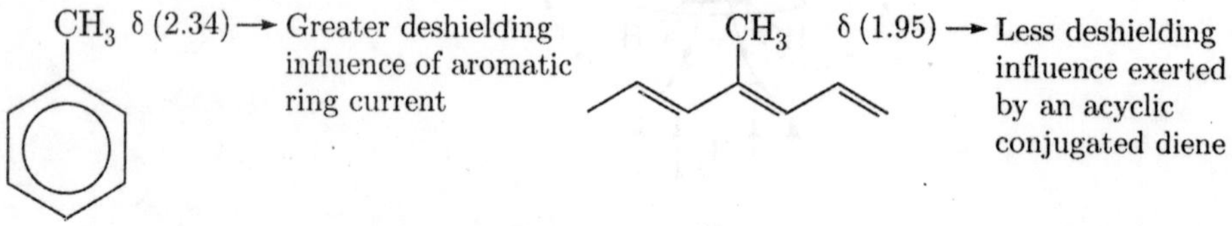

Magnetic anisotropy can even be shown by sigma electrons. The equatorial protons in cyclohexane rings come to resonance about 0.5 ppm higher than the axial protons and this is attributed to anisotropic deshielding by the σ-electrons in the β—γ bond as shown below. This effect is small compared with the anisotropic influence of circulating π-electrons, but is readily observed in rigid systems and also in mobile systems at low temperature.

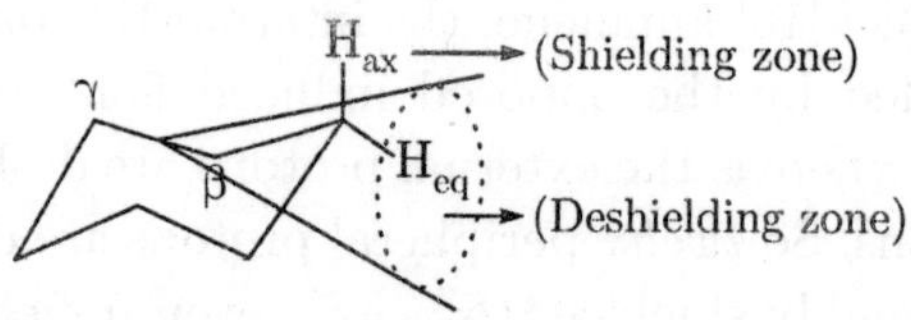

Anisotropic shielding and deshielding in clohexanes

3. **Effect of hydrogen bond and dipolar interaction** : If any proton is attributed by hydrogen bond or by a dipolar molecule, then the proton has less influence by the σ–electrons which form the bond with the proton. As a result, the diamagnetic shielding of σ-electrons becomes less and the proton signal comes at a downfield region. For example, the phenols which are hydrogen bonded internally absorb at a much *downfield* compared to those which are not hydrogen bonded. Chloroform gives proton signal at δ 7.3 in cyclohexane compared to proton signal of chloroform in benzene, which is much upfield (δ=6.74). Benzene molecule behaves as a Lewis base and the proton of chloroform molecule resides in a plane perpendicular to that benzene ring. As a result, the proton of chloroform falls under the diamagnetic shielding zone of benzene and consequently has lower δ value.

Chemical shift positions for protons in organic molecules

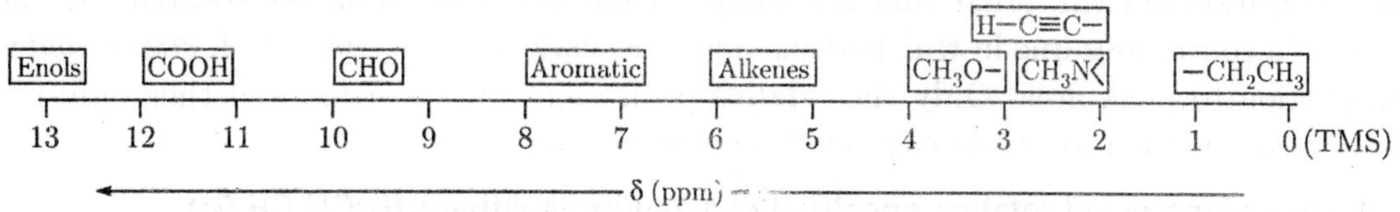

Solvents Used in NMR spectroscopy : Non viscous solution of samples give the sharpest NMR spectra. Sometimes the compound itself is a non viscous liquid, so a *neat* liquid can be used. A solvent in which a solute is dissolved even upto only 10% can be used. But it is advantageous to use an aprotic solvent. Some solvents used in NMR spectroscopy are CCl_4, CS_2, $CDCl_3$, C_6D_6, D_2O, $(CD_3)SO$ or (DMSO–d_6), CD_3CO(acetone–d_6), $(CCl_3)_2CO$ (hexachloroacetone) etc.

NH, SH and particularly OH protons, all have their NMR signals substantially moved on changing to solvents of different polarity. This effect is largely associated with the hydrogen bonding. At low concentrations, intermolecular hydrogen bonding is diminished in simple OH, NH and SH compounds. Since hydrogen bonding involves electron-cloud transfer from the hydrogen atoms to a neighbouring electronegative atom (O, N or S), the hydrogen experiences a net deshielding effect, when hydrogen bonding is strong and is less deshielded when hydrogen bonding is diminished. Thus, at high concentrations (strong hydrogen bonding, strong deshielding) OH, NH and SH protons appear at higher δ than in dilute solution. Increased temperature also reduces intermolecular hydrogen bonding, so the resonance positions for these protons are temperature dependent (higher temperatures mean lower δ values). Intramolecular hydrogen bonding is unchanged by dilution and the NMR spectrum from such systems is virtually unaltered by varying concentration. Salicylates and enols of β-dicarbonyl compounds are examples of such systems. Chelates such as the salicylates show the OH resonance at very high δ (10–12) and enol OH appears higher (δ 11–16).

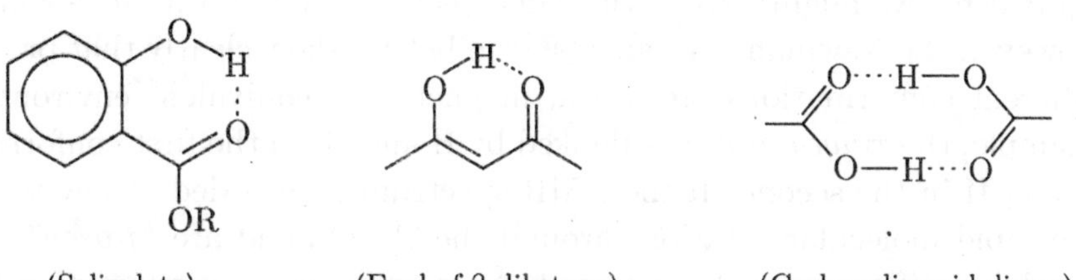

(Salicylate) (Enol of β-diketone) (Carboxylic acid dimer)

Intramolecular H-bonding; δ values largely unaffected by concentration changes

Carboxylic acid are a special case of hydrogen bonding because of their stable dimeric association, which persists even in very dilute solution. Carboxylic OH appears between δ 10–13, usually nearer δ 11–12.

Integrals in proton NMR spectra : NMR peak area

The area under each NMR signal in that spectrum is proportional to the number of hydrogen atoms in that environment. The two peaks in *toluene spectrum* (one for $-CH_3$ group and another for *five* aromatic protons) have relative areas 5:3 corresponding to C_6H_5 and CH_3 respectively.

Measurement of peak area is carried out automatically on the NMR spectrometer by integration of each signal, and the integral value is indicated on the spectrum in the form of a continuous line in which steps appear as each signal is measured, *step height* is proportion to peak area. Only the *relative* peak areas are recorded and thus only the *ratio* between the protons in each environment is given.

Influence of restricted rotation spectrum of 1,2–dibromoethane ($BrCH_2CH_2Br$) and N, N–dimethylformamide ($HCONMe_2$)

(a) The NMR spectrum of N, N–dimethylformamide, $HCONMe_2$) recorded around room temperature, shows *two* signals for the methyl groups, although it might have been expected that the two methyl groups would be in magnetically equivalent environments. DMF is represented by the two resonance forms shown below, and the result of conjugation between the carbonyl group and the nitrogen non-bonding pair is to increase the double bond character of C—N bond sufficiently to restrict the rotation at room temperature; one methyl group is *cis* to oxygen and the other is *trans* and anisotropy of the carbonyl group is sufficient to influence the chemical shift position for the *cis* group.

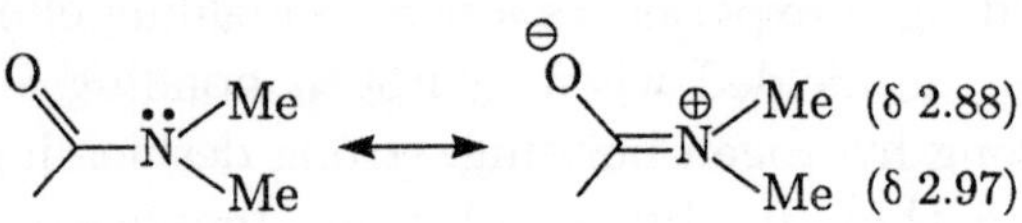

At high temperature (~130°C), the spectrum shows only one signal for the methyl groups. At elevated temperatures, rotation around the C—N bond is so rapid that each methyl group experiences the same time-averaged environment.

(b) The four protons in 1,2–dibromoethane ($BrCH_2CH_2Br$) are chemically indistinguishable, and one might also suppose that they are magnetically equivalent; we might expect the same chemical shift position for all the four. However, the Newman diagrams (shown below) show clearly that protons in the different conformations are *not* in magnetically equivalent environments. For example, the *ringed proton* is flanked by H and Br in the first conformer, but by H and H in the second. If the NMR spectrum is recorded at low temperature, the rapid molecular rotations around the C—C bond are "*frozen*" sufficiently for these differences to be detected. At room temperature, rotation is so rapid that each proton experiences the same time-averaged environment and only one sharp signal appears in the NMR spectrum.

I.

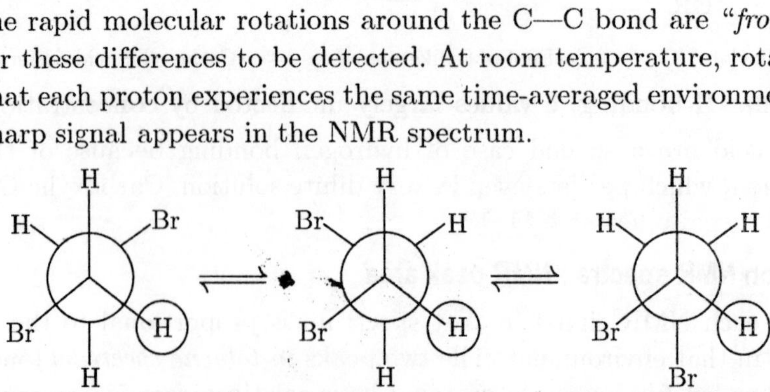

(Rotational isomers of 1,2-dibromoethane)

II. 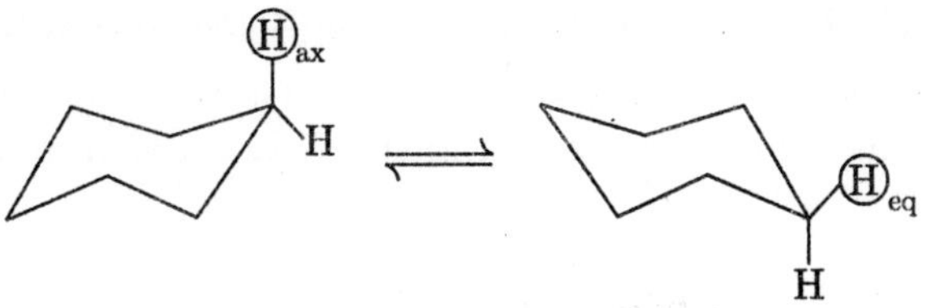

(Cyclohexane ring flips)

Similar effects are found in fluxional molecules and in structures where steric effects can intervene; examples are cyclohexane ring flips, bridged structures (*e.g.*, α-pinene, discussed earlier) etc.

Equivalent and non-equivalent protons

Two or more protons that are in identical magnetic environments have same chemical shift and therefore give only one NMR signal, thus, they are known as equivalent or chemical shift equivalent protons. For example, the *twelve* protons in $(CH_3)_4C$ lie in the same magnetic environment and thus have same chemical shift values. These protons are thus said to be equivalent or chemical shift equivalent protons. Protons that have different chemical shifts are said to be non-equivalent or chemical shift non-equivalent protons. Naturally, these protons lie in different magnetic environments. For example, *p*-xylene exhibits (H_3C–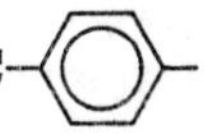–CH_3) *two* peaks in 3:2 ratio. The *six CH_3 protons* are *equivalent* to one another and give rise to a *single signal.* Similarly, the *four aryl protons* are equivalent to one another as they are in the same magnetic environment. Thus, the six —CH_3 protons and four aryl protons are non-equivalent with respect to their own category. Six —CH_3 protons give a *sharp* single peak at δ 2.3 and the four aryl protons give another *single peak* at δ 7.1 (characteristic chemical shift for aryl protons). Hence, the spectrum of *p*-xylene contains *two* signals, one for six CH_3 protons and another for four aryl protons in 3:2 ratio.

The ¹H-NMR spectrum of *n*-propane (CH_3—CH_2—CH_3) contains *two* signals, one for six equivalent —CH_3 protons and the other for *two* equivalent —CH_2— protons.

Chemical shift non equivalence can occur when two environments are stereochemically different, *e.g.*, the *two vinyl protons* of 2-bromopropene have different chemical shifts.

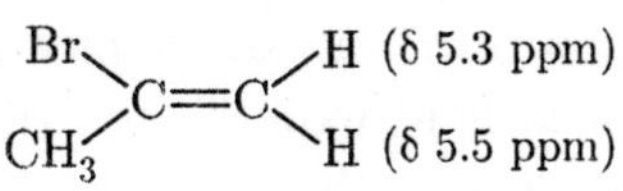

(2-bromopropene)

Generally *diastereotopic* protons give different chemical shifts whereas *enantiotopic* protons give same chemical shift irrespective of field strength.

Peak splitting : Spin-spin coupling : First order spectra

Most NMR spectra do not show simple single peaks but rather group of peaks because of spin-spin coupling and the groups of peaks tend to cluster about certain δ values. The δ value of a signal having a number of peaks is determined by the central position of these peaks. For example, the NMR spectrum of 1,1,2-trichloroethane shows a signal for C-1H with *three* peaks. That is, this proton (C-1H) forms a triplet in the signal. Again C-2H gives a signal with two peaks, *i.e.*, this proton forms a signal as a doublet.

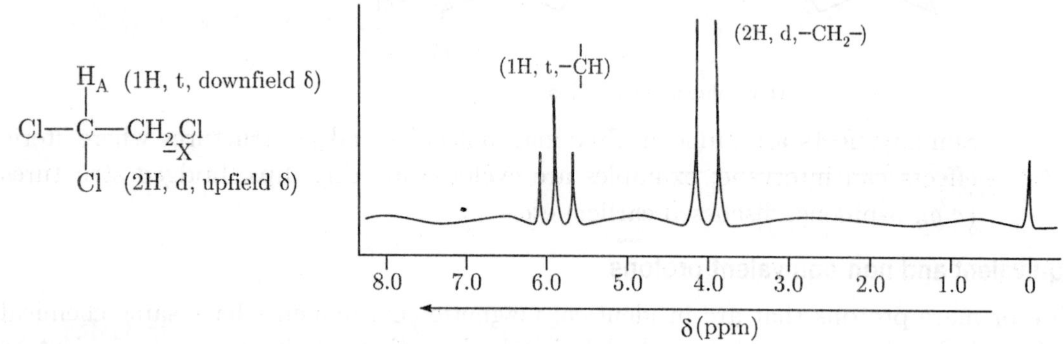

Fig. 1.17 :

The interference of a vicinal proton spinning in a particular direction to the spin of a particular proton, spinning either in the same or in the opposite direction is known as *spin-spin coupling.*

1. **AX Type spin-spin coupling (see also page 96) :** H_A and H_X of cinnamic acid reside in different magnetic environments and come to resonance at different positions

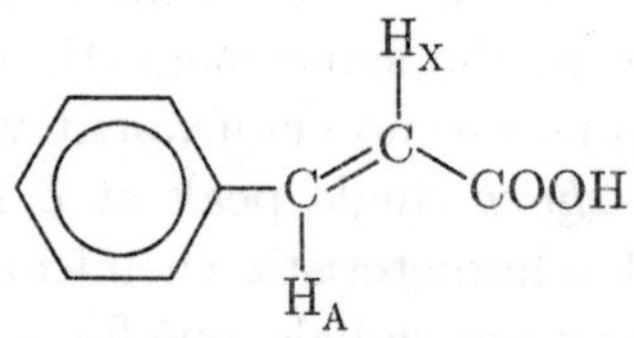

(Cinnamic acid)

in the NMR spectrum. They do not give rise to single peaks (singlets) but doublets. The separation between the lines of each doublet is equal. This spacing is called the *coupling constant, J.* The resonance position for A depends on its total magnetic environment, part of its magnetic environment is the nearby proton X. Which is itself magnetic. The proton X can have its nuclear magnet either *aligned with* proton A or *opposed to* proton A. Thus, proton A can either *increase* the net magnetic field experienced by A (X aligned) or decrease it (X opposed). In fact, it does both. The two spin orientations of X create two different magnetic fields around proton A; in roughly half of the molecules, the spin orientation of X creates a shielding field around proton A, and in the other half, a deshielding field. Therefore, proton A comes to resonance, *not once, but twice* and proton A gives rise to a doublet. Similarly, proton A is a magnet having two spin orientations with respect to X and A creates two magnetic fields around X. Proton X comes to resonance *twice* in the NMR spectrum.

The mutual magnetic influence between protons A and X is not transmitted through space but via the electrons in the intervening bonds. The nuclear spin of A couples with the electron spin of C—H_A bonding electrons, these, in turn, couple with C—C bonding electrons and then with the C—H_X bonding electrons. This coupling is eventually transmitted to the spin of the H_X nucleus. This electron-coupled spin interaction operates strongly through one bond or two bonds, less strongly through three bonds and weakly and only in unusual cases through four or five bonds.

We can represent the possible spin orientations of coupling protons. Proton A can see proton X as *aligned (parallel ↑)* or *opposed (antiparallel ↓)*. These two spin orientations correspond effectively to two different magnetic fields. Therefore, proton A comes to resonance twice. The same argument explains why proton X appears as a doublet. The A and X protons of cinnamic acid give rise to this characteristic pair of doublets, caused by two protons undergoing spin coupling. Such spectrum is called an *AX spectrum*. Since the probability of the two spin orientations of A and X arising is equal in molecules througout the sample, the two lines in each doublet are of equal intensity.

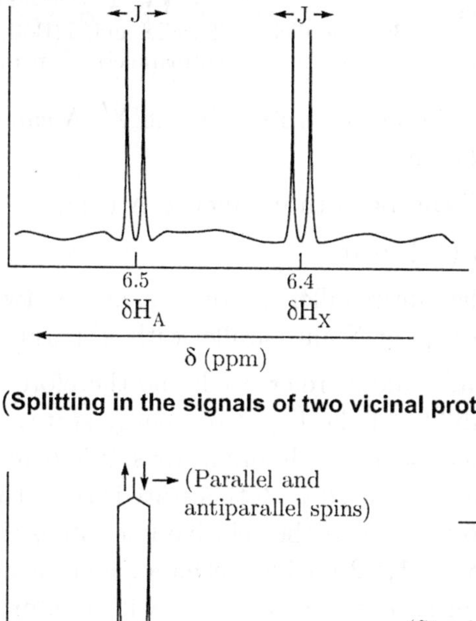

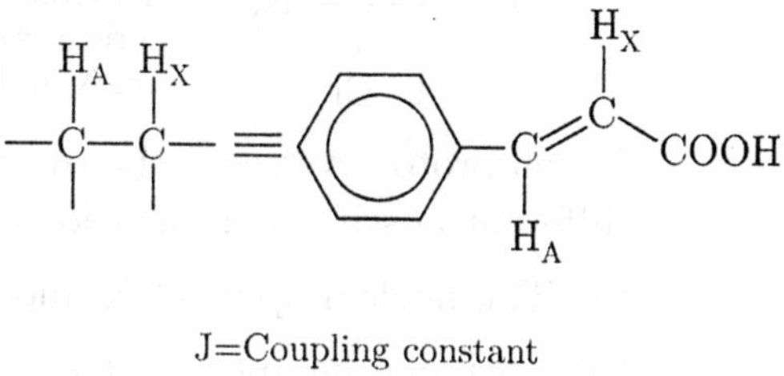

(Splitting in the signals of two vicinal protons of cinnamic acid)

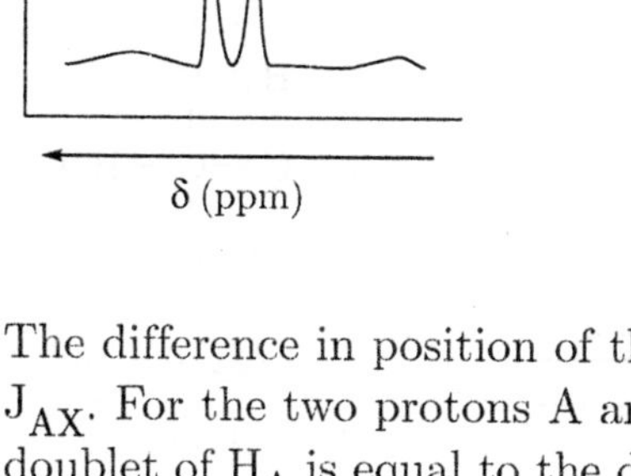

(Simulation of spin-coupling between a proton A and neighbouring proton X)

Fig. 1.18 :

The difference in position of the two peaks is known as the coupling constant, J_{AX}. For the two protons A and X, J_{AX} is a constant. So the difference in the doublet of H_A is equal to the difference in the doublet peaks of H_X. The centre

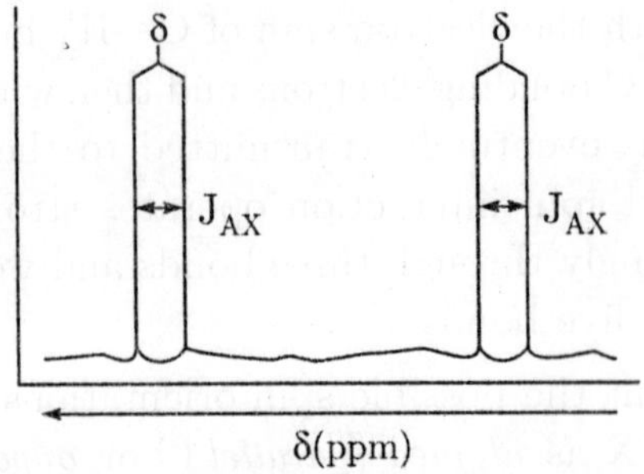

Fig. 1.19 :

or mid point of each doublet gives the chemical shift (δ) value of that signal. Coupling constant can be expressed either in *cps* or in *Hertz*.

2. **AX_2 Type spin-spin coupling (see also page 97)** : Let us examine the spectrum of 1,1,2-trichloroethane.

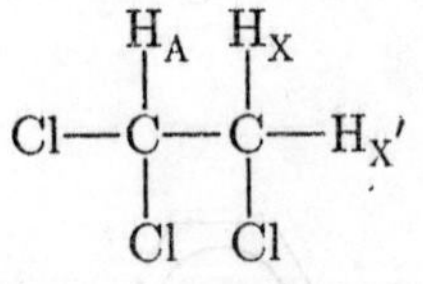

For proton A:			
Possible spin orientations of X and X′	↑↑ (Both parallel)	↑↓ ↓↑ (Parallel and antiparallel)	↓↓ (Both anti-parallel)

When proton A "sees" the two neighbouring protons X and X′, A can see *three* different possible combinations of spin:

(a) The nuclear spins of X and X′ can be both parallel to A (↑↑),

(b) Both can be antiparallel to A (↓↓), and

(c) One can be parallel and the other antiparallel and this can arise in two ways— X parallel with X′ antiparallel (↑↓) or X antiparallel with X′ parallel (↑↓).

Three distinct energy situations, a,b, and c are created, and therefore proton A gives rise to a *triplet.* The probability of the first two energy states arising is *equal,* but since the third state can arise in two different ways, it is *twice* as likely to arise. The intensity of the signal associated with this state is *twice* that of the lines associated with the first two states and the relative line intensities in the triplet are 1:2:1. The spectrum of 1,1,2-trichloroethane, consisting of the characteristic *doublet* and *triplet* of two protons coupling with one proton, can be called an AX_2 spectrum.

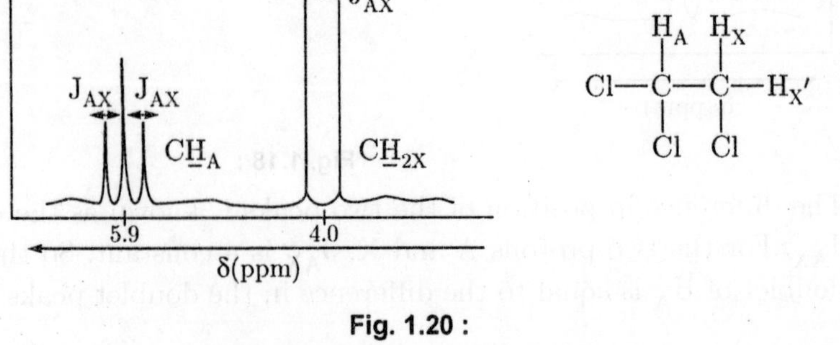

Fig. 1.20 :

More complex spin-spin splitting systems

The two examples of spin coupling, namely AX and AX_2 cases show virtually undistorted multiplets, with the multiplicity following the (n+1) rule and signal intensities almost exactly 1:1 and 1:2:1. Such spectra are described as *first-order* spectra.

Multiplicity rule : The number of peaks into which the signal for a particular proton splits is called its "*multiplicity*".

The number of lines (multiplicity) observed in the NMR signal for a group of protons is not related to the number of proton(s) in that group, the multiplicity of lines is related to the number of protons in neighbouring groups.

(n+1) rule : The simple rule is to find out the multiplicity of the signal from a group of protons, count the number of neighbours (n) and add 1.

Example : The spectrum of CH_3CHBr_2

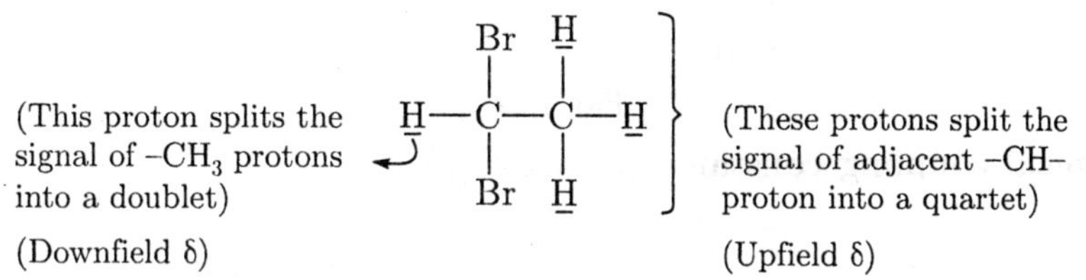

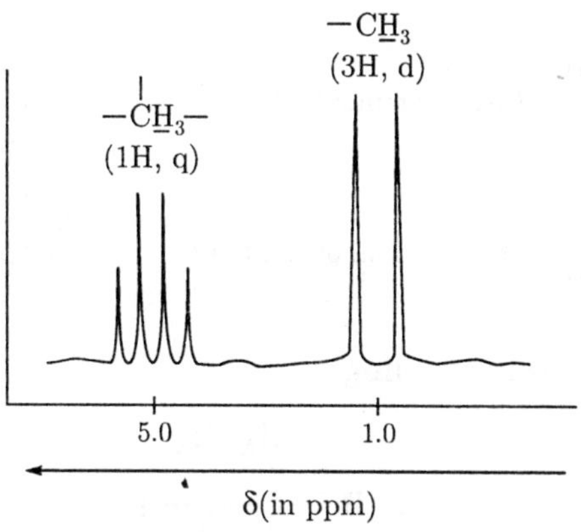

Fig. 1.21 :

Splitting is not observed for equivalent protons, e.g., the signals for $BrCH_2CH_2Br$ at room temperature or

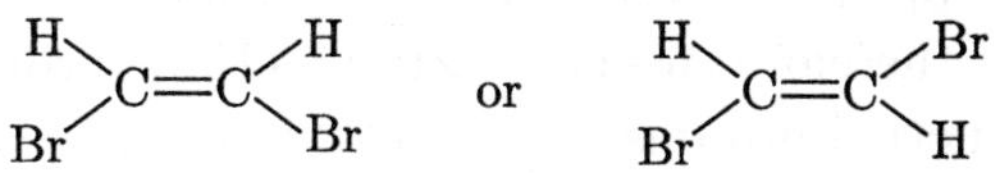

do *not split* because all the *hydrogen* atoms are *equivalent.*

Deuterium does not give a signal in the ^{1}H–NMR nor does it split nearby proton(s). Thus $\overset{a}{CH_3}\overset{b}{CH}DBr$ has only a'*doublet*' for H^a and a more downfield '*quartet*' for H^b. Fluorine (F) atom couples with protons in the same way as do other protons, *e.g.*, in

$\overset{a}{CH_3}CF_2\overset{a}{CH_3}$, the two F atoms split H^a signal into a 1:2:1 triplet, the fluorine atom if detected would be a '*septet*'.

Coupling constant (J) : The spacing between lines within a multiplet is typically a constant and this spacing in each multiplet is called the '*coupling constant*', J and is expressed in cps or in Hertz. The coupling constant J is independent of field strength but depends on stuctural relationship of the coupled protons.

For $\overset{a}{CH_3}\overset{b}{CH_2}Br$,

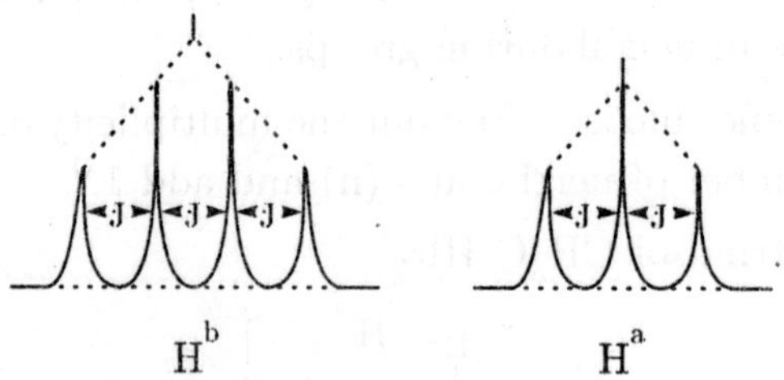

Fig. 1.22 :

Some typical coupling constants (J in Hertz)

H—C≡C—H (~7)

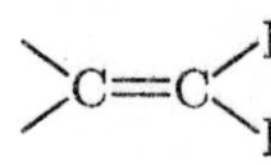

(1-4)

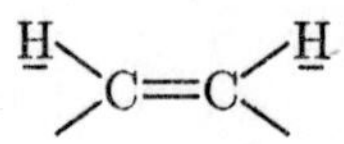

(5-14, commonly 6-8)

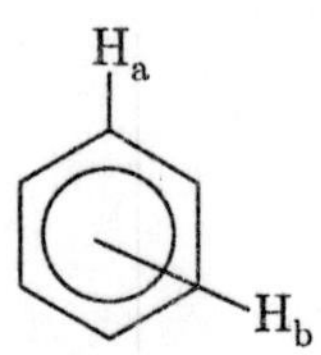

Ortho 7-10

Meta 2-3

Para 2-3

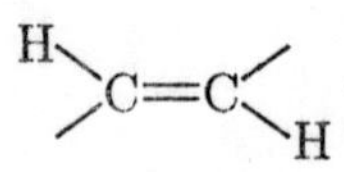

(11-19, commonly 14-16)

3. AX_3 Type spin-spin coupling :

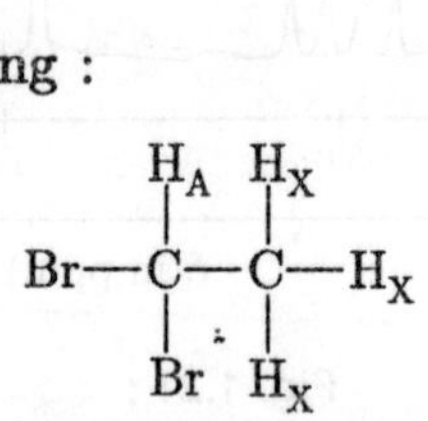

It contains a doublet and a quartet (J=8Hz) corresponding to the coupling of one proton with *three* neighbours. This is an AX_3 spectrum. The methyl protons have one neighbour and therefore appear as a doublet. The methine proton has three neighbours on the methyl group and therefore (n+1) is 4. For methine proton, the various ways of spin orientations of the methyl protons are as follows:

(a) All the three spins of methyl protons parallel (↑↑↑).

(b) Two spins parallel, one spin antiparallel (↑↑↓ or ↑↓↑ or ↓↑↑).

(c) Two spins antiparallel, one spin parallel (↓↑↓ or ↓↓↑ or ↑↓↓).

(d) All the three spins antiparallel (↓↓↓).

Four different energy combinations are produced, therefore, the methine proton comes to resonance four times, appearing as a quartet. The relative probabilities of the above *eight* states arising are in the ratio 1:3:3:1 and the line intensities in the quartet have the same ratio.

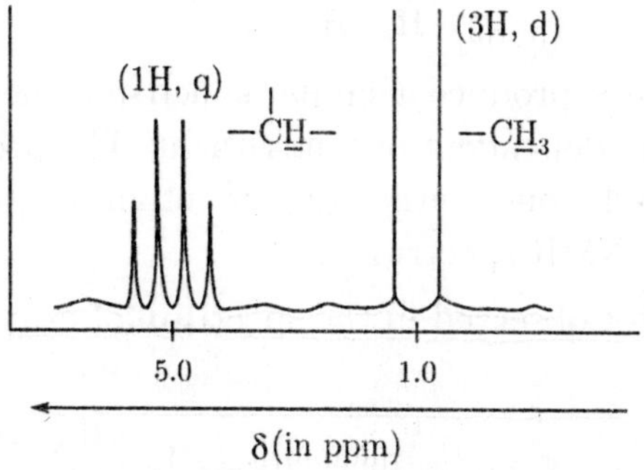

Fig. 1.23 : (^{1}H-NMR spectrum of CH_3CHBr_2)

Another example of AX_3 spectrum is 2-chloropropanoic acid.

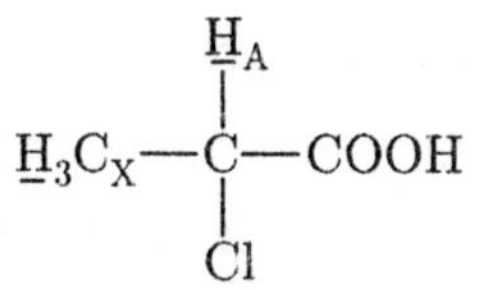

(^{1}H-NMR spectrum of 2-chloropropanoic acid)

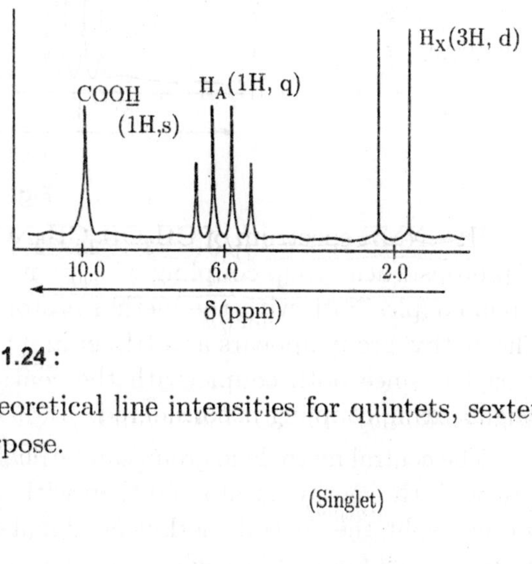

Fig. 1.24 :

One can go further and predict the theoretical line intensities for quintets, sextets etc. **Pascal's famous triangle** serves the purpose.

1 (Singlet)

1 1 (Doublet)

1 2 1 (Triplet)

1 3 3 1 (Quartet)

1 4 6 4 1 (Quintet)

1 5 10 10 5 1 (Sextet)

(Pascal's Triangle)

The outer lines in substantial multiplets are of such low intensity that they may be all but unobservable.

4. A_2X_3 Type spin-spin coupling :

Spectrum of CH_3CH_2Br ≡ 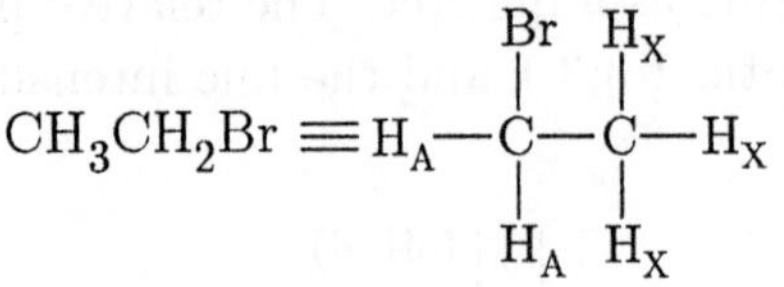

All isolated ethyl groups produce a similar spectrum, the chemical shift positions of the —CH_2— protons being dependent on substituent. The presence of such ethyl groups (as in ethyl esters, ethyl ketones, ethyl ethers, ethanol etc.) is quite unequivocally identifiable from the ^1H—NMR spectrum.

The triplet and quartet observed in the spectrum of ethyl bromide is an example of A_2X_3 case.

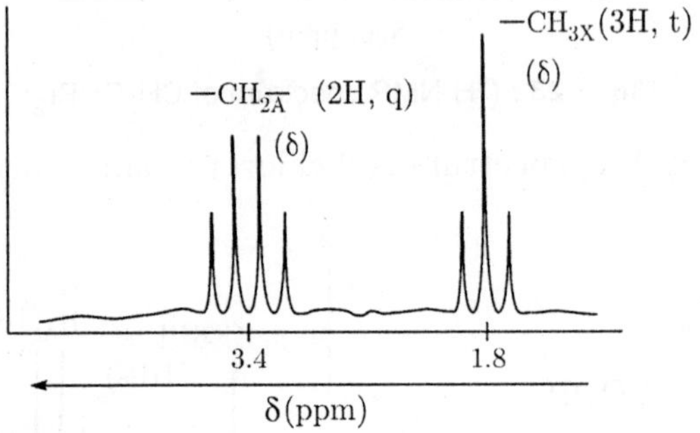

Fig. 1.25 :

^1H—NMR spectrum of $CH_3CH_2CH_2NO_2$ (1–Nitropropane) : There are three groups of protons, each group coupling with its near neighbours, so that the central methylene group couples both with the methyl protons and with the terminal methylene protons. The methyl group appears as a triplet and the terminal methylene group also appears as a triplet, since both couple with the central methylene group (n+1)=(2+1)=3. Only neighbouring coupling is considered.

The central methylene group can be dealt with by considering the successive coupling, first with the methyl group and then with the terminal methylene protons. The methyl protons split the central methylene signal into a quartet, the two terminal methylene protons should now split each line of this quartet into a triplet, giving twelve lines in all. In the spectrum, only *six* lines are observed showing that considerable overlapping of the

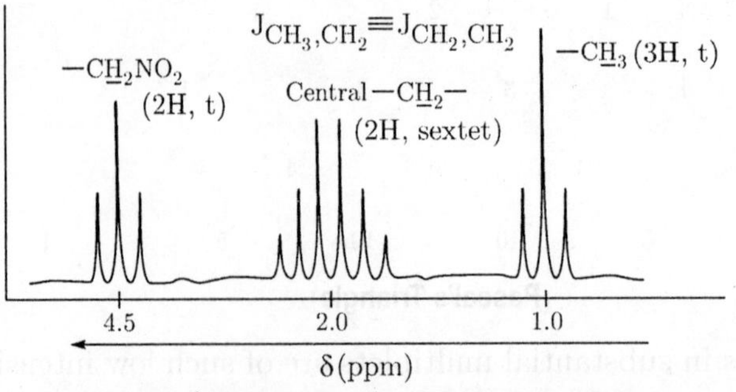

Fig. 1.26 : (^1H-NMR spectrum of $CH_3CH_2CH_2NO_2$)

predicted twelve lines has taken place. In fact, the two coupling constants involved (J_{CH_3, CH_2} and J_{CH_2,CH_2}) are equal and an easier way to consider the central —CH_2— group is to add the *total* number of neighbours with which it couples (CH_3 and CH_2) and then apply (n+1) rule. There are five coupling neighbours, therefore the multiplicity is 6. This simplified approach only succeeds when the two coupling constants are equal. If the two coupling constants had been different, it might have been possible to observe all twelve predicted lines.

5. AMX Type spin-spin coupling : The three groups of protons A, M and X each can couple with the other two as is frequently observed in unsaturated systems and aromatic systems. For such as system to be first order, the chemical shift positions of the protons must be relatively well separated, just as A, M, and X are separated in the alphabet.

Example : ^{1}H–NMR spectrum of furan–2–aldehyde

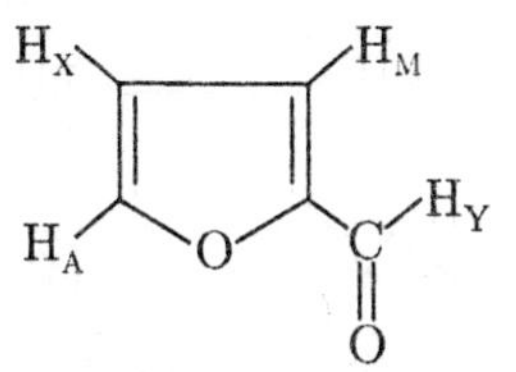

The three nuclear protons each give rise to four-line signal, so that twelve lines in all are observable, the aldehydic proton appears as a singlet. *Proton A* couples with *X*, which splits the A signal into a doublet; but A also couples with M so that each line of A is further split into *two*, giving *four* lines in all. *The signal for proton A* shows two splittings J_{AM} and J_{AX} and is therefore a *double doublet* (rather than a quartet). Similarly, the M signal is split into two by coupling with X, and each line is further split into two by coupling with A; two coupling constants are again seen, J_{AM} and J_{MX} and *M* appears as a *double doublet.* Lastly the X signal is split into a double doublet by two successive couplings J_{MX} and J_{AX}. The NMR spectrum of many compounds, e,g *vinyl* acetate *show AMX coupling system.*

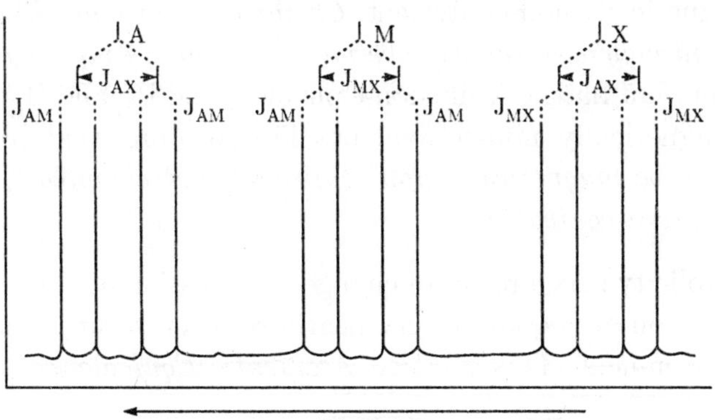

Fig. 1.27 : Coupling constants in an AMX system

Chemical and magnetic equivalence in NMR : Two protons are defined as being chemically equivalent if by virtue of symmetry within the molecule, their electronic environments are indistinguishable, and therefore they possess the *same value of chemical shift.*

Examples :

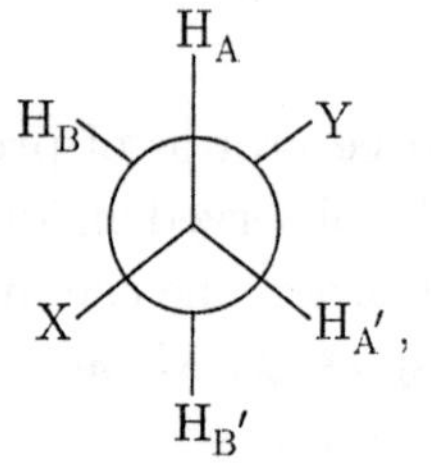

(I)

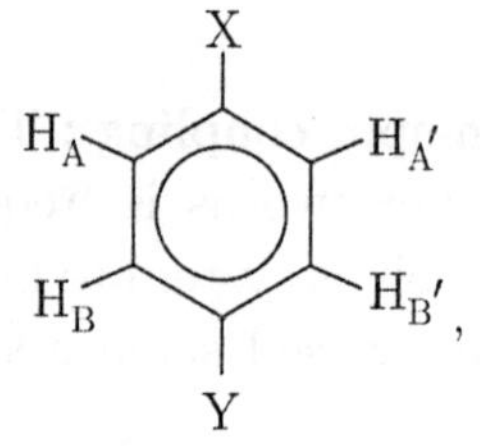

(II)

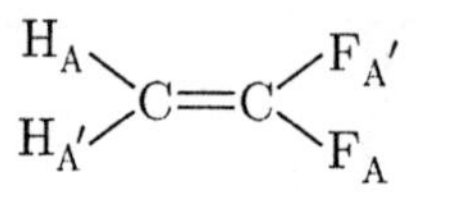

(III)

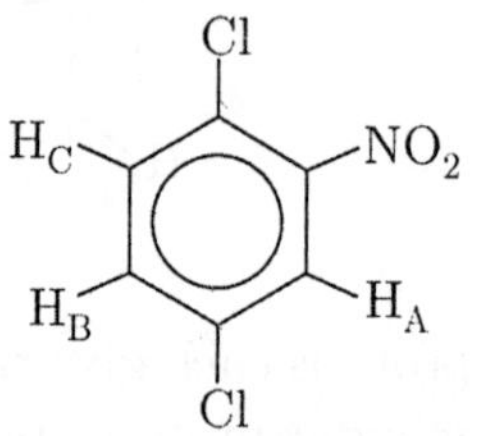

(IV)

The two protons are defined as being magnetically equivalent if each couples equally to a third neighbouring proton, otherwise they are magnetically non equivalent.

The labels A, B, C and so on are allocated to each separate group of chemically equivalent nuclei; if two protons H_A are magnetically non-equivalent, this is indicated by the use of primes (thus H_A and H_A'). Similarly protons H_B and H_B' must be chemically equivalent but magnetically non-equivalent. *Chemical equivalence simply means chemical shift equivalence and magnetic equivalance means coupling equivalence.* H_A and H_A' are chemically equivalent but magnetically non-equivalent and H_B and H_B' are also chemically equivalent but magnetically non-equivalent. Two protons that are *chemically non-equivalent must also be magnetically non-equivalent, but chemically equivalent protons can be magnetically non-equivalent.*

Deceptive simplicity : As a result of change, it occassionally arises that the chemical shifts of the two proton are equal or very nearly so, even though they do not have the same chemical environment. This is called ***Accidental Equivalence.***

Example : 2,5–Dichloronitrobenzene

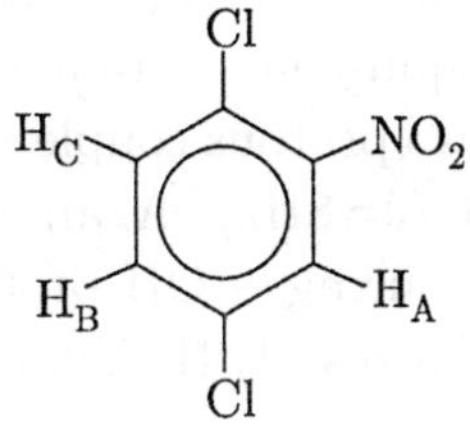

H_B and H_C have *near identical chemical shifts.* The ^1H—NMR spectrum of this molecule is superficially first order, with a doublet for H_B and H_C as they couple with H_A (δ 7.5) and a triplet for H_A (coupling with H_B and H_C) (δ 7.9), J_{AB} (meta)=2–3 Hz and J_{AC}(para)=0.

Proton exchange reactions : If the ^1H—NMR spectrum of ethanol is recorded on a slightly impure sample and then compared with the spectrum of a high purity sample., *two* different spectra are found. *The spectrum of commercial grade sample is easily explained by use of the multiplicity predictions of an A_2X_3 case as for ethyl bromide.* Clearly the OH proton is not involved in coupling with —CH_2— group. The spectrum for the pure sample does show this coupling and we can explain the multiplicity using the arguments developed for 1-nitropropane system.

Why is the OH coupling not observed in the spectrum recorded on the contaminated sample of ethanol?

Exchange of the OH protons among ethanol molecules is normally so rapid that one particular proton does not reside for a sufficiently long time on a particular oxygen atom for the nuclear coupling to be observed.

$$R—O—H + R'—O—H^* \rightleftharpoons R—O—H^* + R'—O—H$$

If there is a rapid proton exchange, the residence time will be short and the coupling will not be observed. The rate of exchange is related to the coupling constant (here it is 6Hz). If we are unable to resolve the coupling, the rate of exchange must be greater than $6\ s^{-1}$. The exchange is acid and base–catalysed and only in samples that are acid- or base free is the residence time sufficiently long for the coupling to be observed between OH and CH_2. Rapid proton exchange occurs in carboxylic acids, phenols, amines and thiols. In the case of alcohols, it is relatively easy to see the OH coupling if the sample is pure, or if the spectrum is recorded with a low temperature sample (when the exchange is retarded) or if the sample is dissolved in a highly polar solvent such as Me_2SO, when strong solvation presumably stabilises individual molecules and reduces the exchange.

^1H—NMR spectrum of ethanol (CH_3CH_2OH)

Case 1 : Pure ethanol : The ^1H—NMR picture of pure ethanol shows three signals at δ 1.2, δ 3.7 and δ 5.0 respectively. From the ratio of height of integration, the ratio of protons at these positions is 3:2:1. The signals corresponding to δ 5.0 and δ 1.2 are *two triplets.* The signal corresponding to δ 3.7 is a multiplet, (actually a double quartet). The proton of OH has δ at 5.0 and forms a triplet.

The proton of OH group undergoes spin-spin coupling with the —CH_2— group protons (J=6Hz) to form this triplet. The signal at δ1.2 is another triplet for —CH_3 protons which is formed by the spin-spin coupling at δ3.7 is the signal for the two protons of —CH_2— group. These two protons couple with the neighbouring three protons of —CH_3 group to give a quartet (J=8Hz). Again, these methylene protons undergo spin-spin coupling with the neighbouring —OH proton (J=6Hz) and each peak of this quartet divides into a doublet. As a result, the signal appears as a *multiplet.* (Double-Quartet).

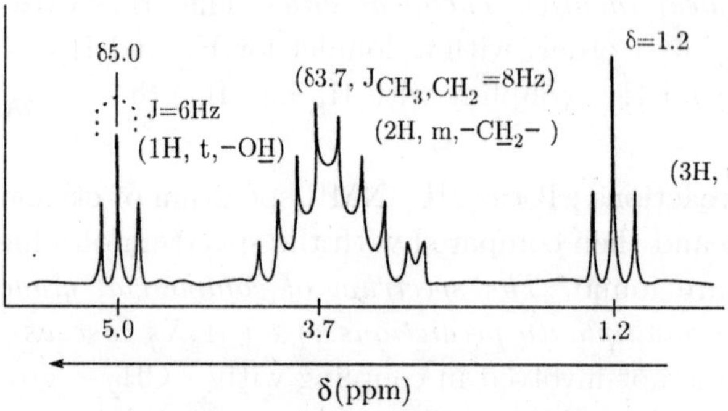

Fig. 1.28 : (^{1}H–NMR spectrum of pure ethanol)

Case 2 : ^{1}H—NMR spectrum of ethanol (Ordinary grade), CH_3CH_2OH : When ethyl alcohol contains acidic or basic impurities, a rapid exchange of proton occurs from one molecule to another. This reduces the time for the OH proton to get resolved by spin-spin coupling. So the OH proton can not couple either with the neighbouring —CH_2— protons nor the —CH_2— protons can couple with OH proton. As a result, the signal of OH proton in an impure sample of ethanol appears as a singlet. The methylene —(CH_2)— protons couple with the neighbouring —CH_3 protons and appear as a *quartet.* Again, the methyl protons (—CH_3) couple with —CH_2— protons to give rise to a triplet.

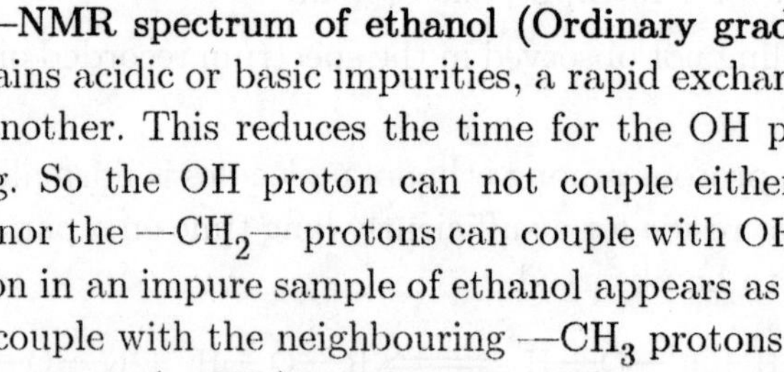

Fig. 1.29 : (^{1}H–NMR spectrum of ordinary grade ethanol)

In D_2O, the hydrogen atom of —OH (of alcohol) gets replaced by D as follows.

$$CH_3CH_2OH + D_2O \rightleftharpoons CH_3CH_2OD + HOD$$

As a result, **the signal for —OH proton at δ5.0 vanishes.** A quartet appears at δ 3.7 for —CH_2— protons and a triplet appears at δ 1.2 for —CH_3 protons in the integration ratio 2:3.

Deuterium Exchange : D_2O exchanges with labile protons such as OH, NH and SH. ROH becomes ROD; RCOOH becomes RCOOD; $RCONH_2$ becomes $RCOND_2$ etc.

$$R—O—H + D—O—D\ (D_2O) \rightleftharpoons R—O—D + H—O—D$$

Peaks previously observed for the labile protons disappear (or are diminished) and a peak corresponding to H—O—D appears around δ5.0.

The technique of deuteriation is widely used to detect the presence of OH groups etc. and is easily carried out. The NMR spectrum can be recorded conveniently in a solvent other than D_2O and then a few drops of D_2O are shaken with the sample and the spectrum is rerun. Peaks diminish or disappear for OH, NH etc. signals. The method can be extended to detect *reactive methylene* groups, such as those flanked by carbonyl. The spectrum is recorded normally and then a small amount of D_2O and NaOD is added to the sample tube; base catysed deuterium exchange occurs only on reactive sites. For example,

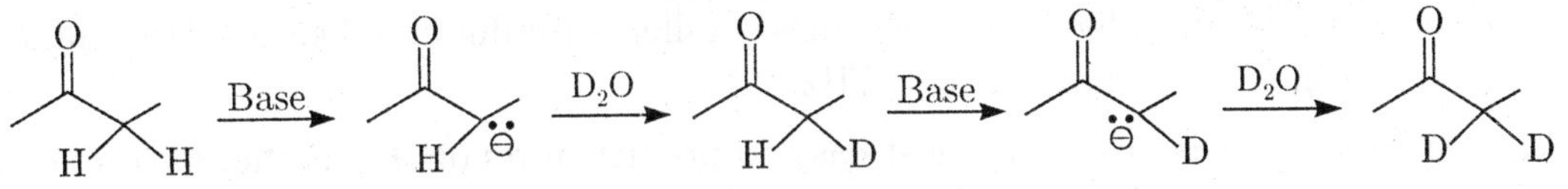

When the spectrum is rerun, signals from protons previously on these sites disappear.

Factors influencing the coupling constant, (J.) : (see also page 93)

1. *Geminal coupling* : Involving protons on $—CH_2—$ groups is strong, J being typically 10–18 Hz, but it will only be observed where the geminal protons have different chemical shift positions.

2. Vicinal coupling (three bonds separating the protons) varies from J=0 to J=12 Hz in rigid systems, but in freely rotating carbon chains (alkyl groups) it is usually around 8 Hz.

3. Long range coupling in alkane systems (extending over more than three bonds) is usually vanishingly small, but is observed within rigid systems where the *W-shaped* zigzag of bonds is nearly to being coplanar.

4. *Trans coupling* in alkene groups (J=11–19Hz) is stronger than *cis-coupling* (J=5–14Hz). Typical values, 16Hz and 8Hz respectively.

5. Aromatic coupling depends on whether the coupling protons are *ortho*, *meta* or *para* to each other and in simple cases, the coupling constant is definitive in deciding the orientation, J_{ortho}=7–10Hz; J_{meta}=2–3Hz; J_{para}=0–1Hz.

6. *Allylic coupling* : J is very small (0–2Hz) as it is a four bond coupling. The analogous coupling in aromatic systems (for example, between methyl protons and the ortho protons in the ring) is *not* normally large enough to be measured.

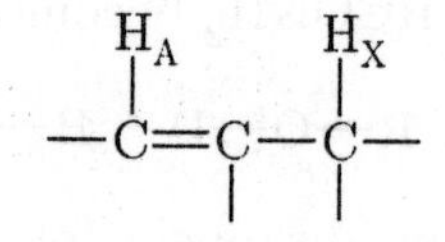

(J_{AX}, allylic coupling, 0–2 Hz)

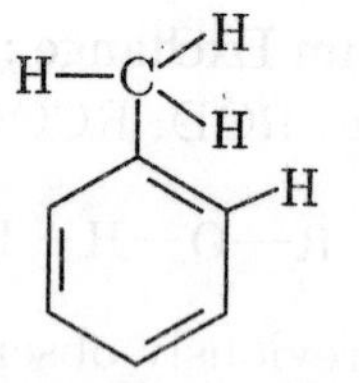

(No coupling between $-CH_3$ and ortho protons observable)

The electronegativity of an attached substituent alter the values of *gem*–coupling. In $—CH_2—X$, the *gem*–coupling will range from 12Hz to 9Hz as the electronegativity of X is increased. The magnitude of J_{gem} also varies with the C—C—C bond angle, being of greatest magnitude (10–14Hz) in the strain–free cyclohexanes and cyclopentanes. With increasing angular strain, the value of J_{gem} drops being 8–14Hz in cyclobutanes and 4–9Hz in cyclopropanes.

Factors influencing Vicinal coupling : The more electronegative is the attached substituent (s), the value of vicinal coupling gets altered. With increase in electronegativity of the substituent, the value of J_{vic} becomes smaller. In unhindered ethane, the value of J=8Hz but in halogenoethane, it is 6–7Hz.

The factor that is obviously most easy to predict in its on J_{vic} is the *dihedral angle* ϕ, between the two vicinal C—H bonds, the equation due to Karplus gives frequent agreement with the observed value.

Karplus Equation

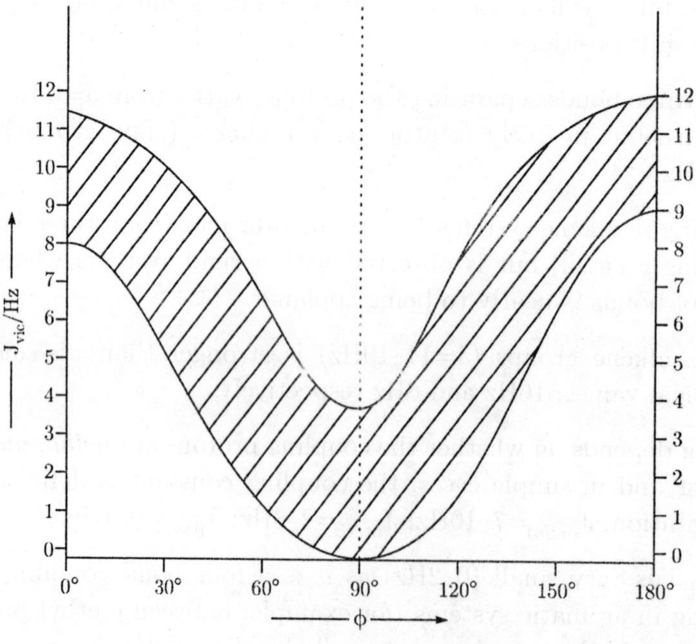

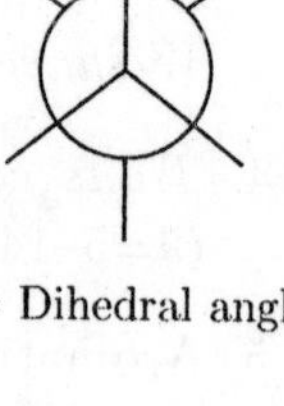

(ϕ= Dihedral angle)

Fig. 1.30 :

The largest vicinal coupling arises with protons in *trans coplanar positions* (ϕ=180°) and vicinal couplings for *cis-coplanar* protons (ϕ=0°). Very small couplings arise between protons at 90° to each other. These are all conclusions from Karplus equation.

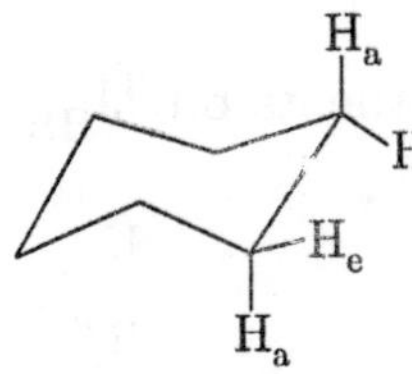

Diaxial protons have coupling constants J=10–13Hz and this correlates with their 180° orientation. Diequatorial protons or those with axial/equatorial relationship have coupling constants around 2–5Hz corresponding to about 60° orientations.

Coupling constant (J) depends upon three factors.

1. Through bond distance between the protons.
2. Angle between the two C—H bonds.
3. Electronegative substituents.

The coupling through three bonds (H—C—C—H) is designated as $^3J_{H\text{-}H}$. These coupling constants $^3J_{H\text{-}H}$ are usually about 7Hz in an open chain, freely rotating system; C—C bond might be in a single or double bond. Couplings $^3J_{H\text{-}H}$ across the double bonds are usually 11Hz. $^3J_{H\text{-}H}$ couplings are called vicinal couplings because the protons concerned are neighbouring atoms. In an open chain system, we have a time average of all rotational conformations. Across a double bond, there is no rotation and the angle between the two C—H bonds is fixed because they are in the same plane. In the plane of alkenes, the C—H bonds are either at 60° (*cis*) or at 180° (*trans*) to each other. Coupling constants in benzene rings are slightly less than those across *cis*–alkene because the bond is *longer* (bond order is 1.5 rather than 2).

$^3J_{H\text{-}H}$ Coupling constants (Vicinal coupling)

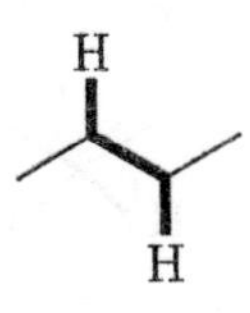

Free rotation (open chain single bond), J ≅ 7Hz

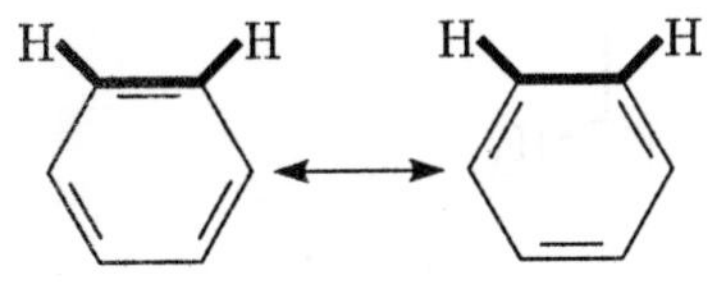

Benzene ring (longer bond, ≅ 0.5 π bond) 60° angle, J=8–10 Hz

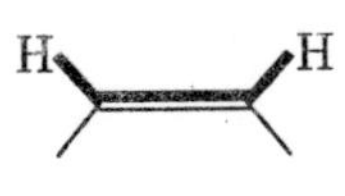

(*Cis-alkene*) (double bond) (60° angle, J=10-12 Hz)

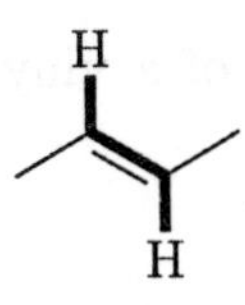

(*Trans-alkene*) (double bond) (180° bond angle J=14-18 Hz)

Regarding electronegativity, alkene enol ethers have smaller coupling constants than the alkenes containing only phenyl group. The more electronegative oxygen atom is withdrawing electrons from the C—H bond in the enol ethers and weakening communication through the bonds.

Effect of Electronegative substituents on $^3J_{HH}$

($^3J_{cis}$=11.5 Hz) ($^3J_{trans}$=16.0 Hz) ($^3J_{cis}$=6.0 Hz) ($^3J_{trans}$=12.0 Hz)

← Alkenes → ← Enol ethers →

$^4J_{HH}$ or W–coupling

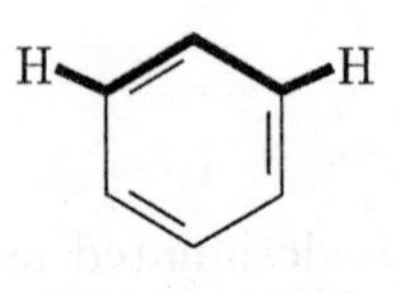

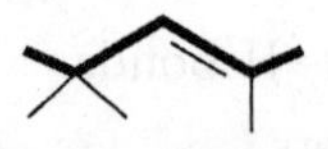

($0 < {}^4J_{HH} < 3$ Hz)

(*Meta* coupling) (Allylic coupling)

When the through bond distance gets longer, coupling is not usually seen. Four bond coupling $^4J_{HH}$ is usually zero. In some cases, like *meta* coupling in aromatic rings and allylic coupling in alkenes $^4J_{HH}$ becomes inportant. The four bonds arrange like a word 'W' and this sort of coupling is called *W–coupling.* The *magnitude* of *W–coupling* is small about 1–3Hz.

***Examples* :**

I.

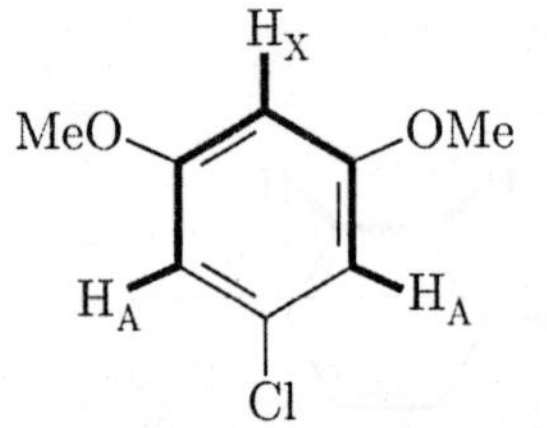

($^4J_{HH}$ coupling) J ≅ 2.5 Hz

H_X (1H, t), H_A (2H, d)

II.

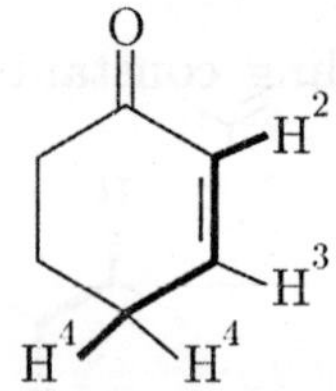

($^4J_{HH}$ coupling) J ≅ 2 Hz

H^2=double triplet

Coupling constants of a vinyl group :

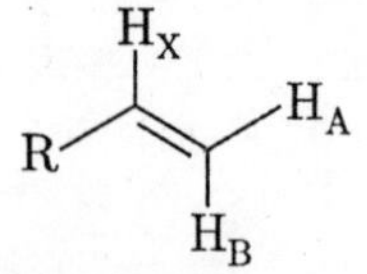

J_{AB} very small (0-2 Hz), J_{AX} (*cis*) large (10-13 Hz) J_{BX} (*trans*) very large (14-18 Hz).

Typical coupling constants :

1. **Geminal $^2J_{HH}$ (Intervened by two bonds)**

a. Saturated 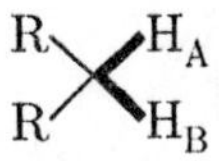 (10-16 Hz)

b. Unsaturated 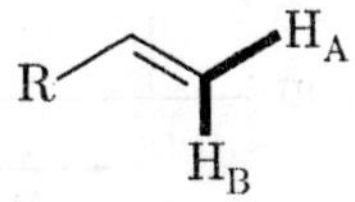 (0-3 Hz)

2. **Vicinal $^3J_{HH}$ (Intervened by three bonds)**

a. Saturated 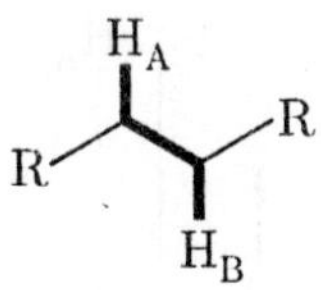 (6-8 Hz)

b. Unsaturated *trans* 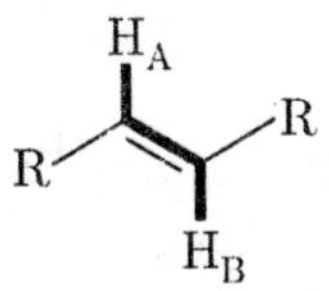 (14-16 Hz)

c. Unsaturated *cis* 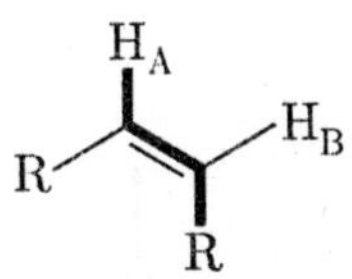 (8-11 Hz)

d. Unsaturated aromatic 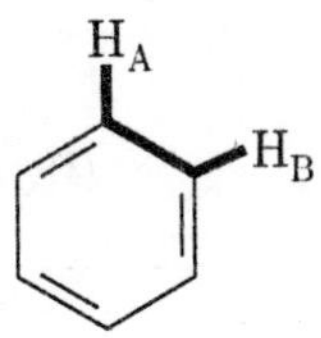 (6-9 Hz)

3. **Long range $^4J_{HH}$ (Intervened by four bonds)**

a. *Meta* 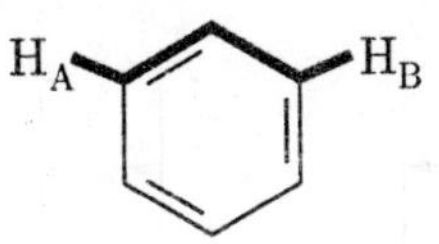 (1-3 Hz)

b. Allylic 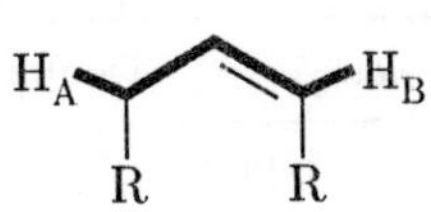 (1-2 Hz)

Summary :

AX Spectrum

Resultant Spectrum

Spectrum with no interaction

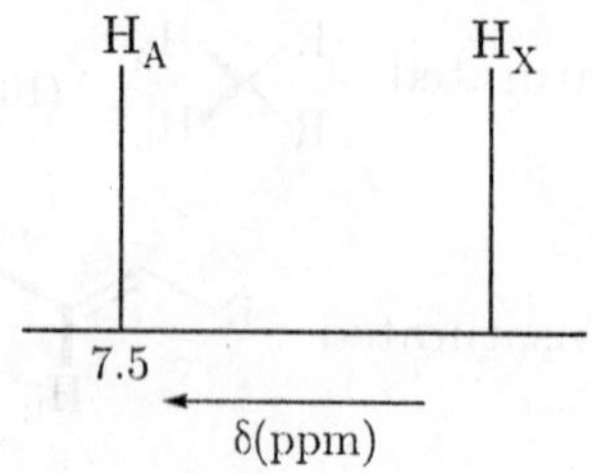

Effect of H_X and applied field acting together on H_A.

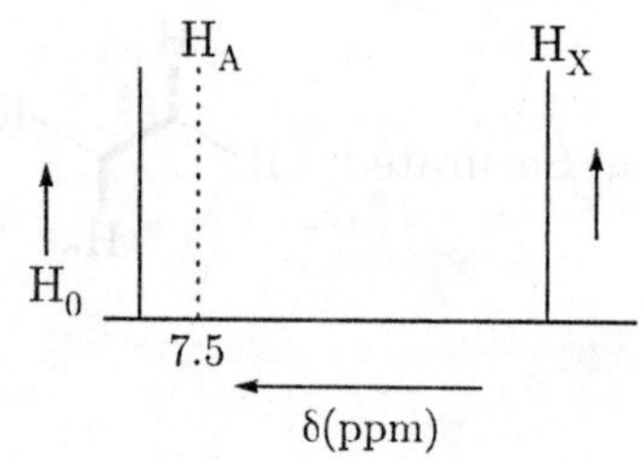

(H_X aligned with the applied field)

Effect of H_X and applied field acting in opposition on H_A.

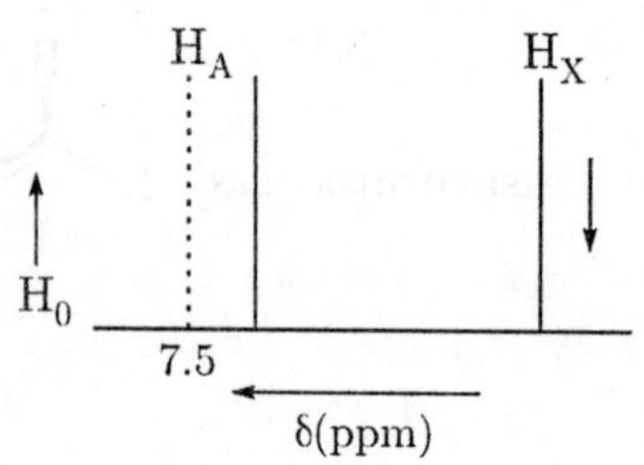

(H_X applied opposed to the applied field)

Effect of H_X on H_A and H_A on H_X

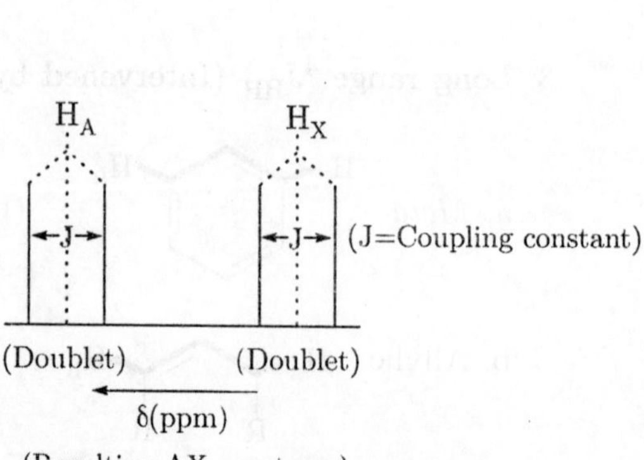

(Resulting AX spectrum)

AX_2 Spectrum

Resultant Spectrum

Spectrum with no interaction

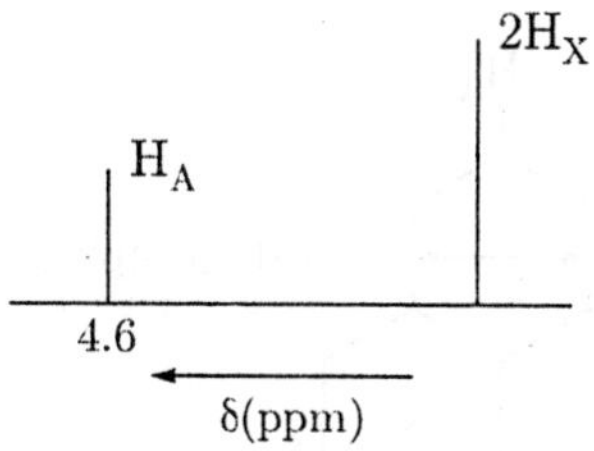

Effect of H_X and applied field acting together on H_A

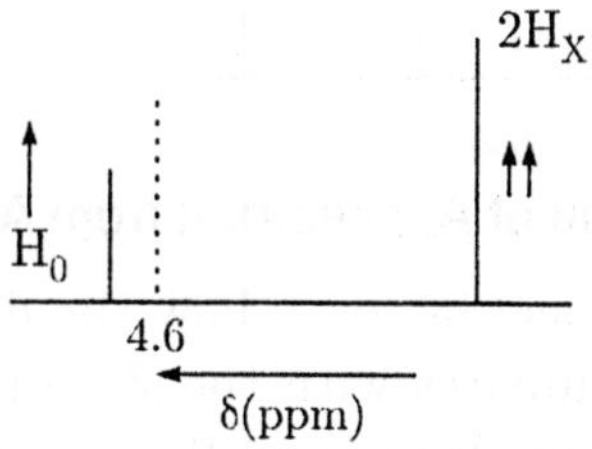

(Both H_X aligned with the applied field)

Two H_X cancel out double intensity signal at true position

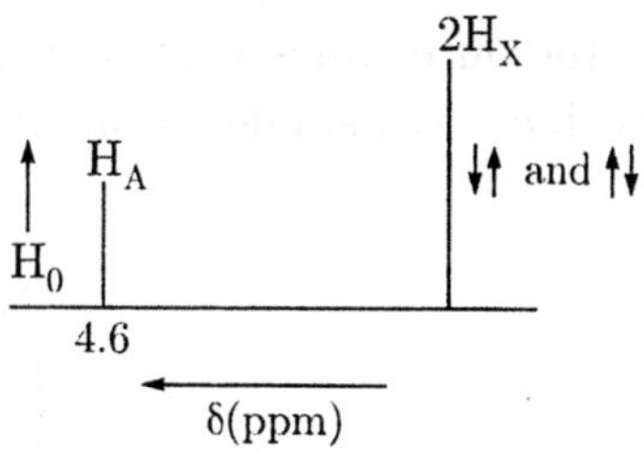

[One H_X aligned with applied field and one H_X against (two ways)]

Effect of H_X and applied field acting in opposition on H_A.

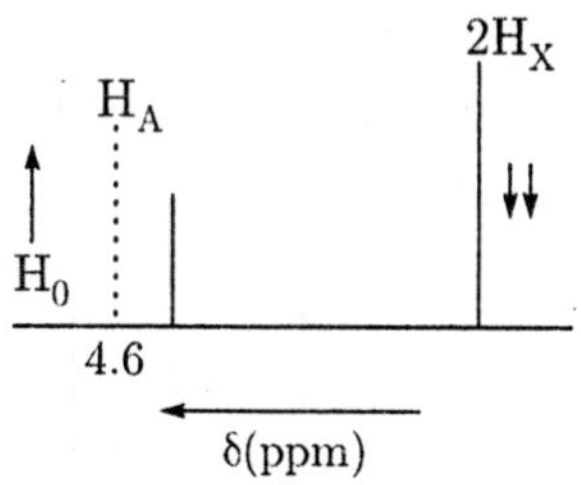

(Both H_X'S aligned against the applied field)

Effect of H_X on H_A and of H_A on H_X.

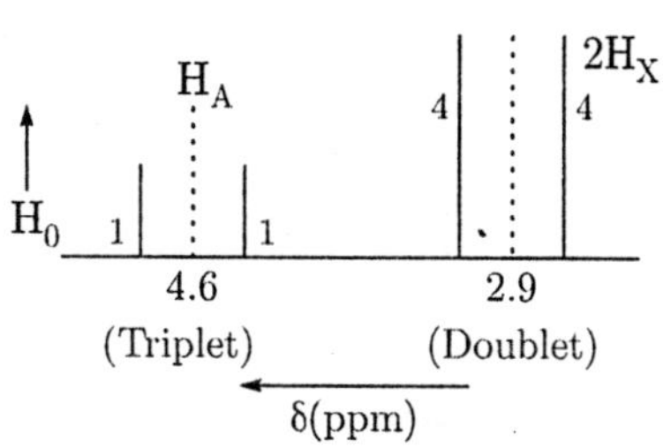

(Resulting AX_2 spectrum)

Coupling in an AX_2 system

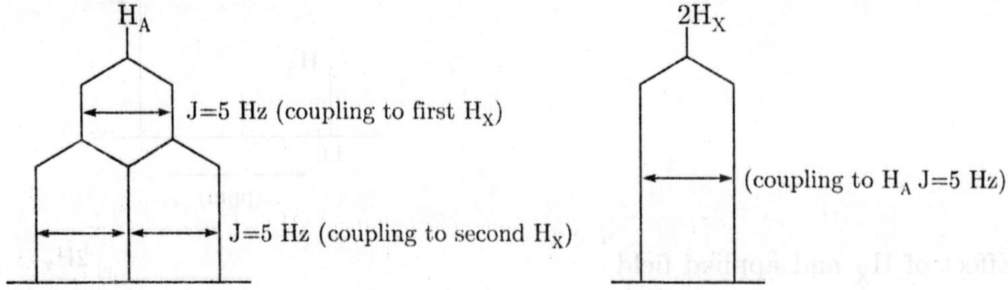

Evolution of A_2 spectrum from AX spectrum

The critical factor is how the difference between the chemical shifts of the two protons ($\Delta\delta$) compares with the size of the coupling constant (J). If $\Delta\delta$ is much larger than J, there is no distortion. If $\Delta\delta$ is 4 ppm and the normal coupling constant is 7Hz (normal value), we will have an AX spectrum of two 1:1 doublets. As $\Delta\delta$ approaches J in size, the inner lines of the two doublets increase and the outer lines decrease until when $\Delta\delta$ is zero, the outer lines vanish away altogether and we are left with the two superimposed inner lines — a singlet or an A_2 spectrum.

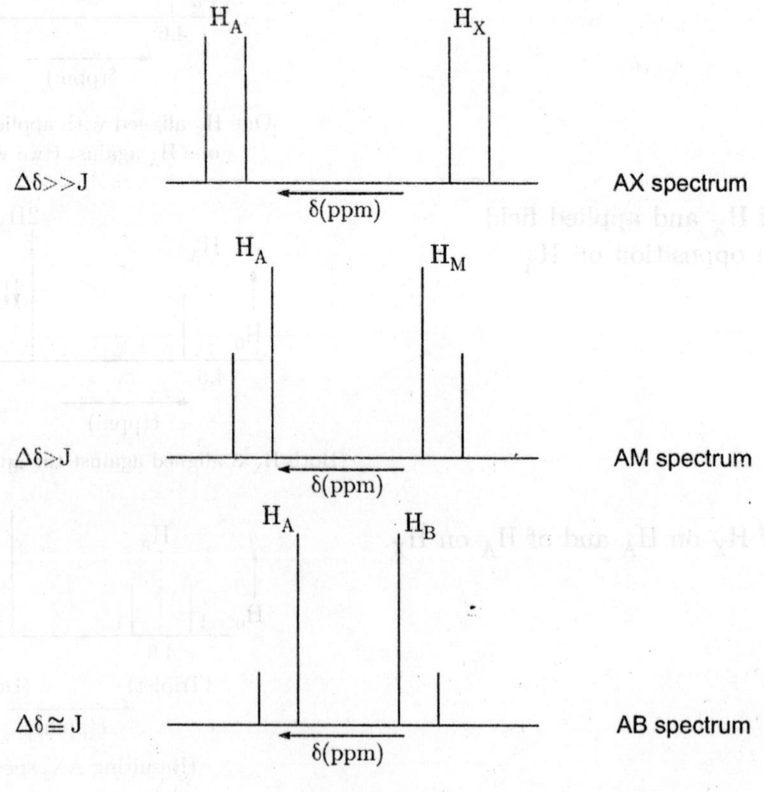

$\Delta\delta < J$

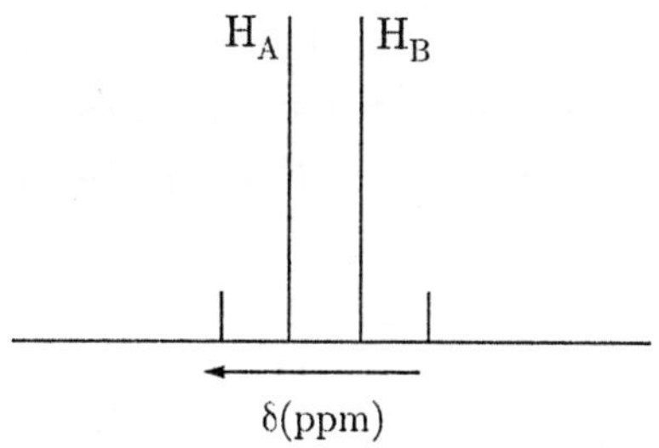

AB spectrum

$\Delta\delta = O$

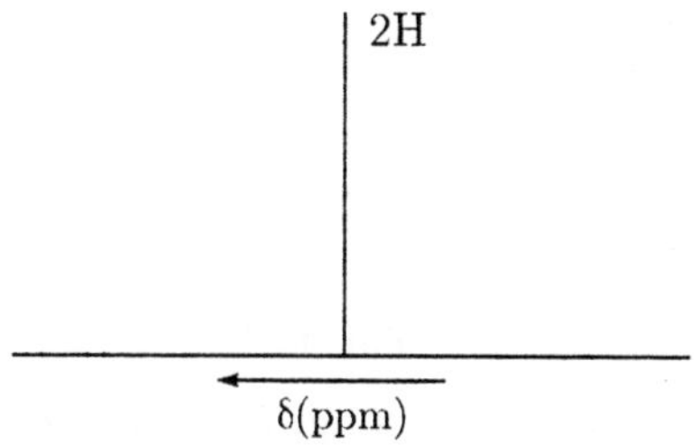

A_2 spectrum

Non-First order spectra

In general, first order spectra will only arise if the separation between multiplets (the chemical shift difference between the signals) is much larger than the coupling constant, J, if $\Delta\delta \geq 6J$, then fairly unperturbed spectra will arise.

If the signals from coupling protons are closer together on the spectrum, and the chemical shift difference is small, distortion of the signals arises. For example, in the AX case, (*e.g.*, cinnamic acid) the signals move together, and the inner peaks become larger at the expense of outer peaks and the chemical shift positions lie approximately at the "*centre of gravity*" of the doublets instead of at the mid point of the doublets. Such spectra are usually called *AB spectra* indicating that the chemical shift values are closer than in AX cases. In the ultimate case, $\Delta\delta=0$ (*e.g.* geminal protons of many —CH_2— groups), the spin interaction is not observable in the NMR spectrum and a *singlet peak* is produced.

In the AX_2 case of 1,1,2–trichloroethane, only five lines appear as predicted by (n+1) first order rules. If the chemical shift values of A and X are closer together, the spectrum becomes *non-first order*, actually an AB_2 case. Altogether nine lines may appear and δ value is determined from the centre of gravity of the spectrum.

For three coupling environments, the first order appearence is *AMX.* If two of the original chemical shift positions are closer than in a true AMX case, then ABX system results which in many cases like AMX exhibits *twelve lines.* If all the coupling environments are close together in chemical shift terms, ABC systems arise, in which upto fifteen lines can be observed. Chemical shift in this case is evaluated on an approximate basis only.

Aromatic Coupling

The majority of aromatic coupling systems are *non–first order spectra* and belong to *long range coupling.*

Case 1 : Unsplit signals are produced by several monosubstituted benzenoid derivatives, provided that the substituent has no strong shielding or deshielding effect. This is an example of "*Accidental Equivalence*". *Toluene* is a classical example in this respect.

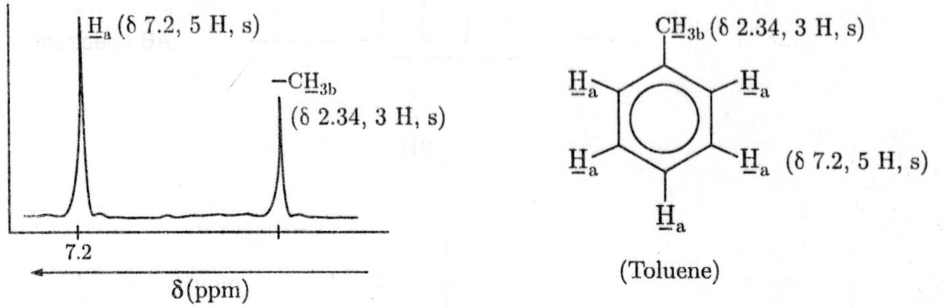

Fig. 1.31 :

Such an absorption is found, i,e, a **singlet** for benzenoid hydrogens with **ethyl benzyl ether**.

Case 2 : ^{1}H—NMR spectra of nitrobenzene or halobenzene (X=Br, Cl)

Nitro, chloro or bromo group has strong (–I) and (–R) effects, so the protons ortho to these groups show *downfield δ values* (δ=8.2 for the two hydrogens *ortho* to —NO_2 group). These two *ortho* hydrogens couple with *meta* and *para* protons to give a complicated spectrum. Nevertheless, the protons at *meta* and *para* to —NO_2 group absorb at a comparative upfield compared to the two protons at the *ortho* positions.

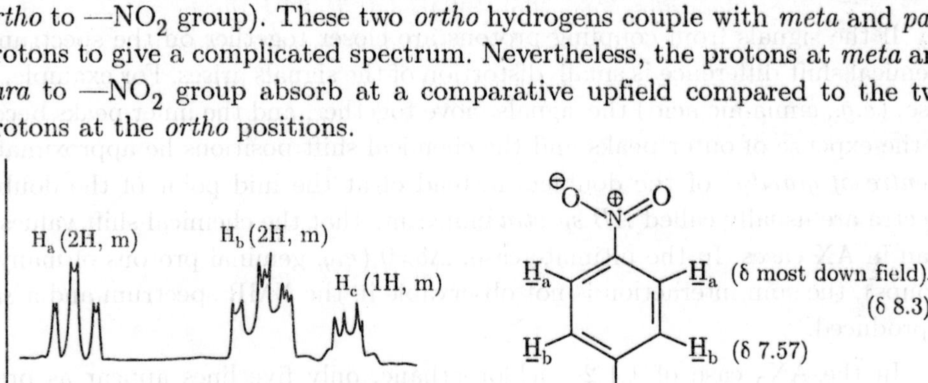

Fig. 1.32 :

Two H_a protons *ortho couple* (J=9.0Hz) with two H_b protons and *meta couple* with H_c (J=3.0Hz) and produce a multiplet. Two H_b protons *ortho* couple with two H_a protons and also with H_c proton (J=9.0Hz) to produce a multiplet. H_c proton *ortho couples* with two H_b (J=9.0Hz) protons and *meta couples* with two H_a (J=3.0Hz) to produce a *multiplet.* Bromobenzene shows analogous spectrum.

Case 3 : *ortho*-dichloro- or *ortho*-dinitrobenzene (AA′BB′ system)

- Considerable symmetry is introduced in the benzene ring by the presence of identical groups *ortho* to each other and the spectrum of such compounds shows complex splitting patterns. Thus there are twenty four lines in the spectrum of o-dinitro- or o-dichlorobenzene. However, though complex, the multiplet is symmetrical about the mid point. The aromatic protons may be chemically equivalent but they are magnetically non equivalent.

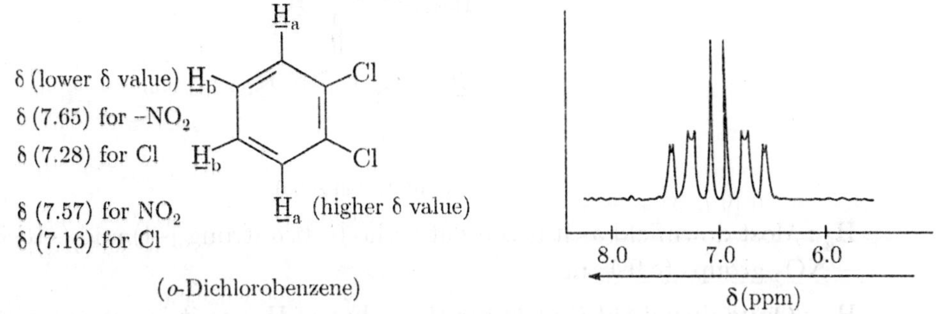

Fig. 1.33 :

H_a protons come at downfield δ values as they reside *ortho* to the electronegative group Cl (or $—NO_2$). H_b protons, as they do not reside *ortho* to Cl atoms (or $—NO_2$ groups) come at lesser downfield region (lower δ values). The mid point of the NMR spectrum shows a double doublet due to strong *ortho* coupling between H_a and H_b and between two H_b protons. The spectrum is symmetric about the mid point. *o*-dinitrobenzene shows similar pattern in its ^1H—NMR spectrum. The only difference is that, $—NO_2$ group being more (–R) and (–I) in nature shows more downfield δ value for the *ortho* protons.

Case 4 : ^1H—NMR spectrum of o-nitrochlorobenzene

The symmetry present in the benzene ring when it is substituted by identical substituents (*e.g.*, o-dichlorobenzene) is not same as when the benzene ring is substituted by non identical *ortho* substituents.

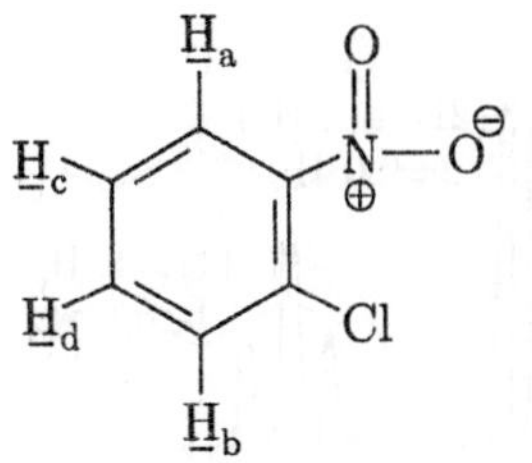

(o-Nitrochlorobenzene)

H_a : Higher δ value compared to H_b as H_a is present ortho to more electronegative (also–R) substituent $—NO_2$ group.(δ 8.2)

H_b : Lower δ value compared to H_b as H_b is present *ortho* to less electronegative substituent that is Cl atom.(δ 7.44)

H_c and H_d : Lower δ values compared to H_a and H_b as they are not present at the *ortho* positions— neither to NO_2 group, nor to Cl atom.(δ H_c.7.56; δ H_d.7.63)

The spectrum is otherwise quite complex.

Case 5 : *m*-dichloro – or *m*-dinitrobenzene

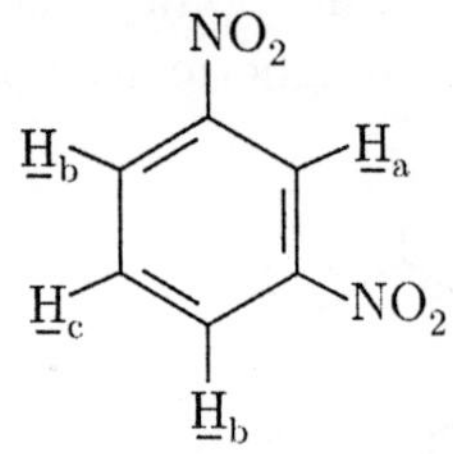

(*m*-dinitrobenzene)

H_a : Most downfield as it is present ortho to *two* strong (–I) and (–R) containing —NO_2 groups.(δ 9.1, m)

H_b : Quite downfield (but lesser than that of H_a) as it is present ortho to only one —NO_2 group.(δ 8.6, dd)

H_c : Comparatively upfield as it is not present-*ortho* to any —NO_2 group.(δ 7.87, m).

The spectrum otherwise shows a complex pattern which is as follows.

H_a : *Triplet* due to *meta coupling* with two H_b protons and extent of *para* coupling is too small (only broadening of triplet).

H_b : *Double doublet* due to *o*-coupling (J=9.0Hz) with H_c proton followed by *meta* coupling (weak) with H_a proton.

H_c : *Triplet* due to *o*-coupling (J=9.0Hz) with two H_b protons which is broadened by weak *p*-coupling with H_a proton.

The ^1H—NMR spectrum of *m*-dichlorobenzene shows a similar pattern.

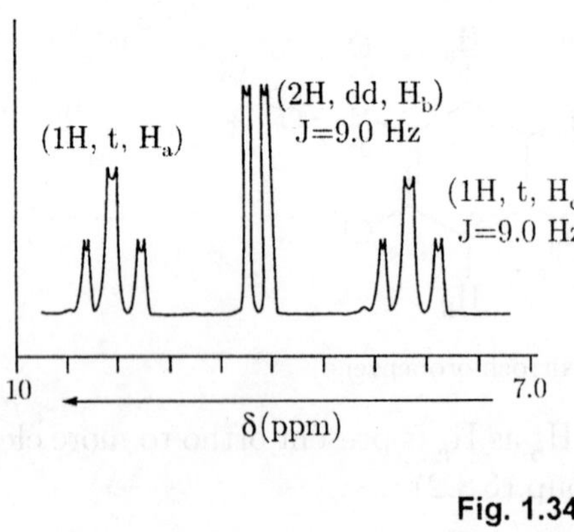

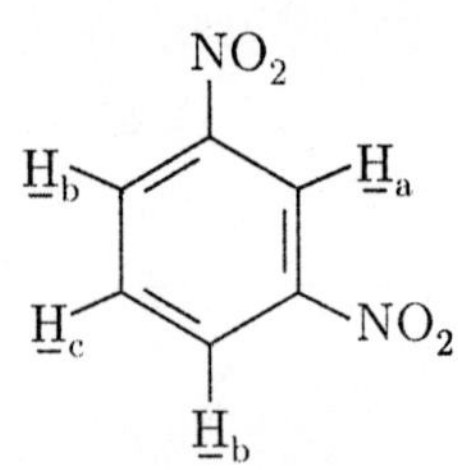

(*m*-dinitrobenzene)

Fig. 1.34 :

Case 6 : *m*-nitrochlorobenzene 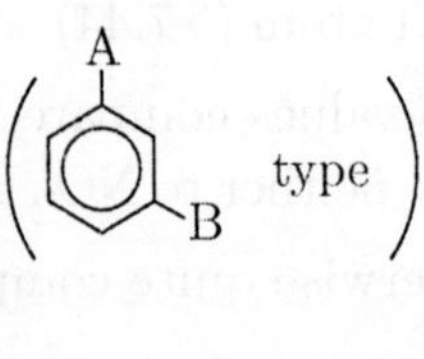

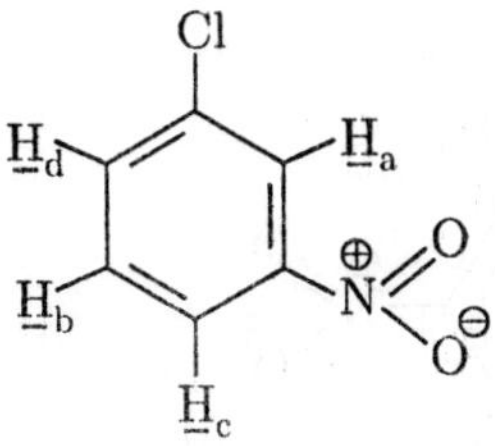

(*Meta* nitrochlorobenzene)

H_a : Most downfield (highest δ) as H_a is flanked by two electron withdrawing groups —NO_2 and Cl.(δ 8.25, dd)

H_c : Quite downfield as it is present *ortho* to —NO_2 group but the value of δ is less than that of H_a.(δ 8.15, m).

H_d : δ value comparatively upfield as H_d is present *ortho* to Cl (Cl has less (–R) effect compared to —NO_2.(δ 7.68, m).

H_b : Most upfield (lowest δ value)(δ 7.5, m).

The splitting pattern is complex which is as follows.

H_a : Froms *double doublet* coupling with two *meta* protons H_d and H_c followed by peak broadening with H_b proton by weak *p*–coupling.

H_c : *Multiplet, ortho* coupling with H_b (J=9Hz) followed by *meta* coupling with H_d and H_a.

H_d : *Multiplet, ortho* coupling with H_b (J=9Hz) followed by *meta* coupling with H_c and H_a.

H_b : Strong *double doublet,* due to *ortho* coupling with H_d and H_c, followed by peak broadening with *para* H_a proton.

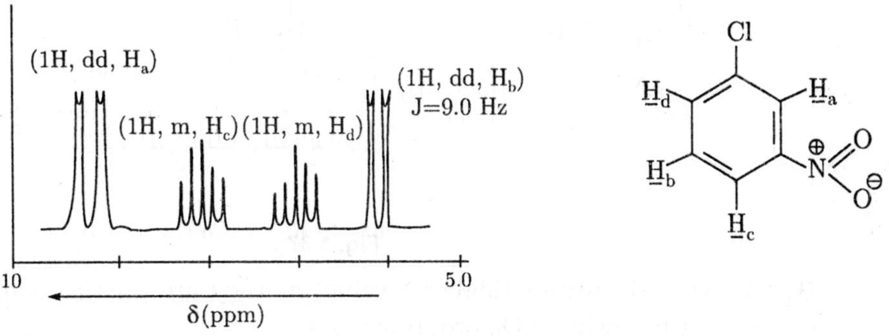

Fig. 1.35 :

Case 7 : *p*-dinitro– or *p*-dichlorobenzene (A–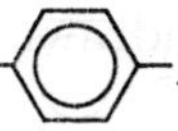–A type)

Compounds with identical *para* substituents, whatever their electronegativities, give single line spectra because of the molecular symmetry. All the four protons in the ring are magnetically equivalent.

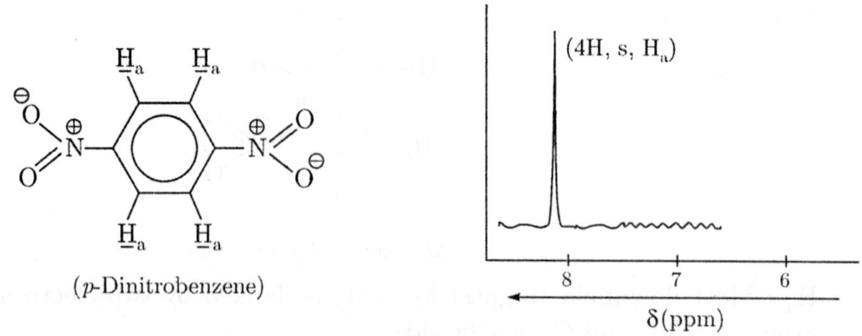

Fig. 1.36 :

Four H_a protons show downfield δ value (~8.0) as they are present *ortho* to NO_2 group which contains both (–I) and (–R) effects.

All the *identically para disubstituted* benzenes show a single line in ^1H—NMR spectra, irrespective of the electronic nature of the substituent, *i.e.*, for both electron donating (—OCH_3) or electron withdrawing substituents. *p*-xylene (CH_3–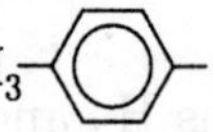–CH_3) shows a similar pattern in its ^1H—NMR spectrum.

Case 8 : *p*-Nitrochlorobenzene (A–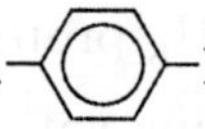–B type) (Approximation has been done; $H_a \cong H_a'$ and $H_b \cong H_b'$)

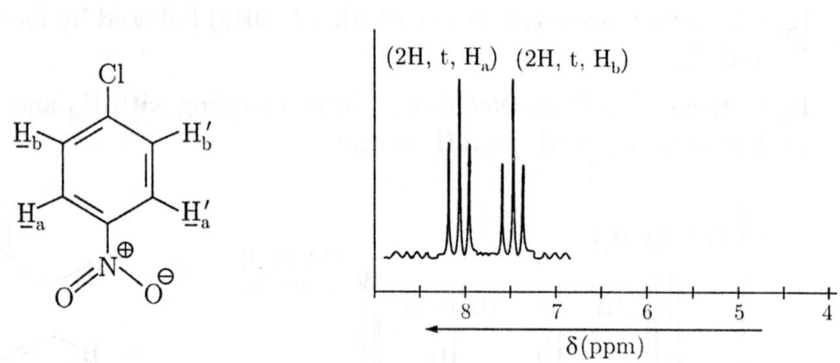

Fig. 1.37 :

H_a : Downfield protons (higher δ value) as they are present *ortho* to strongly electron withdrawing NO_2 group.(δ 8.2, t).

H_b : Comparatively upfield protons (lower δ value) as they are present *ortho* to less electron withdrawing Cl atom.(δ 7.56, t).

Approximate splitting pattern :

H_a : 2H, t, due to strong *o*-coupling with two H_b protons (J=9Hz).

H_b : 2H, t, due to strong *o*-coupling with two H_a protons (J=9Hz).

Case 9 : *o*-Xylene

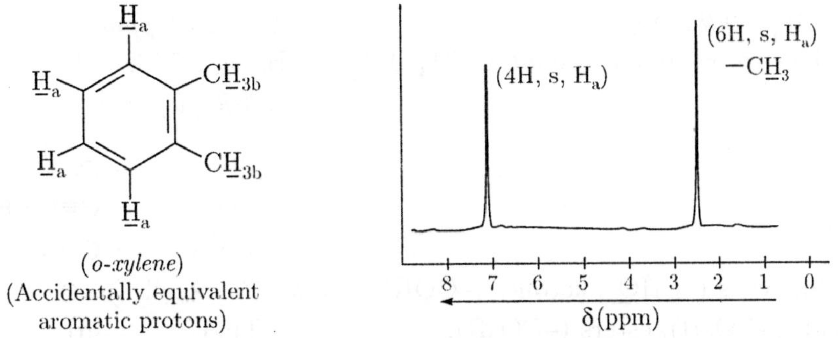

Fig. 1.38 :

—CH_3 is an alkyl substituent which has neither strong deshielding nor strong shielding effect. So the aromatic protons show *accidental equivalence (all four H_a protons).* So only a *singlet* appears for four benzenoid protons at δ 7.2. Six equivalent methyl (—CH_3) protons show a singlet at around δ 2.5.

Case 10 : *p*-Nitroanisole (Approximation has been done; $H_a \cong H_a'$ and $H_b \cong H_b'$)

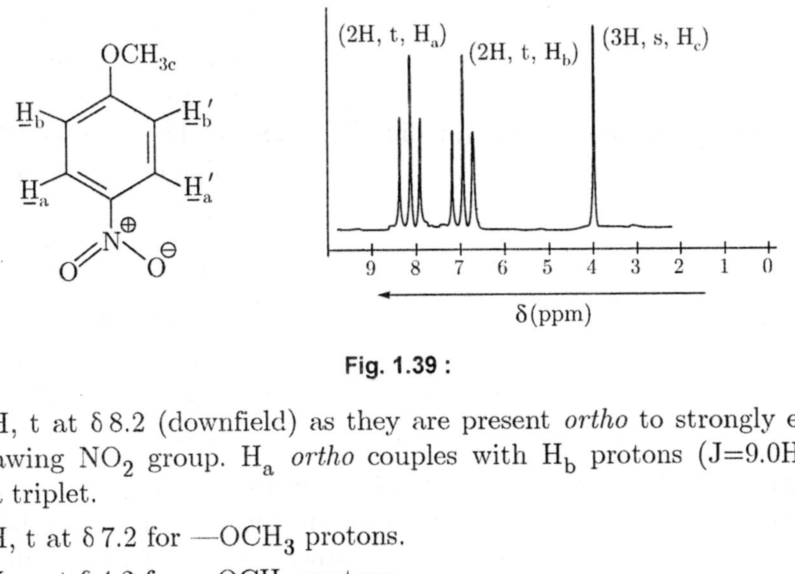

Fig. 1.39 :

$\mathbf{H_a}$: 2H, t at δ 8.2 (downfield) as they are present *ortho* to strongly electron withdrawing NO_2 group. H_a *ortho* couples with H_b protons (J=9.0Hz) and forms a triplet.

$\mathbf{H_b}$: 2H, t at δ 7.2 for —OCH_3 protons.

$\mathbf{H_c}$: 3H, s at δ 4.2 for —OCH_3 protons.

Summary Chart of Proton NMR Shifts :

Standard values :

—CH_3 : *0.9 δ ppm*, —CH_2 : *1.3 δ ppm*, –CH : *1.7 δ ppm*

Values to be added to 0.9 for CH_3, 1.3 for CH_2 or 1.7 for CH.

← ***Shift (1 ppm)***

alkene –C=C–

alkyne –C≡C–R

nitrile –C≡N

[Aldehydes (–CHO), ketones (–COR), acids (–CO_2H), esters (–CO_2R), amides (–$CONH_2$)] ⟹ Carbonyl >C=O

Thiol –SH

sulphide –SR

← ***Shift (1.5 ppm)***

[*Benzene –Ar, heterocycles e.g.*, pyridine] ⟹ Aryl ring –Ar

Amine –NH_2

sulphoxide –S(=O)–R

← ***Shift (2.0 ppm)***

Alcohol –OH

ether –OR

amide –NHCOR

[Chloride (Cl), bromide (Br), iodide (I)] ⟹ halide –Hal (X)

sulphone –SO_2R

← ***Shift (2.5 ppm)***

Aryl ether –OAr

← ***Shift (3.0 ppm)***

Nitro –NO_2

ester –OCOR

fluoro –F

Example : There are just three signals and the integration alone distinguishes the two methyl groups from the –CH_2– group. One methyl group has been shifted from 0.9 ppm by about 1 ppm (0.9+1.0≅2.0 ppm) and the other by more than 3 ppm (0.9+3.0≅3.9 ppm).

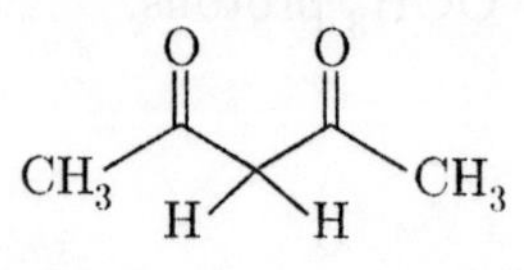

(Ethyl acetoacetate, a ketoester)

The first must be next to C=O and the second next to oxygen. The –CH_2– group is just next to an ester and a ketone carbonyl group, and so we expect it at (1.3+1.0+1.0=3.3 ppm). The molecule actually shows δ values for different protons at these chemical shift values.

2 Chemistry of Carbonyl Compounds

Synthesis of Aldehydes and Ketones

Reactants	Reagents and Reaction	Products
1. a. RCH_2OH (primary alcohol)	$K_2Cr_2O_7/\overset{\oplus}{H}$; $KMnO_4/\overset{\ominus}{O}H$; dil HNO_3 (OXIDATION)	RCHO (Aldehyde)
b. $R^1R^2>CHOH$ (Secondary alcohol)	Conc.HNO_3/Δ; $K_2Cr_2O_7$/conc.H_2SO_4/Δ (OXIDATION)	$R^1R^2>C{=}O$ (Ketone)
2. $R^1R^2>CH(OH)$ (Secondary alcohol)	$Me_3C–O–Al/_3$ (aluminium tertiarybutoxide/reflux), CH_3COCH_3 (OPPENAUR OXIDATION)	$R^1R^2>C{=}O + Me_2CH—O—Al/_3 + Me_2COH$ (Ketone)
3.a. $R^1(H)C{=}C(R^2)H$ (Alkene)	O_3, ozone $(\bar{O}–O–\overset{+}{O})$; 1,3-dipolar cycloaddition reaction (OZONOLYSIS)	$R^1(H)C{=}O$ + $R^2(H)C{=}O + H_2O_2$ (Aldehydes)
b. $R^1R^2C{=}CR^3R^4$ (Alkene)	O_3, ozone $(\bar{O}–O–\overset{+}{O})$; 1,3-dipolar cycloaddition reaction (OZONOLYSIS)	$R^1R^2>C{=}O$ + $R^3R^4>C{=}O + H_2O_2$ (Ketones)

Contd....

Reactants	Reagents and Reaction	Products
4.a. 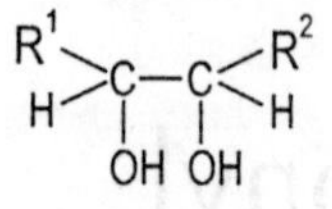 (1,2-Glycol)	$Pb(OAc)_4$ or HIO_4 (OXIDATION)	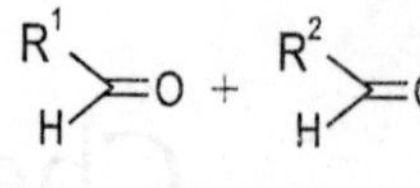 (Aldehydes) + $[Pb(OAc)_2 + 2AcOH]$ or $[HIO_3 + H_2O]$
4.b. 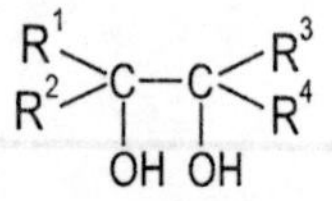 (1,2-Glycol)	$Pb(OAc)_4$ or HIO_4 (OXIDATION)	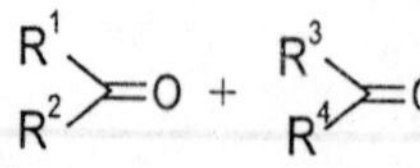 + $[Pb(OAc)_2 + 2AcOH]$ or $[HIO_3 + H_2O]$
5.a. $H-C\equiv C-H$ (Acetylene)	Hot dilute H_2SO_4, $\overset{II}{Hg}SO_4$ (catalyst) (HYDRATION REACTION)	CH_3CHO (Acetaldehyde) + Hg^{2+}
b. $R^1-C\equiv C-H$ (Homologue of acetylene)	Hot dilute H_2SO_4, $\overset{II}{Hg}SO_4$ (catalyst) (HYDRATION REACTION)	$R^1-CH_2-\underset{\underset{O}{\Vert}}{C}-CH_3 + Hg^{2+}$ (Ketone)
6. 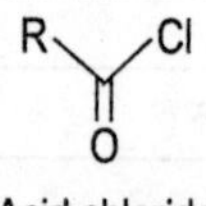 (Acid chloride)	H_2/Pd (poisoned by $BaSO_4$ or quinoline/s) (ROSENMUND REDUCTION)	R–CHO (ALDEHYDE) NO KETONE can be synthesised
7. $R-C\equiv N$ (Alkyl cyanide)	$SnCl_2/HCl$; refluxed in Et_2O or EtOAc or HCO_2Et (STEPHEN'S REDUCTION)	R–CHO (ALDEHYDE) NO KETONE can be synthesised
8.a. HCO_2R (Ethyl formate) + RMgX (G.R.)	GRIGNARD REACTION followed by dilute acid	RCHO (aldehyde) + EtOH
b. $R^1-C\equiv N$ (Alkyl cyanide) + R^2MgX (G.R.)	GRIGNARD REACTION followed by dilute acid	$R^1-\underset{\underset{O}{\Vert}}{C}-R^2 + NH_3$ (Ketone)
9. $CH_3-\overset{\overset{O}{\Vert}}{C}-\underset{\underset{R}{\vert}}{CH}-\overset{\overset{O}{\Vert}}{C}-OEt$ (Substituted E.A.A.)	KETONIC HYDROLYSIS followed by acid	$CH_3-\overset{\overset{O}{\Vert}}{C}-CH_2R$ (KETONE), NO ALDEHYDE is produced
10.a. 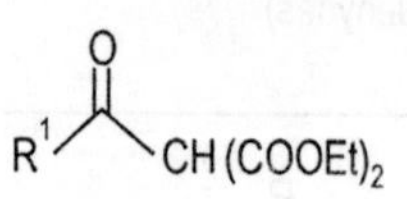 (Substituted DEM)	ALKALINE HYDROLYSIS followed by dilute acid	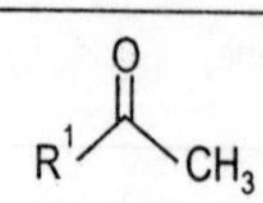 (Methyl ketone)
b. 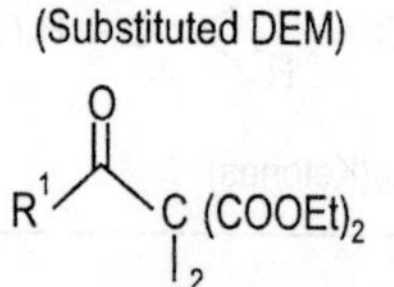	ALKALINE HYDROLYSIS followed by dilute acid	$R^1-\overset{\overset{O}{\Vert}}{C}-CH_2R^2$ (Ketone) (NO ALDEHYDE can be produced)

Contd....

Reactants	Reagents and Reaction	Products
11. $CH_3(CH_2)_5NH_2.HCl$ *n*-Hexylaminohydrochloride + $(CH_2)_6N_4$ Hexamethylenetetramine	SOMMELET'S REACTION	$CH_3(CH_2)_4CHO$ (aldehyde) NO KETONE can be produced
12.a. $ClCH_2COOEt$ (Ethyl chloroacetate) (α-haloester) + aldehyde (R^1CHO)	$NaNH_2$ or NaOEt/EtOH DARZEN'S GLYCIDIC ESTER or 1,2-epoxyester reaction	$R^1CH_2CHO + CO_2\uparrow$ (Aldehyde)
b. $Cl-CH(R^1)CO_2Et$ + 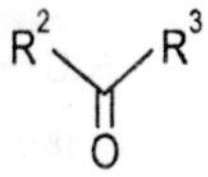 (α-Haloester) (Ketone)	$NaNH_2$ or NaOEt/EtOH DARZEN'S GLYCIDIC ESTER or 1,2-epoxyester reaction	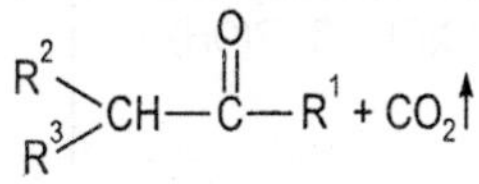 (Ketone)
13. 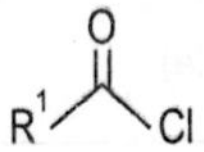 (Acid chloride)	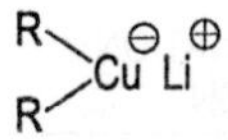 (Lithium dialkyl cuprate)	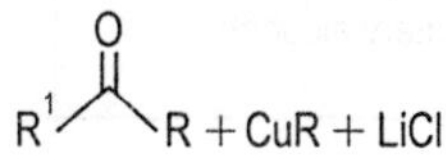
14.a. $(R\overset{\alpha}{C}H_2COO)_2Ca$ (Ca-salt of carboxylic acid) + $(HCOO)_2Ca$ (Calcium formate)	Strong heat passes via ALDOL TYPE CONDENSATION reaction	$2RCH_2CHO + CaCO_3$ (Aldehyde)
b. $(RCH_2COO)_2Ca$ Ca-salt of carboxylic acid	Strong heat passes via ALDOL TYPE CONDENSATION reaction	$RCH_2-\overset{O}{\overset{\|\|}{C}}-CH_2R + CaCO_3$ (Ketone)
15. 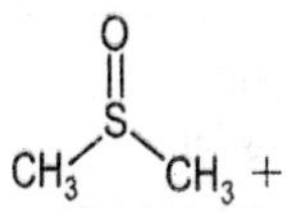 + 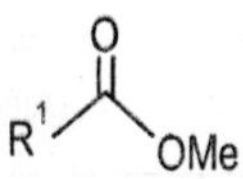 (Dimethyl sulphoxide) (Methyl ester)	NaH,/followed by Al/Hg in THF/H_2O (by COREY *et al*)	$CH_3-\overset{O}{\overset{\|\|}{C}}-R^1$ (Methyl ketone)
16.a. $R^1-C\equiv C-H$ (1-Alkyne)	Controlled addition of disimylborane ($Si\alpha_2BH$) in THF followed by $H_2O_2/\overset{\ominus}{O}H$(HYDROBORATION/ OXIDATION of alkynes)	$R^1CH_2-\overset{O}{\overset{\|\|}{C}}-H$ (Aldehyde)
b. $R^1-C\equiv C-R^2$ (Alkyne)	Controlled addition of disimylborane ($Si\alpha_2BH$) in THF followed by $H_2O_2/\overset{\ominus}{O}H$	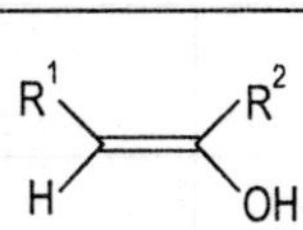 $\rightleftharpoons$ $RCH_2-\overset{O}{\overset{\|\|}{C}}-R^2$ (Ketone)
17. 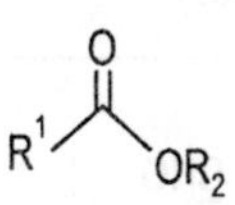 (Ester)	DIBAL-H (diisobutyl aluminium hydride), –78°C followed by water	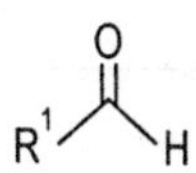 (Aldehyde)

Contd....

Reactants	Reagents and Reaction	Products
18. $R^1-C\equiv N$ (Alkyl cyanide)	DIBAL-H, hexane; followed by water	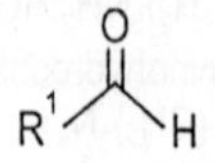 (Aldehyde)
19. $RCHX_2$ (Dihaloalkane)	ALKALINE HYDROLYSIS followed by heat	RCHO (Aldehyde)
20. RRC(OH)–CRR(OH)	Dilute acid and heat PINACOL/PINACOLONE REARRANGEMENT	$R_3C-\overset{\overset{\displaystyle O}{\parallel}}{C}-R$ (Ketone)
21. RCH_2OH (Primary alcohol)	Cu or Ag/Δ DEHYDROGENATION REACTION	RCHO (Aldehyde)
22. RCOOH + HCOOH (Carboxylic acid) (Formic acid)	ThO_2/MnO at 300°C	RCHO (Aldehyde)
Synthesis of Aromatic Carbonyl Compounds		
23. $PhCH_2Cl$ (Benzyl chloride)	Aqueous $Cu(NO_3)_2$ or Aqueous $Pb(NO_3)_2$	PhCHO (Aldehyde)
24. $PhCH_3$ (Toluene)	CrO_2Cl_2 ETWARD REACTION	PhCHO (Aldehyde)
25. $PhCH_3$ (Toluene)	Metal oxides, CrO_3/Ac_2O, Δ OXIDATION REACTION	PhCHO (Aldehyde)
26. PhH	HCl + $HCN/ZnCl_2$ GATTERMANN ALDEHYDE Synthesis	PhCHO (Aldehyde)
27. PhH	CO + HCl /$AlCl_3$ GATTERMANN –KOCH aldehyde synthesis	PhCHO (Aldehyde)
28. $Ph\overset{+}{N}_2\overset{-}{Cl}$	1. CH_2=NOH, 2. H_2O	PhCHO (Aldehyde)
29. PhH	PhN(Me)CHO/$POCl_3$ VILSMEIER HAACK REACTION	PhCHO (Aldehyde)
30. PhOH	1. $CHCl_3/\overline{O}H$, 2. $H_3\overset{+}{O}$ REIMER-TIEMANN REACTION	HO–C_6H_4 CHO (*o*-and *p*-isomer)

General Methods of synthesis of aldehydes and Ketones

Aldehydes : General formula $C_nH_{2n}O$ with $\mathrm{H}\!>\!C{=}O$ group.

Ketones : General formula $C_nH_{2n}O$ with $>\!C{=}O$ group.

1. **Oxidation reaction.**

(a) $$\underset{\text{(Primary alcohol)}}{RCH_2OH} \xrightarrow{K_2Cr_2O_7/\overset{+}{H} \text{ or } KMnO_4/\overline{OH} \text{ or dil. } HNO_3} \underset{\text{(Aldehyde)}}{RCHO}$$

Mechanism : $$\overset{VI}{K_2Cr_2O_7} + \overset{+}{H} \longrightarrow \overset{VI}{H_2Cr_2O_4}$$

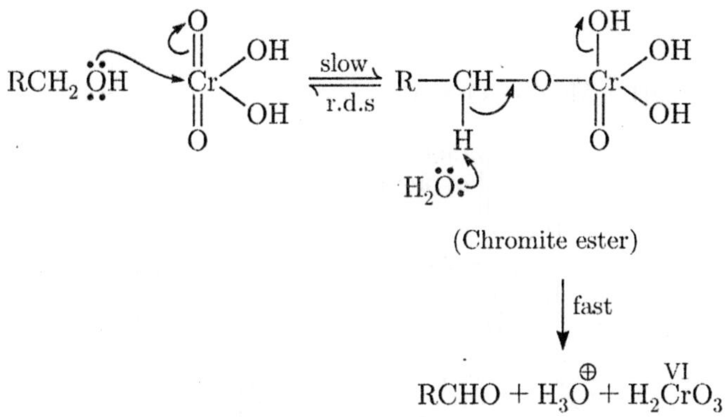

(b) $$\underset{\substack{(R^1=R^2 \text{ or } R^1 \neq R^2)\\ \text{(Secondary alcohol)}}}{R^1R^2CHOH} \xrightarrow[\text{or } K_2Cr_2O_7/\text{conc. } H_2SO_4/\Delta]{\text{conc. } HNO_3/\text{prolonged heating}} \underset{\text{(Ketone)}}{R^1R^2C{=}O}$$

Mechanism : $$\overset{VI}{K_2Cr_2O_7} + \overset{\oplus}{H} \longrightarrow \overset{VI}{H_2Cr_2O_4}$$

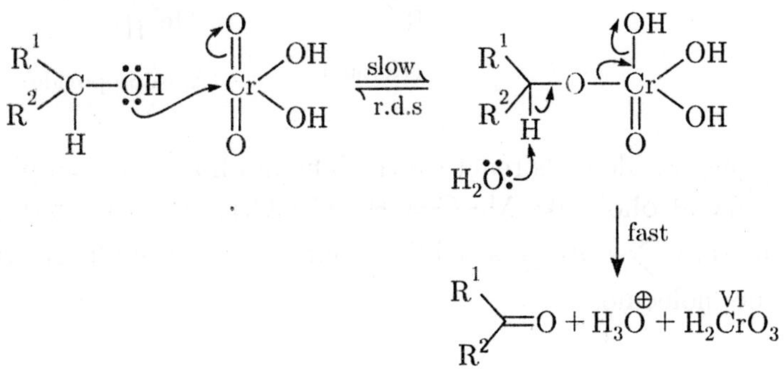

2. 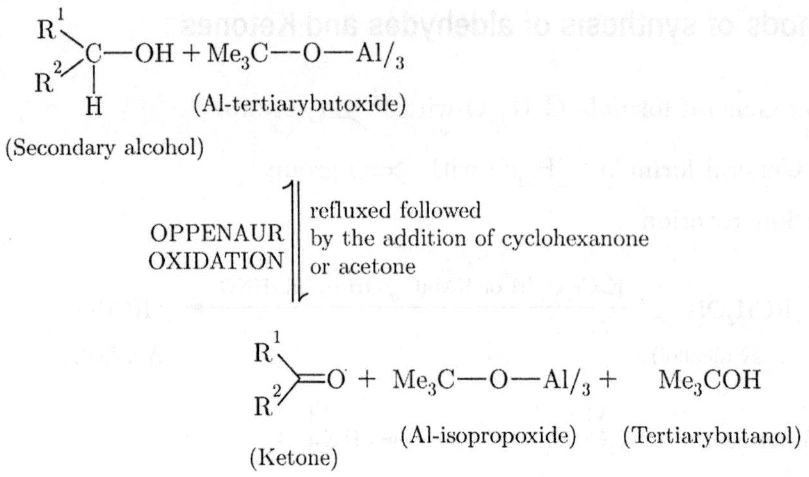

Mechanism :

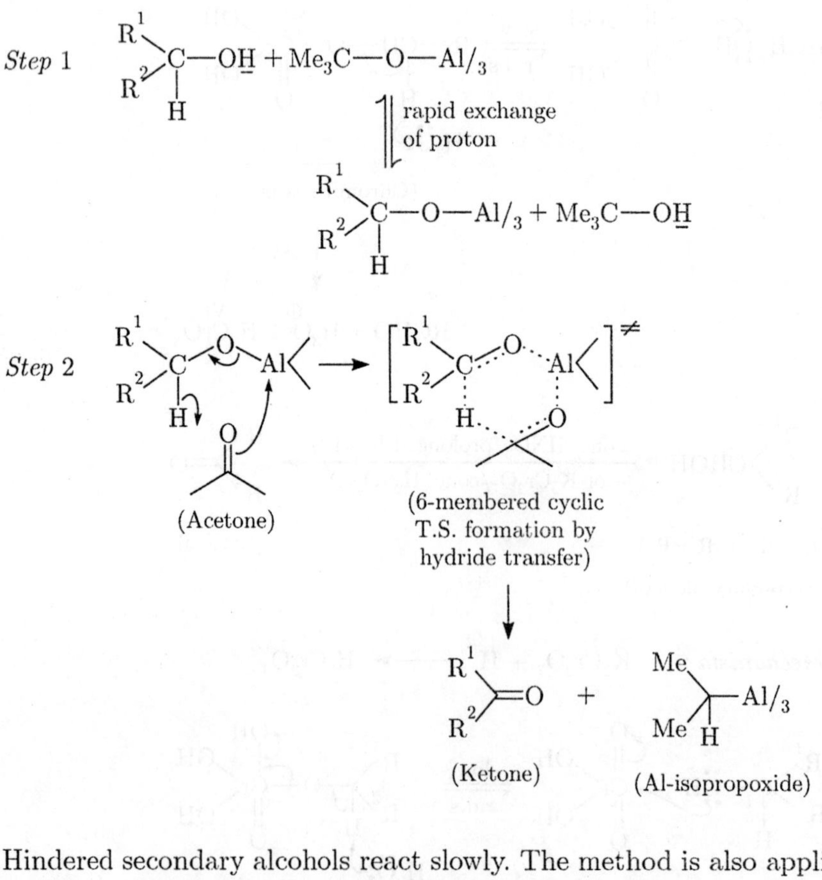

Hindered secondary alcohols react slowly. The method is also applicable to low boiling primary alcohols like $Me_2C{=}CH—CH_2CH_2OH$. The oxidising agent is *mild*, so that only $>$—OH gets oxidised but not the double or triple bond if present in the molecule.

3. Ozonolysis reaction

(a) 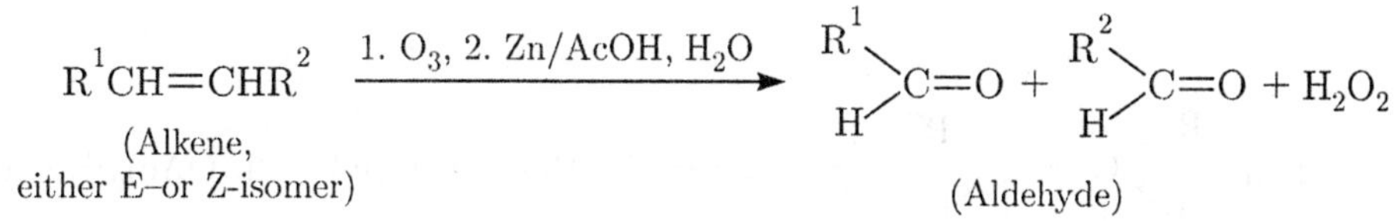

Mechanism :

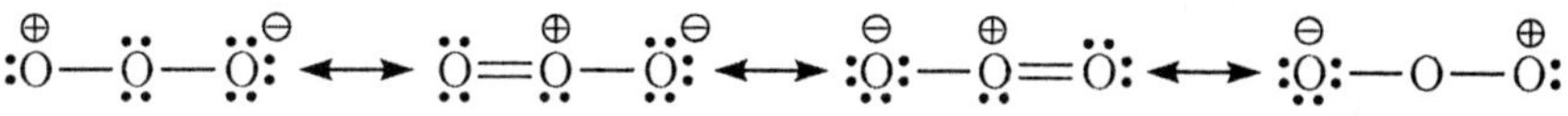

Resonating structures of ozone

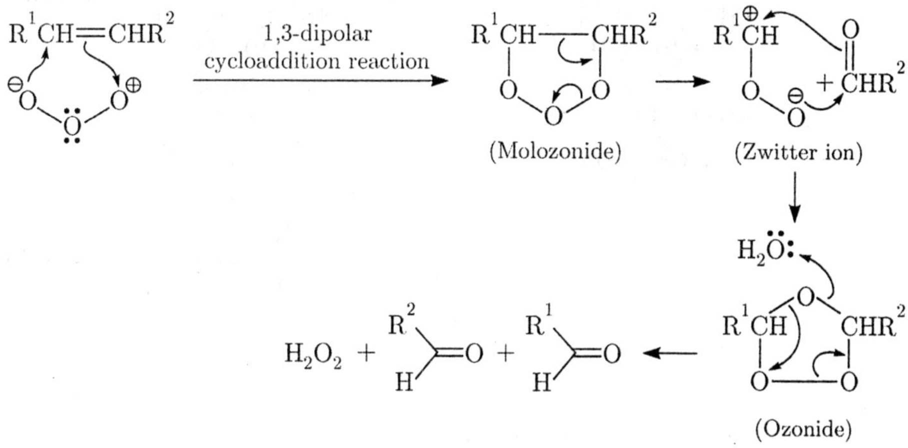

(b) 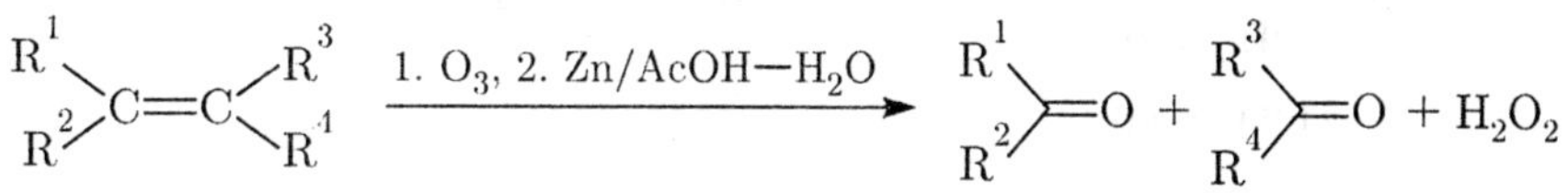

Mechanism :

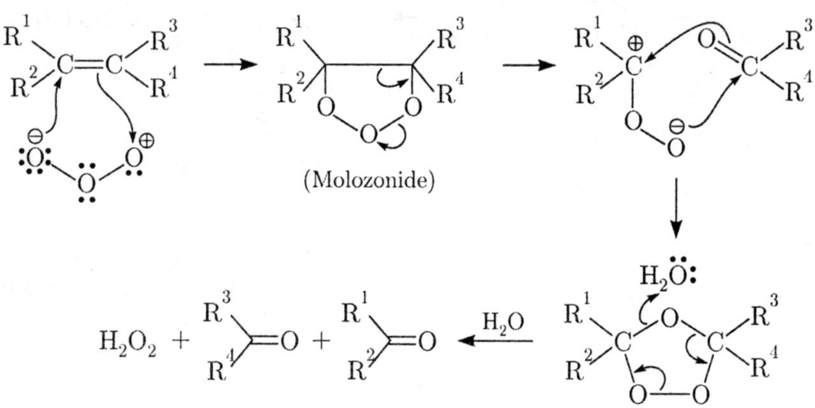

4. Oxidation of 1,2-glycols by $\overset{VII}{HIO_4}$ or $\overset{IV}{Pb(OAc)_4}$

I.(a)

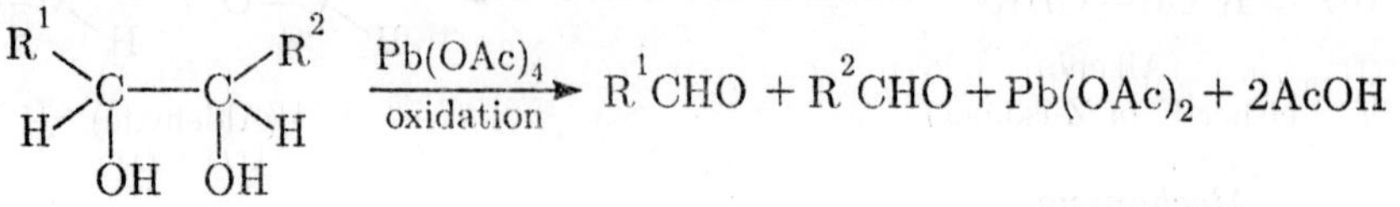

(1,2-Glycol)

Mechanism :

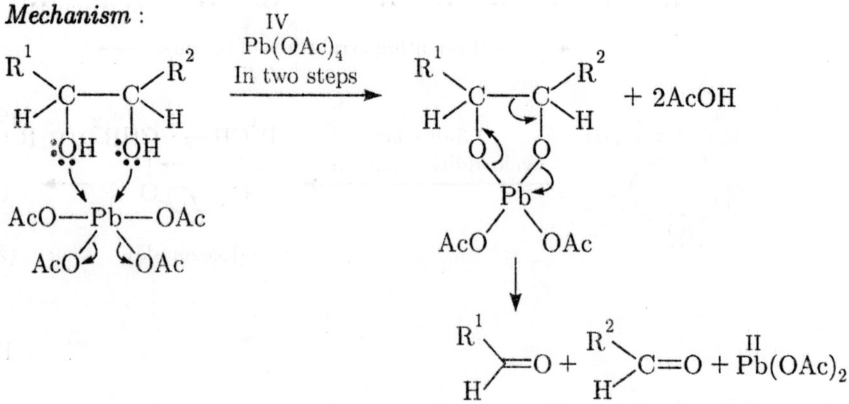

(b)

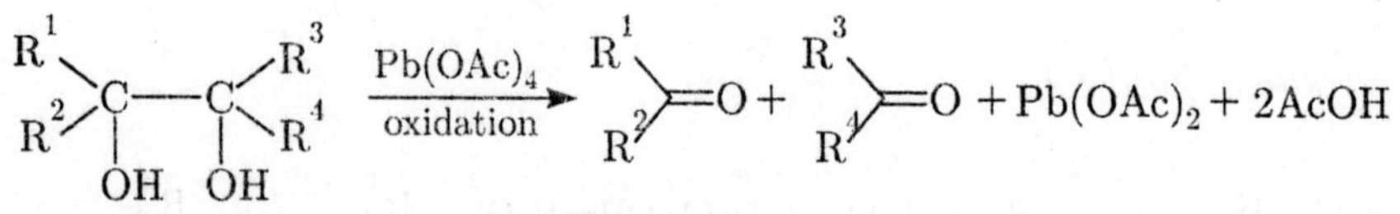

(1,2-Glycol)

Mechanism :

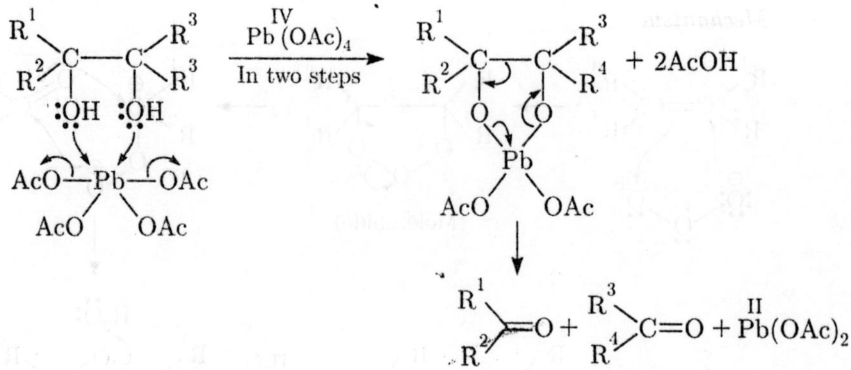

II.(a)

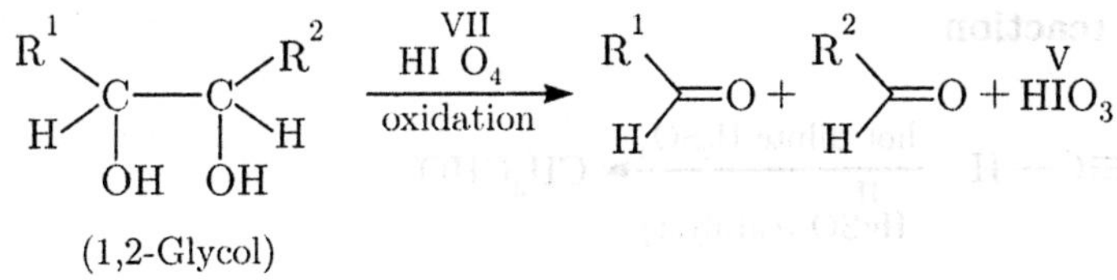

Mechanism :

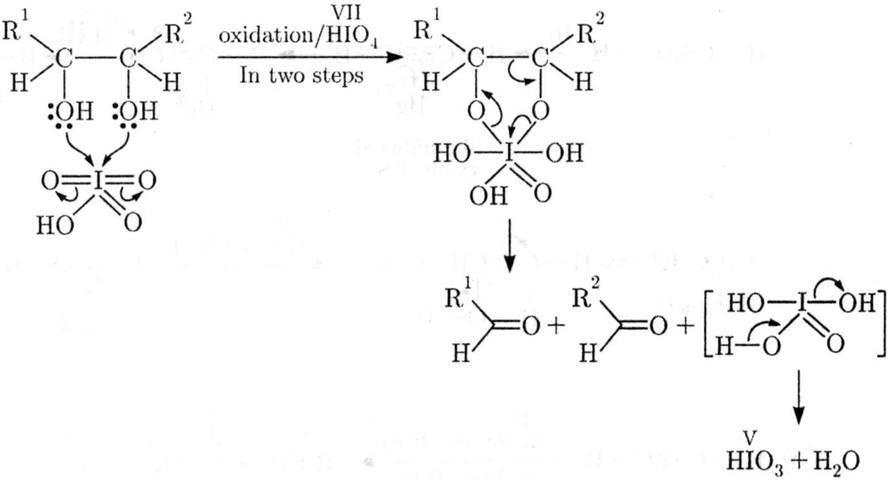

(b)

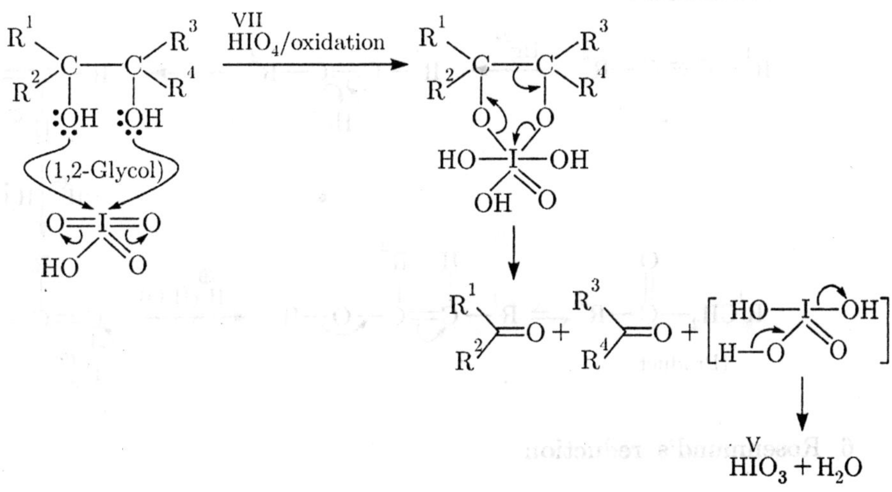

5. Hydration reaction

(a) $H-C\equiv C-H \xrightarrow[\text{II}\ HgSO_4\text{(catalyst)}]{\text{hot dilute } H_2SO_4} CH_3CHO$

Mechanism :

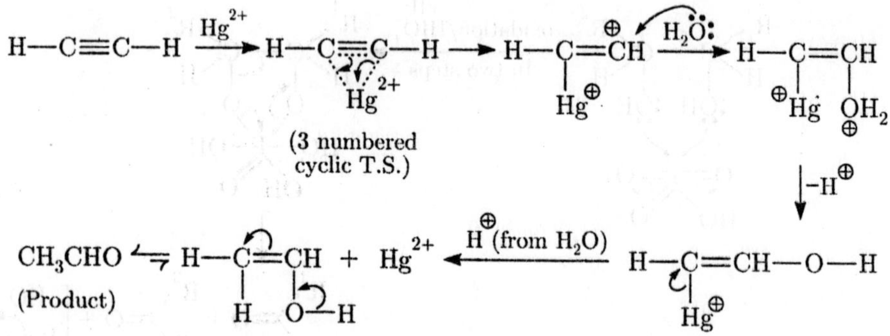

(b) $R^1-C\equiv C-R^2 \xrightarrow[\text{hot dilute } H_2SO_4]{\text{II}\ HgSO_4\text{(catalyst)}} R^1CH_2-\overset{O}{\overset{\|}{C}}-R^2$ or $R^1-\overset{O}{\overset{\|}{C}}-CH_2R^2$

Mechanism :

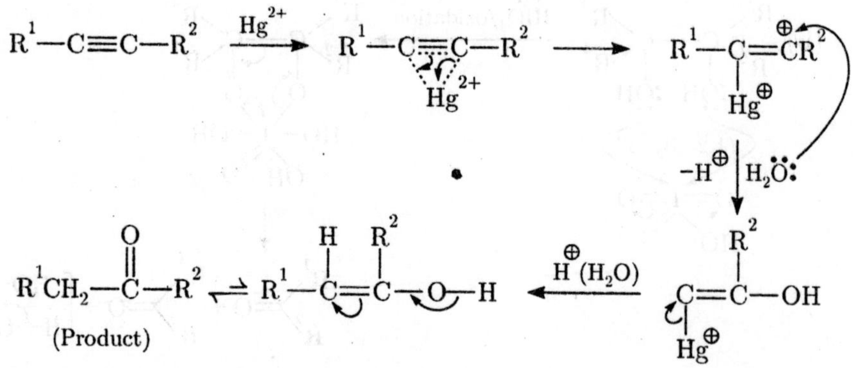

6. Rosenmund's reduction

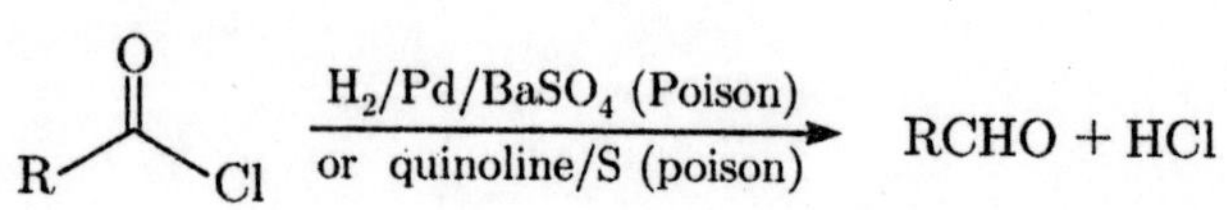

It is an exclusive method for the preparation of *aldehydes.* Aldehydes are more readity reduced than acid chlorides. So $BaSO_4$ or quinoline/sulphur is used which act as an inhibitor (poison) for the further reduction of aldehydes to alcohols. There is no analogous method for the synthesis of ketones.

7. **Stephen's reduction :** This is an exclusive method for the preparation of aldehydes. An alkyl cyanide is dissolved in ether or ethyl formate or ethyl acetate as solvent and reduced with $SnCl_2$ and HCl and then steam distilled.

$$R—C\equiv N \xrightarrow[SnCl_2/HCl,\ reduction]{Et_2O\ or\ EtOAc\ or\ HCO_2Et\ (solvent)} RCHO$$

***Mechanism* :**

$$SnCl_2 + 4Cl^- \text{ (form HCl)} \longrightarrow SnCl_6^{2\ominus}$$

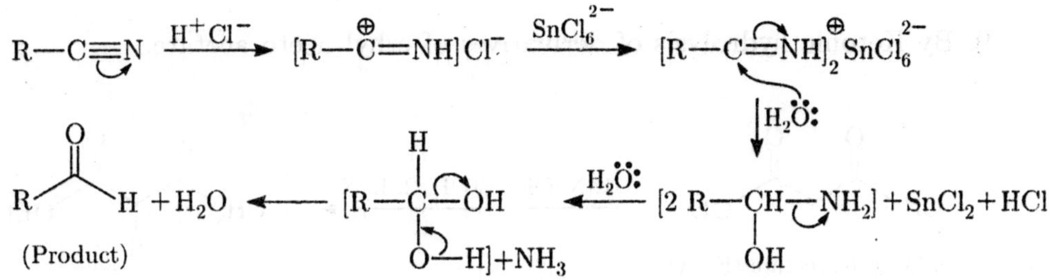

8. **By Grignard reagent**

(a) $$H(EtO)C{=}O + RMgX \xrightarrow{H_3O^\oplus} RCHO + EtOH$$

(Formate ester)

***Mechanism* :**

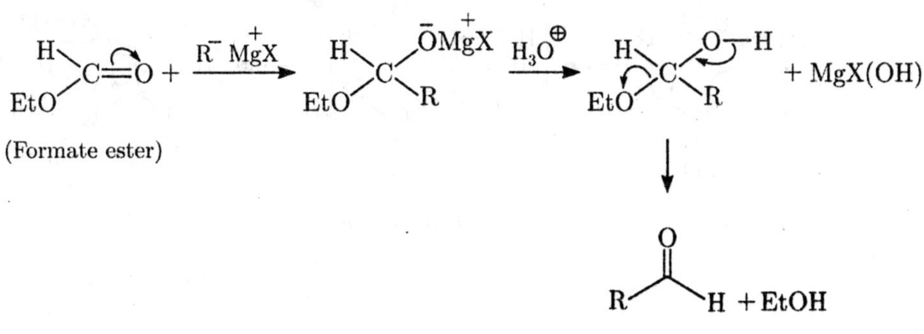

(Aldehyde)

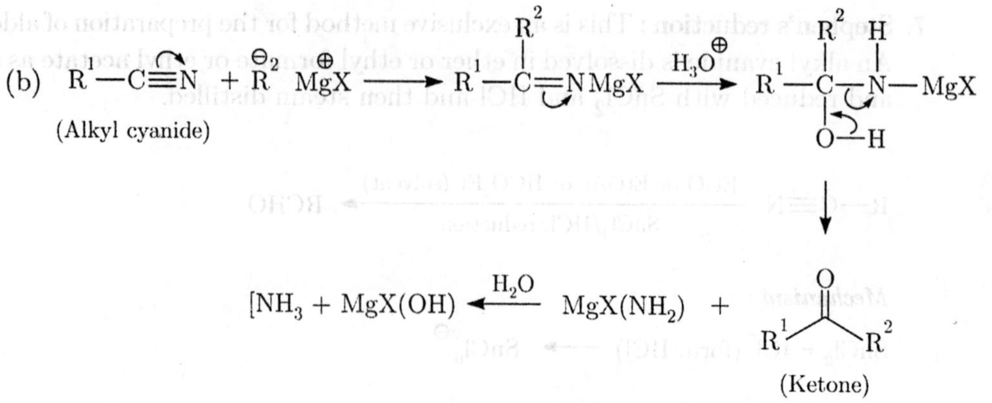

9. By Ketonic hydrolysis of derivatives of ethyl aceto acetate.

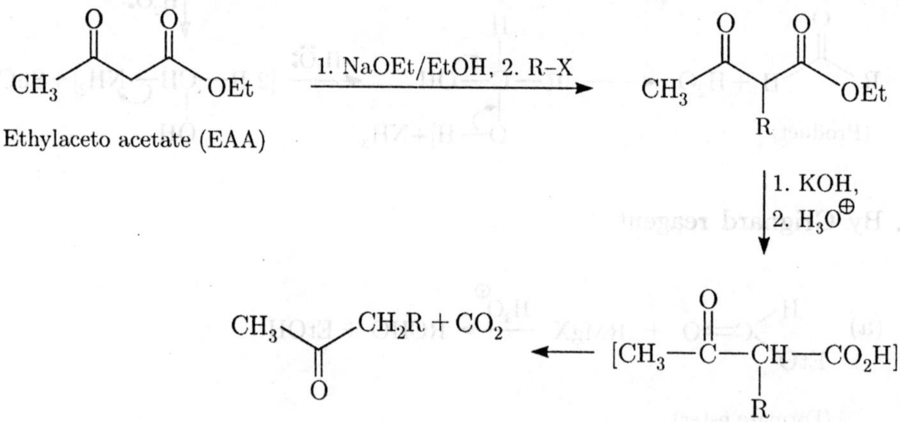

Mechanism of decaboxylation :

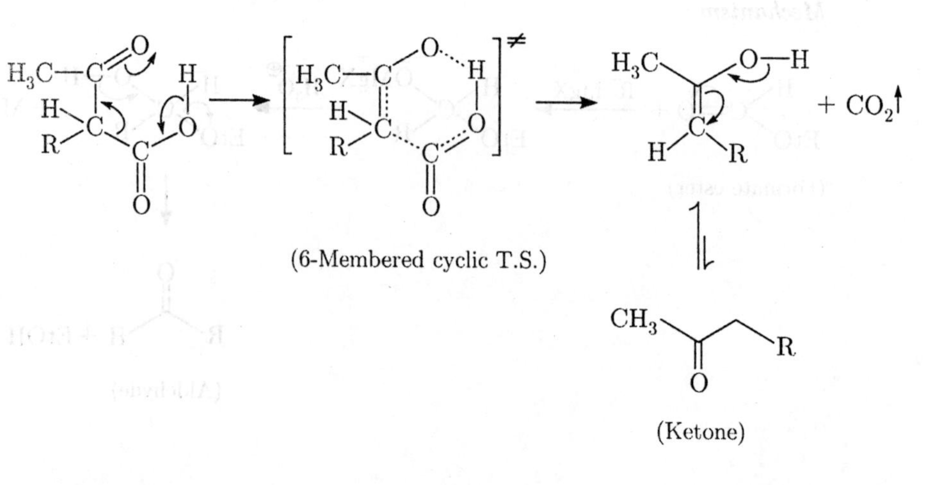

No aldehyde can be prepared by this method.

10. From substituted diethylmalonate (DEM)

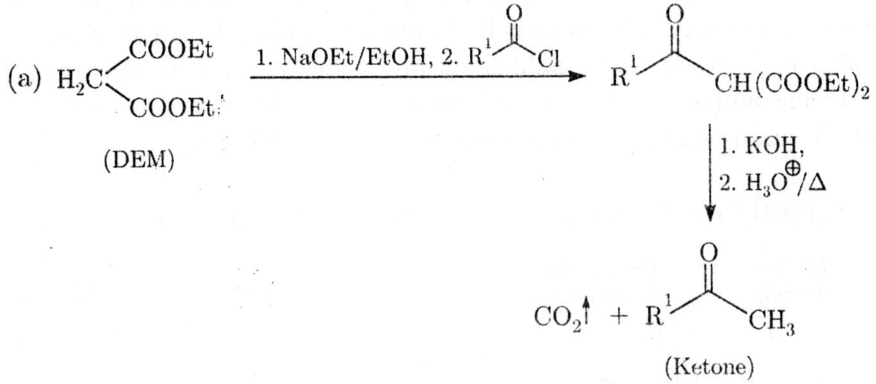

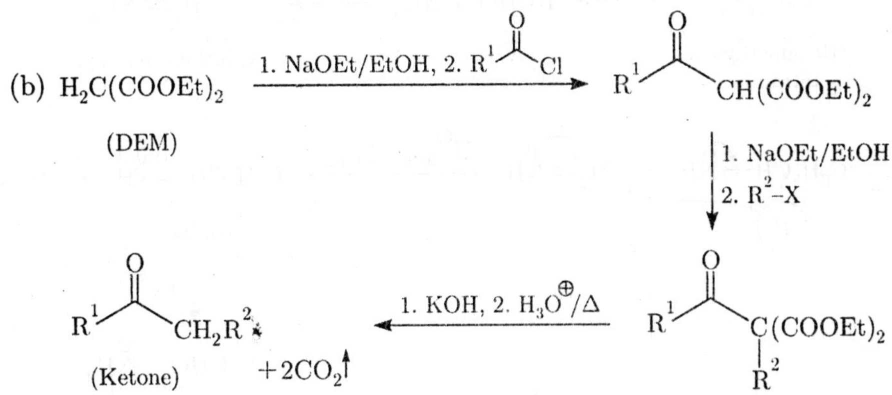

11. Sommelet's reaction : It is an exclusive method for the preparation of *aldehydes.* Sommelet reaction involves the oxidation of chloromethyl group (–CH_2Cl group) to an aldehyde functionality by the use of hexamethylenetetramine ($C_6H_{12}N_4$) and subsequent hydrolysis in acidic medium (pH 3.00–6.5). The reaction is also successful with benzylic halide $C_6H_5CH_2Cl$ or $ArCH_2Cl$.

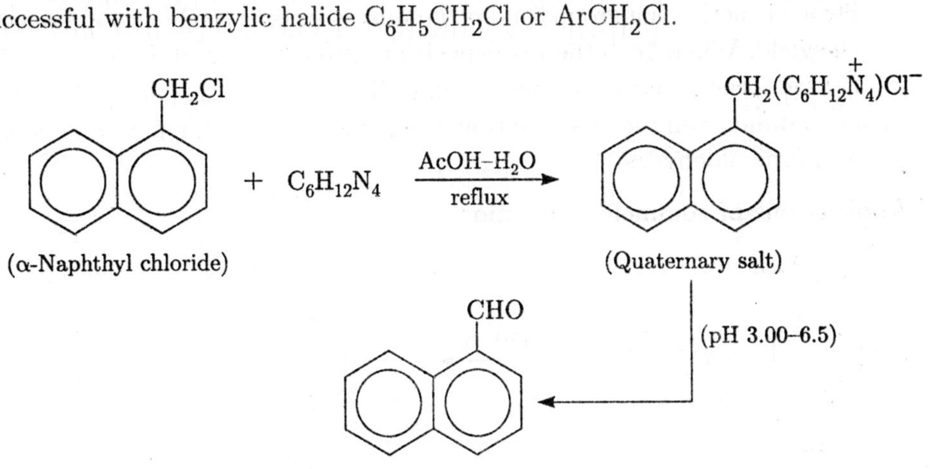

Mechanism : The mechanism of the reaction is not clearly understood. According to Angyal and coworkers, the halide reacts with hexamethylenetetramine to form a quaternary salt which is hydrolysed to amine. Hexamethylenetetramine is also hydrolysed to formaldehyde and ammonia which subsequently form methylene amine. The amine then transfers a hydride ion to methylene amine to form an imine which is finally hydrolysed to an aldehyde.

$$\underset{\text{(Benzyl chloride)}}{C_6H_5CH_2Cl} + \underset{\text{(Hexamethylene tetramine)}}{C_6H_{12}N_4} \longrightarrow C_6H_5CH_2(C_6H_{12}\overset{+}{N}_4)Cl^- \longrightarrow \underset{\text{(Amine)}}{C_6H_5CH_2NH_2}$$

$$\underset{\text{(Hexamethylene tetramine)}}{C_6H_{12}N_4} \xrightarrow{H_3O^{\oplus}} HCHO + NH_3 \longrightarrow \underset{\text{(Methylene amine)}}{CH_2{=}\overset{\oplus}{N}H_2}$$

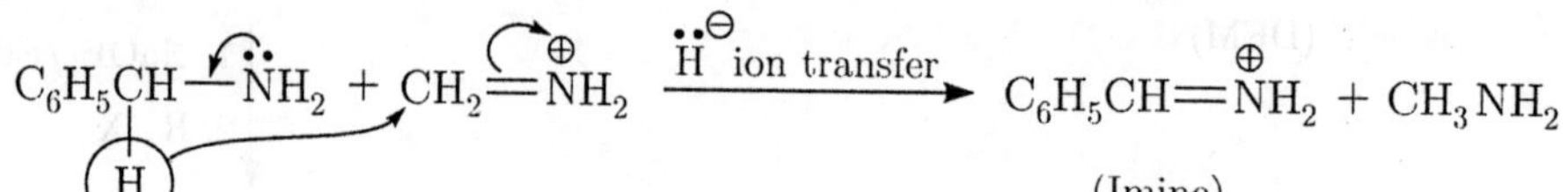

$$\underset{\text{(Imine)}}{C_6H_5CH{=}\overset{\oplus}{N}H_2} \xrightarrow{H_3O^{\oplus}} C_6H_5CHO + \overset{\oplus}{N}H_4$$

Reaction of benzylamine with excess of $C_6H_{12}N_4$ to produce aldehyde is the actual *sommelet's reaction.* When benzylamine is refluxed with hexamethylenetetramine in acidic medium, benzaldehyde is obtained. This observation supports the above said mechanism.

Strong deactivating groups and *ortho* substituents in the benzene nucleus decrease the yield. When both the *ortho* positions are substituted, as in 2,4-dinitrobenzyl chloride, the reaction completely fails. The yield is also very poor with phenolic compound. Sommelet's reaction is particularly useful for the preparation of aromatic aldehydes.

Applications of sommelet's reaction :

(a)

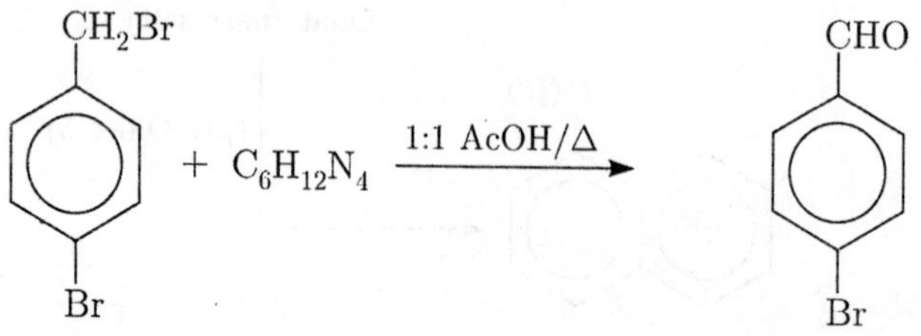

(*p*-Bromobenzaldehyde)

(b) 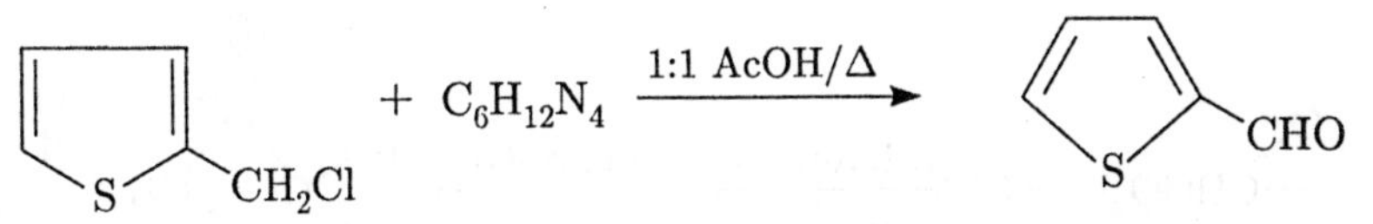

(Thiophene-2-aldehyde)

(c) 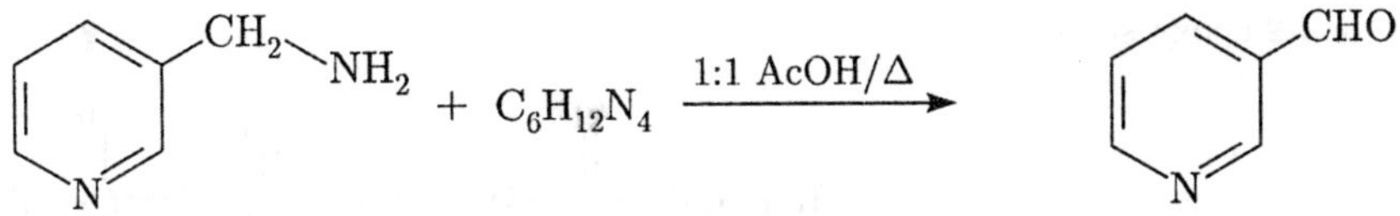

(Pyridine-3-aldehyde)

(d) $CH_3(CH_2)_4CH_2NH_2 + C_6H_{12}N_4 \xrightarrow{HCl/\Delta} CH_3(CH_2)_4CHO$

(n-Hexylamine) (n-Hexanal)

(e) $C_6H_5CH_2Cl + C_5H_5N \longrightarrow [C_6H_5CH_2\overset{\oplus}{N}C_5H_5]Cl^-$

(Benzyl chloride) (Pyridine)

1. p-$NO_2C_6H_4NMe_2/\bar{O}H$
2. $H_3O^{\oplus}$

KRÖHNKE REACTION (modified sommelet's reaction)

$\downarrow$

C_6H_5CHO

(Product)

12. Darzen's glycidic ester condensation method

Aldehydes like R^1CHO can also be used in place of 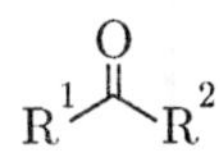

(a) 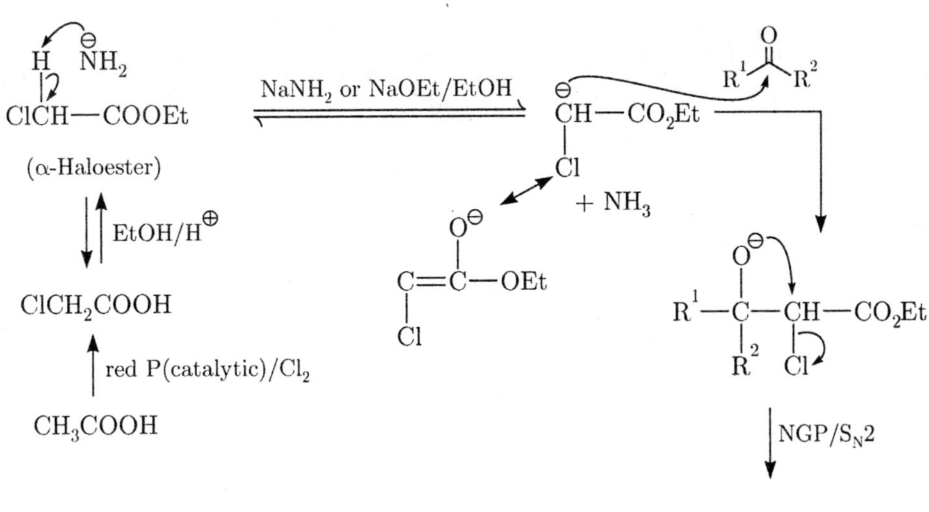

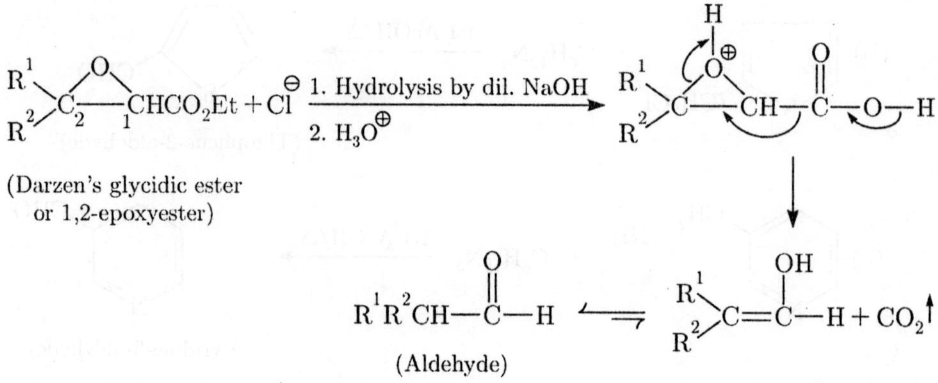

(b)

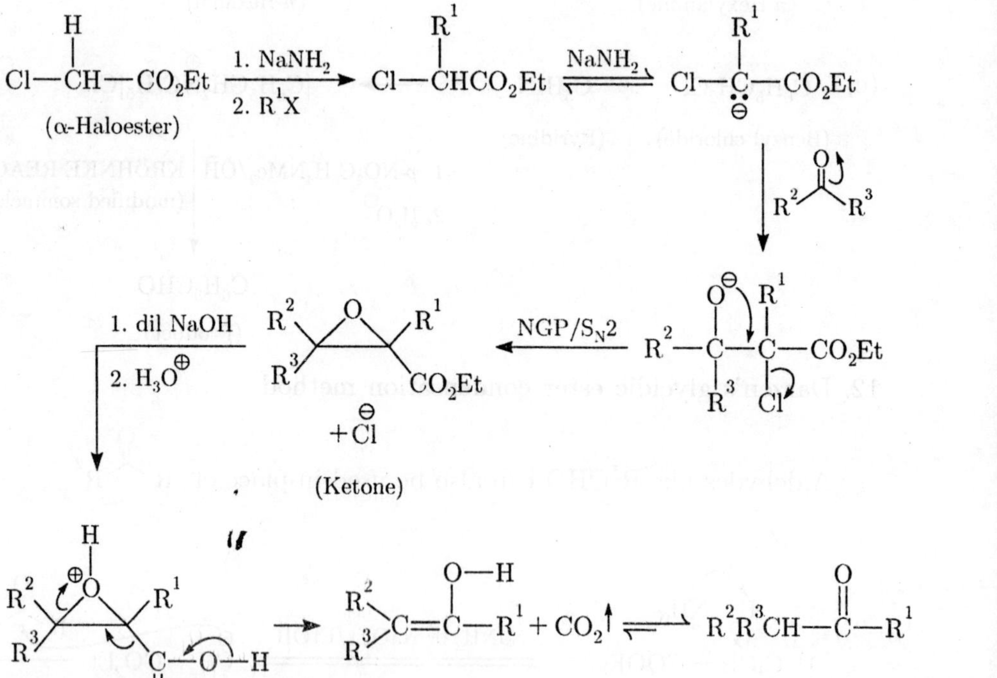

13. Preparation of ketones using organocopper reagents

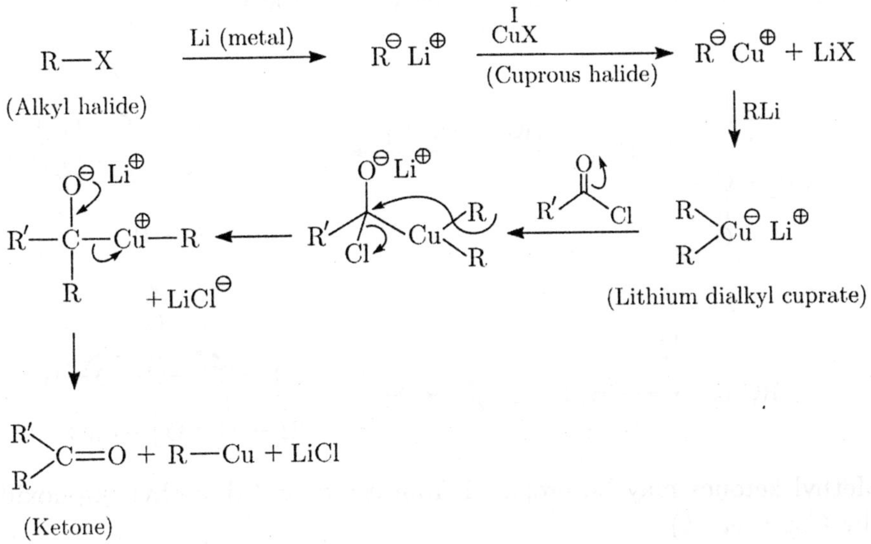

14. By heating a mixture of calcium salt of formic acid and one of its homologue

(a) $(RCH_2COO)_2Ca + (HCOO)_2Ca \xrightarrow{\Delta} 2RCH_2CHO + 2CaCO_3$

(Aldehyde)

Mechanism :

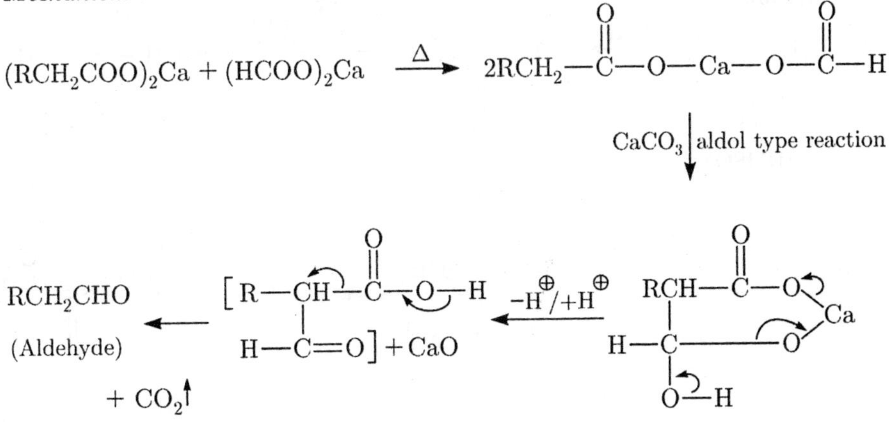

(b) $(RCH_2COO)_2Ca \xrightarrow{\Delta} RCH_2-\overset{O}{\overset{\|}{C}}-CH_2R + CaCO_3$

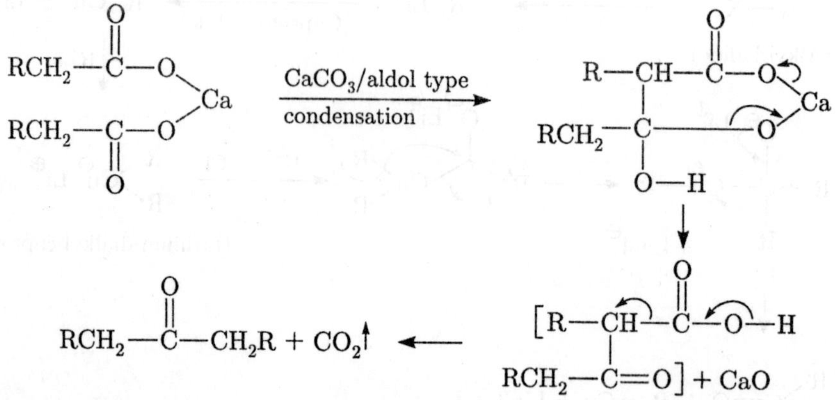

15. Methyl ketones may be prepared from esters and dimethyl sulphoxide (by Corey *et al.*)

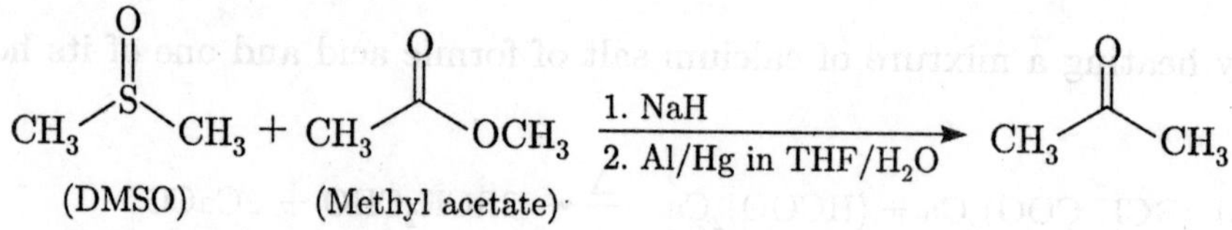

Instead of CH_3COOCH_3, RCOOMe may be used.

Mechanism :

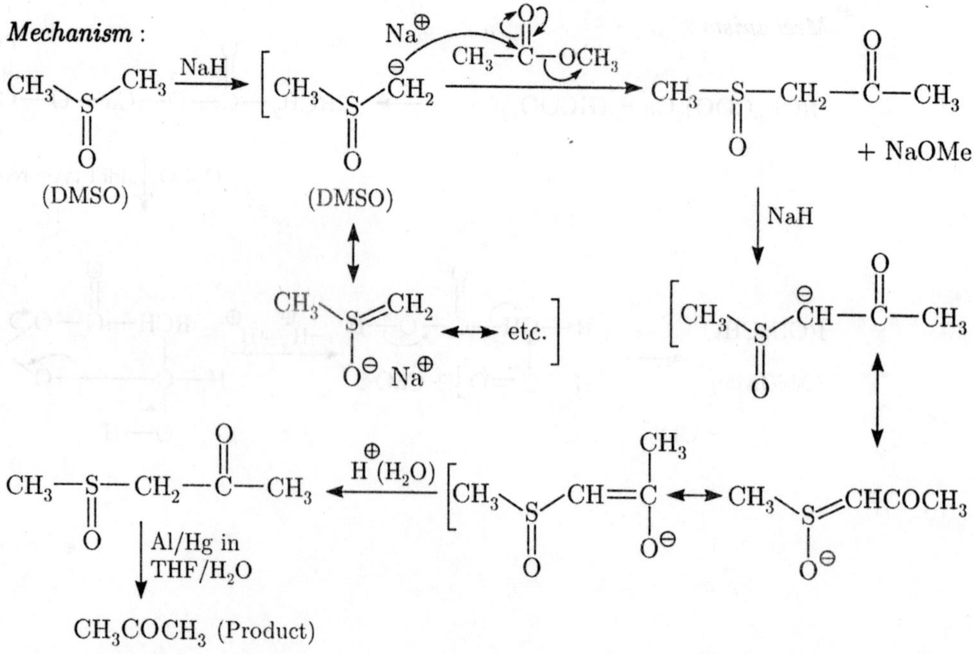

16. Hydroboration–oxidation of alkynes

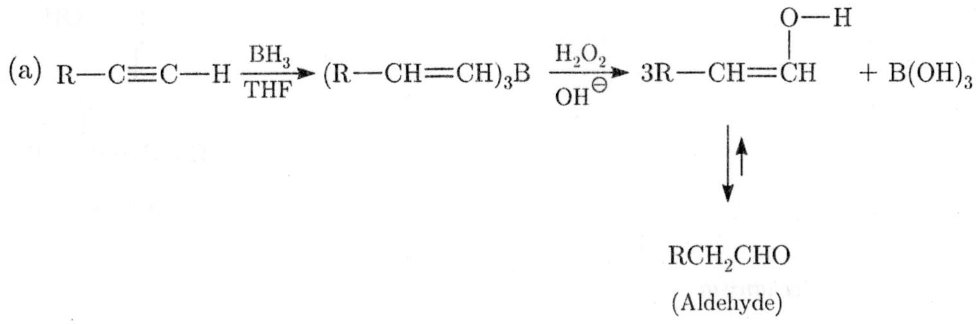

Mechanism :

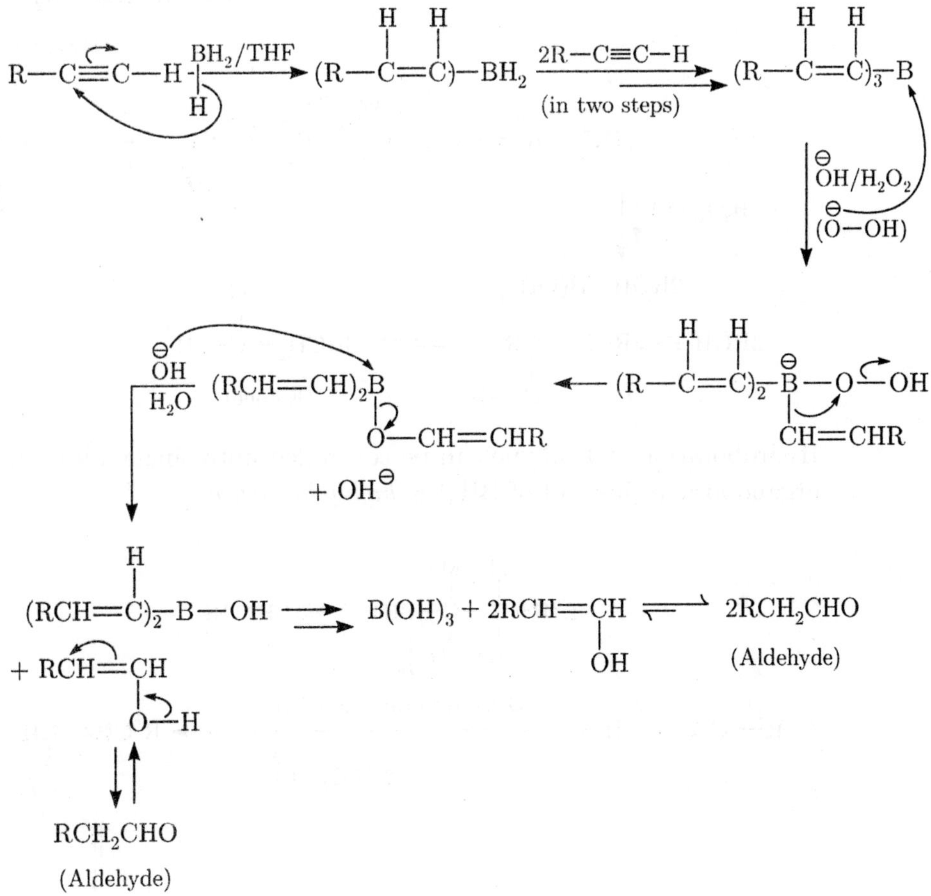

(b) 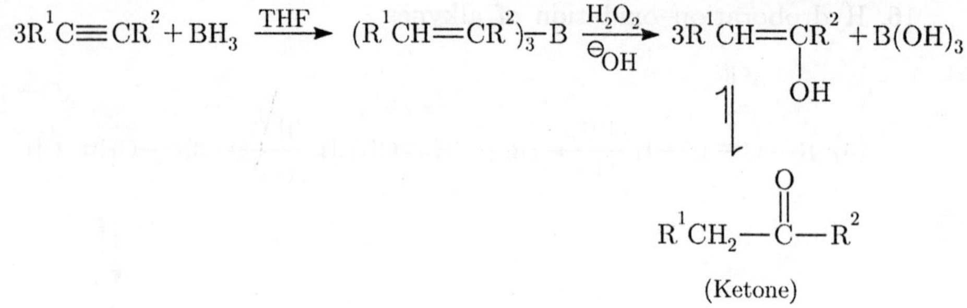

Mechanism :

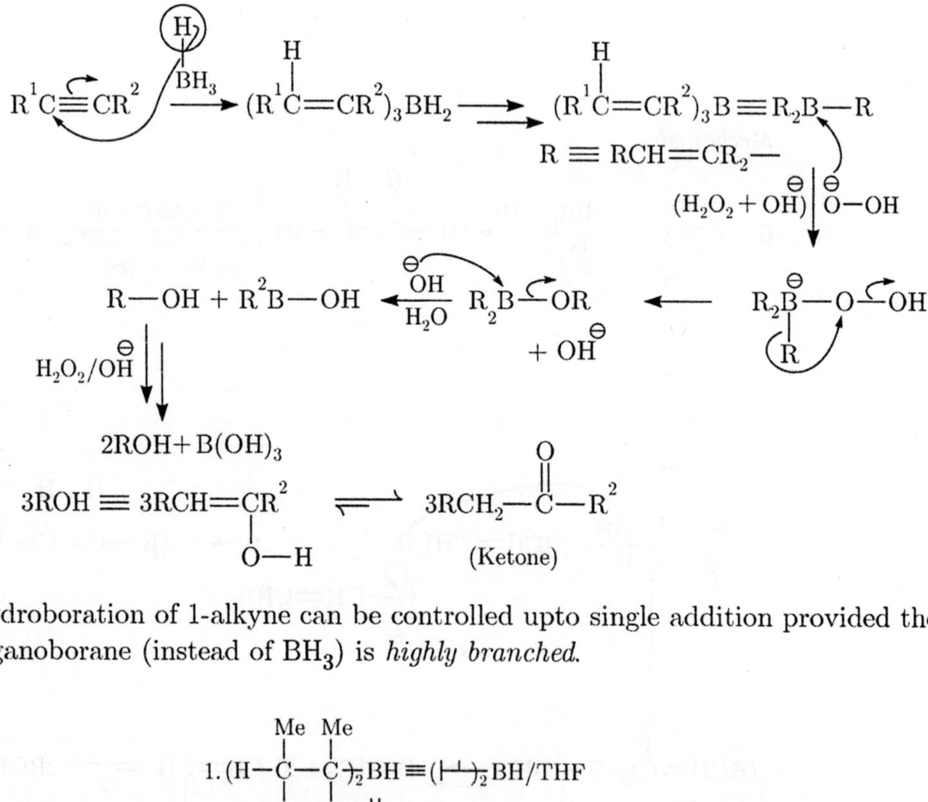

Hydroboration of 1-alkyne can be controlled upto single addition provided the organoborane (instead of BH_3) is *highly branched.*

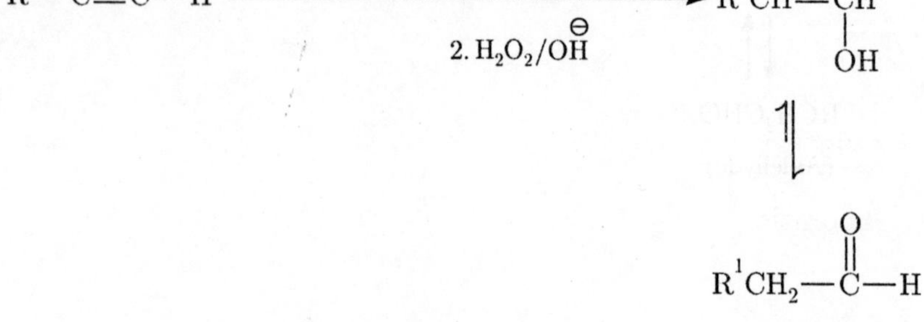

17. Aldehydes from esters by DIBAL-H

The reducing agent used here is 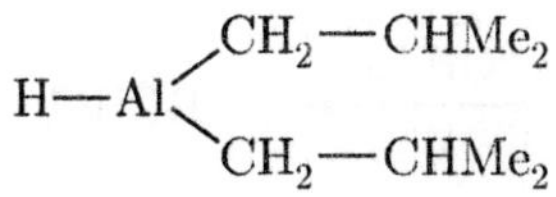

(Diisobutyl aluminium hydride)
(iBu_2Al–H or DIBAL–H)

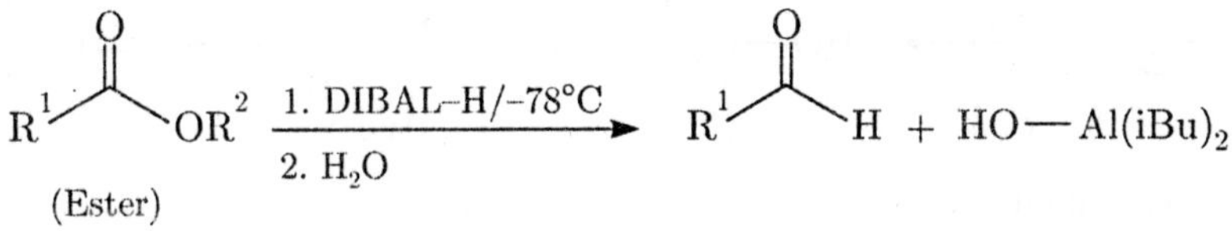

Mechanism :

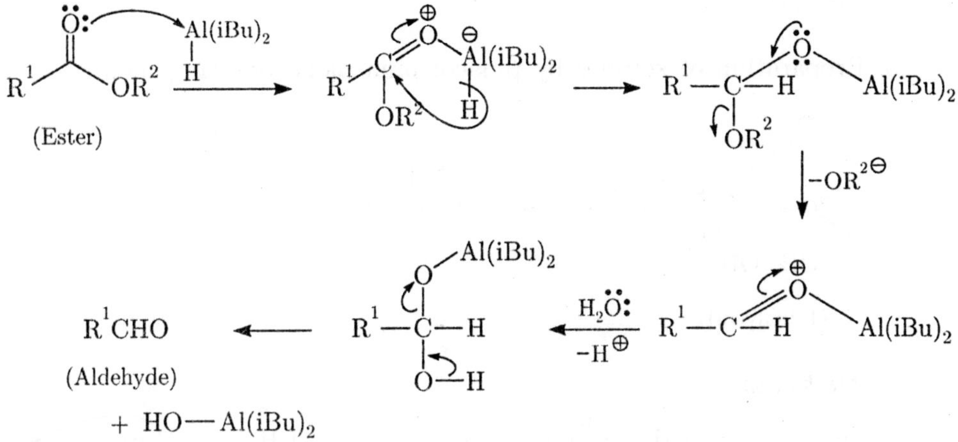

18. Aldehydes from nitriles by DIBAL-H

$$R{-}C{\equiv}N: \xrightarrow[2.\ H_2O]{1.\ \text{DIBAL-H}} RCHO + H_2NAl(iBu)_2$$

(Alkyl cyanide) or (Alkyl nitrile) → (Aldehyde)

Mechanism :

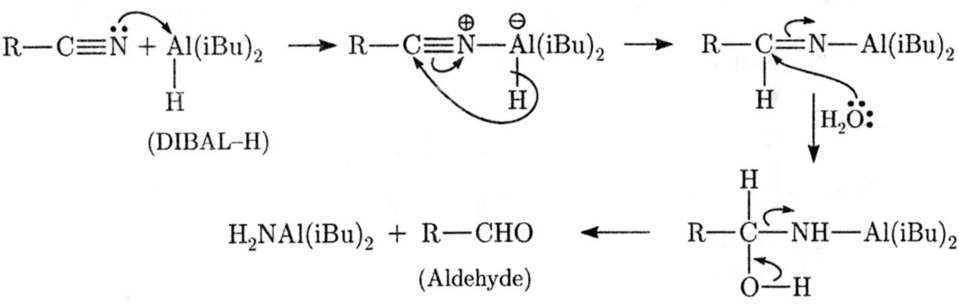

19. Alkaline hydrolysis of dihaloalkanes to aldehydes

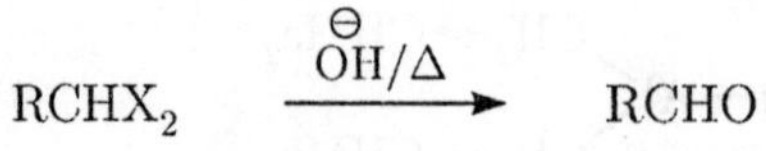

(Dihaloalkane) (Aldehyde)

Mechanism :

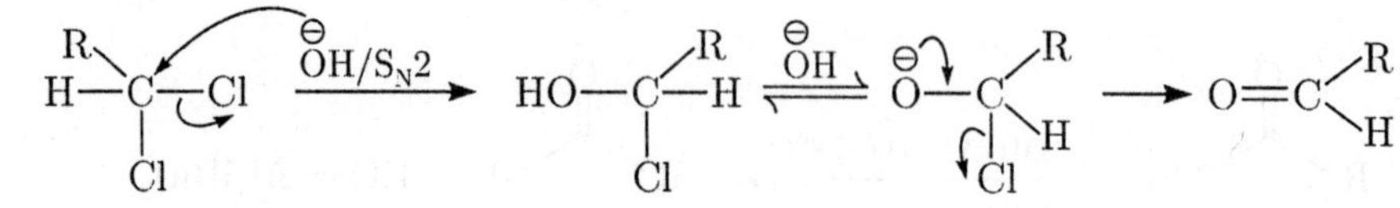

(Terminal geminal dihalide)

(R=alkyl or aryl)

20. Preparation of ketones by pinacol pinacolone rearrangement

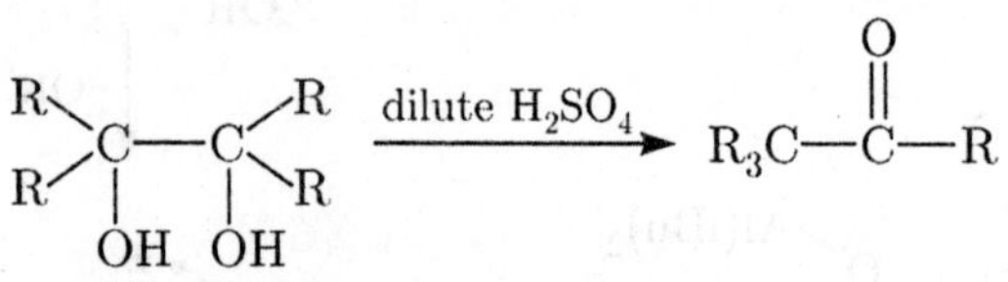

(1,2-Glycol)

Mechanism :

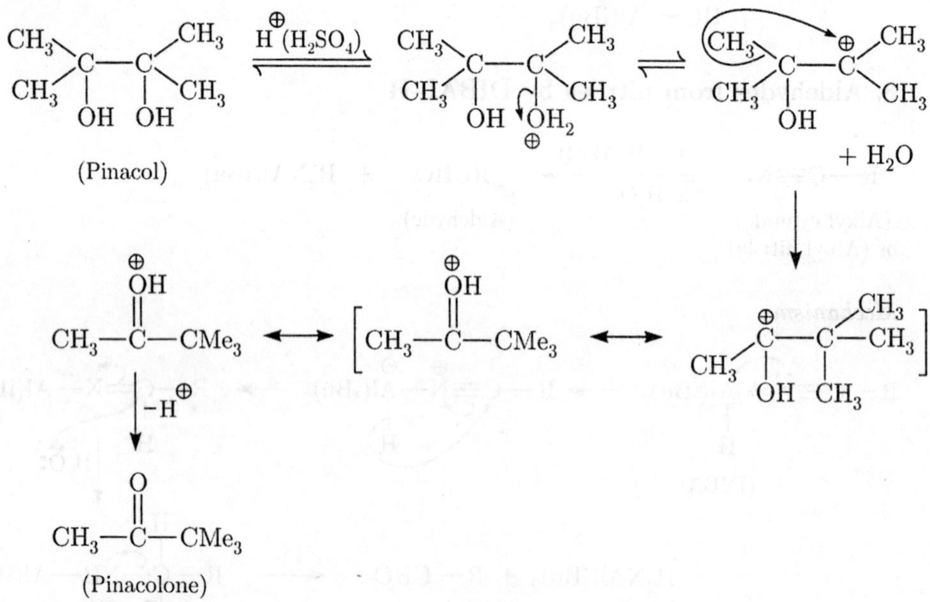

(Pinacol)

(Pinacolone)
(Product)

21. $$\underset{\text{(Primary alcohol)}}{RCH_2OH} \xrightarrow[\frac{1}{2}O_2]{\text{Cu or Ag/600°C}} RCHO + H_2O$$

(Dehydrogenation reaction)

Mechanism :

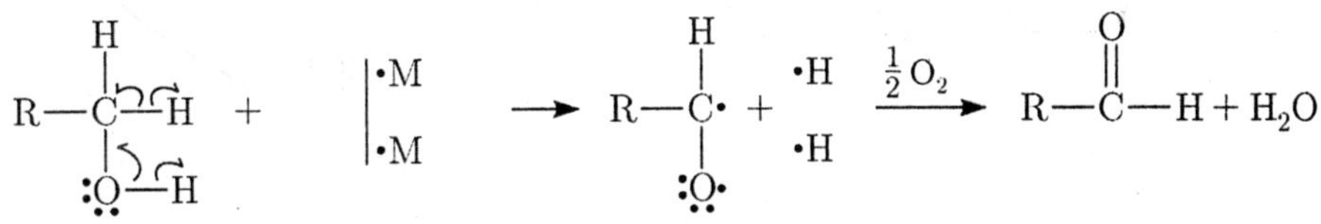

(1°-Alcohol) (Metal surface)

22. Preparation of aldehydes from carboxylic acids

$$\underset{\substack{\text{(Fatty acid)}\\\text{(Vapour)}}}{RCOOH} + \underset{\substack{\text{(Formic acid)}\\\text{(Vapour)}}}{HCOOH} \xrightarrow[\text{or MnO (manganous oxide)}]{\text{300°C/thoria }(ThO_2)} \underset{\text{(Aldehyde)}}{RCHO}$$

Synthesis of Aromatic carbonyl compounds

23. **By the oxidation of chloromethyl group :** When benzyl chloride is oxidised by the aqueous cupric nitrate or lead nitrate solution in a current of CO_2, benzaldehyde is formed.

$$\underset{\text{(Benzyl chloride)}}{PhCH_2Cl} \xrightarrow[\text{oxidation reation}]{\text{aq. }Pb(NO_3)_2\text{ or }Cu(NO_3)_2} \underset{\text{(Benzaldehyde)}}{PhCHO}$$

Mechanism :

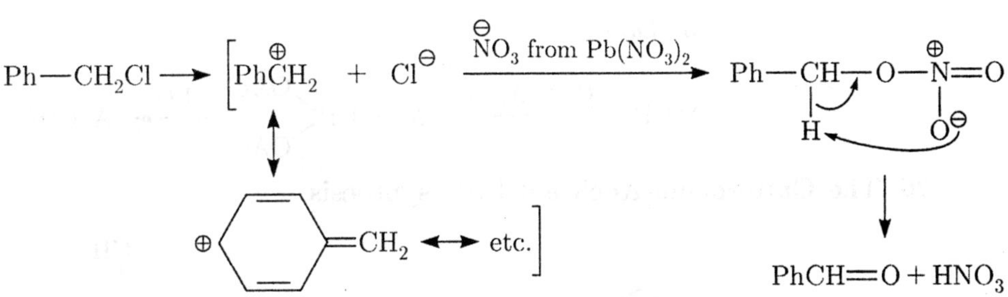

(Resonance stabilised)

(Benzaldehyde) (Product)

24. Preparation of aldehydes by Etard reaction : When toluene is treated with chromyl chloride in carbon tetrachloride solvent, a complex is formed, which on treatment with water gives benzaldehyde and the reaction is called **Etard reaction**.

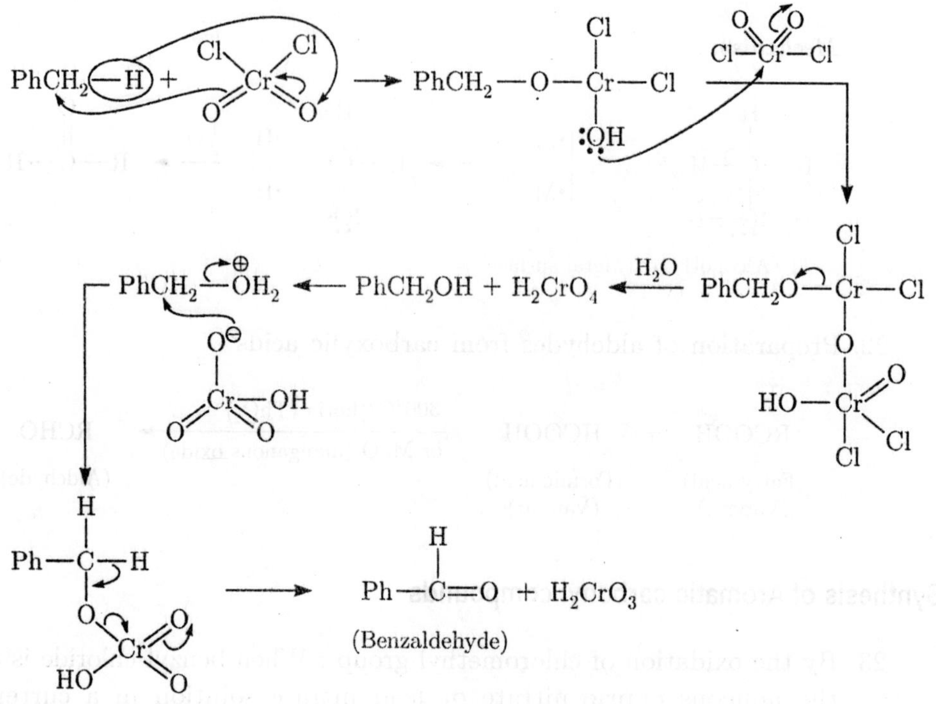

25. Preparation of aldehydes by the oxidation of side chain of arenes : The side chain of an arene may also be oxidised to the aldehyde by chromium trioxide in acetic anhydride.

$$\underset{\text{(Toluene)}}{ArCH_3} \xrightarrow{CrO_3/Ac_2O,\ \Delta} ArCHO$$

***Mechanism* :**

$$ArCH_3 \xrightarrow{CrO_3/Ac_2O} Ar-CH(OAc)_2 \xrightarrow{H_2O} ArCHO$$

26. The Gattermann-Koch aldehyde synthesis

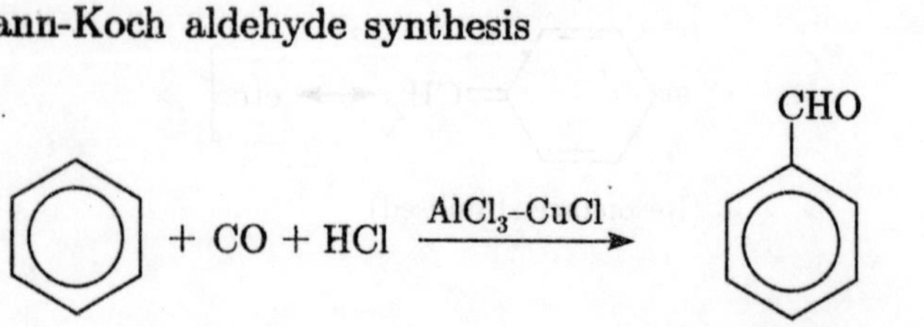

(Benzaldehyde)

The reaction is carried out by passing a mixture of CO and HCl through a solution of the substrate and the catalyst (CuCl is taken in very small amount) in nitrobenzene or ether, when aromatic aldehydes are formed. Phenols, phenolic ethers, amines and *m*-substituents retard the reaction.

Mechanism :

$$HCl + AlCl_3 \rightleftharpoons \overset{+}{H}\,\overset{-}{Al}Cl_4$$

$$:\overset{-}{C}\equiv\overset{+}{O} + \overset{+}{H}\,\overset{-}{Al}Cl_4 \rightleftharpoons [H-C\equiv\overset{\oplus}{O} \longleftrightarrow H-\overset{+}{C}=O]\,\overset{-}{Al}Cl_4$$

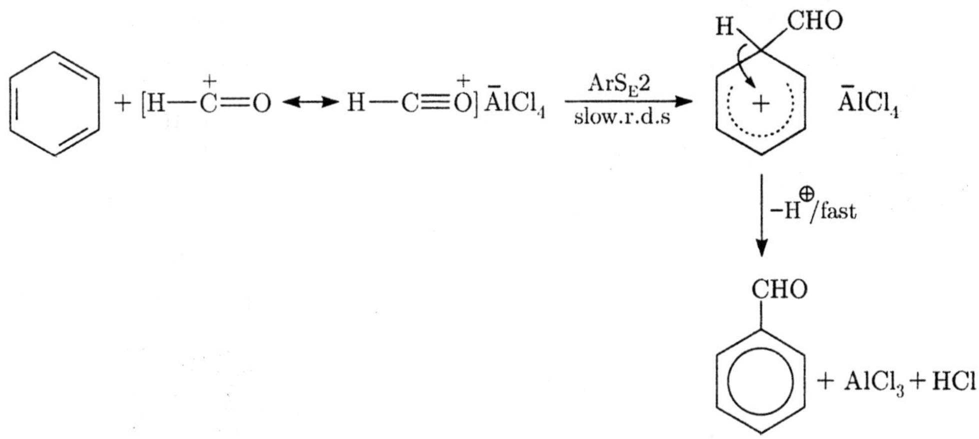

CuCl coordinates with CO and thereby increases the effective concentration of the latter.

27. The Gattermann aldehyde synthesis

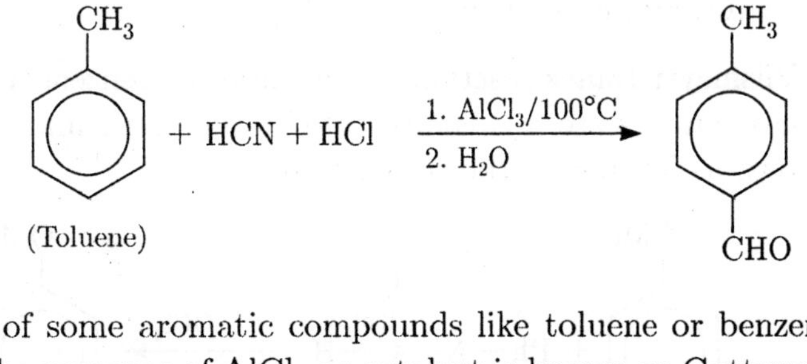

Formylation of some aromatic compounds like toluene or benzene with HCN and HCl in the presence of $AlCl_3$ as catalyst is known as Gattermann aldehyde synthesis. The reaction may be carried out by passing HCl through nitrobenzene containing the substrate and $Zn(CN)_2$ in the solution while $ZnCl_2$ and HCN are formed *in situ*. $ZnCl_2$ acts as a catalyst. *m*-Directing groups retard the reaction.

Mechanism :

$$Zn(CN)_2 + 2HCl \rightleftharpoons ZnCl_2 + 2HCN$$

$$ZnCl_2 + HCl \rightleftharpoons \overset{\ominus}{Zn}Cl_3\ H^{\oplus}$$

$$H{-}C{\equiv}N + H^{\oplus}\ \overset{\ominus}{Zn}Cl_3 \rightleftharpoons [H{-}C{\equiv}\overset{\oplus}{N}H \longleftrightarrow H{-}\overset{\oplus}{C}{=}NH]Cl^- + ZnCl_2$$

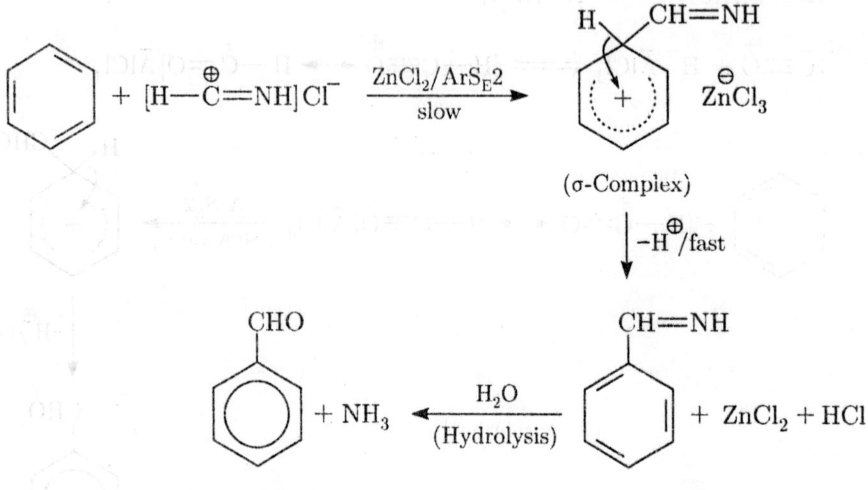

(σ-Complex)

(Benzaldehyde)

28. From arenediazonium salts to aldehydes

$$Ph{-}\overset{\oplus}{N}{\equiv}N\overset{\ominus}{Cl} \xrightarrow{H_2C=NOH} PhCH{=}NOH \xrightarrow{H_2O} PhCHO$$

(Benzene diazonium chloride) (Benzaldehyde oxime) (Benzaldehyde)

When arenediazonium salts are treated with formaldoxime, followed by hydrolysis with water, aromatic aldehydes are formed.

29. The Vilsmeyer-Haack reaction : Formylation of benzene, phenols, phenolic ethers, aromatic amines etc. by disubstituted formamides and phosphorus oxychloride is known as Vilsmeyer-Haack reaction.

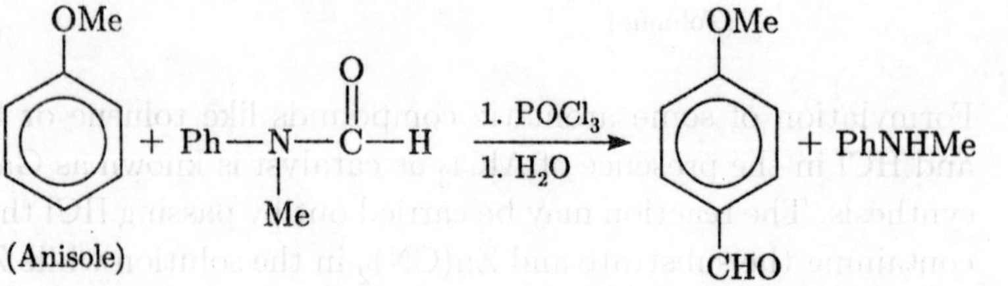

(Anisole)

This is by far the best method for the formylation of activated aromatic compounds. There are reactions where $COCl_2$ is used in place of $POCl_3$.

Mechanism :

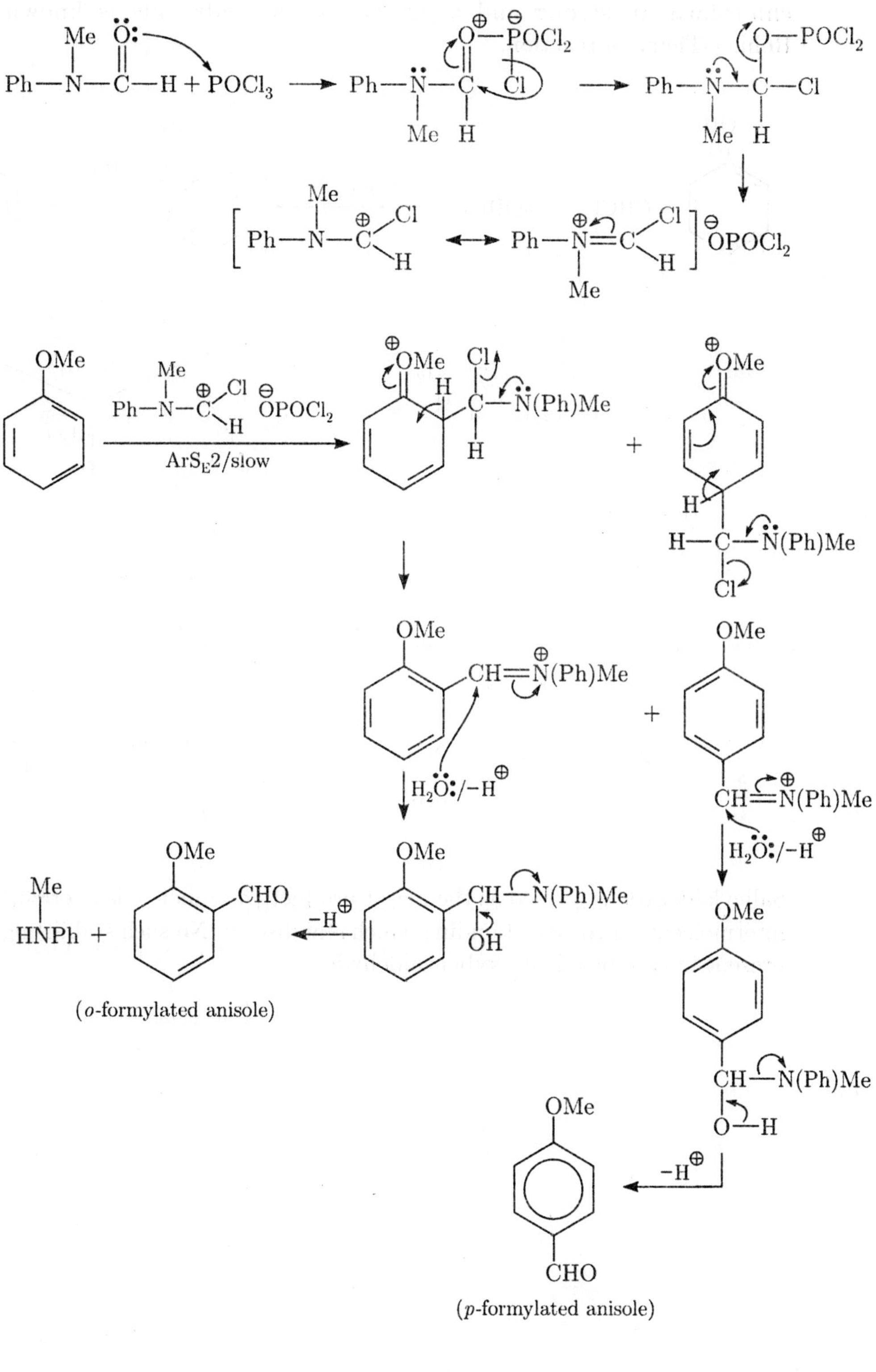

30. The Reimer-Tiemann reaction : Formylation of phenols by the reaction with chloroform in strong and aqueous sodium hydroxide is known as the Reimer-Tiemann reaction.

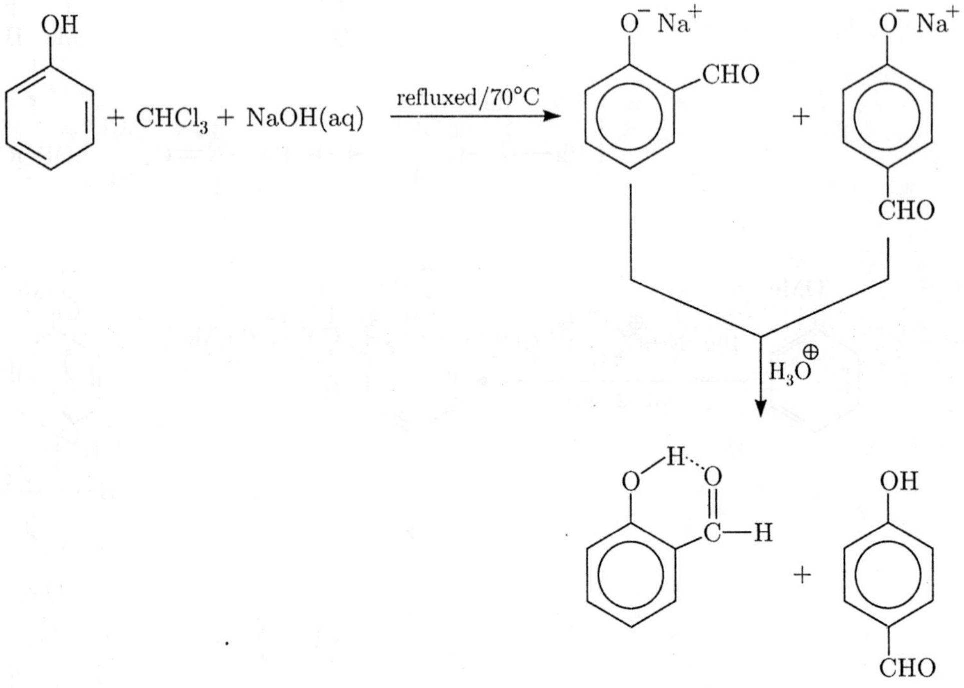

(Salicyladehyde) (*p*-Hydroxy-benzaldehyde)

4 : 1

Salicylaldehyde is formed as the major product (*o*-isomer: *p*-isomer=4:1) due to intermolecular hydrogen bonding which stabilises it. No such stabilising effect is present in case of *p*-hydroxybenzaldehyde.

Mechanism :

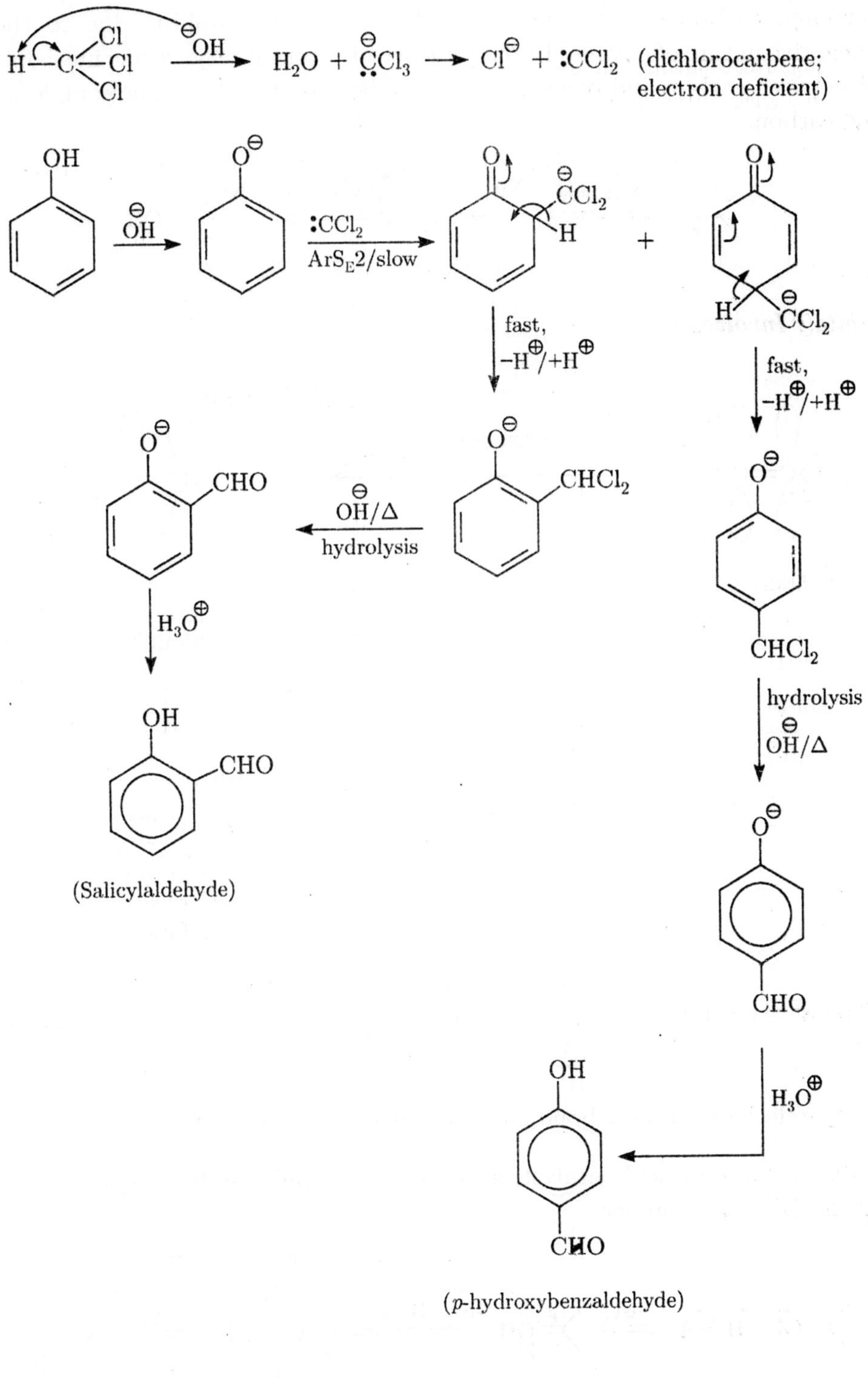
OH
H—C—Cl
Cl
Cl
H_2O + $\ddot{C}Cl_3$ → $Cl^{\ominus}$ + :CCl_2 (dichlorocarbene; electron deficient)
:CCl_2
ArS_E2/slow
fast,
$-H^{\oplus}/+H^{\oplus}$
$CHCl_2$
$\overset{\ominus}{O}H/\Delta$
hydrolysis
$H_3O^{\oplus}$
CHO
(Salicylaldehyde)
(p-hydroxybenzaldehyde)

Nucleophilic Addition to Carbon-Oxygen Double Bond (C=O)

The carbonyl carbon of an aldehyde or ketone is electrophilic due to the more electronegative nature of oxygen. In the presence of external reagent like nucleophile, the π bond between carbon and oxygen gets easily polarised and the nucleophile joins the carbonyl carbon.

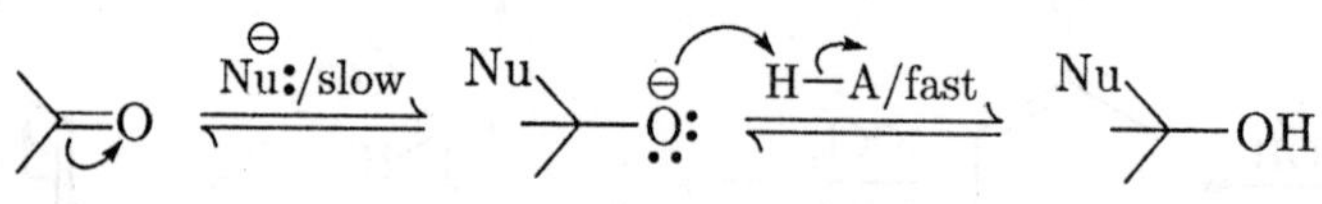

(Adduct)

Orbitals Involved :

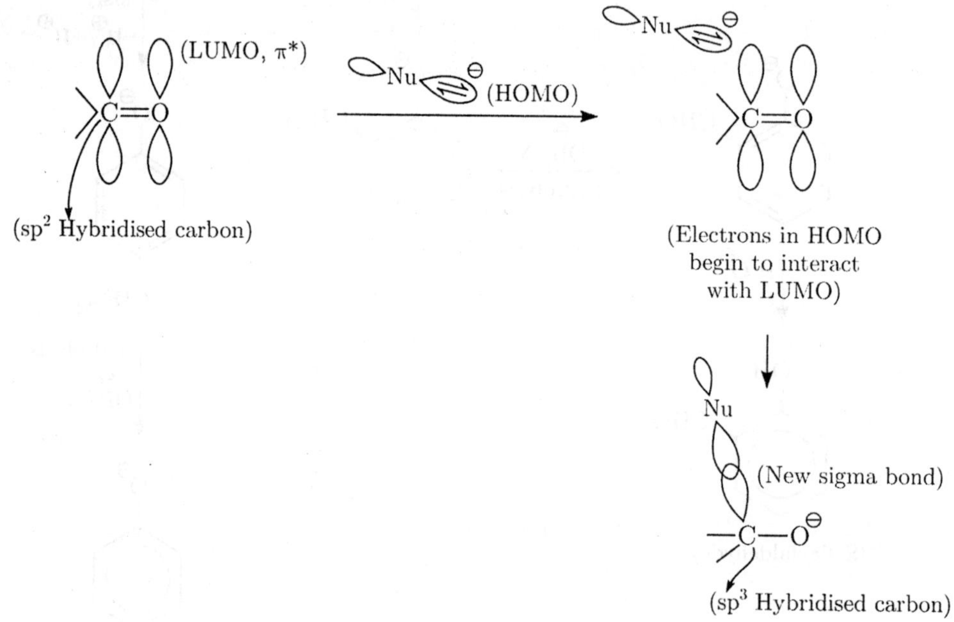

While at the same time, 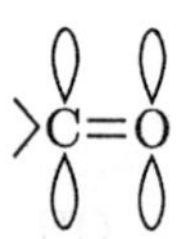 (filling up of π* causes π bond to break) to form

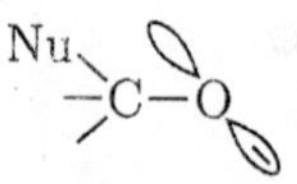 (electrons from π-bond end up as negative charge on oxygen).

In the presence of acid catalyst, a neutral nucleophile adds to a carbonyl carbon atom in the following manner.

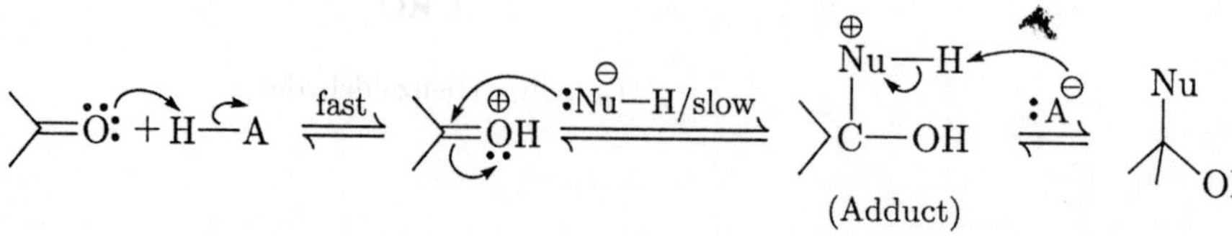

(Adduct)

This type of reaction pathway is called Ad_N2. Although a quick equilibrium is established between the reagents and the adduct, the extent of adduct formed is dependent on the $\Delta G°, \Delta H°$ and $\Delta S°$ of the reaction. So Ad_N2 is an example of thermodynamically controlled reaction.

If the nucleophile contains electronegative atoms like N,O, halogens etc., $\Delta H°$ of reaction becomes positive and the equilibrium shifts to the reactant side. Adduct breaks up into carbonyl compound and the product (adduct) becomes minor in the equilibrium.

Specific Examples

(a) 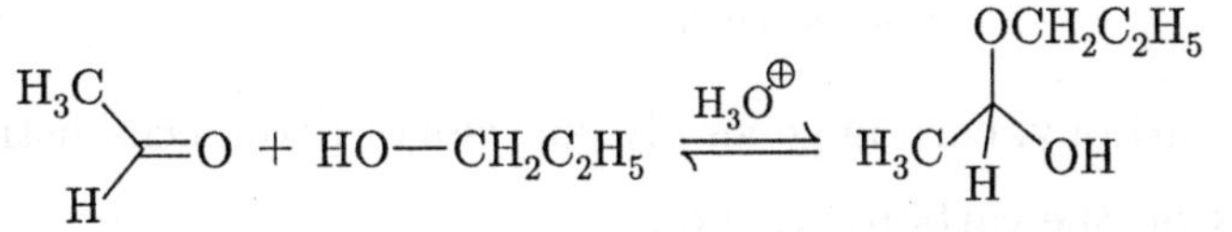

(a Hemiacetal)

(b) 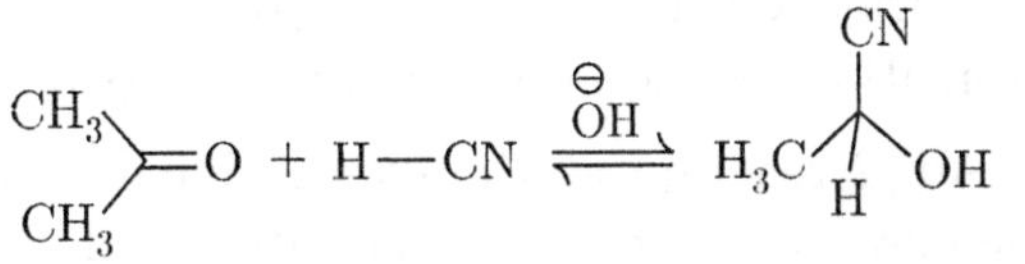

(a cyanohydrin)

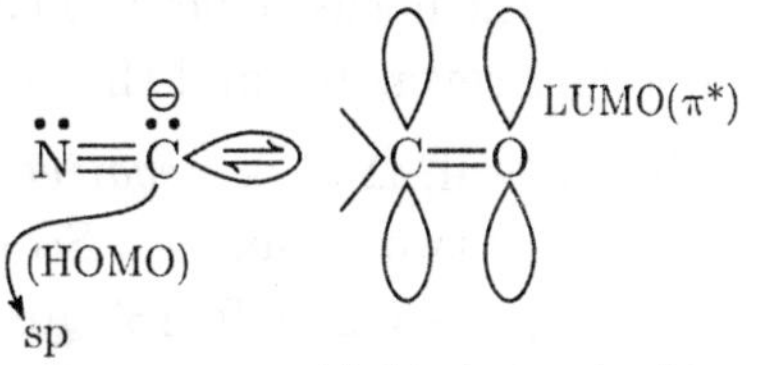

(Orbitals involved in addition of cyanohydrin)

Some equilibrium constants

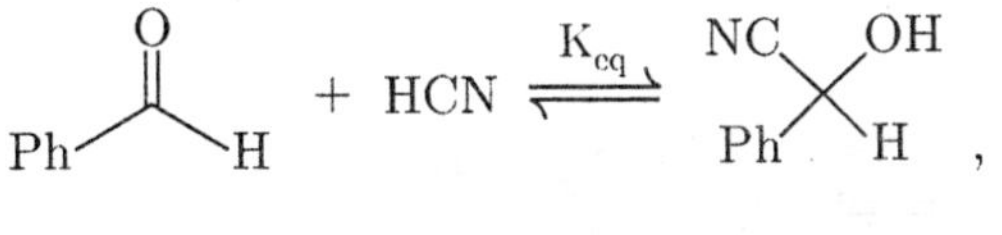

K_{eq}=212

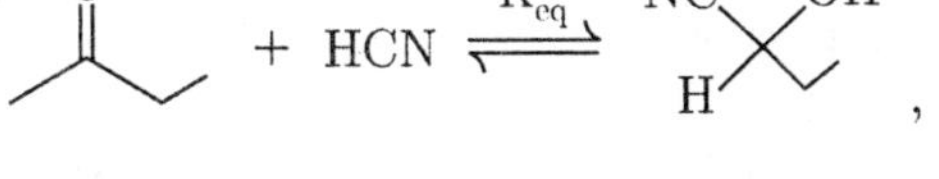

K_{eq}=28

The angle of nucleophilic attack on aldehydes and ketones

The nucleophiles approach the carbonyl group at a particular angle, not classically anticipated at an angle 90° (*i.e.*, perpendicular to the plane of carbonyl group). This angle is **107°** to the >C=O group and is known as **Bürgi-Dunitz trajectory**, after the authors of the elegant crystallographic methods that revealed it. This angle of attack is a result of compromise between maximum orbital overlap of the HOMO with π* and minimum repulsion of the HOMO by the electron density in the carbonyl π bond.

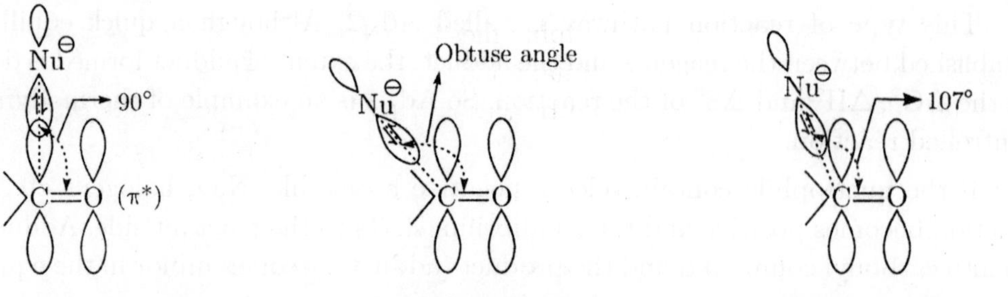

(Maximum overlap with π*, perpendicular to C=O bond)

(Repulsion from filled π-orbital forces nucleophile to attack at obtuse angle)

(Nucleophile attacks C=O at 107° angle (combined effect))

Note : Addition to the carbonyl carbon generally consists of two mechanistic steps.

1. Nucleophilic attack on the carbonyl carbon.
2. Protonation of the anion that results.

When the nucleophiles used are like hydrides cyanides and carbanions etc. the reaction is no longer reversible and the adduct fromation reaction becomes an irreversible process.

In general, $\Delta S°$ is *negative* for an Ad_N2 reaction as the translational randomness decreases for two molecules. So with increase in temperature, the rate of Ad_N2 reaction decreases ($\Delta G° = \Delta H - T\Delta S°$ and $\Delta S°$ is negative in this case). But if the carbonyl compound contains an *inbuilt* nucleophile and if either 5- or 6-membered adduct is formed by internal nucleophilic addition, then only rotational randomness decreases. As a result, the $\Delta S°$ becomes comparatively *less* negative. In other words, internal nucleophilic addition reaction has a higher rate than that of bimolecular nucleophilic addition.

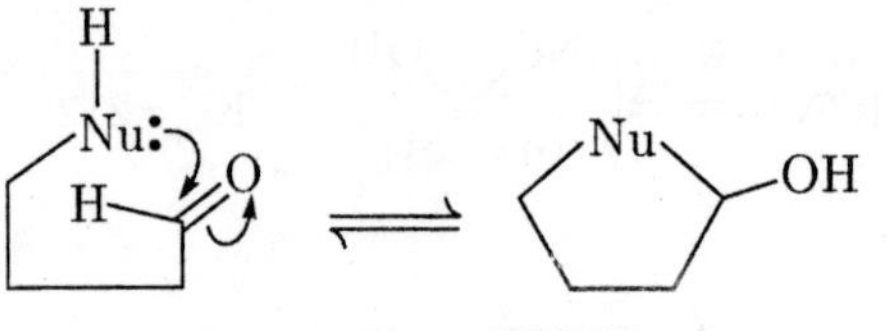

(Adduct)

Intramolecular Ad_N2 reaction

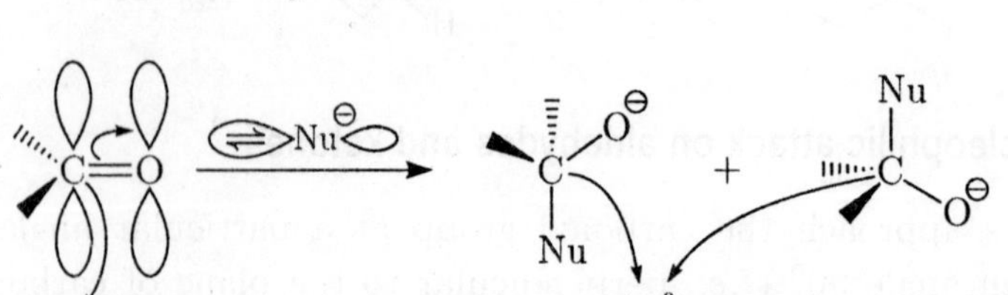

(Tetrahedral products)

If the two faces of carbonyl group is either *homotopic* or *enantiotopic*, then an *achiral reagent* attacks the two faces with equal probability(as the two transition states formed bear same energy content). But if the face be diasterotopic, the two transition states will bear non-mirror image relationship and the transition state having lower energy content will predominate.

The rate of Ad_N2 reaction depends on:

1. ***Concentration*** : The rate of Ad_N2 reaction increases with increase in concentration of substrates, or nucleophile or both. (the reaction is bimolecular in nature).
2. ***Electrophilicity of the carbonyl carbon*** : The electrophilicity of the carbonyl carbon increases with substituents having (–I, –R) effects, and the rate of Ad_N2 reaction increases. On the other hand, substituents with (+I, +R) effects decrease the rate of reaction. The presence of an acid catalyst (protic acid or Lewis acid) increases the electrophilicity of the carbonyl carbon and the rate of the reaction increases.

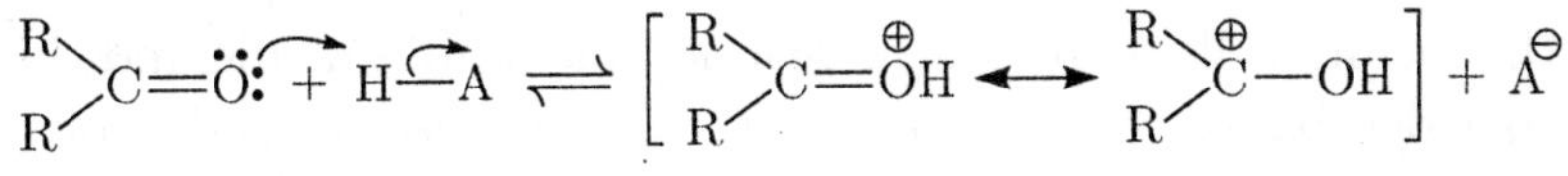

If the nucleophile possess basic characteristics, the rate of the reaction decreases in the presence of an acid, as the nucleophilicity gets decreased.

3. ***Steric effect*** : The state of hybridisation of carbonyl carbon (sp^2, bond angle 120°) changes to sp^3 hybridisation (bond angle 109°28′) by Ad_N2 reaction, and geometry from trigonal planar to tetrahedral. So, if the groups attached to the nucleophile or to the carbonyl carbon are bulky the transition state (which is product like with sp^3 bond angle, 109°28′) becomes *sterically crowded* and $\Delta G^{\neq}$ becomes high. As a result, the rate of the reaction decreases.
4. ***Effect of other strains*** : C=O group in small carbocyclic compounds contains bond angle ($C\hat{C}C$) lower than 120°. This angular strain is relieved in the transition state which is tetrahedral intermediate like. For this reason, the rate of Ad_N2 reaction is more with cyclopropanone and cyclobutanone.

   If the carbonyl substrate contains a dipolar bond at its α-position and exerts a strong dipole/dipole interaction, then nucleophilic addition gives a relief to this dipole-dipole interaction in the transition state As a result, $\Delta G^{\neq}$ becomes less and the rate of nucleophilic addition increases.

   The rate of cyanohydrin formation is more with chloral (Cl_3CCHO) than that with CH_3CHO. Apart from the (–I) effect of three Cl atoms, the strong dipole/dipole interaction becomes less in the tetrahedral intermediate.

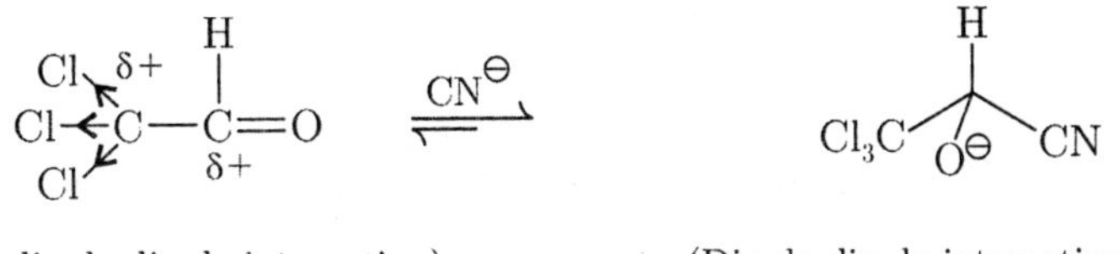

(Strong dipole-dipole interaction) (Dipole-dipole interaction is less in the tetrahedral intermediate interaction)

5. ***Relative stability of substrate and intermediate*** : If the substrate gets extra stability due to resonance, hyperconjugation etc., $\Delta G^{\neq}$ increases, and the rate of the reaction decreases. The rate of nucleophilic addition is less for aromatic ketones compared to aliphatic ketones. The carbonyl group is in resonance with the phenyl group in the aromatic ketones which is lost in the tetrahedral intermediate (and also in the transition state) and the reaction rate becomes less.
6. ***Reactivity of the nucleophiles*** : The π-bond of carbonyl group (C=O) is highly polarisable. So, at the very first stage of breaking up of a π-bond, the nucleophile starts forming bond with carbonyl carbon. In other words, the reactivity of a nucleophile is determined from the overlap factor. With increase in the energy level of HOMO, the rate of the reaction increases. In other words, the rate of Ad_N2 reactions increases with nucleophiles having big size, less electronegativity and more polarizability. The reactivity of the nucleophile depends on the pH of the medium. If the pH of the reaction medium is acidic and the nucleophile has considerable basicity, the reaction rate decreases considerably.

Summary of Ad_N2 reaction

1. When the reagent is a strong nucleophile ($\overset{\ominus}{Nu}$:), addition converts trigonal planar (sp^2 hybridised) aldehyde or ketone into a tetrahedral product.

   Mechanism :

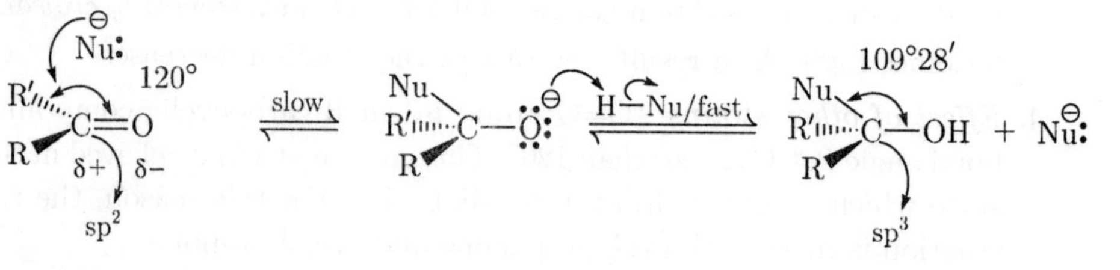

(Trigonal planar substrate) (Tetrahedral intermediate) (Tetrahedral product)

   Alkoxide oxygen being strongly basic removes a proton from H–Nu or from some other acid. The hybridisation state of carbonyl carbon changes from sp^2 to sp^3 and carbonyl oxygen accomodates the electron pair of C=O bond. In the second step, more basic alkoxide anion accepts a proton.

2. A second general mechanism that operates in nucleophilic addition to C=O double bond is an acid catalysed mechanism.

   Mechanism :

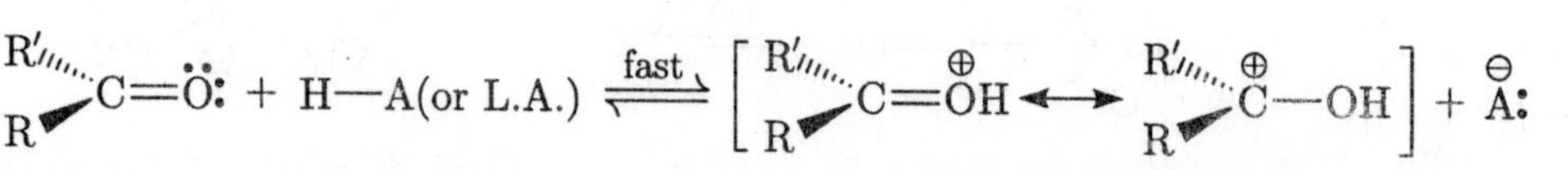

(Oxonium cation)

The carbon of oxonium cation is more succeptible to nucleophilic attack, than the carbonyl of the starting ketone.

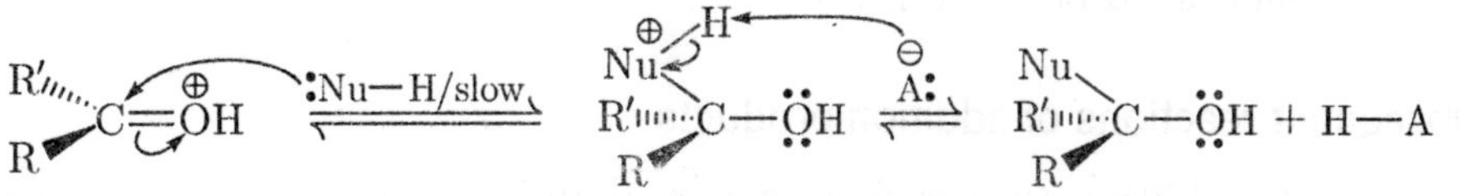

The oxonium ion accepts the electron pair of the nucleophile. Lastly a base (may be the conjugate base of the acid used) removes a proton from the positively charged atom, regenerating the acid.

This mechanism operates when carbonyl compounds are treated with strong acids in the presence of weak nucleophiles. Acid donates a proton to the electron pair of carbonyl oxygen atom. The protonated carbonyl compound, an oxonium cation, is highly reactive toward the nucleophilic attack at the carbonyl carbon atom because the carbonyl carbon carries more positive charge than it does in the unprotonated compound.

Reversibility of nucleophilic additions to the carbon-oxygen double bond

Many nucleophilic additions to C=O double bonds are reversible, the overall results of these reactions therefore depend on the position of the equilibrium. This behaviour contrasts markedly with most electrophilic additions to C=C bouble bonds and with nucleophilic substitutions at saturated carbon atoms. The latter reactions are essentially irreversible.

Relative reactivity : Aldehydes versus ketones

In general, aldehydes are more reactive in nucleophilic addition than are ketones. Both steric and electronic factors favour aldehydes. With one group being the small hydrogen atom, the central carbon of the tetrahedral product formed from an aldehyde is less crowded and the product becomes more stable. Formation of product is therefore favoured at equilibrium. With ketones, the two alkyl substituents at the carbonyl carbon cause greater steric crowding in the tetrahedral product and make it less stable. So, a small concentration of product is present at equilibrium.

Because alkyl groups are electron releasing, aldehydes are more reactive on electronic grounds. Aldehydes have only one electron releasing group to partially neutralise and therefore stabilise the positive charge at their carbonyl carbon atom, ketones have two electron releasing groups and are stabilised more. Greater stabilisation of the ketone (reactant) relative to its product means that the equilibrium constant for the formation of the tetrahedral product from a ketone is smaller and the reaction is less favourable.

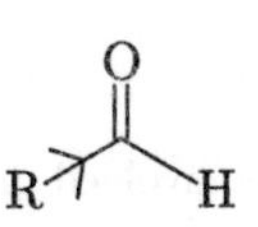

(Carbonyl carbon is more positive for aldehyde)

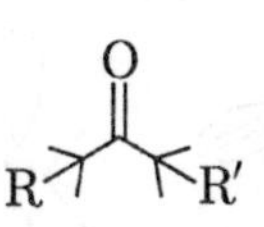

(Carbonyl carbon is less positive for ketones)

Electron withdrawing substituents like CF_3 or CCl_3 groups cause the carbonyl carbon to be more positive (starting compound becomes less stable) and cause the addition reaction to be more favourable.

Subsequent reactions of addition products

Nucleophilic addition to a carbon-oxygen double bond may lead to a product that is stable under the reaction conditions employed. If this be the case, the following product can be isolated.

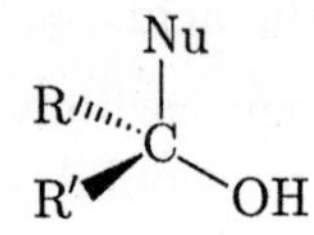

Examples of Ad_N2 reaction

1. **The addition of hydrogen cyanide** : Hydrogen cyanide adds to the carbonyl group of aldehydes and most ketones to form compounds called cyanohydrins. Ketones in which the carbonyl group is highly hindered do not undergo this reaction.

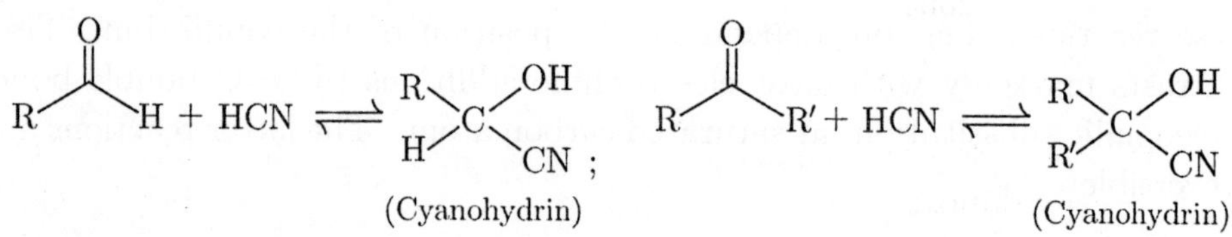

The reaction is usually carried out in the acidic medium (pH $\cong$ 4) to yield α-hydroxynitriles called aldehyde or ketone cyanohydrins. Sometimes the reaction is carried out in slightly basic medium also. The presence of acid in the former is needed to protonate the resulting alkoxide anion to produce final cyanohydrin. The addition of hydrogen cyanide itself takes place very slowly because HCN is a poor source of nucleophile (HCN is partially a covalent compound). The addition of KCN or NaCN or any base that can generate cyanide ions from the weak acid HCN, causes a dramatic increase in the rate of reaction.

Mechanism :

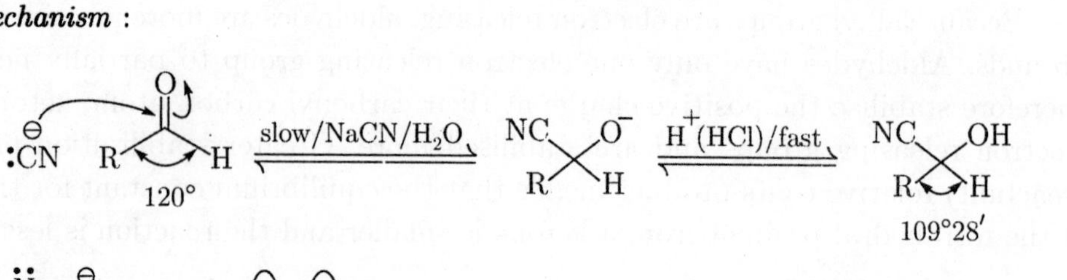

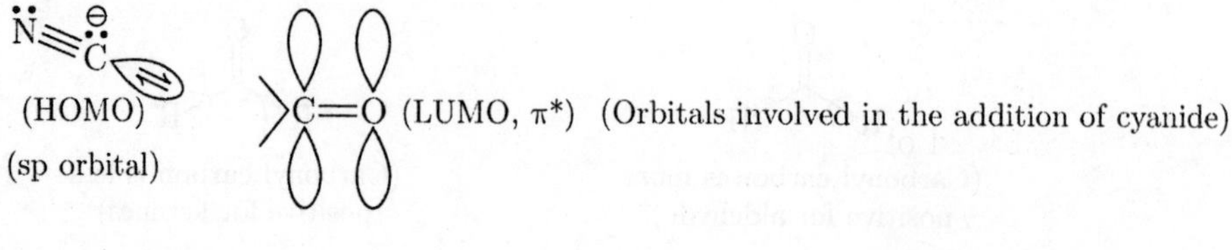

The base catalysed reaction follows a second order kinetics. Rate=k [substrate] [CN⊖], the addition of cyanide being slow and the protonation step is a fast step. This is a reversible reaction and the back reaction follows the E1cB pathway. The reversibility of cyanohydrin formation reaction is due to the fact that, it is a leaving group. The cyanide ion being a very strong nucleophile is able to attack the carbonyl carbon rapidly and once the addition of cyanide ion has taken place, the strongly basic alkoxide oxygen atom of the intermediate removes a proton from any available acid. If this acid be HCN, this step generates cyanide ion. Bases stronger than cyanide ion catalyse the reaction by converting HCN ($pk_a \cong 9$) to cyanide ion in an acid-base reaction. The cyanide ions, thus formed can go on attack the carbonyl group.

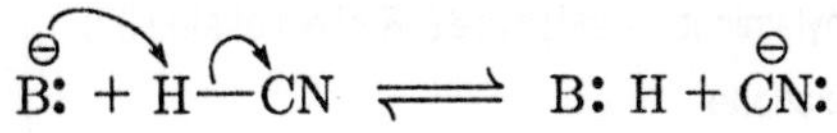

HCN (a gas) is generated in the reaction mixture, as it is toxic and volatile. This can be done by mixing the aldehyde or ketone with aqueous NaCN and then slowly adding H_2SO_4 to the mixture. Cyanohydrins are useful intermediates in organic synthesis.

1. 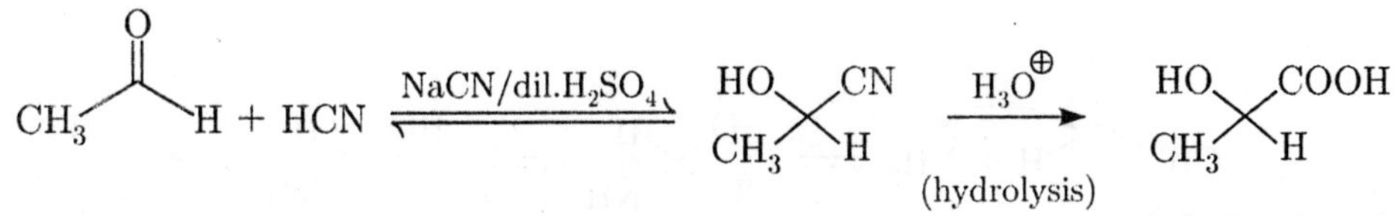

(±)- Lactic acid

2. 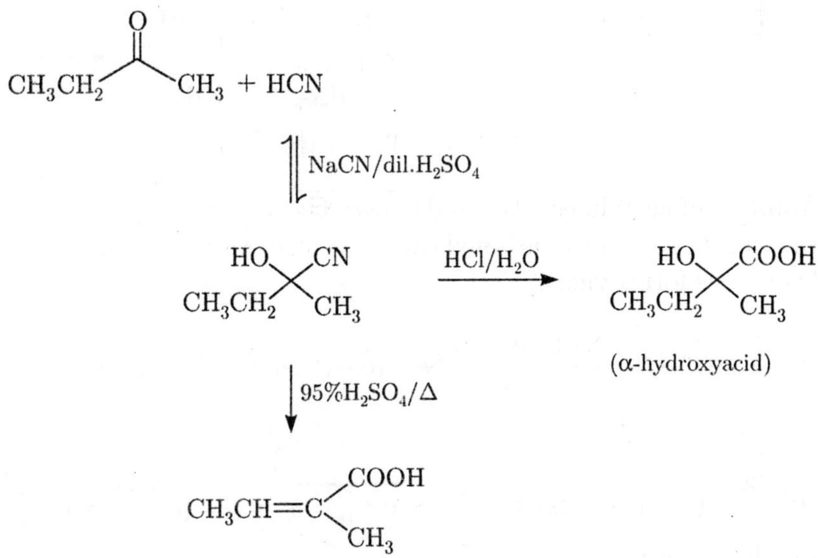

(α-hydroxyacid)

(α,β-unsaturated acid)

3. 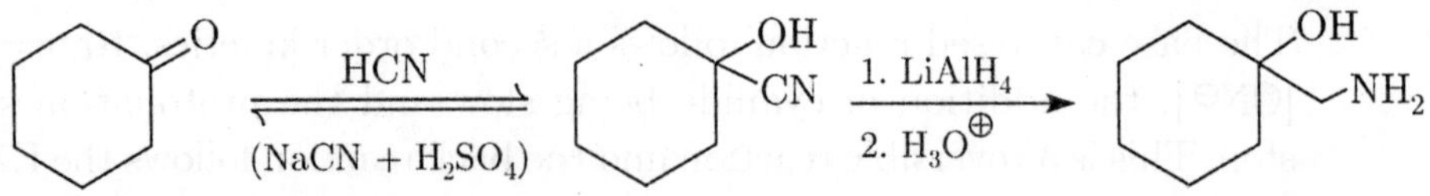

High acid concentration suppresses the dissociation of hydrocyanic acid since it is a weak acid and consequently has low cyanide ion concentration.

Carbonyl compounds	K formation of cyanohydrin
1. Acetaldehyde (no steric congestion)	Immeasurably high
2. *p*-nitrobenzaldehyde (–R and –I effect of $-NO_2$ group)	1430
3. *p*-Methoxybenzaldehyde (+R effect of $-OCH_3$ group)	210
4. *p*-dimethylaminobenzaldehyde (+R effect of Me_2N)	2.5
5. Cyclohexanone	10,000
6. Ethyl methyl ketone (steric congestion)	38
7. Acetophenone (steric congestion)	0.77
8. Benzophenone (steric congestion)	Immeasurably low

1. Addition of ammonia to acetaldehyde

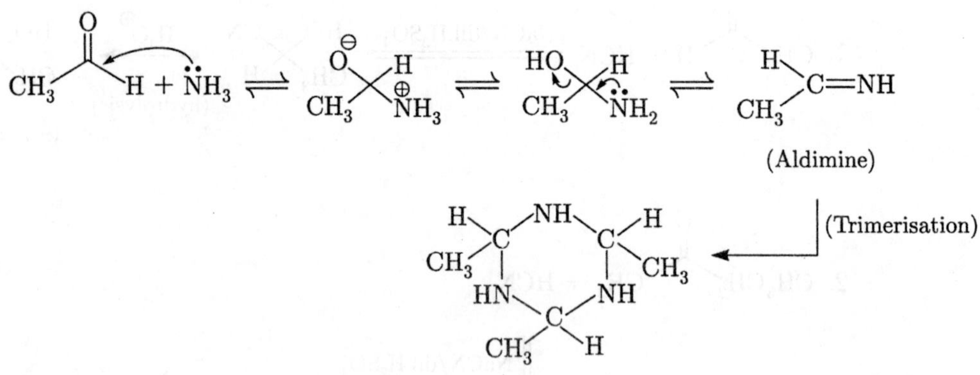

2. Addition of acetylides : Acetylide ions are strong nucleophiles and readily attack the electron-deficient carbonyl carbon centre. Metal ynolate is formed which on hydrolysis forms ynols.

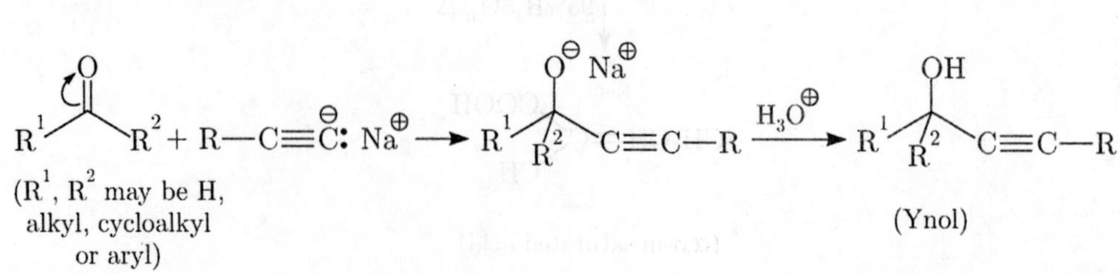

Ynols may be converted to other compounds of synthetic value.

Example :

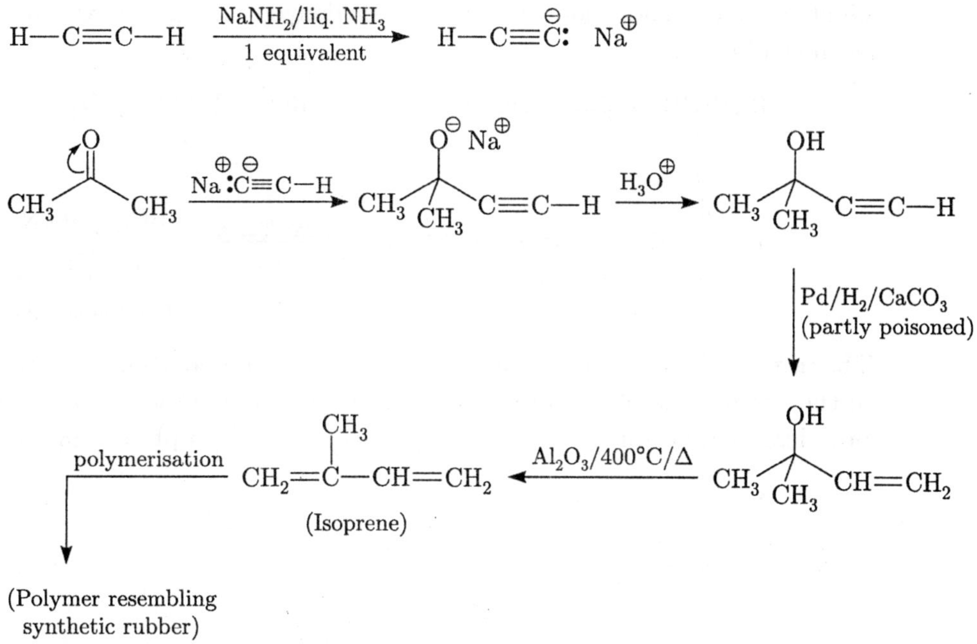

3. **Addition of sodium bisulphite ($NaHSO_3$)** : When aldehydes and ketones are shaken with an aqueous solution of saturated sodium bisulphite, slightly soluble bisulphite addition compounds, called aldehyde bisulphite and ketone bisulphite addition compounds are formed. The reaction is a *reversible* one.

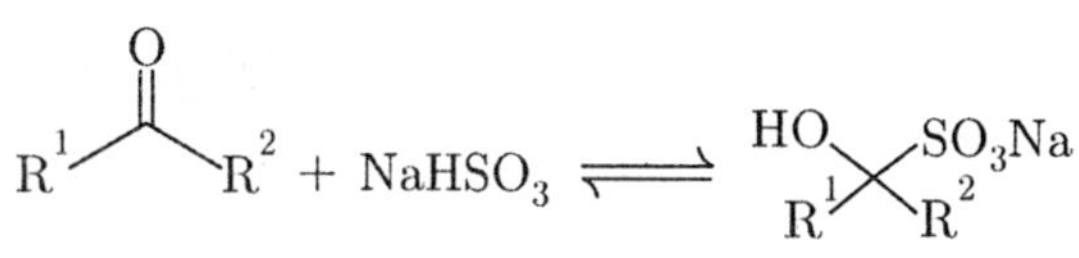

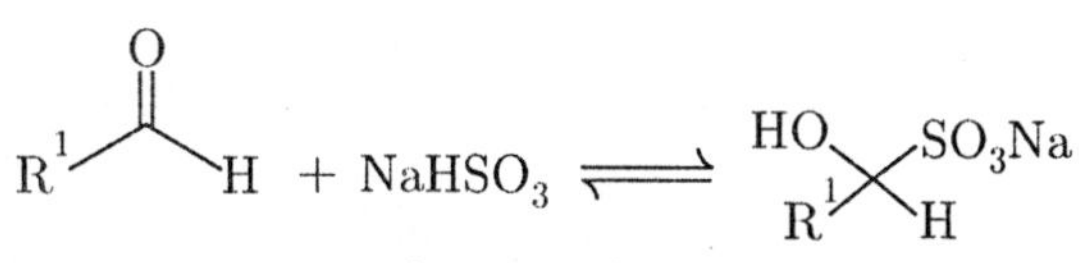

It is important to note that, if R^1 and R^2 groups are larger than methyl, the addition compounds are formed with difficulty. The main importance of bisulphite addition compounds is their use to separate carbonyl compounds from their mixtures with other organic compounds. Since, bisulphite addition compounds are salts, they become insoluble in organic solvents, and can be separated from other organic compounds by filtering and washing with ether. The bisulphite adduct formation being a reversible reaction, the carbonyl compound is regenerated by any reagent that reacts irreversibly with the bisulphite adduct. Usually, alkalis are used to regenerate the ketones and acids to regenerate the aldehydes. However, the position of equilibrium for the reaction of formaldehyde with bisulphite is more to the right than with any aldehyde or ketone, the carbonyl compound can be regenerated by heating a bisulphite adduct with a slight excess of an aqueous solution of formaldehyde through an exchange reaction as shown below.

$$RCH(OH)SO_3Na + HCHO \rightleftharpoons RCHO + H_2C(OH)SO_3Na$$

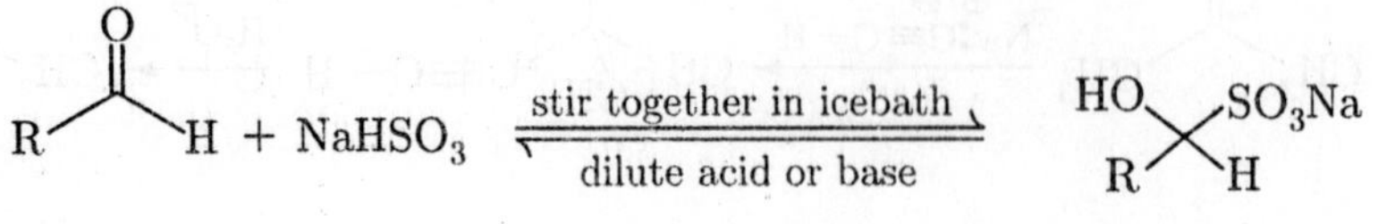

(Crystalline solid)

The reversibility of the reaction makes bisulphite compounds useful intermediates in the synthesis of other adducts from aldehydes and ketones. For example, one practical method for making cyanohydrins involve bisulphite compounds.

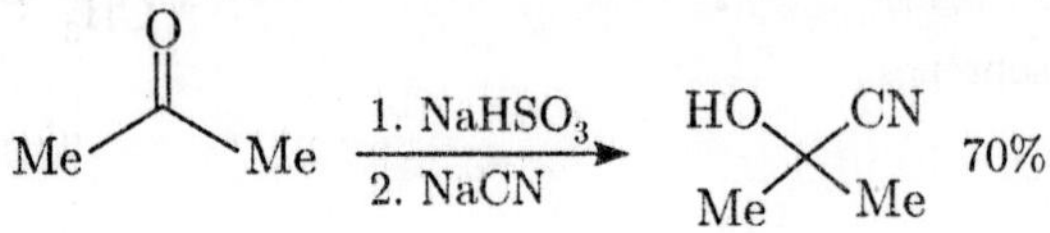

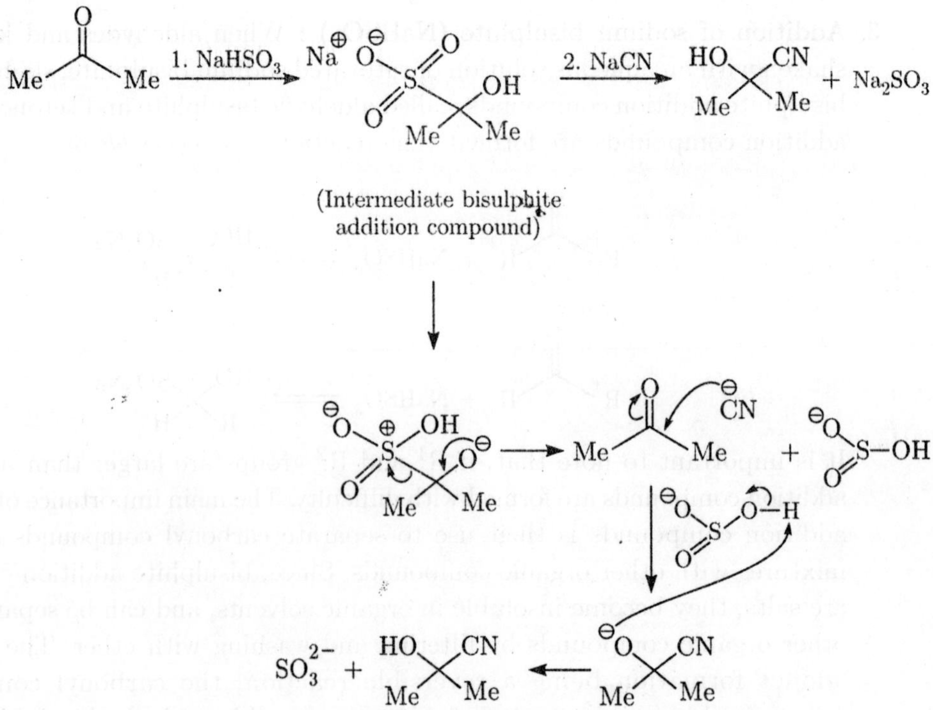

(Intermediate bisulphite addition compound)

(Cyanohydrine of acetone)

Mechanism of bisulphite addition reaction :

$$NaHSO_3 \longrightarrow Na^{\oplus} + HSO_3^{\ominus}; \quad H_2O + HSO_3^{\ominus} \rightleftharpoons H_3O^{\oplus} + \underset{\text{(Sulphite ion)}}{SO_3^{2-}}$$

***Step* 1** : Nucleophilic attack by the sulphite ion through sulphur (S being more nucleophilic than O) on the electron-deficient carbonyl carbon.

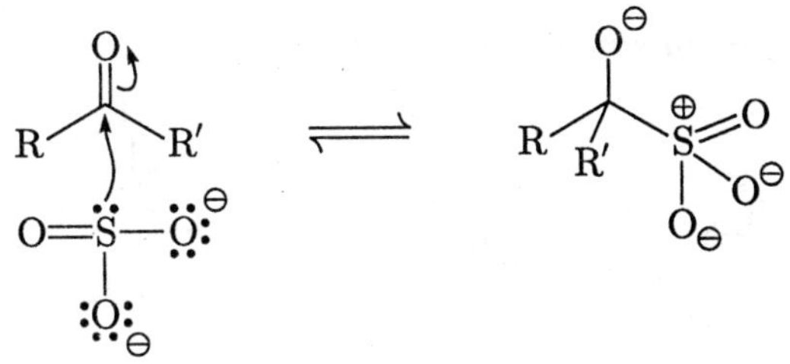

***Step* 2** : Protonation of alkoxide oxygen.

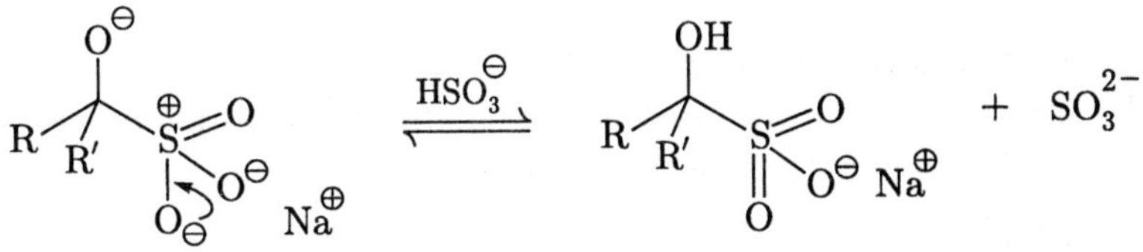

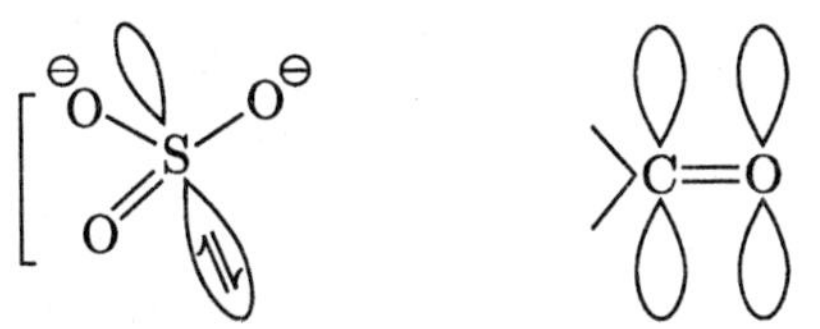

(HOMO=sulphur hybrid contains lone pair)

LUMO (π*)

[Orbitals involved in the addition of bisulphite]

4. **Addition of alcohols** : Alcohols add to aldehydes and ketones in the presence of specific acid catalysts to yield acetals via hemiacetals. Acetals are 1,1-diethers and hemiacetals are ether alcohols, *i.e.*, half acetals. Acetal formation reaction is also an equilibrium related reaction, where a slow equilibrium is established between aldehyde or ketone and hemiacetal.

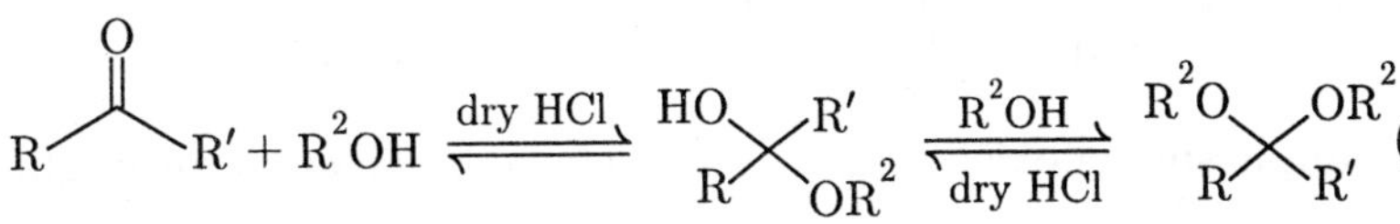

(R and R′=H or alkyl) (Acetal) (ΔH=20–40 kJ/mol)

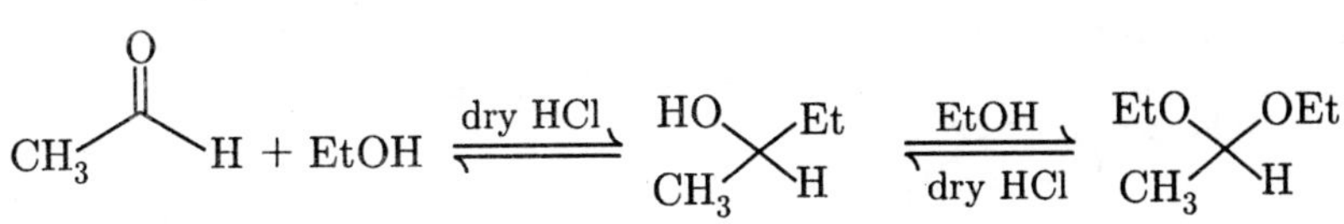

Names for functional groups

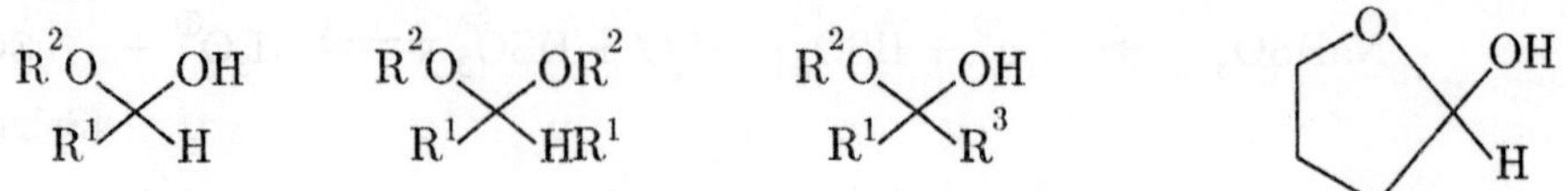

(Hemiacetal) (Acetal) (Hemiacetal from ketone or hemiketal) (A cyclic hemiacetal or lactol)

Mechanism of formation of hemiacetals :

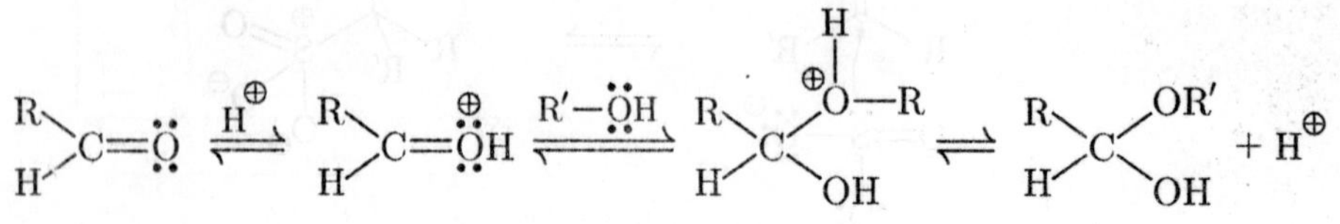

(Aldehyde) (Ketone also may be taken) (Hemiacetal) (usually unstable to be isolated)

The essential structural features of a hemiacetal are an –OH and an –OR group attached to the same carbon atom. Most open chain hemiacetals are too unstable to be isolated. Cyclic hemiacetals with 5- or 6- membered rings are comparatively more stable.

A stable hemiacetal :

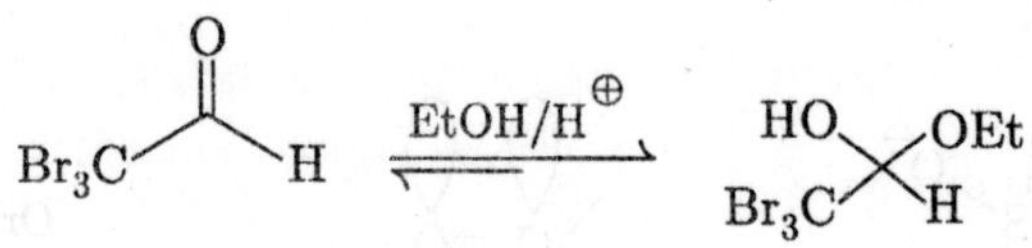

(a) 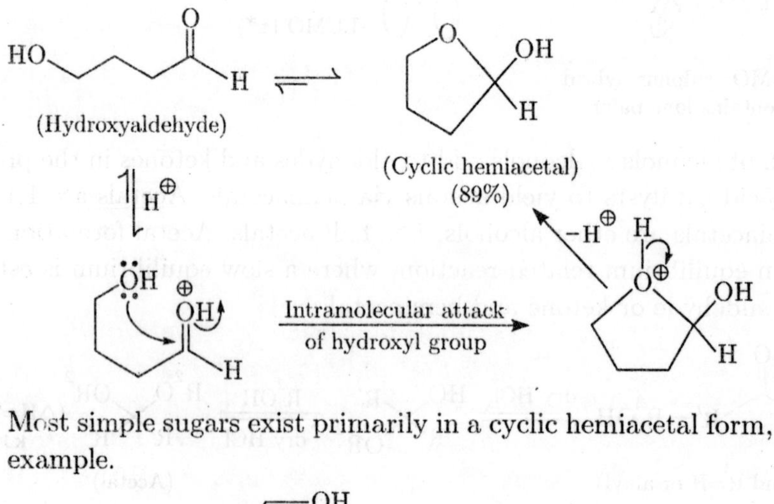

(b) Most simple sugars exist primarily in a cyclic hemiacetal form, glucose being an example.

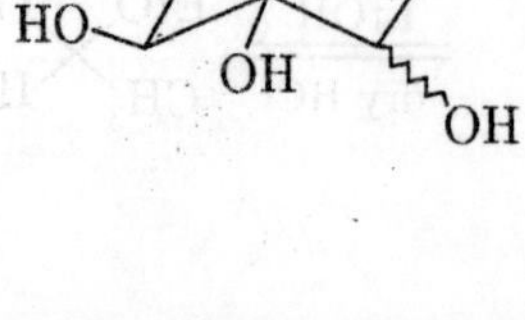

(+)– Glucopyhanose (*a cyclic hemiacetal*)

(c) $HO(CH_2)_4CHO \rightleftharpoons$

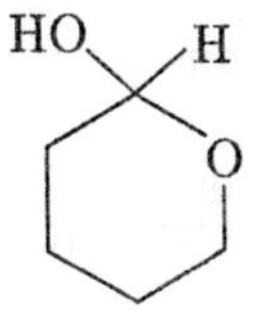

(Cyclic hemiacetal, 99%)

(d) $HO(CH_2)_8CHO \rightleftharpoons$

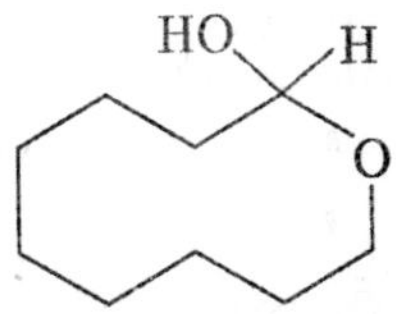

(10–membered ring, 9%)

(e) $3 \times CH_3CHO + H^{\oplus} \rightleftharpoons$

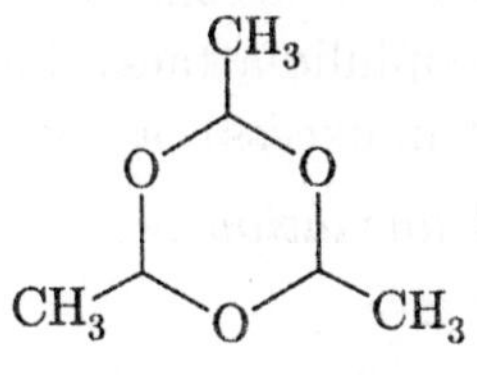

(Paraldehyde)

Part of the reason for the stability of cyclic hemiacetals concerns entropy. Formation of an acyclic hemiacetal involves a decrease in entropy (ΔS° negative) because two molecules are consumed for everyone produced. This is not the situation for the formation of a cyclic hemiacetal, where one molecule of hemiacetal is produced from one molecule of hydroxyaldehyde and only rotational randomness is decreased with no change in translational randomness. The cyclic hemiacetal formation reactions may be viewed as intramolecular hemiacetal formation reaction. Ketones undergo similar reactions when they are dissolved in an alcohol. The *unstable* products are sometimes called hemiketals, which is no longer recommended by IUPAC. The preferred usage is to call them hemiacetals as well.

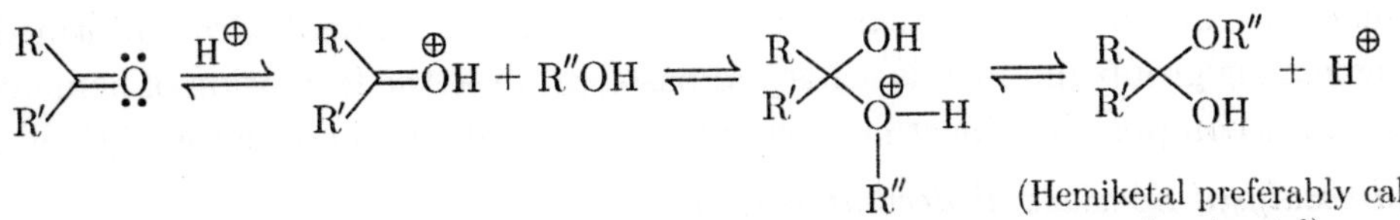

(Hemiketal preferably called hemiacetal)

Acid or base catalysts increase the rate of equilibration of hemiacetals with their aldehyde and alcohol parents.

Acid-catalysed hemiacetal formation

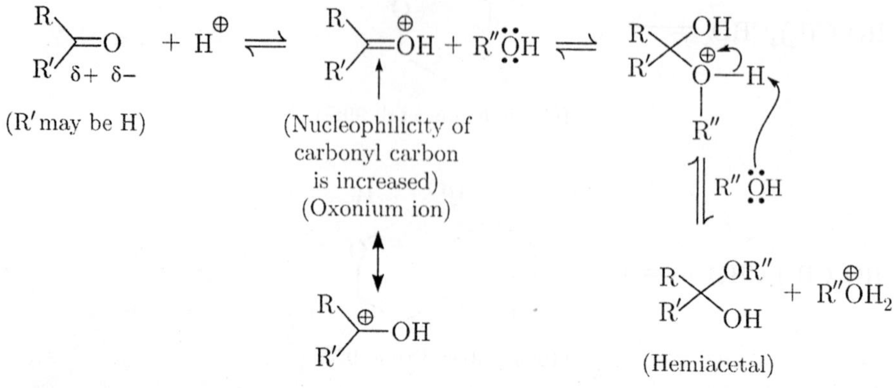

Protonation of the aldehyde or ketone oxygen atom makes the carbonyl carbon atom more succeptible to nucleophilic attack. The protonated alcohol results from the reaction of the alcohol (present in excess) or with the acid catalyst, *e.g.*, HCl.

Base-catalysed hemiacetal formation :

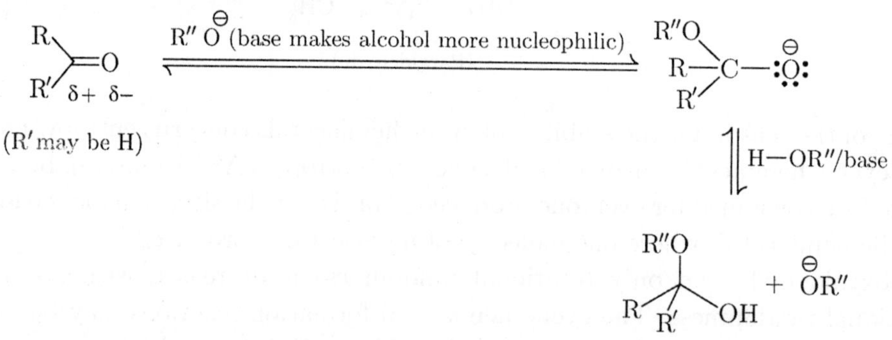

The alkoxide anion acting as a nucleophile, attacks the carbonyl carbon atom. An electron pair shifts onto the oxygen atom producing a new alkoxide anion, which abstracts a proton from an alcohol molecule to produce the hemiacetal and regenerates an alkoxide anion.

Hemiacetals are unstable because they are essentially tetrahedral intermediates containing leaving group and just as acids and bases catalyse the formation of hemiacetals, they also can decompose hemiacetals back into starting aldehyde or ketone and alcohol.

Acid-catalysed hemiacetal decomposition :

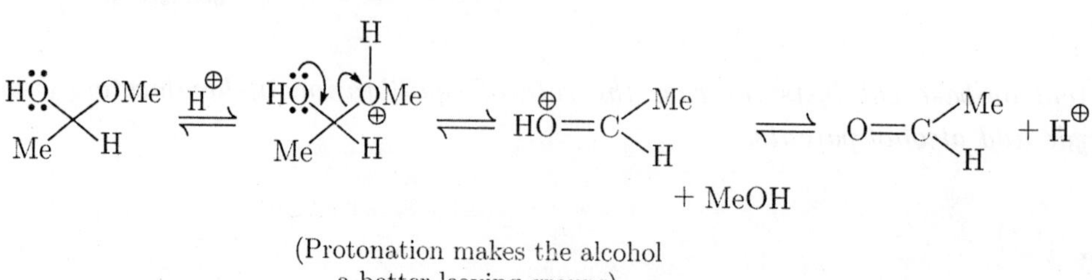

Base-catalysed hemiacetal decomposition :

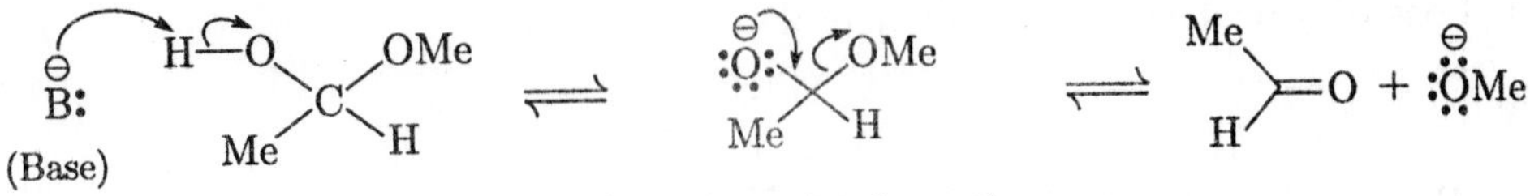

(Deprotonation forces the alcohol to leave as an alkoxide)

Summary : Hemiacetal formation and decomposition are catalysed by acid or base.

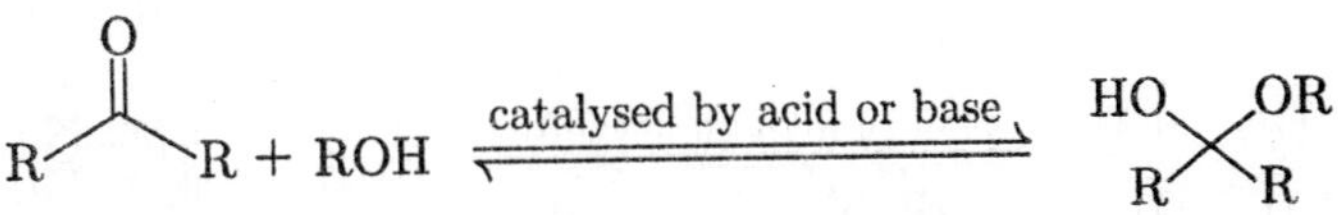

(Hemiacetal)

Acetals and cyclic acetals are formed from aldehydes or ketones with alcohols in the presence of acid :

When a small amount of gaseous HCl or *p*-TsOH is passed into an alcoholic solution of an aldehyde, hemiacetal is formed first and then a second reaction takes place. The hemiacetal reacts with a second molar equivalent of the alcohol to produce an acetal (or ketal). An acetal has two –OR groups attached to the same carbon atom. Usually aldehydes undergo the acetal formation reaction readily since the equilibrium lies to the right at room temperature. The position of equilibrium of the reaction between ketones and monohydric alcohols at room temperature is so far to the left that ketals do not form appreciably. At a low temperature, however, the reaction between methyl alcohol and unhindered ketones is somewhat favourable. For example, acetone reacts with methyl alcohol at –27°C in the presence of strong acid ion-exchange resin as catalyst.

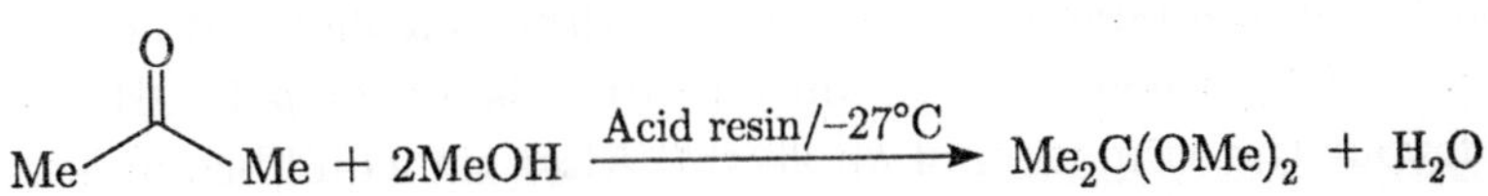

Acetal formation reaction is *acid-catalysed*, it can not be done in the presence of base.

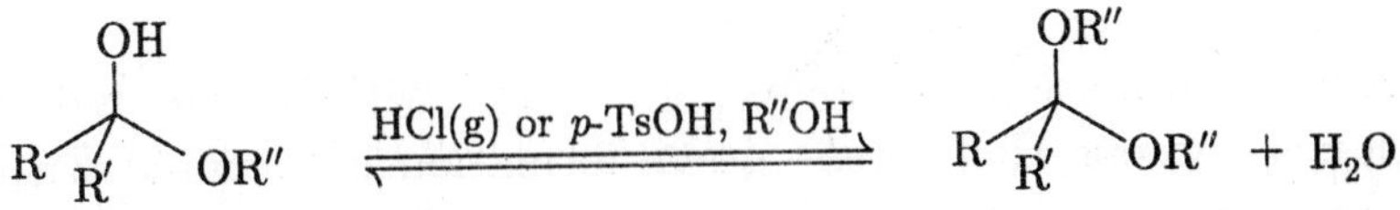

(Hemiacetal) (Acetal)

(R′ may be H)

The stages of acetal formation reaction are as follows.

1. Protonation of the hydroxyl group of hemiacetal.
2. Loss of water by elimination. This elimination leads to an unstable and highly reactive oxonium ion.

3. Addition of methanol to the oxonium ion.
4. Loss of a proton to give the acetal.

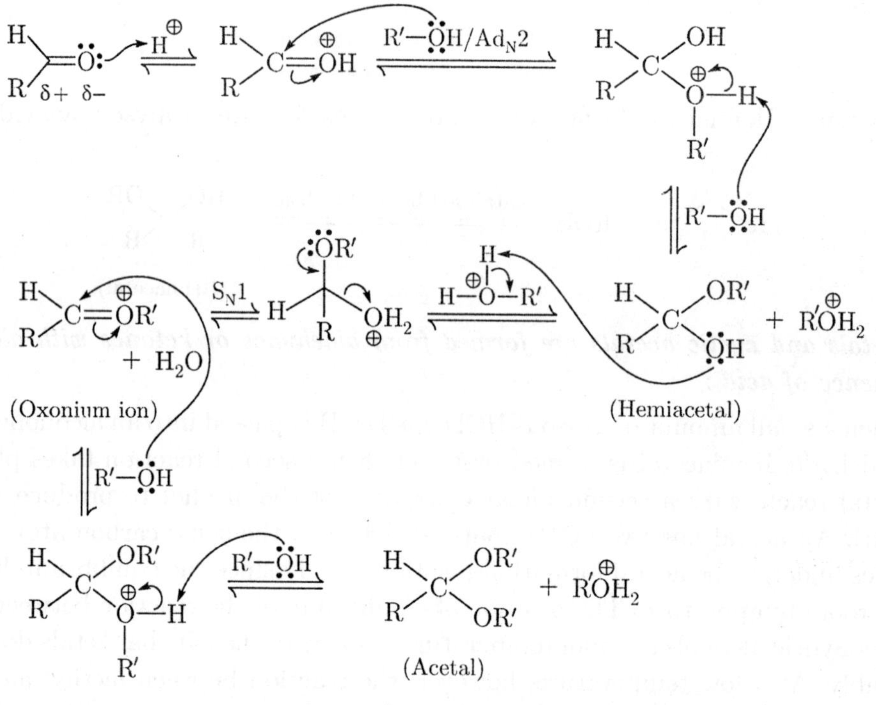

All the steps in the formation of an acetal from an aldehyde are *reversible.* If we dissolve an aldehyde in a large excess of an anhydrous alcohol and add a small amount of an anhydrous acid (gaseous HCl or concentrated H_2SO_4 or *p*-TsOH), the equilibrium will strongly favour the formation of an acetal. After the equilibrium is established, we can isolate acetal by neutralising the acid and evaporating the excess alcohol. In the preparation of ethyl acetals, the water is removed by adding benzene since water, ethyl alcohol and benzene form a constant boiling mixture at 65°C.

Although acetal formation reaction is not favoured with ketones and simple alcohols in the presence of gaseous HCl, *cyclic acetal* formation is favoured when a ketone is treated with an excess of 1,2-diol and a trace of acid.

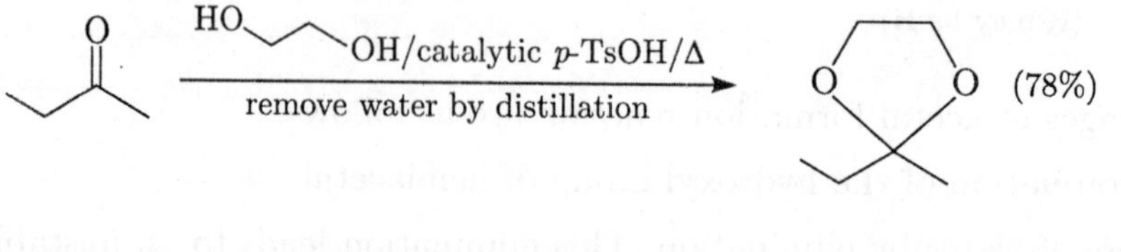

Mechanism :

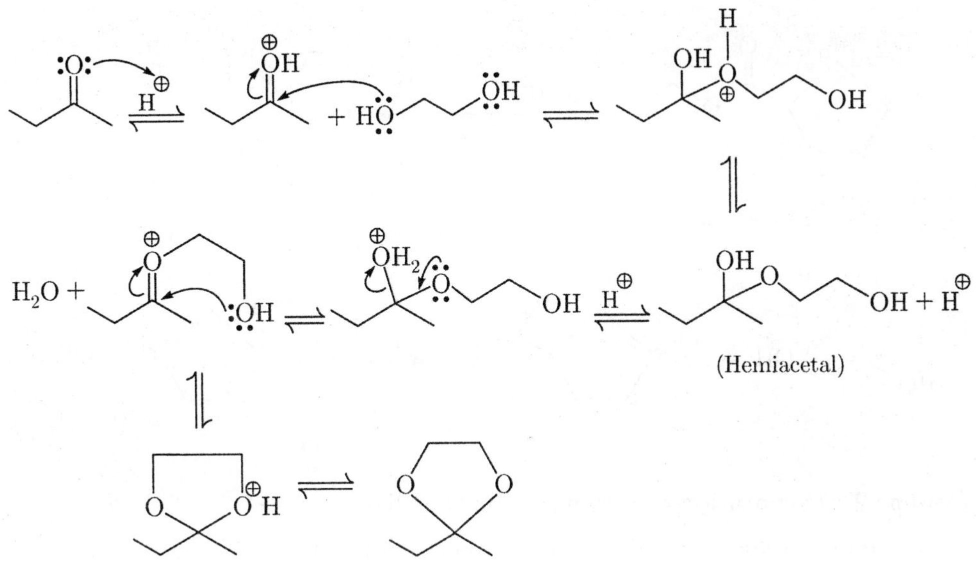

(Dioxolane, a cyclic acetal)

Cyclic acetals are more resistant to hydrolysis and easier to make than the acyclic ones. Again the entropy factors to thank for their stability. For the formation of a cyclic acetal, two molecules go in (ketone + diol) and two molecules go out (acetal+water) and so the unfavourable ΔS° factor is no longer against this.

Acetals as protecting group

Acetals are hydrolysed in aqueous acid, but they are stable towards bases. Acetals do not contain any active H atom which can be abstracted by a base, so the acetals can not be hydrolysed by bases. Moreover, alkoxide anion is a poor leaving group, so base catalysed hydrolysis of acetals does not occur.

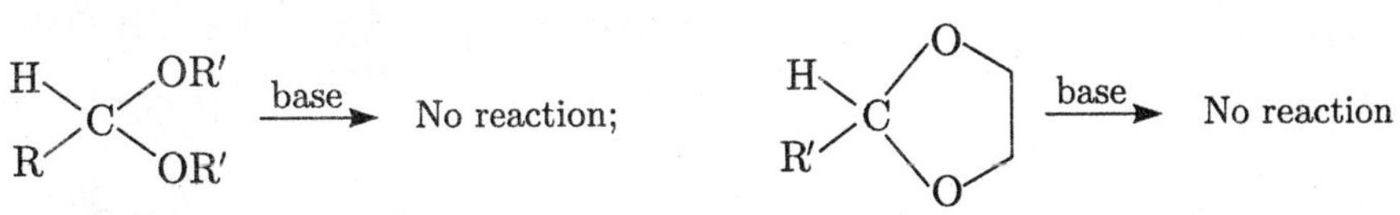

Because of this property, acetals give us a convenient method for protecting aldehyde and ketone functionalities from undesired reactions in basic solutions. Acetals are geminal diethers and like other ethers, they are unreactive towards bases.

Example 1 : Conversion of 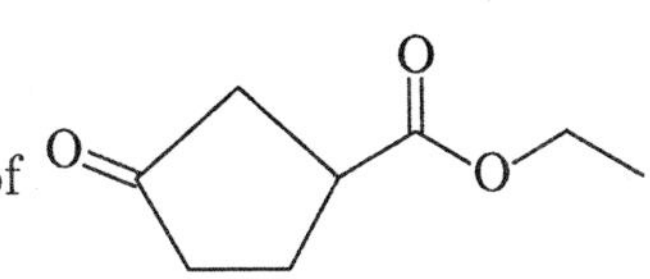 to 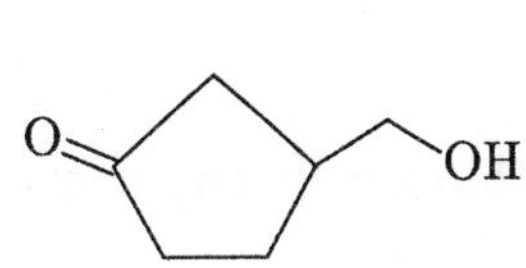

Keto groups are more readily reduced than the ester groups. Any reducing agent ($LiAlH_4$ or H_2/Ni) that can reduce ester group can reduce carbonyl group as well. But if the keto group is protected by a cyclic acetal (the ester group does not react) we can reduce the ester group in basic solution without affecting the cyclic acetal.

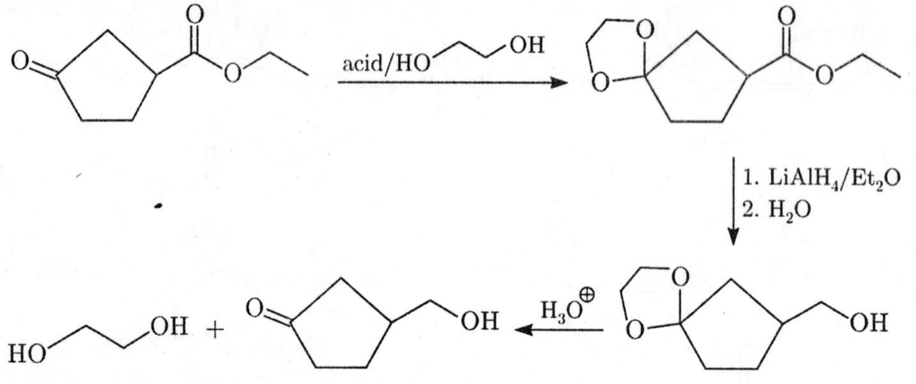

Exampe 2 : Preparation of Grignard Reagent like 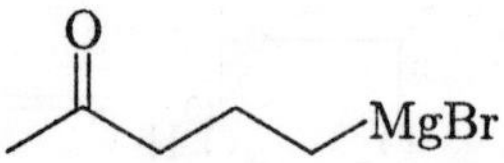

This Grignard reagent is impossible to synthesise as it would react with itself. But the same Grignard Reagent can be prepared by protecting the keto group with acetal-forming step.

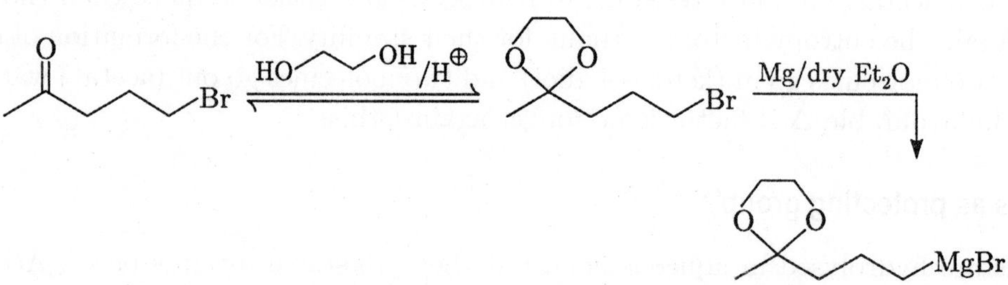

Example 3 :

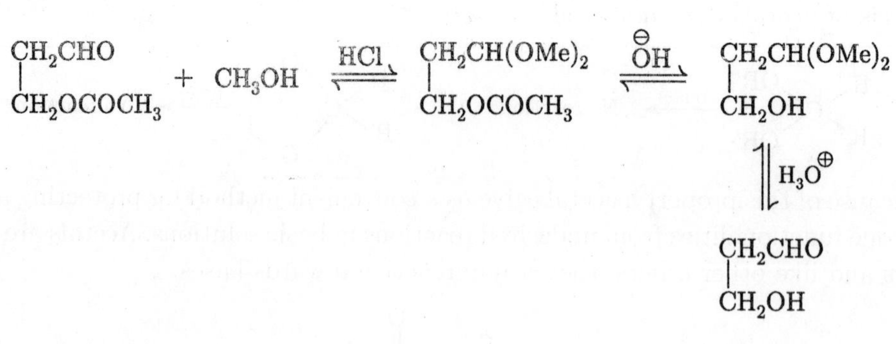

Thioacetals and cyclic thioacetals

Aldehydes and ketones react with thiols to form thioacetals. The nucleophilicity of sulphur being greater than that of oxygen, thiols undergo the acetal formation reaction more readily than the alcohols. The thioacetals are relatively stable to dilute acids and bases.

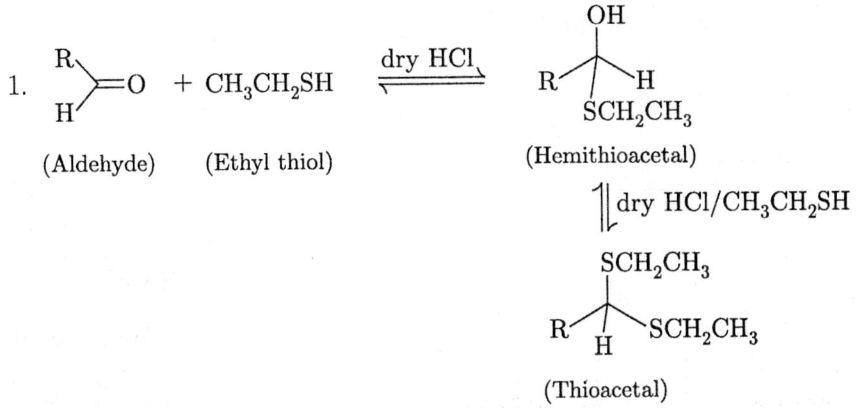

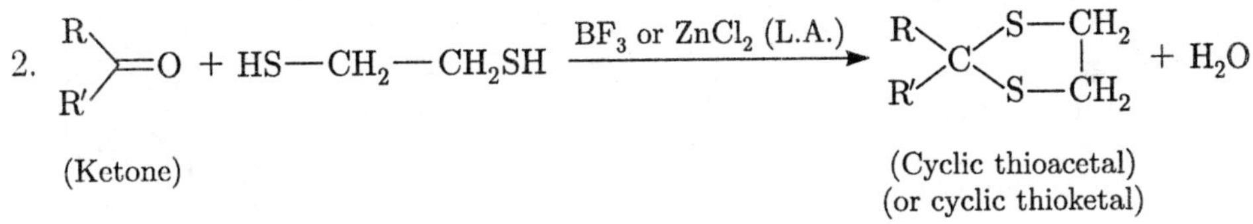

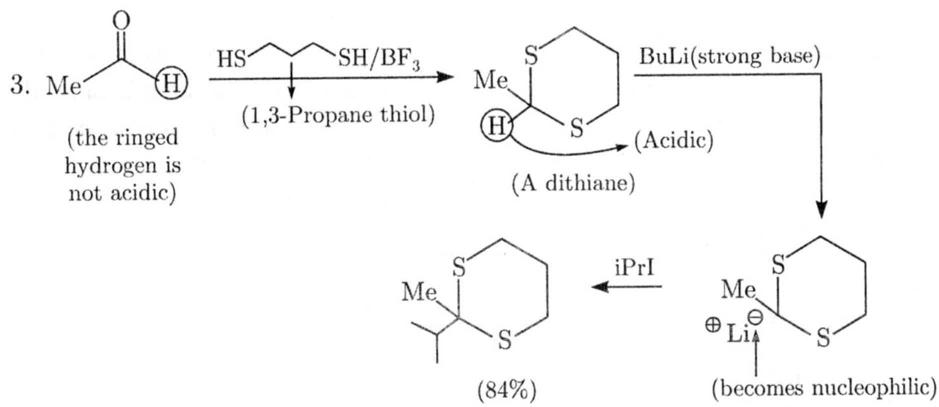

Dithianes are extremely important compounds in organic synthesis because going from ketone to thioacetal inverts the polarity at the functionalised carbon atom. This is a case of UMPOLUNG and dithianes are one of the most important umpolung reagents.

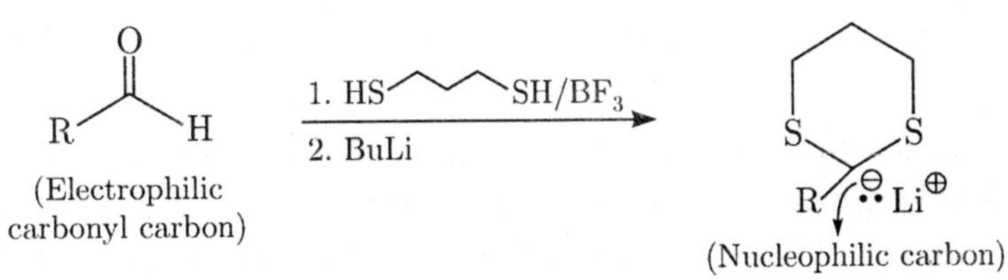

Dithianes are more stable than acetals, being stable in dilute acids. A mercury reagent ($HgCl_2/CdCO_3$ mixture) has to be used to assist their hydrolysis. Hg (II) and sulphides form strong coordination complexes and Hg (II) catalyses the reaction by acting as a sulphur selective Lewis acid.

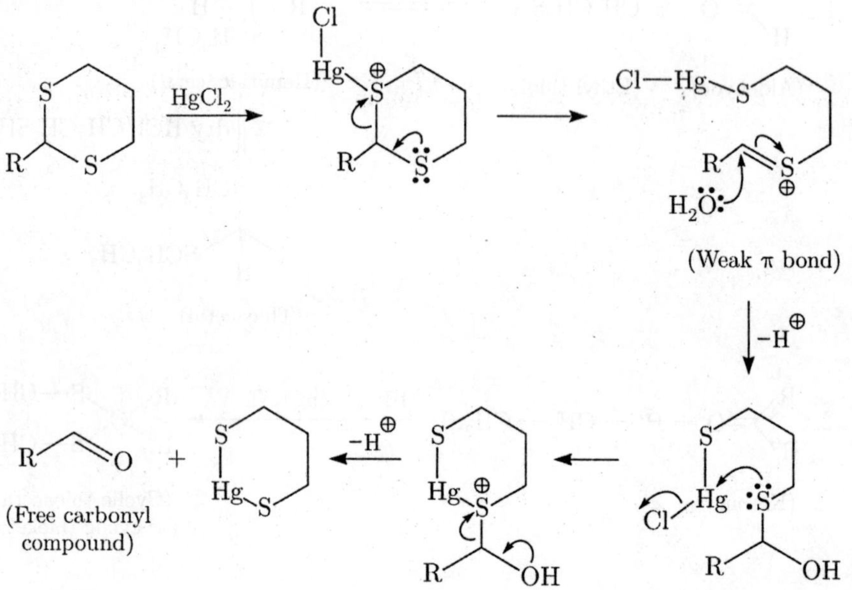

There are two reasons why the normal acid-catalysed hydrolysis of acetals usually fails with thioacetals. Sulphur is less basic than oxygen, so the protonated species is lower in concentration at a given pH, and the sulphur 3p lone pairs are less able to form a stable π-bond to carbon than are the oxygen 2p lone pairs.

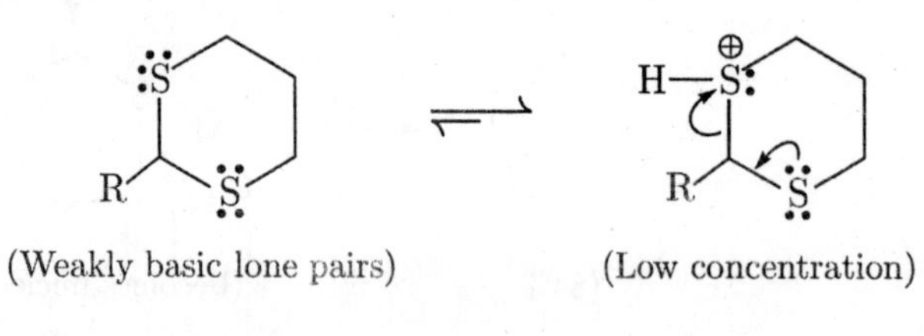

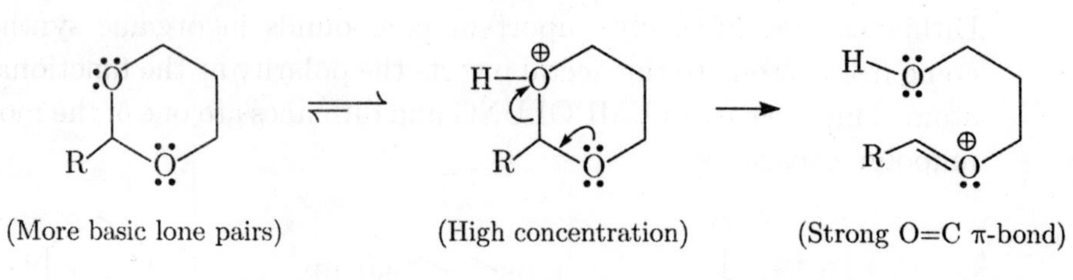

Thioacetals are important in organic synthesis, as they react with Raney Ni to yield hydrocarbons. Raney Ni is a special nickel catalyst that contains adsorbed hydrogen. Thioacetal formation and desulphurisation provides an additional method for converting carbonyl groups of aldehydes and ketones to —CH_2— groups.

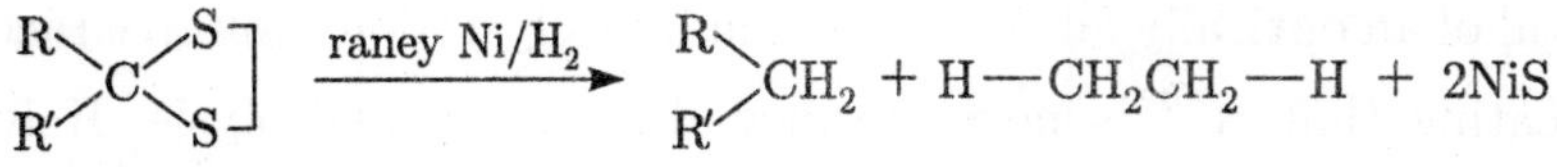

Hydrolysis of acetals

The acetal formation reaction is reversible and the hydrolysis of the acetal back to the starting carbonyl compound may be effected with dilute acid. $H_3O^{\oplus}$ protonates OR group and the latter becomes $R\overset{\oplus}{O}H$, which is a good leaving group. On the other hand, there is no active H present in an acetal to be abstracted by a base and $\overset{\ominus}{O}R$ is a poor leaving group. So like ethers, acetals (geminal diethers) are stable in alkali.

Mechanism of hydrolysis of acetals :

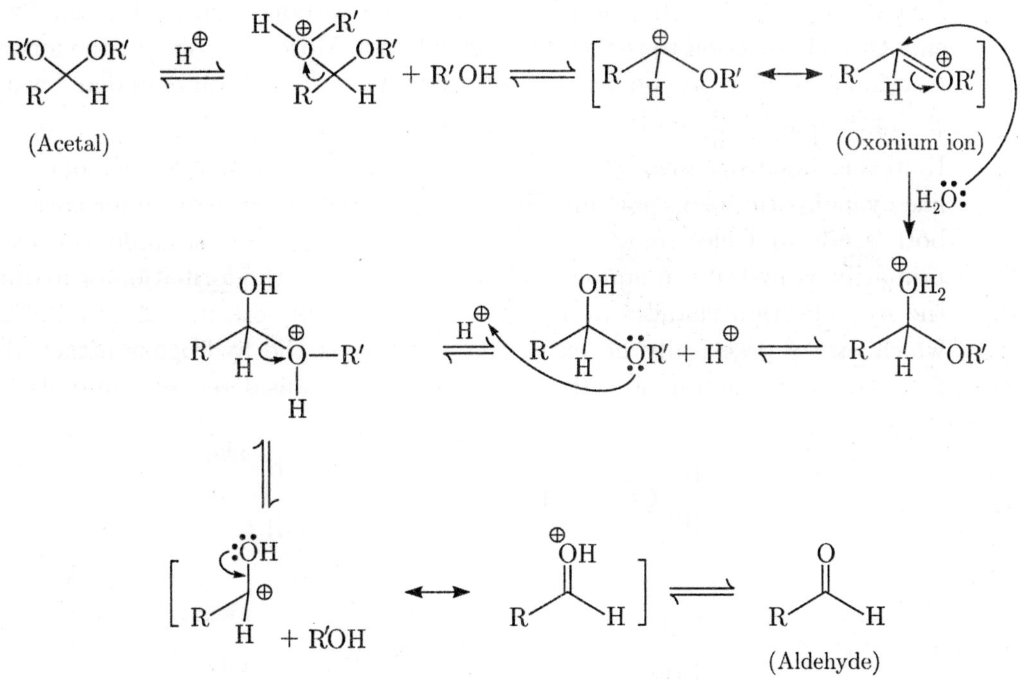

Since the hydrolysis of acetals and formation of acetals are reverse reactions, the mechanism follows the principle of *microscopic reversibility.*

The following facts support the mechanism of hydrolysis of acetals

1. The reaction proceeds with specific acid catalyst $H_3O^{\oplus}$.
2. The reaction is faster with D_2O.

3. R′—O bond *does not* break even when R′=*t*-butyl, which is proved by O^{18} labelling. Only C—OR′ bond breaks.
4. Acetal of an optically active alcohol on hydrolysis does not give racemic alcohol, indicating that $R'^{\oplus}$ is never formed during the hydrolysis. If $R'^{\oplus}$ has been formed, we would get racemic R′OH, which is never found.
5. Acetals are diethers and likely to be cleaved by acids but stable towards alkalis.

5. **Addition of water (formation of hydrates) :** The addition of water to a carbonyl group is a reversible reaction and the equilibrium lies over to the left as shown below.

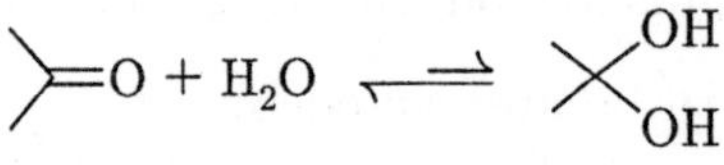

ΔH=20 kJ/mol

(Hydrate, a gemdiol)

We know that C=O bond dissociation energy is more than twice C—O bond formation energy. So the addition of water to a carbonyl function is usually an endothermic reaction to the extent of 20 kJ/mol. Moreover, ΔS° for the forward reaction is negative as two molecule of reactants (carbonyl compound and water) give rise to only one molecule of product.

However, aldehydes give hydrates readily than those by ketones. Ketones, just like cyanohydrin formation, are not favourable regarding hydrate formation on both steric and electronic ground. Some aldehydes like formaldehyde exists primarily as hydrate in aqueous solution because on the formation of hydrate, the hybridisation changes from sp^2 to sp^3 (bond angle from 120° to 109°28′) which exerts practically no extra steric strain as the hydrogens attached to C=O are very small in size. Hydrates can also be considered as gem diols.

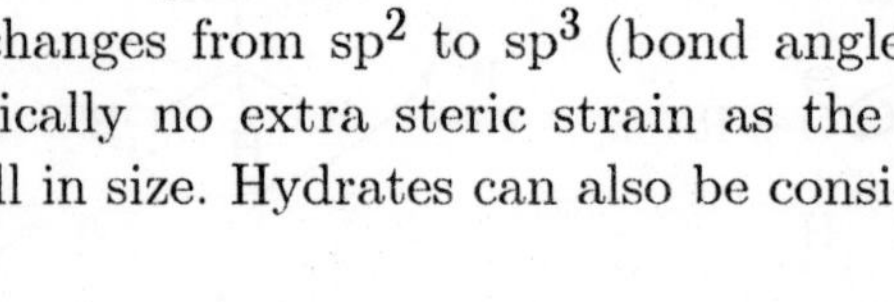

(*gem*-diol)

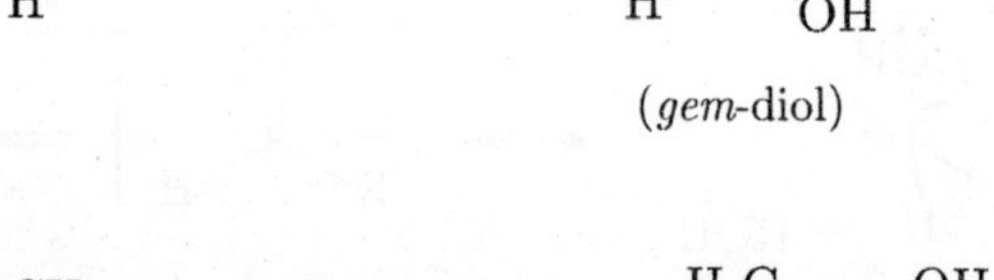

(*gem*-diol)

The reaction of formation of hydrated acetaldehyde is very slow at pH 7.00 but occurs readily at pH 4.00 and 11.00. This means that, the acid or base catalysed hydration is rapid.

Mechanism of hydrate formation reaction :

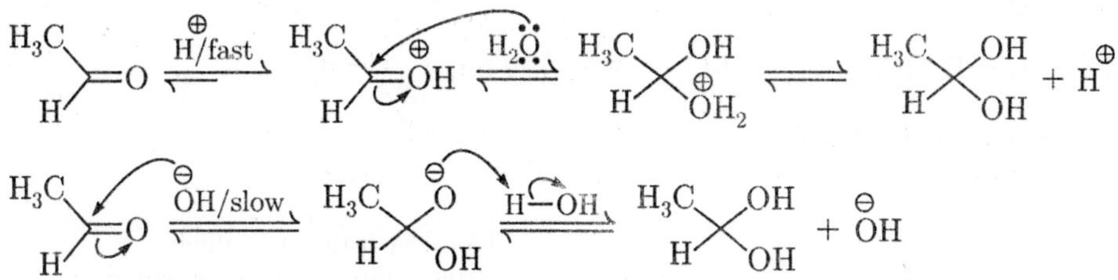

Orbitals involved in addition of water :

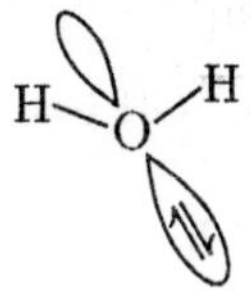

(HOMO=oxygen sp^3 containing lone pair)

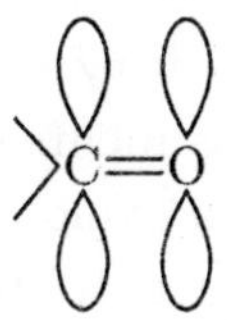

π^*(LUMO)

Gem-diols can not be isolated from aqueous solutions in which they are formed. Evaporation of water displaces the overall equilibrium to the right and the *gem*-diol reverts to the carbonyl compound.

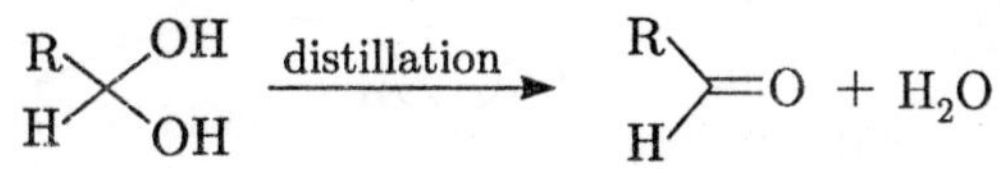

Electronic effects can also favour reaction with nucleophiles, electronegative atoms such as halogens attached to the carbon atoms next to the carbonyl group can increase the extent of hydration according to the number of halogen substituents and their electron withdrawing power.

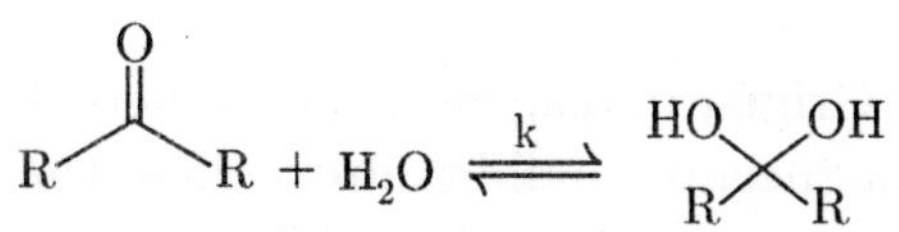

Acetone (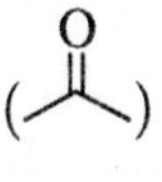) — 0.001 (Equilibrium constant, K)

Acetaldehyde (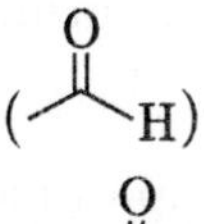) — 1.06 (K)

Formaldehyde (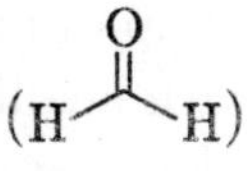) — 2280 (K)

Chloral (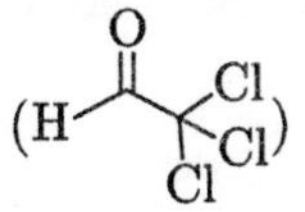) — 2000 (K)

Hexafluoroacetone (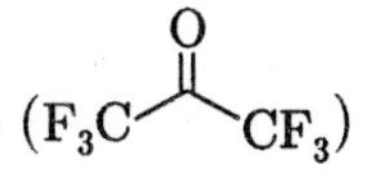) — 1,200,000 (K)

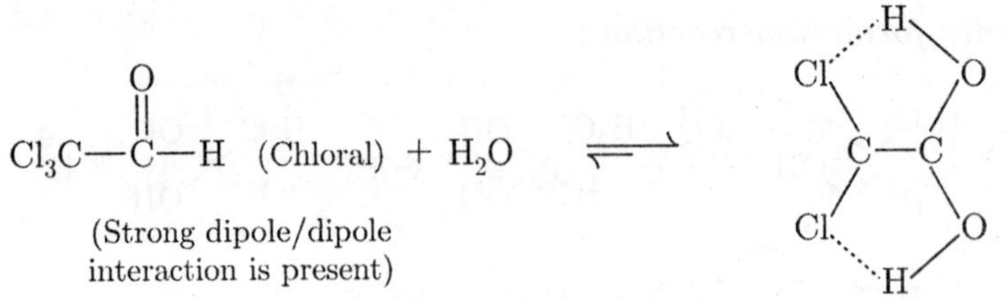

(Strong dipole/dipole interaction is present)

(Chloral hydrate, crystalline)
(Stabilised by internal hydrogen bonding, chloral hydrate is used as annesthetic. IR spectrum shows no absorption between 1700-1800 cm^{-1} for C=O, instead we have tell-tale broad –OH peak at 3400 cm^{-1}

Cyclopropanones are also hydrated to a considerable extent. Cyclopropanones and other small ring ketones prefer small bond angle because their substituents are already confined within a ring. A three-membered ring is very strained, the bond angles are forced to be 60°. For the sp^2 hybridised ketone, this means the angle of deviation is 60° (120° normal sp^2 bond angle)- 60° (bond angle in a cyclopropanone ring)=60°. But for the sp^3-hybridised hydrates, the bond angles have to be distorted by only 49°28′ (109°28′–60°=49°28′). So addition to the C=O group allows some of the strain inherent in the small ring to be released; hydration is favoured and indeed cyclopropanone and cyclobutanone are reactive electrophiles.

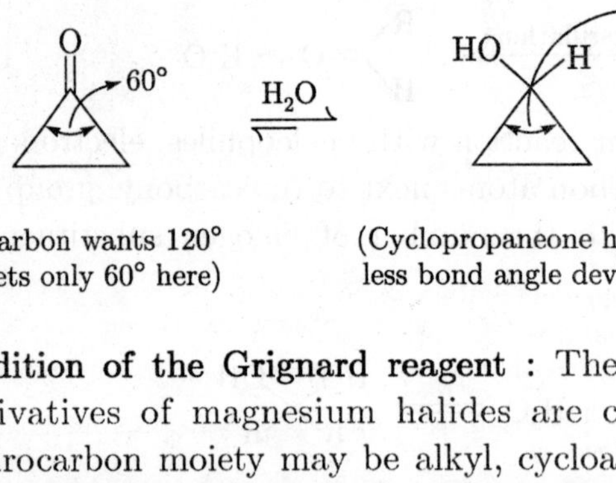

[should be 109°28′(sp^3 bond angle) but actually is only 60°]

(sp^2 carbon wants 120° but gets only 60° here)

(Cyclopropaneone hydrate, less bond angle deviation)

6. **Addition of the Grignard reagent** : The ethereal solutions of hydrocarbon derivatives of magnesium halides are called the Grignard reagents. The hydrocarbon moiety may be alkyl, cycloalkyl, allyl, aryl etc. and the halides may be Cl, Br or I. The ether medium may be Et_2O, THF or diglyme (DG). Grignard reagents are depicted by the general formula RMgX where R is hydrocarbon and X is Cl, Br or I.

   The Grignard reagents add to the carbonyl group of aldehydes and ketones to yield addition products which on hydrolysis with acidified water give alcohols. Formaldehyde gives primary alcohol, other aldehydes yield secondary alcohols and ketones give tertiary alcohols.

Examples :

1. 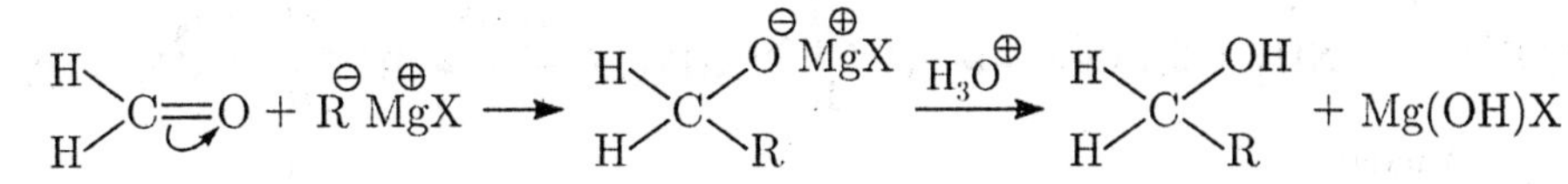

(Formaldehyde) (primary alcohol)

2. 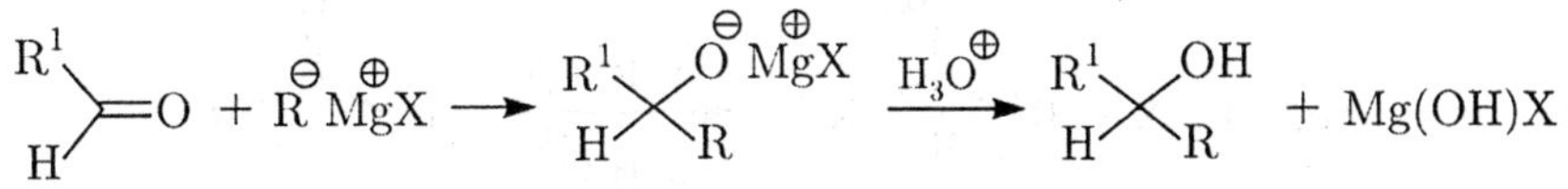

(Aldehyde) (secondary alcohol)

3. 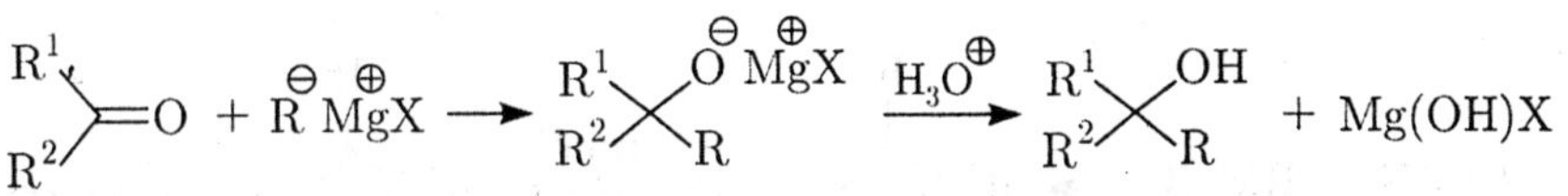

(Ketone) (tertiary alcohol)

Acid halides, esters amides, cyanides etc. undergo nucleophilic substitution reaction with the Grignard reagents to form ketones. The ketones may then undergo the addition reactions to yield tertiary alcohols.

4. 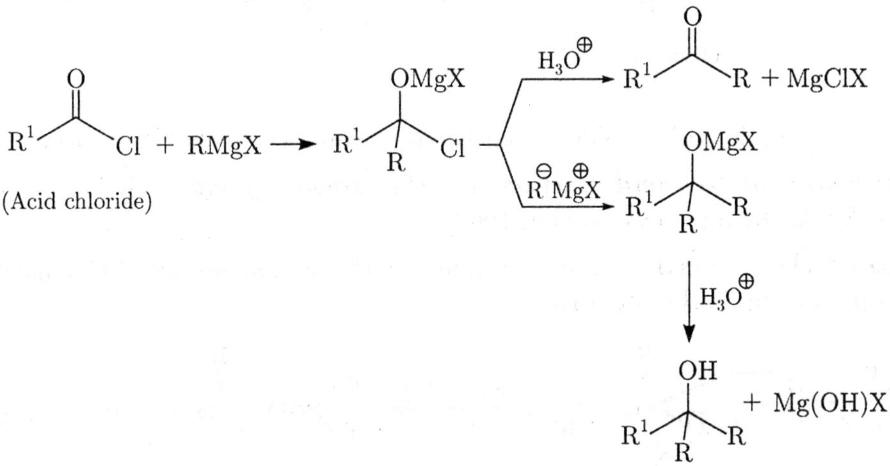

(Acid chloride)

(tertiary alcohol)

5. 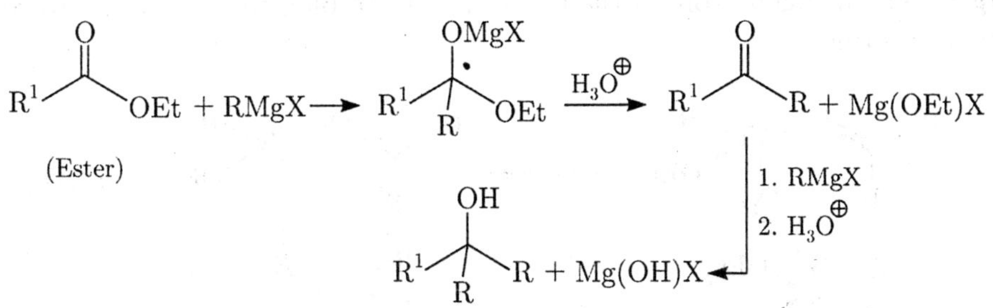

(Ester)

(tertiary alcohol)

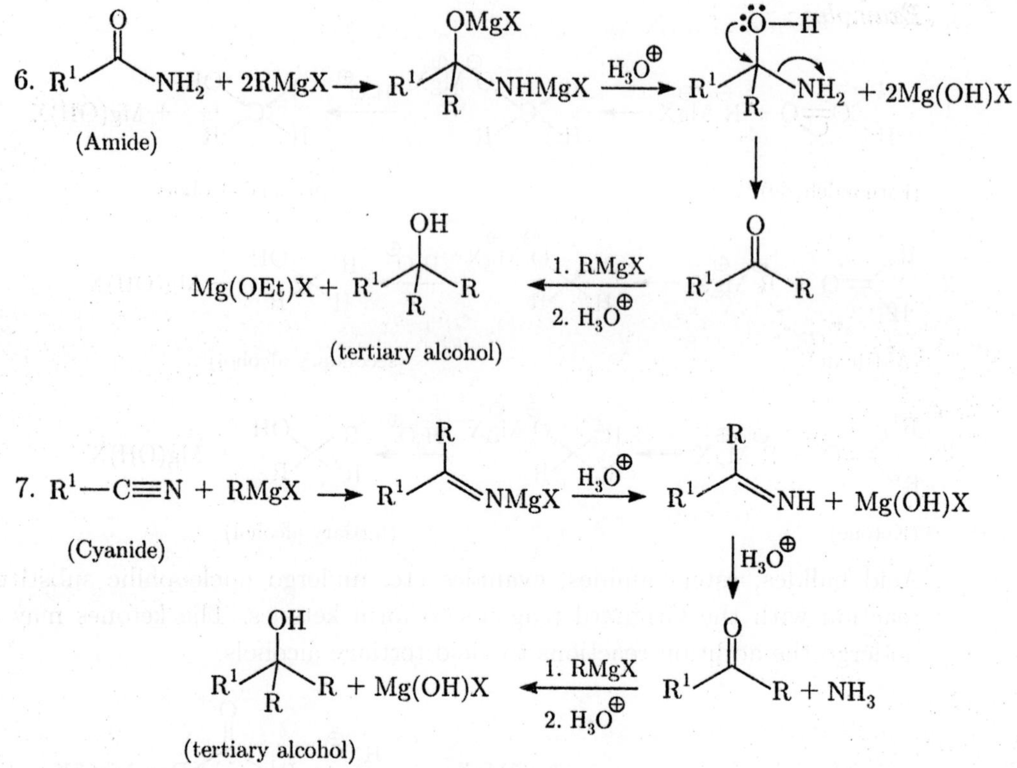

With amide and cyanide, when R′=H, secondary alcohols are formed.

Mechanism of Grignard reaction towards carbonyl group : The mechanism was proposed by Ashby and coworkers in 1967.

***Step* 1** : The carbonyl oxygen coordinates with the magnesium of Grignard reagent which is present in dietherate form.

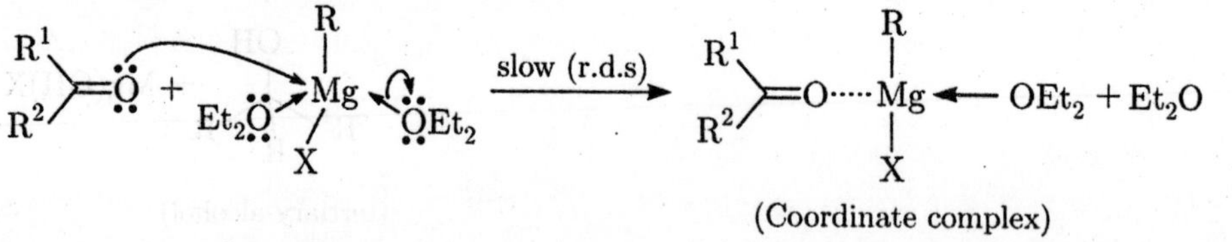

***Step* 2** : The halogen atom of the coordinated complex then of Grignard reagent in the dietherate form.

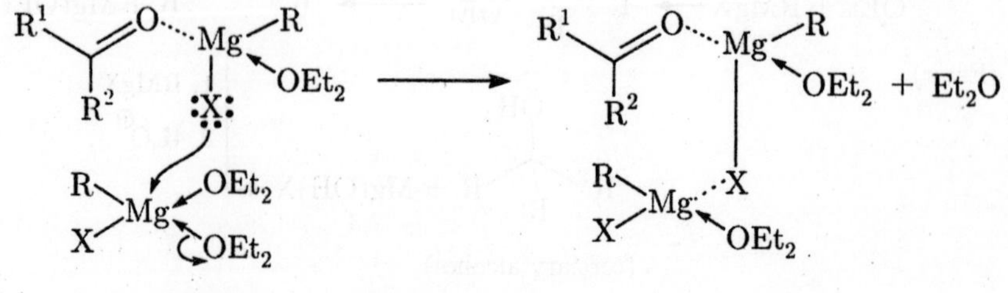

***Step* 3** : Formation of a six-membered cyclic transition state

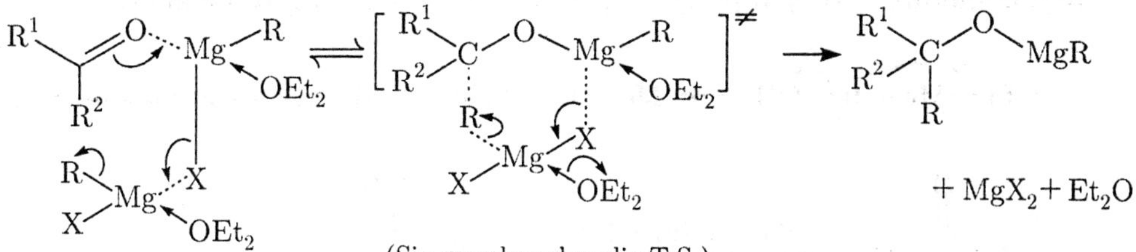

(Six-membered cyclic T.S.)

***Step* 4** : Formation of a four-membered cyclic transition state

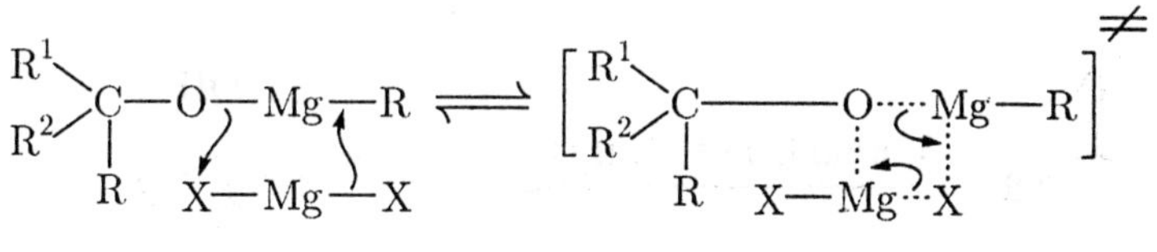

(Four-membered cyclic T.S.)

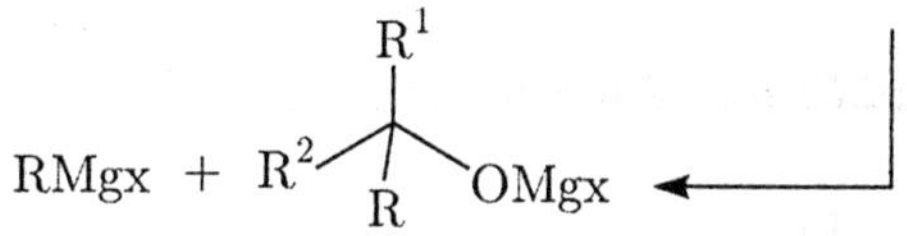

***Step* 5** : Hydrolysis in an acid medium.

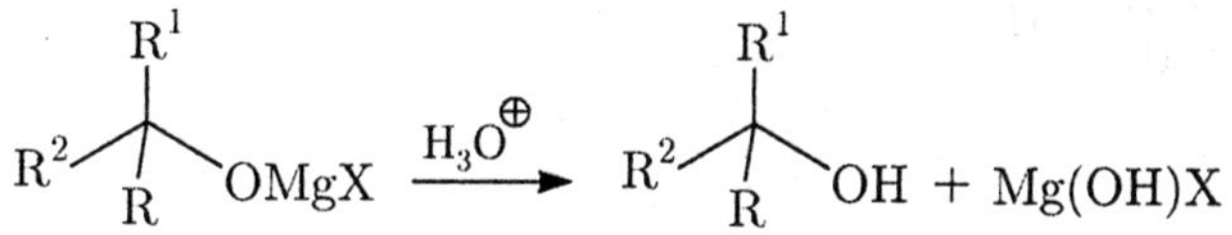

(tertiary alcohol)

Evidences in favour of the mechanism

1. The rate of the reaction decreases when half the Grignard reagent has been used up. This supports the participation of two RMgX units in the reaction.
2. The rate of the reaction increases when $MgBr_2$, a better Lewis acid than RMgX is added. This supports the step 1 as slow and r.d.s.
3. When R_3COMgR and $MgBr_2$ are taken together in the ether medium, $R_3COMgBr$ forms. This supports the steps 2 and 3.

7. Addition of organolithium

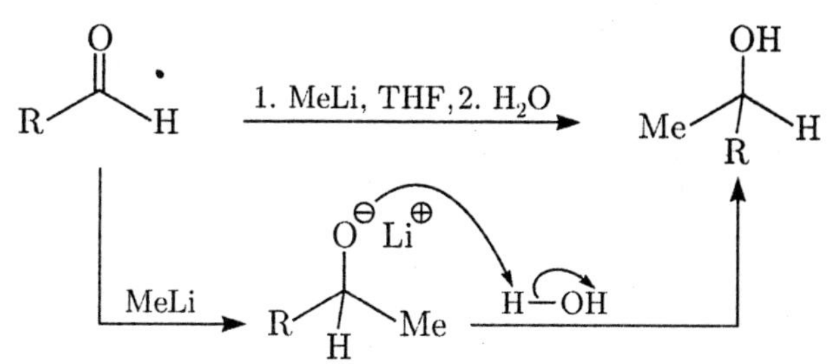

Water must not be present during the addition of MeLi, as water destroys organometallics very rapidly by protonating them to give alkanes.

$$\text{Li—Me} + \text{H—OH} \longrightarrow \text{Me—H} + \text{LiOH}$$ (Exothermic and fast reaction)

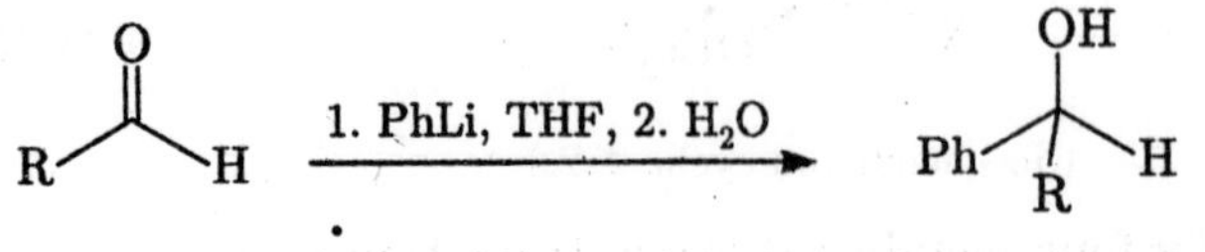

(Secondary alcohol)

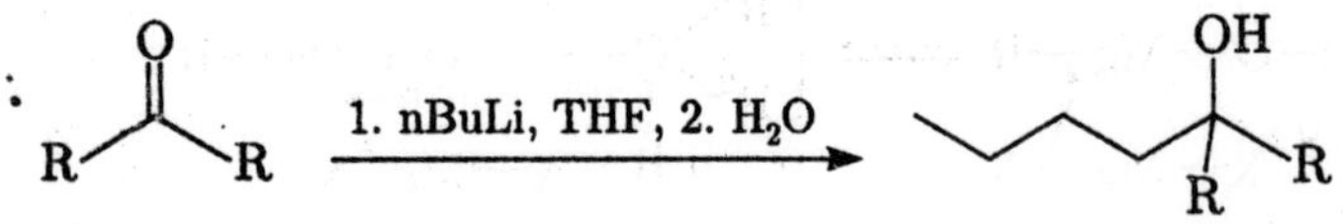

(Tertiary alcohol)

Orbitals involved in the addition of methyllithium :

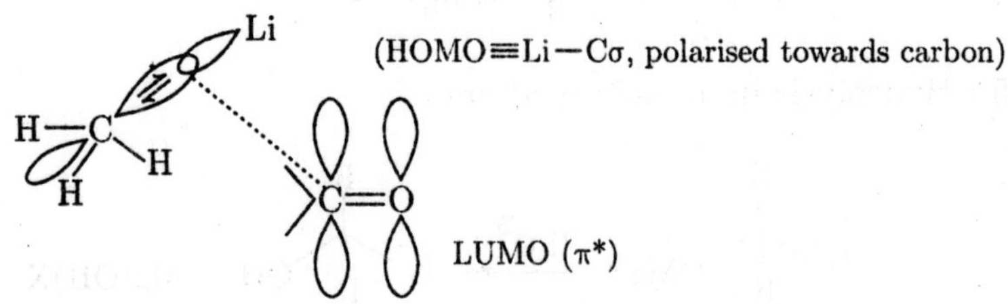

8. **The addition of organozinc reagent : The Reformatsky reaction :** The Grignard like addition of an α-haloester to an aldehyde or a ketone in the presence of *metallic zinc* to yield a β-hydroxyester is known as the Reformatsky reaction.

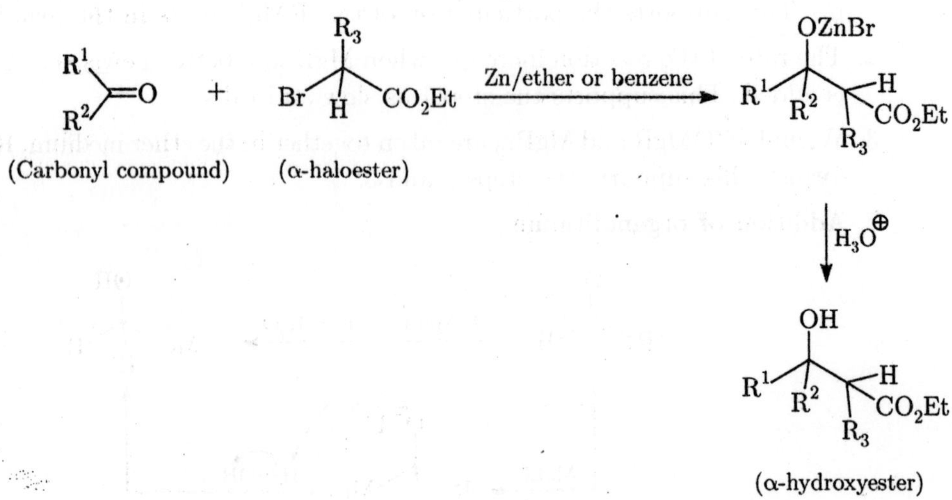

(α-hydroxyester)

α-Haloesters used in most cases is either α-bromoester or its vinylogue –RCH (Br)–CH=$CHCO_2Et$. However the reaction is also carried out with α-bromonitriles or α-halo-N,N-disubstituted amides.

In practice, the carbonyl compound, α-bromoester and zinc in dry benzene are carefully heated under reflux when zinc dissolves. Zinc may be activated by adding traces of iodine or $Hg^{I}Br$ or copper powder. The mixture is then treated with ice-cold dilute sulphuric acid and benzene layer separates out. Benzene is distilled off when β-hydroxyester is obtained.

Mechanism of Reformatsky reaction :

Step 1 : Formation of zinc enolate. Zinc, like magnesium is a two electron donor and forms Zn(II) from Zn(O).

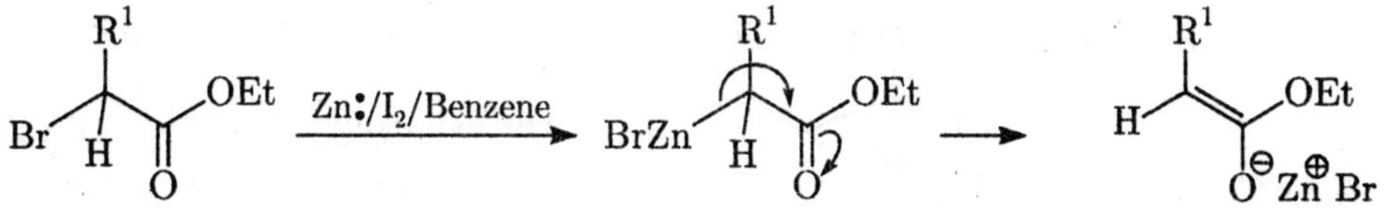

(Zinc bromide enolate)
(Insertion of Zn is similar to Mg in G.R. formation)

There is no danger of self condensation with zinc enolates as they do not react with esters.

***Step* 2** : Addition of zinc bromide enolate to the carbonyl group.

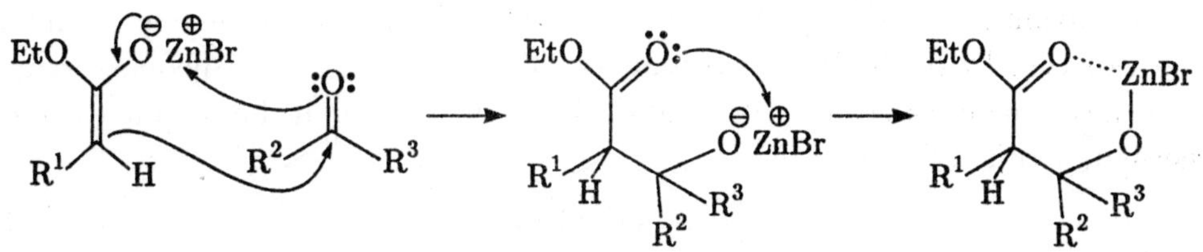

***Step* 3** : Hydrolysis of the adduct by dilute acid.

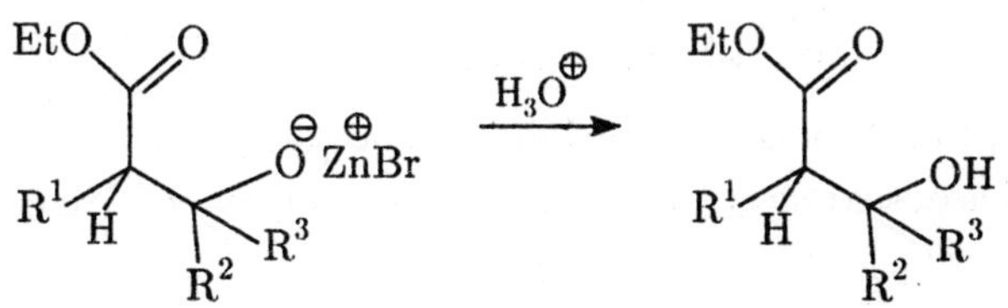

(β-hydroxyester)

The β-hydroxyester product is generally dehydrated to an α, β-unsaturated acid as dehydration yields a *conjugated system.*

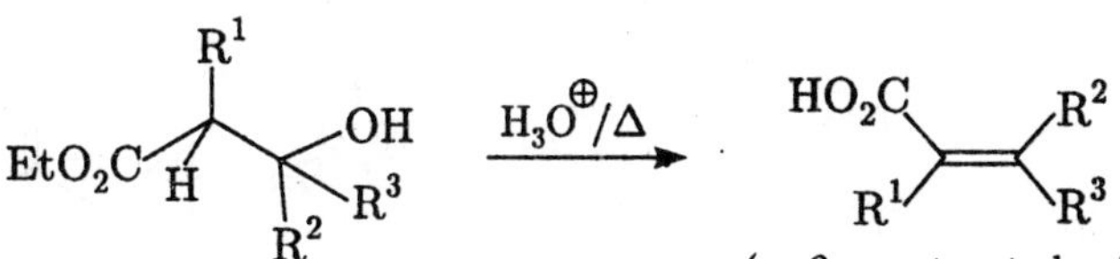

(α, β-unsaturated acid)

Alternative Mechanism of Reformatsky reaction

This mechanism is widely accepted now.

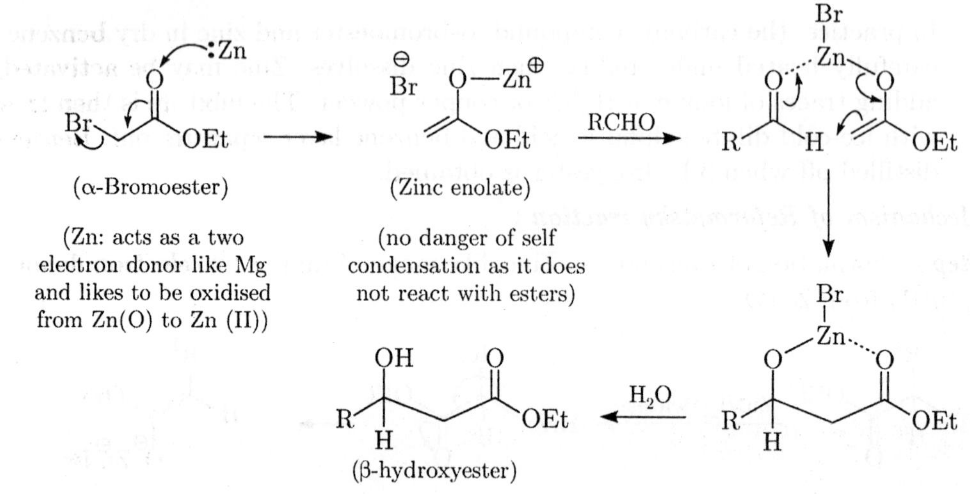

The zinc enolate is often called *Reformatsky reagent* after its inventor. Zinc enolate should not be written as 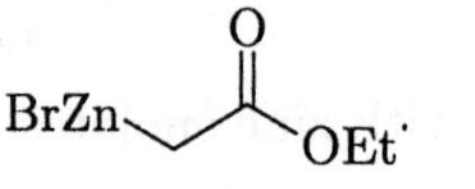.

Organozinc compounds are less reactive than the Grignard reagents. Organozinc compounds react very slowly with esters but readily with aldehydes and ketones. By taking the advantage of this preferential reactivity of organozinc halides, β-hydroxy-esters are prepared by the Reformatsky reaction. The structure of intermediate organozinc bromides have been isolated (1966) and the structure of it has been established (Zimmerman and Traxler).

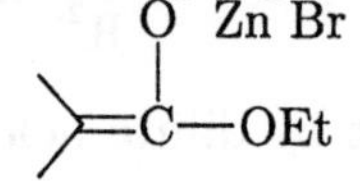

(Structure of organozinc compound)

Organozinc compounds of α-bromoesters can not add to sterically hindered carbonyl compounds. In that case, two molecules of α-bromoester react with each other to produce a β-ketoester.

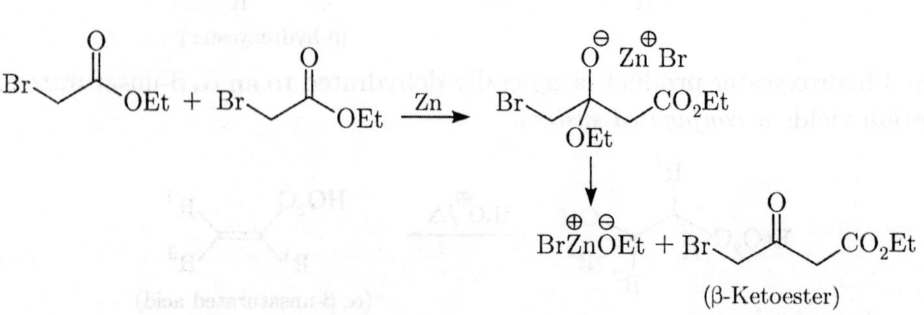

(β-Ketoester)

The reaction may be extended to the vinylogous compounds of α-bromoesters.

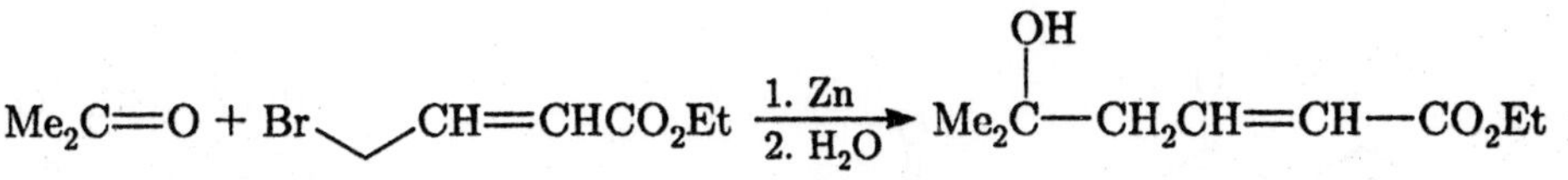

Reformatky reaction proceeds well with aldehydes, methyl ketones and cyclic ketones. Reactivity order of haloesters is as follows.

Iodo > bromo > chloro

—— Reactivity decreases ——→

The β-and γ-haloesters are less reactive.

Applications of Reformatsky reaction :

1. *Preparation of β-hydroxy esters, α, β-unsaturated ester and saturated carboxylic acids*

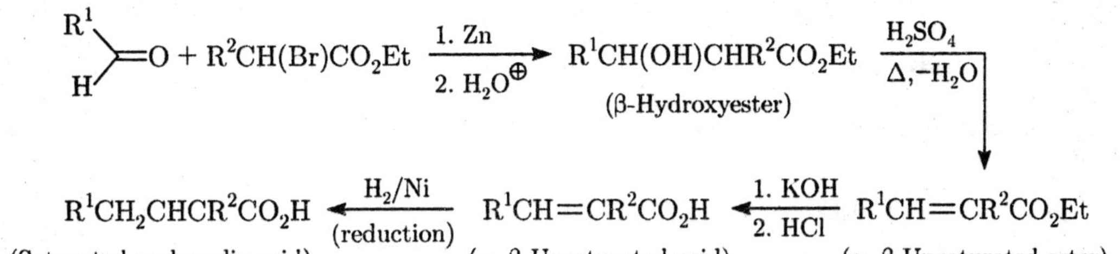

2. 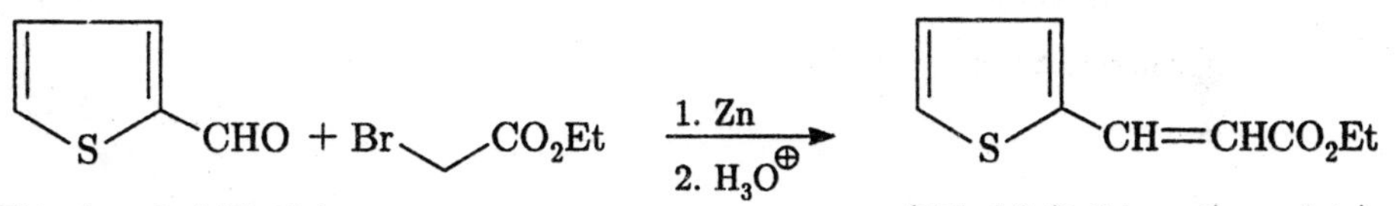

(Thiophen-2-aldehyde) (Ethyl-β-(2-thioenyl) acrylate)

3. *Lengthening of the carbon chain*

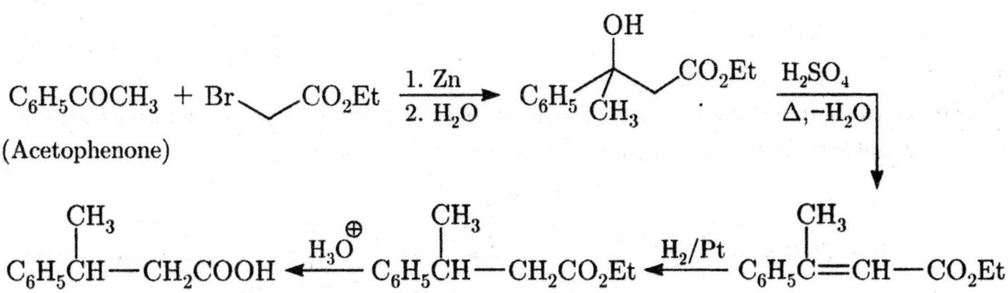

Unsaturated or saturated acids or esters with branching at α- and β-carbon can be synthesised.

4. *Synthesis of arylacetic acid*

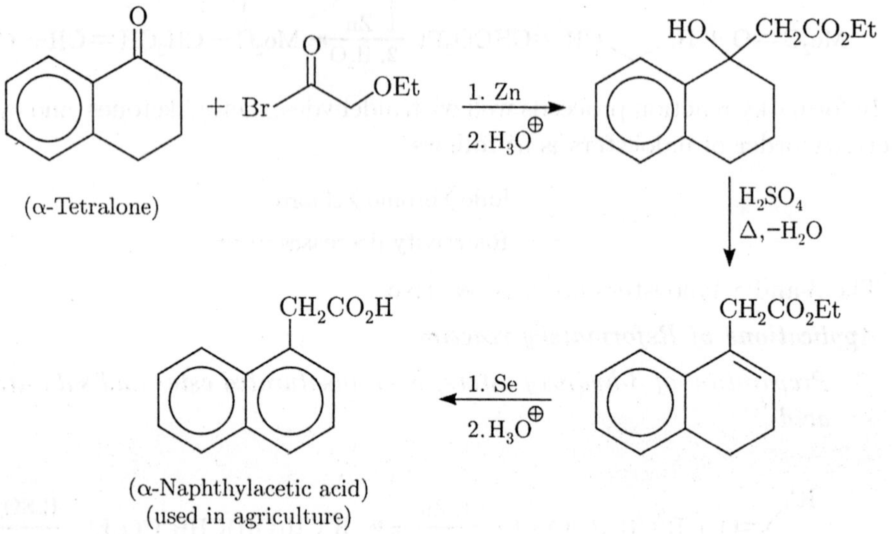

5. *Synthesis of citric acid*

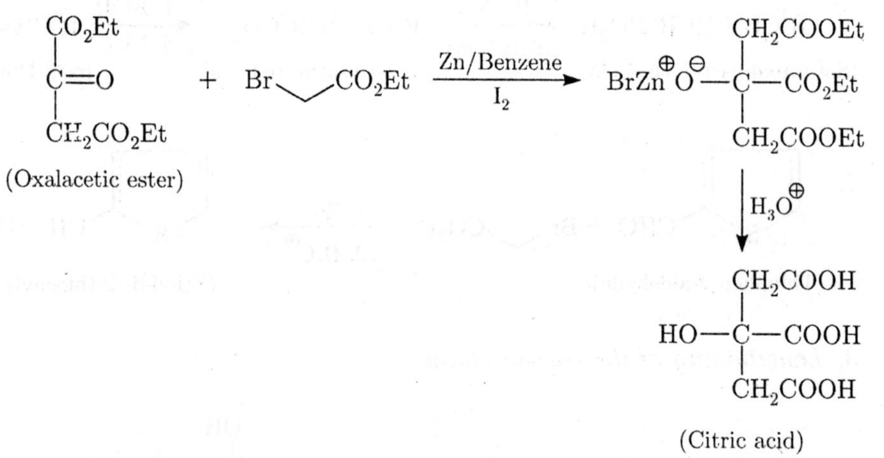

6. Reaction between a nitrile and α-bromoester in the presence of zinc is a similar reaction. In this case, a β-ketoester is formed.

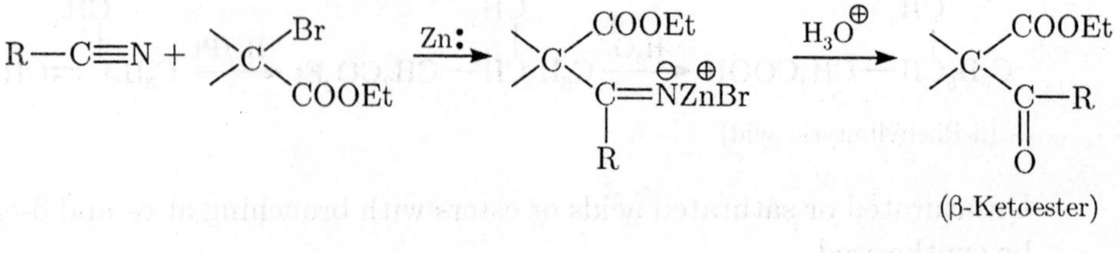

9. Reactions involving hydride ion transfer

(a) ***The Nystrom and Brown reduction by $LiAlH_4$*** : $LiAlH_4$ (may be prepared by the reaction between LiH and $AlCl_3$) is a good hydride ion donor and compounds containing carbonyl moiety are good hydride ion acceptors. For this reason, the latter compounds are reduced very often by $LiAlH_4$ or its derivatives. The polar nature of carbonyl moiety makes the carbon atom electrophilic toward the uncleophilic hydride ion and enables the compounds containing carbonyl moiety to be reduced by $LiAlH_4$ (or similar compounds). Thus, aldehydes, ketones, carboxylic acids, esters, amides, acid halides, nitriles, nitro-compounds etc. get reduced on treatment with $LiAlH_4$ in ether medium. $LiAlH_4$ does not reduce C=C or C≡C bonds. However, $LiAlH_4$ reduces,

1. An aldehyde to a primary alcohol
2. A ketone to a secondary alcohol
3. A carboxylic acid to a primary alcohol
4. An ester to a primary alcohol
5. An amide to an amine
6. An acid halide to an alcohol etc.

Examples :

1. $4CH_3CHO \xrightarrow{LiAlH_4/Et_2O} (CH_3CH_2O)_4\overset{\ominus}{Al}Li^{\oplus} \xrightarrow{4H^{\oplus}} 4CH_3CH_2OH + Li^{+} + Al^{3+}$

2. $4CH_3COCH_3 \xrightarrow{LiAlH_4/Et_2O} (Me_2CHO)_4\overset{\ominus}{Al}Li^{\oplus} \xrightarrow{4H^{\oplus}} 4Me_2CHOH + Li^{+} + Al^{3+}$

3. $CH_3COOH \xrightarrow[2.\ H_3O^{\oplus}]{1.\ LiAlH_4/Et_2O} CH_3CHO \xrightarrow[2.\ H_3O^{\oplus}]{1.\ LiAlH_4/Et_2O} CH_3CH_2OH$

4. $PhCOOCH_3 \xrightarrow{LiAlH_4/Et_2O} 4PhCHO + 4CH_3O^{-} \xrightarrow{H^{\oplus}} 4CH_3OH$

$$4PhCHO \xrightarrow{LiAlH_4/Et_2O} (PhCH_2O)_4\overset{\ominus}{Al}Li^{\oplus} \xrightarrow{H_3O^{\oplus}} PhCH_2OH$$

$LiAlH_4$ being soluble in ether, the reaction is usually carried out in ether, THF etc. At first a lithium aluminium alkoxide type complex is formed which on acidification liberates the reduction product, since $LiAlH_4$ does not usually reduce carbon-carbon multiple bonds, unsaturated alcohols are prepared from unsaturated carbonyl compounds, acids and esters.

$$CH_3CH{=}CH{-}CH_2CHO \xrightarrow{LiAlH_4/THF} \xrightarrow{H^{\oplus}} CH_3CH{=}CH{-}CH_2CH_2OH$$

However, when a carbon-carbon multiple bond is in conjugation with an aromatic system on one side and a carbonyl group on the other side gets reduced by $LiAlH_4$.

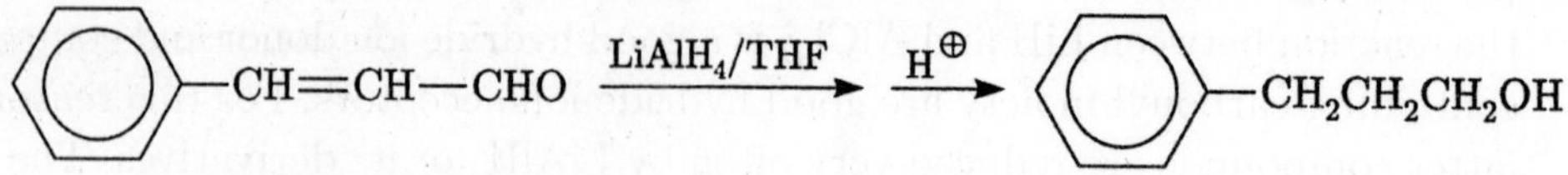

Since $LiAlH_4$ neutralises a carboxylic acid, the reduction of a carboxylic acid requires a large excess of the reagent. To avoid it, the sodio salt of carboxylic acid is usually treated with the reagent.

$LiAlH_4$ is one of the most useful reducing agents in organic chemistry. It serves generally as a source of hydride ion ($H:^{\ominus}$). Hydrogen being more electronegative than aluminium, the Al–H bonds in $\overset{\ominus}{Al}H_4$ ion carry a substantial fraction of negative charge.

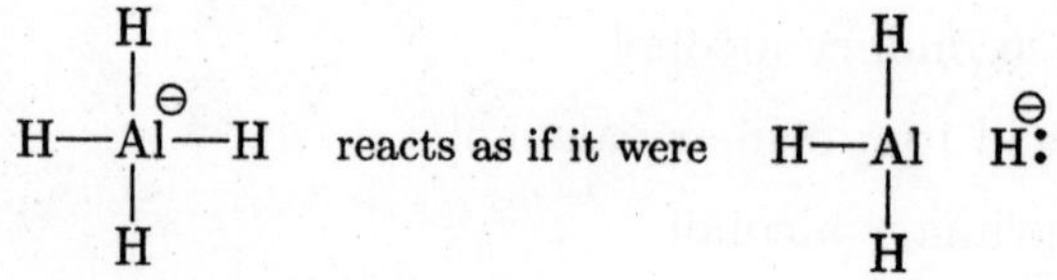

The hydride ion in $LiAlH_4$ is very basic. For this reason, $LiAlH_4$ reacts violently with water and therefore must be used in dry solvents like dry ether or THF.

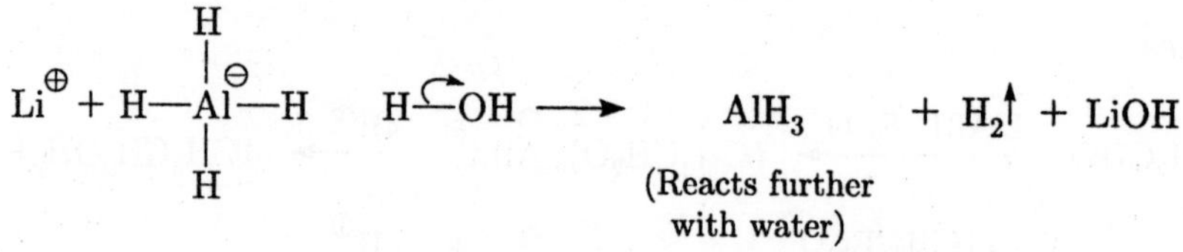

Like many other strong bases, the hydride ion in $LiAlH_4$ is a good nucleophile and $LiAlH_4$ contains its own built in Lewis acid, *lithium ion.* The reaction of $LiAlH_4$ with aldehydes and ketones involves the nucleophilic attack of hydride (derived from $\overset{\ominus}{Al}H_4$) on the carbonyl carbon. *The lithium ion* ($Li^{\oplus}$ ion) *acts as a Lewis acid catalyst by coordinating to the carbonyl oxygen.*

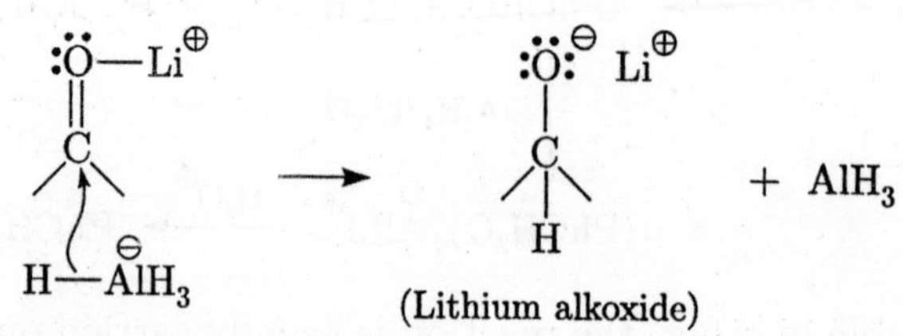

The addition product, an alkoxide salt can react with AlH_3, and the resulting product can also serve as a source of hydride.

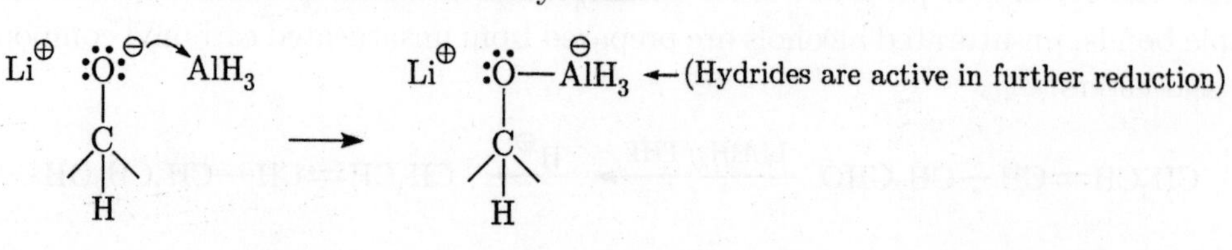

Similar processes occur at each stage of the reduction until all the hydrides are consumed. All the four hydrides of $LiAlH_4$ are active in the reduction, and it takes one fourth of a mole of $LiAlH_4$ to reduce a mole of aldehyde or ketone. After the reduction is complete, the alcohol product exists as an alkoxide addition compound with the aluminium. This is converted by protonation in a separate step into the alcohol product. The proton source can be an aqueous hydrochloric acid or even an aqueous solution of a weak acid such as ammonium chloride.

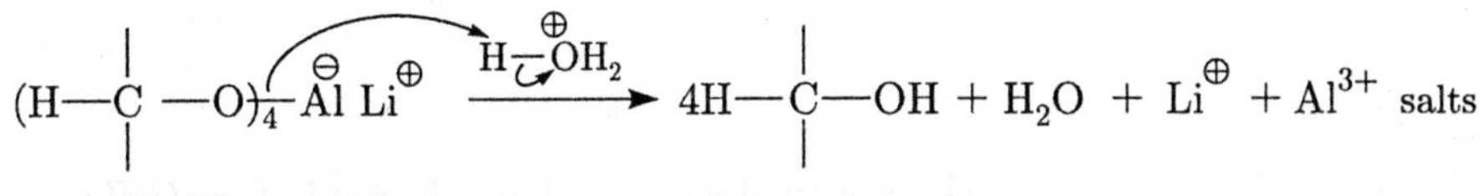

(Aluminium alkoxide) (Addition product) (Alcohol product)

Reduction of acids to primary alcohols by $LiAlH_4$:

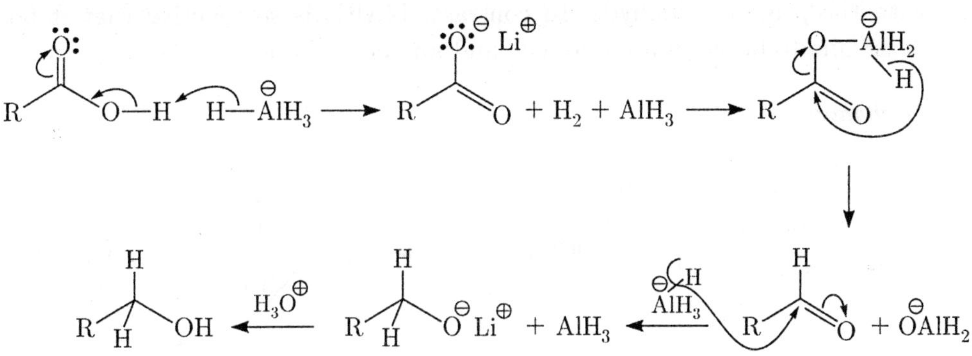

$LiAlH_4$ reduction of aldehydes and ketones is an example of nucleophilic addition, but it is *irreversible*. Because the reverse process process involves expulsion of $\overset{\ominus}{H}$**:** ion, which is a very strong base and thus the reverse process is not allowed as strong bases are poor leaving groups.

1. ***Derivatives of lithium aluminium Hydride (cousins of $LiAlH_4$)***

(a) *Lithium tri (tertiarybutoxy) aluminium hydride*

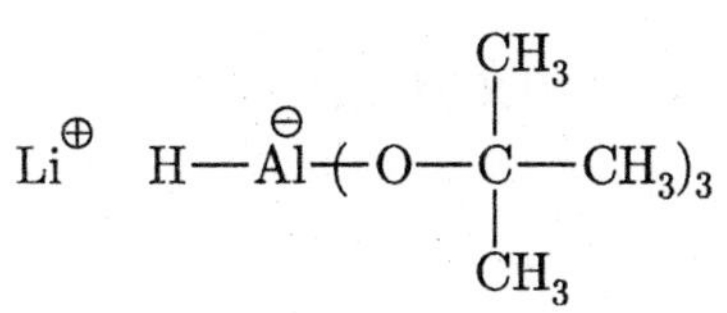

Preparation of the reagent

$$Li^{\oplus}\ \overset{\ominus}{Al}H_4 + 3Me_3C{-}OH \longrightarrow Li^{\oplus}\ H{-}\overset{\ominus}{Al}[O{-}CMe_3]_3 + 3H_2\uparrow$$

The hydride reagent used in this reduction is derived by the replacement of three hydrogens of $LiAlH_4$ by tertbutoxy groups. As the hydrides of $LiAlH_4$ are replaced successively with alkoxy groups, less reactive reagents are obtained. The one remaining hydride reduces only the *most reactive functional group*.

Example 1 :

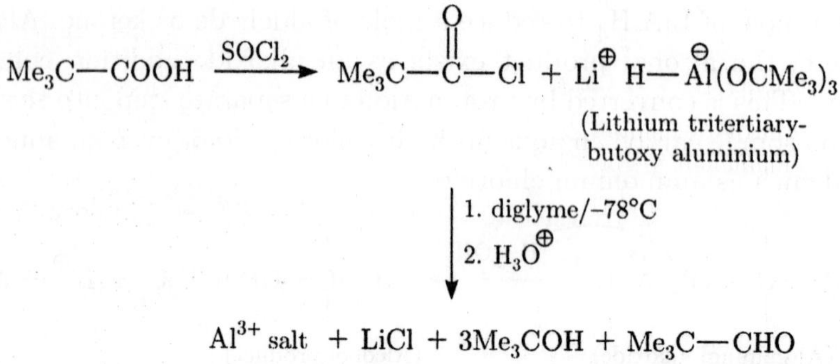

Acid chlorides are much more reactive than aldehydes toward the nucleophiles. The reagent reacts preferentially with the acid chloride reactant rather than with the product aldehyde. In contrast, $LiAlH_4$ is so reactive that it fails to discriminate between an aldehyde and an acid chloride.

Mechanism :

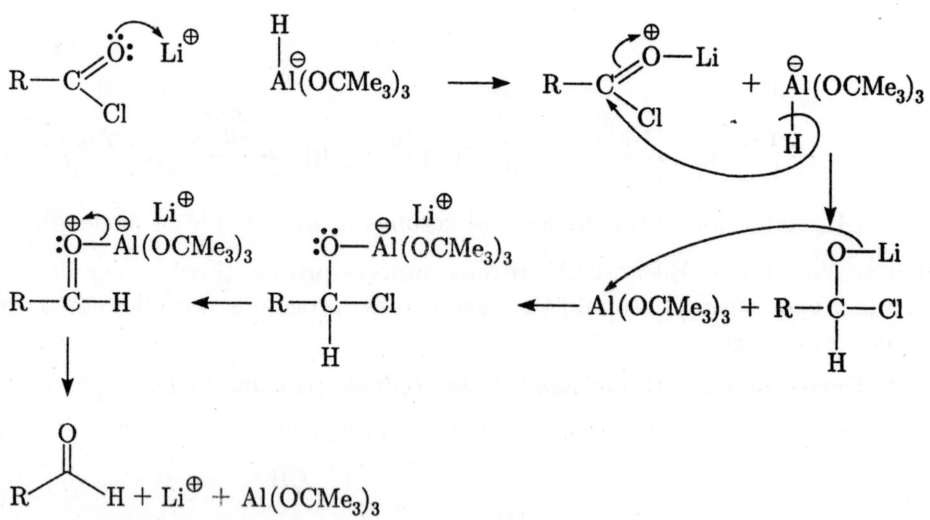

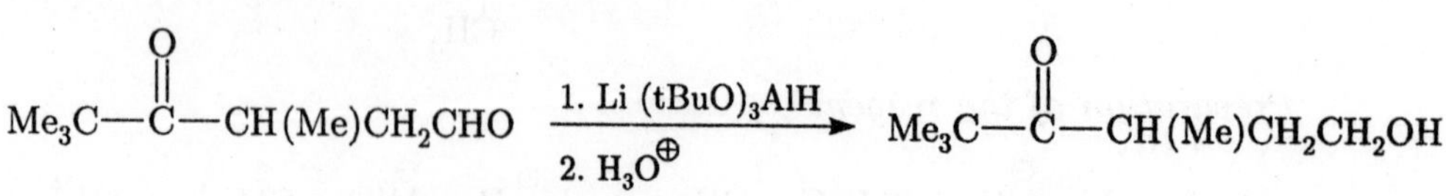

Here, lithium (tritertiarybutoxy) aluminium hydride successfully reduces a specific carbonyl group in a dicarbonyl compound. The less sterically hindered carbonyl group gets reduced proferentially over the more sterically hindered one.

(b) *Diisobutyl aluminium hydride* (iBu_2AlH or DIBAL–H)

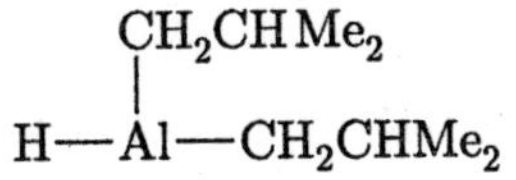

(DIBAL–H)

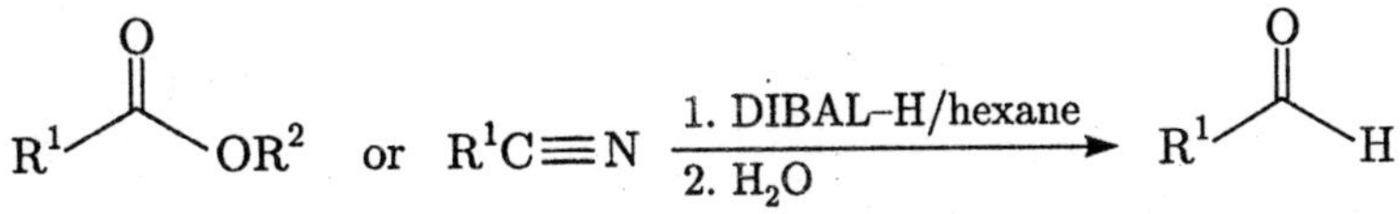

a. 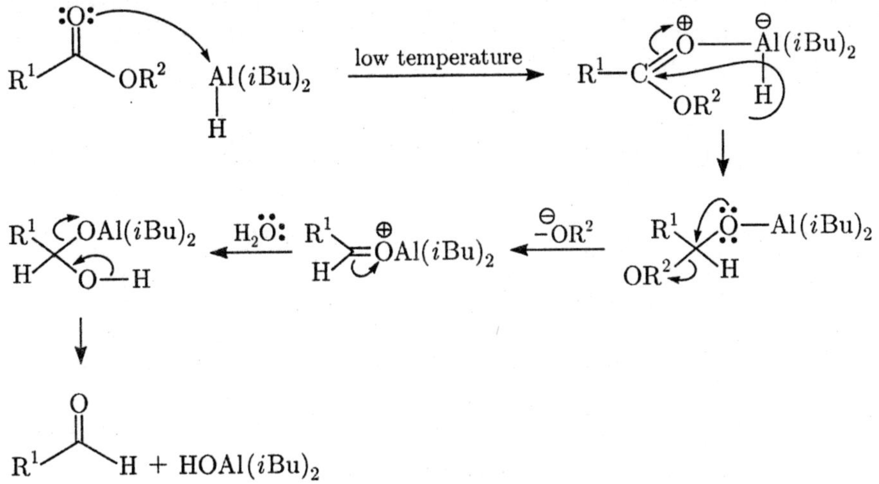

Ester reduction must be carried out at low temperature with precaution so that over reduction is not done.

b. 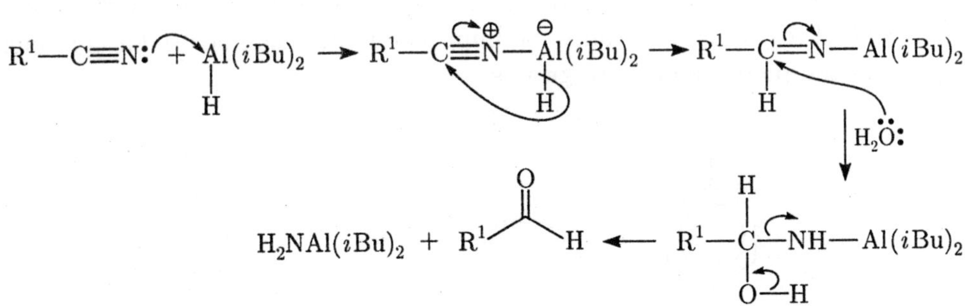

2. ***Reduction by sodium borohydride ($NaBH_4$)*** : The reduction of sodium borohydride with aldehydes and ketones is conceptually similar to that of $LiAlH_4$. The sodium ion is a much weaker Lewis acid than the lithium ion. For this reason, $NaBH_4$ reductions are carried out in protic solvents such as alcohols. Hydrogen bonding between the alcohol solvent and the carbonyl group serves as a weak acid catalyst

that activates the carbonyl group. Unlike $LiAlH_4$, $NaBH_4$ reacts only slowly with alcohols and can be used in water if the solution is not acidic.

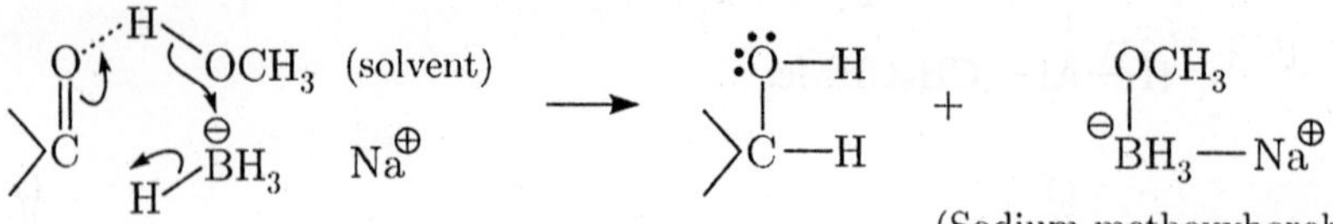

(Sodium methoxyborohydride, active in further reductions)

All four hydride equivalents of $NaBH_4$ are active in the reduction. Reduction by $NaBH_4$ is also an example of nucleophilic addition which essentially is a hydride transfer reaction. In case of $LiAlH_4$ reduction, proton is delivered at the last step from an acid added, whereas in case of $NaBH_4$, it is the solvent alcohol which supplies the proton.

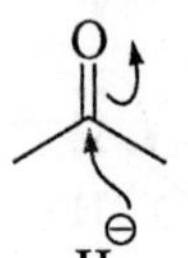

$\overset{\oplus}{H}$ (from acid in case of $LiAlH_4$ and from solvent in case of $NaBH_4$)

$\overset{\ominus}{H}$ (from $\overset{\ominus}{AlH_4}$ or $\overset{\ominus}{BH_4}$)

In case of $NaBH_4$ reduction also, the nucleophilic addition is not a reversible reaction. Because reversal of the addition would expel a hydride ($\overset{\ominus}{H}$:) ion to get back the starting material. But hydride ($\overset{\ominus}{H}$:) ion is a very strong base and is not easily expelled as a leaving group (strong bases are poor leaving groups). Hence hydride reduction of aldehydes and ketones is not reversible, they go to complition.

$NaBH_4$ can reduce aldehydes, ketones, esters, acid chlorides etc. to alcohols, but it does not reduce $CONH_2$, CN, NO_2, COOH, C=C, and C≡C, alkyl halides, alkyl tosylates etc. groups. Sodium borohydride can be used as a reducing agent in the presence of these groups.

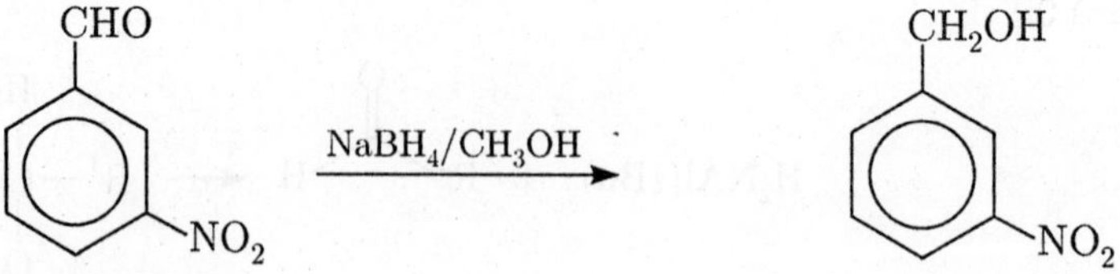

(3-Nitrobenzaldehyde)

(3-Nitrophenylbenzaldehyde)
($-NO_2$ group is net reduced by $NaBH_4$)

$NaBH_4$ is much less hazardous reagent than $LiAlH_4$. The greater selectivity and safety of $NaBH_4$ make it the preferred reagent in many applications.

Mechanism of $NaBH_4$ reduction :

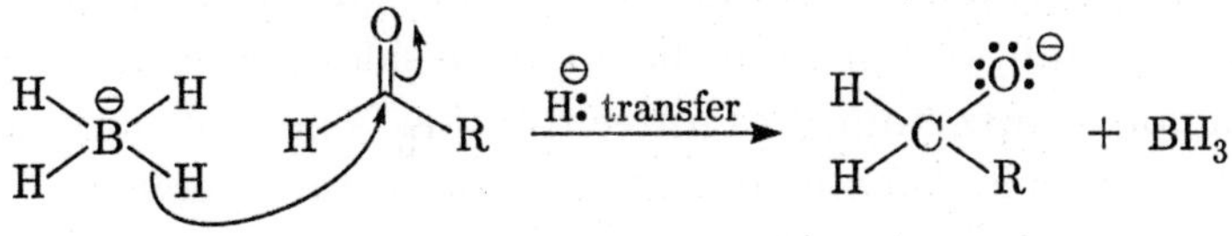

The oxyanion produced in the first step can help stabilise the electron-deficient BH_3 molecule by adding electron to its empty *p* orbital. Now, we have a tetravalent boron anion again, which could transfer second hydrogen atom (with its pair of electrons) to another molecule of aldehyde.

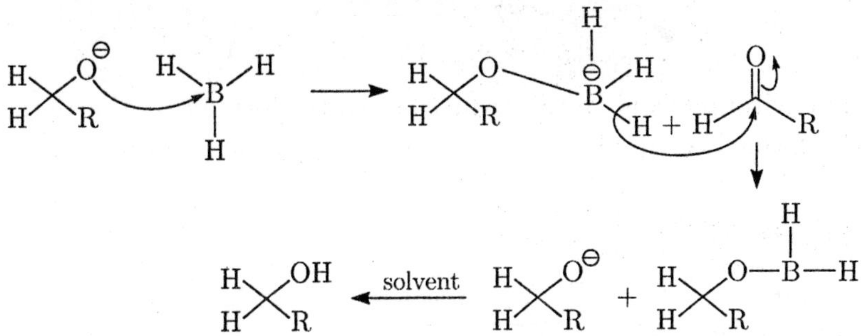

When any molecule contains both an aldehyde and an ester, **only the aldehyde** group will be reduced.

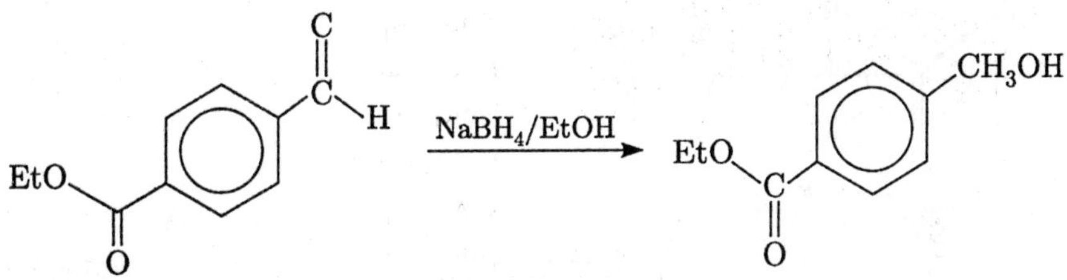

Nucleophilic attack by the hydride ion (say from NaH) is not a known reaction.

hydride ($\overset{\ominus}{H}$:) ion is too small and with high charge density it only ever reacts as a base. The reason is that, its filled 1s orbital is of an ideal size to interact as the hydrogen atom's contribution to the σ* orbital of an H–X bond (X can be any atom), but too small to interact easily with carbon's more diffused 2p orbital contribution to the LUMO (π*) of the C=O group. The orbitals involved in borohydride reductions are the π* of the C=O group as the LUMO and B–H σ orbital as the HOMO. So there is a much better orbital match.

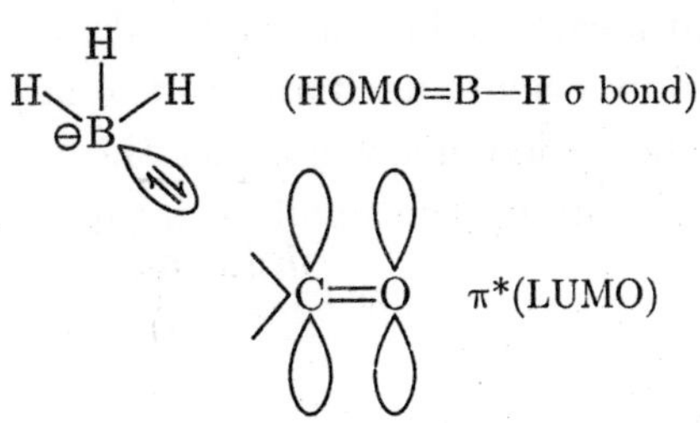

The stereochemistry of the nucleophilic addition to the carbonyl group : The addendum (Y–Z) may add to the carbonyl (C=O) group either from the same side of the double bond (*cis*-addition) or from the opposite sides (*trans*-addition). But the mode of addition can not be ascertained as a free rotation is possible around the carbon-oxygen single bond axis to adopt a stable conformation instanteneously.

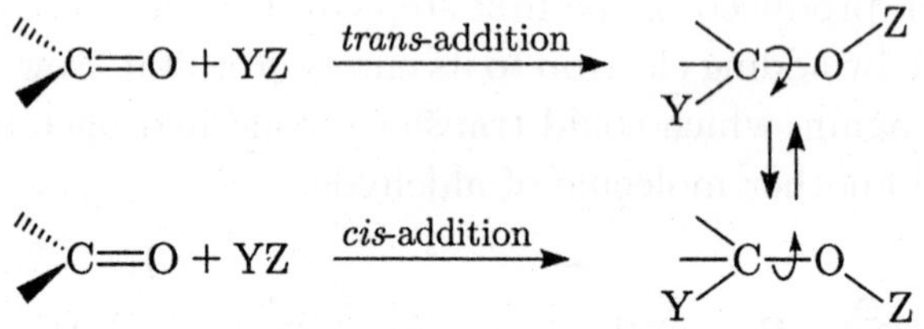

If the environment is chiral, transition states formed by the pathways (a) and (b) will not be formed in equal amounts. One form will be predominant over the other.

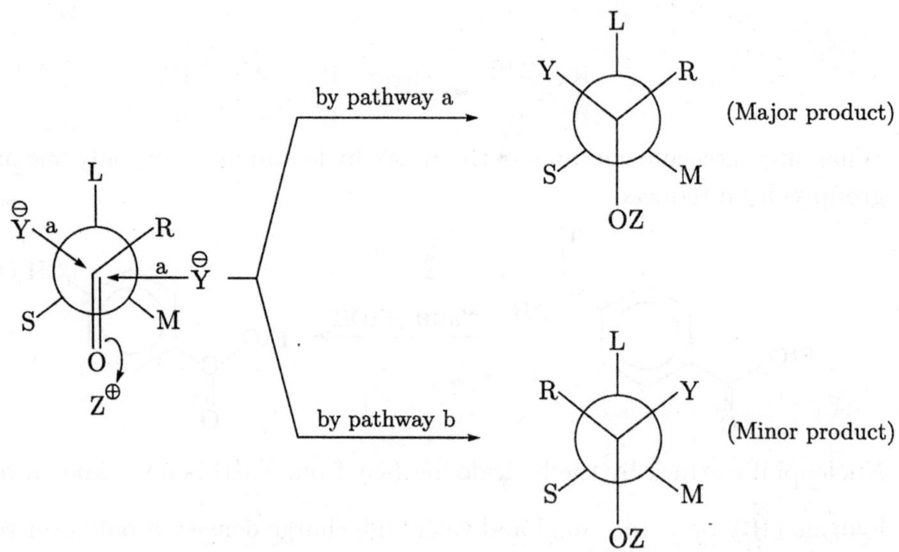

When the α-carbon atom is asymmetric in a carbonyl compound, the predominant product formed may be assumed by applying *Cram's Emperical Rule* of "steric control of asymmetric induction". This rule considers only steric effects and nothing about the electronic effects. So sometimes Cram's rule fails to predict the formation of the predominant product.

The rule states that a carbonyl compound will react in that formation in which the O atom of the C=O group orients itself anti to the largest of the three substituents on the *α-carbon* atom and the nucleophile will attack the carbonyl carbon atom preferentially from the side of plane containing the smallest group.

Example : *Addition* of *HCN to 2-methylbutanal*

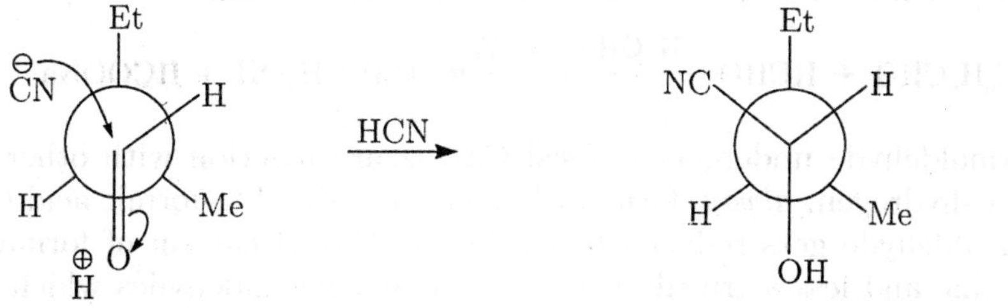

(More stable diastereo isomer)
($\phi_{\,Et/CN=60°}$, $\phi_{\,OH/Me=60°}$)

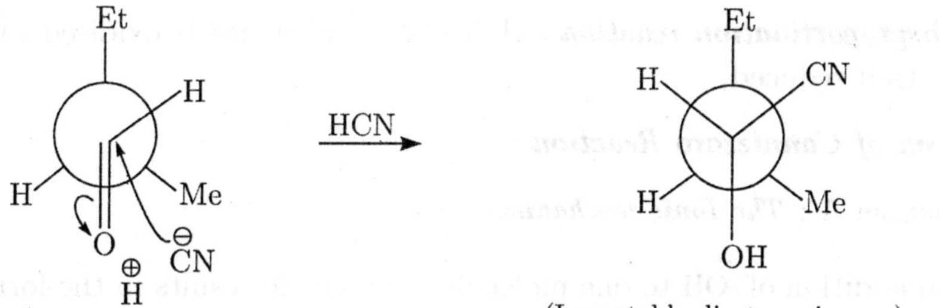

(Less stable diastereo isomer)
($\phi_{\,Et/CN=60°}$, $\phi_{\,CN/Me=60°}$, $\phi_{\,Me/OH=60°}$)

Hydride transfer reactions–the Cannizzaro reaction : In the presence of a *strong base*, aldehydes without α-hydrogen atoms i,e non-aldolisable aldehydes undergo self-oxidation-reduction, i,e *disproportionation reaction.* This is known as *Cannizzaro reaction.* Thus aromatic aldehydes (ArCHO), formaldehyde (HCHO), trialkylacetaldehyde (R_3CCHO) heterocyclic aldehydes like 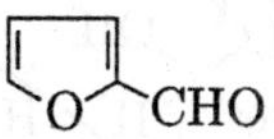 (furfuraldehyde) etc. which contain no α hydrogen atom undergo Cannizzaro reaction.

$$2C_6H_5CHO + NaOH(conc.) \xrightarrow{\Delta} \underset{\text{(Benzyl alcohol)}}{C_6H_5CH_2OH} + \underset{\text{(Sodium benzoate)}}{C_6H_5CO\overset{\ominus}{O}\,Na^{\oplus}}$$

$$2HCHO + NaOH(conc.) \xrightarrow{\Delta} \underset{\text{(Methyl alcohol)}}{CH_3OH} + \underset{\text{(Sodium benzoate)}}{HCOONa}$$

The reaction best proceeds with aromatic aldehydes, although the reaction is known to occur with aldehydes containing *no* α-hydrogen atom. A few aliphatic aldehydes are known which undergo Cannizzaro reaction.

$$\underset{\text{(Trimethylacetaldehyde)}}{Me_3CCHO} + NaOH(conc.) \xrightarrow{200°C} \underset{\text{(2,2-Dimethylpropanol)}}{Me_3CCH_2OH} + \underset{\text{(Sodium salt of 2,2-dimethylpropanoic acid)}}{Me_3CCO\overset{\ominus}{O}\,Na^{\oplus}}$$

The reaction may also occur between two different aldehydes having no a-hydrogen. This type of reaction is known as *Crossed Cannizzaro Reaction.*

$$C_6H_5CHO + HCHO \xrightarrow{NaOH(conc.)/\Delta} C_6H_5CH_2OH + HCOONa$$

When formaldehyde undergoes crossed Cannizzaro reaction with other aldehydes containing no α-hydrogen, *always* formaldehyde gets oxidised to formic acid (sodio salt) and the other aldehyde gets reduced to alcohol. Carbonyl carbon of formaldehyde is more electrophilic and less sterically congested than other aldehydes which makes the attack of hydroxide ($\overset{\ominus}{O}H$) ion facile to this centre. This gives rise to $HOCH_2\overset{\ominus}{O}$, which transfers hydride ($\overset{\ominus}{H}$) directly and thus formic acid is formed as its sodio salt.

Note : *Disproportination reaction* : Half of the substrate is oxidised by the other half, which is itself reduced.

Mechanism of Cannizzaro Reaction :

1. **Mechanism A** : ***The Ionic mechanism***

   Rapid addition of $\overset{\ominus}{O}H$ to one molecule of aldehyde results in the formation of a hydroxy alkoxide ion which like aluminium isopropoxide (MPV reduction for example) acts as a hydride ion donor to the second molecule of aldehyde. In the last step of the reaction, the acid and the alkoxide ion exchange proton between themselves.

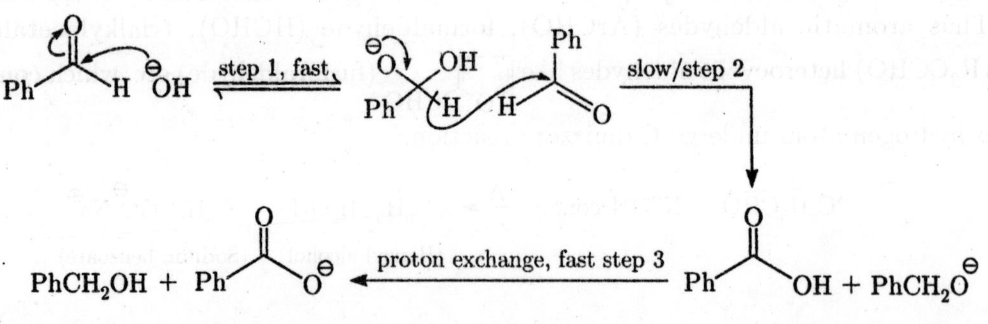

Proton exchange is spontaneous as acyl anion is resonance stabilised which is not present with alkoxide anion.

In presence of a *very strong* concentration of alkali, aldehyde first forms a doubly charged anion from which a hydride ion is transferred to the second molecule of the aldehyde to form acid and an alkoxide anion. Subsequently, the alkoxide anion acquires a proton from the solvent.

Mechanism B :

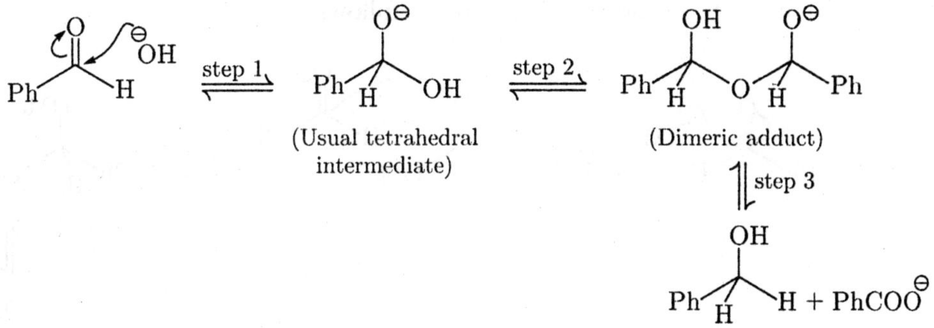

This is proposed *mechanism B* where an *intermediate dimeric adduct* is formed.

Evidences in support of the mechanism

1. The reaction follows third order law (second order with respect to aldehyde and first order with respect to base).

$$\text{Rate}=k_3[\text{aldehyde}]^2.\ [\overset{\ominus}{\text{OH}}]\ (k_3=\text{third order rate constant})$$

This suggests that the reaction between the first formed anion (from base and aldehyde) and another molecule of aldehyde is the rate determining step.

In the presence of a high concentration of base, the reaction follows fourth order law, (second order in both the aldehyde and the base).

$$\text{Rate}=k_4 \times [\text{aldehyde}]^2.[\overset{\ominus}{\text{OH}}]^2\ (k_4=\text{fourth order rate constant})$$

The rate law suggests that the reaction between the doubly charged anion (formed from one molecule of aldehyde and two molecules of base) and another molecule of aldehyde is the rate determining step.

At lower concentrations of base, it is a mixture of both third and fourth order reactions.

$$\text{Rate}=k_3[\text{aldehyde}]^2\ [\overset{\ominus}{\text{OH}}] + k_4[\text{aldehyde}]^2\ [\overset{\ominus}{\text{OH}}]^2$$

The mechanism B which involves the formation of an intermediate dimeric adduct and follows the fourth order rate law is *ruled out* by the following experiment.

The Cannizzaro reaction should work well if methoxide is used as a nucleophile in a mixture of methanol and water. If the mechanism B were correct, the reaction with methoxide would be as follows.

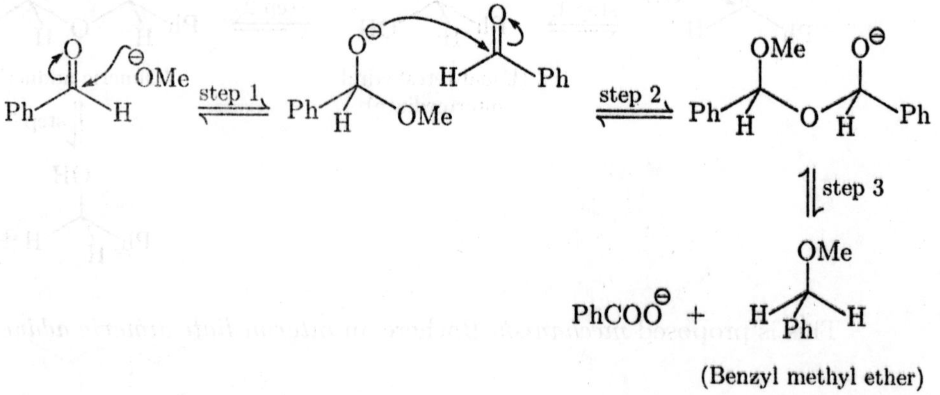

One of the products would be benzyl methyl ether instead of benzyl alcohol. None is observed experimentally. Under the conditions of the experiment, benzyl methyl ether does not react to form benzyl alcohol, so it can not be the case that the ether is formed but then reacts to form the products. Mechanism B can therefore be ruled out.

2. ***Isotopic labelling*** : Hydride ion is directly transferred from one molecule of aldehyde to the other and does not become free in the solution. This has been proved by the observation that there is *no C–D bond* in the products, when the reaction is carried out in D_2O instead of water (H_2O). This tells us that the hydrogen must come from the aldehyde and not from the solvent.

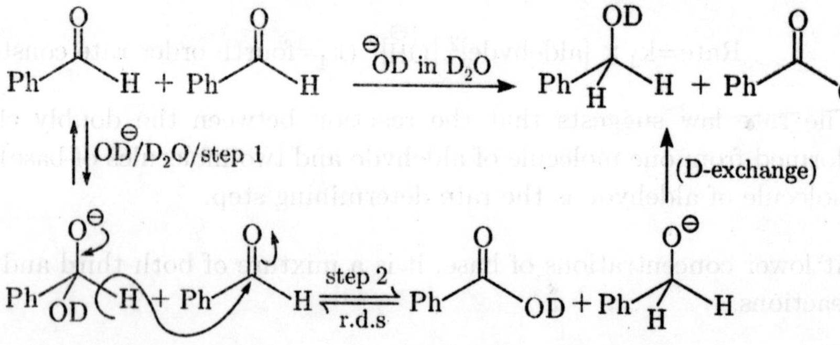

If the reaction is carried out in water labelled with ^{18}O, the oxygen in the benzaldehyde exchanges with the ^{18}O from the solvent much faster than the Cannizzaro reaction takes place.

This can only be because of a rapid equilibrium in step 1 and so step 1 can not be rate limiting. Naturally step 2 (mechanism A) becomes the rate limiting step.

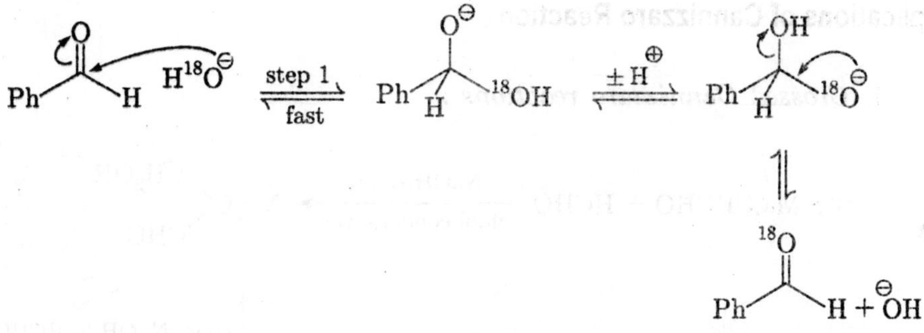

3. The reaction rate depends on the nucleophilic attack on the carbonyl carbon. Hence the factors which reduce the positive charge of the carbonyl carbon retard the reaction rate, *e.g.*, +I effect on the carbonyl carbon. In extreme cases, the reaction may not occur, *e.g.*, N,N-dimethylaminobenzaldehyde does not undergo Cannizzaro reaction at all.

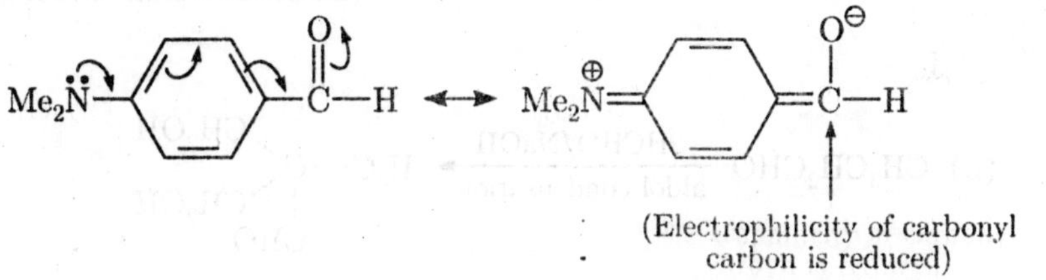

Similarly, electronwithdrawing group at the *p*-position increases the rate. Also the sterically hindered aldehydes do not undergo Cannizzaro reaction.

Aldehydes	Relative to Benzaldehyde at 25°C	Relative Rate to benzaldehyde at 100°C
1. Benzaldehyde	1	1
2. *p*-methoxybenzaldehyde (electron donating + R effect at the *p*-position due to –OMe group)	0.05	0.05
3. *p*-methylbenzaldehyde (+ R effect at the *p*-position)	0.20	0.20
4. *p*-methylaminobenzaldehyde (strong + R effect at the *p*-position)	very slow	very slow
5. *p*-nitrobenzaldehyde (electron-withdrawing –R effect of $-NO_2$ group at the *p*-position)	210	210

Applications of Cannizzaro Reaction

1. ***Crossed Cannizzaro reactions*** :

(a) 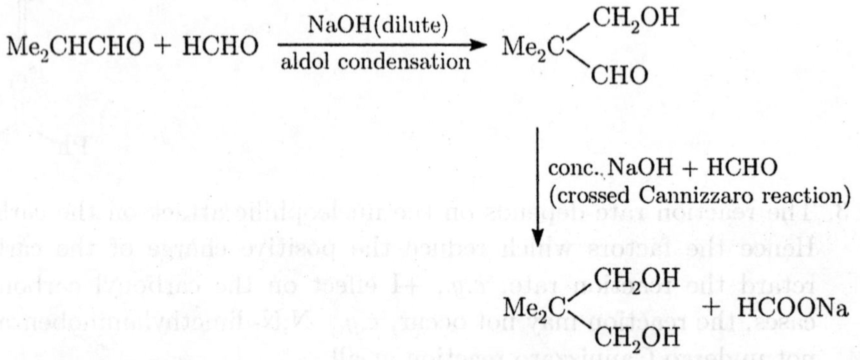

(Substituted trimethyleneglycol)

(b) 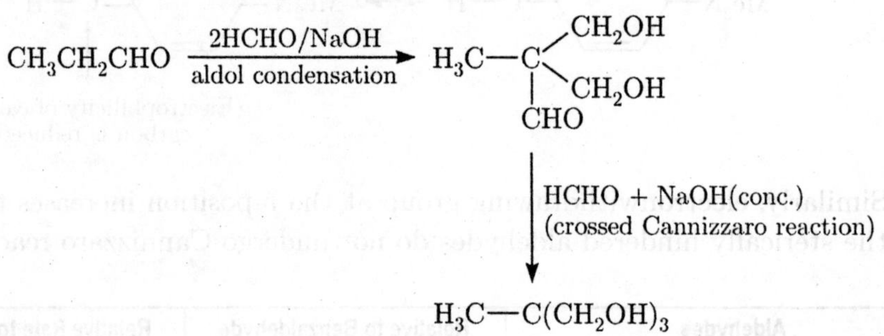

(c) 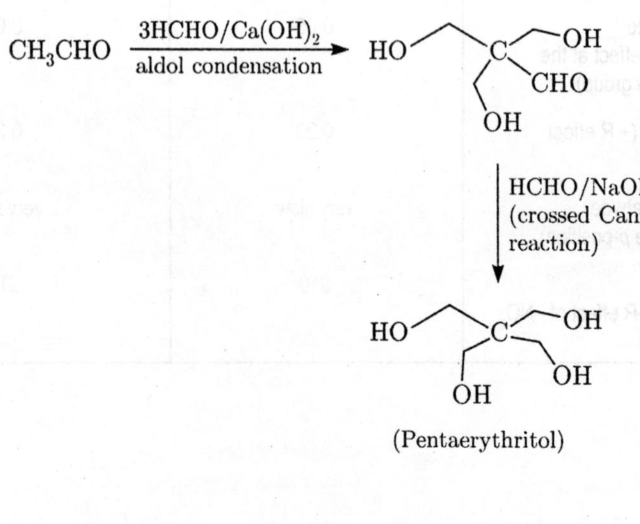

(Pentaerythritol)

2. ***Intramolecular Cannizzaro reaction*** : Dialdehydes and α-ketoaldehydes undergo intramolecular Cannizzaro reaction giving various valuable products.

(a) 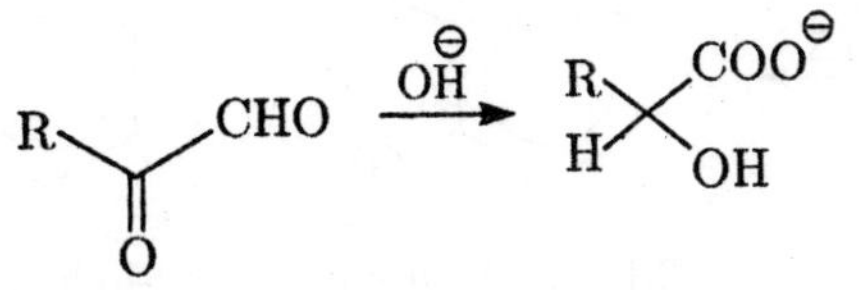

(b) 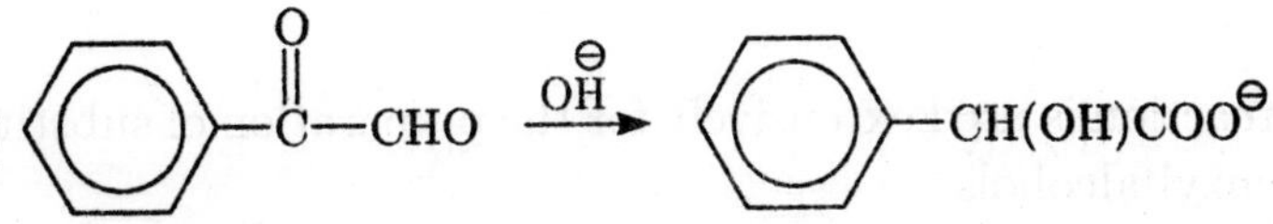

(Phenylglyoxal)

Mechanism :

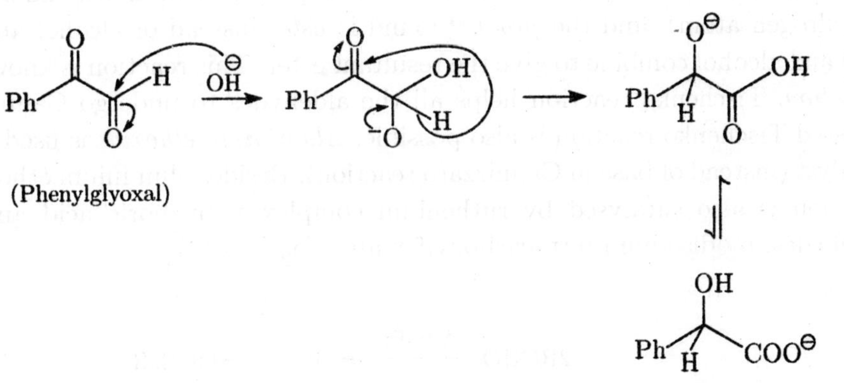

(Phenylglyoxal)

(Salt of mandelic acid)

3. ***Synthesis of various types of alcohols and acids*** :

(a) 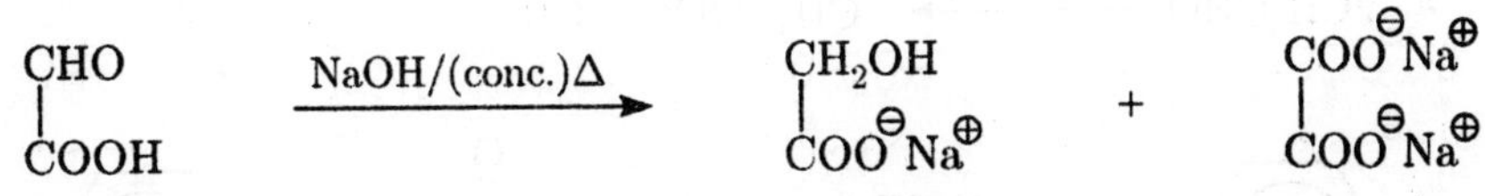

(Glyoxalic acid) (Sodium glyoxalate) (Sodium oxalate)

b. 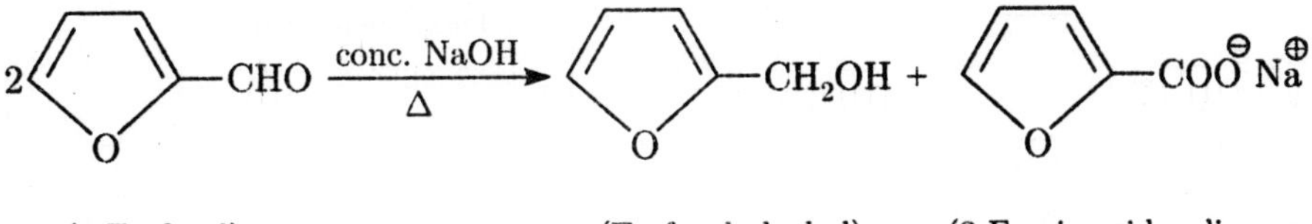

(2-Furfural) (Furfuryl alcohol) (2-Furoic acid sodium salt)

c. 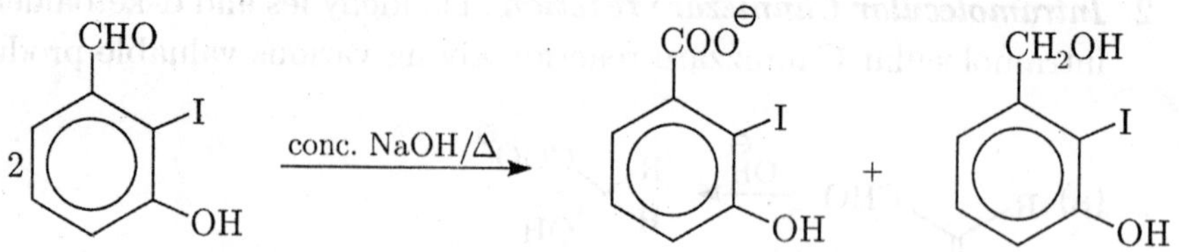

(2-Iodo-3-hydroxy-benzaldehyde) (2-Iodo-3-hydroxy-benzoic acid salt) (2-Iodo-3-hydroxy-benzyl alcohol)

Cannizzaro reaction is used extensively for the preparation of substituted benzoic acids and benzyl alcohols.

The Tischenko Reaction (Tischenko Aldehyde-Ester Disproportionation)

When aldehydes, with or without α-hydrogen, are treated with aluminium ethoxide, one molecule is oxidised and the other reduced (compare Cannizzaro reaction where disproportionation reaction occurs between aliphatic or aromatic aldehydes having no α-hydrogen atom), and the *product* found is *ester* instead of alcohol and acid. In fact, acid and alcohol combine to give the resultant ester. This reaction is known as *Tischenko Reaction.* Tischenko reaction helps all the aldehydes to undergo Cannizzaro reaction. Crossed Tischenko reaction is also possible. *Aluminium ethoxide* is used as a Lewis acid catalyst (instead of base in Cannizzaro reaction). Besides aluminium ethoxide, Tischenko reaction is also catalysed by ruthenium complexes, by boric acid and for aromatic aldehydes, by disodium tetracarbonylferrate, $Na_2Fe(CO)_4$.

$$2RCHO \xrightarrow{Al(OEt)_3} R-\overset{O}{\overset{\|}{C}}-OCH_2R$$

(Ester)

Examples :

a. $2CH_3CHO \xrightarrow{Al(OEt)_3} CH_3COOCH_2CH_3$

b. 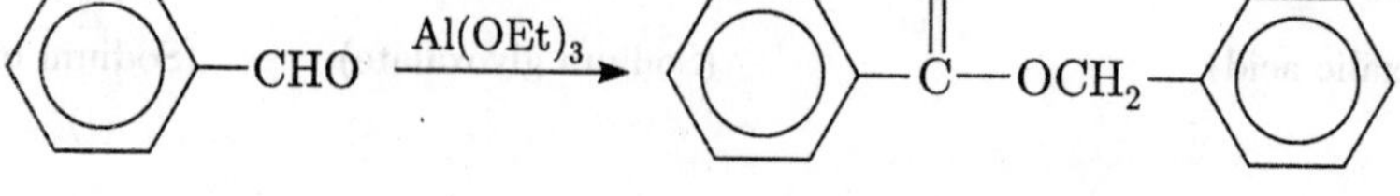

(Benzyl benzoate)

Mechanism of Tischenko reaction :

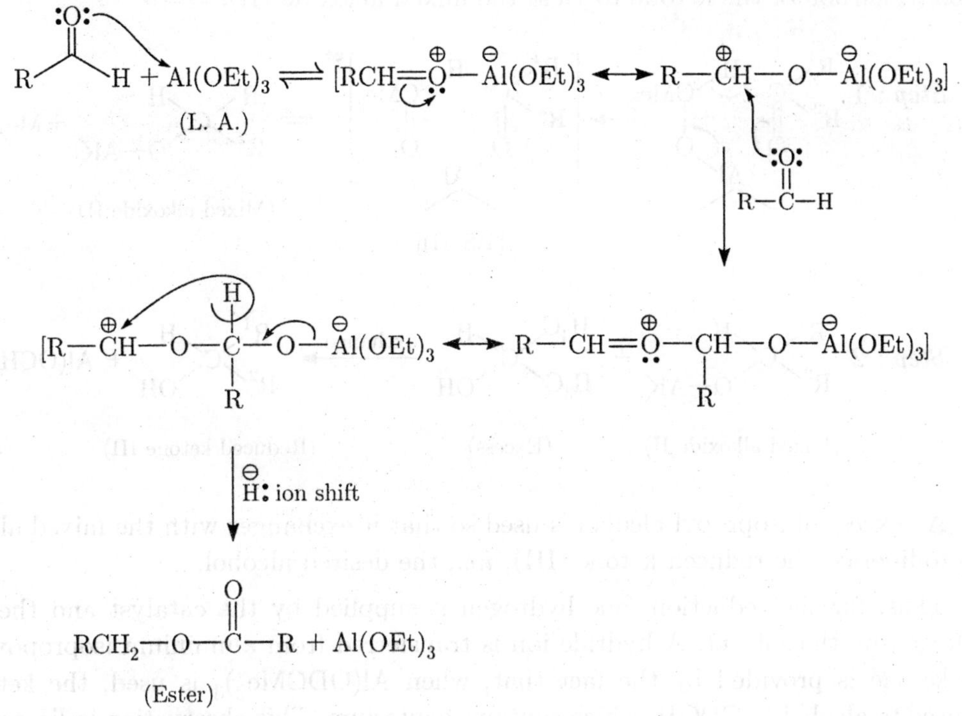

Hydride Transfer Reactions

Meerwein-Pondorf-Verley reduction (MPV reduction)

The reaction involves the reduction of aldehydes or ketones to alcohols by treatment with aluminium isopropoxide in the presence of excess of isopropyl alcohol.

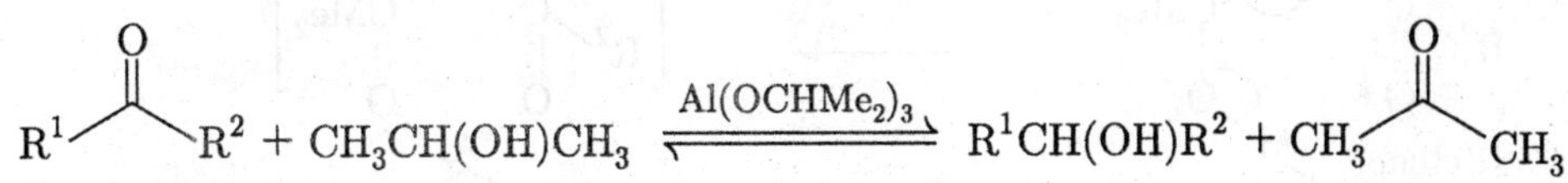

The reaction is reversible. The reverse reaction is called Oppenaur oxidation, which is employed for the oxidation of alcohols, using aluminium tertiarybutoxide as catalyst in the presence of excess acetone.

The reaction shifts in the forward direction by the removal of acetone by distillation. The reaction occurs under mild conditions, rapid, side reactions negligible and the yield is high. The reaction is specific for carbonyl group, other reducible groups such as olefinic bond, $-NO_2$, –C≡C– etc. remain unaffected. If a compound contains two carbonyl groups, one may be protected by acetal formation and the other is then reduced. Ketones with high enol content, *e.g.*, β-diketones, β-ketoners etc. do not respond to this reaction.

Mechanism of MPV reduction : The reaction probably involves a cyclic transition state (I) in which a hydride ion from the α-*C–H* bond of the alkoxide migrates to the carbonyl carbon of the ketone to yield the mixed alkoxide (II).

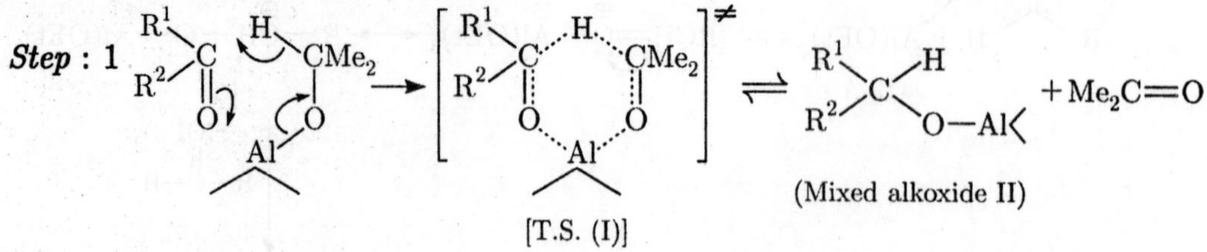

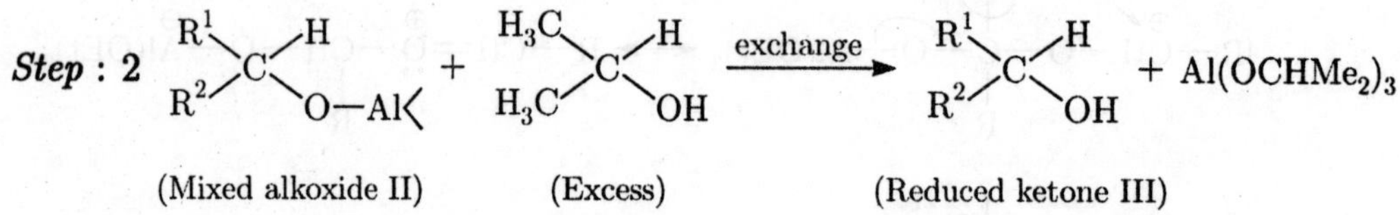

An excess of isopropyl alcohol is used so that it exchanges with the mixed alkoxide (II) to liberate the reduced ketone (III), *i.e.*, the desired alcohol.

Thus, for the reduction, one hydrogen is supplied by the catalyst and the other hydrogen by the solvent. A hydride ion is transferred from aluminium isopropoxide to the ketone is provided by the fact that, when $Al(ODCMe_2)_3$ is used, the ketone is reduced to alcohol R_2CDOH, which contains deuterium. This observation indicates that, the reaction is proceeding *via* cyclic transition state.

Isotope labelling experiment :

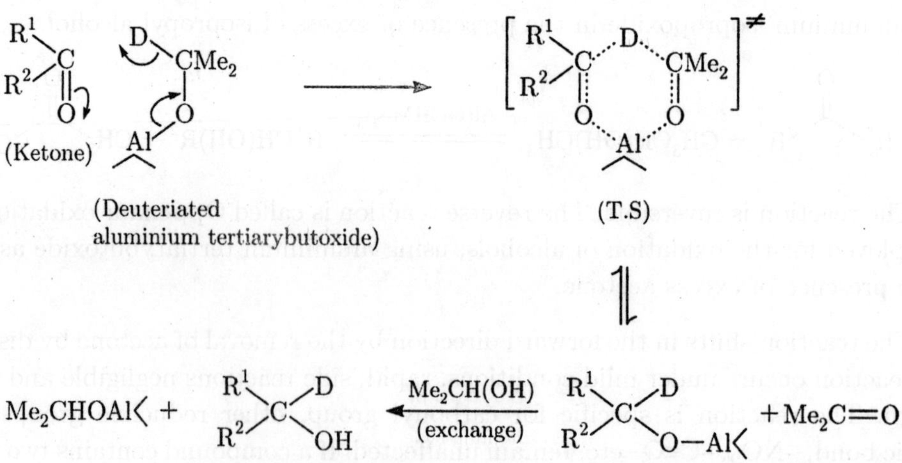

Specificity of aluminium isopropoxide : A number of metal alkoxides have been used, but aluminium isopropoxide is found to be the best reagent. Aluminium alkoxides are less polar than alkali metal alkoxides, since **Al–O bond** is nearly **covalent** in nature. Hence, this undergoes very little dissociation to give alkoxide ion which generally cause some polymerisation of the carbonyl compounds, specially the sensitive aldehydes. Thus, the side reactions are negligible. The boiling point of aluminium isopropoxide is 140°–150°C at 12 mm of Hg. This enables acetone to be distilled over as to shift the equilibrium in the formward direction.

Applications of MPV reduction :

1. 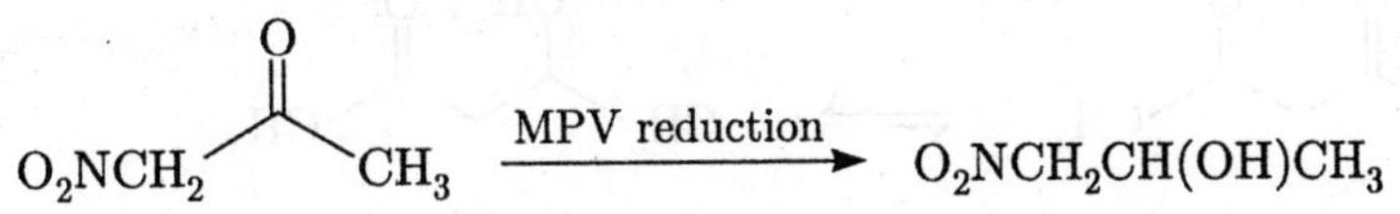

2. **Selective reduction of a carbonyl group of a dicarbonyl compound via acetal formation.**

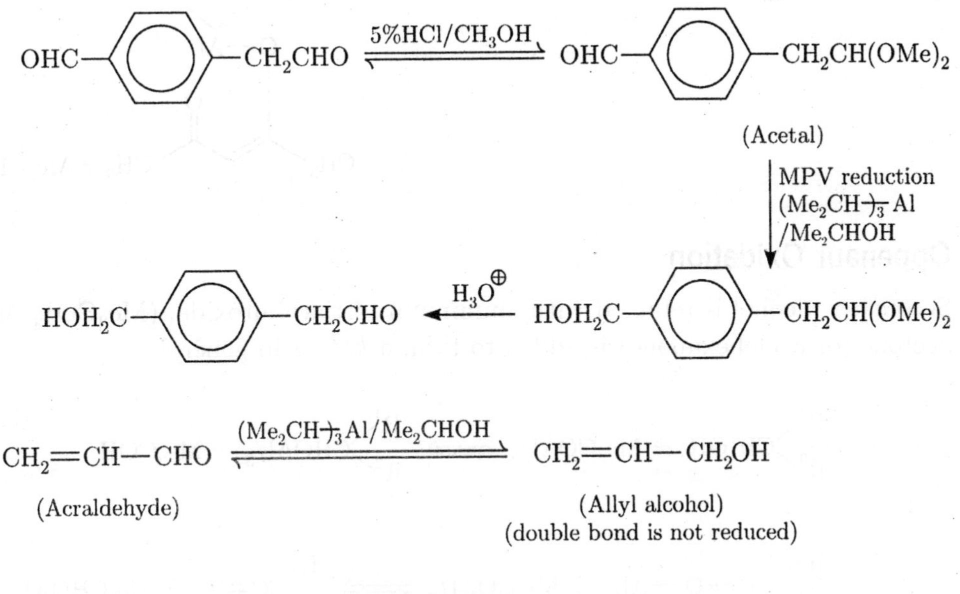

3. $CH_2{=}CH{-}CHO \xrightleftharpoons{(Me_2CH)_3Al/Me_2CHOH} CH_2{=}CH{-}CH_2OH$

(Acraldehyde) (Allyl alcohol) (double bond is not reduced)

4. $C_6H_5COCH_3 \xrightleftharpoons{(Me_2CHO)_3Al/Me_2CHOH} C_6H_5CH(OH)CH_3$

(Aromatic ketone)

5. 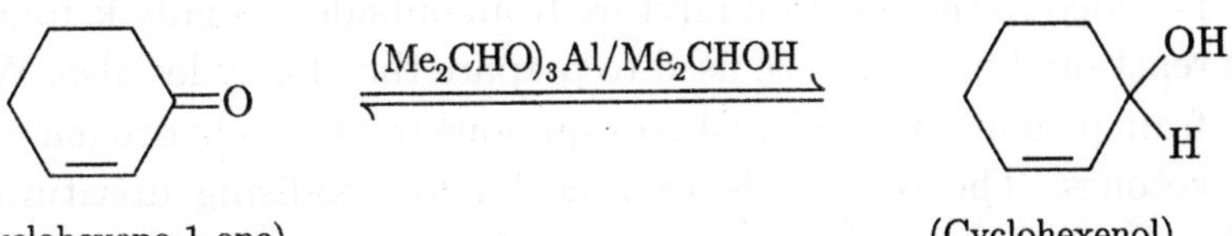

(2-Cyclohexene-1-one) (Alicyclic ketone) (Cyclohexenol)

6. 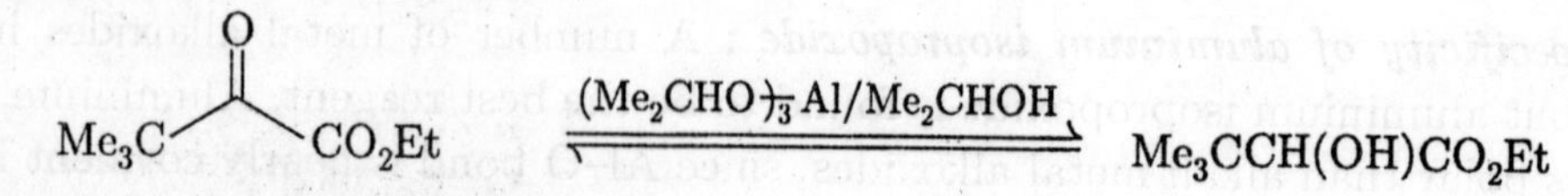

(Ethyl trimethyl pyruvate)
(Ketoester)

Carbonyl compounds containing high percentage of enol, such as β-diketones. β-ketoesters etc. do not undergo MPV reduction. Perhaps, aluminium isopropoxide gets converted to isopropyl alcohol by the action of enol.

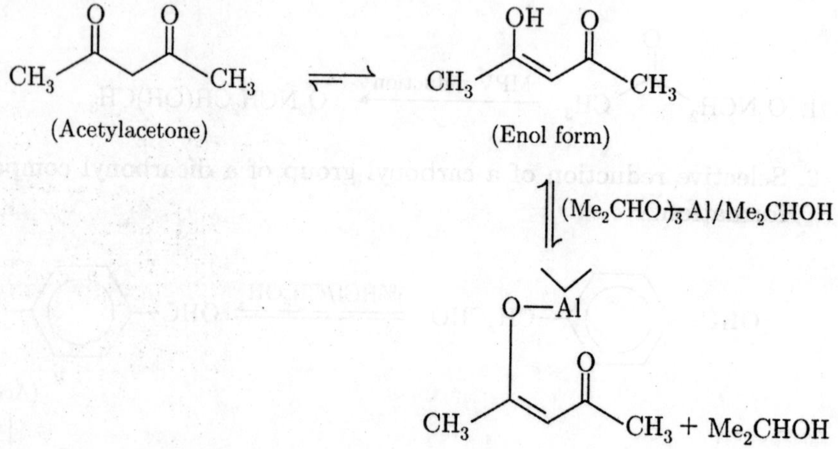

(Acetylacetone) (Enol form)

Oppenaur Oxidation

Secondary alcohol is refluxed with aluminium tertiarybutoxide, $(Me_3CO)_3$ Al and then acetone (or cyclohexanone) is added to form a *ketone* in general.

$$\begin{matrix}R^1\\R^2\end{matrix}\!\!>CH(OH) + Me_3COAl/_3 \rightleftharpoons \begin{matrix}R^1\\R^2\end{matrix}\!\!>CHOAl/_3 + Me_3COH$$

$$\begin{matrix}R^1\\R^2\end{matrix}\!\!>CH{-}O{-}Al/_3 + Me_3COAl/_3 \rightleftharpoons \begin{matrix}R^1\\R^2\end{matrix}\!\!>C{=}O + Me_2CHOAl/_3$$

Aluminium tertiarybutoxide is used as the reagent since the tertiarybutanol produced is not oxidised under these conditions. Acetone (Me_2CO) cannot be prepared by this method as it is added in the reaction mixture from outside. Usually ketones are prepared through this reaction, but it may be used to prepare the aldehydes also. When aldehydes are prepared from primary alcohols, *p*-benzoquinone is used as hydrogen acceptor instead of aliphatic ketones. The process is very useful for oxidising unsaturated secondary alcohols to ketones.

$$CH_3CH{=}CHCH(OH)CH_3 \xrightleftharpoons{\text{Al-}t\text{-butoxide in }p\text{-benzoquinone}} CH_3CH{=}CH{-}\overset{\overset{\displaystyle O}{\|}}{C}{-}CH_3$$

$$CH_3CH{=}CHCH_2OH \xrightleftharpoons{\text{Al-}t\text{-butoxide in }p\text{-benzoquinone}} CH_3CH{=}CH{-}CHO$$

Double bond is *not* reduced during the reaction.

Mechanism of the reaction : The mechanism of Oppenaur oxidation is the reverse of that of MPV reduction. So, this also involves hydride ion transfer through a cyclic transition state.

Step **1** : $\begin{matrix}R^1\\R^2\end{matrix}\!\!>\!CH(OH) + Me_3COAl/_3 \xrightleftharpoons{\text{rapid exchange}} \begin{matrix}R^1\\R^2\end{matrix}\!\!>\!CHO{-}Al/_3 + Me_3COH$

Step **2** : The aluminium derivative then forms with acetone a cyclic transition state which undergoes internal hydride transfer, resulting in the formation of ketone.

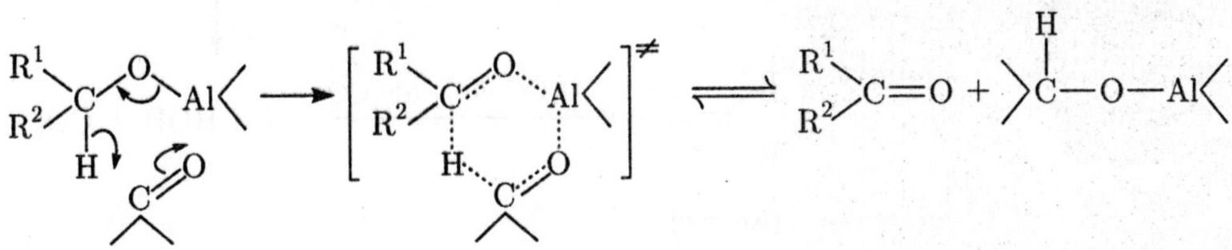

Since the initial attack is on the alcoholic hydroxyl group, hindered alcoholic groups react less readily.

Applications of Oppenaur oxidation :

1. The reagent is particularly useful for oxidising unsaturated alcohols because it does not affect the double bond.

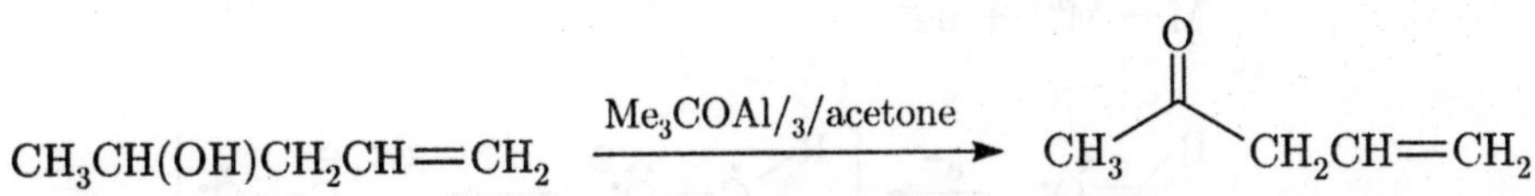

2. The reaction is successful with low boiling aldehydes as they can be distilled off.

$$\underset{\text{(Primary unsaturated alcohol)}}{Me_2C{=}CH{-}CH_2CH_2CH_2OH} \xrightarrow[\text{(}p\text{-benzoquinone is a good hydrogen acceptor)}]{Me_3COAl/_3,\ p\text{-benzoquinone}/60°C/3\text{–}4h} Me_2C{=}CH(CH_2)_2CHO$$

3. β–γ-unsaturated alcohols undergo oxidation with migration of double bond to form α, β-unsaturated ketone.

$$R{-}\overset{\gamma}{C}H{=}\overset{\beta}{C}H{-}CH_2CH(OH)R \xrightarrow[p\text{-benzoquinone}]{Me_3COAl/_3,} RCH_2{-}\overset{\beta}{C}H{=}\overset{\alpha}{C}H{-}\overset{\overset{\displaystyle O}{\|}}{C}{-}R$$

4. Alicyclic alcohols have been oxidised to alicyclic ketones.

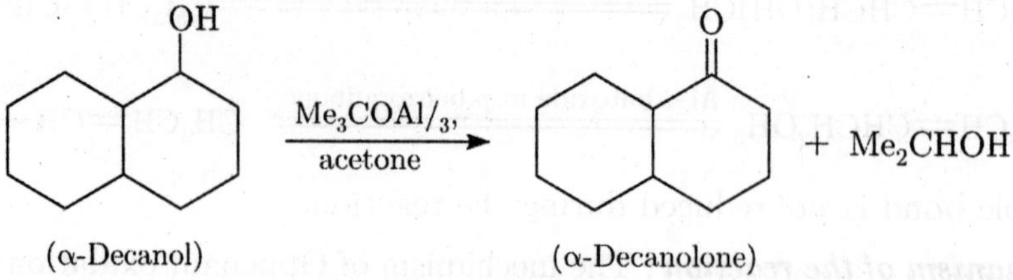

Sensitive alcohols can be oxidised under mild conditions using fluorenone as a strong hydrogen acceptor.

5. Formates (but not acetates or benzoates) have been oxidised to the ketones.

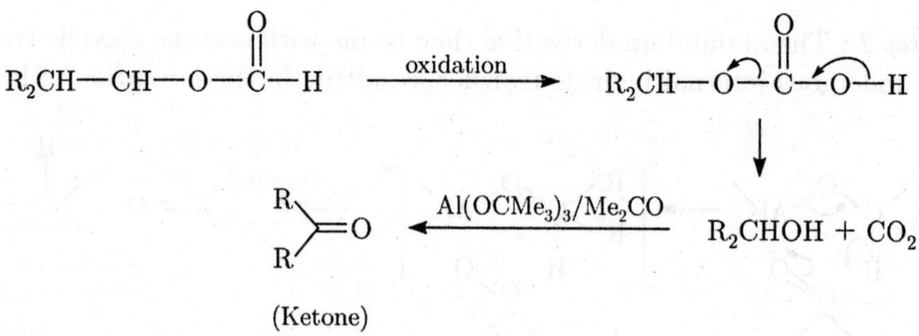

Electrolytic reduction reactions

When carbonyl group reacts with active metals, transfer of electrons takes place and radical anions are formed.

$$M \rightarrow M^{n+} + ne^-$$

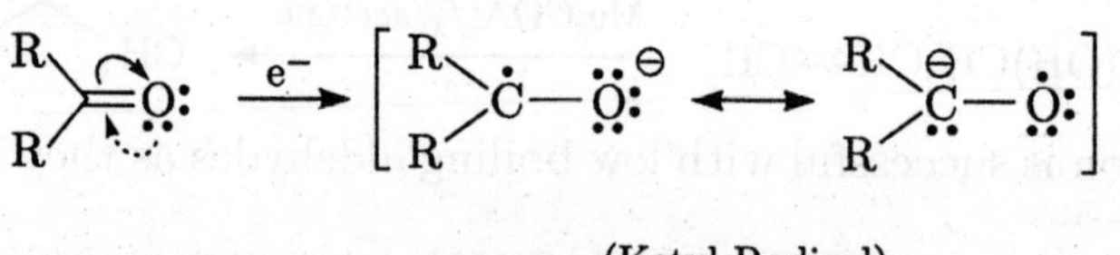

If the reaction medium is aprotic, then the radical anion forms a carbon-carbon bond with another radical anion. No carbon-oxygen or oxygen-oxygen bond is formed. This is due to the fact that, oxygen contains more electron charge density which is adsorbed by the metal cation M^{n+}. Secondly carbon-carbon bond is more stable than carbon-oxygen bond or oxygen-oxygen bond. The destabilising factor is *α-effect* in case of :Ö—Ö: bond (lone pair-lone pair repulsion makes the bond unstable) and lone pair–bond pair repulsion in case of C—Ö: bond. In case of C—C bond, no such destabilisation is present and so becomes most stable according to VSEPR theory.

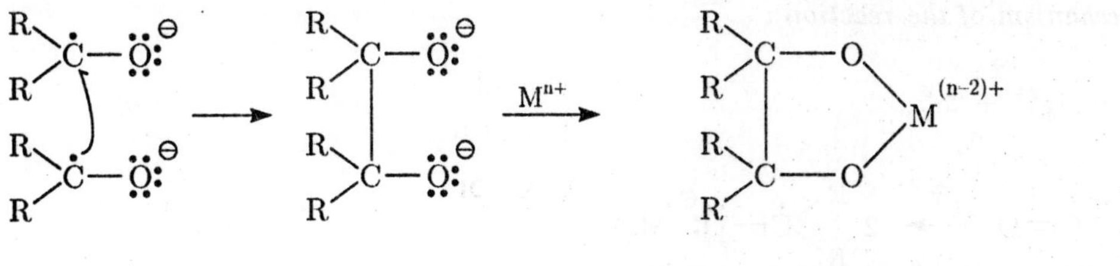

(Strong covalent metal-oxygen bond)

If the reaction medium is protic, the more basic carbanion of the radical anion accepts proton (H^+) from the solvent and the reaction takes place.

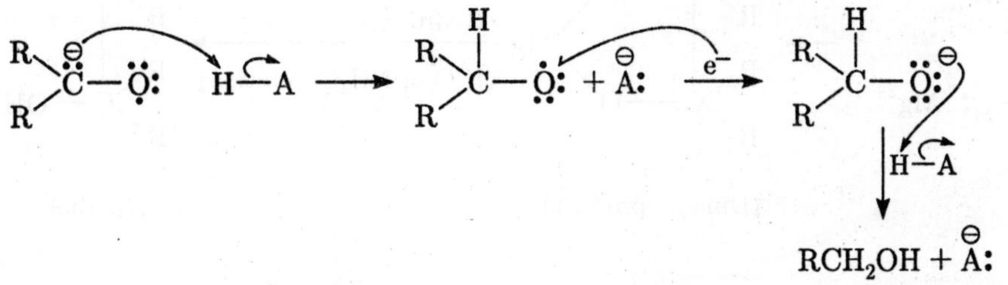

Example of electrolytic reduction–formation of 1,2-diols in protic solvent :

When an aldehyde or a ketone is treated with magnesium or aluminium in ether, two molecules of the carbonyl compound couple to form a dimeric dianion which exists as a metal salt. The salt on treatment with acid or ammonium chloride (NH_4Cl) solution gives 1,2-diol. The diol obtained from acetone is commonly called pinacol.

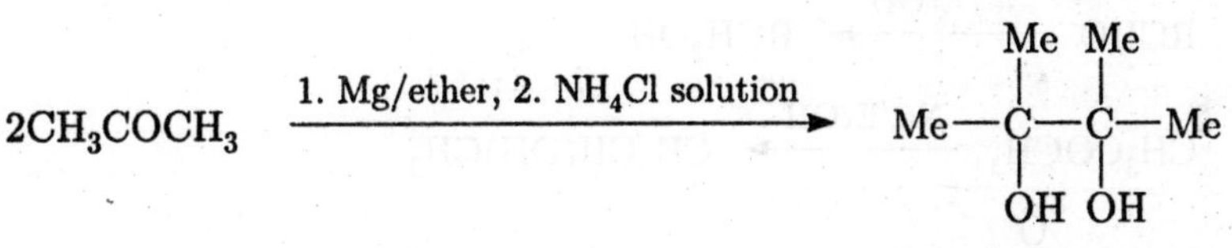

(Pinacol, a 1,2-diol)

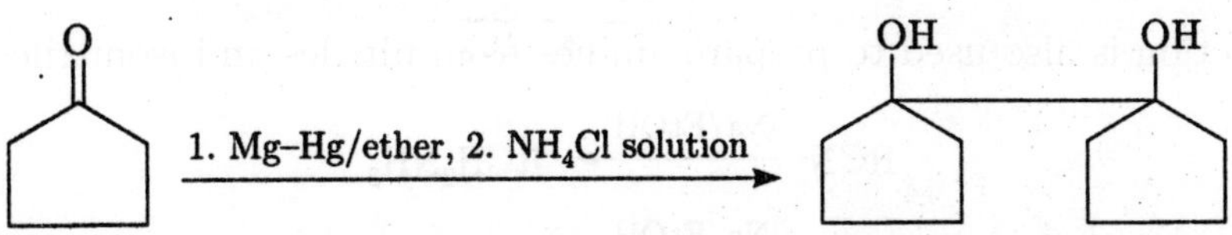

However, the reaction gives better yields with aromatic ketones than that with aliphatic ketones. Cyclic 1,2-diols are prepared from diketones by this reaction.

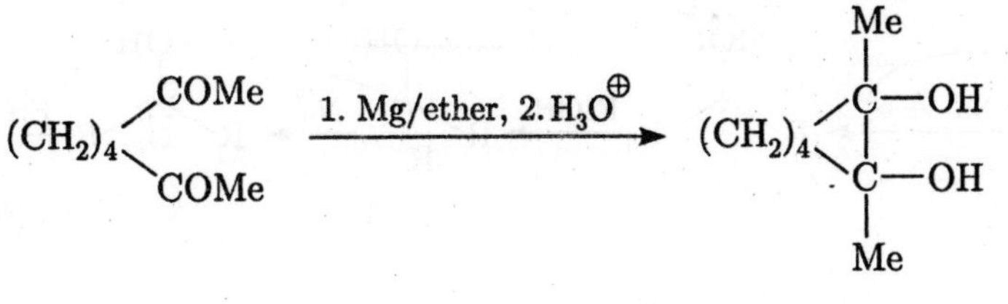

Mechanism of the reaction :

$$Mg \rightarrow Mg^{2+} + 2e^-$$

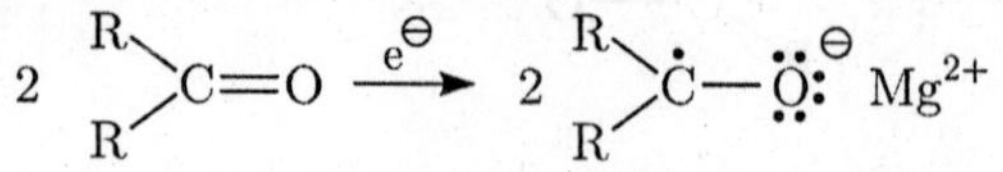

(Anionic Radical)

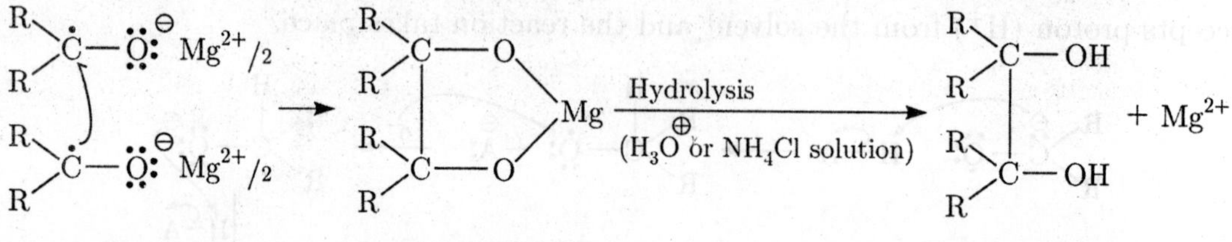

(Dimeric product) (1,2-diol)

Example of electrolytic reduction reaction in protic solvent

The Bouveault-Blanc Reduction : In Bouveault-Blanc Reduction, carbonyl compounds are treated with active metal like sodium in the presence of protic solvents like ethanol or n-butanol. A radical anion is formed where the more basic carbanion abstracts proton from the solvent to make the reduction reaction complete.

$$RCHO \xrightarrow{Na/EtOH} RCH_2OH$$

$$CH_3COCH_3 \xrightarrow{Na/EtOH} CH_3CH(OH)CH_3$$

$$CH_3CH_2\overset{\overset{\displaystyle O}{\|}}{C}—OCH_3 \xrightarrow{Na/EtOH} CH_3CH_2CH_2OH + CH_3OH$$

This reaction is also used to prepare amines from nitriles and isonitriles.

$$RCN \xrightarrow{Na/EtOH} RCH_2NH_2$$

$$RCN \xrightarrow{Na/EtOH} RNHCH_2$$

Mechanism of Bouveault Blanc Reduction :

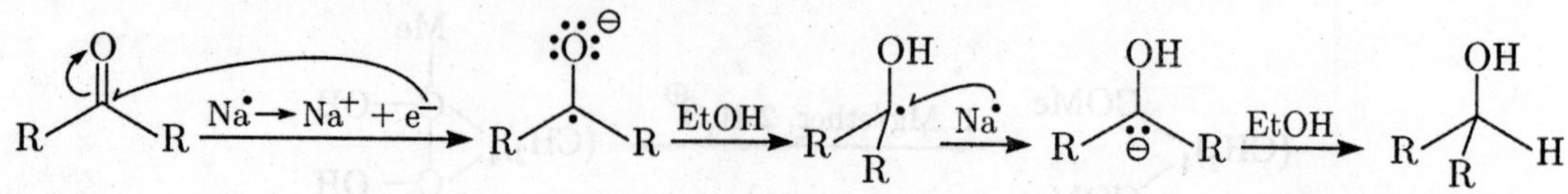

(Secondary alcohol)

Preparation of primary alcohol from ester by Bouveault–Blanc reduction :

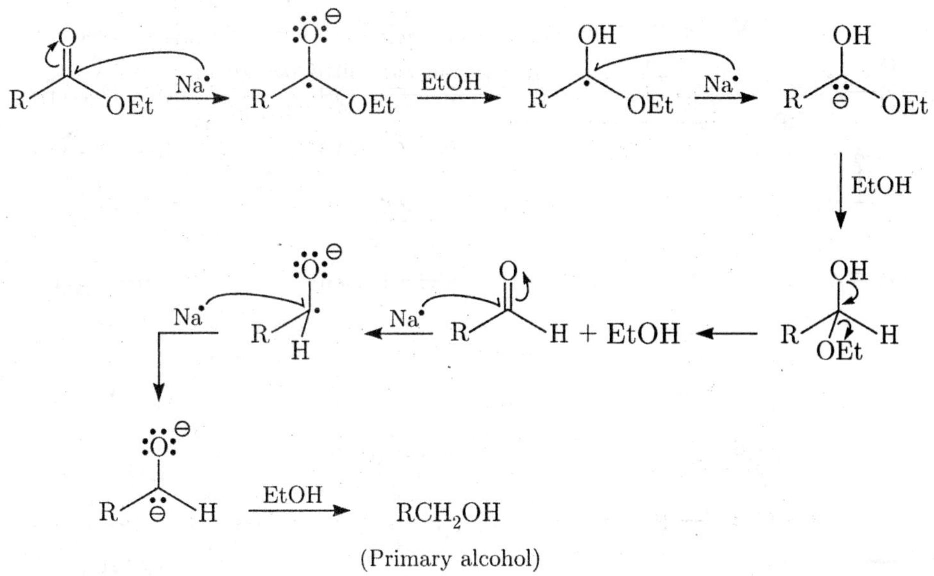

Reductive coupling reactions : *Acyloin Condensation*

When an ester is refluxed with sodium in an inert aprotic solvent such as ether benzene, toluene, xylene etc. in absence of any free alcohol and then the product is treated with an acid or alcohol, a *dimeric α-hydroxyketone* called *acyloin* is obtained and the reaction is called acyloin synthesis or condensation. For example, ethyl propanoate on refluxing with sodium in benzene followed by acidification gives α-hydroxy-3-hexanone.

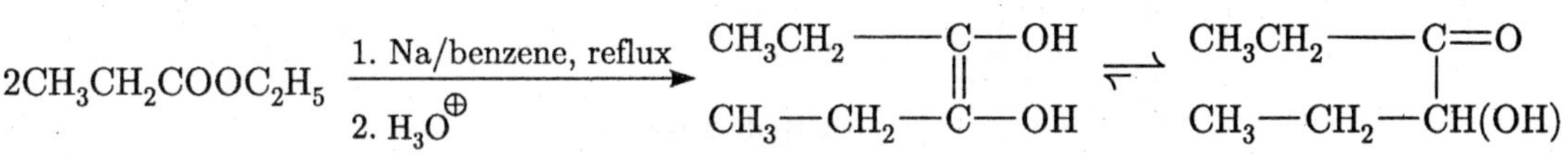

It is a good means for preparing long chain acyloins containing 10-20 carbon atoms. 10-20 membered cyclic acyloins have been prepared from diesters of dicarboxylic acid, *e.g.*, $EtO_2C(CH_2)_nCOOEt$ (n=10-20) using high dilution technique. The yield varies from 60-90%.

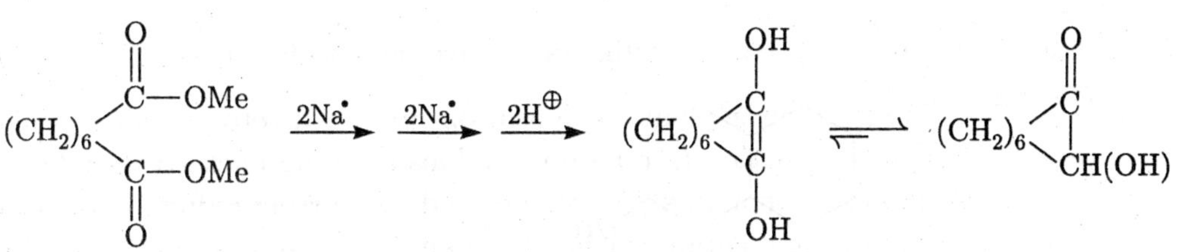

***Mechanism of acyloin condensation reaction* :**

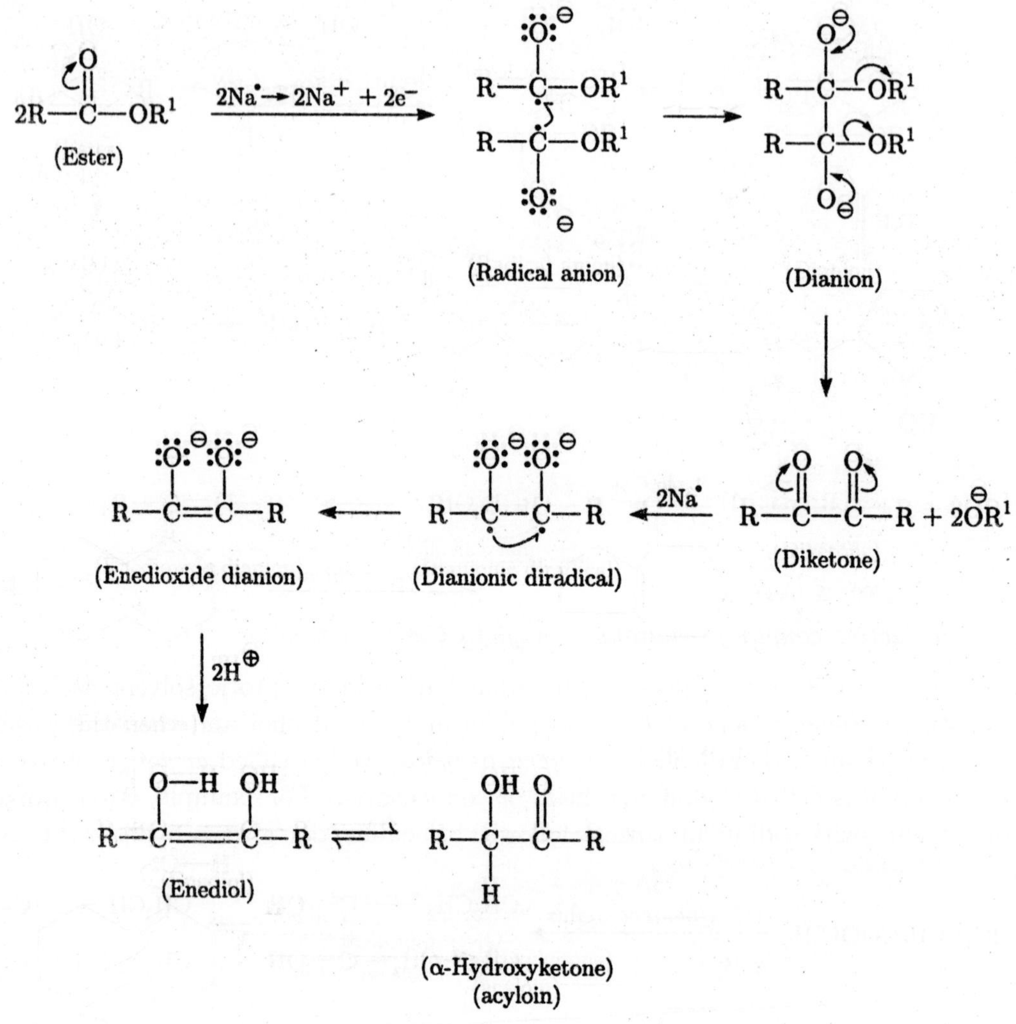

Small traces of oxygen (radical quencher) reduces the yield of the reaction, so an oxygen free environment is needed. A diketone is formed as an intermediate is supported by the following facts.

1. In a number of cases, traces of diketones have been isolated.
2. If an ester, undergoing acyloin condensation gives a diketone which is highly resistant towards reduction (reduction develops a strong back strain (B-strain) in sp^3 hybridised carbon atoms), it does not undergo further reduction to acyloin. So a poor yield of the reaction is generally found. This has actually been found in case of ethyl-2-methylpropanoate. The intermediate diketone being very resistant towards reduction (a high value of B-strain), does not undergo further

reduction to acyloin and the diketone is obtained as the major product of the reaction.

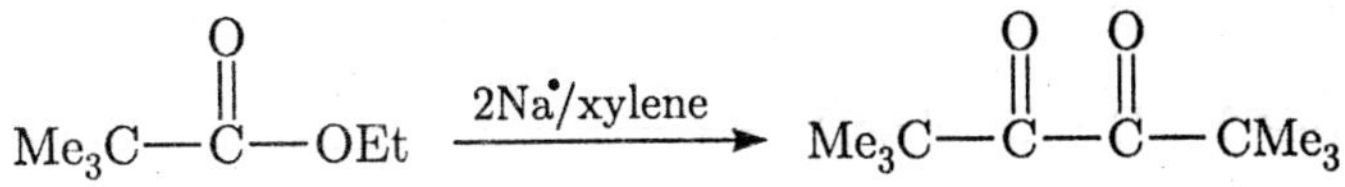

(2,2,5,5-Tetramethyl hexan-3,4-dione)

Since ethoxide (an alkoxide) anion is generated in the acyloin condensation reaction, base catalysed ester condensation reactions can occur in competition. This is especially disadvantageous in the formation of 6–, 7– and 8– membered acyloins, where Dieckmann condensation to give 5–, 6– and 7– membered cyclic β-ketoesters is very efficient. To prevent this competitive reaction, trimethylsilyl chloride (TMS–Cl, Me_3SiCl) is included to trap ethoxide anion as it is formed.

$$Me_3SiCl + EtO^{\ominus} \longrightarrow Me_3SiOEt + Cl^{\ominus}$$

The acyloin dianion is also trapped and the acyloin is released with acid.

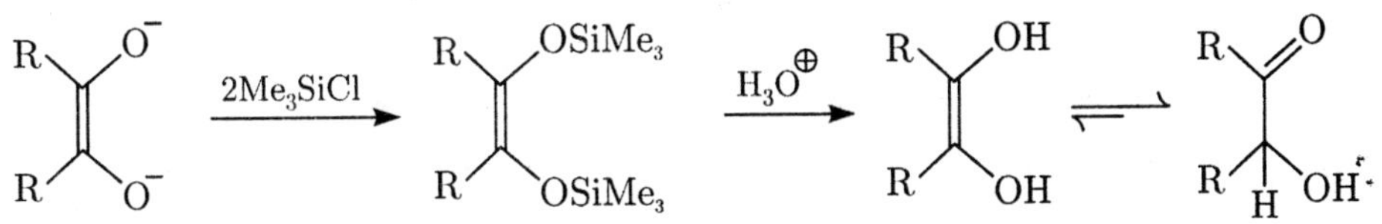

(Acyloin dianion) $+ 2Cl^{\ominus}$ (Acyloin)

It is even possible to make 4-membered cyclic acyloins in this way.

(a) 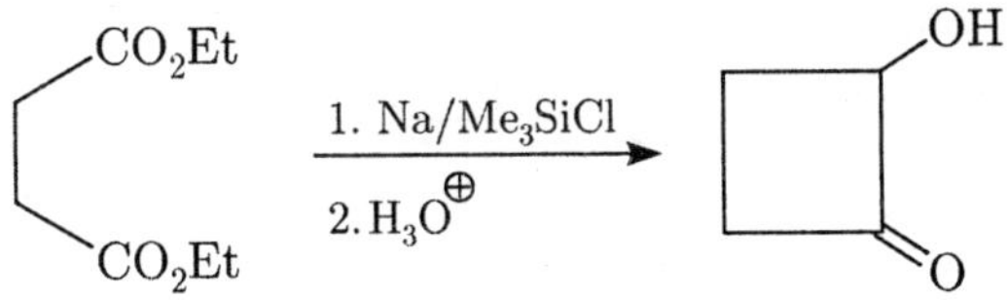

(b) 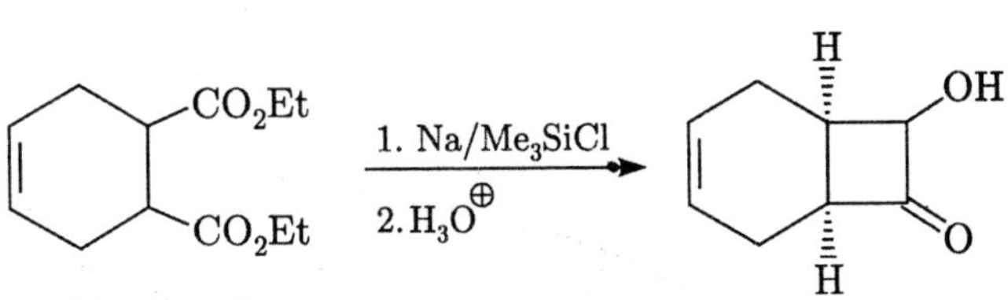

(*Cis*-isomer)

Mechanism of the ring formation reaction :

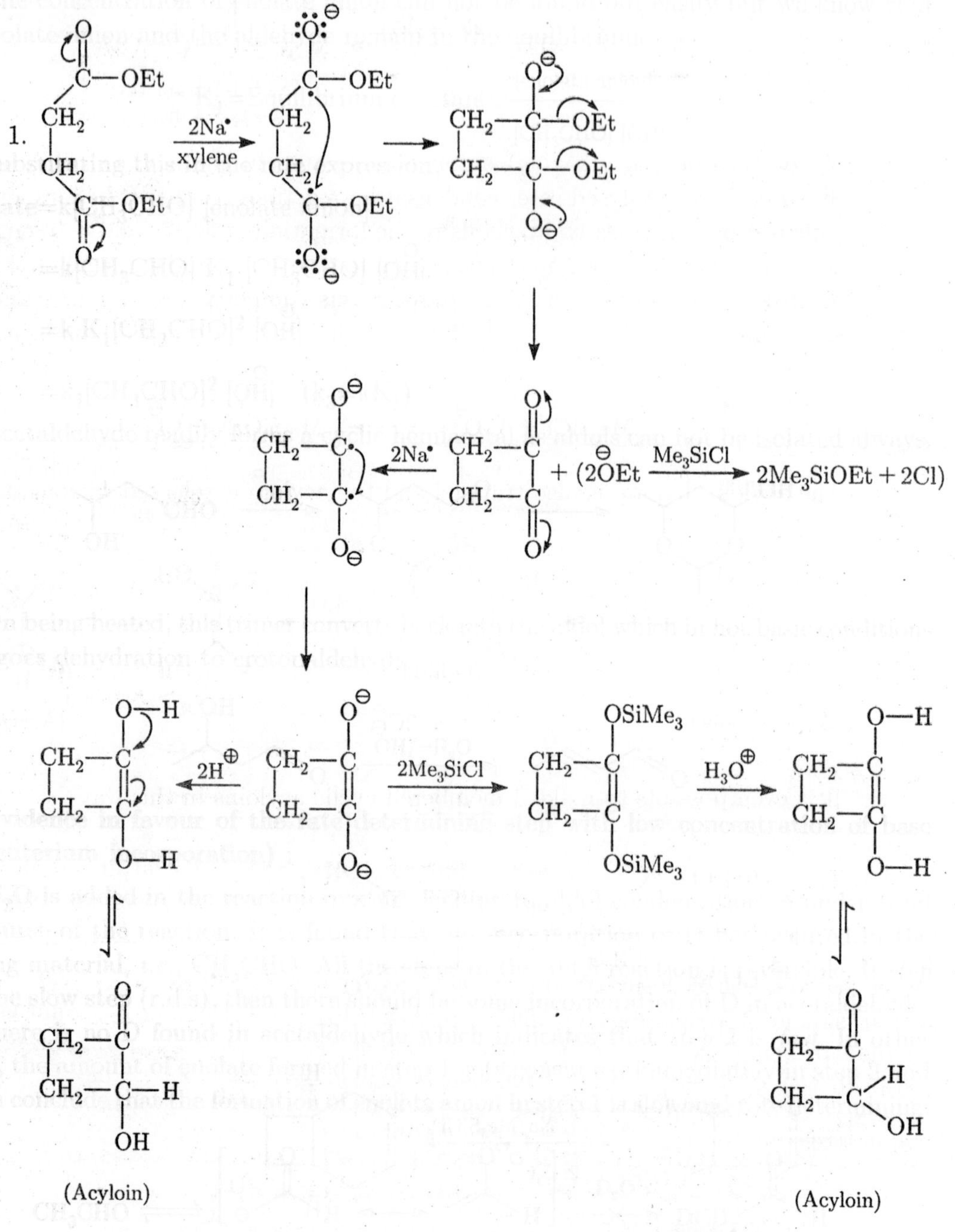

2. 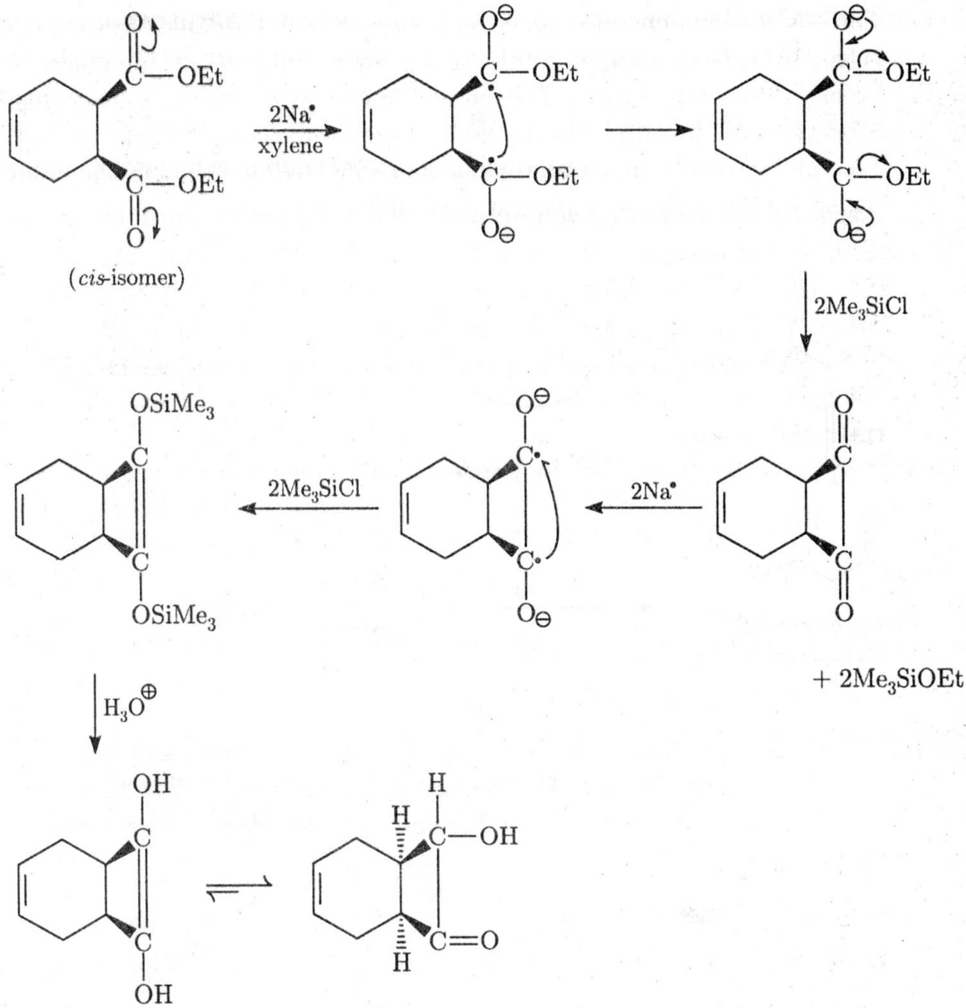

However, the *trans*-isomer of the above ester yields a particularly strained silyl derivative which undergoes a spontaneous electrocyclic reaction.

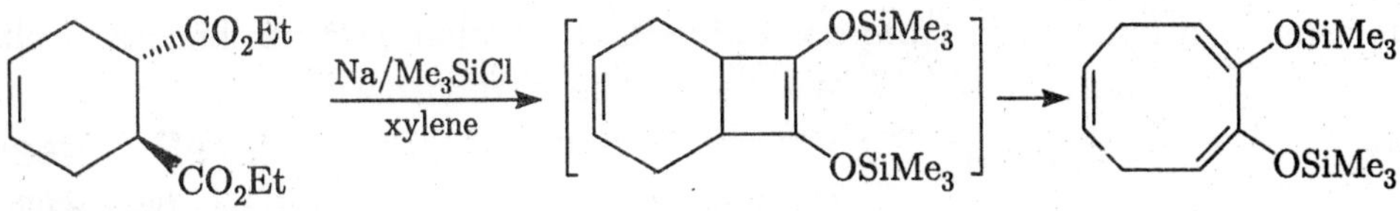

Alternatively the silyl compound can be oxidised with bromine to the α-deketone. For example,

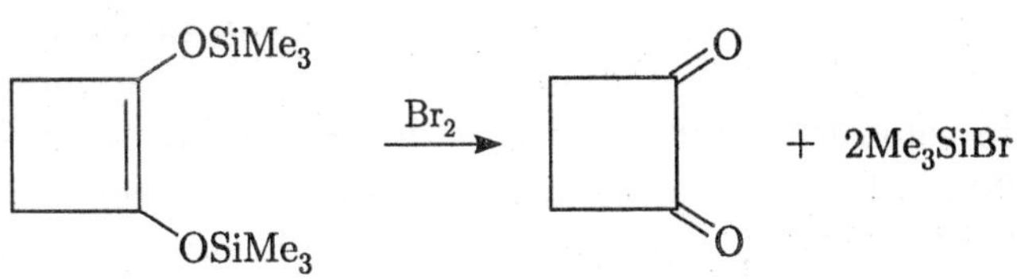

The acyloin condensation reaction is particularly valuable for the synthesis of large rings from dibasic esters. Even rings with 10-13 members (compare Dieckmann condensation, Thorpe nitrile condensation etc.) are formed in fair good yield and for these, the method is superior to those of Ziegler and Blomquist. The intramolecular reaction is possibly facilitated by bringing the polar ends of the substrate molecule on the surface of sodium metal.

In order to account for the ready formation of large rings, which means that the two ends of the chain must approach each other even though this is conformationally unfavourable for long chains, it may be postulated that the two ends become attached to nearby sites on the surface of the sodium metal. Thus the reactive ends are not available for intermediate coupling to compete with cyclisation.

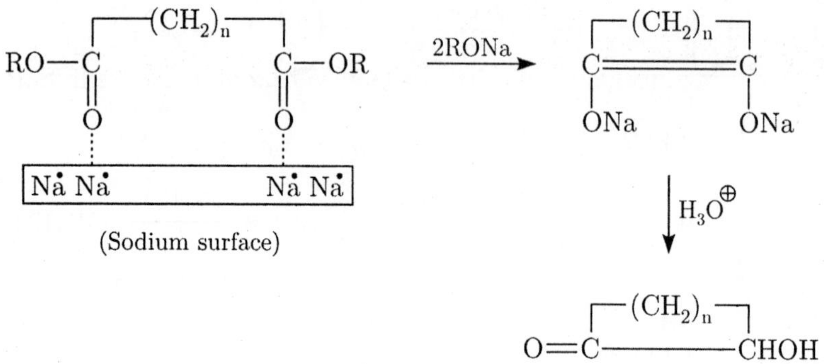

Typical yields are :

Ring size	10	12	13	14	15	16	17	18	20
Yield (%)	45	76	67	79	77	84	85	96	96

Applications of acyloin condensation :

1. *Preparation of cyclic acyloins* : The condensation has been employed with great success for the preparation of cyclic acyloins. Long chain carboxylic esters have been converted to large ring compounds without high dilution technique. The method is best for closing rings of ten members or more.

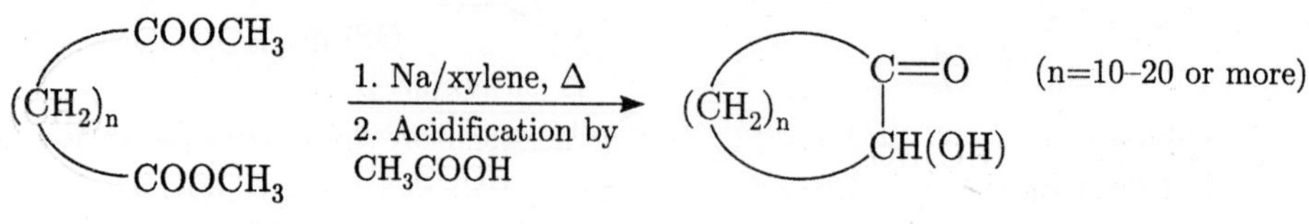

(Yield=60–95%)

2. *Preparation of catenane* : An interesting and unique compound called catenane, a compound with interlocking rings was formed when acyloin condensation was employed for ring closure with ester of 34-carbon dicarboxylic acid.

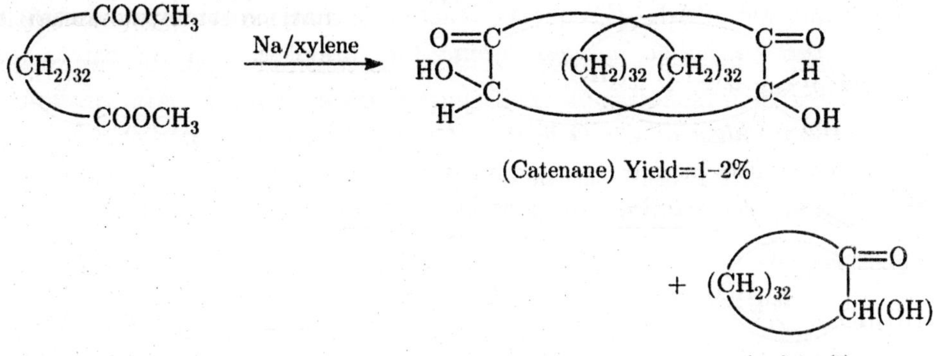

(Catenane) Yield=1–2%

Acyloin (I)

The acyloin (I) is reduced with Zn/Hg–concentrated HCl (Clemmensen Reduction) with DCl in D_2O instead of HCl in H_2O, thus producing a C_{34}– cycloalkane containing D.

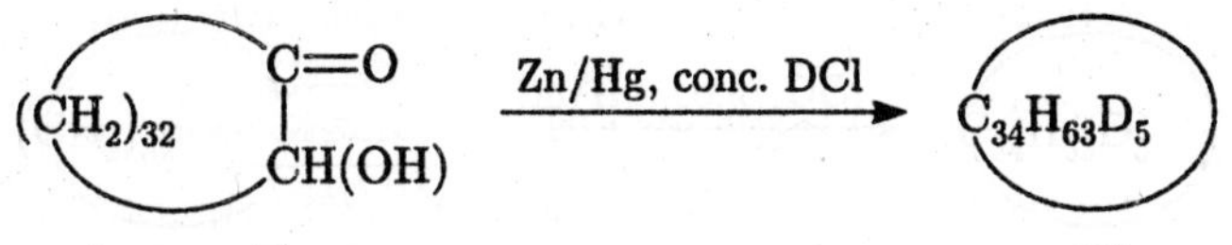

Acyloin (I) (II)

(II) contains about 5 atoms of D. The reaction (acyloin condensation) was then repeated with 1:1 mixture of xylene and (II) as solvent. Some of the molecules of ester would be threaded through (II) before they closed.

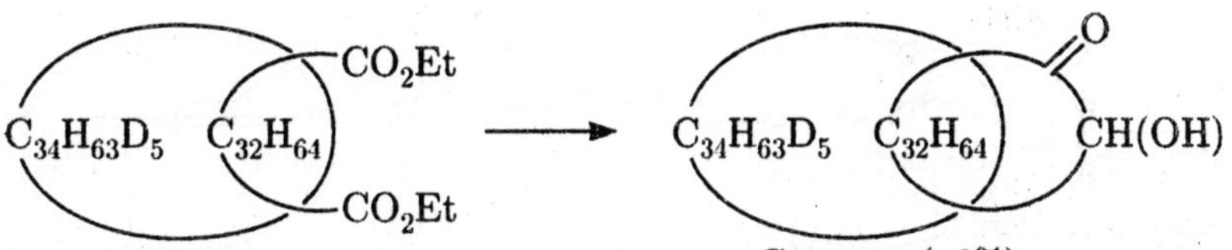

Catenane (~2%)

The compound is very useful in polymer chemistry. But the yield is very poor and it is a chance product depending upon the possibility of threading the diester molecules through the acycloin before it closed.

Condensation Reactions Via Addition-Elimination Sequence (Ad_N–E Sequence)

The stability of the adduct formed by the nucleophilic addition at carbonyl carbon atom (Ad_N2 reaction) depends on the nature of nucleophile taken. Sometimes the adducts formed are unstable and a stable product is only formed following an elimination reaction at the next step.

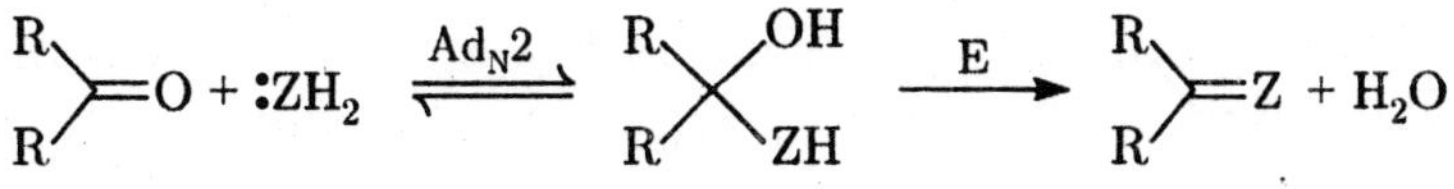

The condition of Ad_N–E sequence reaction is that the attacking nucleophile should contain *at least two active hydrogen atoms.* The rate of elimination reaction depends on the following factors.

1. ***Polarisability of C—O bond*** : If the polarisability of the C—O bond in the tetrahedral product (formed through Ad_N2 reaction) increases, the rate of elimination reaction also increases.

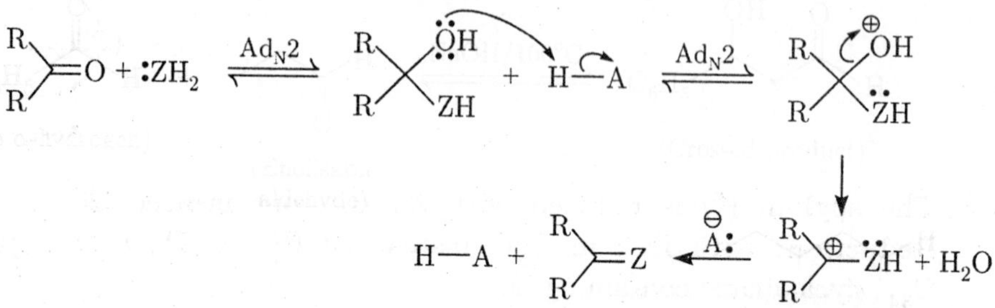

In the presence of acid (H–A), OH group in the tetrahedral adduct gets protonated and the leaving group becomes $\overset{\oplus}{O}H_2$ which is a good nucleofuge. As a result, the $\Delta G^{\neq}$ for the elimination reaction decreases and the rate of the reaction increases.

From the above discussion, it is apparent that, with decrease in pH of the reaction medium, the elimination step becomes fast. But with increasing acidity, the reactivity of the nucleophile decreases as the lone pair of electrons present on it become unavailable upon protonation. As a result, the rate of Ad_N2 reaction decreases. If a particular Ad_N2–E reaction is performed at different pHs, keeping other conditions constant, it is found that, at an *optimum pH*, the rate of that reaction is maximum. Generally nucleophiles containing nitrogen like $H_2\ddot{N}$ (*e.g.*, $\ddot{N}H_2OH$, $\ddot{N}H_2\ddot{N}H_2$, $\ddot{N}H_2NHCONH_2$, $C_6H_5NH\ddot{N}H_2$) undergo addition elimination reaction with carbonyl group at an *optimum pH* between *4.00 to 5.00.*

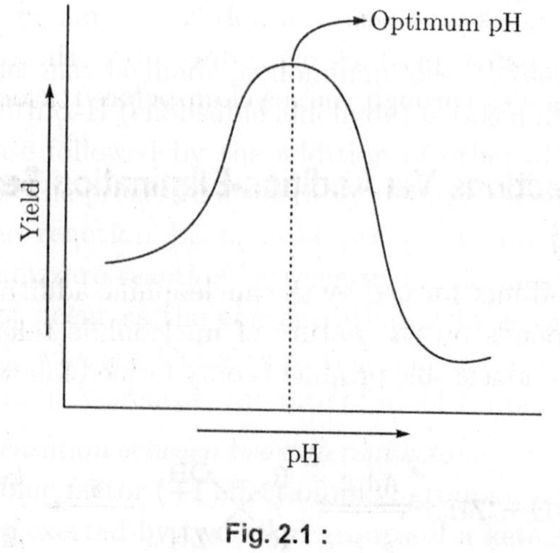

Fig. 2.1 :

2. ***Stability of the adduct*** : The tetrahedral product formed by Ad_N2 reaction experiences more steric strain as the state of hybridisation of carbonyl carbon changes from sp^2 to sp^3. But in Ad_N–E reactions, the hybridisation of carbon again becomes sp^2 upon elimination where steric strain is released. So, regarding relief in steric strain, the rate of elimination reaction increases whereas if the product is intramolecular hydrogen bonded or gets free from dipole dipole interaction, the rate of elimination reaction decreases.
3. ***Stability of the products*** : The rate of the reaction increases with increasing stability of the product formed say by resonance, hyperconjugation etc. In case of isomeric products, the more stable isomer is formed as the major product.

Reactions of aldehydes and ketones with derivatives of ammonia: Certain derivatives of ammonia undergo addition reactions with aldehydes and ketones to yield α-hydroxy derivatives. These, in turn undergo water elimination to yield compounds with C=N bond.

1. ***Reaction with a primary amine*** :

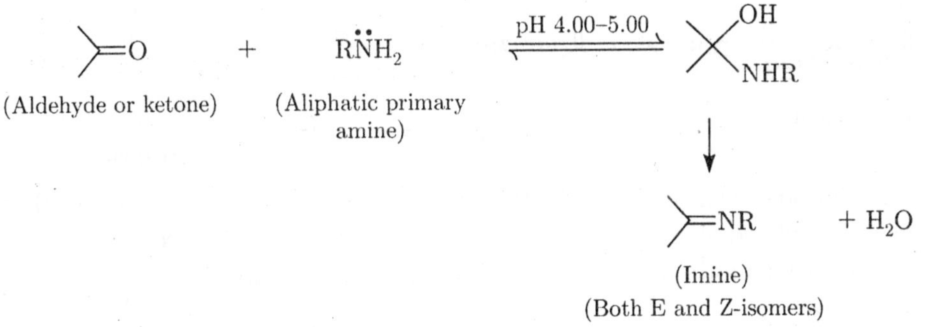

2. ***Reaction with hydroxylamine*** :

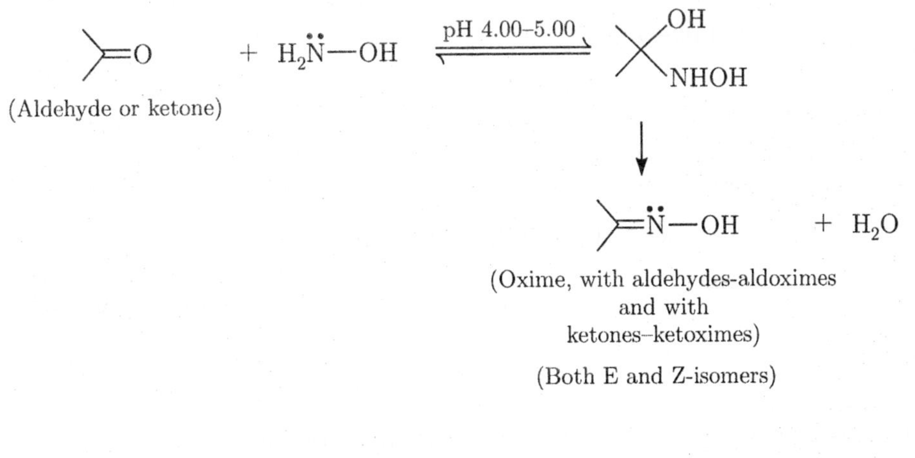

3. ***Reactions with hydrzine*** :

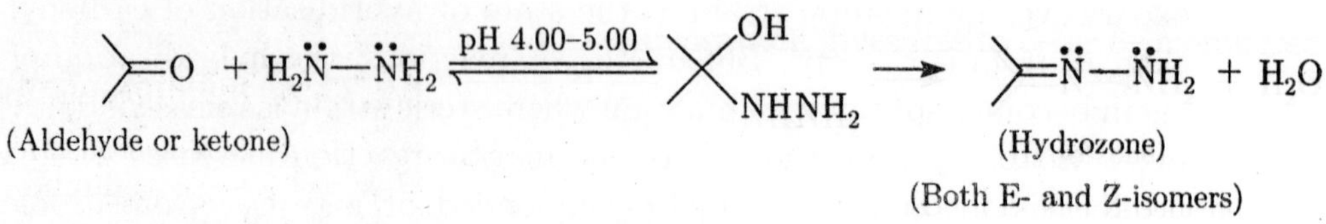

4. ***Reaction with semicarbazide***

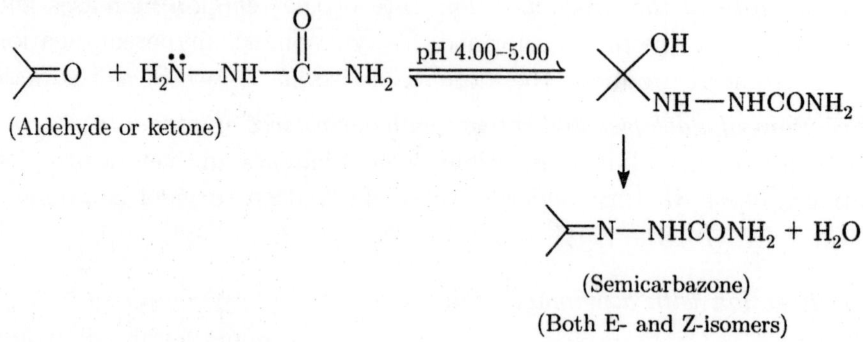

5. ***Reaction with phenylhydrazine*** :

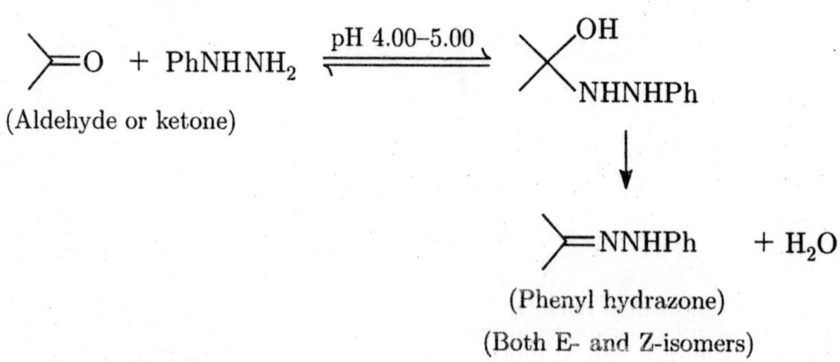

6. ***Reaction with 2,4-dinitrophenylhydrazine (2,4–DNP)*** :

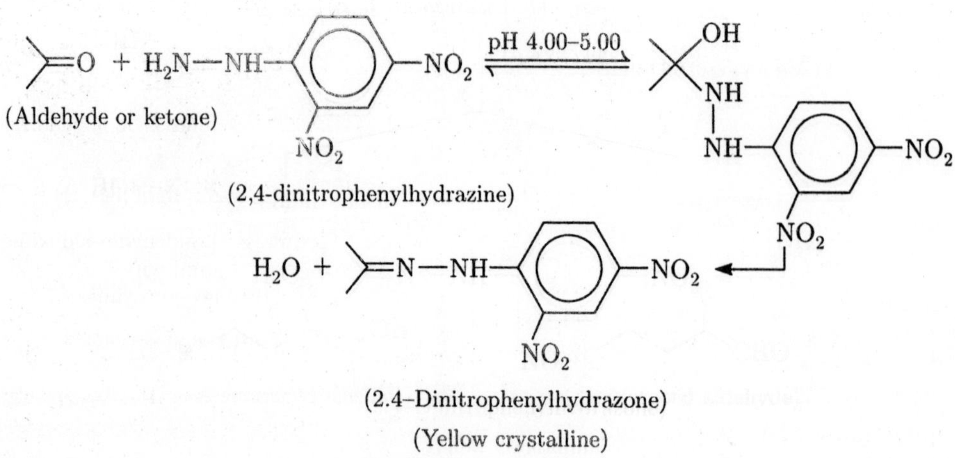

In general, addition-elimination reactions involving derivatives of ammonia may be represented as follows.

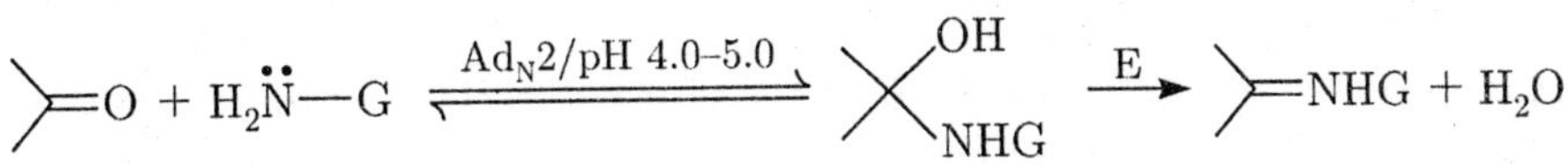

The derivatives of ammonia get easily oxidised by air and for this reason they are stored as their hydrochloride salts. These hydrochloride salts are taken in aqueous sodium acetate buffer where the pH is raised between 4.00 to 5.00, and the reaction proceeds with an appreciable rate. All the reaction products are crystalline and sharp melting which help to identify their parent carbonyl compounds. Hence they have analytical importance.

Ad_N—S_N sequence

The adduct formed through Ad_N2 reaction can have another fate. It is a substitution reaction and generally occurs in the presence of an acid. This type of reactions is known as Ad_N–S_N reactions.

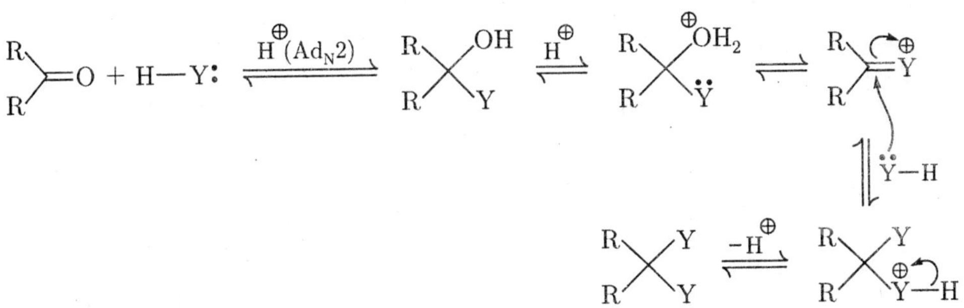

If the reactant contains more than one nucleophilic groups and if there is a possibility of formation of 5- or 6-membered cyclic compounds, the reaction rate becomes appreciable.

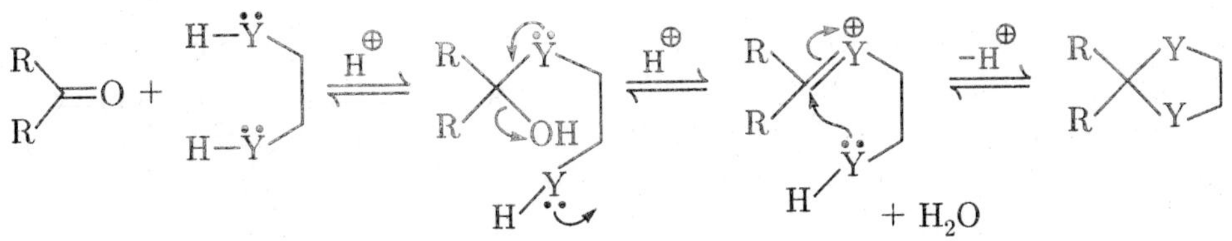

Examples of Ad_N–S_N sequence reactions are acyclic acetal and ketal formation for the first mechanism shown above and the formation of cyclic acetals follow the second mechanism. Acyclic and cyclic thioacetals and thioketals are formed in a similar manner.

Clemmensen Reduction

The reduction of carbonyl groups of aldehydes and ketones to methylene groups with amalgamated zinc and concentrated hydrochloric acid is known as ***Clemmensen reduction.***

$$\underset{\text{(Acetophenone)}}{C_6H_5COCH_3} \xrightarrow{\text{Zn/Hg, conc. HCl, reflux}} \underset{\text{(Ethyl benzene)}}{C_6H_5CH_2CH_3}$$

The reduction is particularly important for ketones containing phenolic or carboxylic acid groups which remain unaffected. Ketones are reduced more often than aldehydes do. The reaction however fails with acid sensitive and high molecular weight substrates. The α,β-unsaturated ketones undergo reduction both to olefinic and carbonyl groups. However the reduction is specific for carbonyl group of aldehydes and ketones containing other functional and reducible groups.

Mechanism of Clemmensen reduction : The reduction (Lakabayaski *et al*) under acid condition involves a protonated carbonyl group to which the electrons are transferred from the zinc metal.

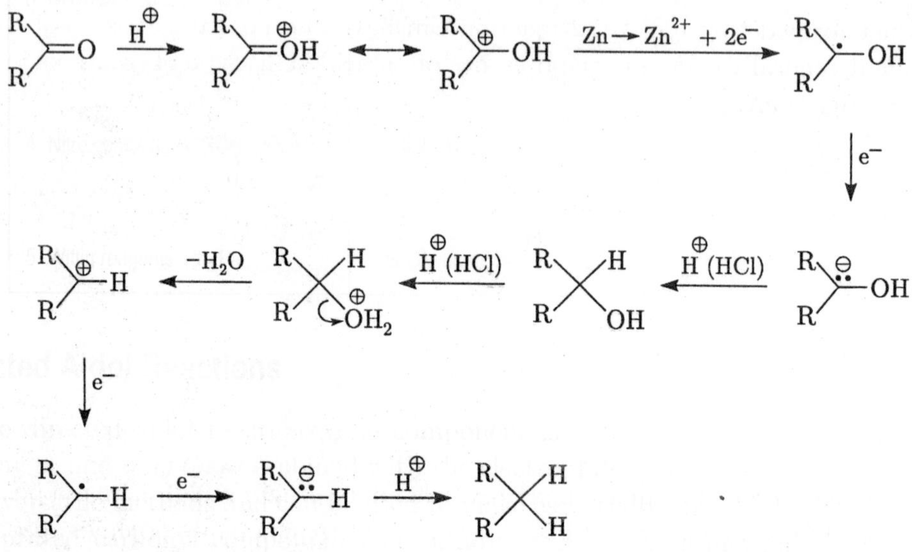

Certain types of aldehydes and ketones do not give the normal reduction products alone. α-Hydroxy ketones give either ketones through hydrogenolysis (cleavage of carbon–hetero atom bond by catalytic hydrogenation) of OH groups or olefins. 1,3-diketones give exclusively monoketones with rearrangement.

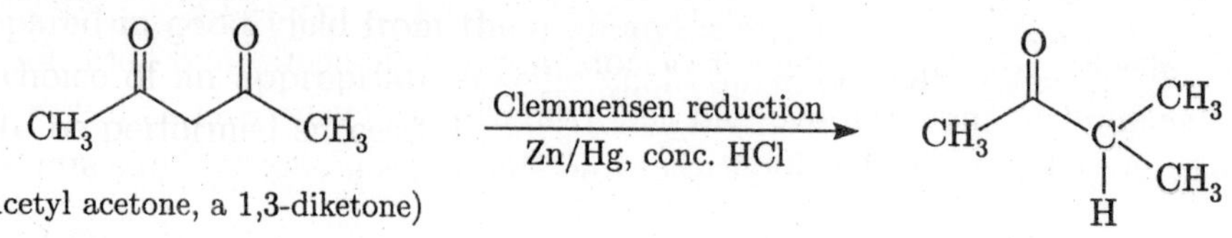

(Acetyl acetone, a 1,3-diketone)

Certain cyclic 1,3-diketones give under Clemmensen reduction conditions a fully reduced product along with a monoketone with ring contraction.

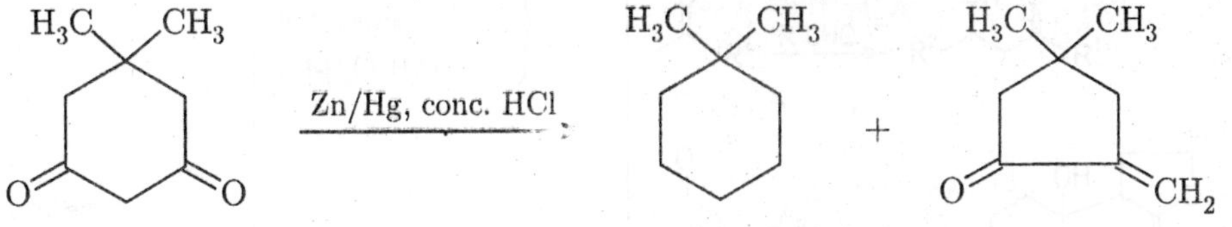

(5,5-Dimethylcyclohexane-1,3-dione) (1,1-Dimethylcyclohexane) (normal product) (Abnormal product)

Mechanism of formation of 2,4,4-trimethylcyclopentanone :

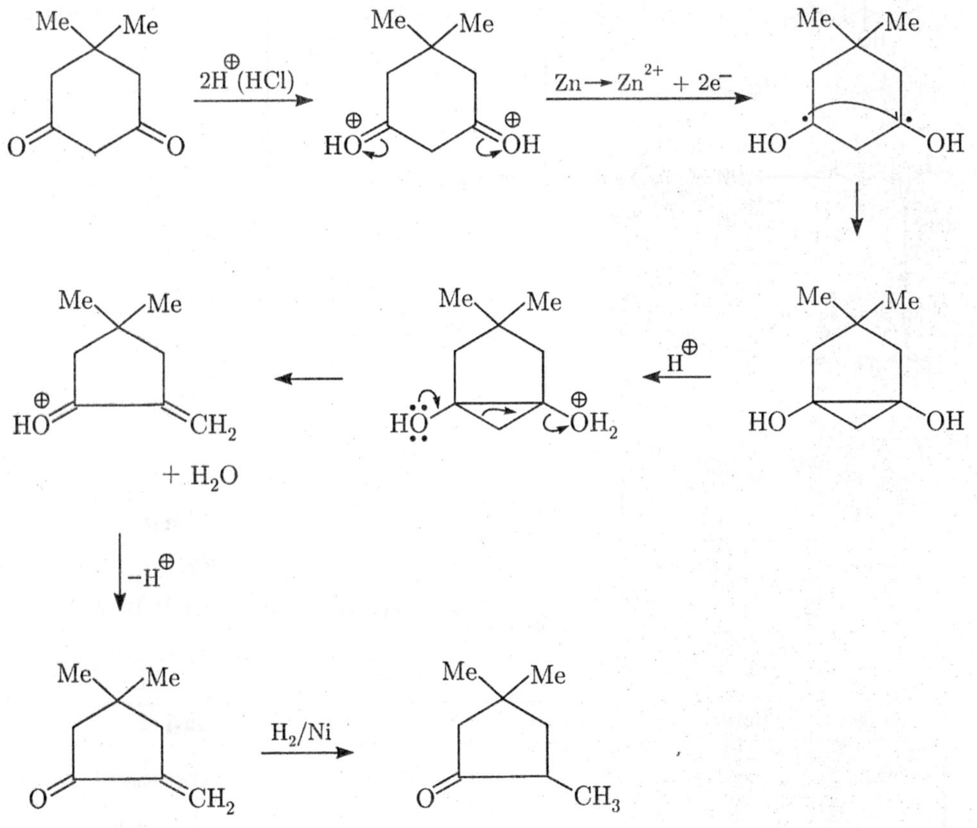

The mechanism resembles pinacol type rearrangement through a diradical with subsequent C—C bond formation.

Applications of Clemmensen Reduction :

1. (a) $CH_3(CH_2)_5CHO \xrightarrow{\text{Zn/Hg, conc. HCl}} CH_3(CH_2)_5CH_3$

(b) $C_6H_5COC_3H_7 \xrightarrow{\text{Zn/Hg, conc. HCl}} C_6H_5CH_2C_3H_7$

(Aromatic ketone)

(c) 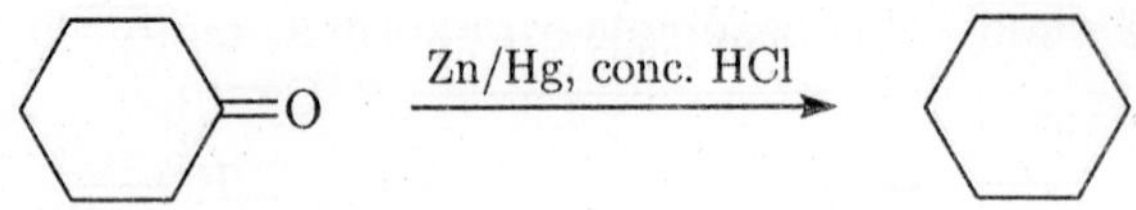

(Cyclic ketone) (Cyclohexane)

2. 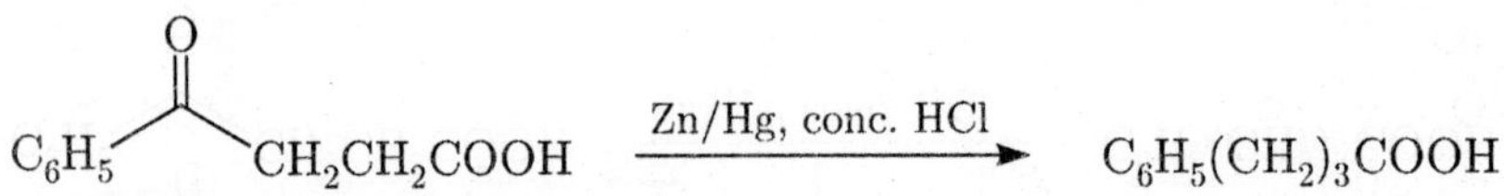

β–Benzoylpropanoic acid (a γ–keto acid) (γ–Phenylbutanoic acid)

α- and β-keto acids are generally not reduced.

3. 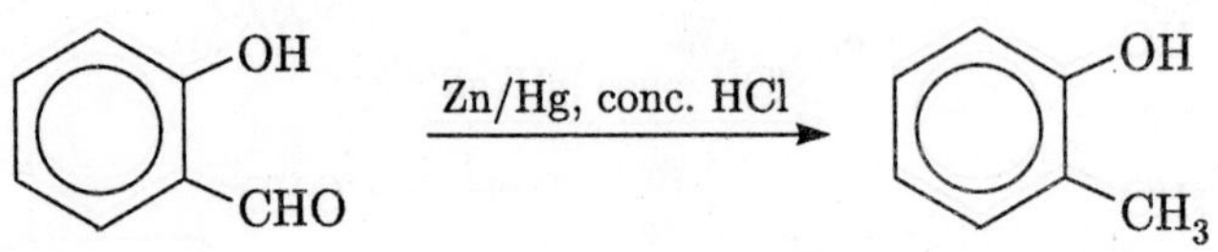

(Salicylaldehyde) (Ortho cresol)

4. Reduction of aromatic ketones :

(a) 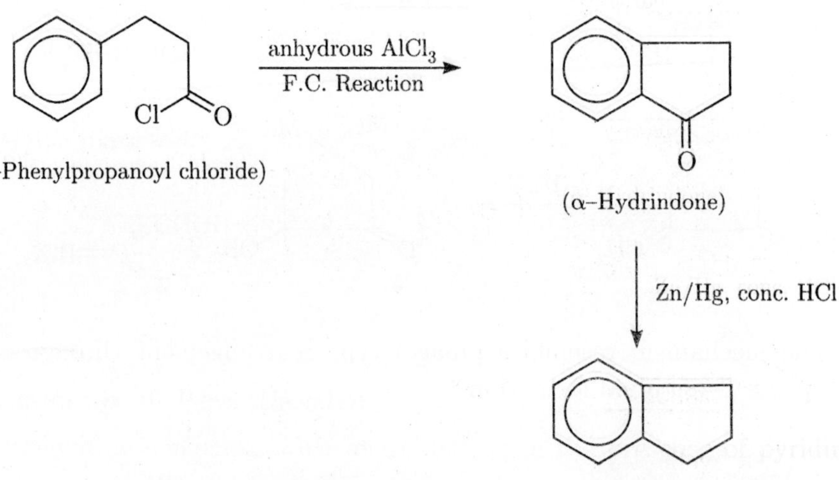

(β–Phenylpropanoyl chloride) (α–Hydrindone) (Indane)

(b)

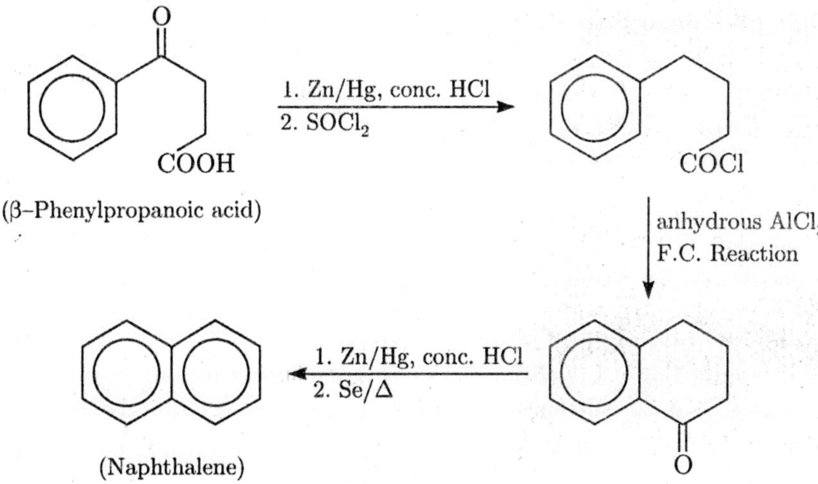

5.

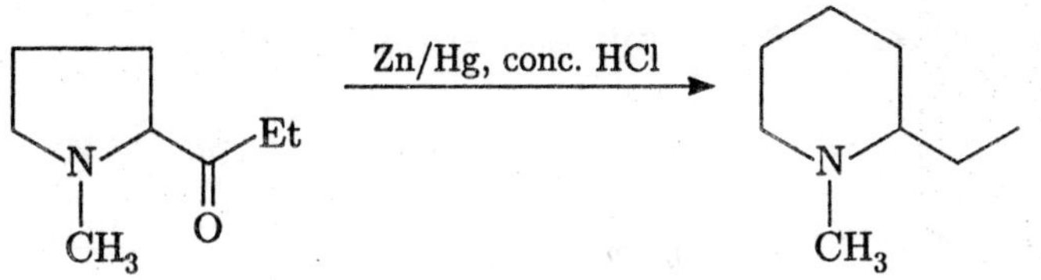

Mechanism :

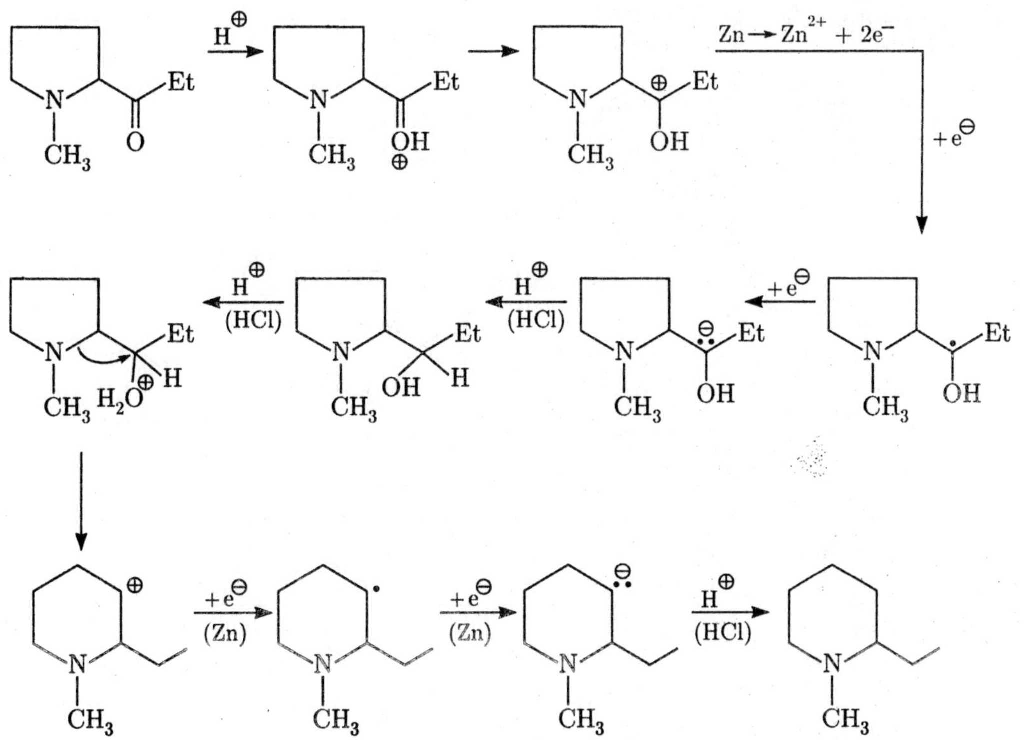

Wolff-Kishner Reduction

Wolf-Kishner reduction involves the conversion of carbonyl groups of aldehydes and ketones to methylene groups by heating their hydrazones, semicarbazones or azines in the presence of strong base such as NaOEt or NaOH.

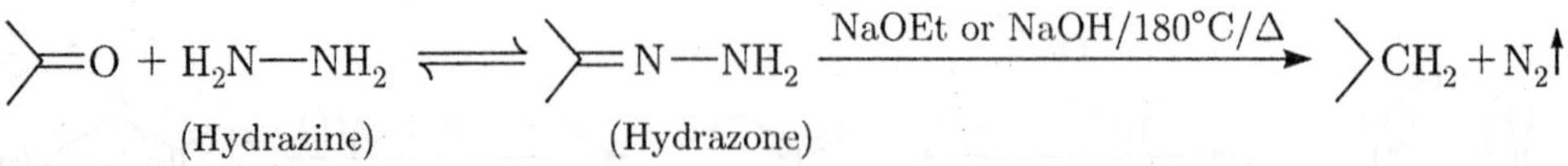

Thus ketones and aldehydes can be conveniently reduced to hydrocarbons by this method. Earlier method of heating the hydrazones of carbonyl compounds with sodium ethoxide at 180°C in an autoclave has since been modified. In the modified procedure, hydrazine hydrate and the carbonyl compound are heated with KOH or NaOH in ethylene glycol for several hours. The water formed escapes and the temperature rises to 200°C when the hydrazone decomposes with the formation of hydrocarbon with the evolution of nitrogen. This is known as **Huang-Minlon** reduction.

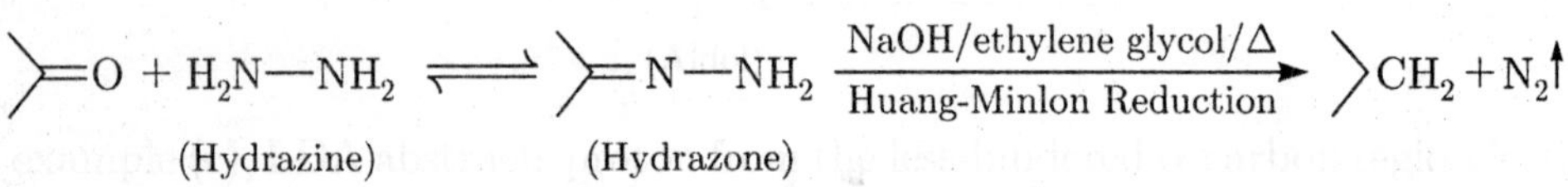

In a further modification, the reduction can be carried out at room temperature by using dimethyl sulphoxide as solvent and potassium tertiary butoxide as base. The yield is excellent. The modification is done by Cram and coworkers.

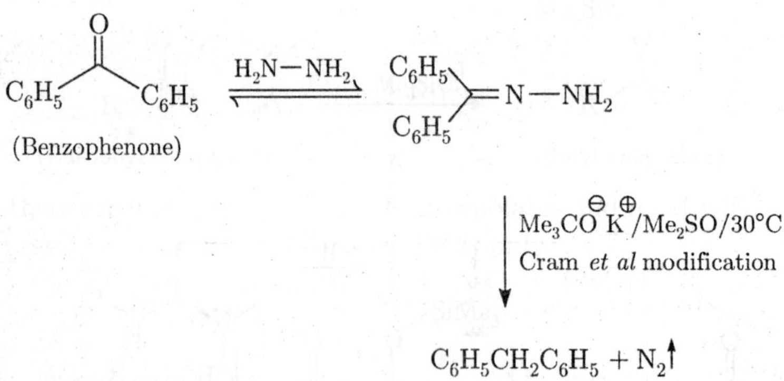

Unlike Clemmensen reduction, this reduction does not fail with high molecular weight or acid sensitive substrates. In general, the yield of reduction is better with Wolff-Kishner and the method is specific for the reduction of the carbonyl group. Other reducible functional groups like NO_2, C=C etc. remain unaffected if present along with the carbonyl group. This method is however not suitable for the reduction of α, β–unsaturated ketones, but the modification by Cram reduces α, β–unsaturated ketones to alkenes. Both Wolff-Kishner and Huang Minlon reductions are satisfactory to reduce *sterically crowded* ketones, which Clemmensen reduction fails to do.

Mechanism of Wolff-Kishner Reduction :

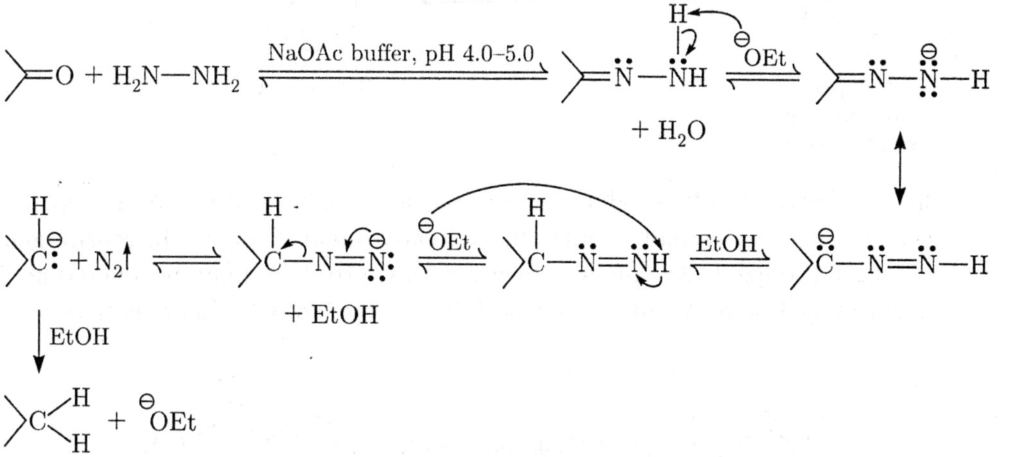

The expulsion of nitrogen makes the last step of the reduction irreversible and the equilibrium shifts to the product side.

Applications of Wolff-Kishner reduction :

1.

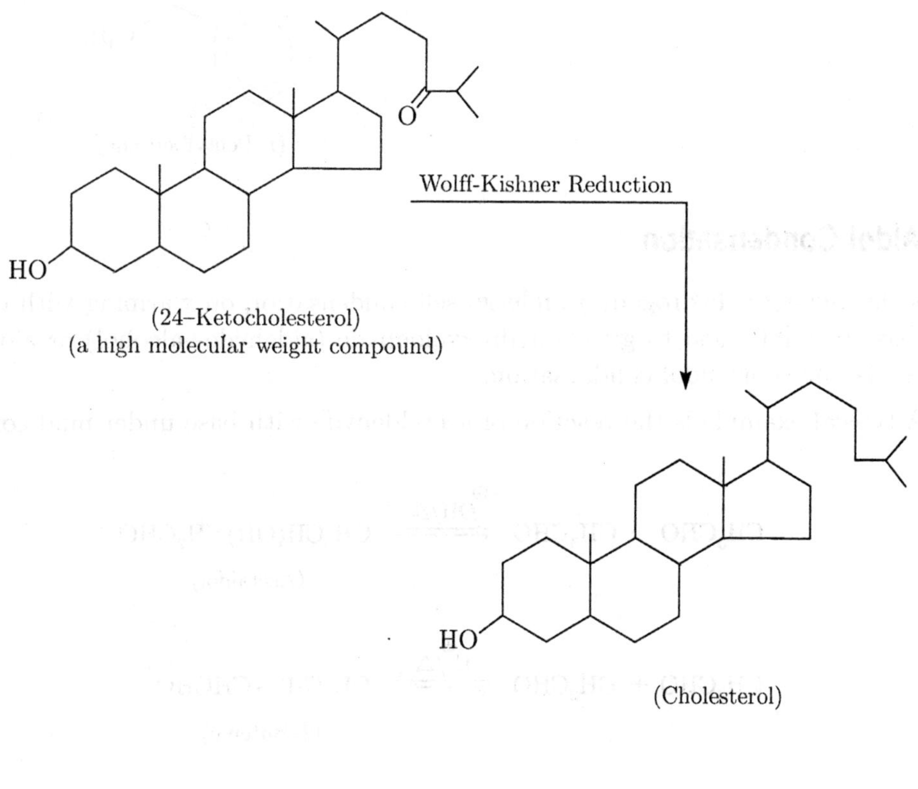

(24–Ketocholesterol)
(a high molecular weight compound)

(Cholesterol)

2. 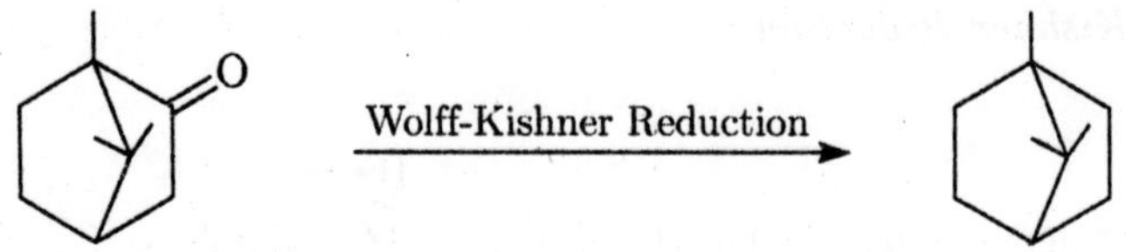

(Camphor) (a high molecular weight ketone) (Camphane)

3. In the Friedal-Craft alkylation reaction, a straight chain alkyl group, longer than ethyl group cannot be introduced in an aromatic ring as the rearrangement of alkyl groups takes place. However this problem may be overcome first performing Friedel-Crafts acylation followed by Wolff-Kishner reduction.

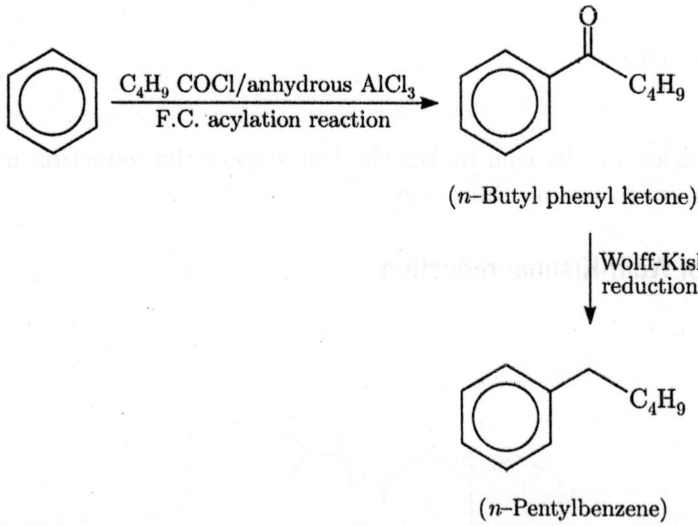

The Aldol Condensation

Aldehydes having α-hydrogen(s) undergo self-condensation on warming with dilute or mild base or dilute acid to give β–hydroxyaldehyde (aldehyde+alcohol) or aldol. This reaction is known as aldol condensation.

A typical example is the reaction of acetaldehyde with base under mild condition.

$$CH_3CHO + CH_3CHO \xrightleftharpoons{\overset{\ominus}{O}H/\Delta} CH_3CH(OH)CH_2CHO$$

(Acetaldol)

$$CH_3CHO + CH_3CHO \xrightleftharpoons{\overset{\oplus}{H}/\Delta} CH_3CH{=}CHCHO$$

(2–Butenal)

Various basic reagents like dilute NaOH, aqueous alkali carbonate, alkalimetal alkoxides (*e.g.*, NaOEt, K^+tBuO^-) etc. may be used. This reaction is not favourable for ketones.

Mechanism of Base-assisted aldol reaction :

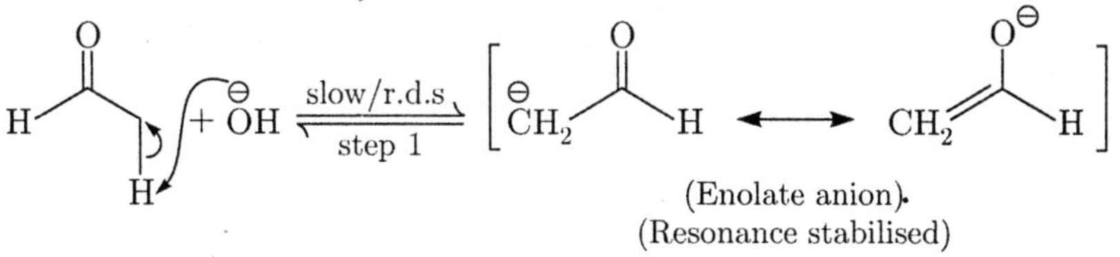

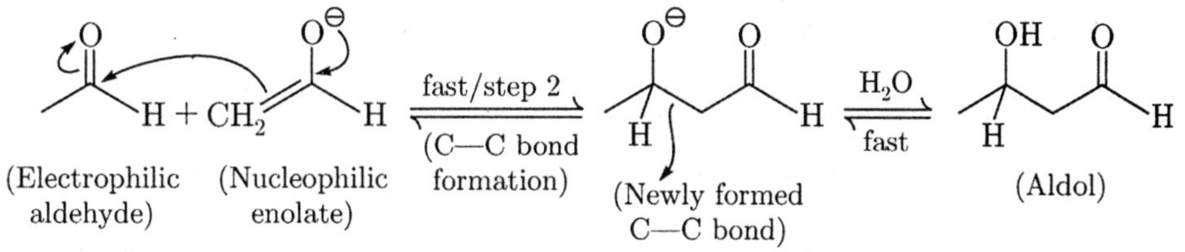

The step involving carbon-carbon bond formation is facilitated by electron withdrawing groups on the carbonyl component and retarded by electron-releasing groups.

Formation of resonance stabilised enolate anion in *step* 1 is slow and hence rate determining at a low concentration of base. Step 2, a nucleophilic attack of the enolate anion to the carbonyl centre of the second molecule of aldehyde is fast followed by a rapid proton transfer from water (solvent), to give the desired aldol.

The Rate-equation for the aldol reaction : At low concentration of base ($\overset{\ominus}{OH}$), the rate expression is found to be, Rate=$k_2[CH_3CHO][\overset{\ominus}{OH}]$, *i.e.*, step 1, the formation of resonance-stabilised enol is rate limiting.

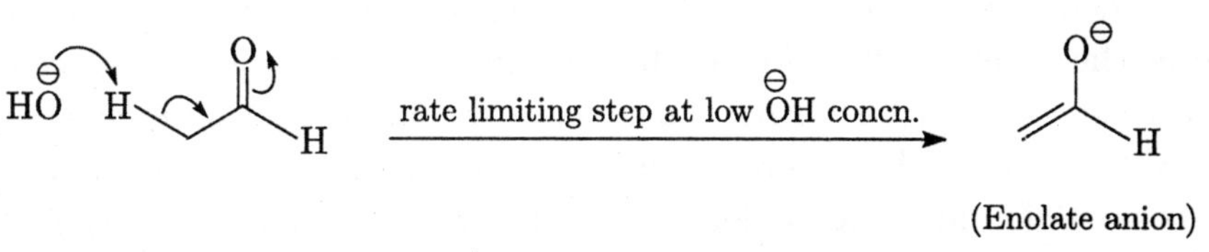

At higher hydroxide concentration, the rate equation becomes termolecular and the rate determining step changes to *step* 2 *not the step* 1.

$$\text{Rate}=k_3[CH_3CHO]^2[OH^-]$$

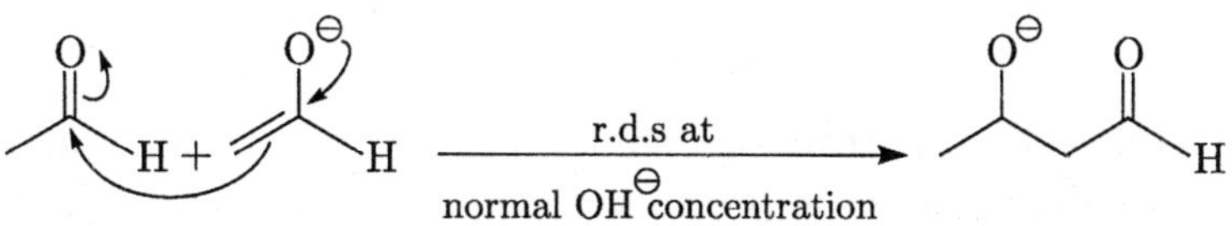

The actual rate expression is,

$$\text{Rate}=k[CH_3CHO][\text{enolate anion}]$$

The concentration of enolate anion can not be found out easily but we know that the enolate anion and the aldehyde remain in the equilibrium.

$$K_1=\text{Equilibrium constant}=\frac{[\text{enolate anion}]}{[CH_3CHO]\,[\overset{\ominus}{OH}]}$$

Substituting this in the rate expression,

$$\text{Rate}=k[CH_3CHO]\,[\text{enolate anion}]$$

$$=k[CH_3CHO]\,K_1\,[CH_3CHO]\,[\overset{\ominus}{OH}]$$

$$=k.K_1[CH_3CHO]^2\,[\overset{\ominus}{OH}]$$

$$=k_3[CH_3CHO]^2\,[\overset{\ominus}{OH}] \quad (k_3=kK_1)$$

Acetaldehyde readily forms a cyclic hemiacetal as aldols can not be isolated always.

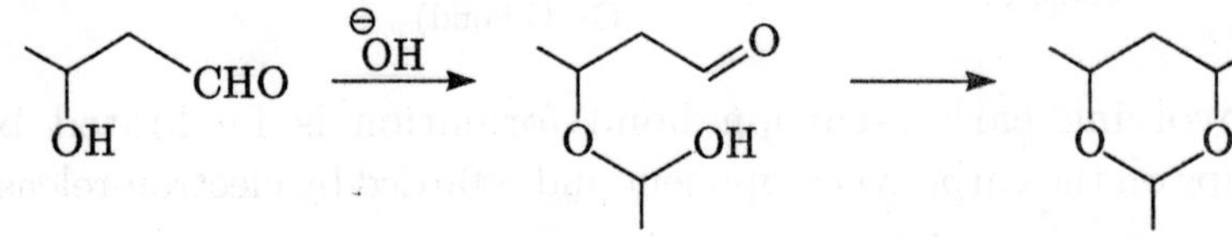

On being heated, this trimer converts back into the aldol which in hot basic conditions undergoes dehydration to crotonaldehyde.

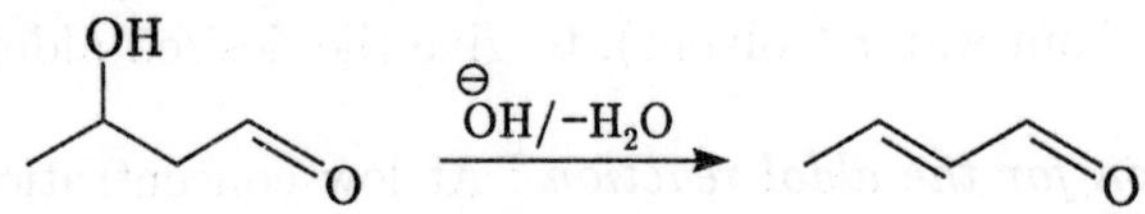

Evidence in favour of the rate determining step with low concentration of base (by deuterium incorporation) :

D_2O is added in the reaction mixture leading to aldol condensation to understand the course of the reaction. It is found that, no incorporation of D has occured in the starting material, *i.e.*, CH_3CHO. All the steps in the aldol reaction is reversible. If *step* 2 be the slow step (r.d.s), then there should be some incorporation of D in acetaldehyde. But there is no D found in acetaldehyde which indicates that *step* 2 is *fast.* In other words, the amount of enolate formed in step 1 gets consumed immediately in step 2 and we can conclude that the formation of enolate anion in step 1 is slow and rate determining.

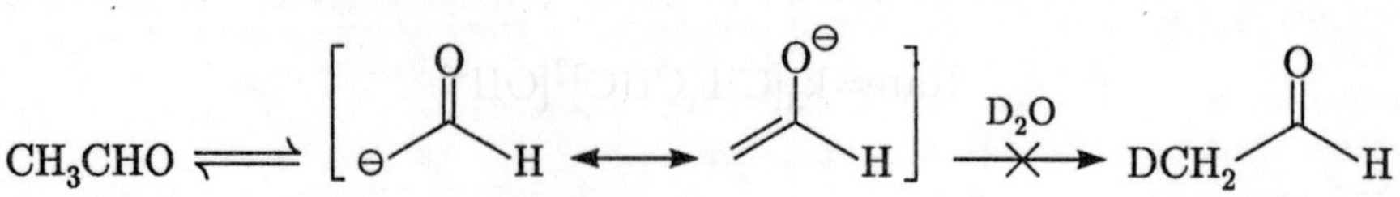

(Enolate anion)

The base catalysed aldol reactions sometimes give the aldol and sometimes the elimination product. The nature of product depends on the conditions (stronger base, higher temperature, higher reaction time etc.) to give the elimination product and also on the structure of the reactants. Some combinations are easy to stop the reaction at the aldol stage.

Aldol condensation between two molecules of ketones

The reaction conditions of aldol condensation are not favourable for ketones.

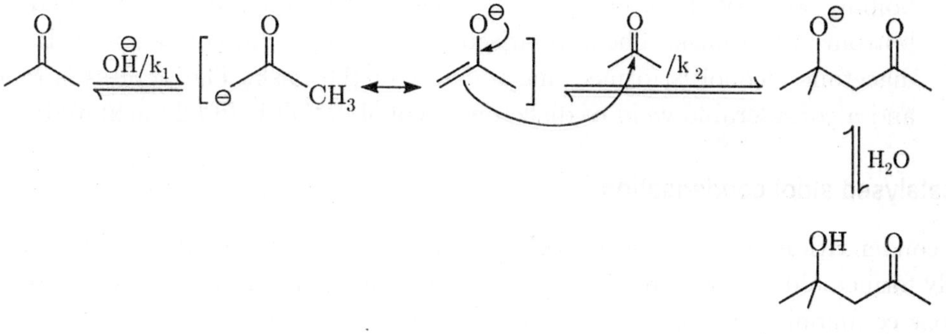

(Diacetone alcohol)
yield ≅ 2%

Diacetone alcohol is stable but dehydration can be brought about by applying acid or base.

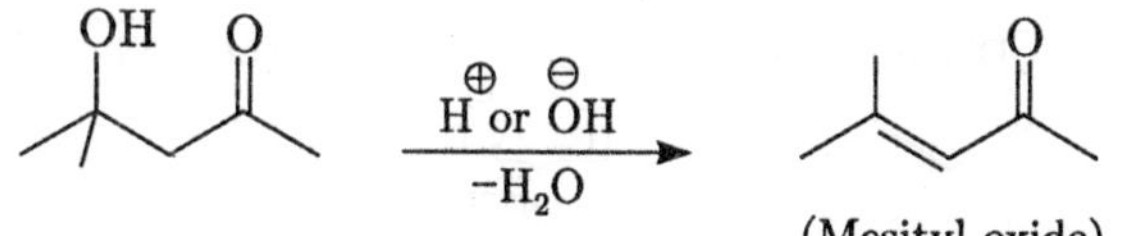

(Mesityl oxide)

The poor yield of diacetone alcohol (≅2%) indicates that the equilibrium of the reaction lies almost to the left. This is because the carbonyl carbon of a ketone is less positive (due to +I effect of two alkyl groups) and more sterically hindered relative to aldehydes. So a ketone is a bad acceptor of carbanion. If D_2O is used in the reaction mixture, some incorporation of D is found in acetone. The enolate anion of acetone approaches a second acetone molecule (carbanion acceptor) in a sluggish manner and the enolate anion can revert back to acetone, i,e the starting material.

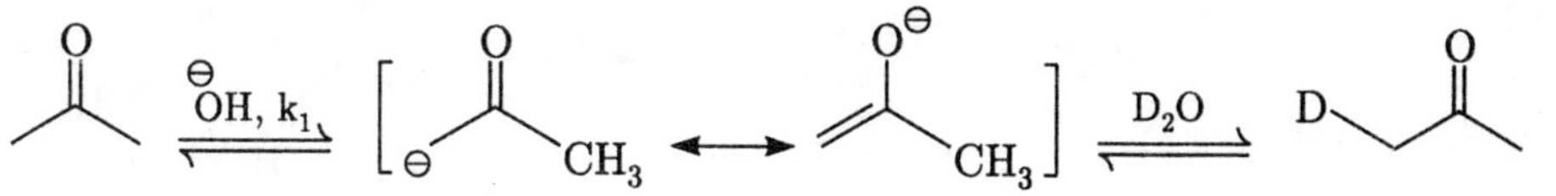

The base catalysed aldol reaction of acetone (or similar ketones) is often referred as *retro aldol condensation*, as the equilibrium is shifted almost towards left, *i.e.*, at the reactant side. Better yield of aldol reaction between two molecules of acetone (base catalysed) can be achieved by the following manner:

1. The aldol product of the ketone formed is removed immediately from the contact of base and thus the equilibrium gets shifted towards right, *i.e.*, to the product side.
2. The condensation product between two molecules of acetone is increased by taking acetone in *soxhlet* apparatus. The apparatus contains $Ba(OH)_2$ as base, and it is heated at 60°C. Acetone comes in contact with $Ba(OH)_2$ and diacetone alcohol is formed. The unreacted acetone gets vapourised (b.p. 56°C) where the boiling point of diacetone alcohol being quite high remains as liquid at the bottom of the flask. The vapourised acetone comes in contact with $Ba(OH)_2$, diacetone alcohol is formed and remains in the flask. The process is repeated and a considerable yield of diacetone alcohol (71%) is finally achieved.

Acid-catalysed aldol condensation

Aldol condensation can also be brought about with acid followed by dehydration of initially formed aldol. The elimination is easier in acid solution and acid–catalysed aldol reactions commonly give unsaturated products instead of aldols.

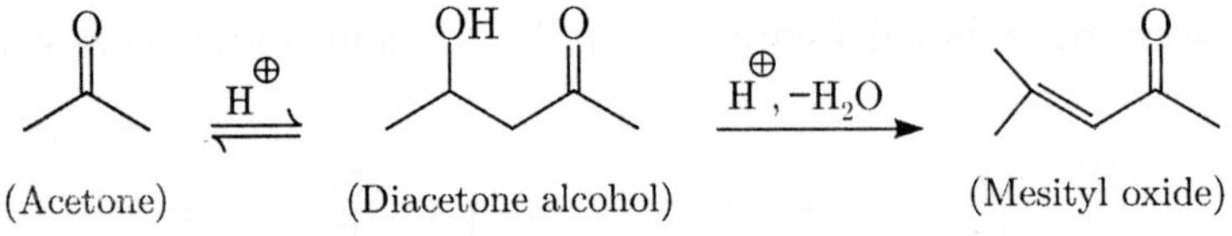

Mechanism :

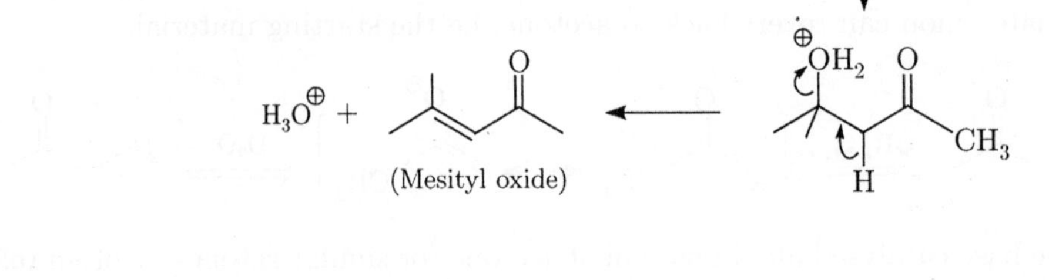

Dehydration of diacetone alcohol shifts the equilibrium to the right as it is not a reversible step and the yield of diacetone alcohol thus gets increased.

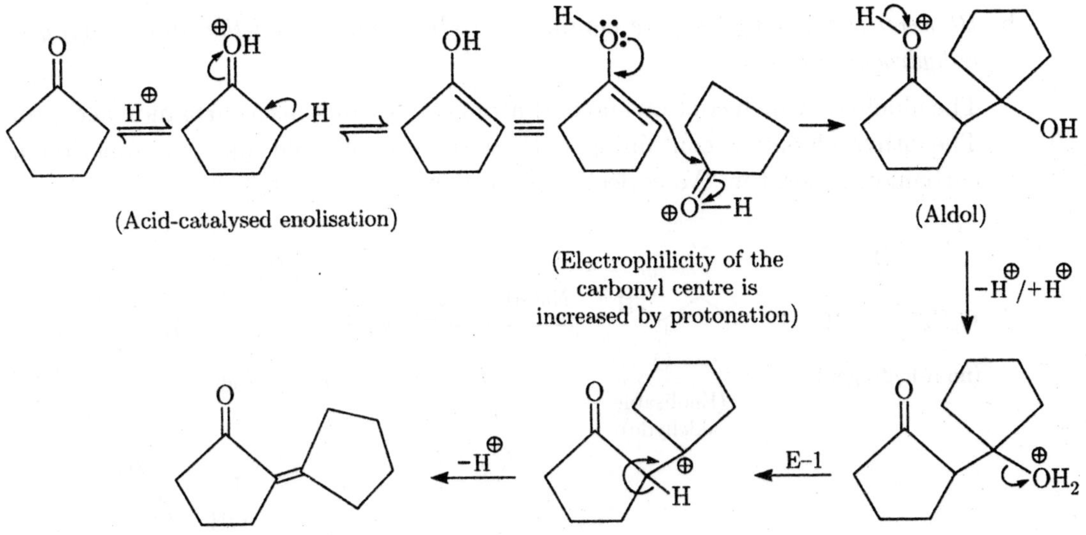

The aldol is a tertiary alcohol and would be likely to eliminate by an E1 mechanism in acid.

Typesof aldol condensation reaction

1. ***Crossed aldol condensation*** : When aldol condensation is done between two different carbonyl compounds, it is known as crossed aldol condensation.

a. *Between two different aldehydes both containing α-hydrogen(s) in the presence of base like dilute sodium hydroxide.*

The reaction is of little synthetic value. Both the aldehydes can act as carbanion generator and carbanion aceptor. So, we expect at least *four* products in the reaction mixture.

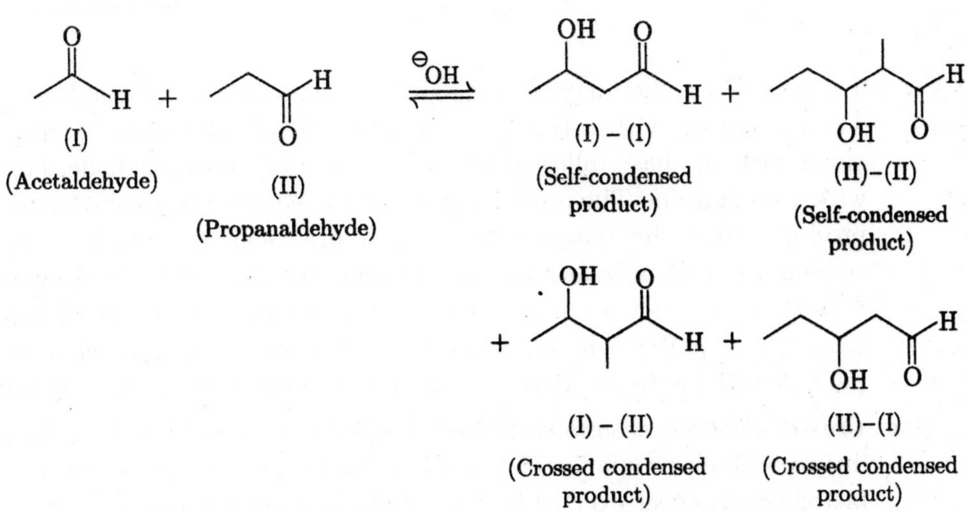

b. *Between two aldehydes, one containing α-H atom (s) and the other having no α-hydrogen atom.*

The aldehyde which contains no α-H atom can act only as a carbanion acceptor. The other aldehyde containing α-H atom is enolisable and can function as carbanion generator. We expect *two* products as shown below.

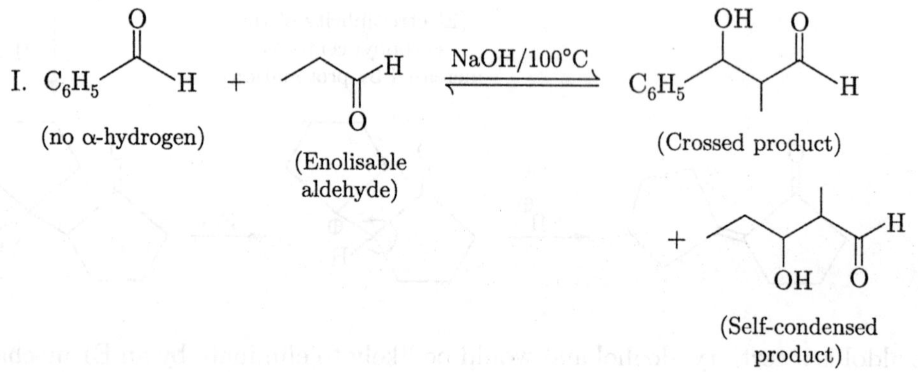

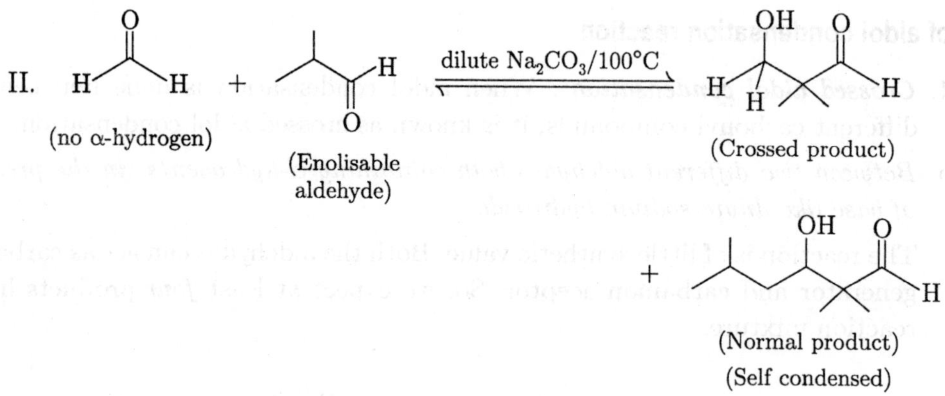

The crossed product may be made predominant over the self-condensed product. The component with α-H (enolisable aldehyde) is taken at a low concentration along with the base followed by the addition of other aldehyde, i,e, aldehyde with no α-H atom. The process considerably reduces the yield of self-condensed product. Now the reaction becomes a practical and viable crossed aldol condensation. Cannizzaro reaction between two molecules of aldehydes with no α-H atom does not occur as the concentration of base employed here is quite mild (20% NaOH), whereas Cannizzaro reaction requires much stronger base (50% NaOH solution). Moreover, the rate of aldol condensation is faster.

c. *Crossed aldol condensation between two different ketones*: This is rarely attempted due to both electronic factor (+I effect of alkyl groups), as well as due to steric factor (steric effect exerted by two alkyl groups of a ketone).

d. *Crossed aldol condensation between an aldehyde and a ketone*

I. Aldol condensation between an enolisable aldehyde (having α-H atom) and a ketone with α-hydrogen atom leads to two products.

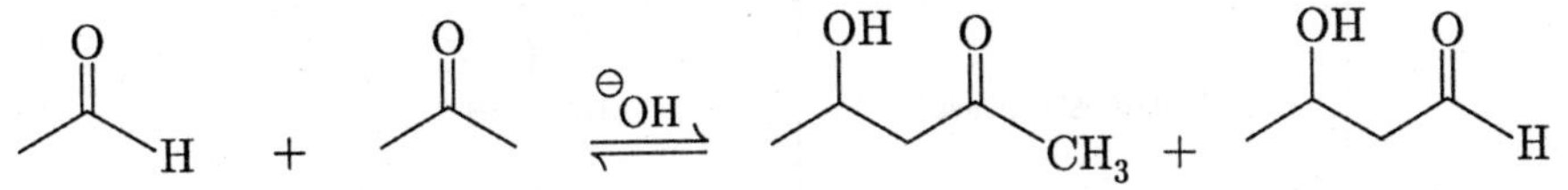

(Acetaldehyde) (Aldehyde) + (Acetone) (Ketone) → (Crossed product) + (Normal product)

Condensation between two molecules of ketone is negligible under basic condition. Here also, the yield of crossed product may be increased by taking a low concentration of acetone (ketone) followed by addition of acetaldehyde.

II. *Between an aldehyde with no α-H atom and ketone with α-hydrogen atom* ***(Claisen-Schmidt*** **or** ***Claisen reaction).***

In Claisen-Schmidt reaction, only *one* product is obtained. So this is an example of viable crossed aldol condensation.

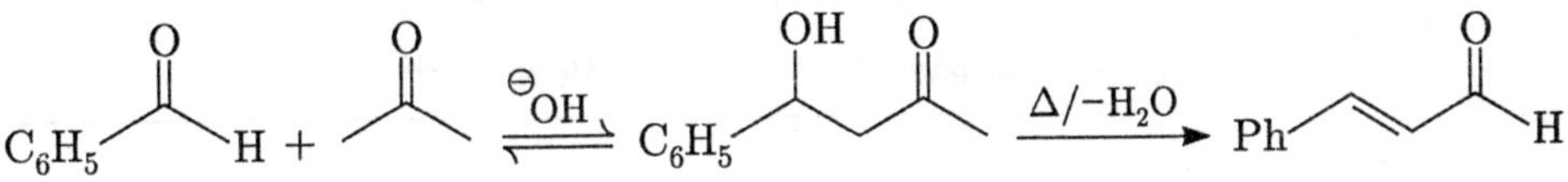

(no α-H; aldehyde part) + (Ketone) → (Benzalacetone)

Base applied is generally dilute NaOH and as ketones generally do not condense under basic condition, which, leads to a single product. If acetone is not in excess, dibenzalacetone can be obtained in about 80% yield.

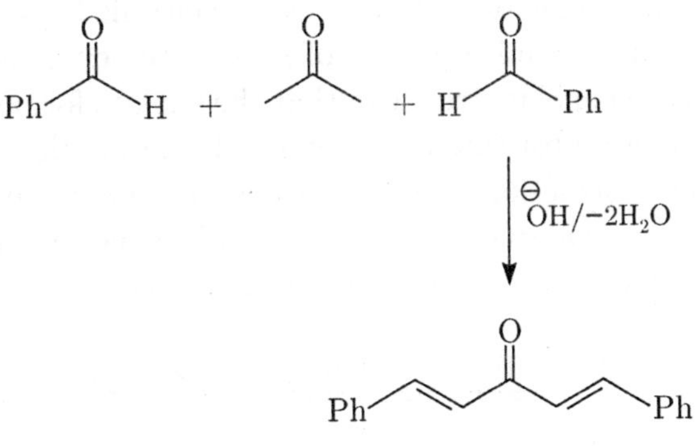

(Dibenzalacetone)

Successful crossed aldol reaction

Conditions :

1. *One partner only* must be capable of enolisation.
2. The other partner must be incapable of enolisation and be *more electrophilic* than the enolisable partner.

List of carbonyl substituents that block enolisation

Substituent	***Typical Compounds***
1. H (most reactive)	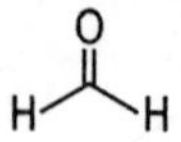
2. Cl_3C, F_3C	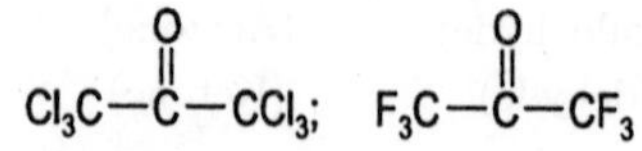
3. *t*–alkyl	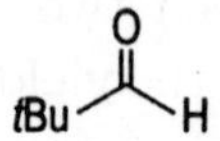
4. Alkenyl	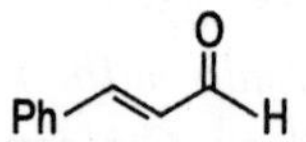
5. Aryl	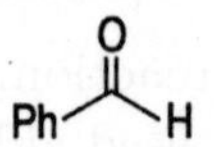
6. NR_2 (least reactive)	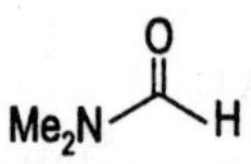

III. *Between an unsymmetrical ketone having α-H atom(s) and an aldehyde with no α-hydrogen atom*

The course of this category of reaction solely depends on the nature of the base used in the reaction.

In presence of bases like NaOH, Na_2CO_3 etc, both thermodynamically controlled enolate and kinetically controlled enolates are formed, the yield of thermodynamically controlled enolate being high. By thermodynamically controlled enolate we mean that the enolate formed on abstraction of proton from more substituted α-carbon and a kinetically controlled enolate is formed by the abstraction of protons from less substituted α-carbon. So the present case is an example of Claisen-Schmidt reaction where small bases like NaOH or Na_2CO_3 are used for a prolonged time.

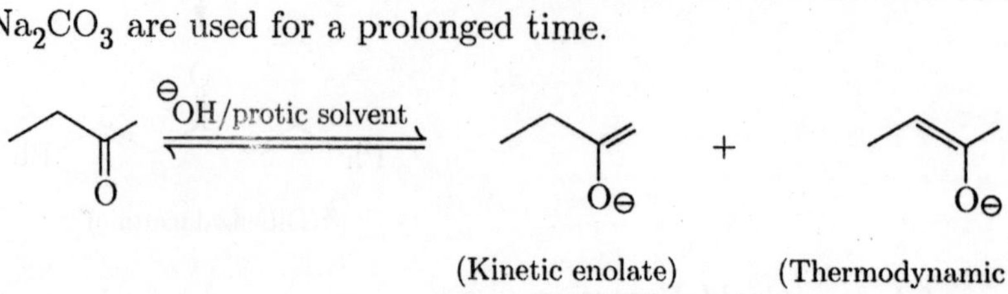

(Kinetic enolate) (Thermodynamic enolate)

On addition of non-enolisable aldehyde (having no α-H atom), *two products* are expected and we get two products in Claisen-Schmidt reaction, if an unsymmetrical ketone is used which can be enolised in two alternative positions.

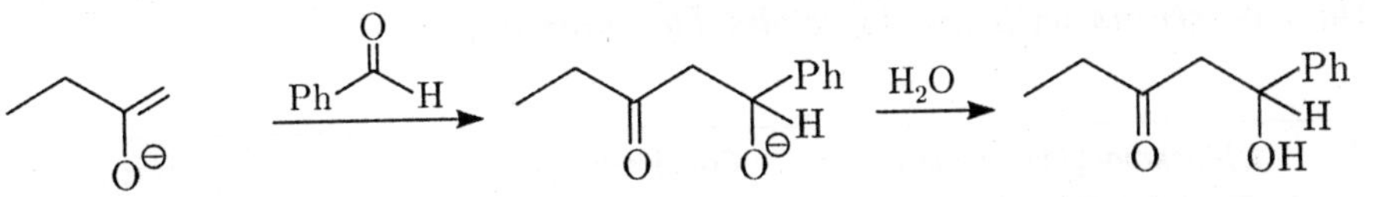

(Kinetic enolate) (Kinetically controlled aldol)

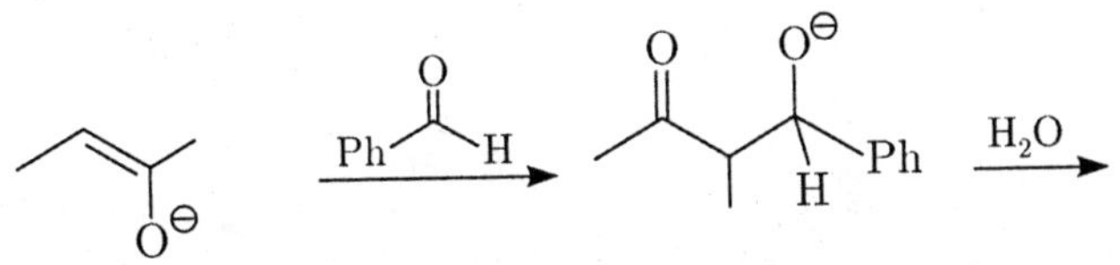

(Thermodynamic enolate) (Thermodynamically controlled aldol)

Summary of equilibrium-controlled aldol reactions : In the equilibrium method, the carbonyl compound(s) must be treated with weak, usually aqueous or alcoholic acid or base and allowed to equilibrate with all possibe enols or enolates. Either only one product is possible (due to symmetry or blocking of α-positions) or some thermodynamic factor (such as formation of a stable conjugated enone) ensures that the reaction goes down one preferred route.

Types of aldol reaction under thermodynamic control

Type of reaction	*Typical conditions*	*Examples*
1. Self condensation of aldehydes	2% NaOH, aq. ethanol	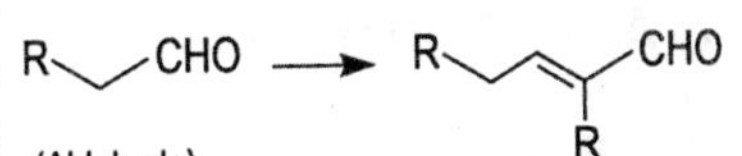 (Aldehyde) (Enal)
2. Self condensation of ketones	HCl, $Al(OR)_3$, NaOH, KOH	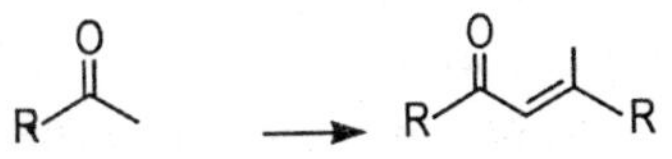 (Ketone) (Enone)
3. Crossed condensations of an enolisable ketone and a non-enolisable aldehyde	NaOH, KOH, Na_2CO_3, HCl or H_2SO_4	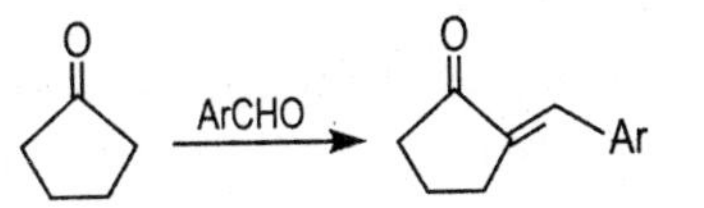
4. Crossed condensations of aryl methyl ketones and non-enolisable aldehydes	dilute HCl or NaOH	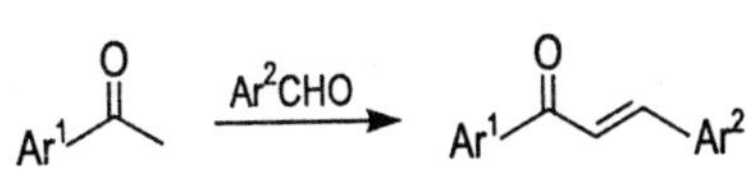
5. Cyclisation reactions	2% NaOH, aq. ethanol, or HCl or H_2SO_4	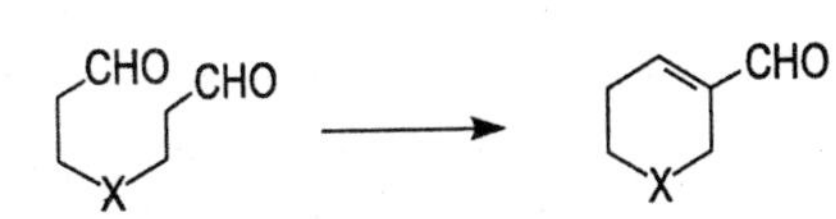 (X=C, O, N, S)

Aldol reactions with highly enolisable compounds

1,3-Dicarbonyl compound	Conditions	Examples
1. $CH_2(COOH)_2$ (Malonic acid)	Piperidine/DMSO	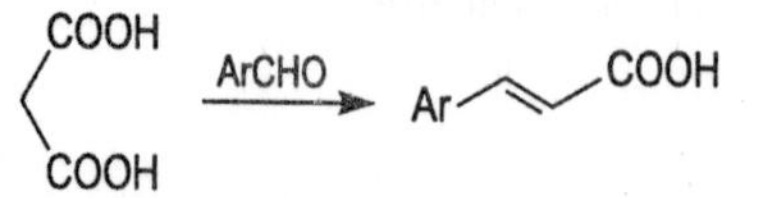
2. $CH_2(COOEt)_2$ (DEM)	$\overset{\oplus}{N}H_4Ac\overset{\ominus}{O}$	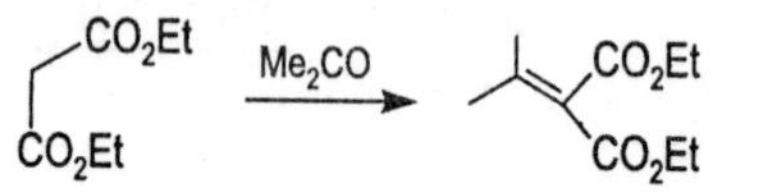
3. $CH_3COCH_2CO_2Et$ (EAA)	Piperidine, EtOH/r.t.	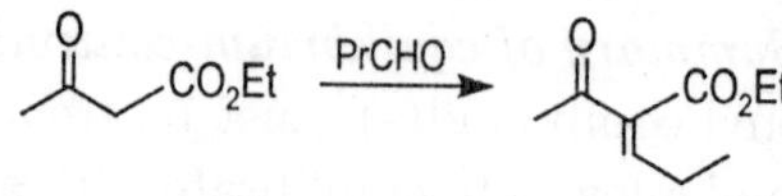
4. Nitro compounds, RCH_2NO_2	NaOH, H_2O	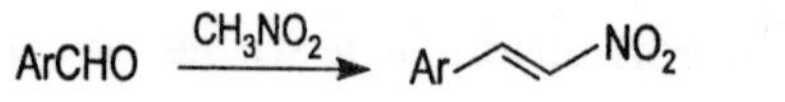
5. Wittig reagents $Ph_3\overset{\oplus}{P}CH_2COR$	NaOMe/MeOH	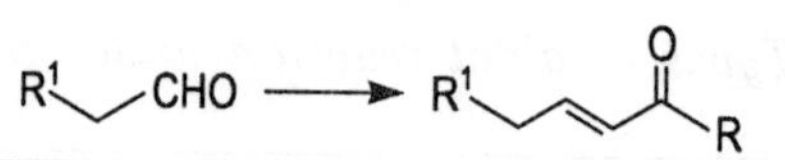

Directed Aldol Reactions

In the directed aldol reactions, one component is first converted into a specific enol equivalent and *only then* combined with the electrophilic partner. The following are the most versatile methods and can be used to make essentially any aldol or any conjugated unsaturated carbonyl compound. One disadvantage of these methods is to make the specific enol equivalent under rigorous anhydrous conditions with strong bases or powerful Lewis bases. Specific enol equivalents are used only when the classical equilibrium methods fail.

Controlling aldol reactions with specific enol equivalents : Specific enol equivalents are intermediates that still have the reactivity of enols or enolates but are stable enough to be prepared in good yield from the carbonyl compound without any aldol reaction. Sensible choice of an appropriate specific enol equivalent will allow almost any aldol reaction to be performed successfully.

Specific enol equivalent	*Conditions*	*Examples*
1. Lithium enolate	a. LDA, THF, –78°C b. Aldehyde c. NH_4Cl, H_2O	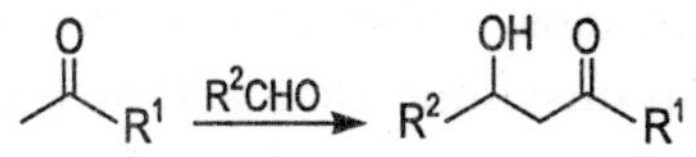
2. Silyl enol ether	$TiCl_4$, CH_2Cl_2, –78°C, 1h under argon atomosphere	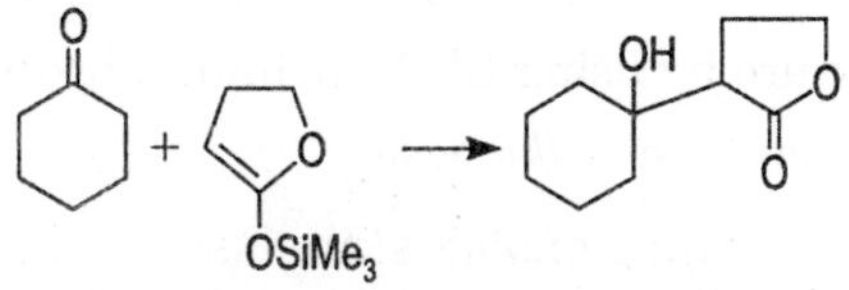
3. Enamine	pyrrolidine (N–H), heat	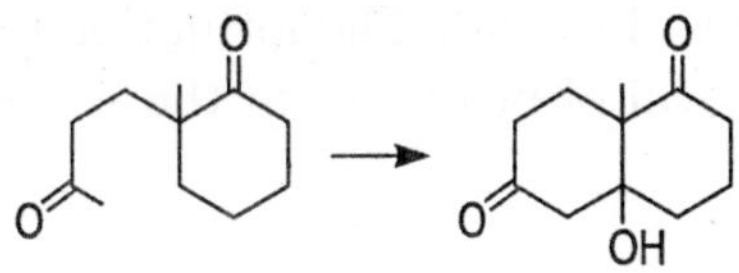
4. Aza–enolate	1. RNH_2, 2. LDA, 3. ketone 4. dilute H_2SO_4	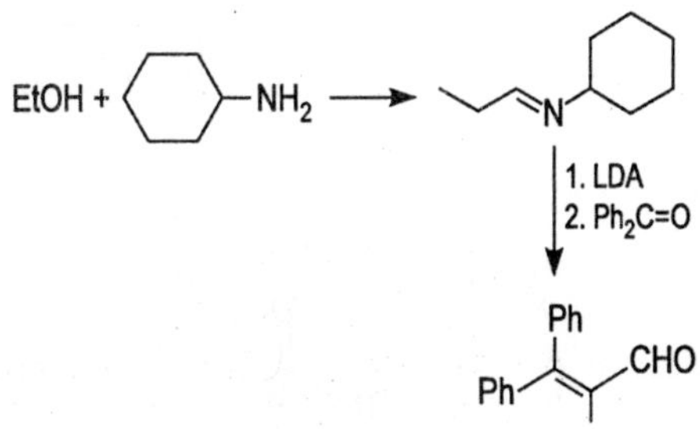
5. Zinc enolate (Reformatsky reaction)	1. Zn, 2. Aldehyde or ketone	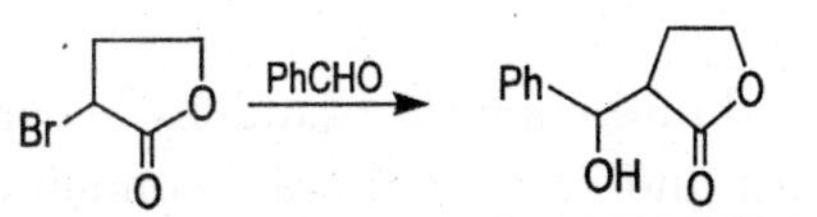

Summary of the specific enol equivalents

Useful enolates for the aldol reaction

Enolate Type	*Aldehyde*	*Ketone*	*Ester*	*Acid*
1. Lithium enolate	×	√	√	√
2. Silyl enol ether	√	√	√	√
3. Enamine	√	√	×	×
4. Aza enolate	√	√	×	×
5. Zinc enolate	×	×	√	×

Silyl enol ethers and lithium enolates have wide applications. Silyl enol ethers are more likely enols. They are more basic and not very reactive, whereas lithium enolates are more like enolate anions, being basic and reactive.

Lithium enolates in aldol reaction

One of the most effective and versatile way to bring about a crossed aldol reaction between an unsymmetrical ketone (enolisable, having α-hydrogens available on both the α-carbon atoms) and an aldehyde (with no α-hydrogen atom) is to use a lithium enolate anion obtained from a ketone. Kinetically controlled enolate is ensured in the reaction mixture by using LDA (lithium diisopropyl amide, $(i\ C_3H_7)_2\ \bar{N}: Li^+$) which is *very strong as well as a bulky base.*

Lithium enolates are usually made at room temperature in aprotic solvents like THF with a hindered base (LDA) and are stable under these conditions because of the strong O—Li bond. The formation of enolate begins with Li—O bond formation before the removal of proton from the α-position by the basic nitrogen atom.

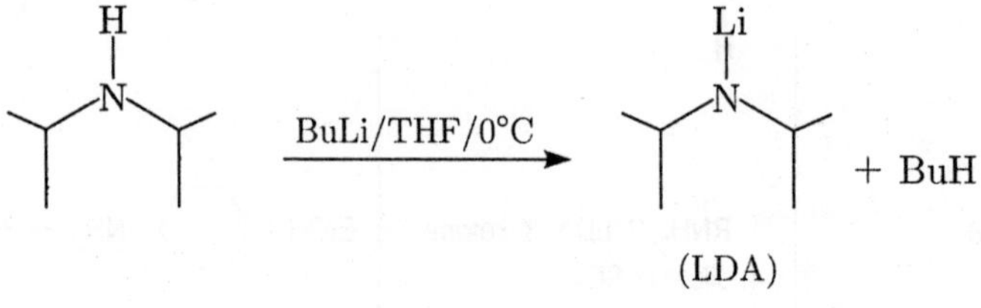

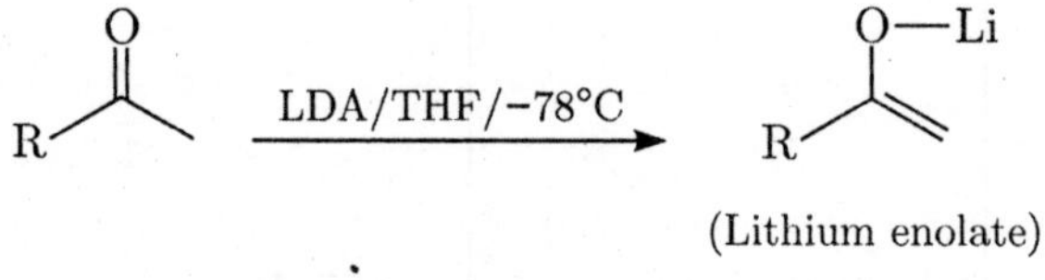

Lithium enolates of aldehydes are generally not done, because self-condensation is too fast and unwanted aldol condensation products are formed.

The tetrahedral structure of lithium-enolate in THF :

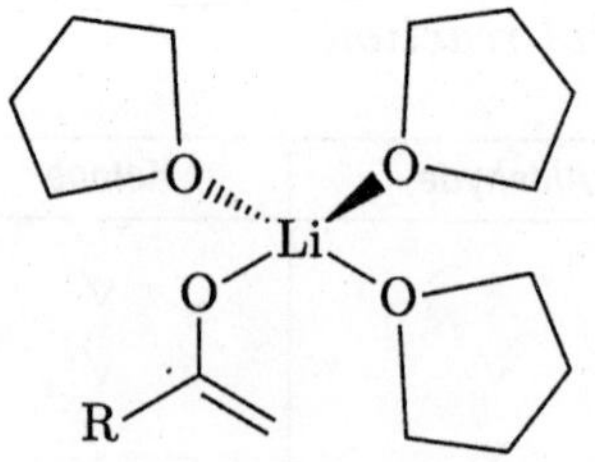

Lithium is tetra-coordinated and before the aldol reaction takes place, one of the THFs must be displaced by electrophilic carbonyl partner.

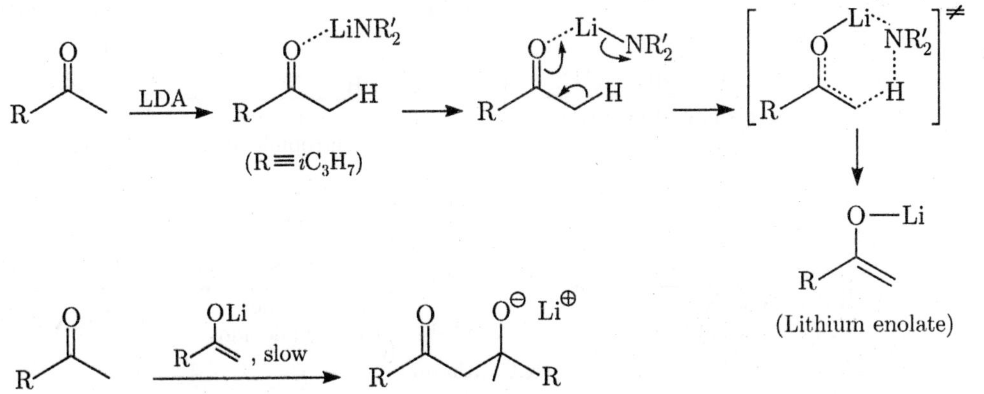

Now, if a second carbonyl compound is added, it too complexes with the same lithium atom. This allows the aldol reaction to take place by a cyclic mechanism in the coordination sphere of the lithium atom.

Aldol reaction with a lithium enolate :

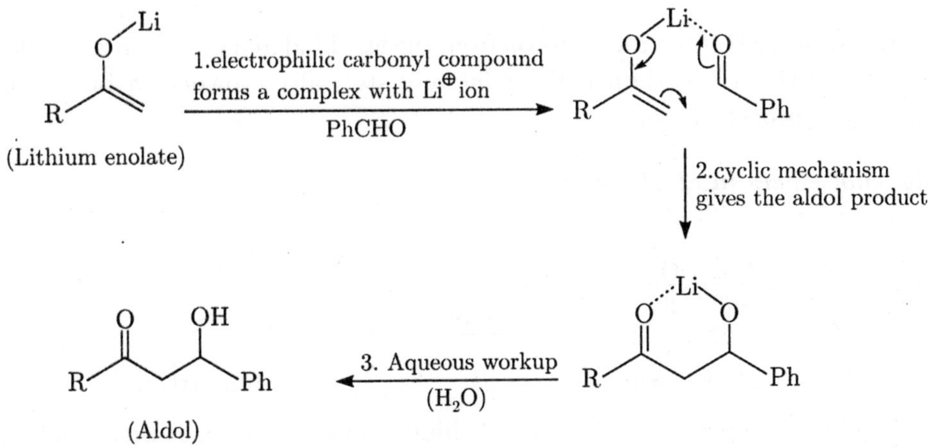

The aldol step itself is now a very favourable intramolecular reaction with a six-membered cyclic transition state. The product is initially the lithium alkoxide of the aldol, which gives the aldol on workup. This is done in two steps, first the specific enol equivalent (here, the lithium enolate) is formed and then electrophile is added. In contrast to the equilibrium methods crossed aldols are formed where enolisable component, base and electrophile are mixed well together.

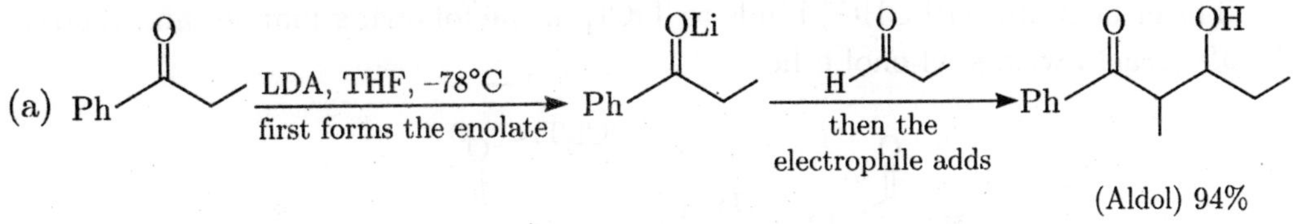

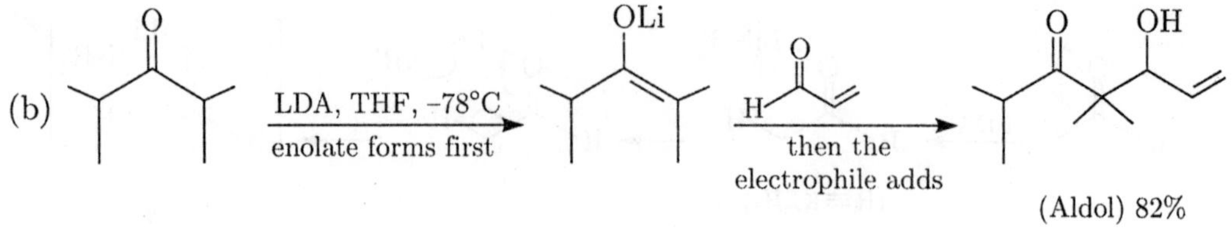

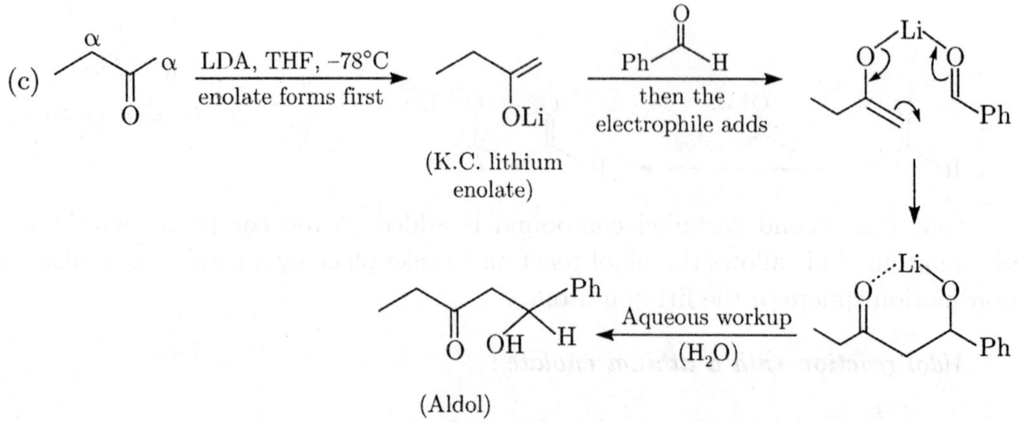

In example (c), LDA abstracts proton from the less-hindered α-carbon regioselectively. The more substituted α-carbon being relatively sterically crowded, a bulky base like LDA can not approach there.

Silyl enol ethers in aldol reactions **:**

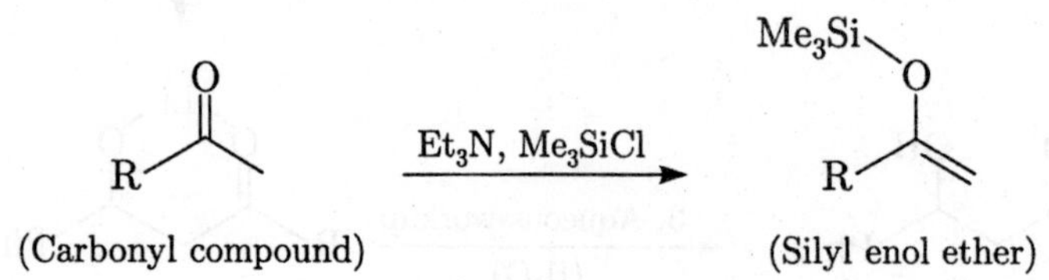

Silyl enol ethers are less reactive than lithium enolates and react with aldehydes and ketones in the presence of *Lewis acid catalyst* $TiCl_4$ *only.*

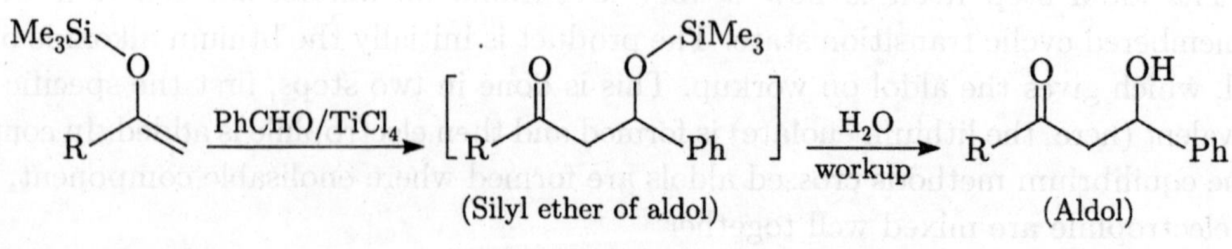

The electrophile (PhCHO) binds to $TiCl_4$ in the following manner and the *resulting complex* reacts with silyl enol ether.

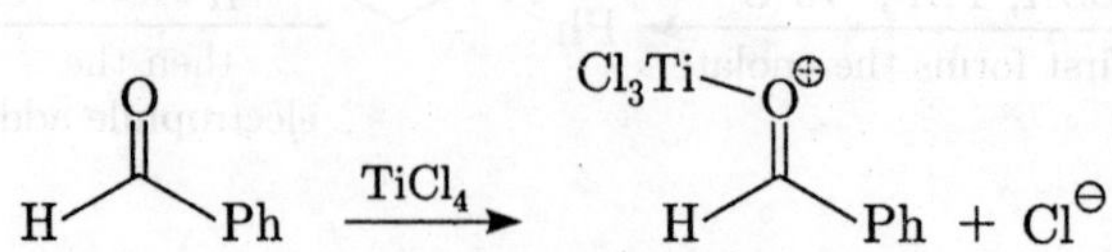

Example :

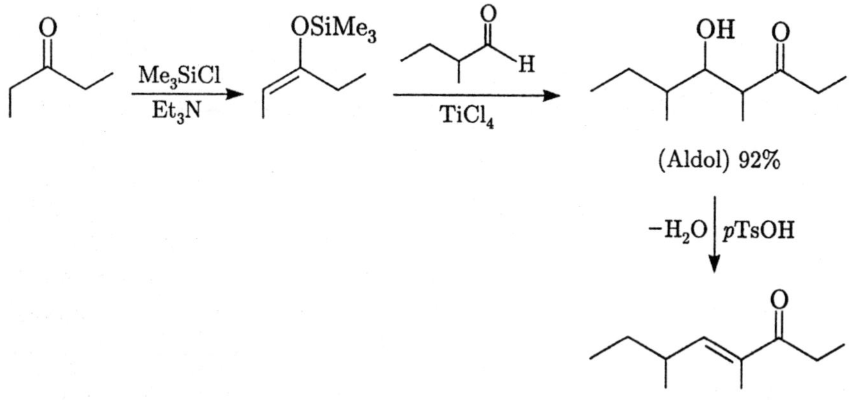

(Aldol) 92%

(Manicone) 83%

A high yield in aldol reaction is found with no significant self condensation of either product.

Intramolecular aldol reactions : Intramolecular aldol condensation reactions offers a convenient way to synthesise molecules with 5-and 6-membered rings rather than those giving strained 3- or 4-membered rings and also the medium rings (8- to 13-membered) are prepared. This can be done by an intramolecular aldol condensation using a dialdehyde, a ketoaldehyde or a diketone.

1. 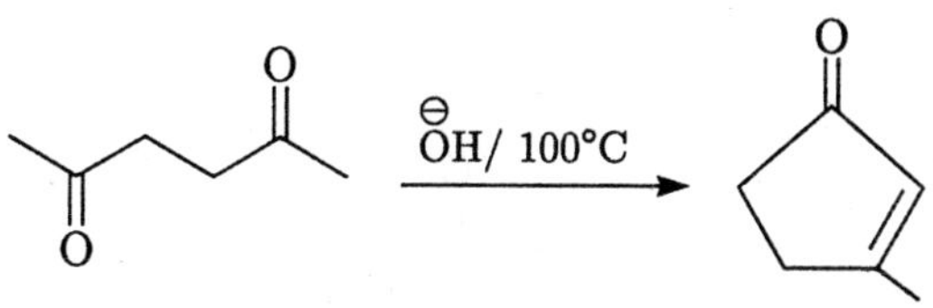

2. 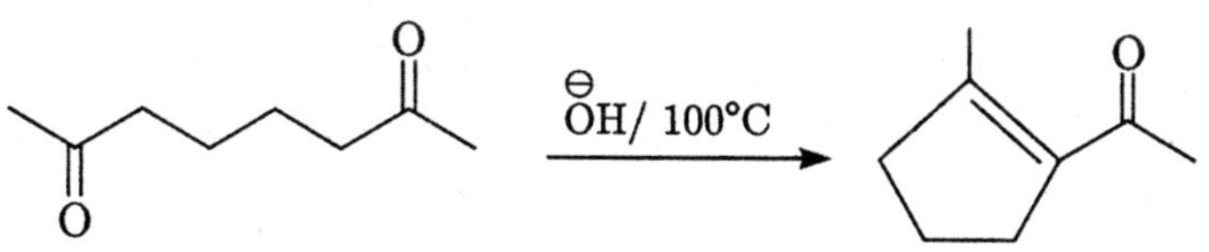

3. 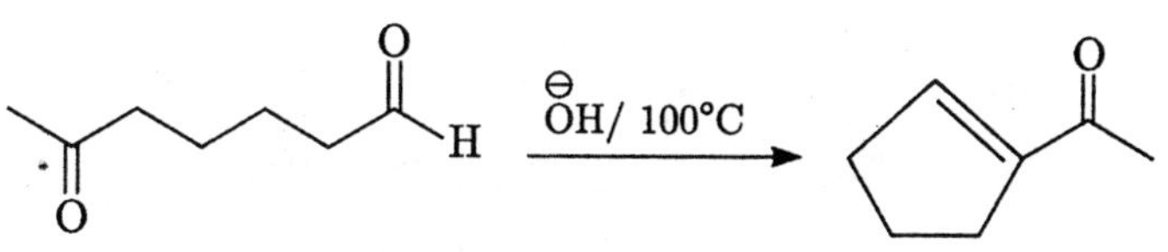

Different enolates may be formed, but enolate from the ketone counterpart adds to the aldehyde part of the molecule.

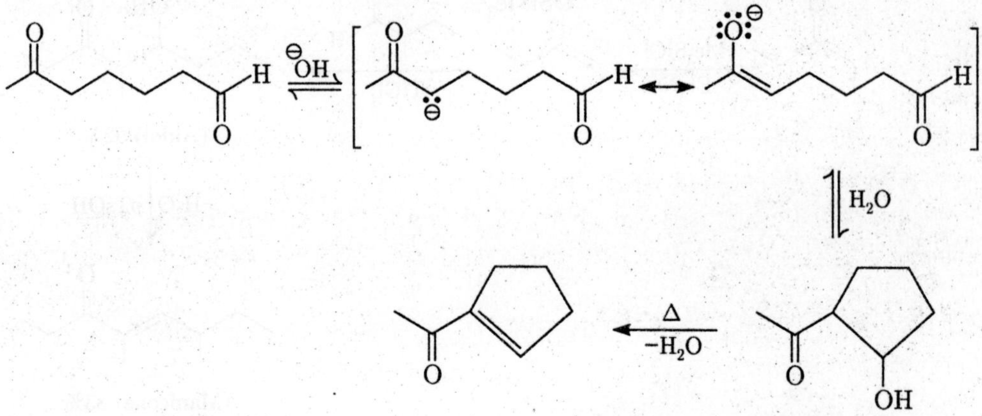

4. 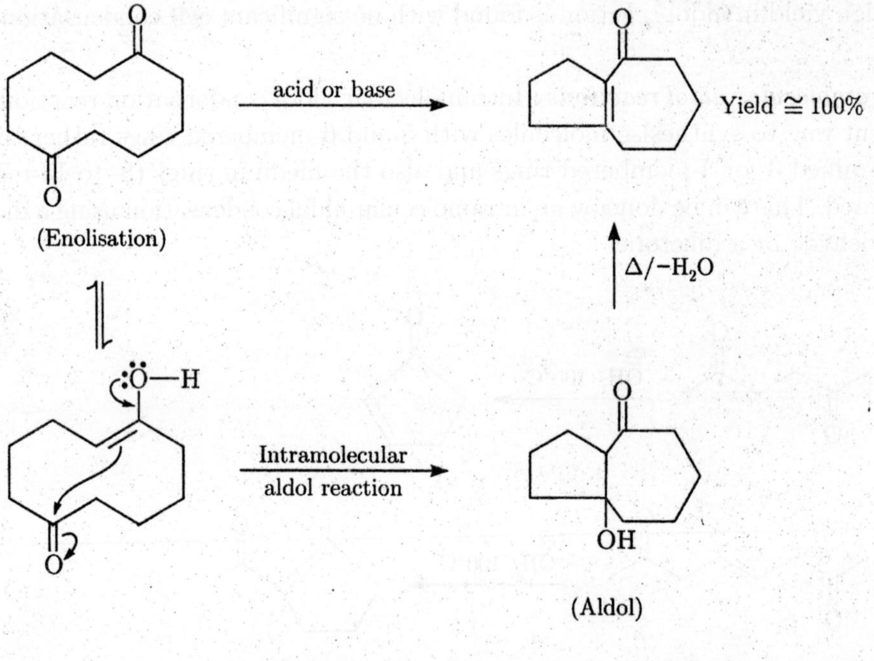

5. 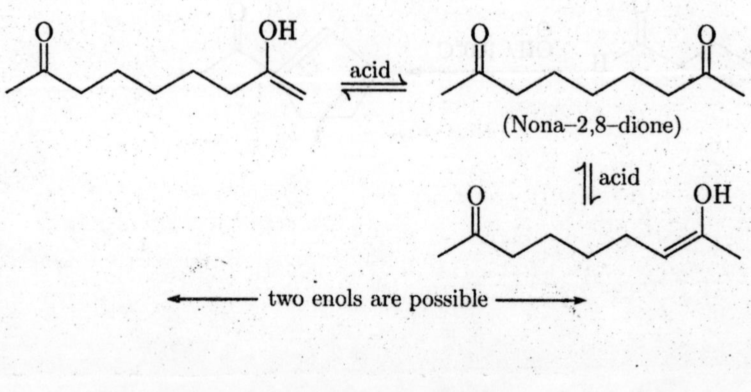

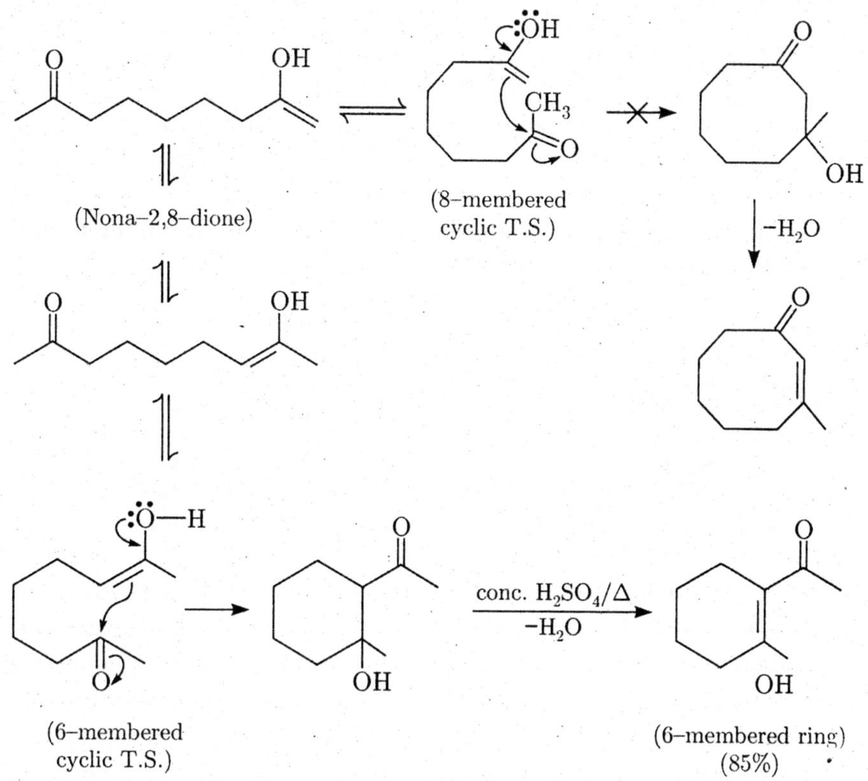

6.

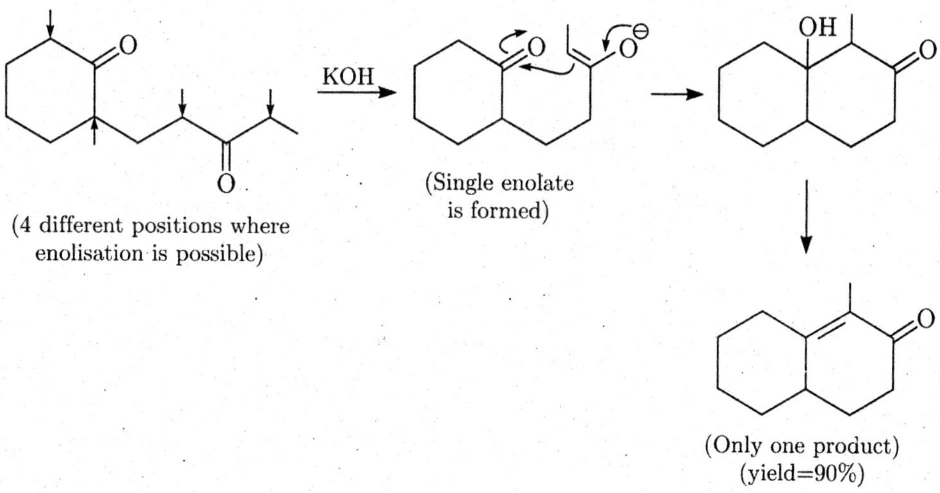

This enolate is not the most stable enolate among the four possibilities (in fact, all the four have comparable stabilities), but this is the only aldol reaction that leads to a stable conjugated enone in a stable six-membered ring. One possibility gives rise to unstable four-membered ring, which would revert to enolate.

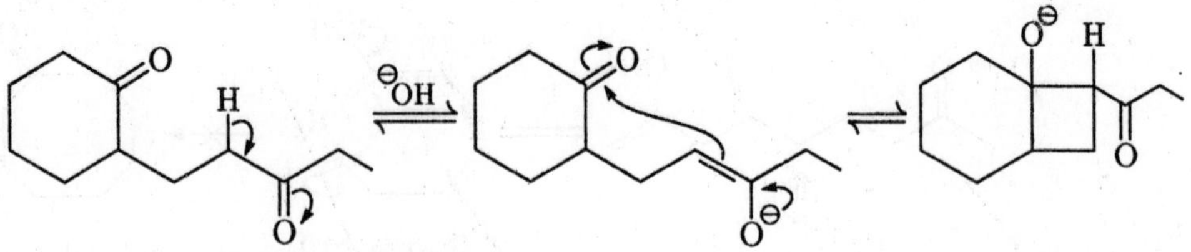

There is one alternative cyclisation to give a six-membered ring and this does not occur due to an interesting reason.

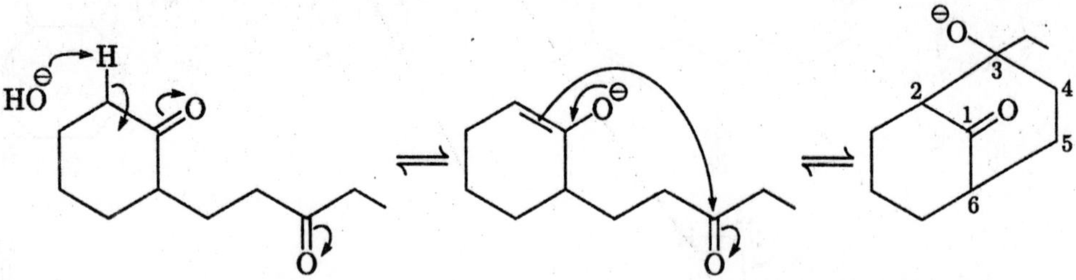

It is a strained bridged compound and dehydration is impossible. No enolate can form at the bridge-head because bridge-head carbons can not be planar and the enone product can not exist for the same reason. The aldol has a perfectly acceptible conformation but that elimination is impossible. The aldol product remains in equilibrium with the alternative aldol products, but only one elimination is possible and that is irreversible, so eventually only one enone is found.

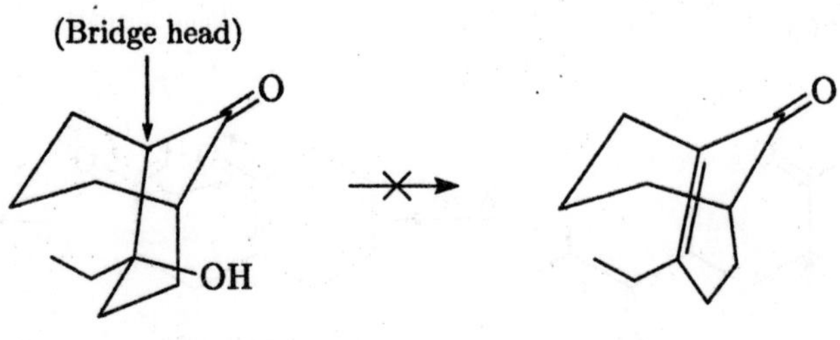

(Aldol product) (Impossible alkene)

7. 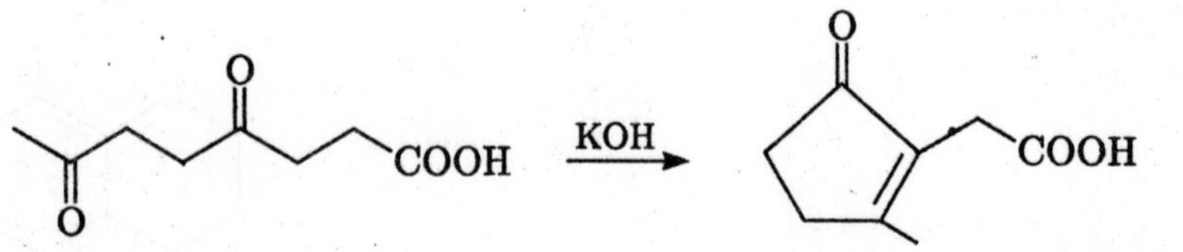

(Single product, yield 97%)

8. 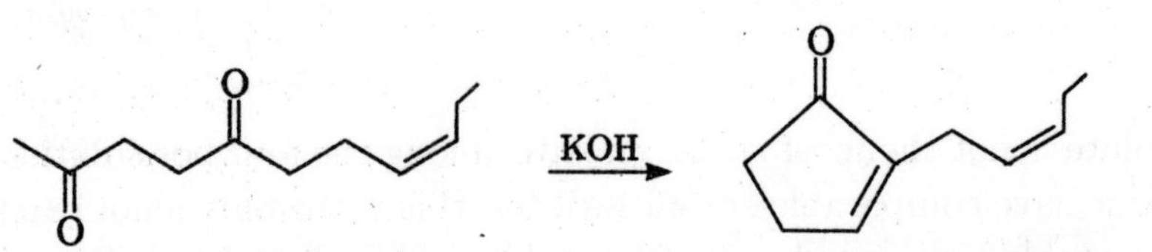

(Z–undeca–8–en–2,5–dione) (*Cis*–jasmone) yield 80%

9. 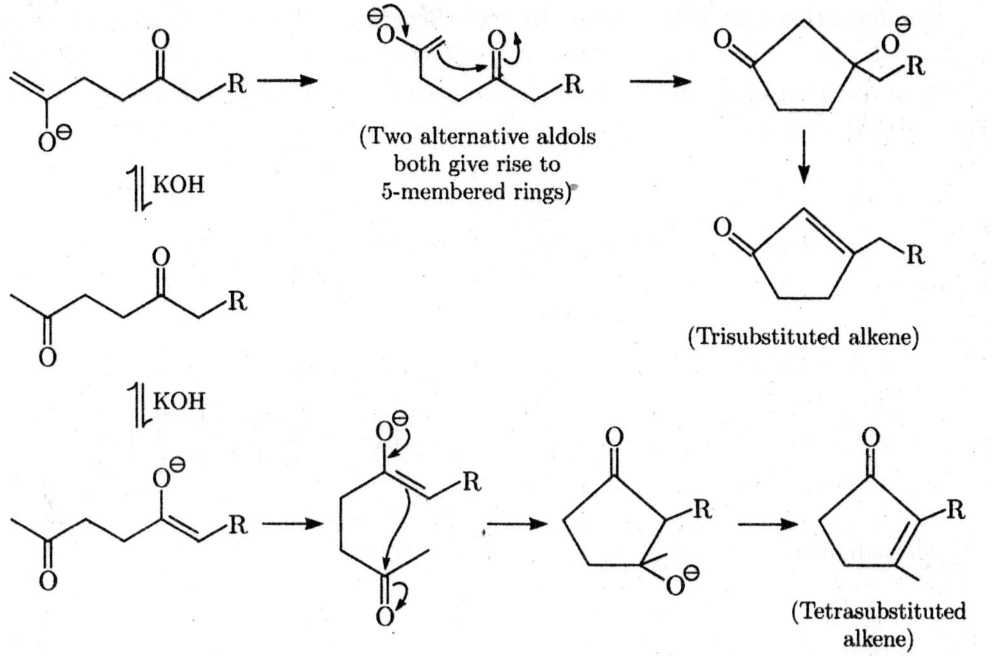

More substituted alkene is the more stable product and found in major amount.

10. 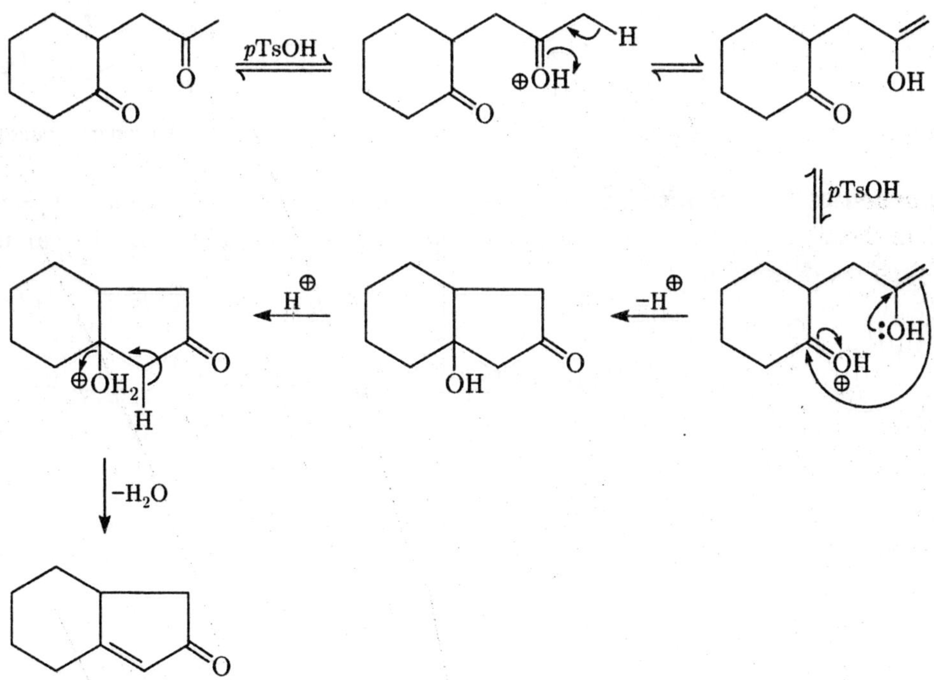

(Only one product is obtained)

Condensation with nitroalkane (Henry's Reaction) : The α-hydrogens of nitroalkanes are appreciably acidic (pK_a=10), more acidic than those of aldehydes and ketones. The acidity of the hydrogen atoms is due to the powerful electron withdrawing effect of $-NO_2$ group and the resonance stabilisation of the anion that is produced.

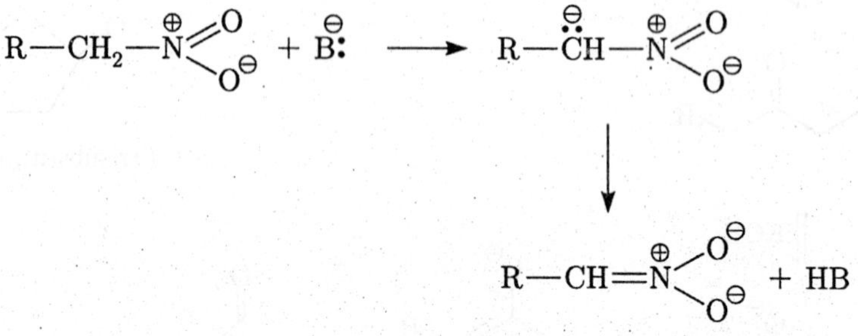

Nitroalkanes having α-H undergo base catalysed aldol reaction.

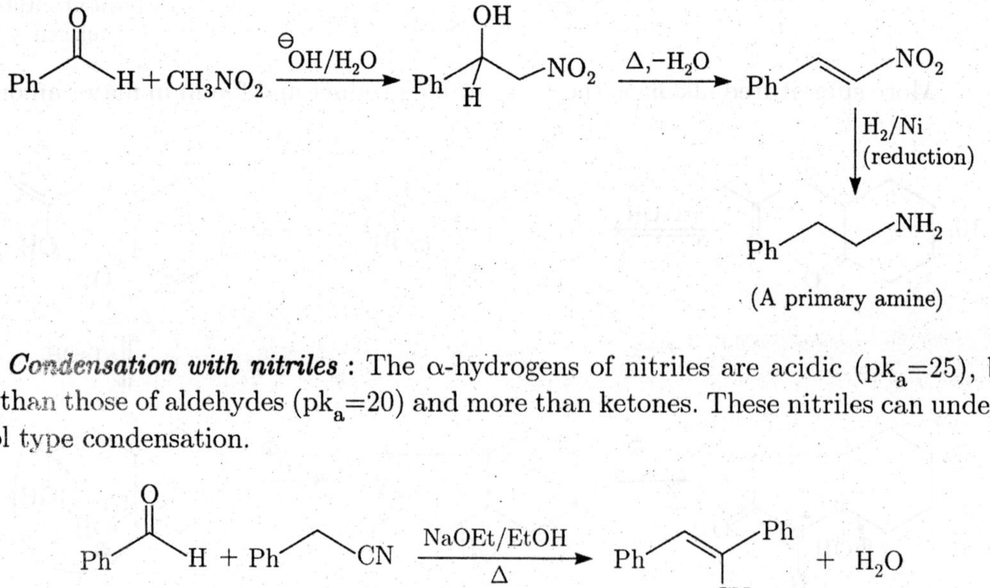

Condensation with nitriles : The α-hydrogens of nitriles are acidic (pk_a=25), but less than those of aldehydes (pk_a=20) and more than ketones. These nitriles can undergo aldol type condensation.

Salient features of aldol reaction :

1. *Dehydration of aldol addition compounds* : Aldols are readily dehydrated to α, β-unsaturated compounds on heating alone or with acid or base.

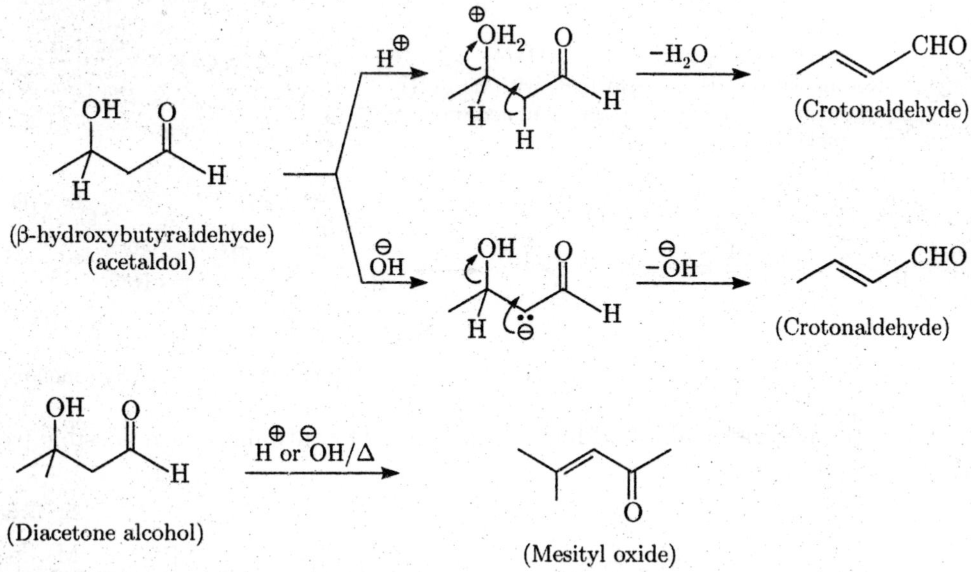

2. When aldol condensation is carried out in the presence of strong alkali, repeated condensation and dehydration results in the formation of resins.

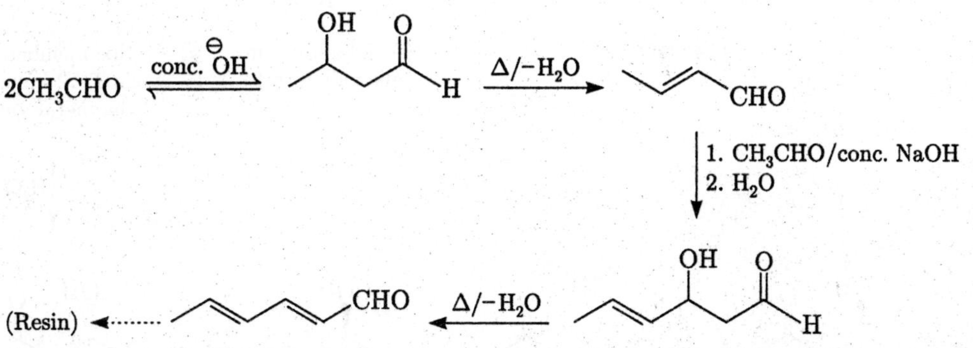

3. The condensation is promoted by –I effect and reduced by +I effect on the carbonyl carbon.

4. The reaction equilibrium is favourable for aldehydes, but less favourable for ketones.

Stereochemistry of Aldol Reaction

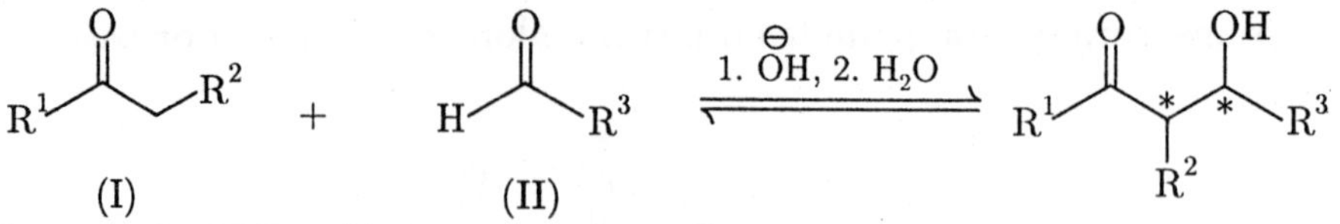

(I) (Ketone with α–H) (Carbanion generator–enolisable)

(II) (Aldehyde with no α–H) (Carbanion acceptor)

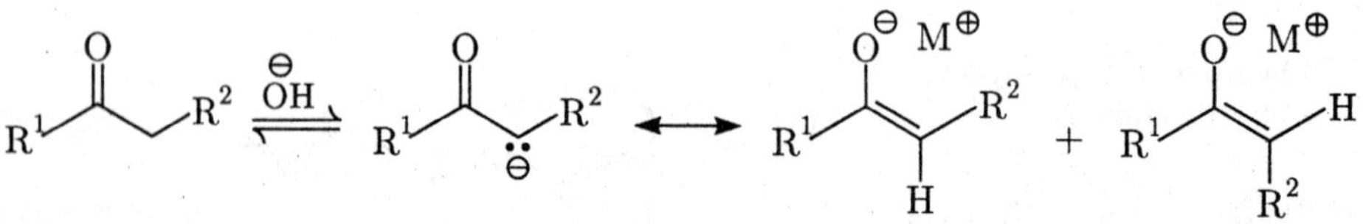

(*Anti* enolate) (*Syn*-enolate)

Four stereoisomeric aldol adducts (two pairs of enantiomers) are possible from *syn*– and *anti*– enolates.

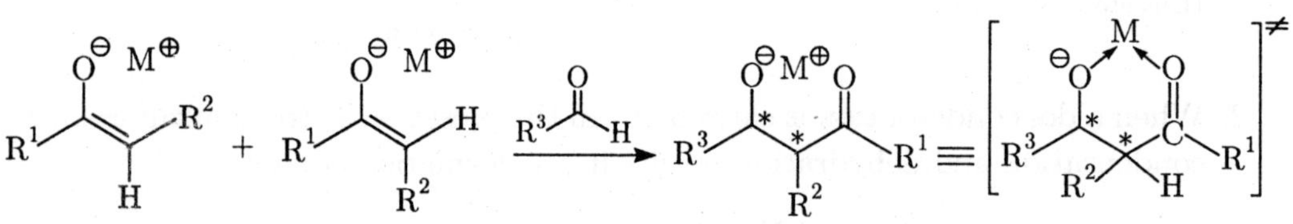

(*Anti* enolate) (*Syn*-enolate) (Aldol adduct in alkoxide form) (Six–membered cyclic T. S. including the metal ion)

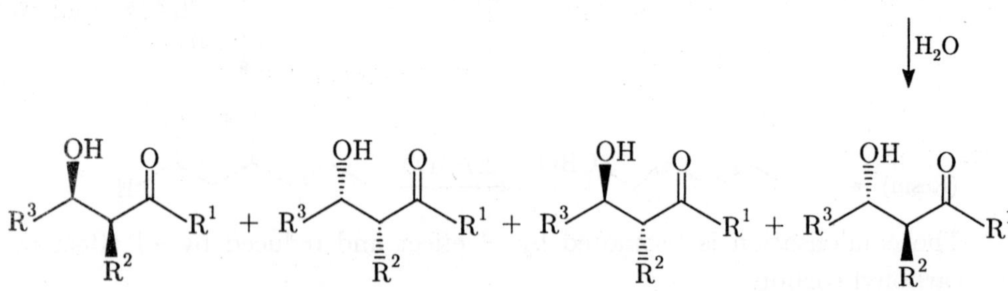

(I) (I′) (II) (II′)

(Z–isomer of aldol) (*dl pair*) (E–isomer of aldol) (*dl pair*)

The predominance of either Z–isomer or E–isomer is governed by the stability of the six–membered transition state formed. From the stability of the corresponding transition state, it is concluded that *trans*–aldol (E–aldol) will predominate in the reaction mixture.

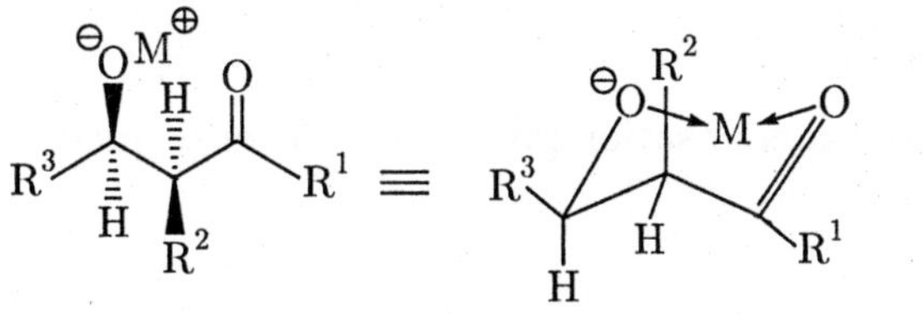

(I)
(Z–isomer)

(*Six* membered cyclic T.S. corresponding to Z–isomer)

(R^2 is in axial position so the T.S of Z–isomer is less stable)

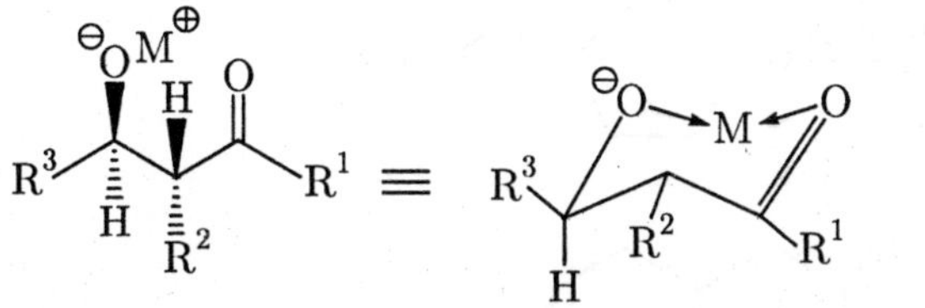

(II)
(E–isomer)

(*Six* membered cyclic T.S. corresponding to E–isomer)

(R^2 is in equatorial position so the T.S of E–isomer is more stable)

A way to increase the diastereoselectivity–Trapping of enolates

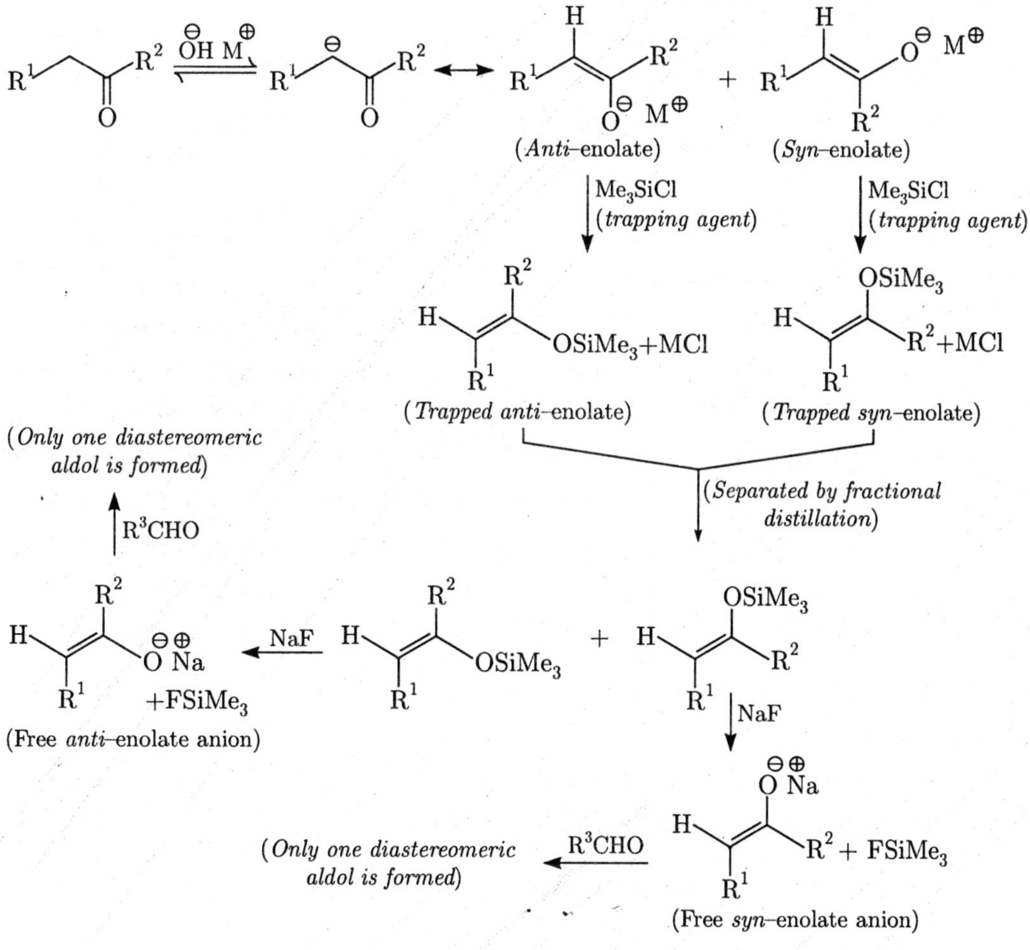

Applications of aldol reaction

1. Cyclisation via intramolecular aldol condensation gives rise to 5– or 6– membered cyclic compounds.

Example :

(a) 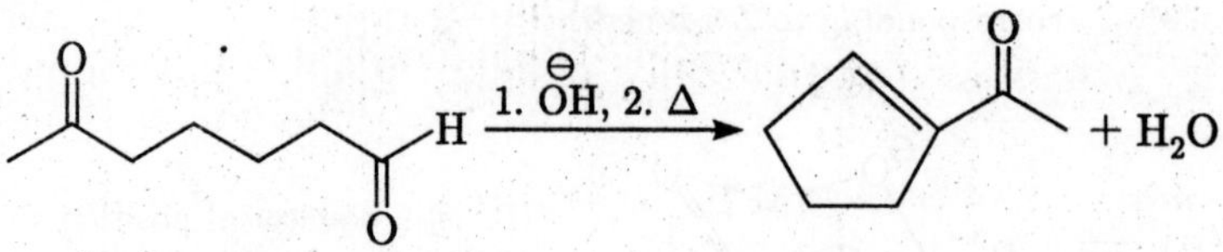

(b) 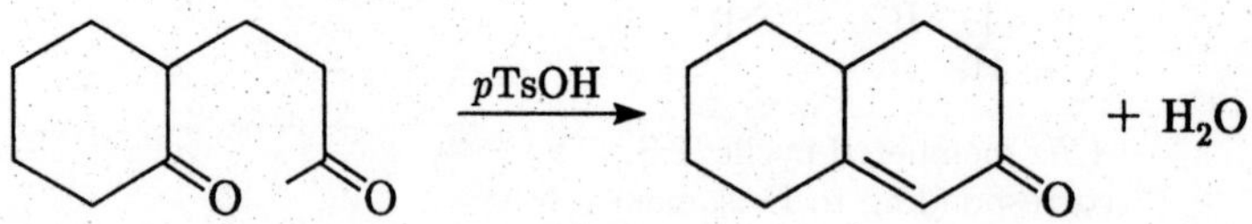

2. ***Increment in carbon chain***

(a) 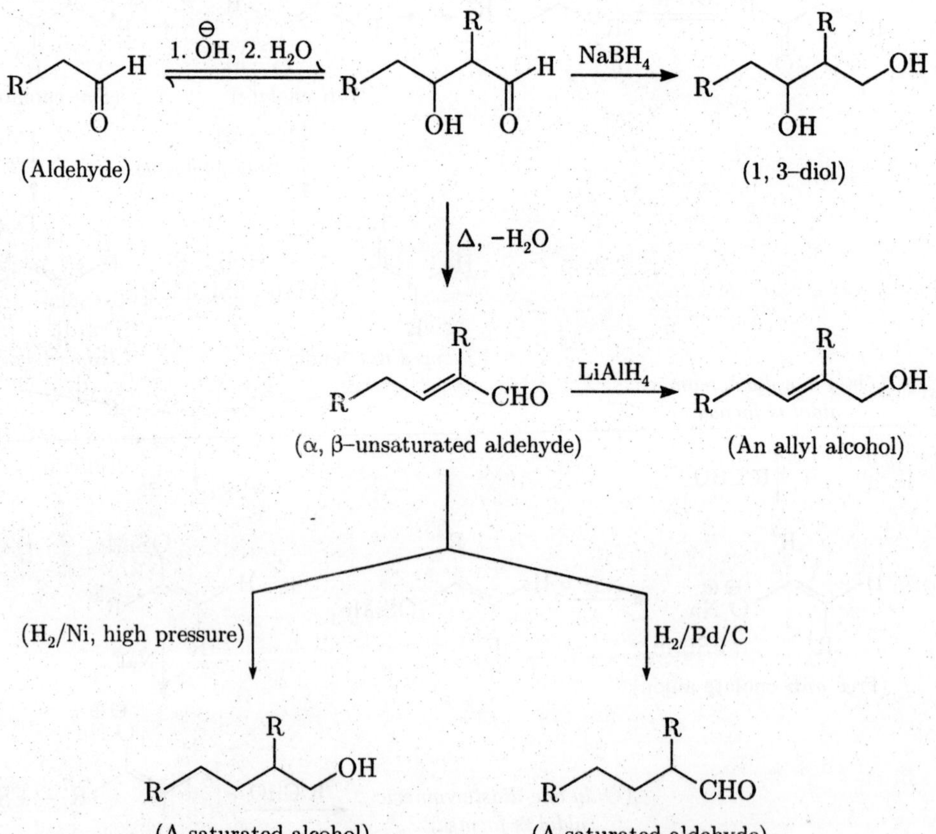

(b) 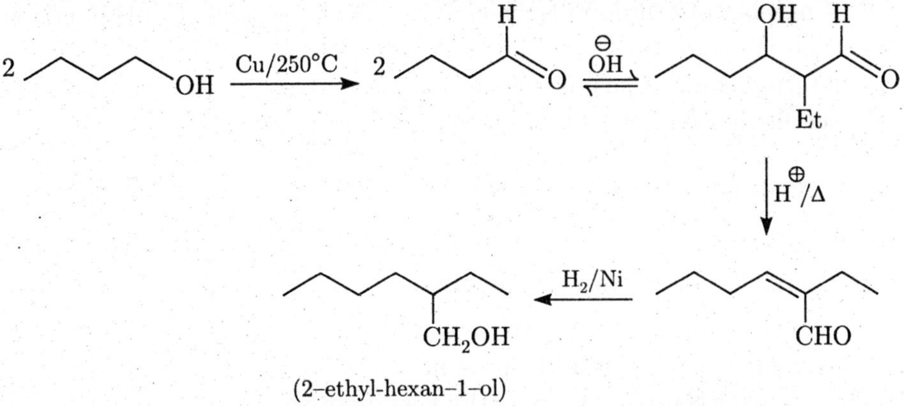
2
OH
Cu/250°C
2
H
O
$\overset{\ominus}{O}H$
OH H
O
Et
$H^{\oplus}/\Delta$
H_2/Ni
CH_2OH
CHO
(2-ethyl-hexan-1-ol)

3. 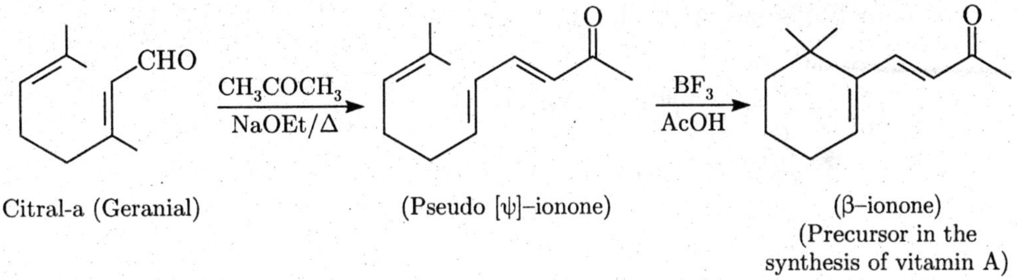
CHO
CH_3COCH_3
NaOEt/Δ
O
BF_3
AcOH
O
Citral-a (Geranial)
(Pseudo [ψ]-ionone)
(β-ionone)
(Precursor in the synthesis of vitamin A)

4. 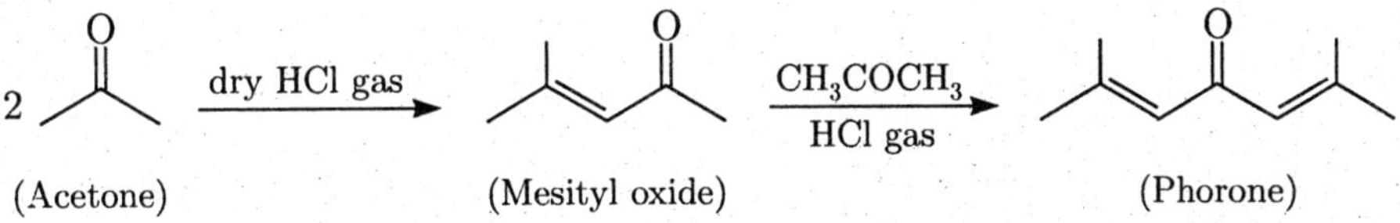
2
O
dry HCl gas
O
CH_3COCH_3
HCl gas
O
(Acetone)
(Mesityl oxide)
(Phorone)

5. 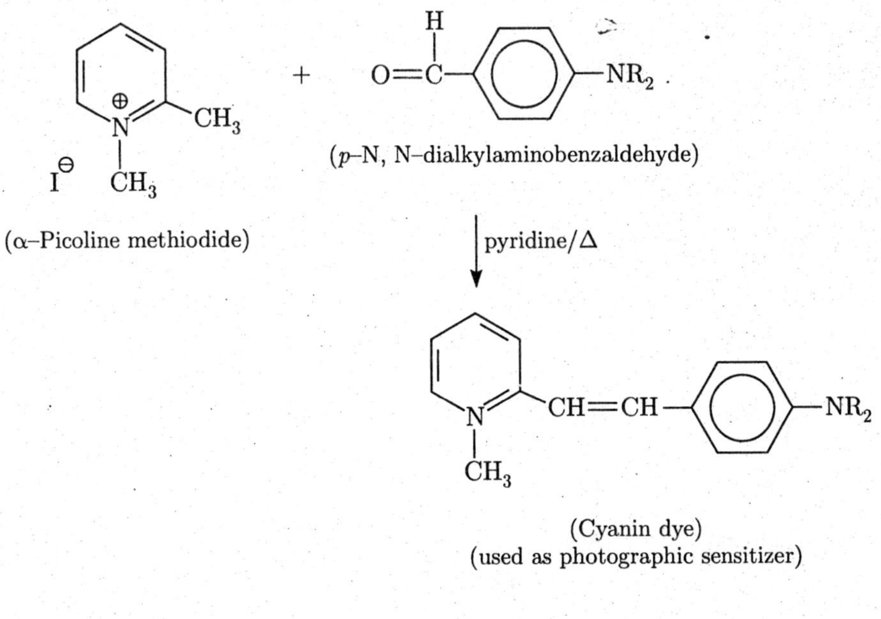
$N^{\oplus}$
CH_3
$I^{\ominus}$
CH_3
+
H
O=C
NR_2
(α-Picoline methiodide)
(p-N, N-dialkylaminobenzaldehyde)
pyridine/Δ
N
CH=CH
NR_2
CH_3
(Cyanin dye)
(used as photographic sensitizer)

6. A number of compounds which have relatively acidic C—H bonds undergo aldol type condensation with aldehydes and ketones to produce valuable synthetic intermediates. Thus, condensation of acetylene with aldehydes or ketones give acetylenic alcohols, which are commercially valuable products.

$$2HCHO + H—C\equiv C—H \xrightarrow[(NaNH_2)]{Na/liq.NH_3} \underset{\text{(2–butyne–1, 4–diol)}}{HOH_2C—C\equiv C—CH_2OH}$$

The process is known as ethynylation.

7. When acetaldehyde is treated with excess formaldehyde (acetaldehyde : formaldehyde = 1:3) in the presence of $Ca(OH)_2$, crossed aldol reaction continues (3 times) until trihydroxymethylacetaldehyde is obtained. The latter having no α–H atom undergoes crossed Cannizzaro reaction to produce a symmetric alcohol, namely pentaerythritol.

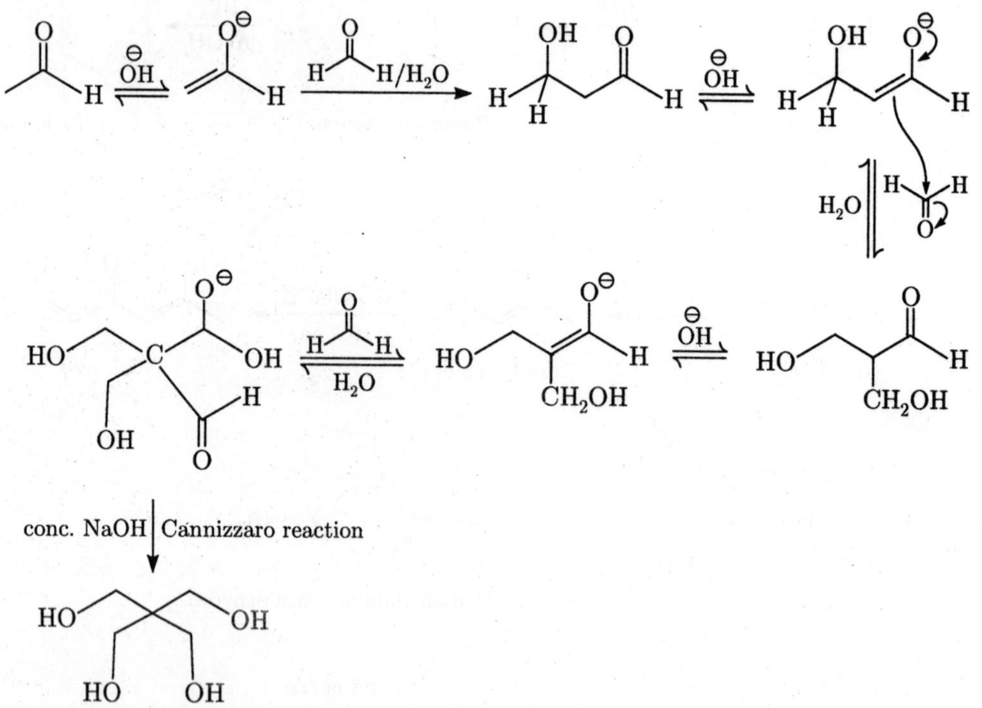

(Pentaerythritol)

8. 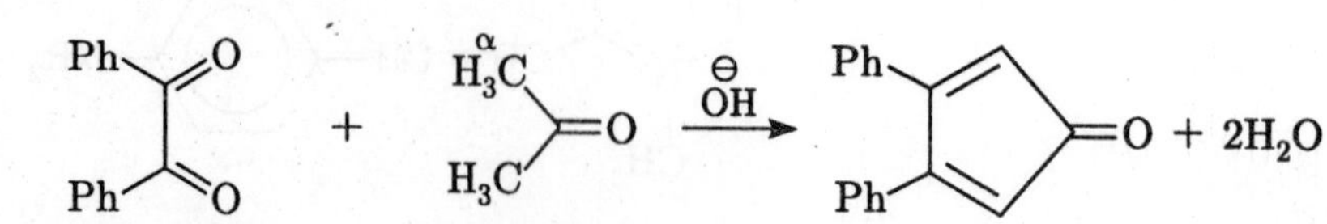

(Biphenyl glyoxal) (no α–H) (Acetone) (contains α–H)

9. Reactions which are closely related to aldol condensation are as follows : (a) Perkin reaction, (b) Claisen ester condensation (c) Knoevenagel reaction, (d) Dieckmann condensation, (e) Doebner reaction, (f) Darzen's glycidic ester condensation etc.

The Perkin Reaction (Condensation)

The aldol type condensation of an aromatic aldehyde with an aliphatic acid anhydride containing *two α–H atoms* in the presence of its carboxylate anion, which acts as a base catalyst to produce the *β–phenylacrylic acid* is said to be Perkin reaction or condensation.

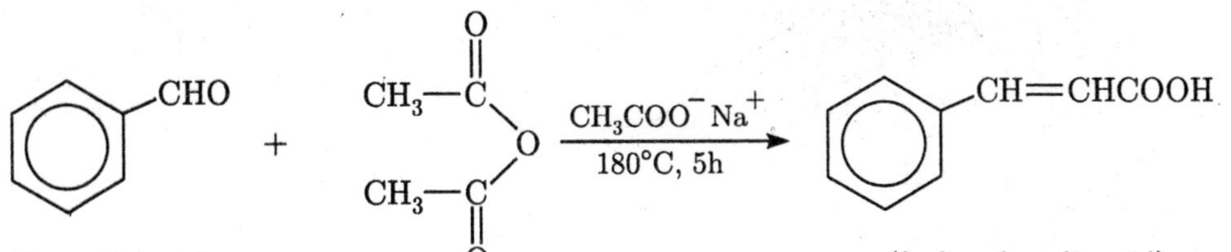

(Benzaldehyde) (Acetic anhydride) (β-phenylacrylic acid) (Cinnamic acid)

Sometimes, instead of carboxylate anion, other bases like triethylamine give better result.

The reaction is carried out by heating the aldehyde with an excess of acid anhydride (which acts as the solvent) centaining corresponding carboxylate salt at 180°C. Usually dehydration takes place under the conditions of the reaction and a mixed anhydride results. The unreacted aldehyde is removed by distillation in steam and the β-arylacrylic acid is obtained by hydrolysis of the mixed anhydride with dilute hydrochloric acid. The condensation is promoted by the presence of electron withdrawing group in the benzene ring and the reaction rate gets retarded by the presence of electron donating group in the ring.

Mechanism of Perkin Reaction :

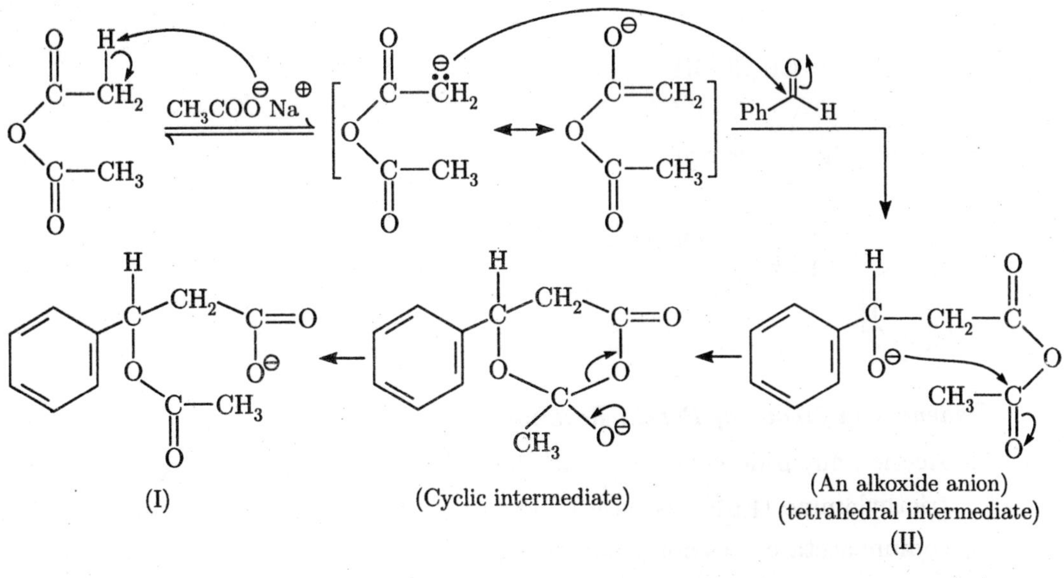

Sometimes, decarboxylative elimination also takes place and a *styrene derivative* is obtained.

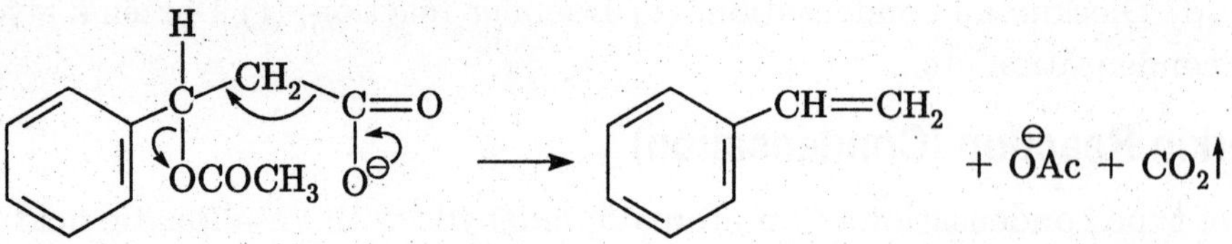

Since *COO^- group is resonance stabilised (I) is more stable over (II).*

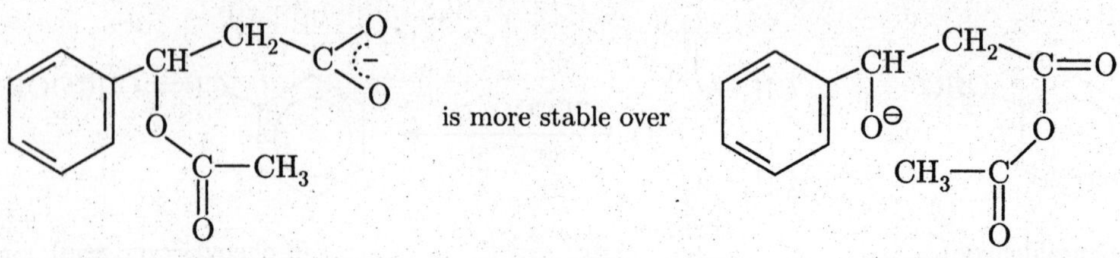

(I) (II)

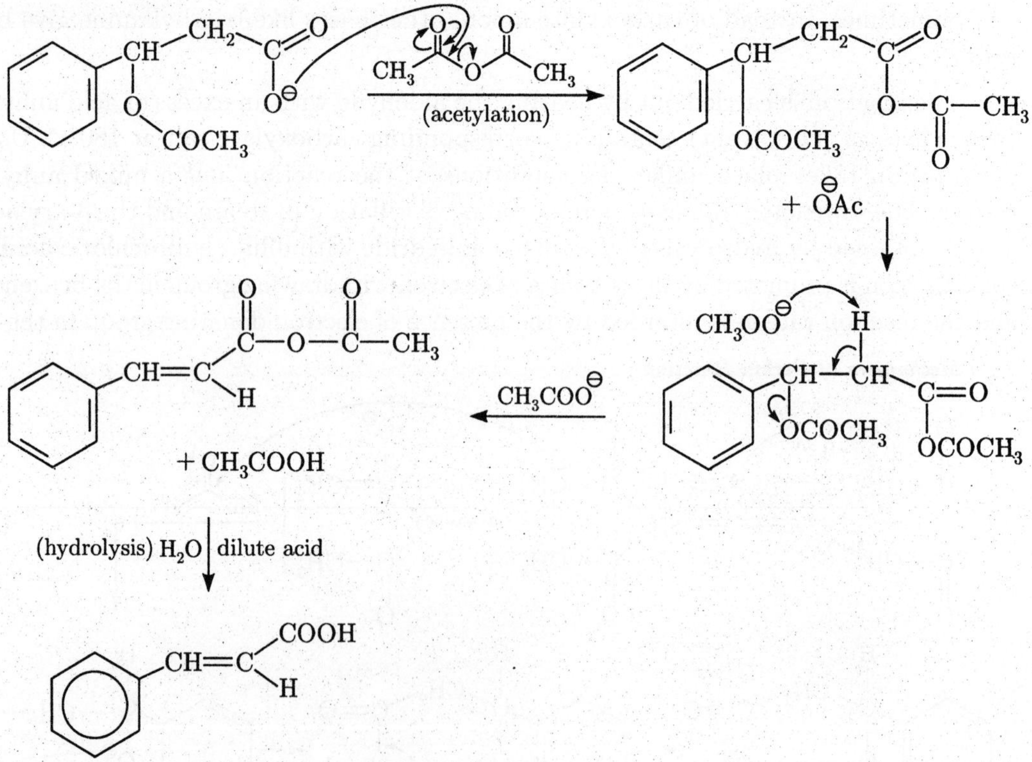

Evidences in favour of Perkin Reaction :

1. Acetic anhydride condenses with benzaldehyde in the presence of pyridine or triethylamine ($Et_3\ddot{N}$) as base to yield cinnamic acid after hydrolysis, whereas sodium acetate does not condense with benzaldehyde in the presence of pyridine.

This supports the formation of carbanion from the *anhydride only* and not from sodium acetate. Sodium acetate acts only as a catalyst in the reaction.

$$\text{PhCHO} + \text{Ac}_2\text{O} \xrightarrow{\text{1. pyridine, 2. } \text{H}_3\text{O}^{\oplus}} \text{PhCH}{=}\text{CHCOOH}$$

$$\text{PhCHO} + \text{Na}^{+}\text{AcO}^{\ominus} \xrightarrow[\times]{\text{1. pyridine, 2. } \text{H}_3\text{O}^{\oplus}} \text{PhCH}{=}\text{CHCOOH}$$

(not formed)

2. Heating is required for a prolonged time (about 5h) at high temperature (140°C) because a weak base (acetate anion) has to react with a weak acid *i.e.*, anhydride.
3. When the acid anhydride contains only one α–H atom, a β-hydroxyacid is formed instead of α, β-unsaturated acid because of the unavailability of the active hydrogen on the α-carbon for subsequent dehydration step.

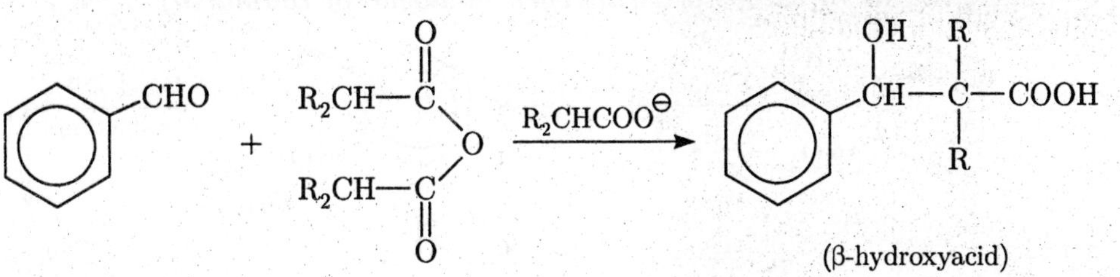

(β-hydroxyacid)

4. *Meta* directing groups in the aromatic ring promotes the reaction. *Ortho* substituted benzaldehyde gives low yield of the product. For example, *o*–methylbenzaldehyde gives only 15% *o*–methylcinnamic acid.
5. Perkin reaction is specific for aromatic aldehydes.

Applications of Perkin's Reaction :

1. ***Preparation of α–substituted unsaturated acids***

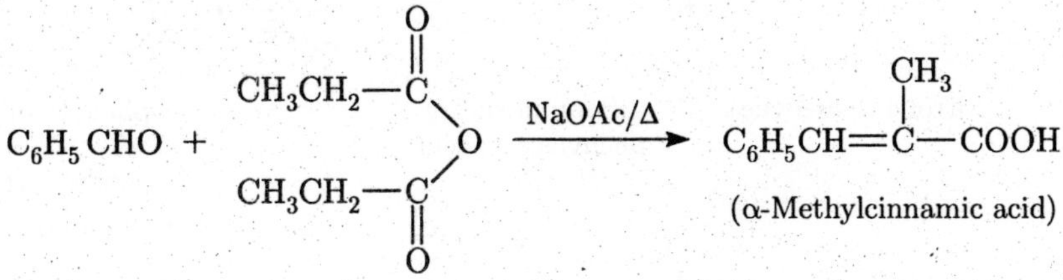

(α-Methylcinnamic acid)

2. ***Synthesis of coumarin***

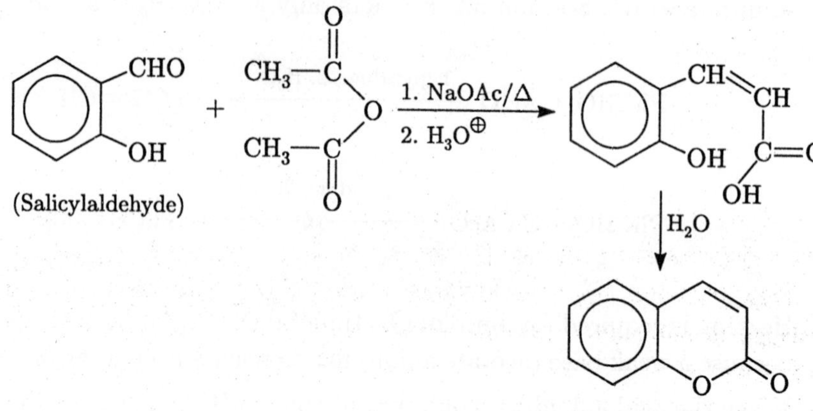

(Salicylaldehyde)

(Coumarin)
(a good flavouring agent)

3. ***Synthesis of carbostyril (nitrogen analogue of coumarin)***

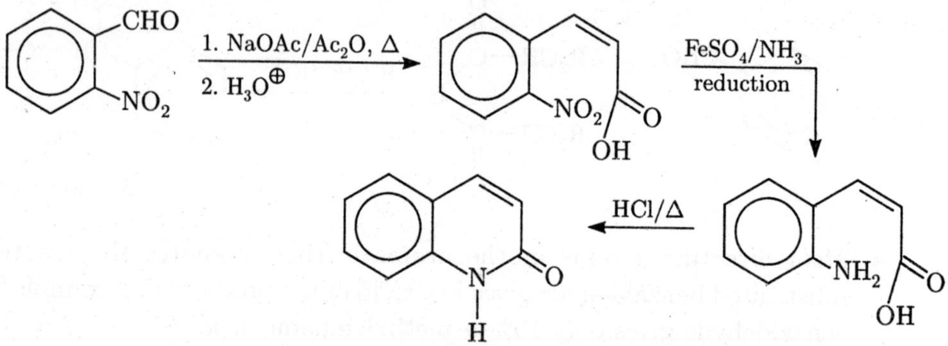

(Carbostyril)

4. ***Synthesis of phenanthrene***

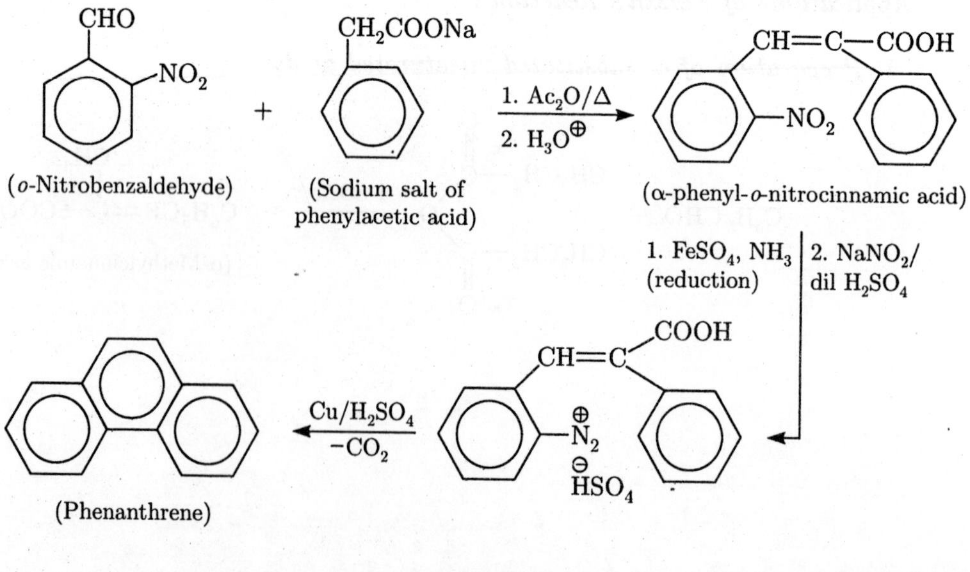

(o-Nitrobenzaldehyde) (Sodium salt of phenylacetic acid) (α-phenyl-o-nitrocinnamic acid)

(Phenanthrene)

5. The reaction occurs with vinylogues of aromatic aldehydes.

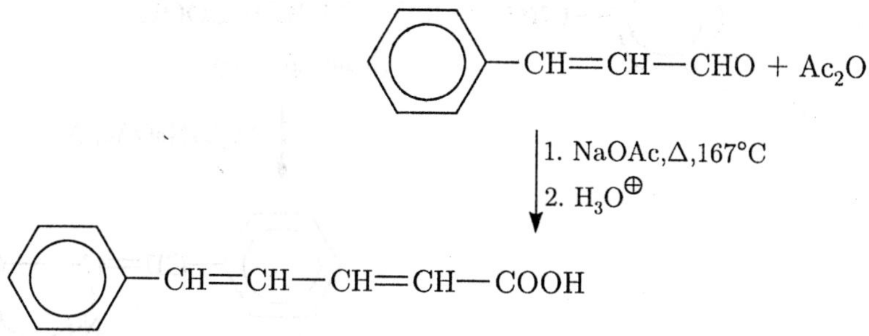

6. ***Preparation of paraconic acid***

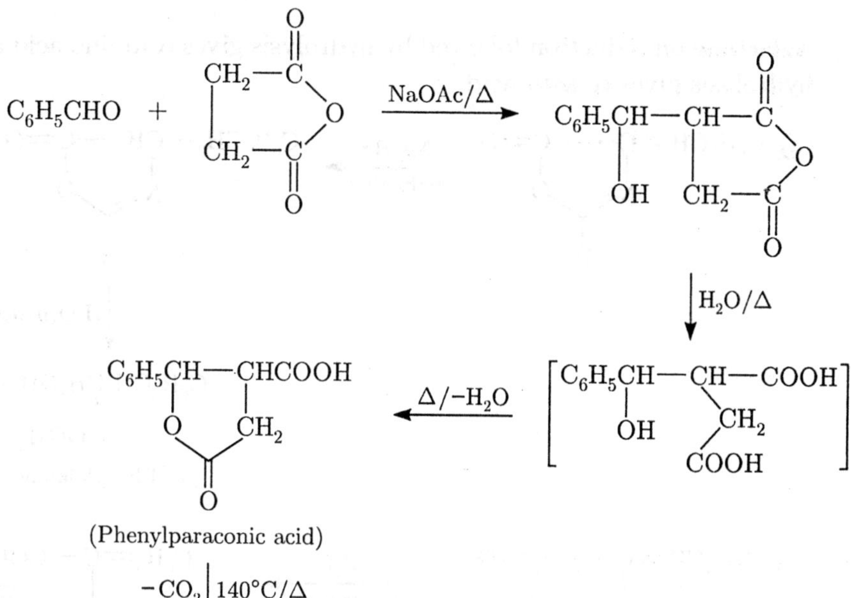

(Phenylparaconic acid)

$C_6H_5CH{=}CHCH_2COOH$

(4-Phenyl-3-butenoic acid)
(β, γ-unsaturated acid)

7. By the Perkin's reaction, aryl substituted acrylic acid is preparaed and followed by hydrogenation, β–aryl derivatives of saturated carboxylic acids are formed.

$$ArCH{=}CHCOOH \xrightarrow{H_2/Ni} ArCH_2CH_2COOH \xrightarrow[2.\ H_3O^{\oplus}]{1.\ LiAlH_4/Et_2O/\Delta} ArCH_2CH_2COOH$$

8. ***Arlenmeyer's azlactone synthesis*** : Aromatic aldehydes are condensed with N–acylglycine in the presence of sodium acetate and acetic anhydride to yield an *azlactone.*

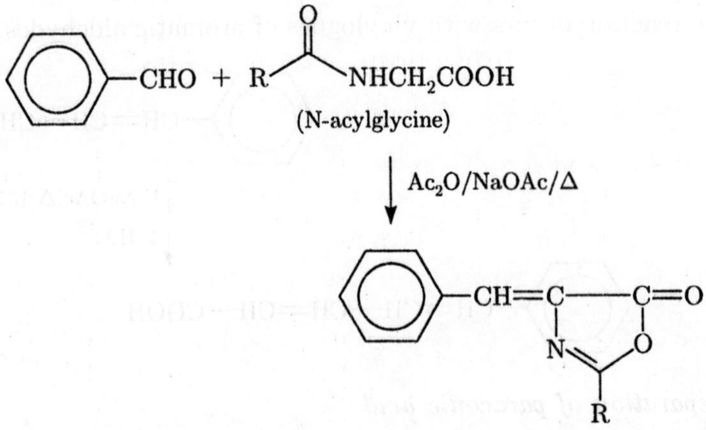

(Azlactone)

Azlactone on reduction followed by hydrolysis gives α-amino acid and on simple hydrolysis gives α–keto acid.

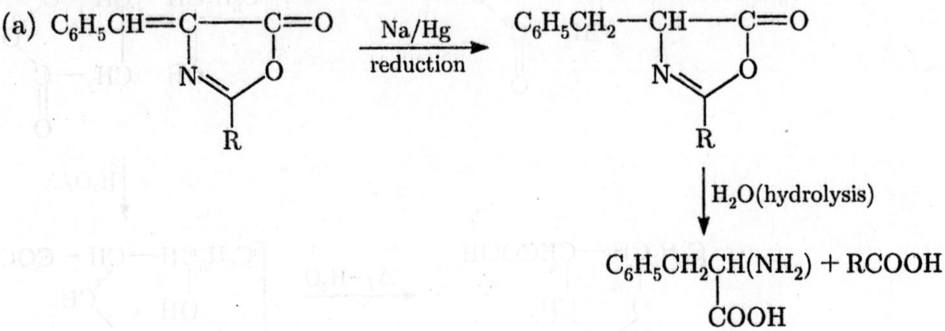

(±) Phenylalanine

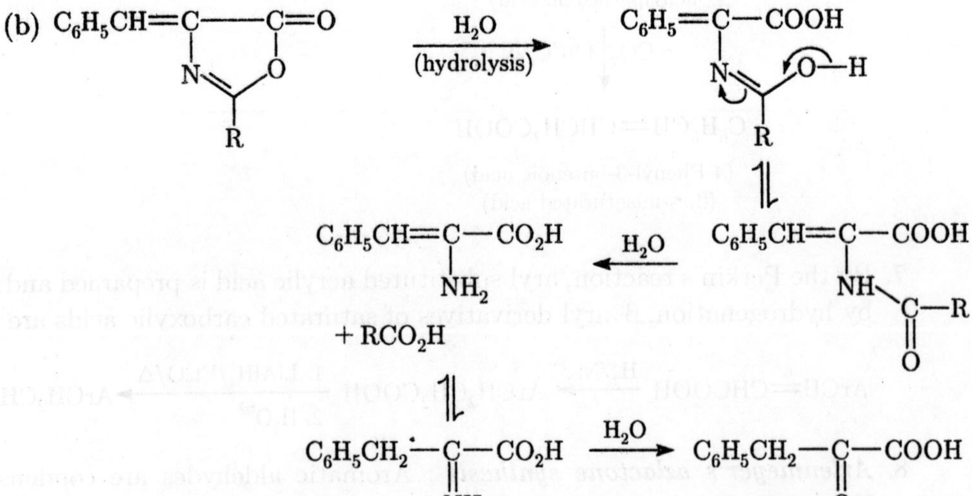

(α-Keto acid)

9. 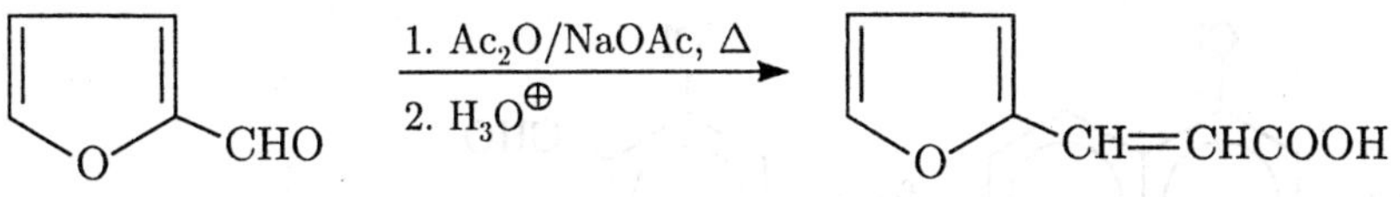

(Furfuraldehyde) 3-(α-Furfuryl)-acrylic acid

10. Aromatic anhydrides in place of aldehydes may be used.

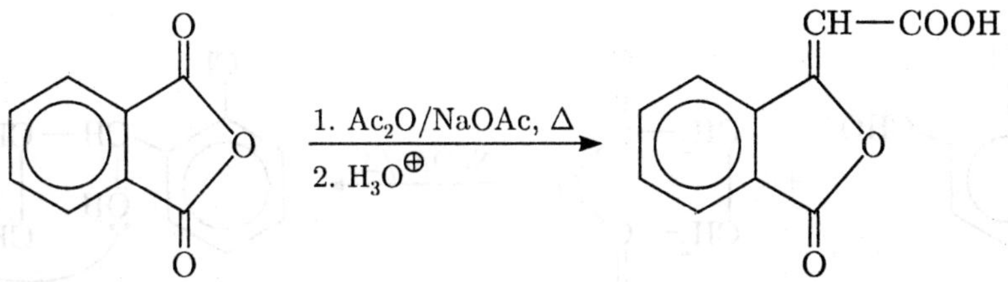

(Phthalic anhydride) (Phthalyl acetic acid)

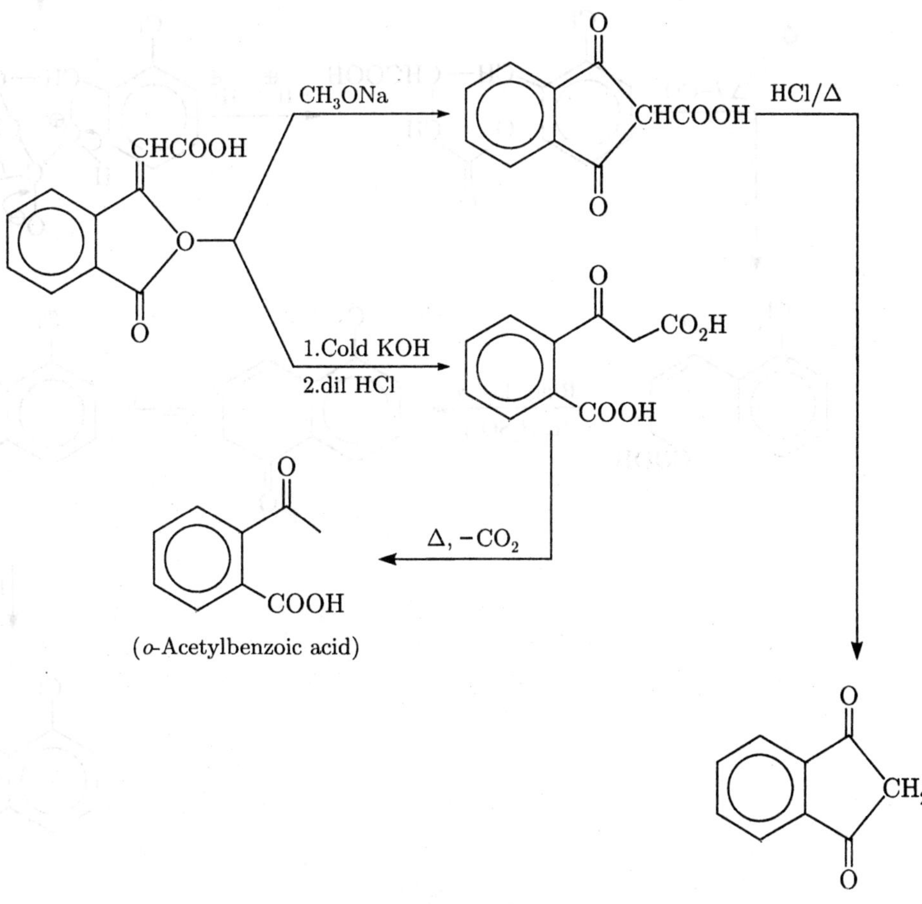

(*o*-Acetylbenzoic acid)

(Indane-1,3-dione)

11. Prepare 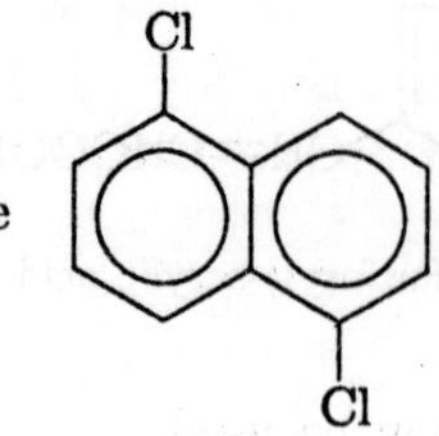 from 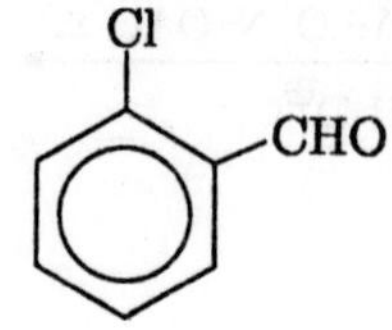

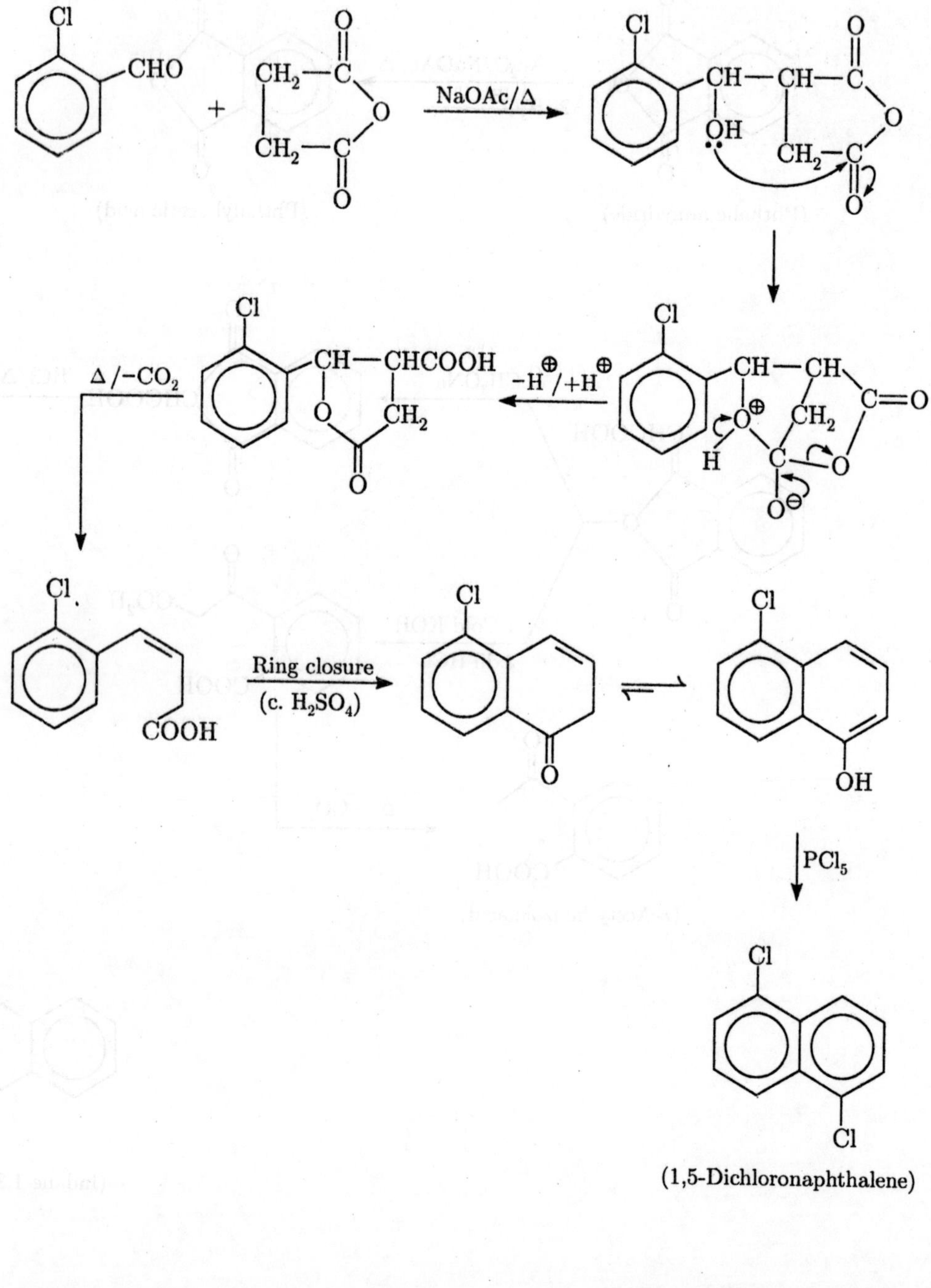

(1,5-Dichloronaphthalene)

12. Prepare 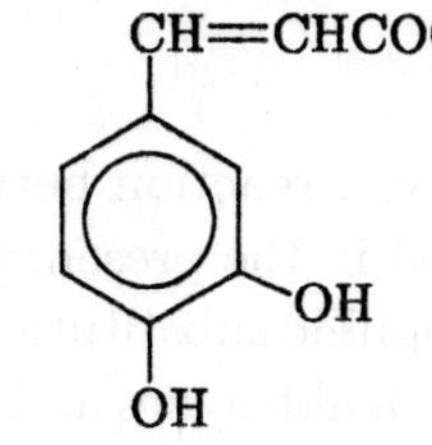 from 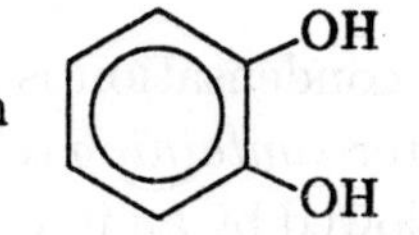

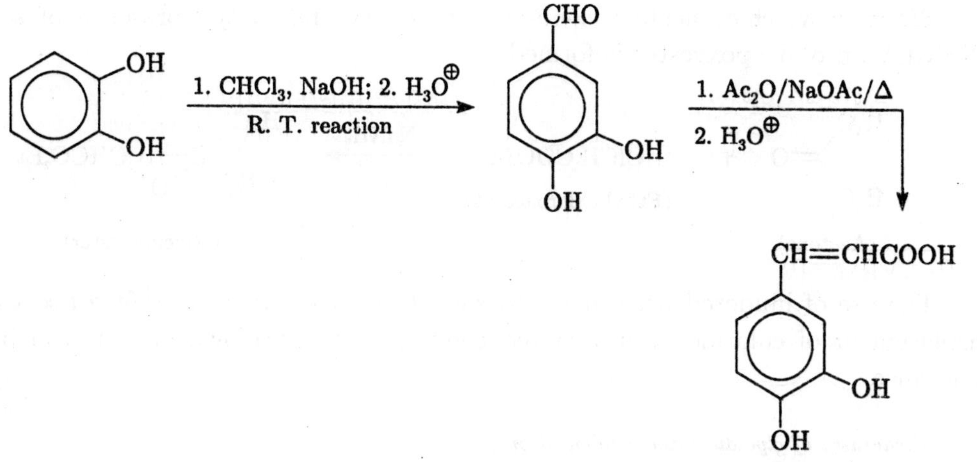

(Caffeic acid)

13. 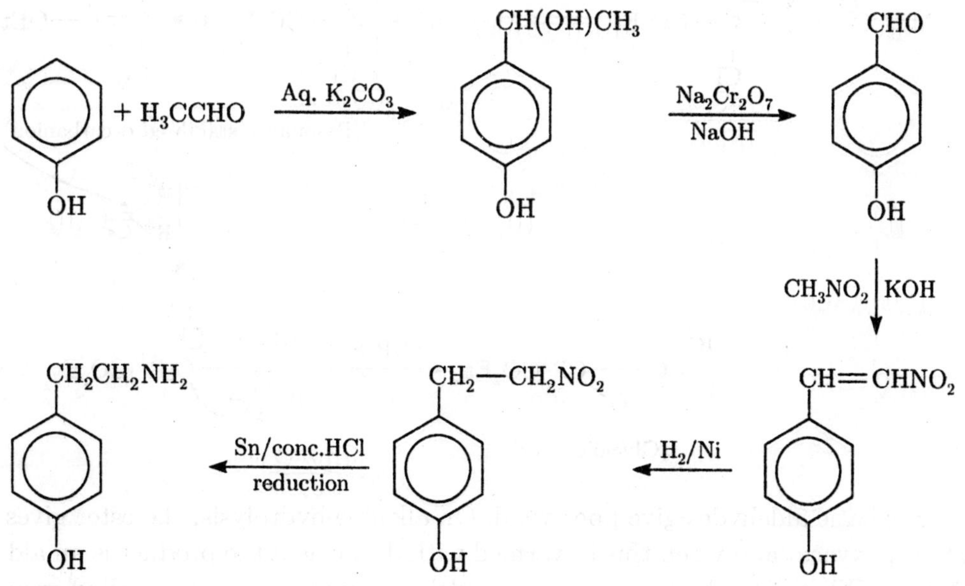

(Tyramine)

Darzen's Glycidic Ester Condensation

The Darzen's glycidic ester condensation is an aldol type reaction between a carbonyl compound and an α–haloester *containing α–H* atoms(s) in the presence of organic base like NaOEt, $NaNH_2$ etc., followed by an internal nucleophilic substitution which leads to the formation of a glycidic ester (an α, β-epoxyester). Both aldehydes and ketones undergo Darzen's glycidic ester condensation.

When ethyl chloroacetate condenses with acetone in the presence of sodamide ($NaNH_2$), an α, β–epoxyester is formed.

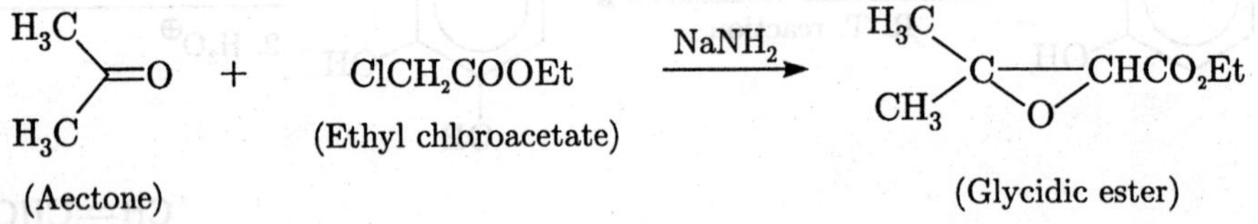

The use of hindered base like *potassium tertiarybutoxide is preferred* so that S_N2 displacement of chloride is disfavoured compared with removal of a proton by steric hindrance.

Mechanism of glycidic ester condensation :

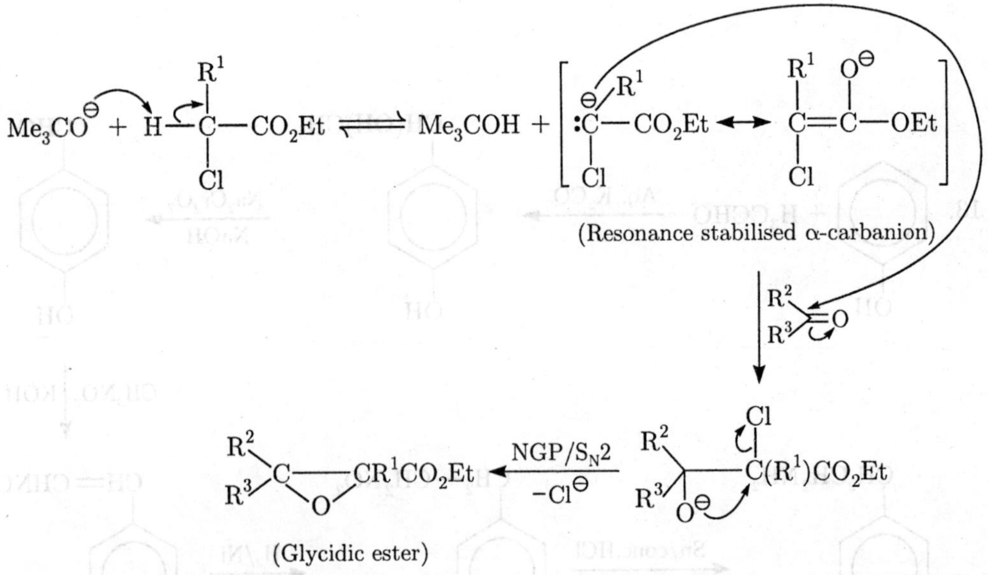

Aliphatic aldehydes give poor yield. On alkaline hydrolysis, the ester gives the salt of the epoxyacid and when this is warmed with dilute acid the product is an aldehyde or a ketone. When R^1 is hydrogen, it is an aldehyde and when R^1 is an alkyl group, it is a ketone.

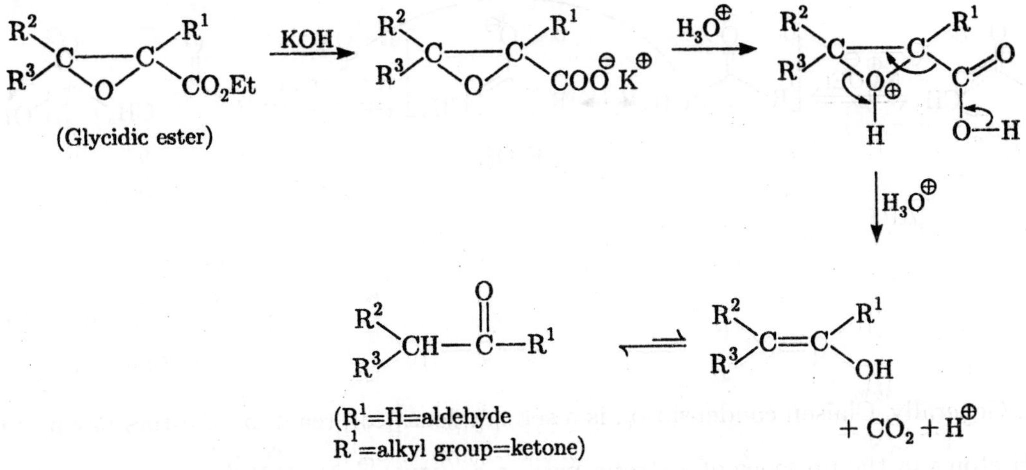

The synthesis can be shortened by using tertiarybutyl glycidates, since the ester on pyrolysis eliminates isobutene to give an aldehyde or ketone.

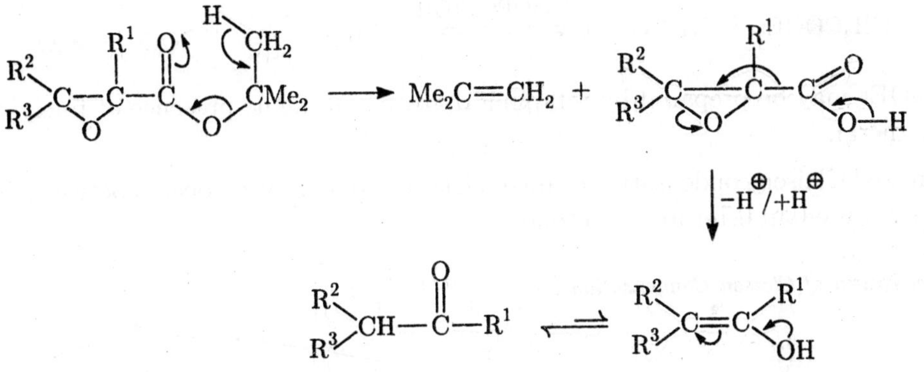

The overall process therefore consists of the addition of one carbon atom as carbonyl group to a carbonyl group.

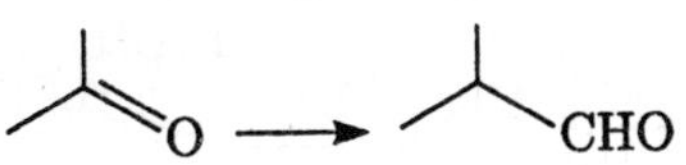

With α-haloacetate, the product is an aldehyde and with substituted α–haloacetate, the product is a ketone.

The Claisen Condensation

An aldol type condensation reaction involving a nucleophilic attack of a carbanion (generated by abstraction of an α–H atom usually from ketones, esters etc. by a strong base, *e.g.*, sodio salt of alkoxide ion, triphenylmethyl anion etc.) on an electron deficient carbonyl carbon atom (usually of esters) followed by loss of an anion leading to a nucleophilic substitution is known as the Claisen condensation reaction.

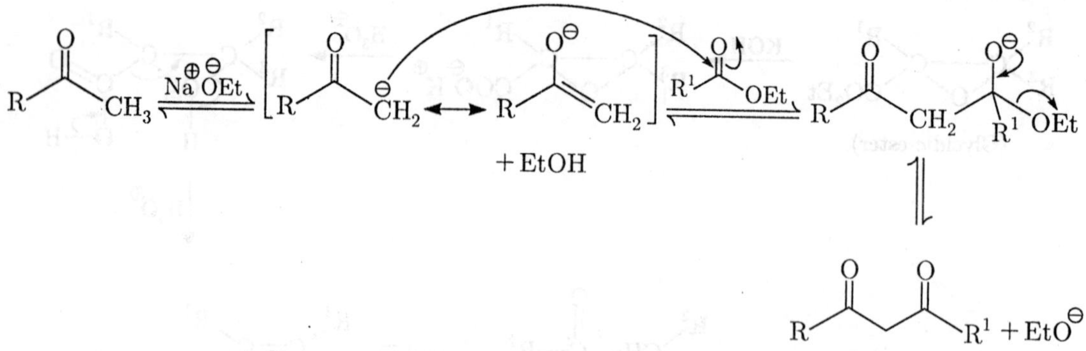

(1, 3-Diketone)

Generally, Claisen condensation is a self condensation reaction of esters having two α–H atoms in the presence of a strong base, *e.g.*, $\overset{\ominus}{O}EtNa^{\oplus}$, $Ph_3\overset{\ominus}{C}Na^{\oplus}$ etc. to give β–keto-esters is the Claisen condensation which may be termed as Claisen ester condensation.

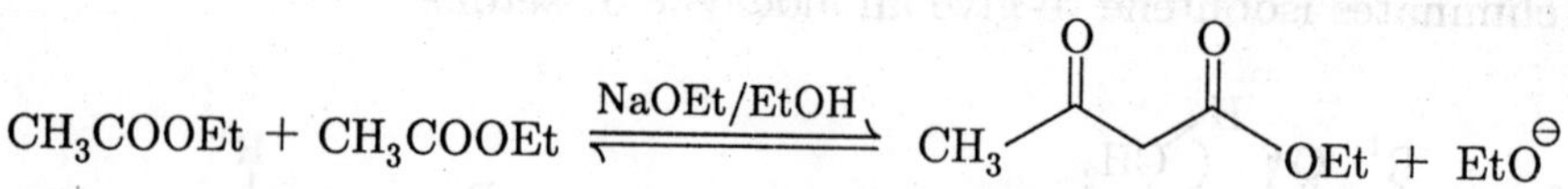

NaOEt may be prepared by refluxing dry ethanol in the presence of finely divided sodium metal.

Crossed Claisen condensation or mixed Claisen condensation occurs between different ester or between an ester and a ketone.

***Mechanism of Claisen Condensation* :**

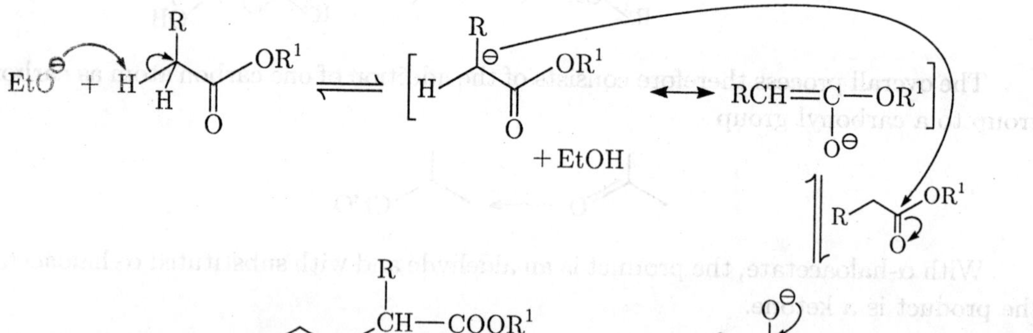

(I)

Reversible formation of the carbanion is proved experimentally by deuterium exchange reaction using a little amount of EtOD in the reaction medium.

$$RCH_2COOR^1 \underset{}{\overset{Et\overset{\ominus}{O}}{\rightleftharpoons}} EtOH + R\overset{\ominus}{\ddot{C}}HCOOR^1 \overset{R^1OD}{\rightleftharpoons} R^1\overset{\ominus}{O} + RCHDCOOR^1$$

How ever, EtOH being a stronger acid than ethyl acetate, the equilibrium of this step lies on the left.

Now the β-ketoester of type (I) is a stronger acid than R′OH. The former dissociates to form resonance stabilised carbanion (II), the conjugate base of the β-ketoesters. This makes the equilibrium of the overall reaction lie on the right by removing $Et\overset{\ominus}{O}$ as EtOH.

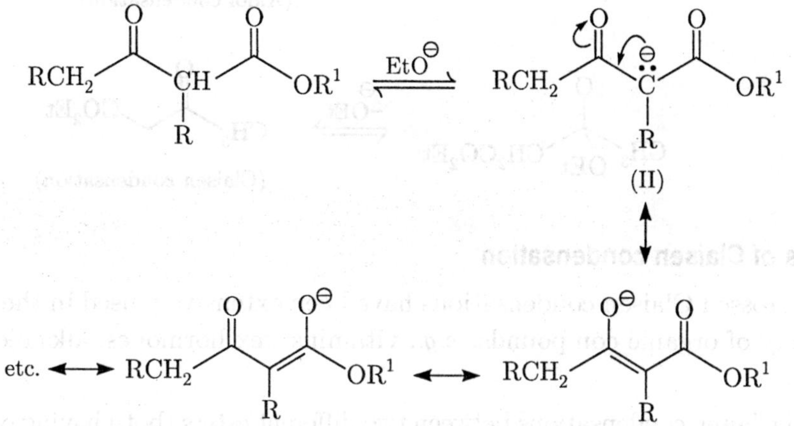

Acid is added finally to neutralise the carbanion salt.

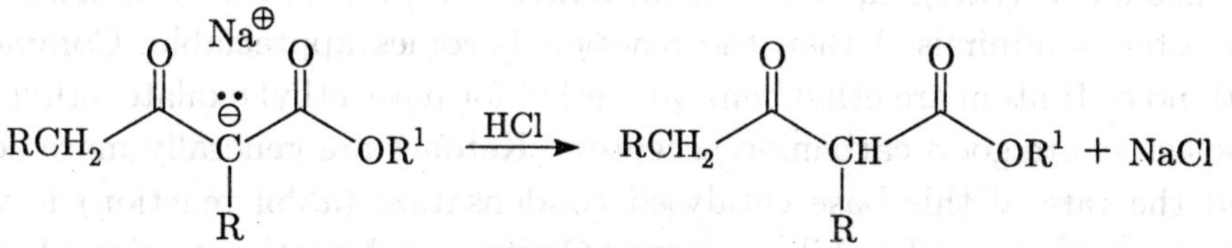

NaOEt is used in excess to force the equilibrium to shift in the forward direction. The mechanism has been proved by the fact that an ester of the type $R_2CHCOOEt$, *i.e.*, containing one α–H atom does not produce β-ketoester ($R_2CHCOCR_2COOEt$) in the presence of NaOEt. Owing to the absence of active α–H on the latter compound, the formation of resonance stabilised carbanion, the conjugate base of the expected product is not possible and thus, the equilibrium of the overall reaction lies to the left almost entirely. However, in the presence of very strong base such triphenylmethyl sodium (instead of NaOEt), the equilibrium of the *step* I lies on the right. Ph_3CH, the conjugate acid, formed by the reaction is a very weak acid ($pK_a \cong 33$) and it is weaker than $R_2CHCOOEt$. In fact, $Ph_3\overset{\ominus}{C}\,\overset{\oplus}{Na}$ withdraws the weakly acidic α–H *irreversibly* from the ester (analogous *step* I is highly *reversible*).

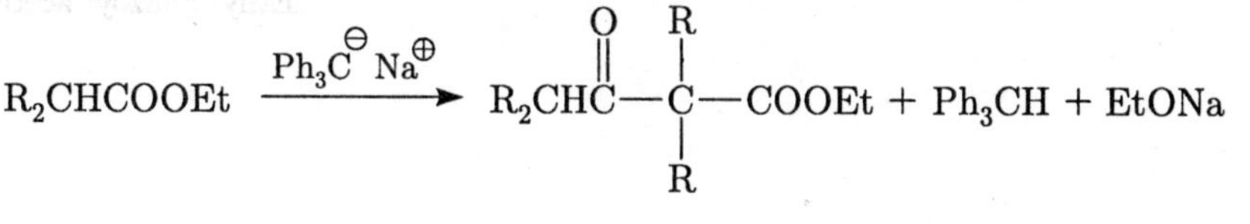

Claisen condensation is very similar to aldol condensation. The only difference is that, in aldol condensation, no group is lost while in Claisen condensation, $\overset{\ominus}{O}R$ (*e.g.*, $\overset{\ominus}{O}Et$) is lost.

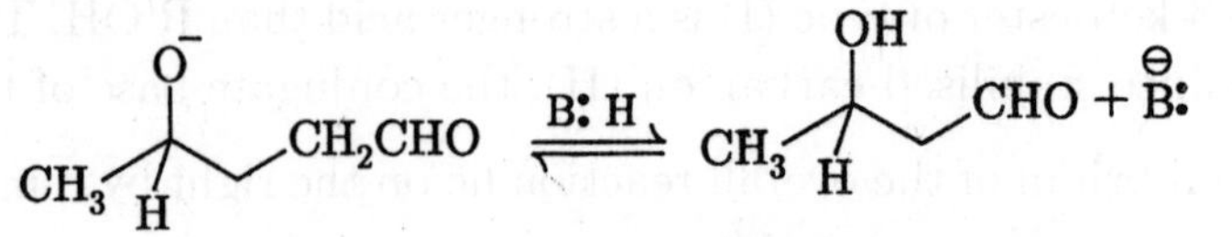

(Aldol condensation)

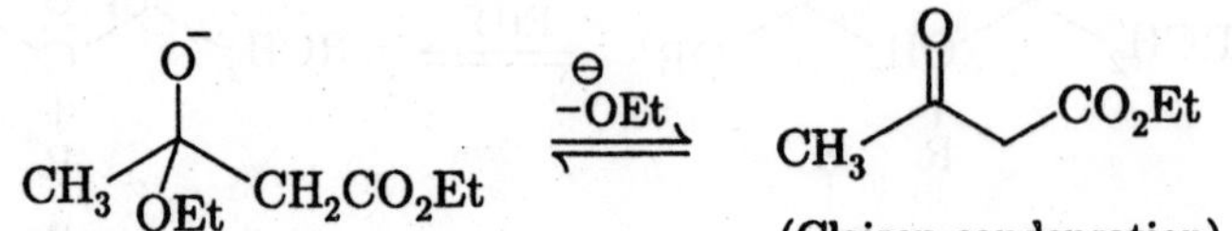

(Claisen condensation)

Applications of Claisen condensation

Simple and crossed Claisen condensations have been extensively used in the synthesis of a wide variety of organic compounds, *e.g.*, vitamins, sex hormones, alkaloids, terpenes, flavones etc.

Crossed Claisen condensations between two different esters (both having α–hydrogens) have little synthetic value, for a mixture of four products are obtained. However if one of the esters has no α–hydrogen, acts as a carbanion acceptor and the self condensation of the other ester is minimised then the reaction becomes appreciable. Commonly used esters with no α–H atom are ethyl benzoate, ethyl formate, ethyl oxalate, ethyl carbonale etc. These esters are good carbanion acceptors. Ketones are generally more acidic than esters and the rate of this base catalysed condensation (aldol reaction) is very slow. Hence ketones serve as nucleophiles in mixed Claisen condensation to give a large variety of products.

1. 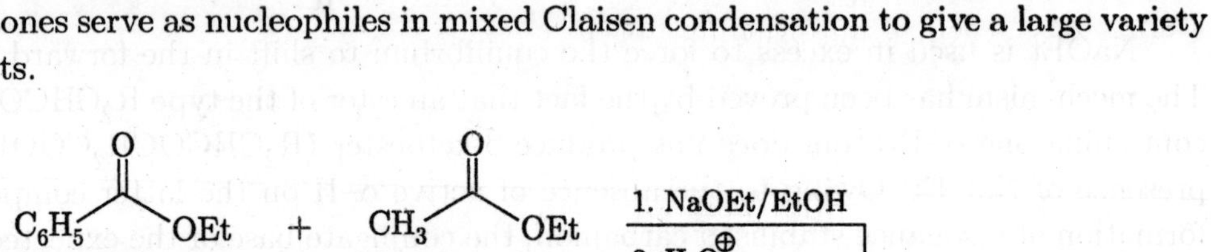

(Ester with no α–H)

(Ethyl benzoyl acetate)

2.

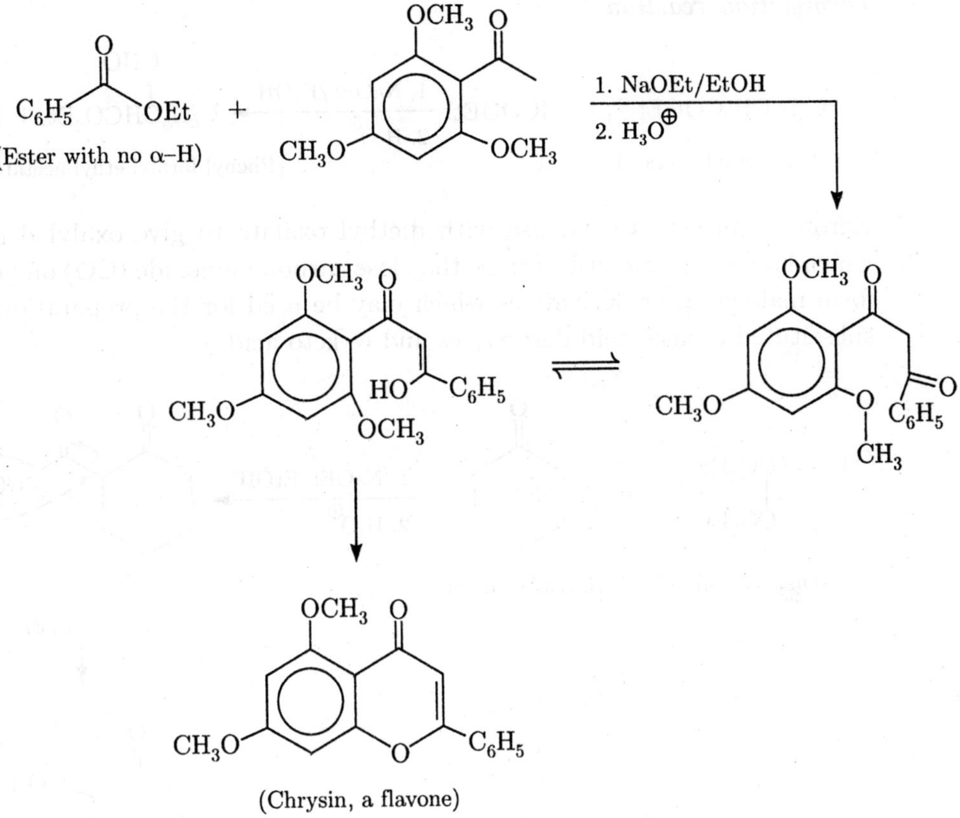
C6H5 OEt
(Ester with no α–H)
OCH3 O
CH3O OCH3
1. NaOEt/EtOH
2. H3O⊕
OCH3 O
HO C6H5
CH3O
OCH3
OCH3 O
CH3O O C6H5
CH3
OCH3 O
CH3O O C6H5
(Chrysin, a flavone)

3.

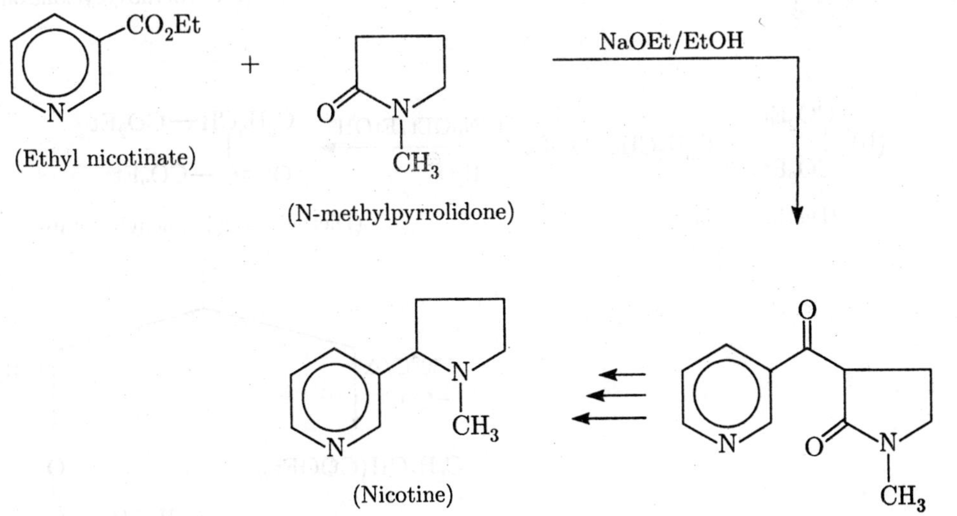
CO2Et
N
(Ethyl nicotinate)
O N CH3
(N-methylpyrrolidone)
NaOEt/EtOH
N CH3
(Nicotine)
O
N O N CH3

4. ***Formylation reaction***

$$\underset{\text{(Phenyl ethyl acetate)}}{C_6H_5CH_2COOEt} + HCOOEt \xrightarrow[\text{2. } H_3O^{\oplus}]{\text{1. NaOEt/EtOH}} \underset{\text{(Phenyl formyl ethyl acetate)}}{C_6H_5\overset{\overset{CHO}{|}}{C}HCO_2Et} + EtOH$$

5. Ketones and esters condense with diethyl oxalate to give oxalyl derivatives, which have synthetic utility since they lose carbon monoxide (CO) on heating to form malonic ester derivatives which may be used for the preparation of aryl-substituted dibasic acid derivatives and α–keto acid.

(a)

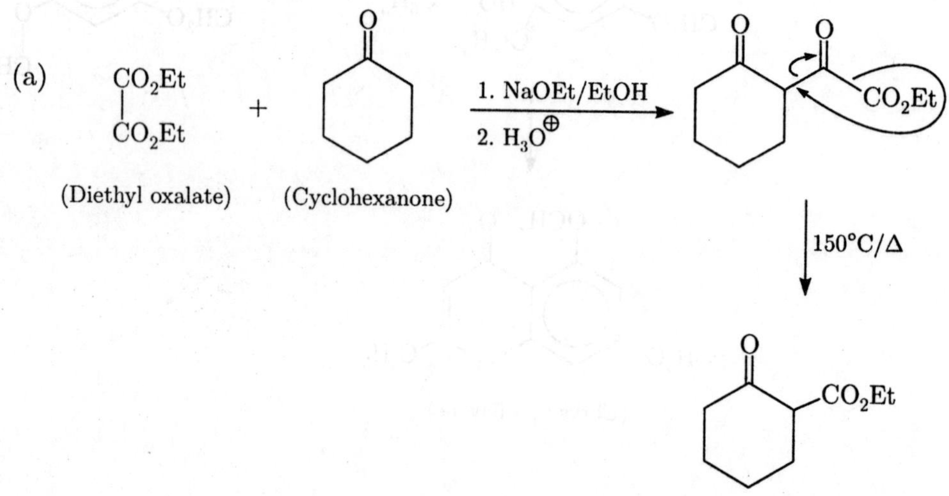

(Diethyl oxalate) (Cyclohexanone)

(2-Carbethoxycyclohexanone)

(b)

$$\underset{\text{(Diethyl oxalate)}}{\begin{matrix} CO_2Et \\ | \\ CO_2Et \end{matrix}} + C_6H_5CH_2COOEt \xrightarrow[\text{2. } H_3O^{\oplus}]{\text{1. NaOEt/EtOH}} \underset{\text{(Diethyl α-oxalylphenyl acetate)}}{\begin{matrix} C_6H_5CH—CO_2Et \\ | \\ O{=}C—CO_2Et \end{matrix}}$$

$$\xrightarrow[-CO]{150°C/\Delta} C_6H_5CH(COOEt)_2$$

$$\xrightarrow{\text{1. } H_2O, \text{ 2.}\Delta} \underset{\text{(Phenylpyruvic acid)}}{C_6H_5CH_2—\overset{\overset{O}{||}}{C}—COOH}$$

6. ***Preparation of camphoric acid***

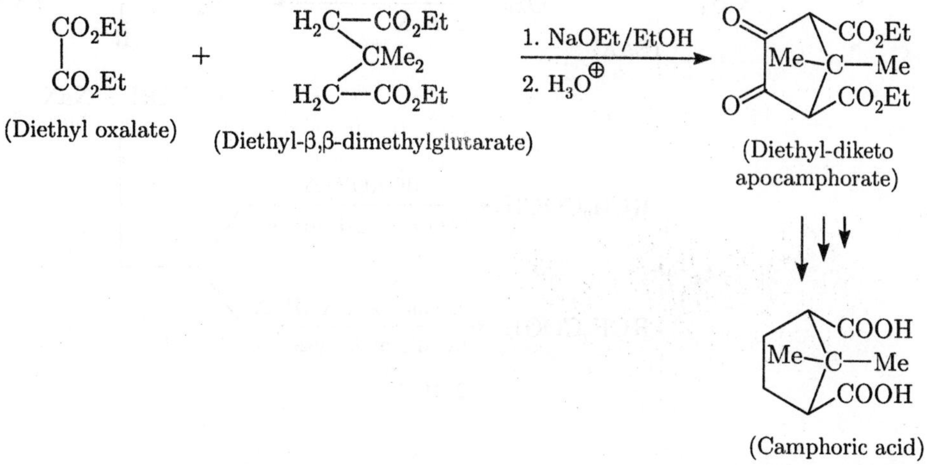

7. ***Condensation with diethylcarbonate*** : Esters condense with diethyl carbonate to form malonic ester derivatives which can be further transformed into various compounds.

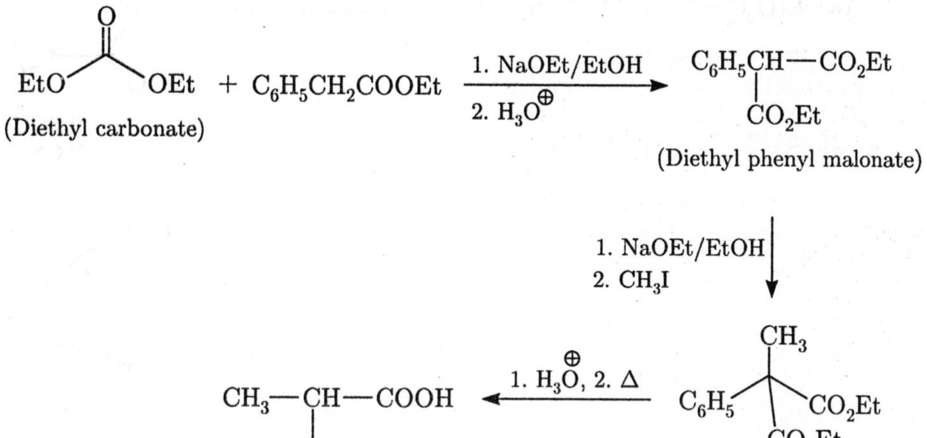

8. A very important product of Claisen condensation is β-ketoester, like ethyl acetoacetate (EAA). It can be easily alkylated. EAA and its alkyl derivatives under different conditions undergo ketonic and acidic hydrolysis to yield ketones and acids respectively.

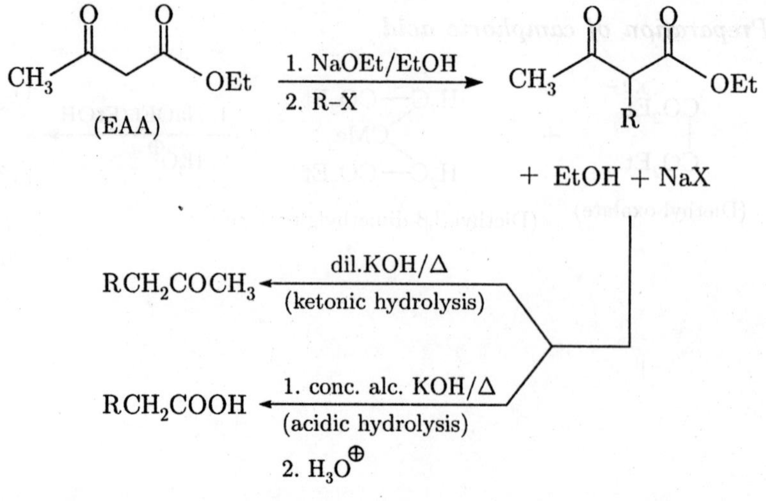

9. ***Crossed intramolecular Claisen condensation***

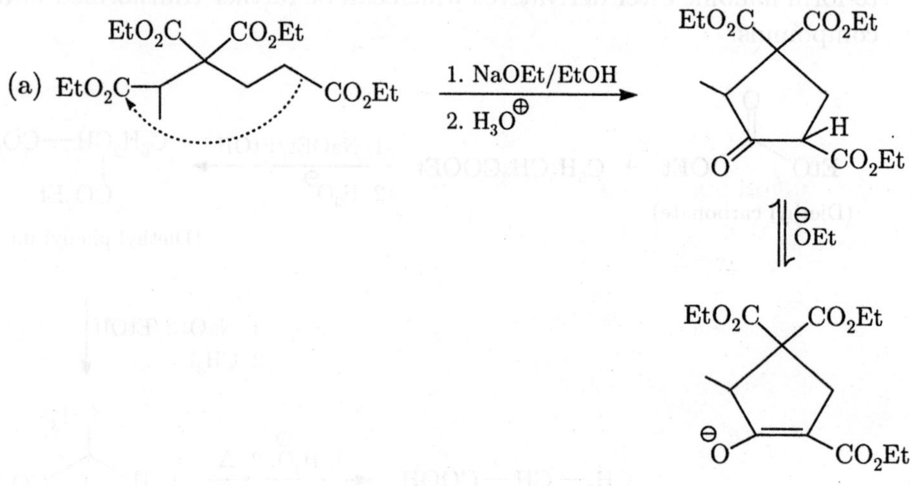

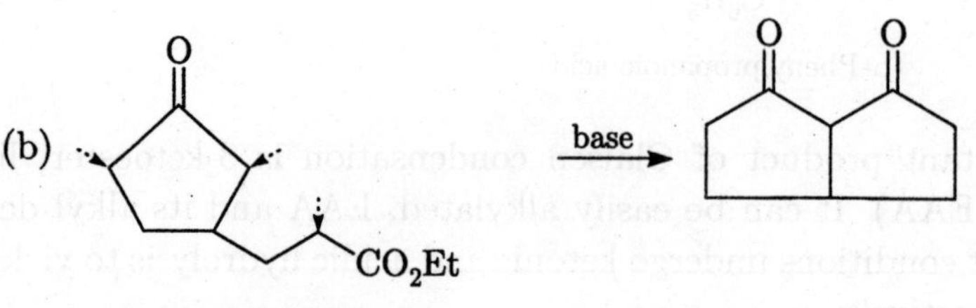

(Three possible sites for enolate formation)

Although there are three possible sites for enolisation, only one product is formed, other two are being unstable.

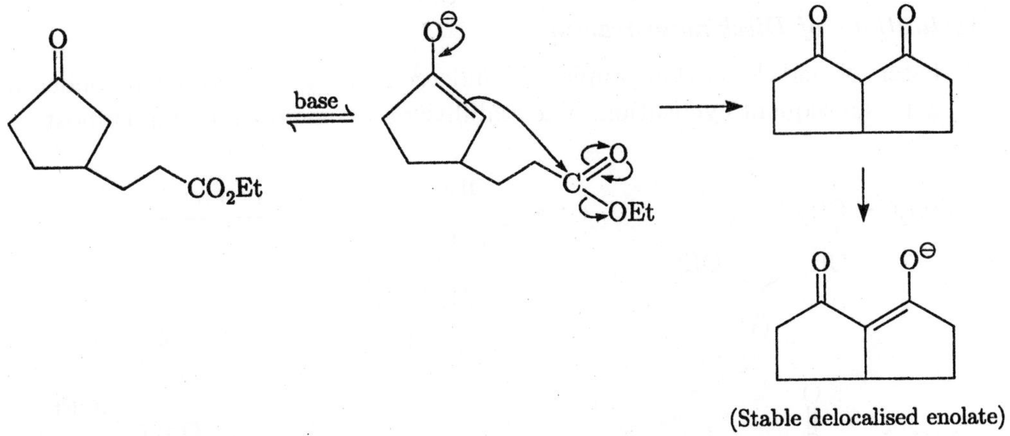

Internal Claisen condensation or Dieckmann Condensation Reaction

Intramolecular or internal Claisen condensation reactions involving esters of dibasic acids containing α–H atoms and 5 to 6 carbon atoms give rise to cyclic compounds (cyclic β-ketoesters) and the reaction is known as *Dieckmann cyclisation reaction.* The condensing bases used are metallic sodium, NaOEt, NaH, $K^{\oplus}tBuO^{-}$ etc.

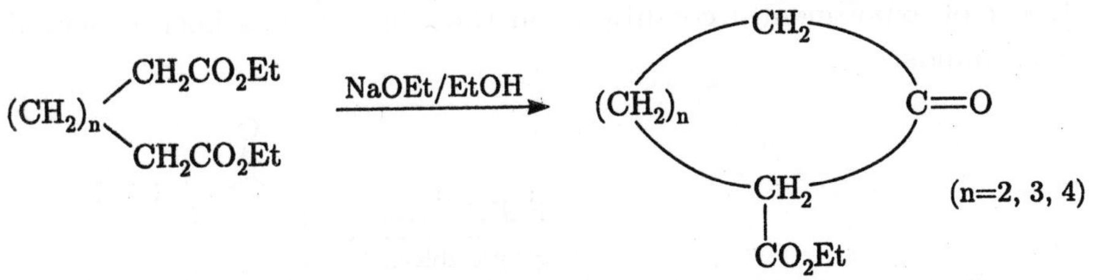

The reaction best proceeds with dibasic acid esters having six, seven or eight carbon atoms which gives stable rings with five, six or seven carbons. Yields of larger ring sizes are very low. High dilution technique is used for the formation of large size rings.

Mechanism of Dieckmann condensation reaction : The mechanism is similar to that of Claisen condensation reaction.

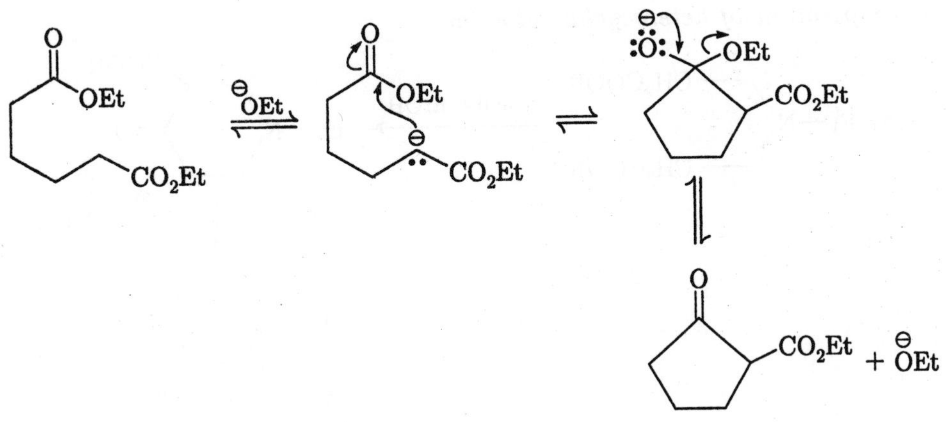

Applications of Dieckmann reaction

1. Esters of acids lower than adipic acid undergo more of intermolecular condensation with subsequent cyclisation. The stability of six–membered ring is most.

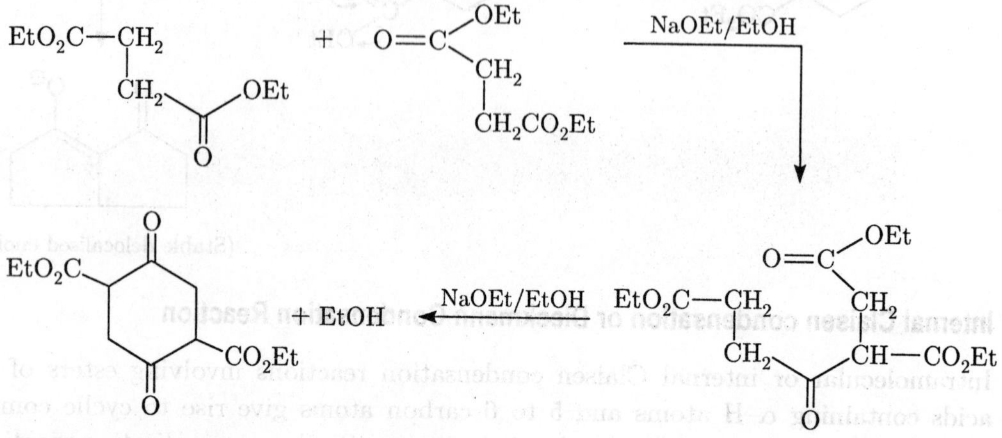

(Cyclohexane-2,5-dione-1,4-dicarboxylic acid

2. Effect of experimental conditions on the ring size has been observed in some compounds.

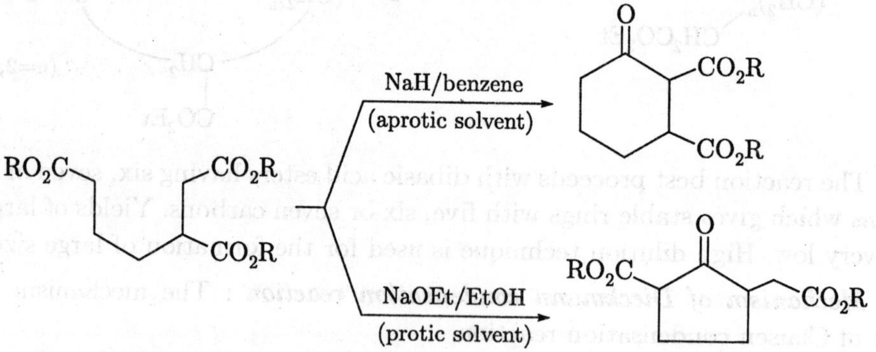

3. *Preparation of heterocyclic ketoesters*

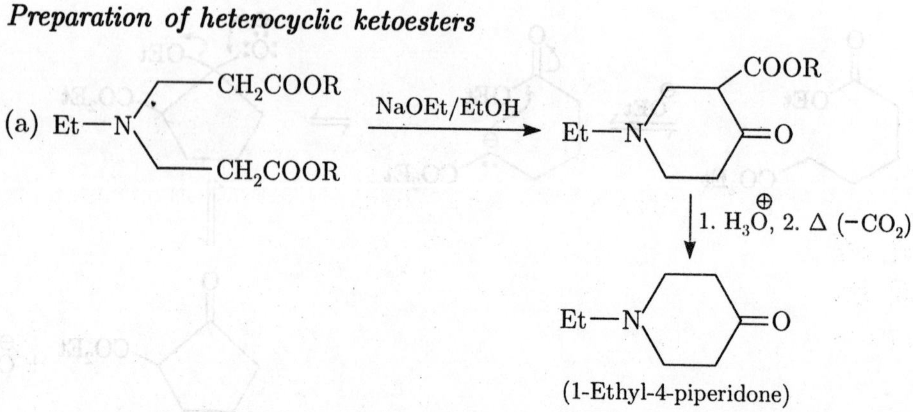

(1-Ethyl-4-piperidone)

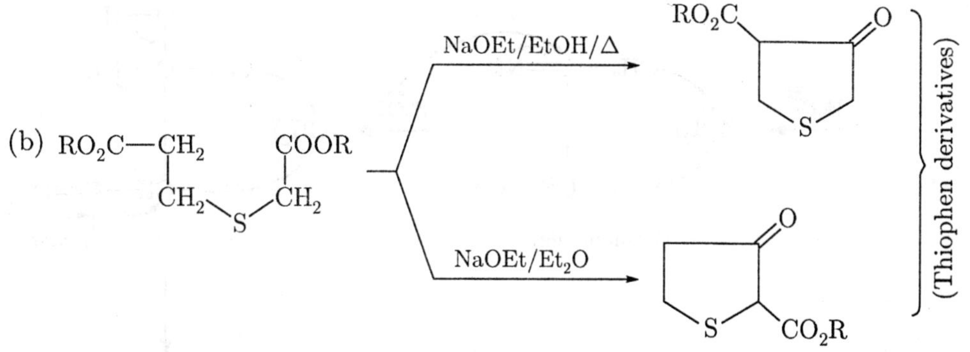

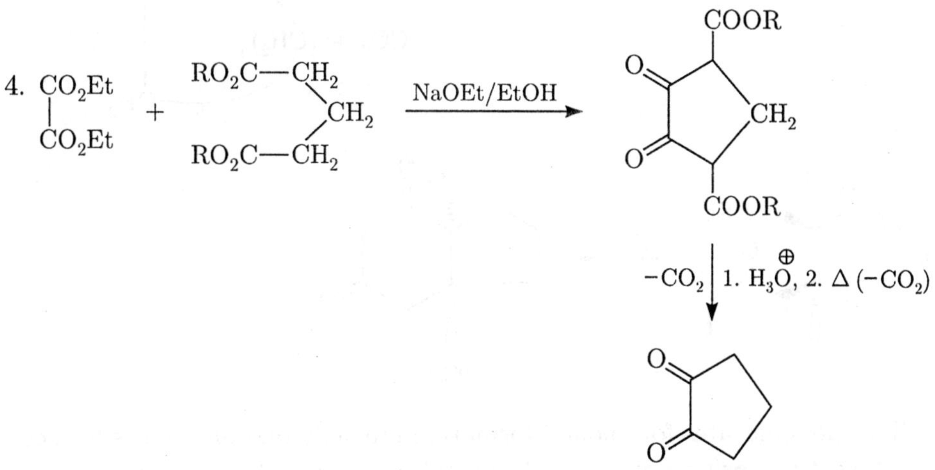

(Cyclopentane-1,2-dione)

5. Ziegler applied Dieckmann reaction on dinitriles to obtain large size rings using lithium ethyl anilide as a base and ***high dilution technique***. On dilution, the intermolecular distance of the reacting groups is greater than the intramolecular distance so that intermolecular distance is minimised.

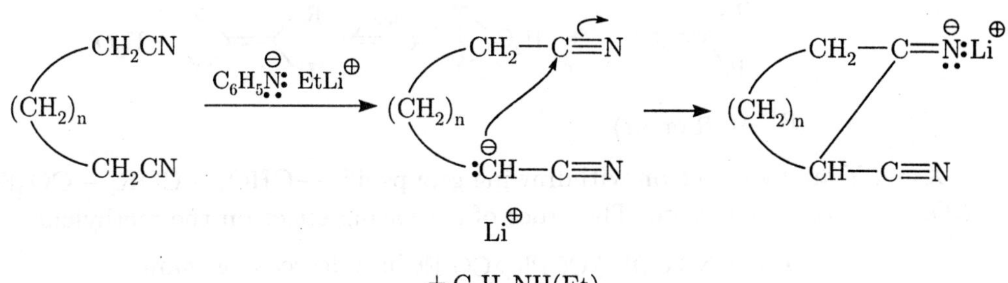

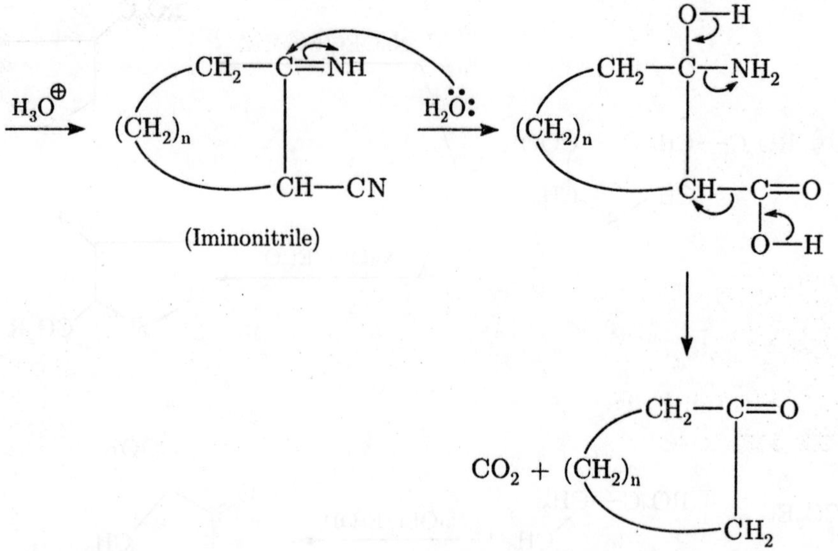

6. 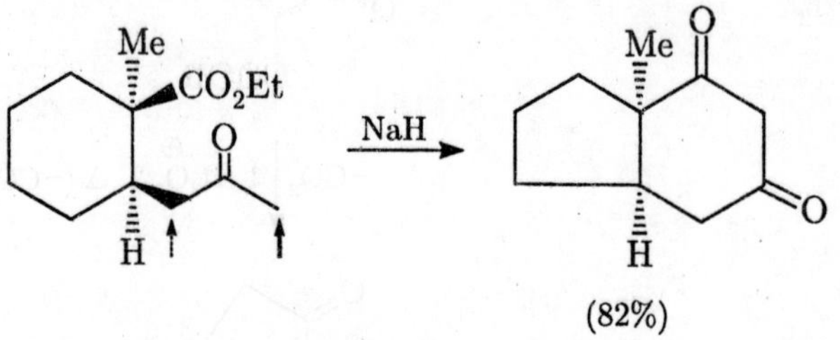

Two possible sites for enolate formation but only one product is formed, as the alternative position gives rise to unstable four-membered ring.

The Knoevenagel Condensation Reaction

Knoevenagel condensation is similar to aldol condensation reaction. The base catalysed aldol type condensation reaction between a carbonyl compound, usually without any α-H atom, and a compound containing an active methylene group is called the Knoevenagel condensation reaction.

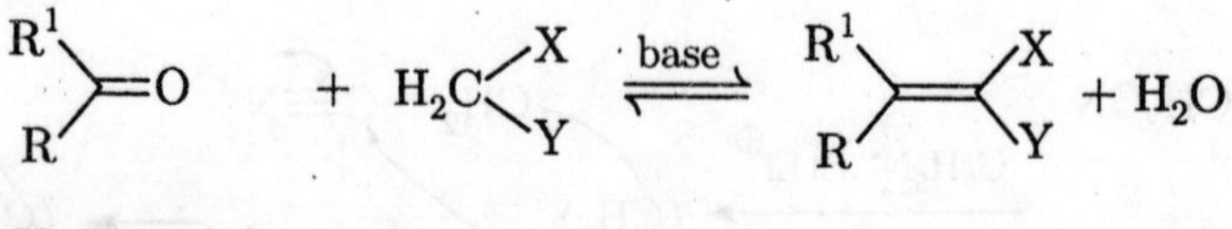

(R^1=H, R or Ar)

X and Y are two electron withdrawing groups like —CHO, —COR, —CO_2R, —CN. —NO_2, —SOR, —SO_2R etc. The order of activating effect on the methylene moiety is,

$O_2N > CN > COR > COPh > CO_2Et$ in a decreasing manner.

However, terminal acetylenes, chloroform, cyclopentadiene etc. also undergo Knoevenagel condensation with the carbonyl compounds because they possess active hydrogen atom.

Usually amines, particularly secondary and tertiary amines are used as catalysis. Other basic catalysis like $\overset{\ominus}{O}R$, $\overset{\ominus}{N}H_2$, $\overset{\ominus}{O}H$ etc. may also be used. However, a few examples of the reaction are given below.

1. $PhCHO + CH_3NO_2 \xrightleftharpoons{NaOH} PhCH{=}CHNO_2$

2. $MeCHO + CH_2(CO_2Et)_2 \xrightleftharpoons{pyridine} MeCH{=}C(CO_2Et)_2$

3. $PhCHO + CH_3COCH_2CO_2Et \xrightleftharpoons{Et_3N} PhCH{=}C(CO_2Et){-}COCH_3$

4. 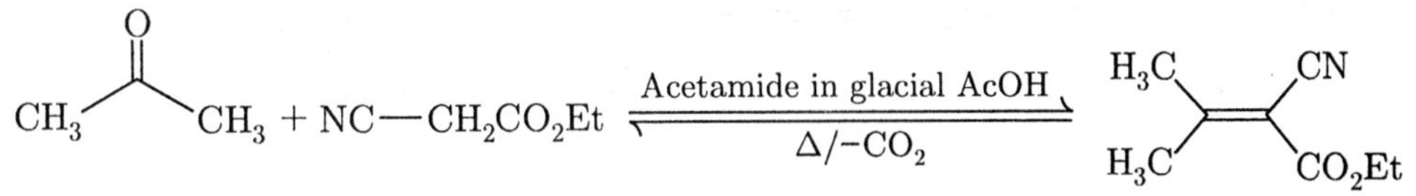

Mechanism of Konevenagel reaction :

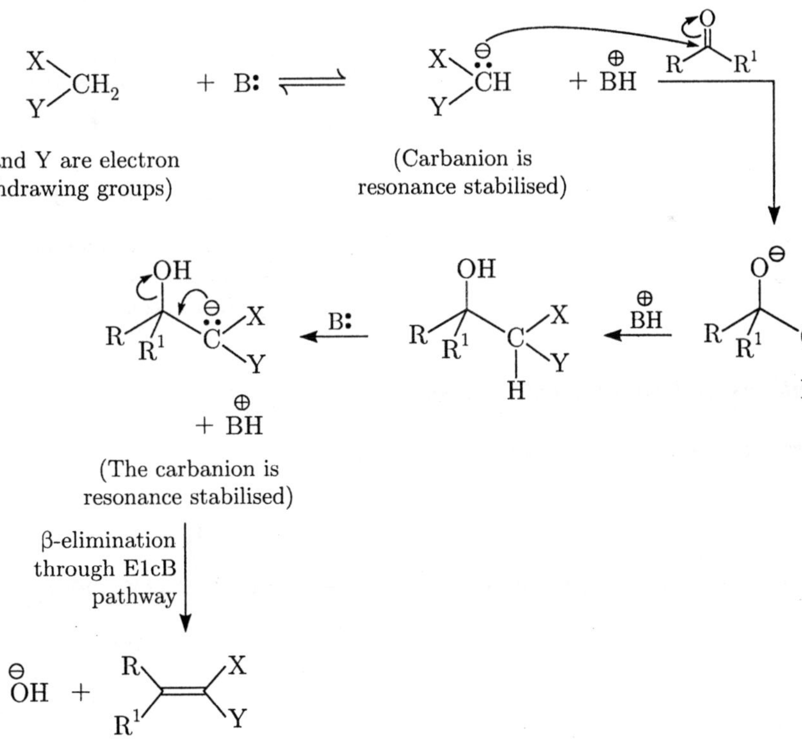

Both aliphatic and aromatic aldehydes undergo Knoevenagel reaction. For steric and electronic reasons, ketones are less reactive than aldehydes. Hence ketones react with compounds having powerful active methylene group only, *e.g.*, ethyl acetoacetate, cyanoacetic acid and its esters but *not* usually with malonic ester for which stronger bases have to be used.

The mechanism of Knoevenagel reaction shows that the reaction is reversible and since the equilibrium favours the reactant side, the yield of Knoevenagel reaction is not satisfactory. Cope modified the procedure by using benzene as a solvent and removing water from the reaction medium as an azeotrope, thus, shifting the equilibrium to the right, *i.e.*, the product side. Consequently, this modification is known as Cope-Knoevenagel reaction.

In some cases, the Knoevenagel condensation product undergo Michael addition with the active methylene compound present in the reaction mixture.

$$CH_3CHO + CH_2(COOEt)_2 \xrightleftharpoons{\text{piperidine}} \underset{\text{(Knoevenagel product)}}{CH_3CH{=}C(COOEt)_2}$$

$$CH_3CH{=}C(CO_2Et)_2 + H_2C(CO_2Et)_2 \xrightarrow[\text{Michael addition reaction}]{\text{piperidine}} CH_3\underset{\displaystyle CH(CO_2Et)_2}{\underset{|}{CH}}{-}CH(CO_2Et)_2$$

$$\Big\downarrow \; 1.\ \overset{\ominus}{O}H \;|\; 2.\ H_3\overset{\oplus}{O}/\Delta;\ -CO_2$$

$$CH_3{-}\underset{\displaystyle CH_2COOH}{\underset{|}{CH}}{-}CH_2COOH$$

(Michael condensation product)

Applications of Knoevenagel reaction :

1. ***Preparation of α, β–unsaturated acids***

$$\text{(a) } H_3C{-}\overset{\displaystyle H}{\overset{|}{C}}{=}O + H_2C(CO_2R)_2 \xrightarrow{\text{piperidine}} H_3C{-}\overset{\displaystyle H}{\overset{|}{C}}{=}C(COOR)_2$$

$$\Big\downarrow \; 1.\ \overset{\ominus}{O}H;\ 2.\ H_3\overset{\oplus}{O},\ 3.\ \Delta\,(-CO_2)$$

$$CH_3CH{=}CHCO_2H$$

(Crotonic acid)

(b)

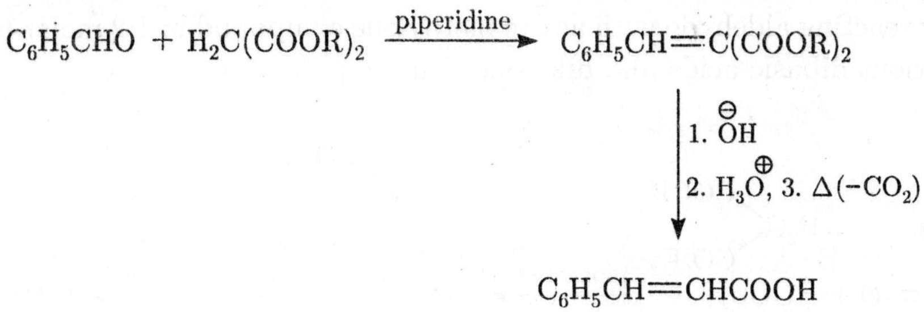

(Cinnamic acid)

(c)

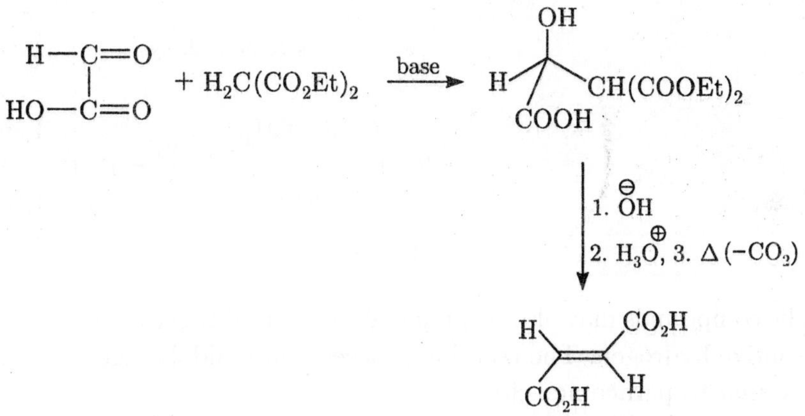

(Fumaric acid)

(d)

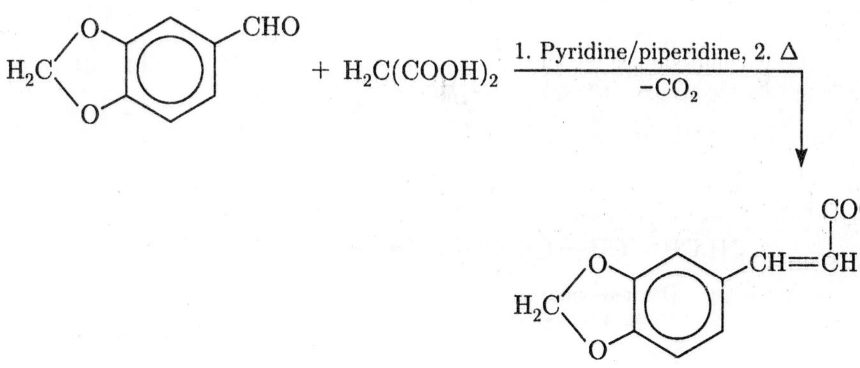

(β-piperonylacrylic acid)

2. By reacting aldehyde with active methylene compound in 1:2 molar proportions, various dibasic acids and diketones can be prepared.

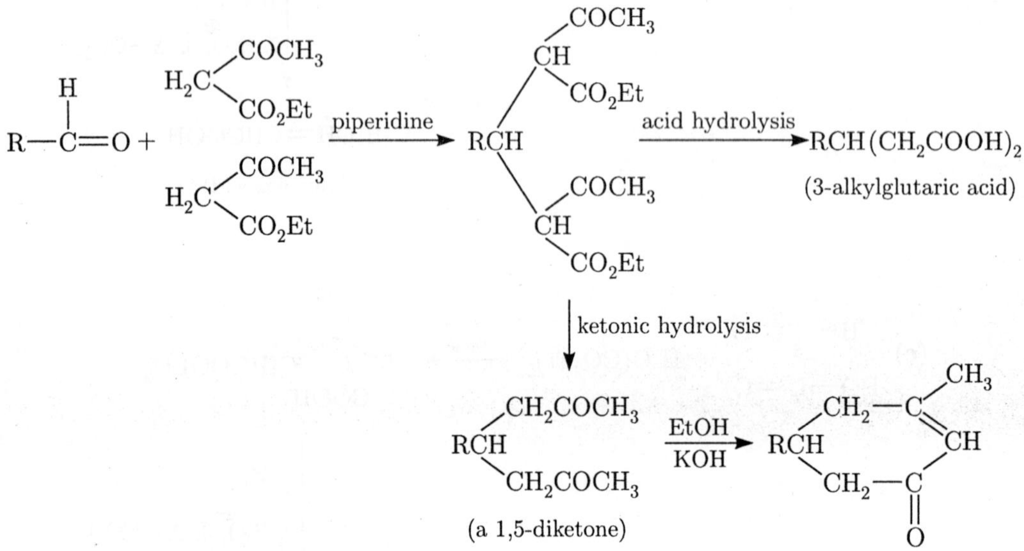

3. Cyclic compounds may also be prepared from suitably selected compounds having one active hydrogen. The reaction proceeds upto aldol stage and then the aldol is cyclised to paraconic acid.

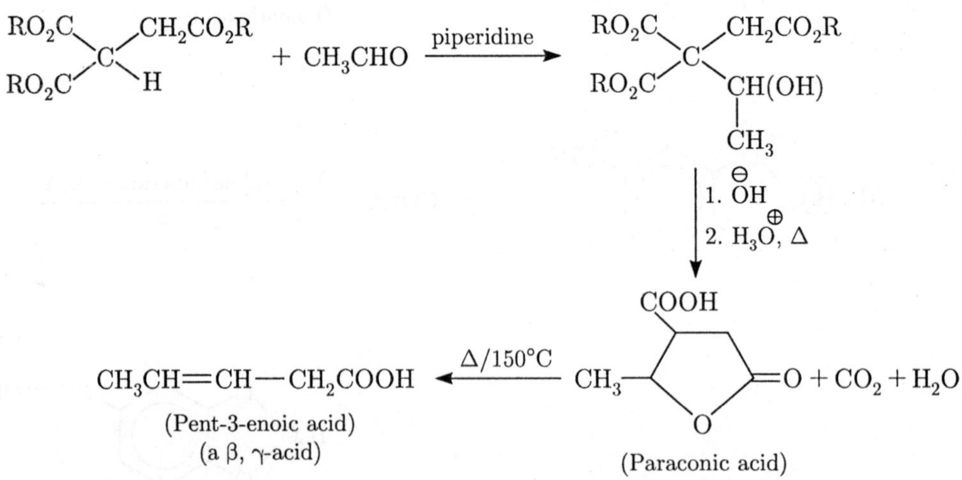

The Doebner condensation reaction

The reaction has similarity with aldol condensation reaction. In Doebner process, a carbanion is generated either from malonic acid or cyanoacetic acid using either pyridine or quinoline as a solvent which acts as a base also. In some cases, a small amount of piperidine is also used.

Mechanism of Doebner condensation reaction :

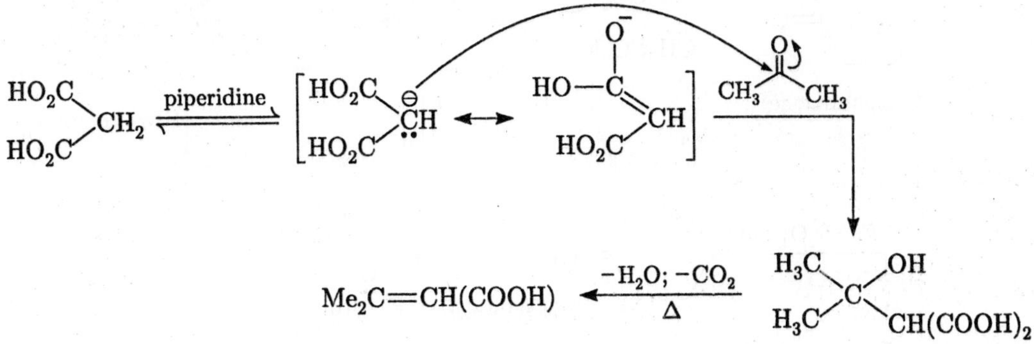

Similarly,

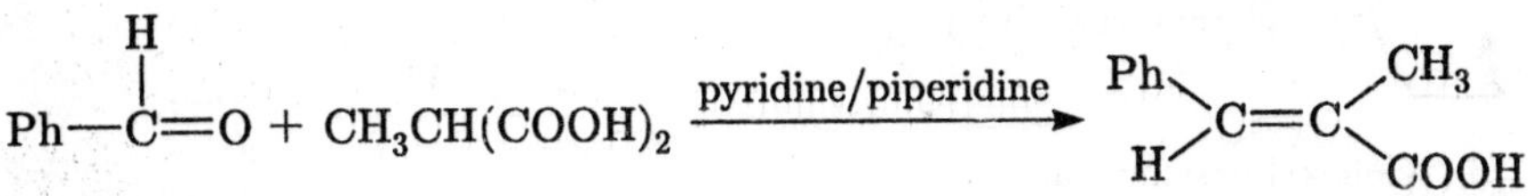

The Stobbe condensation reaction

Stobbe condensation reaction bears close resemblence with aldol condensation reaction. An aldehyde or a ketone undergoes condensation reaction with diethyl succinate in presence of NaOEt or NaH or K^+tBuO^- as bases to produce the salt of an unsaturated ester acid and the reaction is called the *Stobbe condensation.*

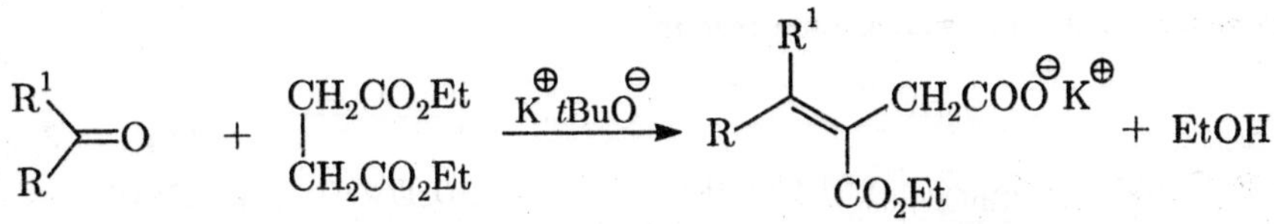

(R, R^1=H or alkyl or aryl)

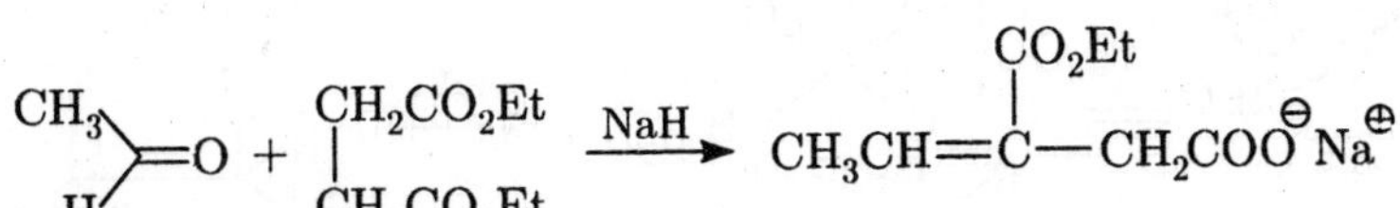

Saturated carboxylic acids may be prepared via Stobbe condensation. When the salt of the unsaturated ester acid is heated with hydrobromic acid in acetic acid, a β, γ–unsaturated acid forms, the latter may be hydrogenated to a saturated acid by copper–chromite catalyst, a mixture of Cr_2O_3 and CuO. For example, cyclohexanone can be converted to 3–cyclohexylpropanoic acid by Stobbe condensation followed by hydrolysis, decarboxylation and hydrogenation steps.

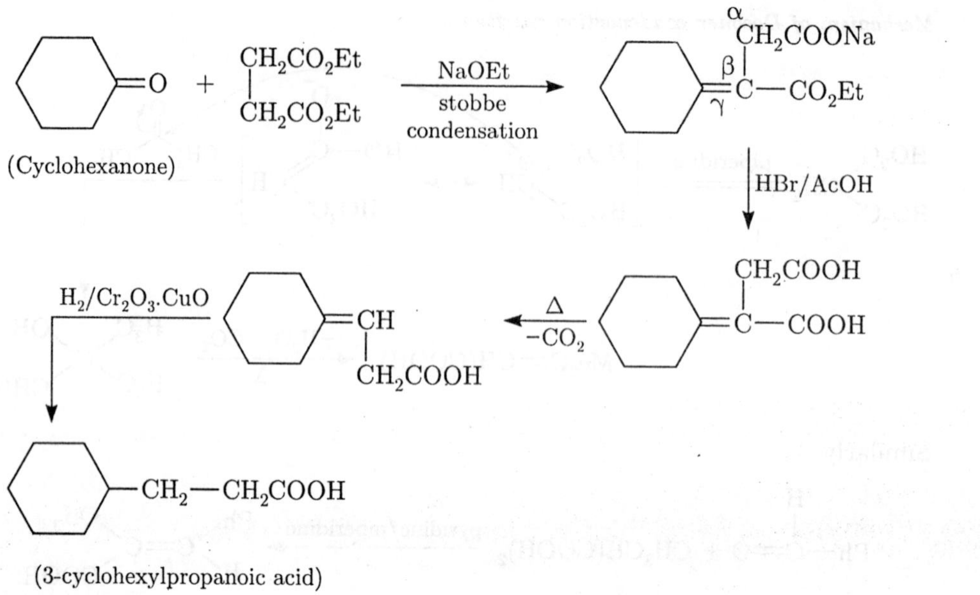

The Stobbe condensation has been extended to ditertiarybutyl esters of glutaric acid.

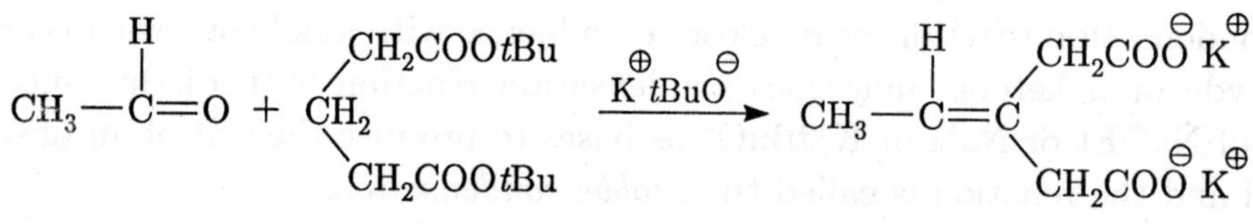

Mechanism of Stobbe condensation reaction :

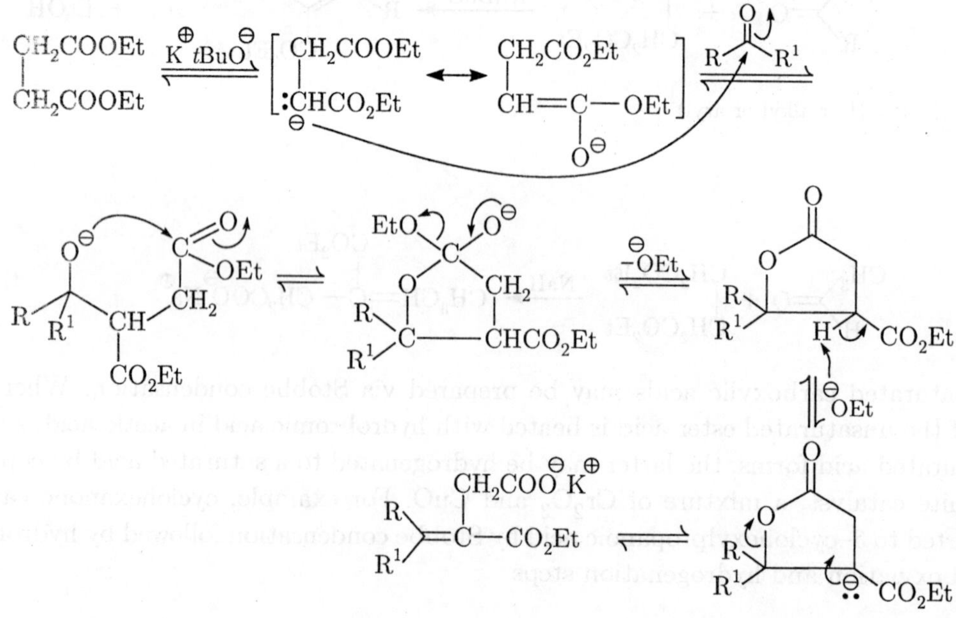

The isolation of the intermediate lactone–ester and the formation of an olefinic compound instead of an alcohol support the mechanism of the Stobbe condensation shown above.

Vinyl Ethers

Vinyl ethers are ethers of vinyl alcohol. ($CH_2{=}CHOH$, vinyl alcohol and $CH_2{=}CH{-}O{-}Et$, ethyl vinyl ether).

Vinyl ethers are considered *derivatives of aldehydes and ketones*, because on hydrolysis they produce aldehydes and ketones in very dilute acid.

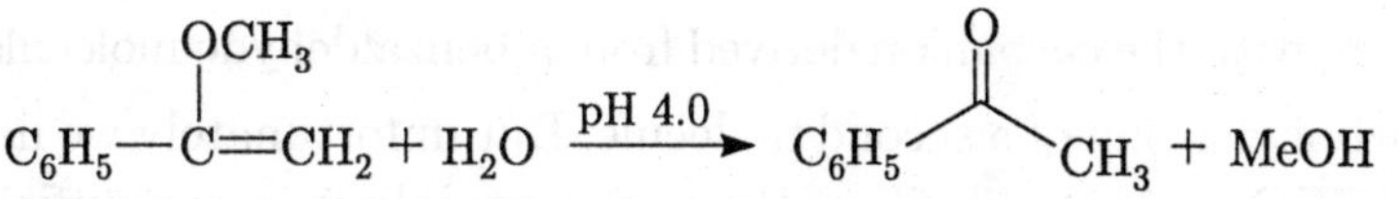

Vinyl ethers hydrolyse much readily in contrast to simple dialkyl ethers (high acid concentration, heat etc. are required for the latter). Vinyl ethers hydrolyse at a rate of 10^{13} times more than any dialkyl ether. So the mechanistic pathway of the hydrolysis of vinyl ethers is different from that of dialkyl ethers.

Mechanism of hydrolysis of vinyl ethers :

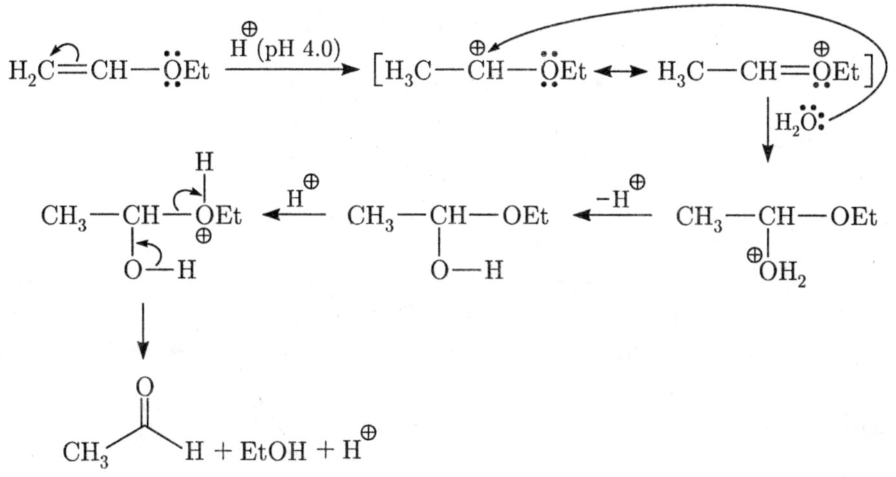

Vinyl ethers and alcohols can react in the presence of anhydrous acid catalysts such as *p*–toluenesulphonic acid to give acetals and ketals.

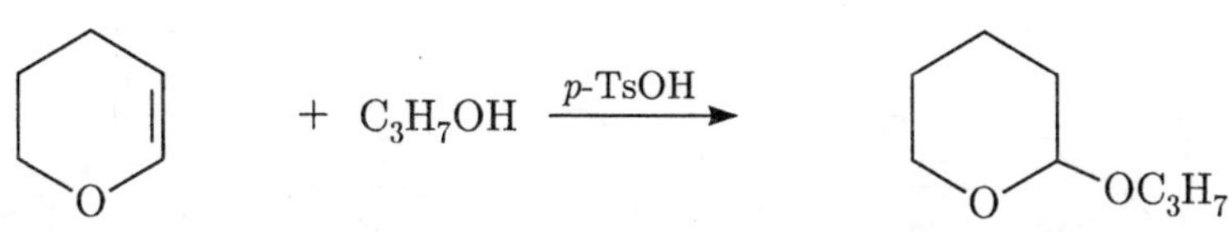

(Dihydropyran)
(a cyclic vinyl ether)

(A tetrahydropyran ether)
(Protected alcohol)

The Benzoin Condensation

The self condensation reaction of an *aromatic aldehyde specifically* catalysed by **cyanide** (CN^-) ion and not by any usual stronger base is referred to a benzoin condensation. An α–hydroxyketone, a dimer, known as *benzoin* is formed by this reaction.

Benzaldehyde on benzoin condensation gives benzoin. The condensation is carried out by boiling the alcoholic solution of the aldehyde containing a small amount of NaCN or KCN. HCN, $Hg(CN)_2$ and nitriles are ineffective catalysts.

Mechanism of Benzoin condensation reaction : Without knowing of the specific cyanide catalysis, we would likely to regard the benzoin condensation as similar to the aldol condensation, with the carbanion derived from a benzaldehyde molecule ($Ph—\overset{\ominus}{\underset{\bullet\bullet}{C}}=O$) attacking the carbonyl group of a second molecule. But unfortunately we have no evidence that the H of —CHO group is significantly acid, certainly it is not sufficiently acidic to be removed by such a weak base as CN^-. However, the cyanide ion can boost the acidity of this hydrogen markedly by converting the aldehyde to the conjugate base of a cyanohydrin (*i.e.*, anion of α–hdroxynitrile), the α–H then becoming similar in character to the α–hydrogens of nitriles or esters.

So the overall reaction becomes,

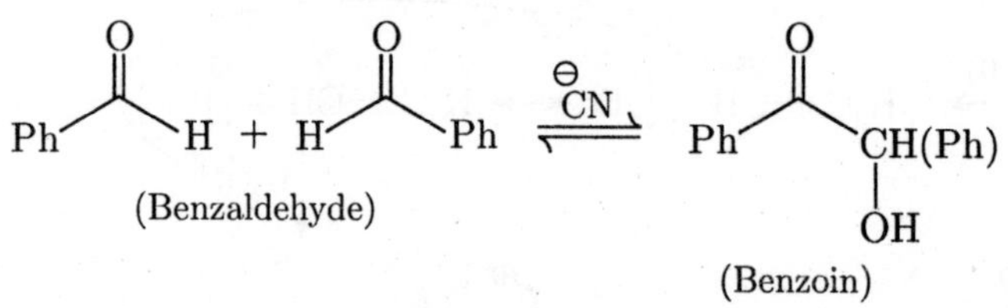

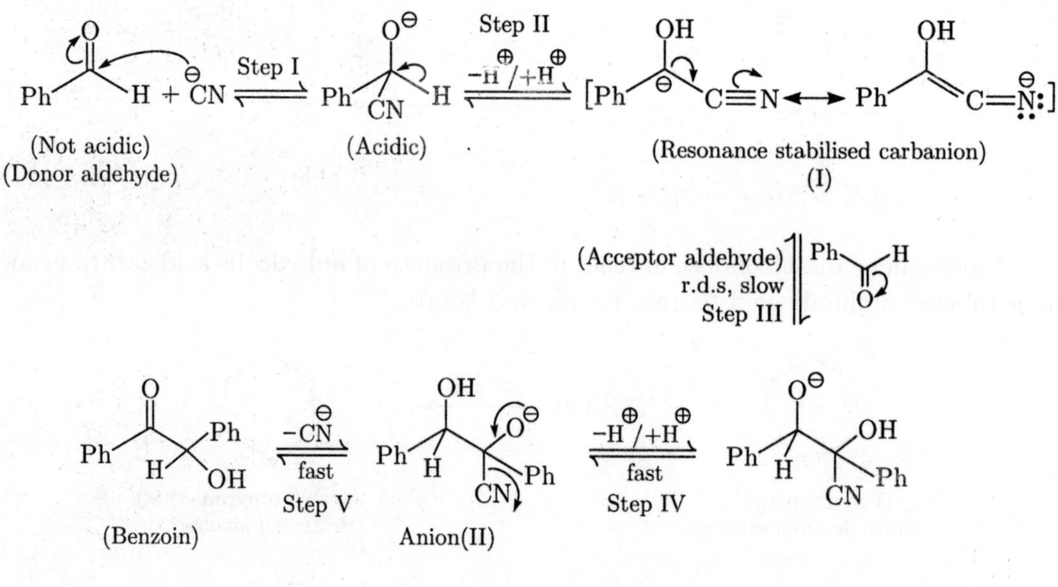

The rate law for the formation of benzoin is,

$$\text{Rate} = k.[\text{PhCHO}]^2\,[\overset{\ominus}{\text{CN}}],\ \textit{i.e.},\ \text{termolecular}$$

The termolecularity of the rate equation tells us that the activated complex in the rate determining step contains two molecules of benzaldehyde and one molecule of cyanide ion. We then may conclude that the carbanion (I) once formed; attack the carbonyl group of a second molecule of benzaldehyde, yielding anion (II)–a cyanohydrin which should be easily converted to benzoin itself. Since the overall condensation is *reversible*, each step must be reversible. The rate law itself does not tell us whether *steps III, IV or V* is rate limiting. But we may assume that *step IV*, a transfer of protons between oxygen atoms is *not*. Furthermore, *step V* is simply the reverse step in a ketone cyanohydrin interconversion, a reaction in which for simple cases, equilibrium is known to be very *rapidly established*. Thus, if the mechanism proposed above is correct, *step III* is certainly *rate determining*.

The reaction is a *completely reversible process*. This has been established by the fact that when a benzoin of an aldehyde is heated with another aldehyde in ethanolic KCN solution, a new benzoin and the aldehyde of original benzoin are obtained.

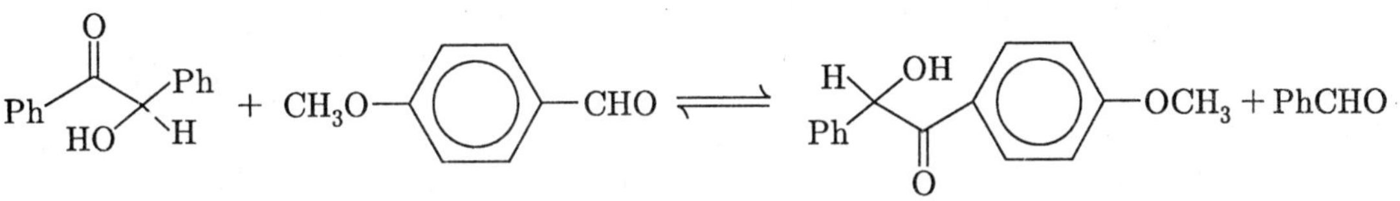

The reaction is unsuccessful with aliphatic aldehydes having α–hydrogen atom. Perhaps the enolisation of the aldehyde inhibits the attack by cyanide ion.

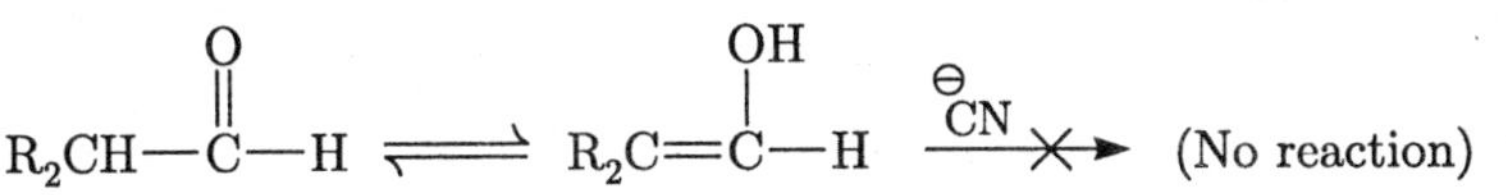

In benzoin condensation, cyanide ion as a specific catalyst has some advantages.

(a) Its ability as a *nucleophile*, (Stronger base of weak acid, HCN)

(b) Its ability as a *leaving group*.

(c) Its ability through electron withdrawal to increase the *acidity* of hydrogen atom and also resonance stabilisation of the carbanion formed.

The limitations of benzoin condensation reaction are of some interest. When a strongly electron donating —NMe_2 group is present para to —CHO group in benzaldehyde, the reaction fails. Due to conjugation from (I) to (II), the carbonyl group acquires additional electron density, *i.e.*, it becomes *less* electrophilic.

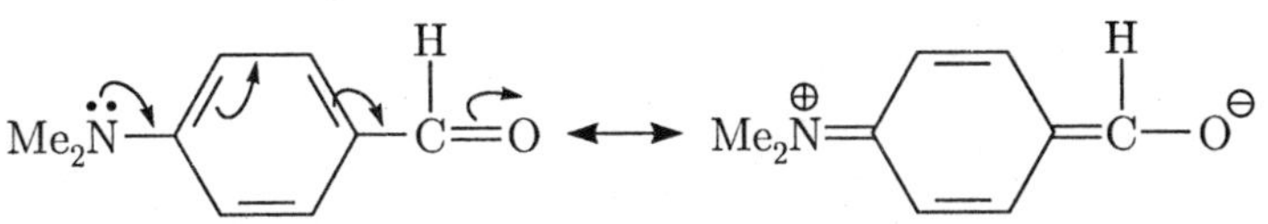

As a result, steps I and III, which involve addition of an anion to the carbonyl group are hindered. Apparently, however, the effect of NMe_2 group on initial cyanohydrin formation is less important than its effect on the rate determing step III; for if a mixture of benzaldehyde and *p*–N,N–dimethylaminobenzaldehyde is treated with NaCN, the "mixed benzoin"; but *not* the "isomeric mixed benzoin" is formed.

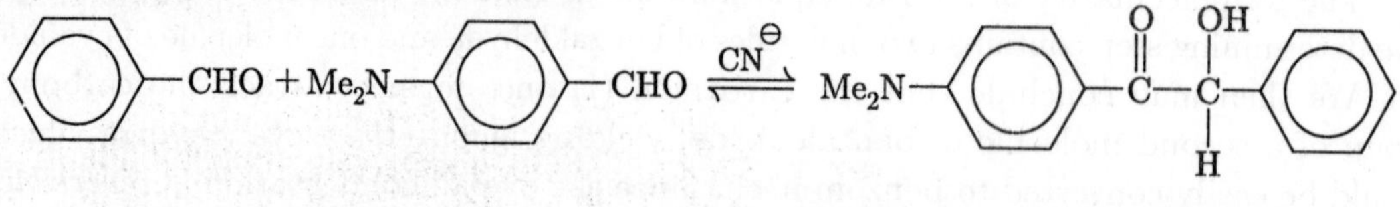

(Single product)

In the mechanism proposed, the carbonyl group on the final product is that involved in the initial cyanohydrin anion formation. We may therefore conclude that the cyanohydrin anion formed from *p*–N,N–dimethyl aminobenzaldehyde may add to benzaldehyde, but that the cyanohydrin anion derived from benzaldehyde will not add to *p*–N,N–dimethylaminobenzaldehyde itself.

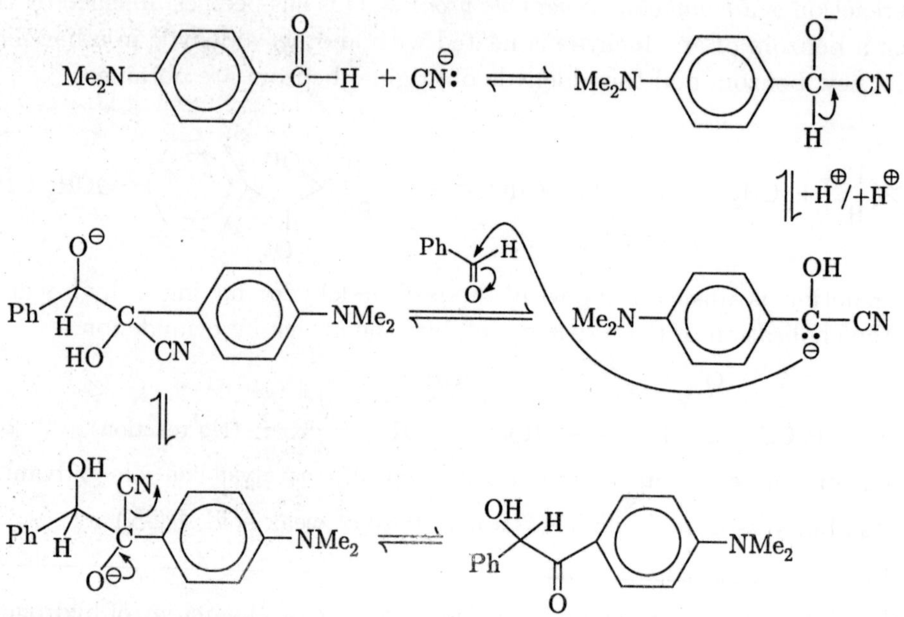

but

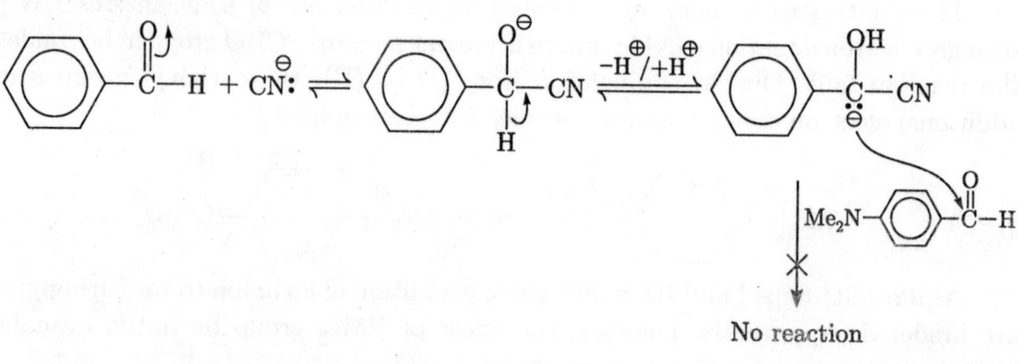

No reaction

The benzoin condensation is also inhibited by strongly electron withdrawing groups, *p*–bromobenzaldehyde forms a benzoin slowly and incompletely and *p*–nitrobenzaldehyde does not undergo benzoin condensation. Both the aldehydes readily form cyanohydrins. But in the anions like

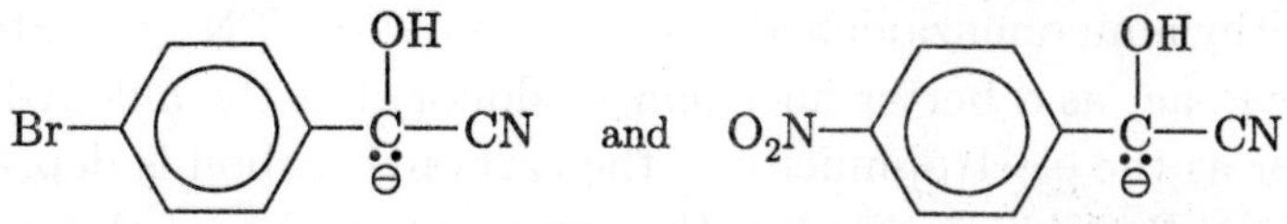

electron density has been pulled away from the attacking carbon, making it far less attacking site.

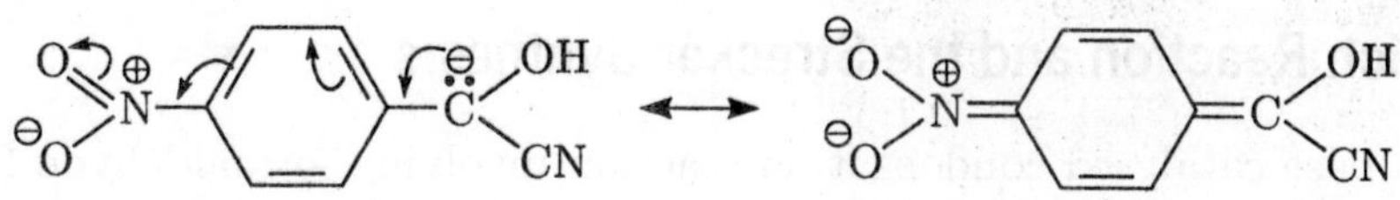

On the other hand, *o*- nitrobenzaldehyde undergoes benzoin condensation, presumably because the conjugation between the —NO_2 group and $-\overset{\ominus}{\ddot{C}}\langle^{OH}_{CN}$ group which prohibits the condensation of the *p*–isomer is rendered ineffective in the anion of the *o*–isomer because coplanarity between the two groups is no longer available.

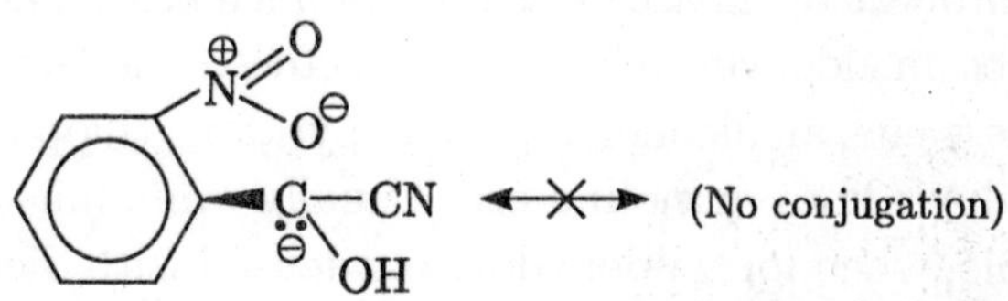

It is now known that, certain thiazolium and imidazolium salts, also act as catalysts for the benzoin condensation. Here, it appears that the condensation proceeds through an intermediate adduct (shown below), in which the α–hydrogen like that in a cyanohydrin, has been rendered acidic by the strongly electron withdrawing character of the ring.

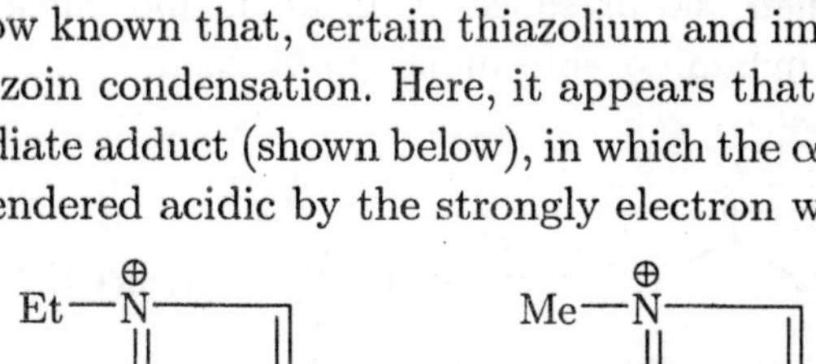

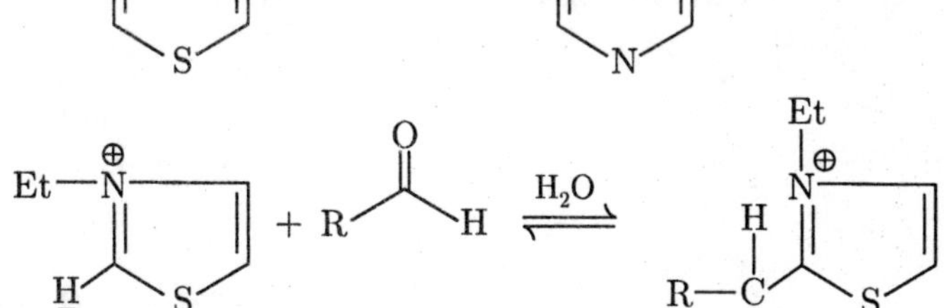

(Acidic hydrogen)

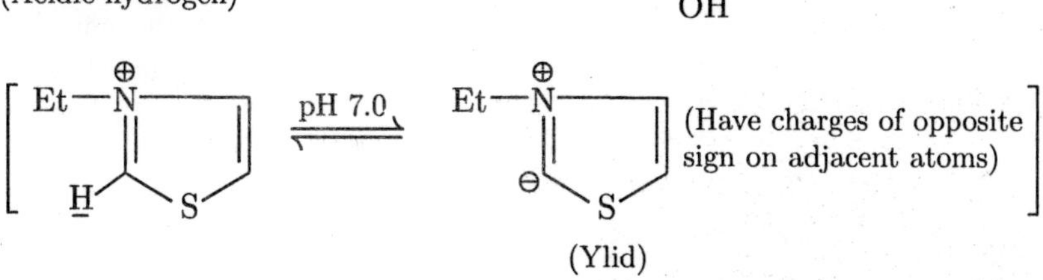

(Ylid)

Problems

p–Dimethylaminobenzaldehyde fails to undergo Benzoin Condensation, but when mixed with benzaldehyde, can carry out Benzoin Condensation smoothly.

Ans. *p*–Dimethylaminobenzaldehyde on reaction with $\overset{\ominus}{C}N$ generates the carbanion and it can act as a better nucleophile (donor) but the aldehyde itself is a weak acceptor as the electrophilicity of the carbonyl carbon is depressed by electron releasing +R effect of the dimethylamino group, hence the condensation fails. But when mixed with benzaldehyde, the mixed benzoin is formed.

The Mannich Reaction and the Strecker Synthesis

The acid or base catalysed condensation reaction involving formaldehyde (or any other aldehyde), ammonia or a primary or a secondary amine and a compound containing at least one active hydrogen to yield amino or substituted amino derivative of the compound originally containing the active hydrogen is called the Mannich reaction.

In the base catalysed reaction, the product, amino or substituted amino derivative is called the *Mannich base.* In the acid catalysed reaction, the salt of Mannich base is obtained which on hydrolysis by a base gives the Mannich base. The compound containing active hydrogen, may be an aldehyde, a ketone, a β–ketoester, a β–cyanoester, a nitroalkane, a monoalkyl or arylacetylene, an alcohol, a phenol, pyridine, thiophen, indole, hydrocyanic acid, α–and γ–methylpyridine, quinoline etc. Usually ammonia or amines are used as their salts. For example, when formaldehyde is condensed with diethylamine (in the form of hydrochloride salt) and acetone in the presence of an acid, and subsequently the product is hydrolysed, 4–(N,N–diethylamino)–butanone is obtained.

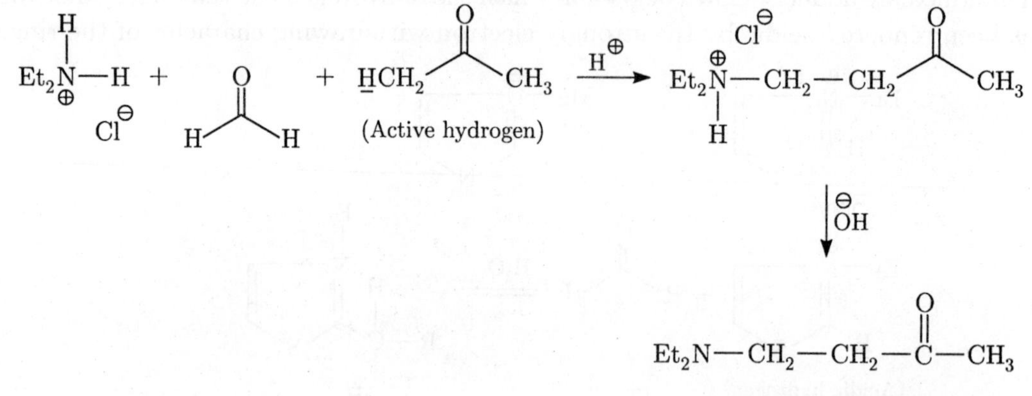

4-(N,N-diethylamino)-butanone
(a Mannich base)

However, the reaction may not stop at this stage. It may further react in three ways.

(a) If the Mannich base is a primary amine, it may further condense with one or two additional molecules of aldehyde and active hydrogen compound.

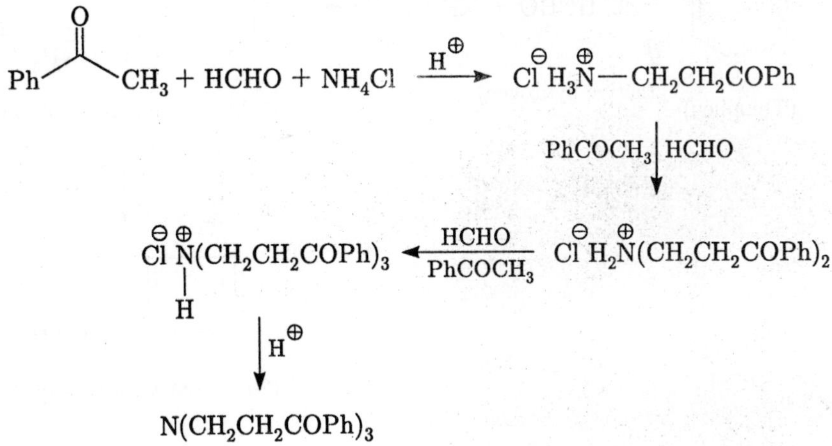

Hence *secondary amine* is *preferred* for this reaction.

(b) If the active hydrogen compound has two or more active hydrogens, stepwise condensation of two or more molecules of the aldehyde and ammonia or amine with one molecule of the active hydrogen compound will take place.

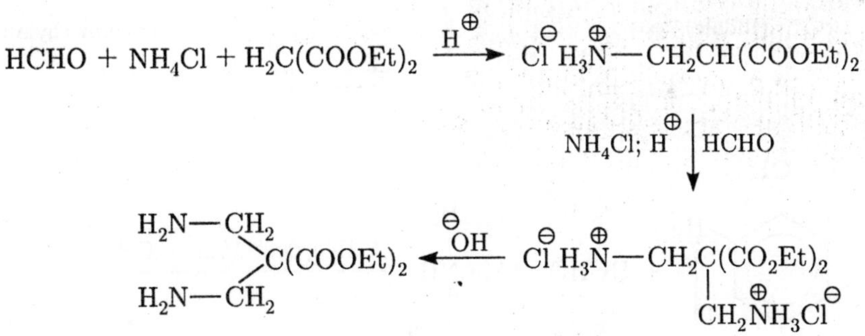

(c) The Mannich base may condense with excess aldehyde.

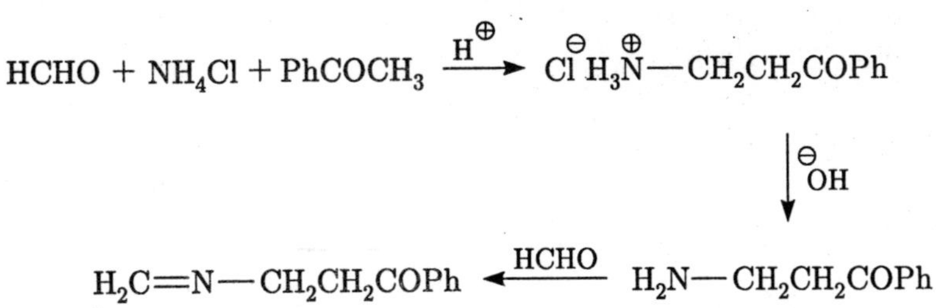

Aryl amines generally do not respond to this reaction.

***Some Examples* :**

1.

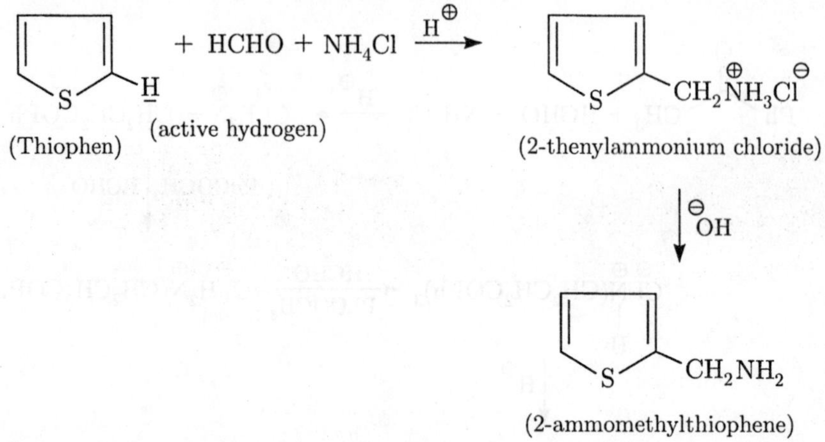

2.

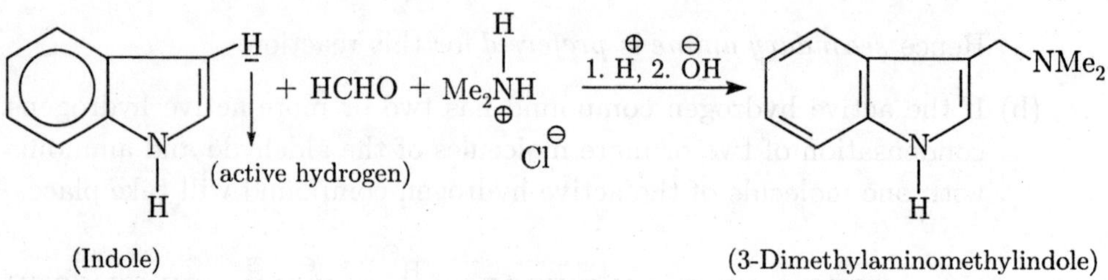

3.

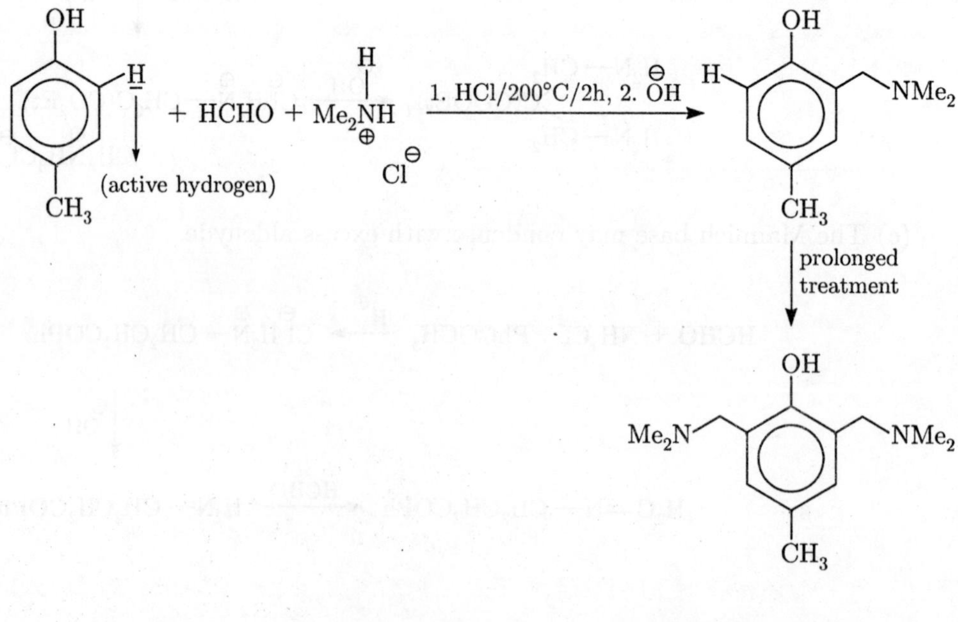

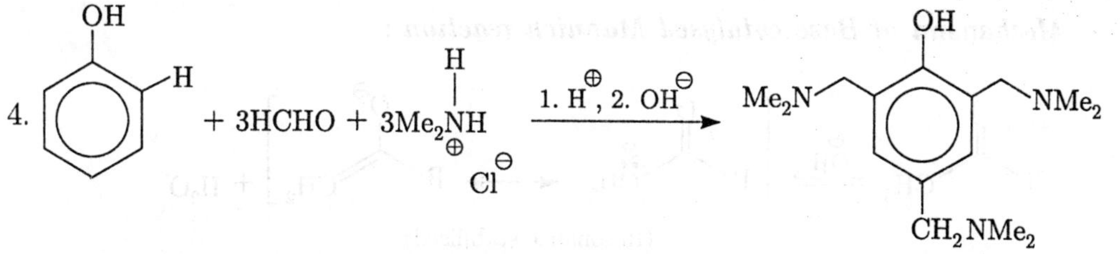

Mechanism of acid-catalysed Mannich reaction : The proposed mechanism tells us that, the amine reacts as a base and not as a salt though the system contains acid catalyst.

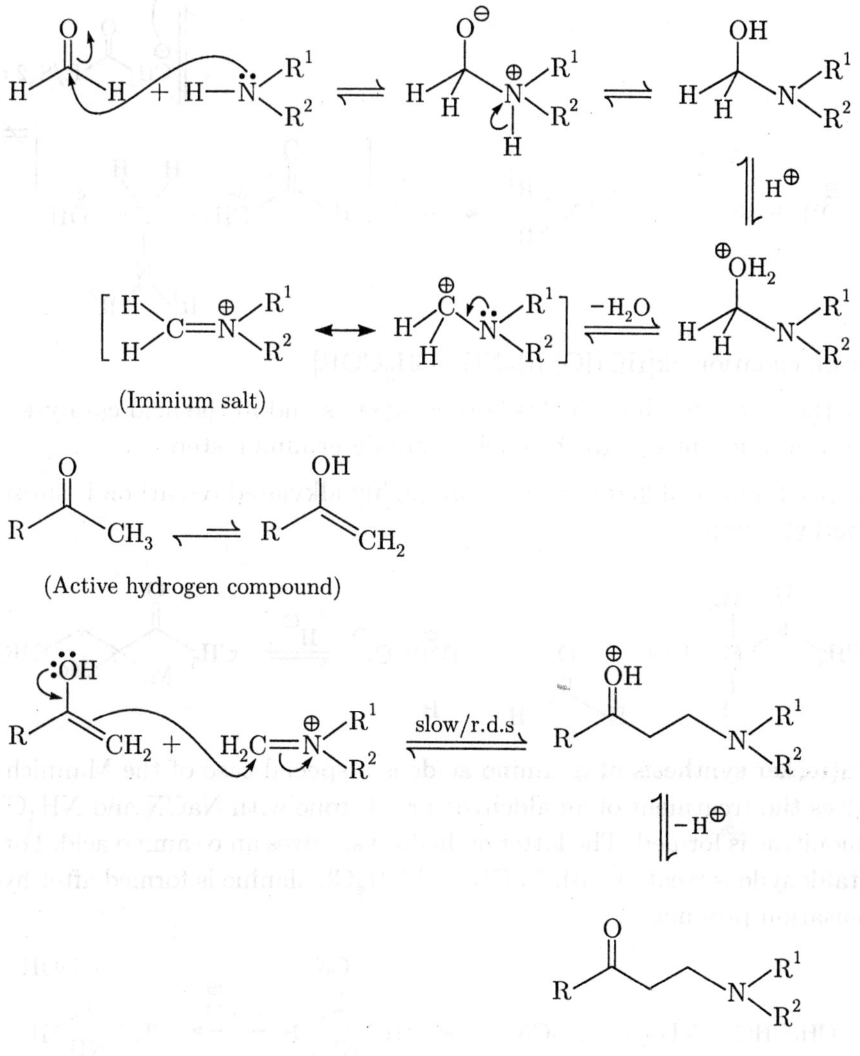

Mechansim of Base-catalysed Mannich reaction :

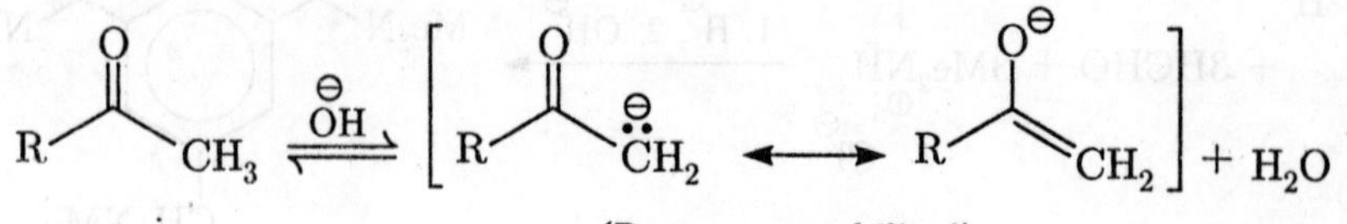

(Resonance stabilised)

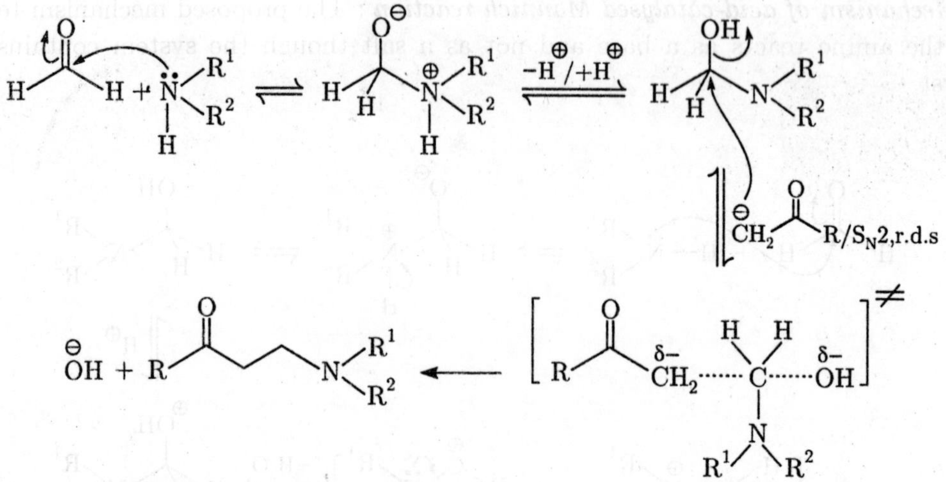

The rate equation=k[HCHO] [R_2NH] [CH_3COR]

Hence the reaction follows a third order kinetics and in the acid catalysed reaction, the addition of iminium salt to the enol is rate determining step.

With unsymmetrical ketones, the more highly alkylated α–carbon is substituted by the aminoethyl group.

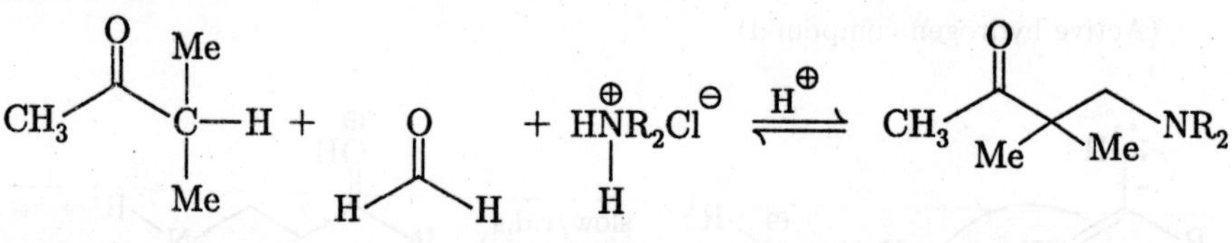

The **Strecker synthesis of α–amino acids** is a special case of the Mannich reaction. This involves the treatment of an aldehyde or a ketone with NaCN and NH_4Cl whereby an α–aminonitrile is formed. The latter on hydrolysis gives an α–amino acid. For example, when acetaldehyde is treated with NaCN and NH_4Cl, alanine is formed after hydrolysing the condensation product.

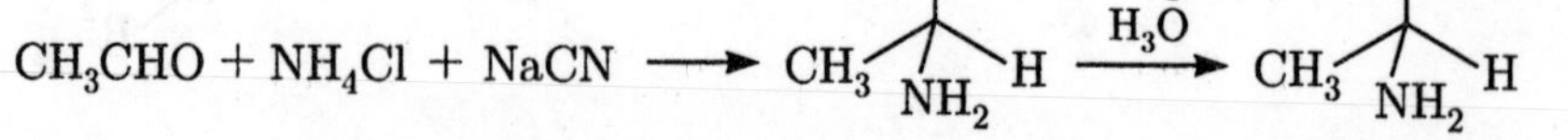

(±)-Alanine

Mechanism of Strecker's synthesis :

$$NH_4Cl + NaCN \longrightarrow NH_4CN + NaCl; \quad NH_4CN \rightleftharpoons NH_3 + HCN$$

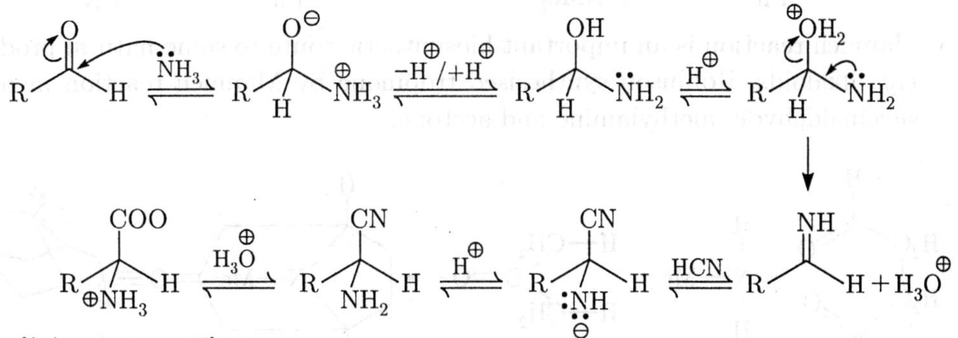

[(±)-α-Amino acid]

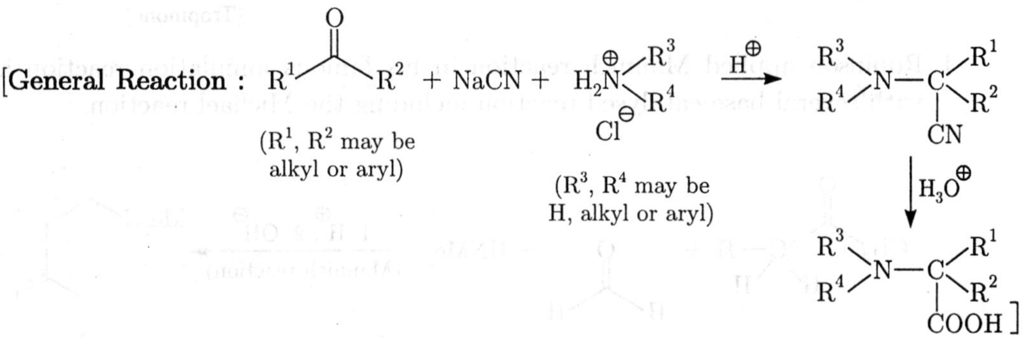

Applications of Mannich reaction :

1. When the Mannich base is a β-aminocarbonyl compound, an α, β–unsaturated carbonyl compound is obtained on heating the Mannich base. This may then be converted to a saturated ketone by the catalytic hydrogenation.

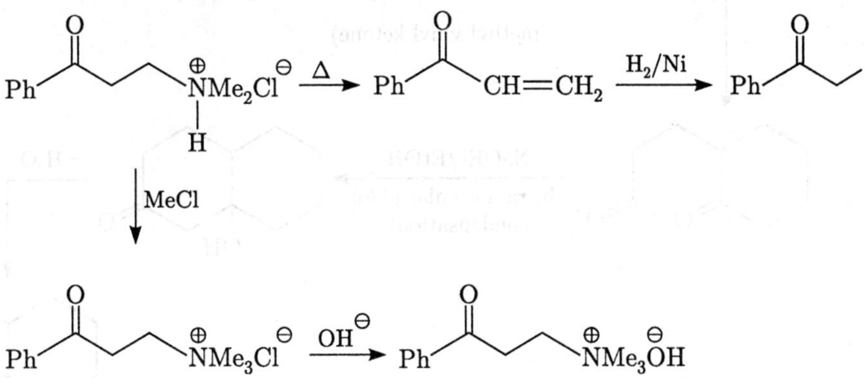

This reaction is useful for the introduction of a vinyl group.

2. The amino group of a Mannich base may be replaced by a nucleophile.

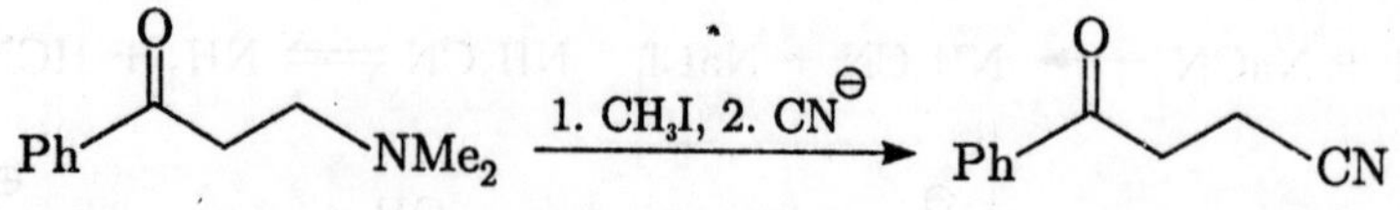

3. Mannich reaction is an important biosynthetic route to some natural products, *e.g.* alkaloids. Robinson synthesised tropinone by Mannich reaction involving succinaldehyde, methylamine and acetone.

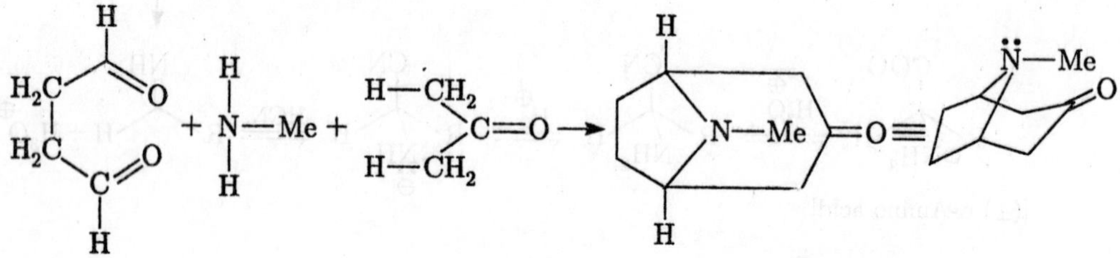

(Tropinone)

4. Robinson applied Mannich reaction in his famous annulation reaction along with several base-catalysed reaction including the Michael reaction.

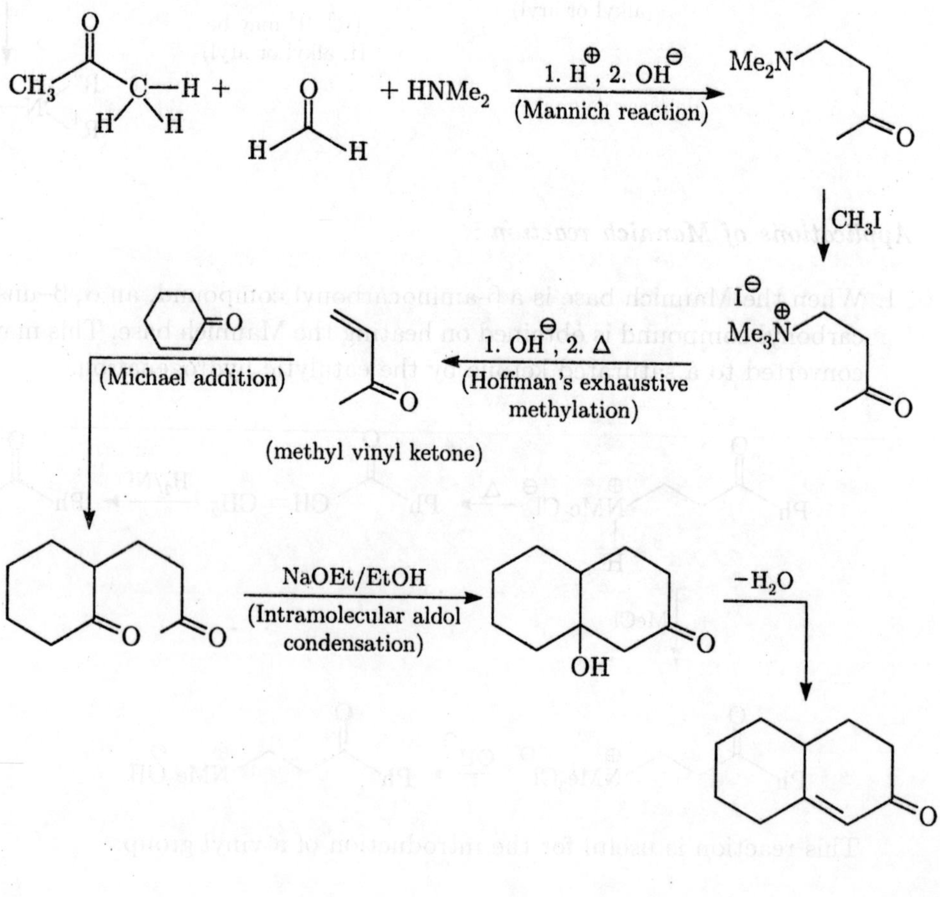

5. The iminium salt being a strong nucleophile, replaces the *active hydrogens* of indole, phenol, nitroalkane etc.

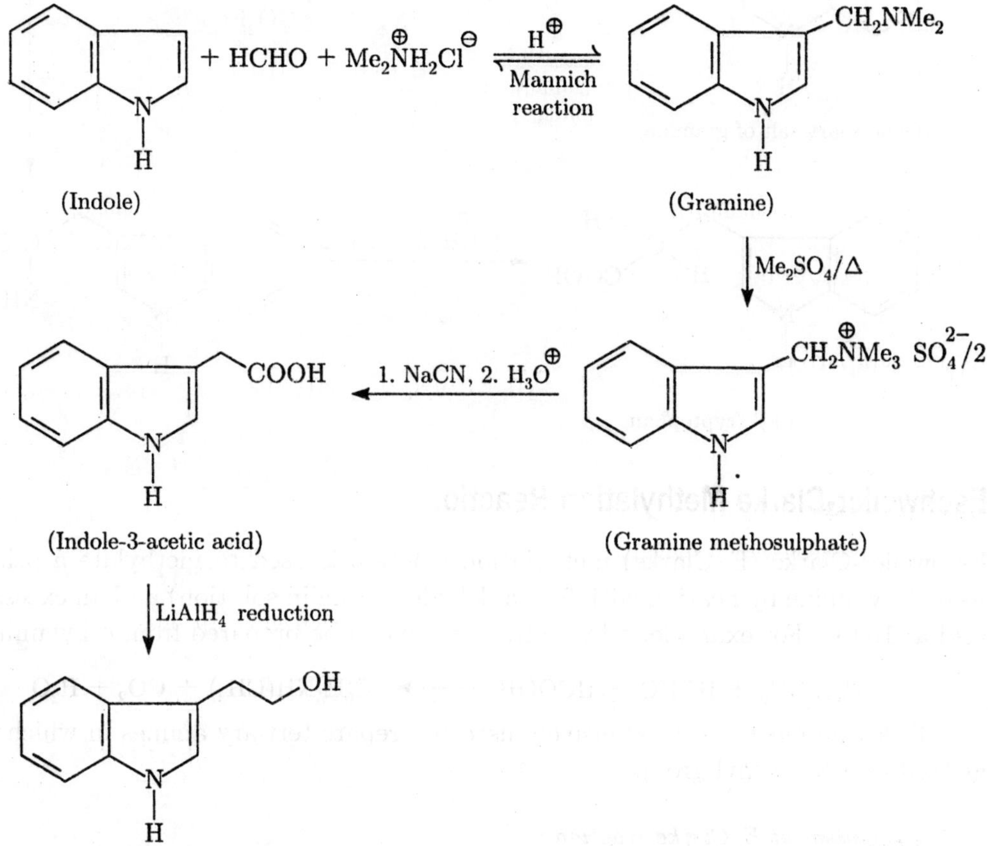

6. Tryptophan may be synthesised from the quaternary salt of gramine and acetamido ester.

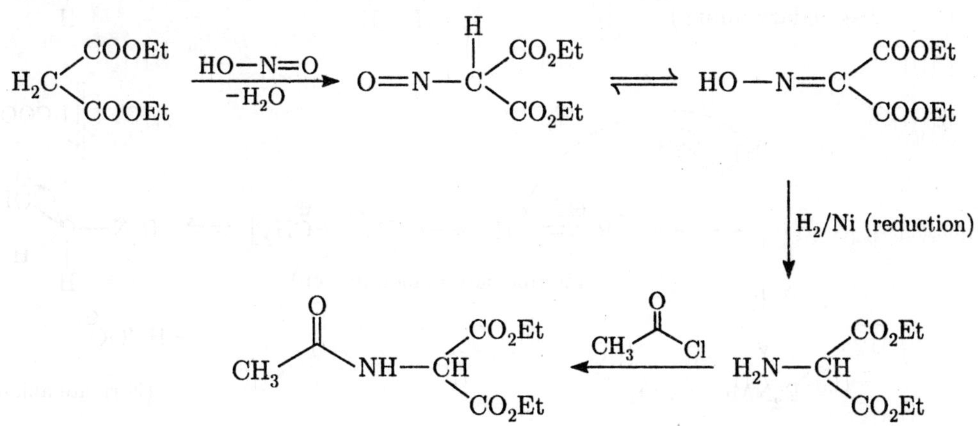

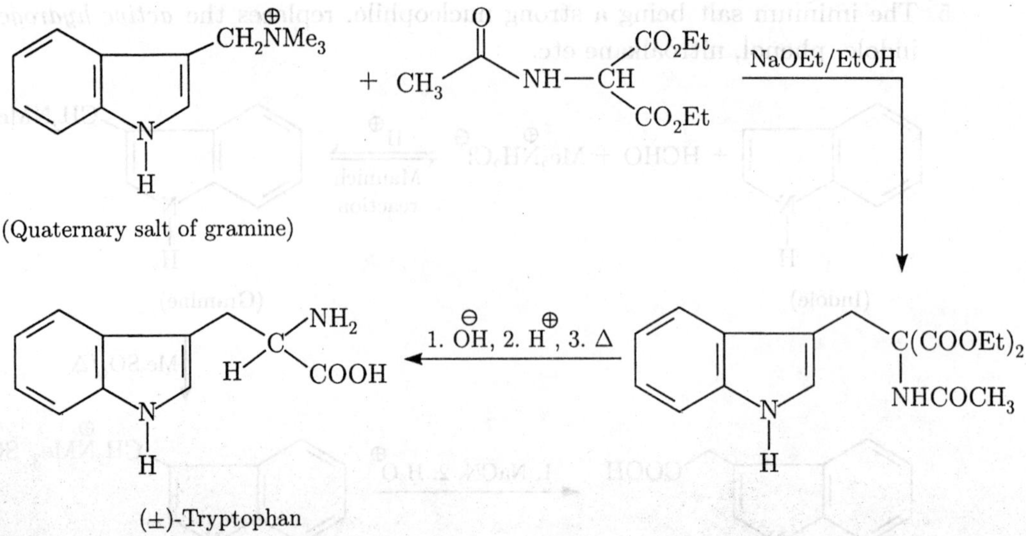

(Quaternary salt of gramine)

(±)-Tryptophan

Eschweiler-Clarke Methylation Reaction

Eschweiler-Clarke (E–Clarke) methylation reaction is used to methylate a primary or secondary amine by heating with formaldehyde (formalin solution) and an excess formic acid at 100°C. For example, ethylmethyl amine can be prepared from ethylamine.

$$C_6H_5NH_2 + HCHO + HCOOH \longrightarrow C_6H_5NH(CH_3) + CO_2 + H_2O$$

This reaction is most extensively used to prepare tertiary amines in which there is at least one N–methyl group.

Mechanism of E–Clarke reaction :

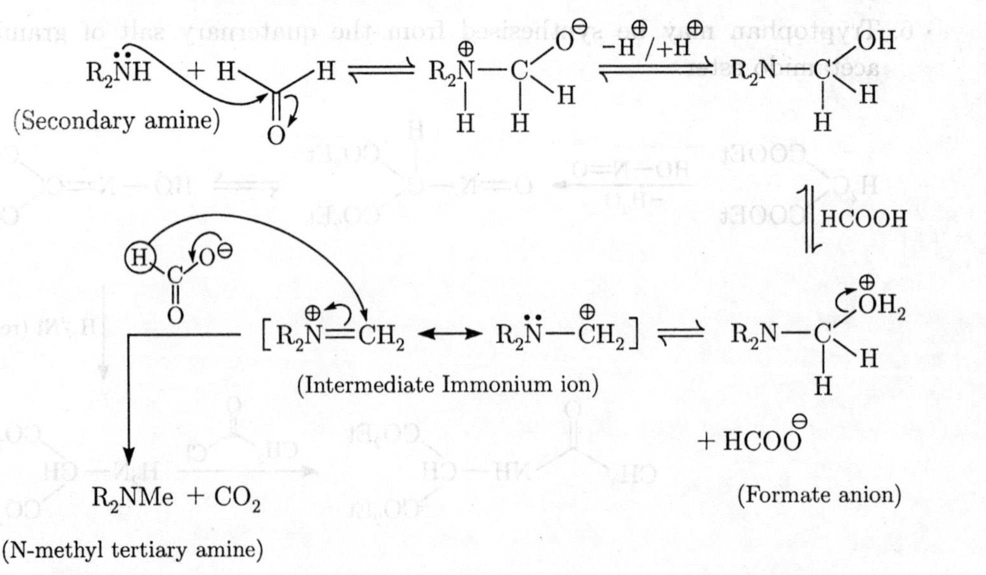

(Secondary amine)

(Intermediate Immonium ion)

(Formate anion)

(N-methyl tertiary amine)

When the starting amine is primary, successive condensations and reductions occur.

$$RNH_2 \xrightarrow{HCHO/HCOOH} RNHMe \xrightarrow{HCHO/HCOOH} RNMe_2$$

For example,

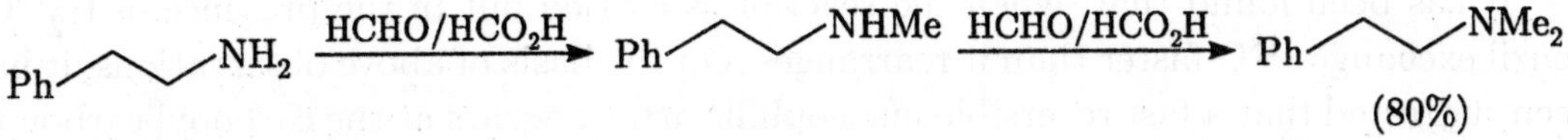

The Leuckart reaction is a variant of E–Clarke reaction, in which aldehydes or ketones other than formaldehyde are heated with ammonium formate or formamide at 180°C–200°C. For example,

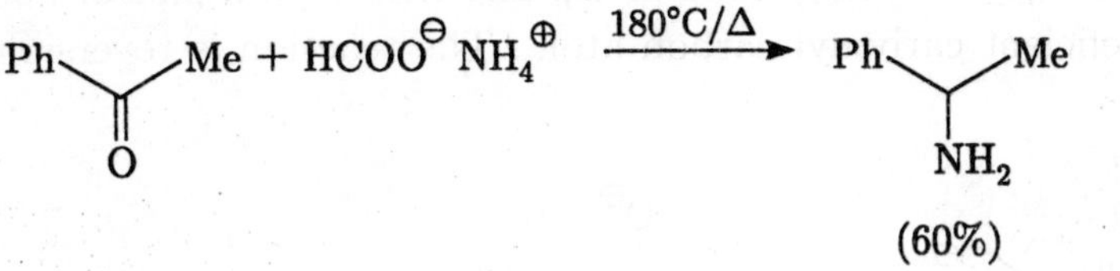

The Benzilic Acid Rearrangement

The base-induced conversion of 1,2–diketones to a salt of 2-hydroxycarboxylic acid is known as the benzilic acid rearrangement. The first studied 1,2–diketone, benzil, on heating with alcoholic alkali gives the anion of benzilic acid through a rearrangement reaction. Any reaction of this kind is named as benzilic acid rearrangement.

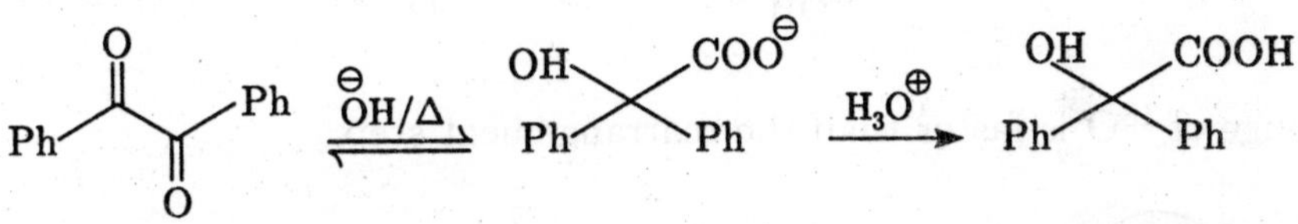

(Benzil) (Benzilic acid)

Barium and thallous hydroxides are more effective than sodium or potassium hydroxides. Alkoxide ions like methoxide, tertiarybutoxide etc. may be used in place of hydroxide ions to yield the *corresponding esters.*

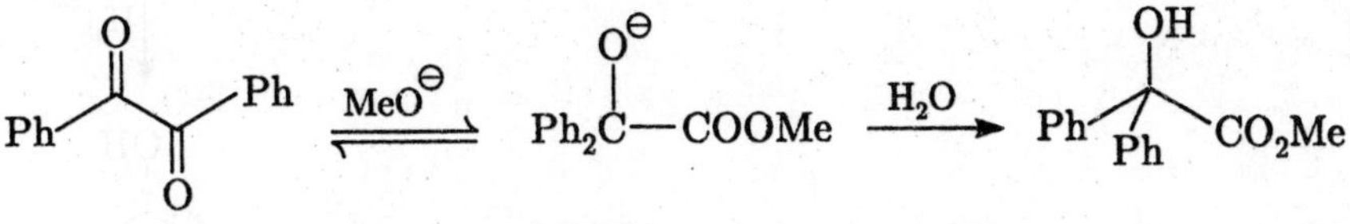

Phenoxide ions are poor nucleophiles to attack. Besides aromatic 1,2–diketones, aliphatic and heterocyclic diketones and *o-* quinones undergo this rearrangement. The yield with aliphatic 1,2–diketones is low, as the aldol condensation competes with this rearrangement.

***Mechanism of Benzilic Acid Rearrangement* :**

The rate of the reaction=k[substrate] [base]

=k[1,2–diketone] [base]

It follows thus a second order reaction.

It has been found that, when the reaction is carried out in the presence of $H_2{}^{18}O$, benzil exchanges ^{18}O faster than it rearranges. On the basis of above observations, it has been suggested that a fast reversible nucleophilic attack occurs at the carbonyl carbon in the first step. The *second step is slow* and hence rate determining in which the migration occurs. Finally a rapid proton transfer completes the process. The rearrangement is essentially a 1,2–carbanionic shift. The migration origin and the migration terminus are the carbon atoms and the migrating group migrates with a pair of bonded electrons to the electron-deficient carbonyl carbon atom. The reaction is reversible and consists of two steps.

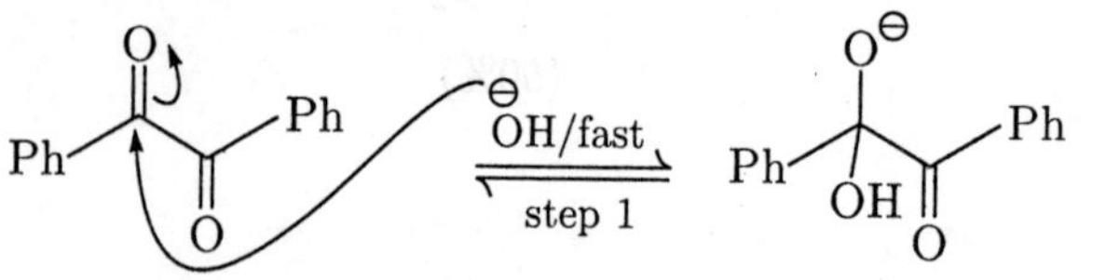

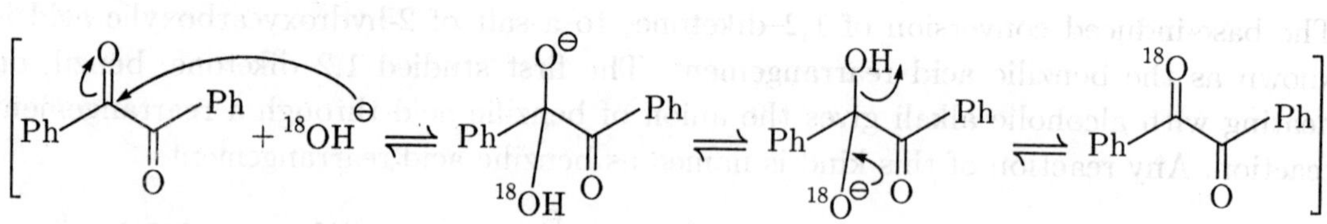

Exchange of ^{18}O is faster than the rearrangement step.

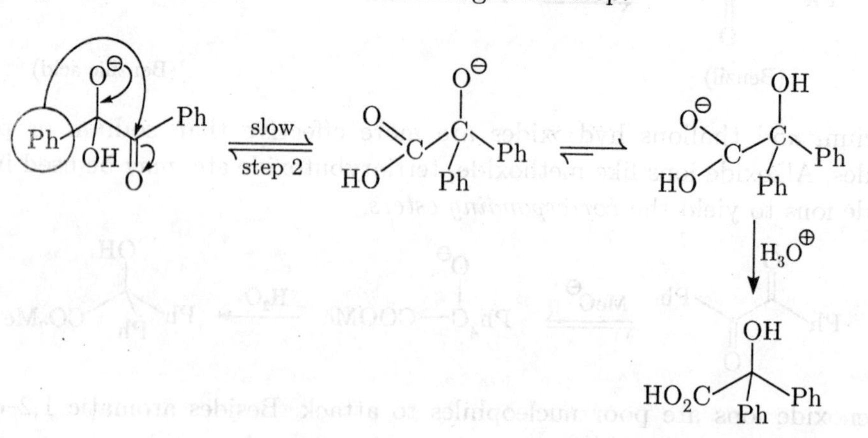

(Benzilic acid)

The rearrangement is analogous to intramolecular Cannizzaro reaction of glyoxal.

The reversibility of the reaction has been established by the *isotope exchange experiment.*

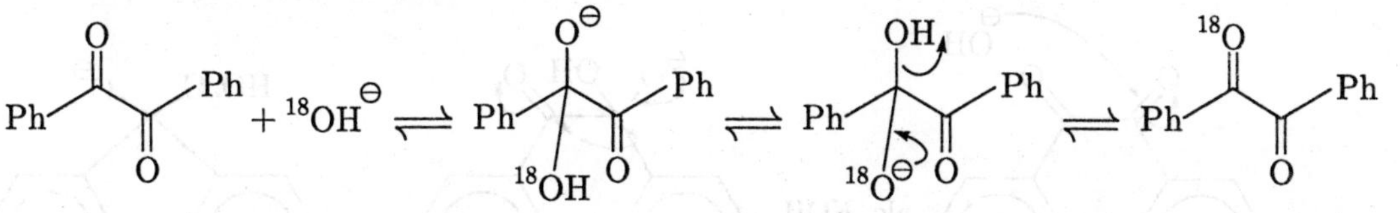

No cross-over products in cross-over experiments have been isolated, which supports the intramolecularity of the reaction.

The carbonyl group which is attached to the less electron releasing group of the two aryl groups (in other words, more electrophilic carbonyl carbon) and hence is attacked by $^{\ominus}OH$ ion.

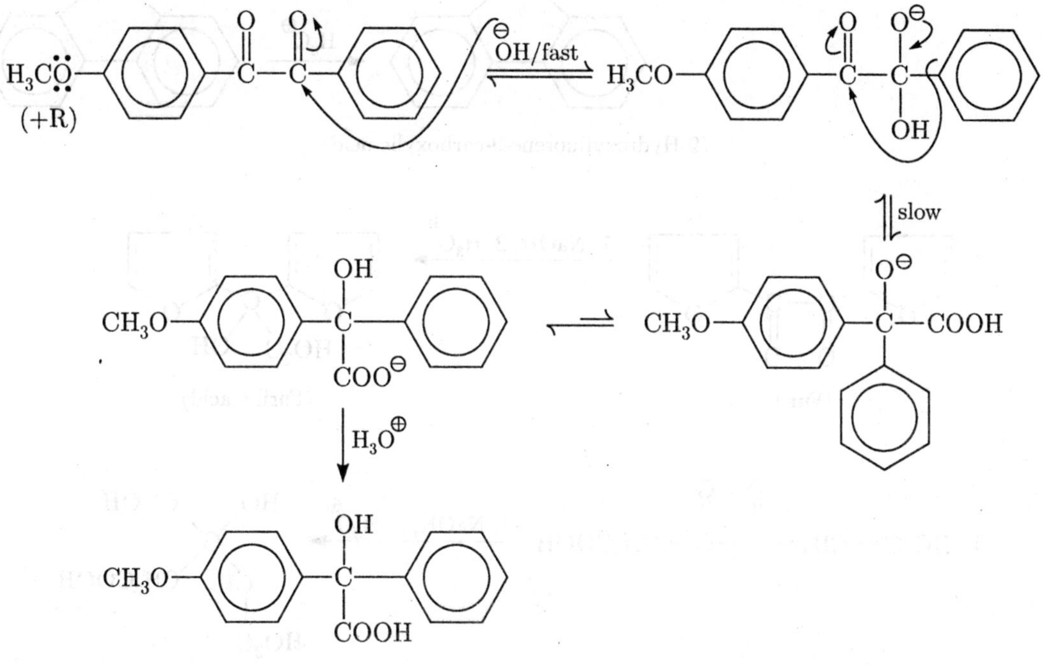

Applications of Benzilic Acid Rearrnagement :

1. 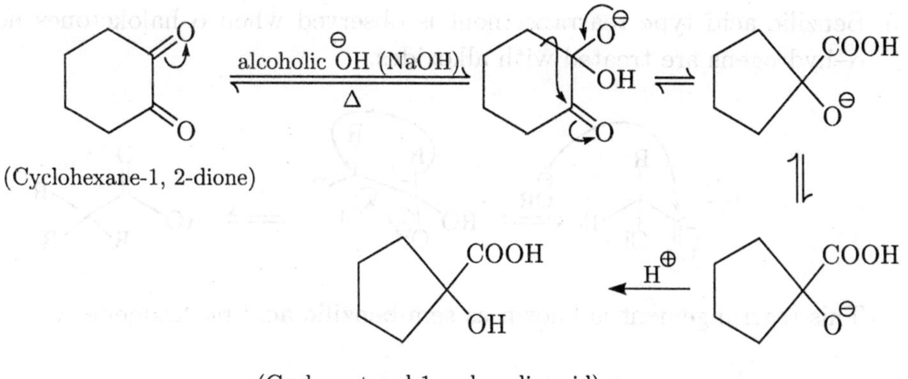

(Cyclopentanol-1-carboxylic acid)

2. 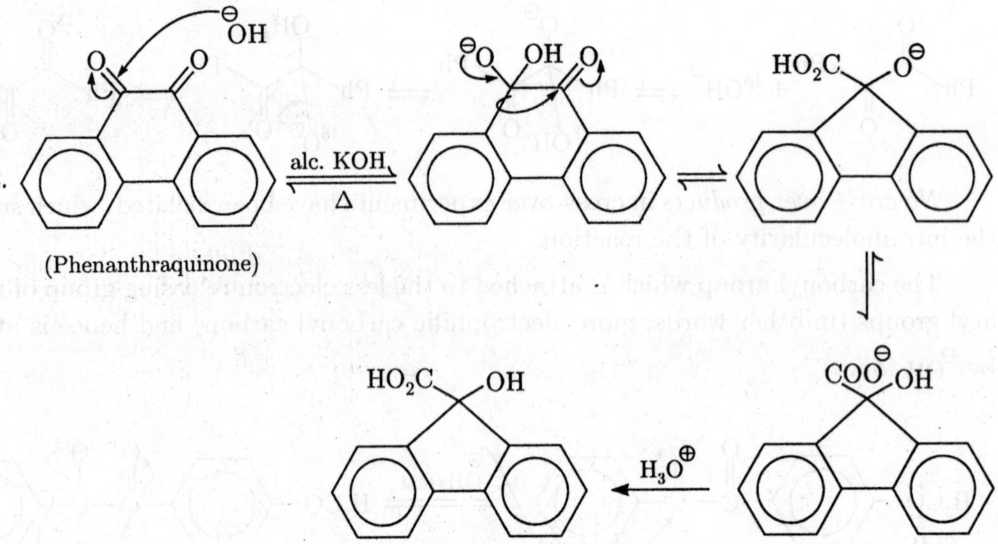

(Phenanthraquinone)

(9-Hydroxyfluorene-9-carboxylic acid)

3. 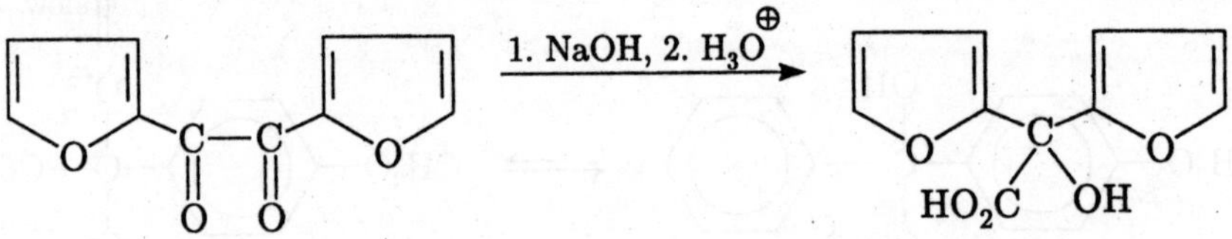

(Furil) (Furilic acid)

4. 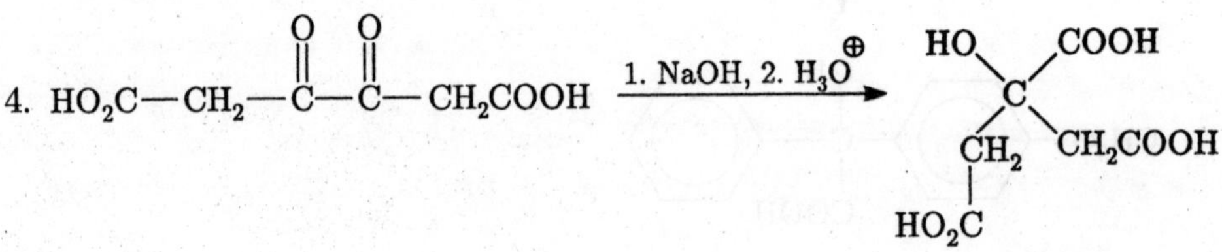

(Citric acid)

5. Benzilic acid type rearrangement is observed when α-haloketones not having α–hydrogens are treated with alkoxides.

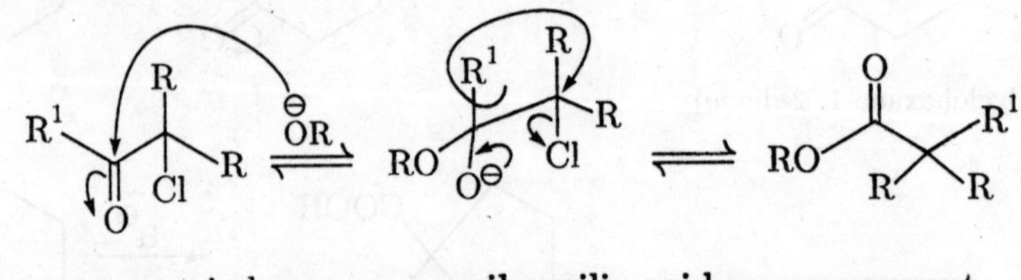

This rearrangement is known as **semibenzilic acid** rearrnagement.

The Wittig Reaction : The Addition of Ylids to Carbonyl Group

Ylids : A species containing an anionic carbon (carbanion) covalently bonded to a positively charged hetero atom, like N, S, P etc. is called a *ylid*, represented by the general formula—

$$-\overset{\ominus}{\ddot{C}}-\overset{\oplus}{X}- \quad \text{where X=N, P or S.}$$

Nitrogen, phosphorus and sulphur ylids are known. When onium salts are treated with strong bases, ylids are formed. Strong bases are usually butyl and phenyllithium in ether or THF, sodium or lithium ethoxides in EtOH or DMF and NaH in DMSO.

$$Ph_3P + MeBr \longrightarrow Ph_3\overset{\oplus}{P}-MeBr^{\ominus} \xrightarrow{PhLi/Et_2O} Ph_3\overset{\oplus}{P}-\overset{\ominus}{C}H_2$$

$$Me_3N + MeBr \longrightarrow Me_3\overset{\oplus}{N}-MeBr^{\ominus} \xrightarrow{PhLi/Et_2O} Me_3\overset{\oplus}{N}-\overset{\ominus}{C}H_2$$

$$Me_2\overset{\oplus}{S}-CH_3\overset{\ominus}{I} \xrightarrow{CH_3-\overset{O}{\overset{\|}{S}}-\overset{\ominus}{C}H_2\ Na^{\oplus}} Me-\overset{\overset{Me}{|}}{\overset{\oplus}{S}}-\overset{\ominus}{\ddot{C}}H_2$$

$$CH_2{=}CH-CH_2Cl + Ph_3P \longrightarrow Ph_3\overset{\oplus}{P}-CH_2-CH{=}CH_2\overset{\ominus}{Cl}$$

$$\xrightarrow{NaOEt/EtOH} Ph_3P{=}CH-CH{=}CH_2$$

Sulphur and phosphorus ylids as more stable over nitrogen ylids since the lone pair of electrons on anionic carbon can form pπ–dπ bonding with the d orbital of sulphur and phosphorus.

$$Ph_3\overset{\oplus}{P}-\overset{\ominus}{\ddot{C}}H_2 \longleftrightarrow Ph_3P{=}CH_2; \qquad Me\overset{\oplus}{S}-\overset{\ominus}{\ddot{C}}H_2 \longleftrightarrow Me_2S{=}CH_2;$$

(Phosphorus ylid)
(Resonance hybrid)

(Sulphur ylid)
(Resonance hybrid)

$$Me_3\overset{\oplus}{N}-\overset{\ominus}{\ddot{C}}H_2 \not\longleftrightarrow Me_3N{=}CH_2$$

(Not possible as N contains no d orbital, maximum covalency being four)

Acyl and aryl derivatives of ylids where α–carbon atom bears the acyl or aryl group gets stabilised through delocalisation.

$$Me_3\overset{\oplus}{P}-\overset{\ominus}{\ddot{C}}H-\overset{\overset{O}{\|}}{C}-CH_3 \longleftrightarrow Me_3\overset{\oplus}{N}-CH{=}\overset{\overset{O^{\ominus}}{|}}{C}-CH_3$$

Groups with (–I) effect, attached to the anionic carbon imports the stability of the ylids. Phosphoranes or ylids are oxidised by air or oxygen to alkene, but with an excess of oxygen, carbonyl compounds are formed.

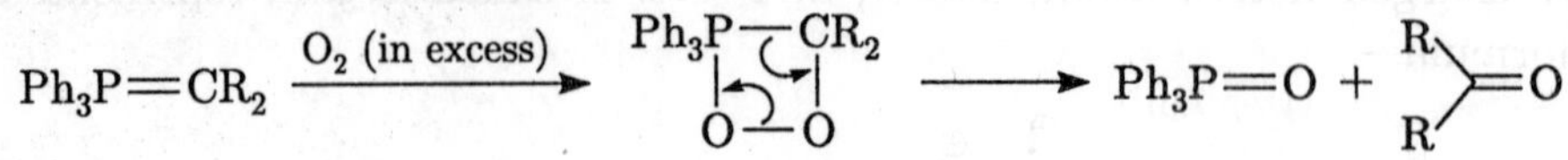

$$2Ph_3P{=}CR_2 \xrightarrow{O_2 \text{ (small amount)}} 2Ph_3P{=}O + R_2C{=}CR_2$$

Ylids are very strong nucleophiles and the anionic carbon is the nucleophilic centre.

The Wittig reaction : Wittig reaction offers an important and useful method for the synthesis of alkenes by the treatment of aldehydes or ketones, with alkylidinetriphenylphosphorane ($Ph_3P{=}CR_2$) or simply phosphorane, commonly known as Wittig reagent.

$$Ph_3P{=}CR_2 + Ph_2C{=}O \longrightarrow Ph_2C{=}CR_2 + Ph_3P{=}O$$

(Triphenylphosphine oxide)
(Strong P=O bond)

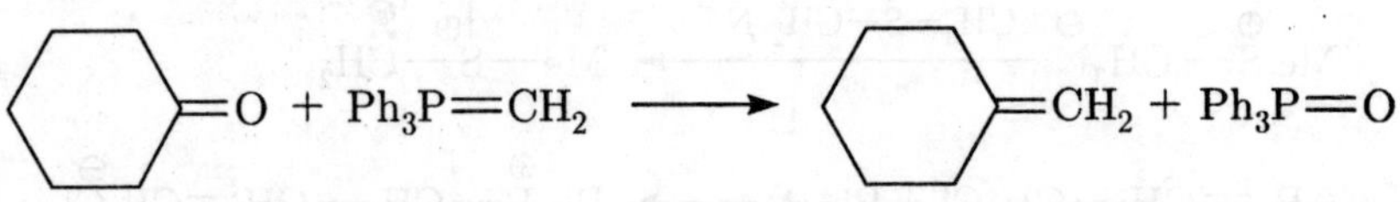

The Wittig reagent (alkylidinetriphenylphosphorane) is prepared by treating trialkyl or triarylphosphine preferably the latter with an alkyl halide in ether solution. The resulting phosphonium salt is treated with a strong base like EtLi, BuLi, $NaNH_2$, NaH, NaOEt etc. The haloacid is removed and the Wittig reagent is recovered. The halide may be primary, secondary or methyl halide.

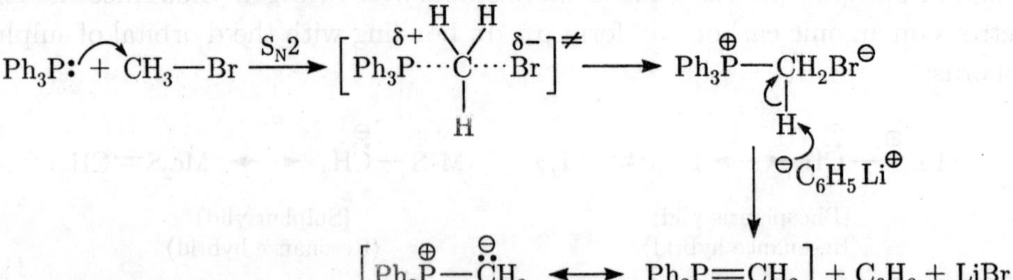

Wittig reagent is stabilised by dπ–pπ bonding in structure (II) and the carbanion in structure (I) is stabilised by the adjacent phosphonium ion. The ylid is generated *in situ* and treated with carbonyl compounds in nitrogen atmosphere because oxygen, water, alcohols, hydrohalic acids etc. react with ylids.

Aliphatic, cyclic and aromatic carbonyl compounds, carbonyl compounds having conjugated double or triple bonds react without interference. Carbonyl compounds containing ester groups may also be used, as ylids react slowly with ester functionality.

Ylids react with the aldehydes containing electron withdrawing groups at α–carbon like —COR, —CHO, —COOR etc. but *slowly* or *not at all* with ketones, containing these electron withdrawing groups.

Stereoselectivity in the Wittig reaction depends on ylids.

We can divide ylids into two types—

1. Ylids with conjugating or anion stabilising substituents adjacent to the negative charge (*e.g.*, carbonyl group)

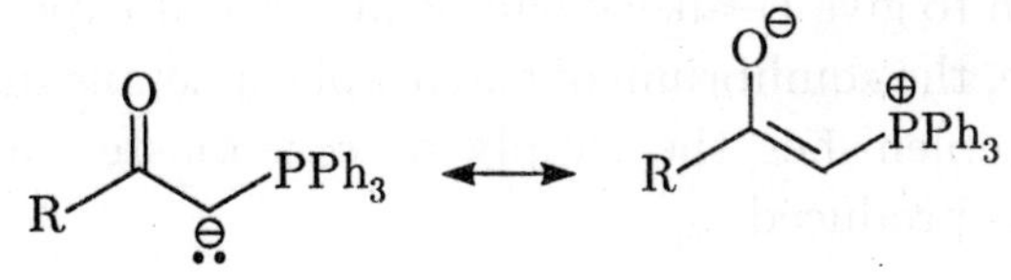

R=H, OR, alkyl

⟵ Stabilised ylids ⟶

2. Ylids with no extra stabilising factor.

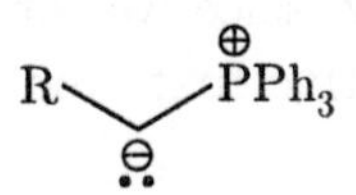

(R=alkyl) (unstabilised ylid)

The stereochemistry of the wittig reaction :

1. ***With stabilised ylids, Wittig reaction is E selective.***

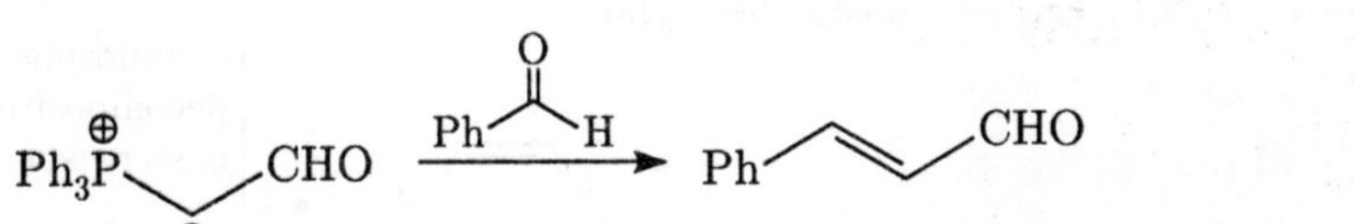

(99% yield, 100% E; T.C. product)

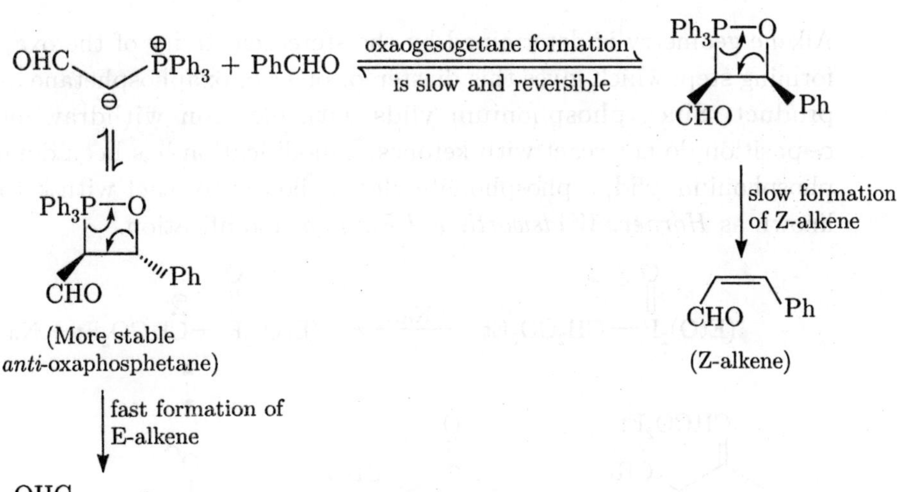

Why change in stereoselectivity from Z to E, when the ylid is stabilised? Stereoselectivity in this step is no longer kinetically controlled but is thermodynamically controlled. New starting materials provide a mechanism by which the oxaphosphetane diastereoisomers can interconvert. Providing the rate of interconversion is faster than the rate of elimination to alkene, the stereospecific step will no longer reflect the initial kinetic ratio of oxaphosphetane diastereoisomers. The *trans*–oxaphosphetane will be the thermodynamically stable diastereoisomer, which on elimination produces E–alkene. Moreover, the rate of elimination to give E–alkene will be faster as it experiences less steric crowding. Meanwhile, the equilibrium of two oxaphosphetane diastereoisomers *via* strating material replenishes the supply of *anti*–diastereoisomer and virtually only E–alkene is produced.

2. ***With unstabilised ylides Wittig reaction is Z–selective*** : If the addition of ylid to the aldehyde produces intermediate oxaphosphetane by an irreversible pathway, the stereospecificity of the alkene formed after elimination is *'syn'*, *i.e.*, Z–alkene is formed. The R group in the following example should not be electron withdrawing or anion stabilising. The Z–selective wittig reaction therefore consists of a *kinetically controlled* stereoselective first step followed by a stereospecific elimination from this intermediate.

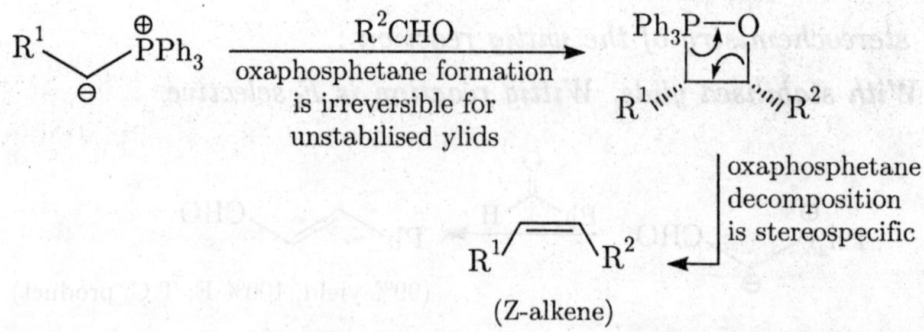

Alkene geometry is determined by the stereoselectivity of the oxaphosphetane forming step, which gives this diastereoisomer of oxaphosphetane as the kinetic product. Since phosphonium ylids with electron withdrawing groups at α–position do not react with ketones, a modification has been done. Instead of phosphonium ylid, a phosphonate ylid is allowed to react with ketones. This is known as *Horner, Wadsworth and Emmons* modification.

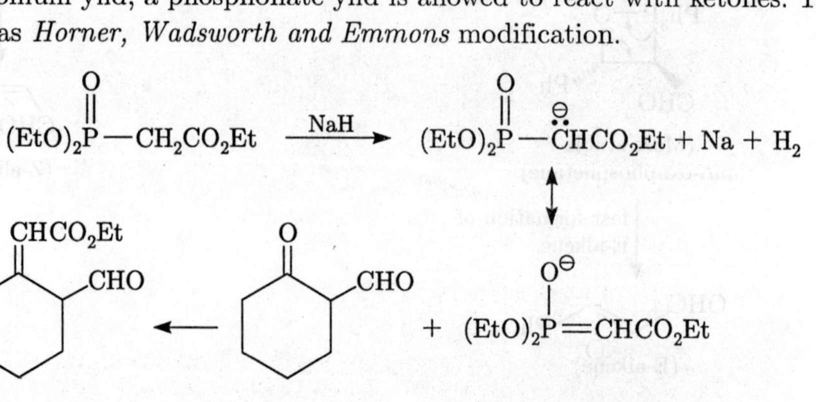

Mechanism of the Wittig reaction :

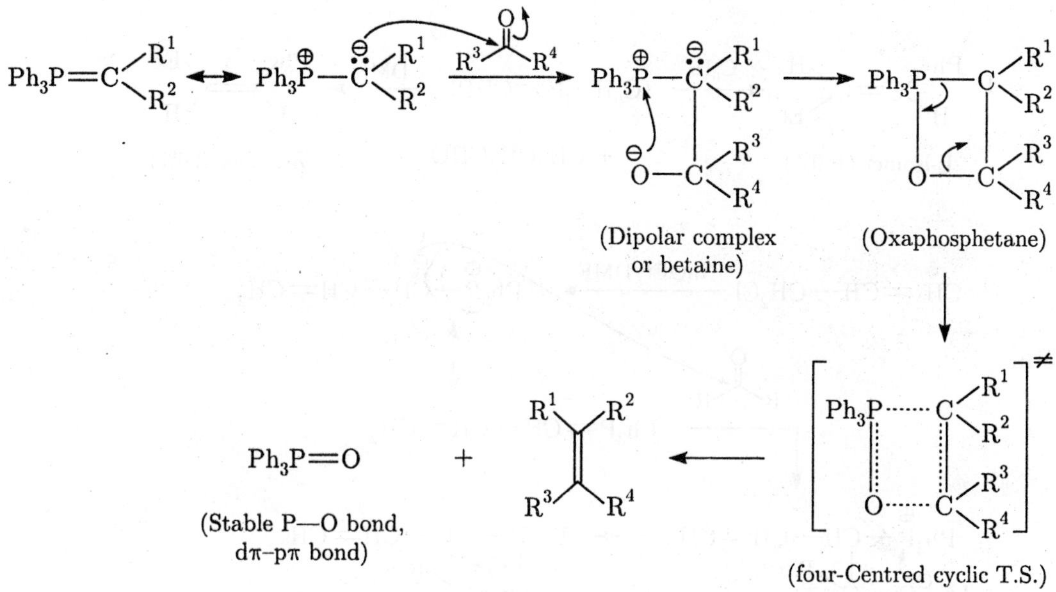

The negative entropy of activation ($\Delta S^{\neq}$) supports the formation of a cyclic intermediate. In some cases, betaines or sometimes even the cyclic transition states are isolated. The mechanism is also supported by the fact that, an optically active phosphonium salt reacts to produce a phosphine oxide with retention of configuration.

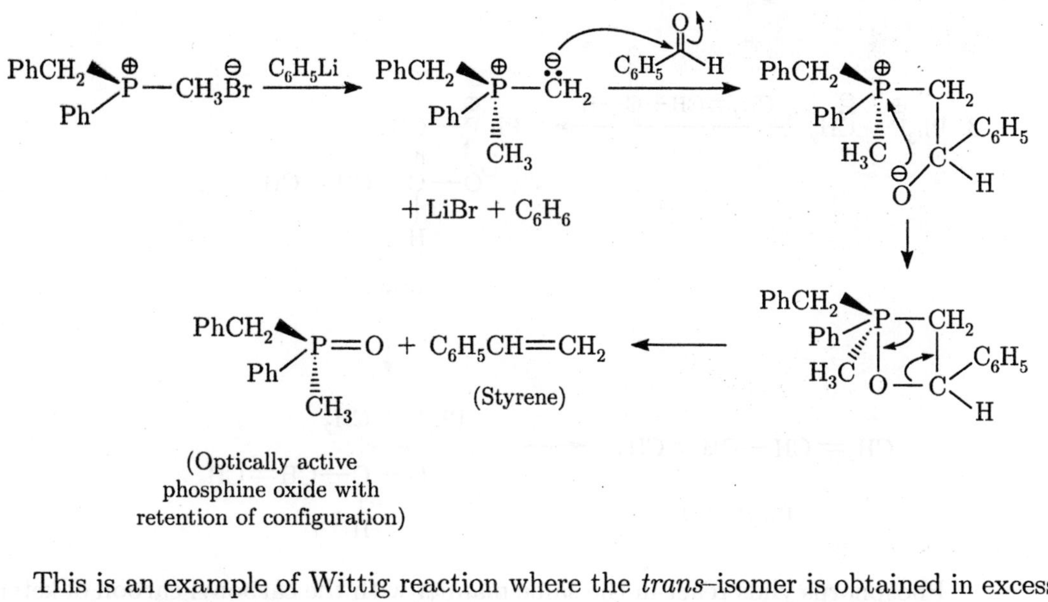

This is an example of Wittig reaction where the *trans*–isomer is obtained in excess when the solvent is non polar whereas in a polar solvent, *cis*–isomer is formed predominantly. Since desired alkyl groups can be introduced in the alkyl halide and the carbonyl compound, it is extremely useful to synthesise *substituted alkenes.* Double or triple bonds even when conjugated with the carbonyl group do not interfere.

1.

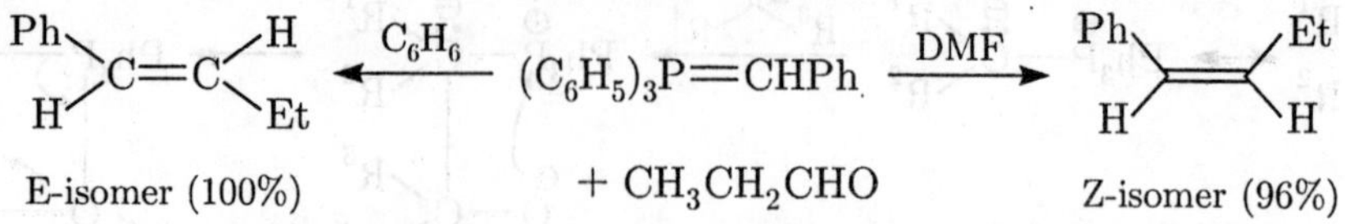

2.

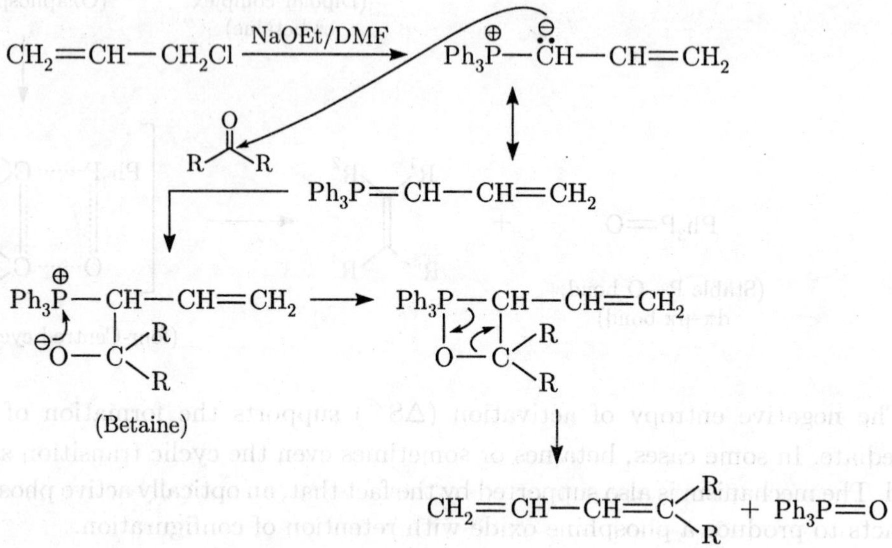

3.

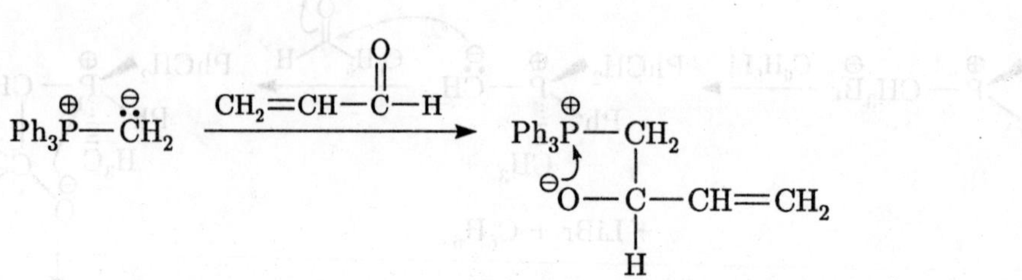

Phosphorus ylids react in the same manner with the carbonyl carbon of ketenes and isocyanates as also with the N=O and C=N groups of nitroso and imine compounds respectively.

(a) 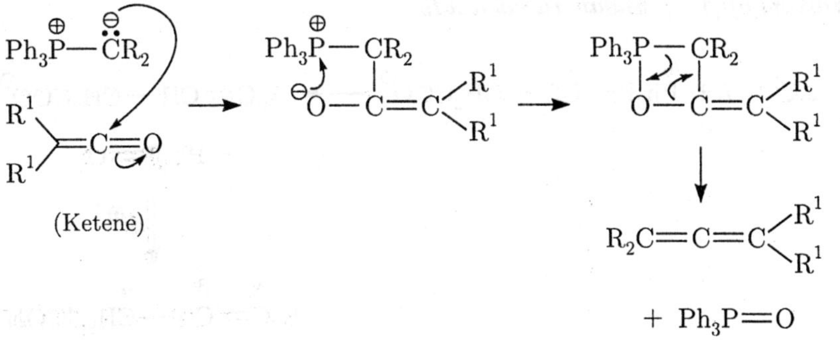

(Ketene)

(b) 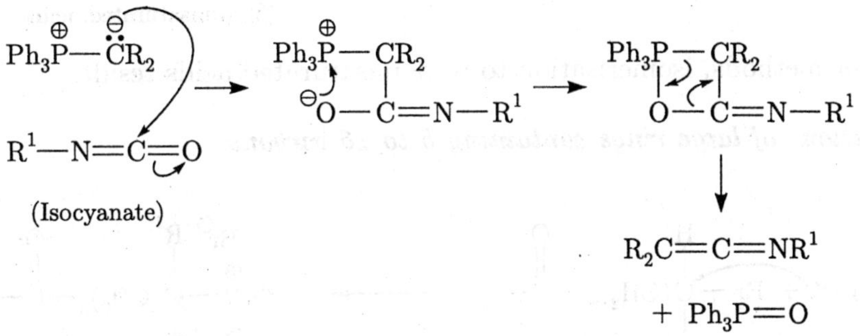

(Isocyanate)

(c) 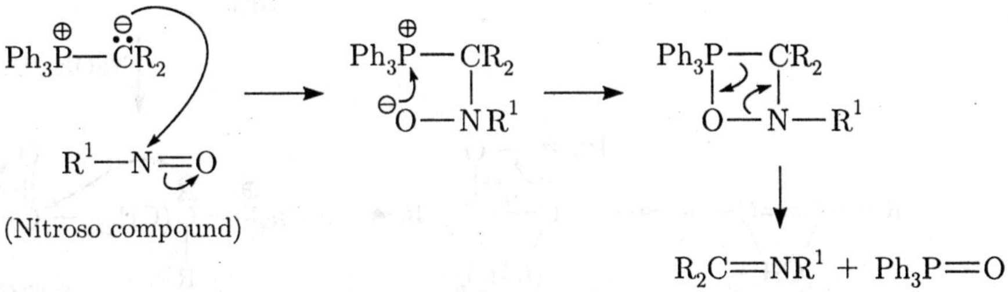

(Nitroso compound)

(d) 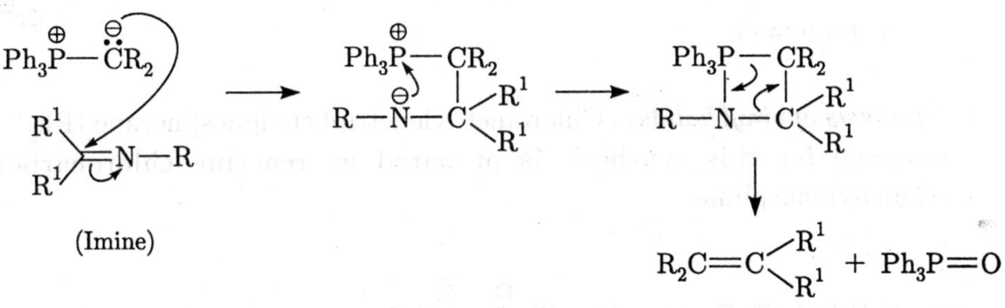

(Imine)

Applications of Wittig reaction :

1. ***Formation of exocyclic double bond***

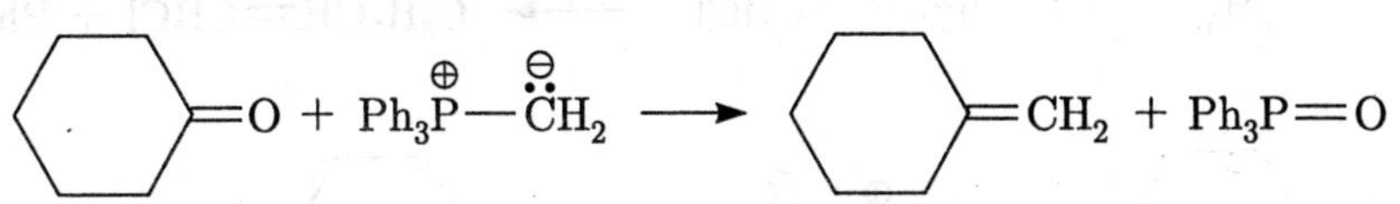

This method of introducing exocyclic methylene group is useful in the synthesis of methylene steroids.

2. ***Preparation of β, γ-unsaturated acids***

$$R_2C{=}O + \overset{\oplus}{Ph_3P}{-}\overset{\ominus}{\ddot{C}H}{-}CH_2COO^{\ominus} \longrightarrow R_2C{=}CH{-}CH_2COO^{\ominus} + Ph_3P{=}O$$

$$\xrightarrow{H^{\oplus}} \overset{\gamma}{R_2C}{=}\overset{\beta}{CH}{-}\overset{\alpha}{CH_2}COOH$$

(β, γ-unsaturated acid)

In other methods, isomerisation to α, β–unsaturated acids result.

3. ***Formation of large rings containing 5 to 16 carbons***

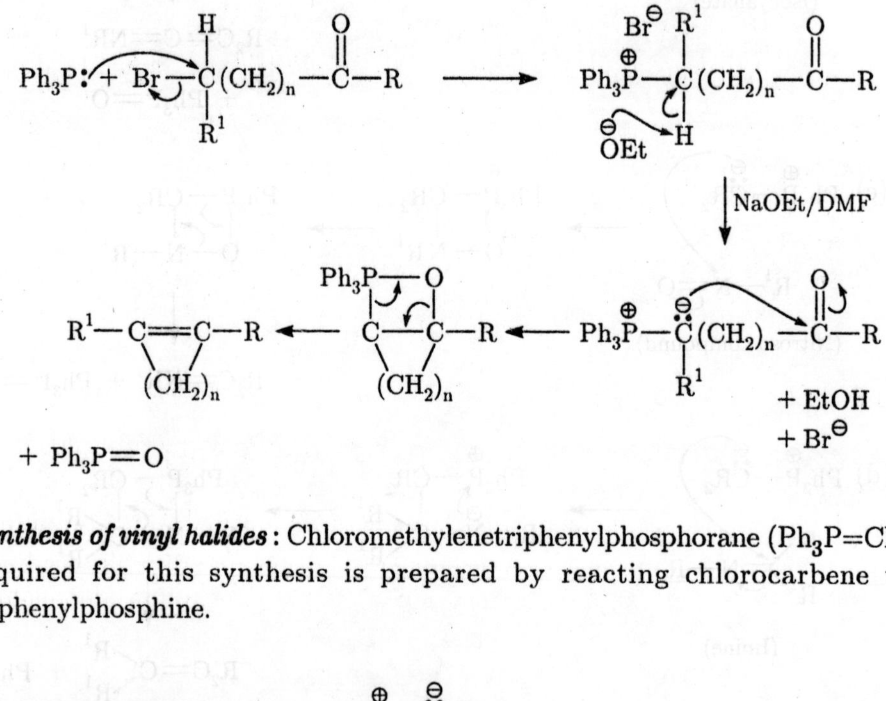

4. ***Synthesis of vinyl halides*** : Chloromethylenetriphenylphosphorane ($Ph_3P{=}CHCl$) required for this synthesis is prepared by reacting chlorocarbene with triphenylphosphine.

(a) $:CHCl + Ph_3P \longrightarrow \overset{\oplus}{Ph_3P}{-}\overset{\ominus}{\ddot{C}HCl}$

(b) 

5. ***Synthesis of ethers*** : Methoxymethyltriphenylphosphorane reacts with carbonyl compounds to give diphenyl substituted vinyl methyl ether.

$$\underset{\text{(Benzophenone)}}{Ph_2C{=}O} + Ph_3P{=}CHOCH_3 \longrightarrow Ph_2C{=}CHOCH_3 \xrightarrow{H_3O^{\oplus}/\text{hydrolysis}} \underset{\text{(Diphenylacetaldehyde)}}{Ph_2CH{-}CHO}$$

6. Triphenylphosphine may be used to convert epoxides to alkenes.

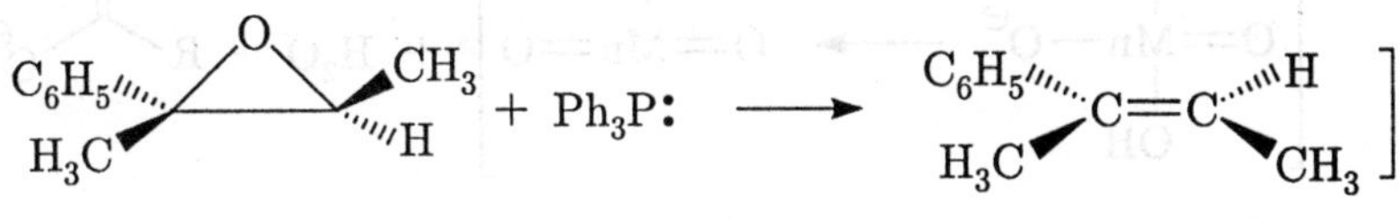

Oxidation of Aldehydes and Ketones

Aldehydes are easily oxidised, ketones are not. The hydrogen atom of the aldehyde molecule is abstracted during oxidation, which is not possible for a ketone, as the abstraction of alkyl or aryl group does not take place.

$$RCHO \text{ or } ArCHO \xrightarrow{Ag(NH_3)_2^{\oplus}\,OH \;/\; KMnO_4/\overset{\ominus}{O}H \;/\; K_2Cr_2O_7/H^{\oplus}} RCOOH \text{ or } ArCOOH$$

These reactions are mainly used for the detection of aldehydes.

$$CH_3CHO + \underset{\substack{\text{(Colourless)}\\ \text{(Tollen's reagent)}}}{2Ag(NH_3)_2^{\oplus}} + 3OH^{\ominus} \longrightarrow \underset{\text{(Silver mirror)}}{2Ag^{\circ}\downarrow} + CH_3COO^{\ominus} + 4NH_3 + 2H_2O$$

Mechanism of $K_2Cr_2O_7$ oxidation of aldehydes in presence of acid :

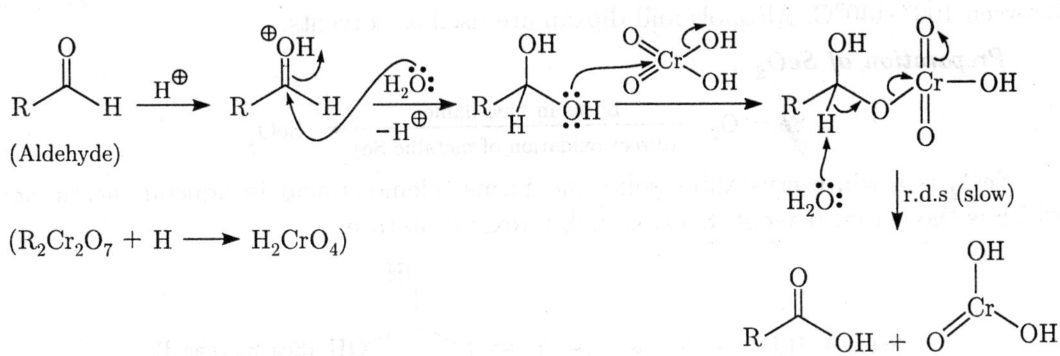

$(R_2Cr_2O_7 + H \longrightarrow H_2CrO_4)$

Mechanism of $KMnO_4/\overset{\ominus}{O}H$ ***oxidation of Aldehydes in presence of alkali*** :

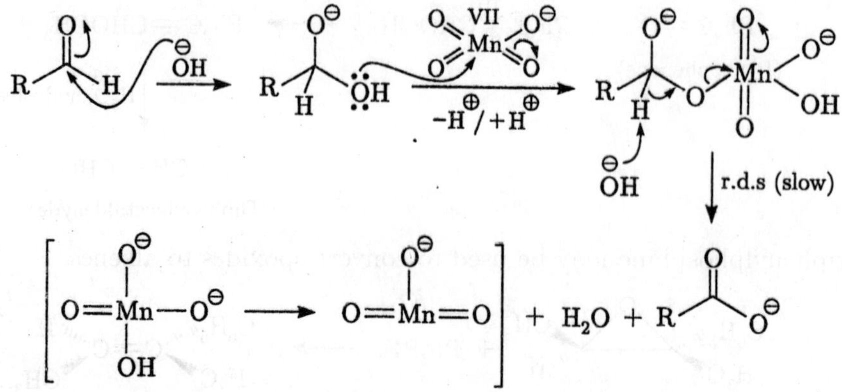

Strong oxidising agents, *e.g.*, acid/dichromate, nitric acid etc. oxidise ketones. Only the carbon atom adjacent to the carbonyl group being attacked and the carbon atom joined to *fewer* number of hydrogen atoms.

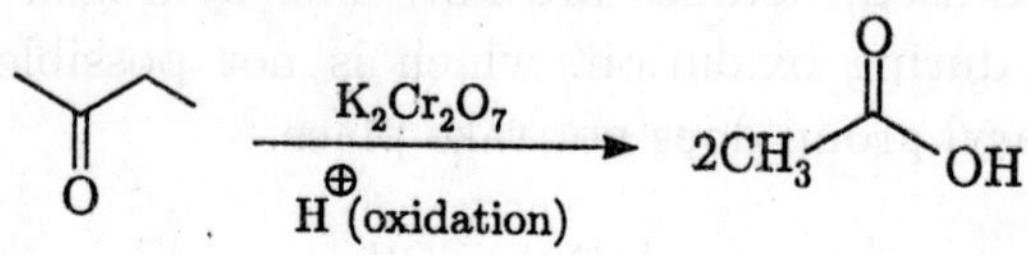

Oxidation of Aldehydes and Ketones by Selenium Dioxide (SeO_2)

Aldehydes and ketones with a methyl or active methylene group adjacent to the carbonyl group are oxidised by SeO_2 at room temperature to dicarbonyl compounds.

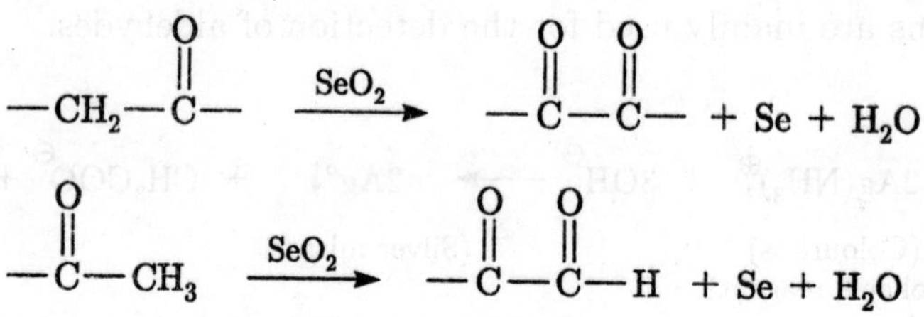

Double bonds, triple bonds and aromatic rings may also activate the methylene group. The reaction is usually carried out in acetic anhydride or acetic acid at a temperature between 100°–140°C. Alcohols and dioxan are used as solvents.

Preparation of SeO_2 :

$$Se + O_2 \xrightarrow[\text{(direct oxidation of metallic Se)}]{\text{burns in blue flame}} SeO_2$$

SeO_2 is a white crystalline solid and forms selenious acid in aqueous acetic acid which is the actual reagent. SeO_2 is highly toxic in nature.

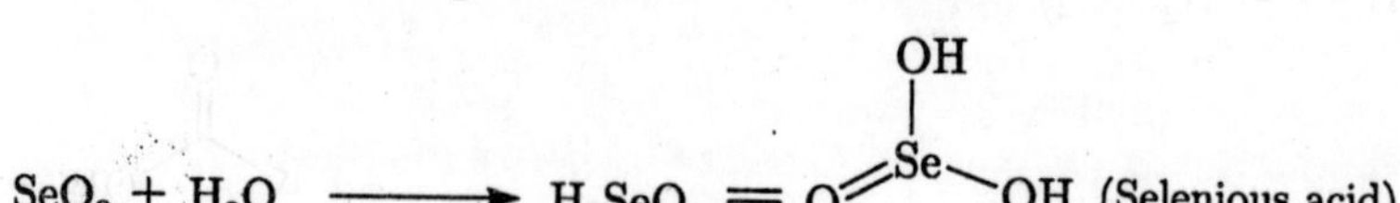

Mechanism of oxidation : The oxidation is carried out in aqueous acetic acid medium and hence the actual reagent is selenious acid, H_2SeO_3.

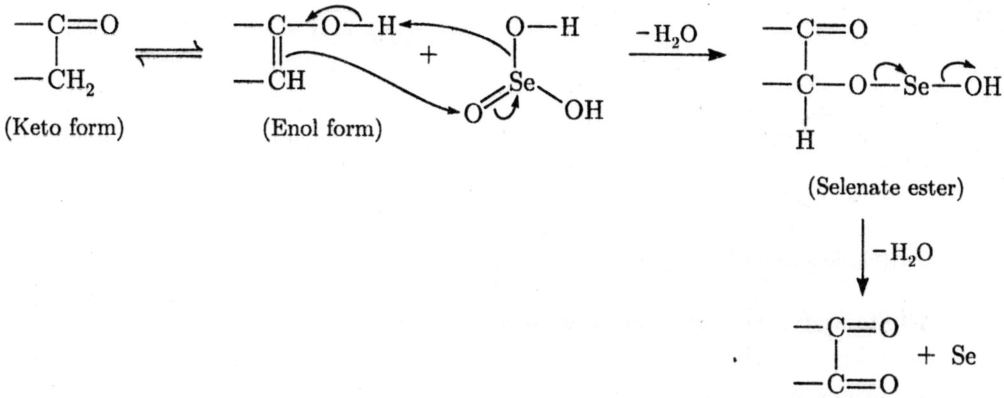

Applications of Use of SeO_2 in Syntheses

1. ***Oxidation*** of ***methyl and methylene groups of carbonyl compounds***

(a) $$CH_3CHO \xrightarrow{SeO_2/AcOH} CHO{-}CHO$$
(Glyoxal)

(b) $$CH_3COCH_3 \xrightarrow{SeO_2/AcOH} CH_3COCHO$$
(Methylglyoxal)

(c) $$PhCOCH_3 \xrightarrow{SeO_2/AcOH} PhCOCHO$$
(Phenylglyoxal)

(d) $$H_2C(COOEt)_2 \xrightarrow{SeO_2/AcOH} O{=}C(CO_2Et)_2$$
(DEM) (Diethyl mesoxylate)

(e) $$CH_3CH_2{-}\overset{\overset{\displaystyle O}{\|}}{C}{-}CH_3 \xrightarrow[AcOH]{SeO_2} CH_3CH_2{-}\overset{\overset{\displaystyle O}{\|}}{C}{-}CHO + CH_3{-}\overset{\overset{\displaystyle O}{\|}}{C}{-}\overset{\overset{\displaystyle O}{\|}}{C}{-}CH_3$$
(Butanone) (Ethylglyoxal, major) (Diacetyl, minor)

(f) 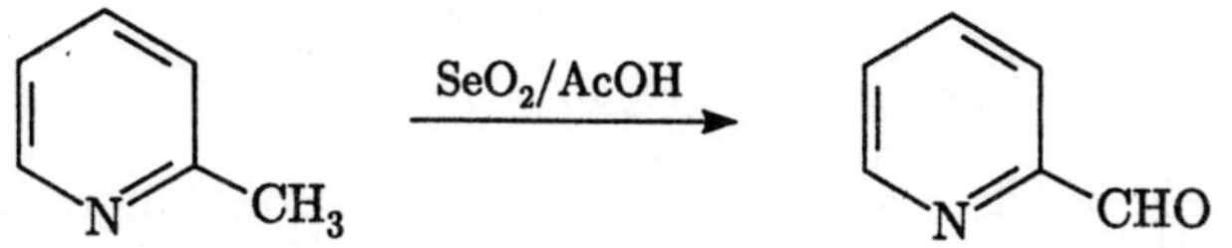

(α-picoline) (α-picolinic aldehyde)

(g) $C_6H_5CH_2C_6H_5 \xrightarrow{SeO_2/AcOH} C_6H_5COC_6H_5$

(Benzophenone)

(h) 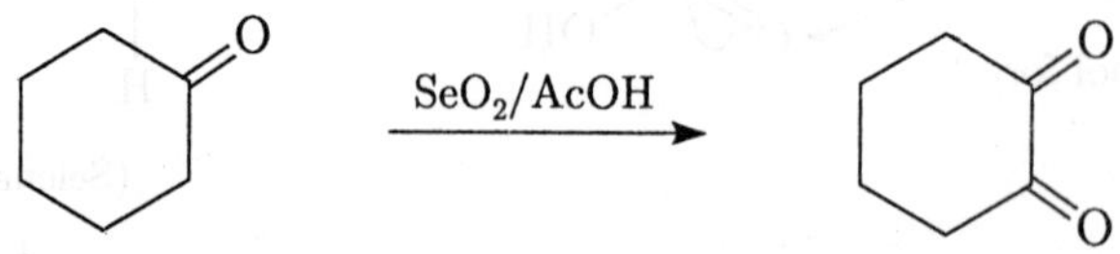

(Cyclohexanone) (Cyclohexan-1,2-dione)

2. ***Allylic hydroxylation and oxidation*** : The methyl or methylene group α–to the most highly substituted end of the double bond is hydroxylated according to the preference of oxidation :$>CH_2> -CH_3> \rightarrow CH$ in a decreasing manner.

(a) $CH_3-CH=C(CH_3)-CH_3 \xrightarrow{SeO_2/AcOH} CH_3CH=C(CH_3)-CH_2OH$

(b) $CH_3CH=C(CH_3)-CH_2CH_3 \xrightarrow{SeO_2/AcOH} CH_3CH=C(CH_3)-CH(OH)CH_3$

(c) $CH_3-C(CH_3)=CH-CH_2CH_3 \xrightarrow{SeO_2/AcOH} CH_3-C(CH_2OH)=CH-CH_2CH_3$

(d) 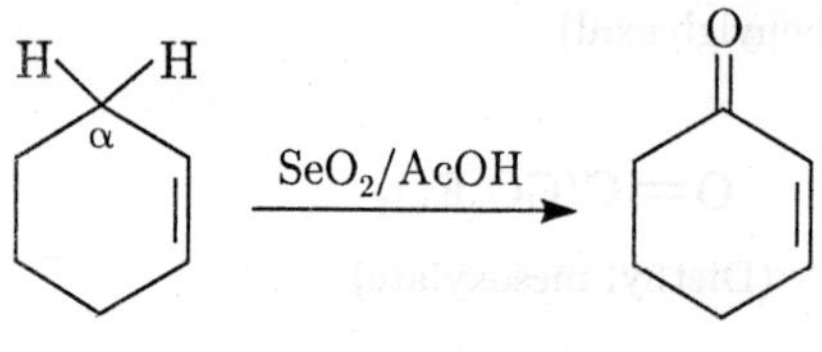

(Ring methylene group at α-position to the double bond is oxidised to ketonic group)

When the cycloalkene is substituted at the double bond, the methylene group at α–position to the substituted end of the double bond is oxidised.

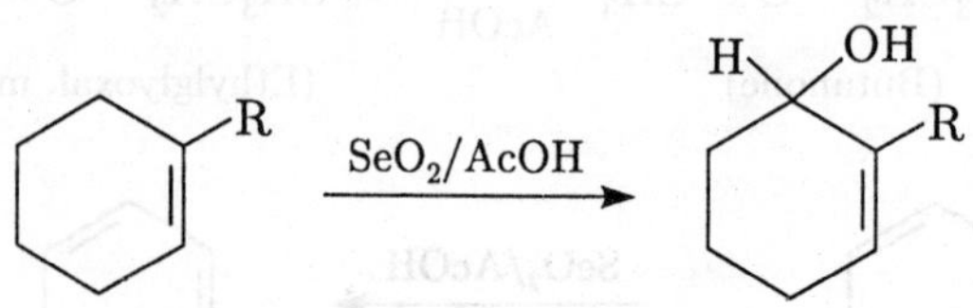

(e) Terminal double bonds are oxidised to primary alcoholic groups along with allylic migration of the double bond.

$$CH_3CH_2CH_2CH=CH_2 \xrightarrow{SeO_2/AcOH} CH_3CH_2CH=CH-CH_2OH$$

3. ***Dehydrogenation*** : SeO_2 is used for dehydrogenation at high temperatures.

(a) $$C_6H_5CH_2OH \xrightarrow{SeO_2/\Delta} C_6H_5CHO$$

(b) $$2CH_3COOH \xrightarrow{SeO_2/\Delta} \begin{array}{l} CH_2COOH \\ | \\ CH_2COOH \end{array}$$

(c) 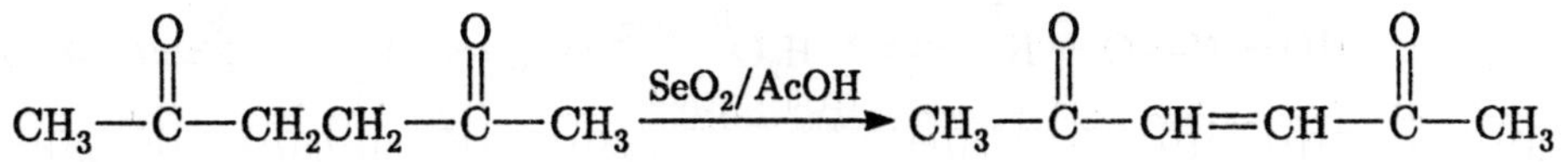

(d) 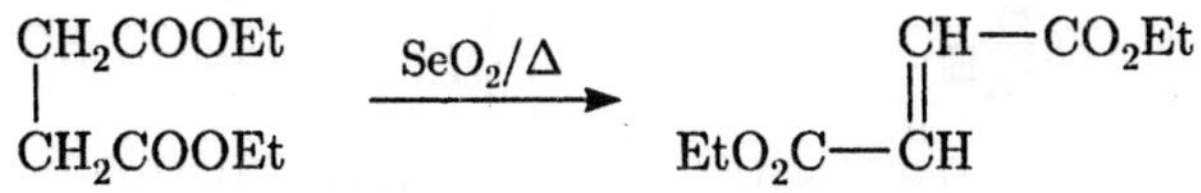

(Diethyl fumarate)

4. ***SeO₂ as a catalyst*** : SeO_2 catalyses the *trans*-hydroxylation of some unsaturated compounds by hydrogen peroxide (H_2O_2).

(a) 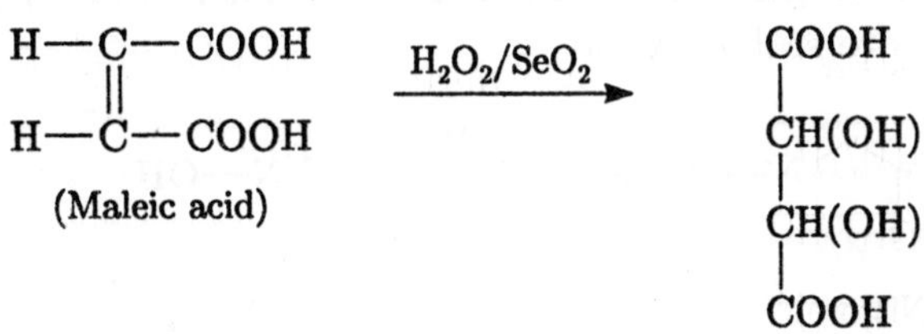

(±)-Tartaric acid

(b) 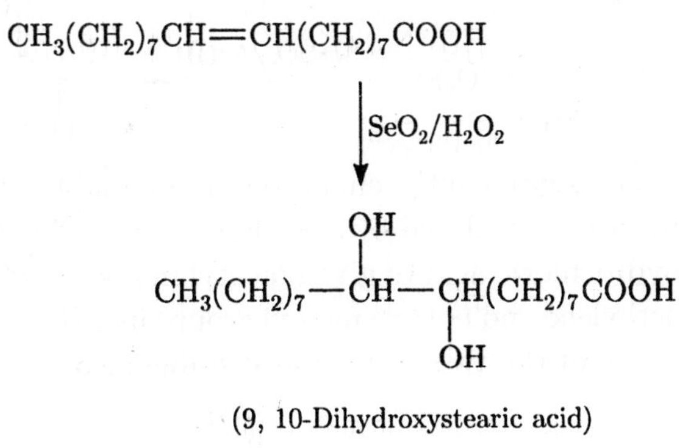

(9, 10-Dihydroxystearic acid)

Substitution at α–Position of Carbonyl Compound by Nitrosation Reaction

The nitroso group may be introduced at the α–position of carbonyl compounds in *two* ways.

1. Carbonyl compounds, which are strongly activated towards electrophiles, react with nitrous acid or an organic nitrile in an acid catalysed process in their *enol forms.* The electrophile is thought to be the nitrosonium ion, $\overset{\oplus}{N}O$.

$$HO-N=O + H^{\oplus} \rightleftharpoons H_2\overset{\oplus}{O}-N=O \rightleftharpoons H_2O + \overset{\oplus}{N}=O \longleftrightarrow N\equiv\overset{\oplus}{O}$$

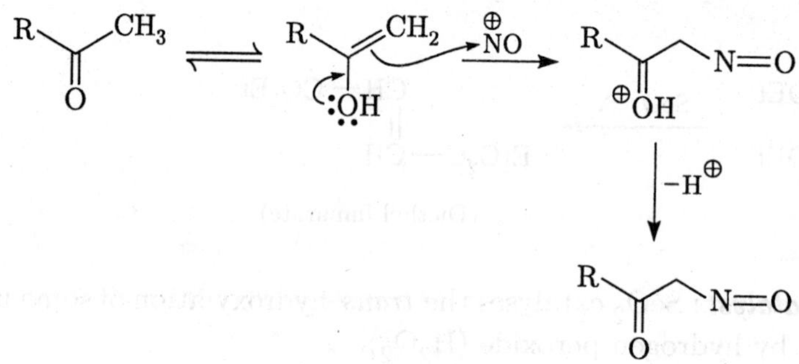

If the product has a hydrogen atom attached to the nitroso bearing carbon, it tautomerises to the more stable oxime.

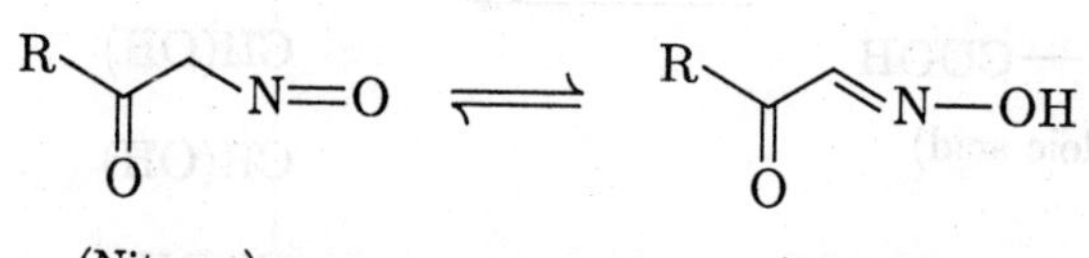

(Nitroso) (Oxime)

For example, acetoacetic ester, when treated in acetic acid solution with aqueous sodium nitrite gives the *oximino derivative.*

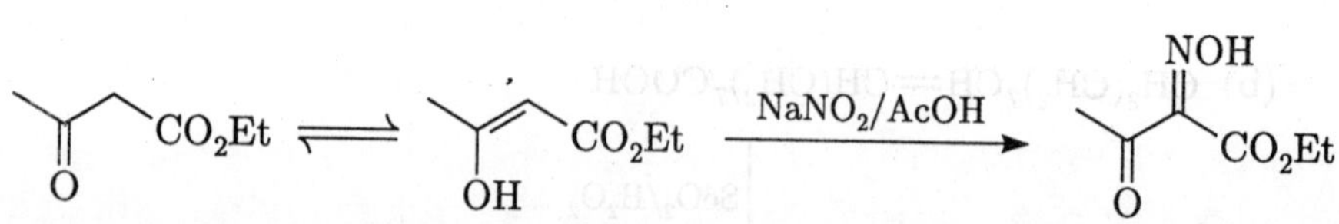

2. Compounds, which are not significantly enolic but are capable of enolisation also react, for the enolisation is catalysed by acid. For example, butanone reacts with ethyl nitrite and hydrochloric acid to give biacetyl in about 70% yield. The reaction occurs at the methylene and not the methyl group since the corresponding enol is formed more readily of the two and is more stable also.

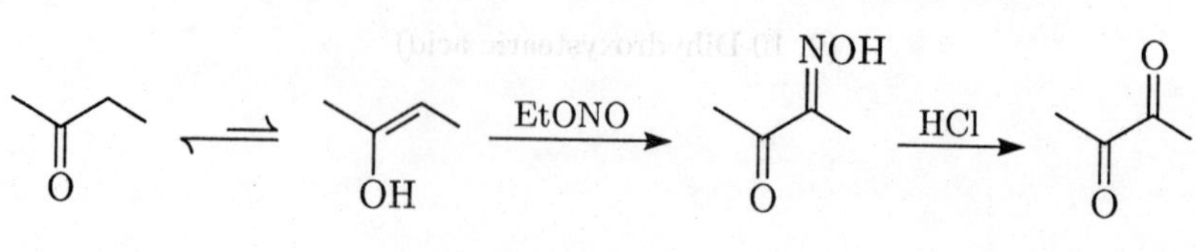

Likewise, nitromethane gives methylnitrolic acid *via* its tautomer.

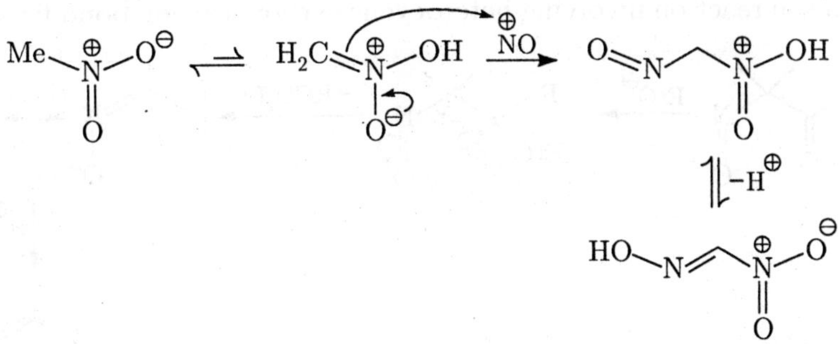

(Methylnitrolic acid)

Preparation of ethyl nitrite

$$NaNO_2 + H^{\oplus} \xrightarrow{\text{aquesus ethanol}} HO—NO$$

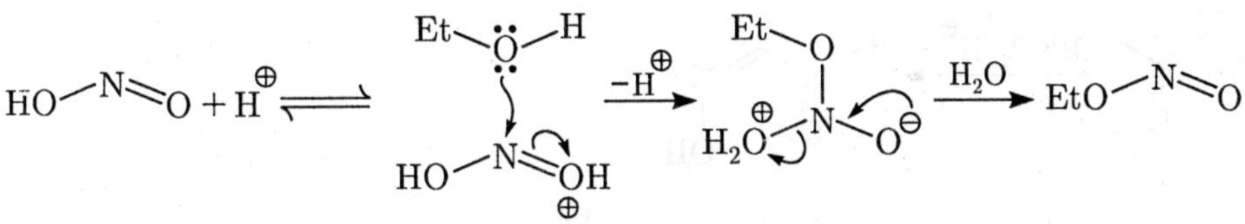

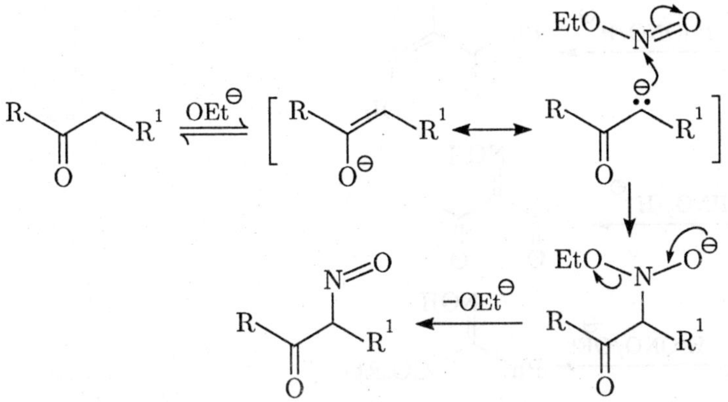

If the product contains a hydrogen atom on the nitrogen leaving carbon, its acidity is such that, it is converted essentially into its delocalised conjugate base. Acidification gives the oxime.

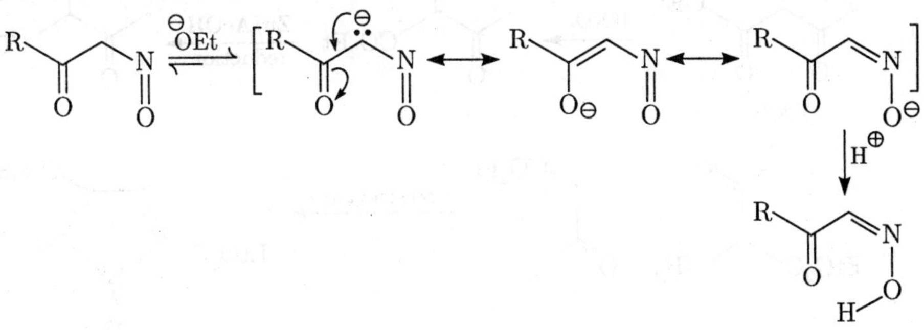

If however, the nitroso product can not be removed from the system in this way, a reverse Claisen reaction involving heterocyclic carbon–carbon bond fission can take place.

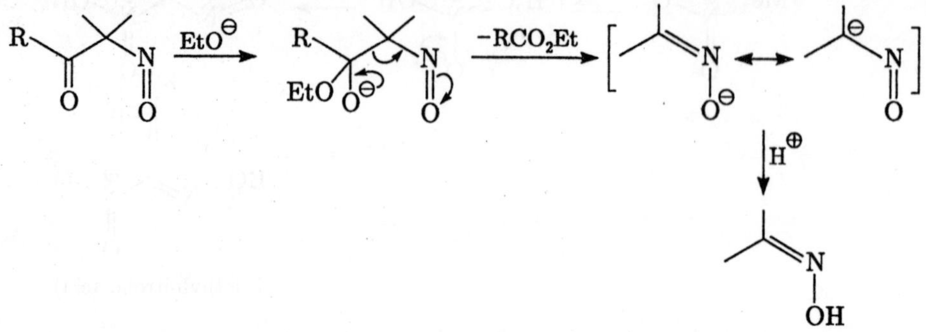

Enols and partially enolic compounds are also those which are capable of giving enolates, so that the acid and base–catalysed methods are alternative procedures. The following examples include both methods.

(a) 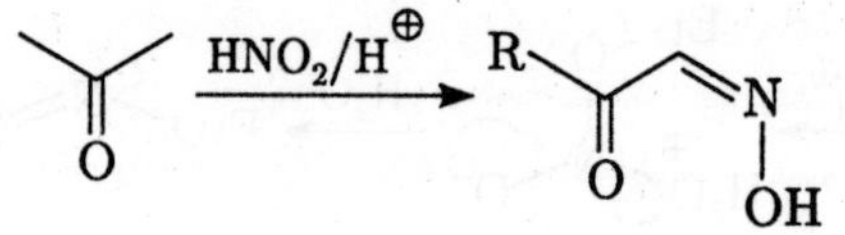

(b) 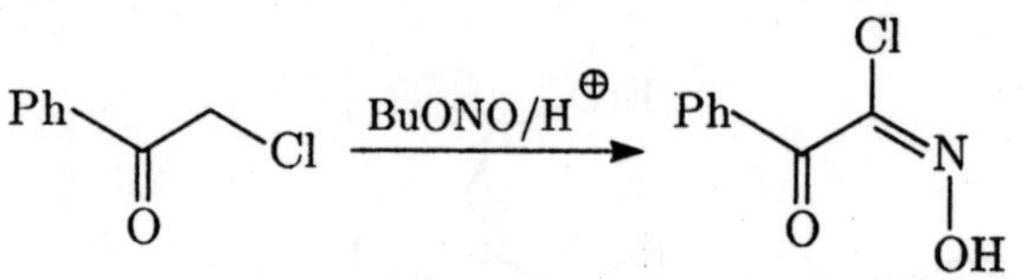

(c) 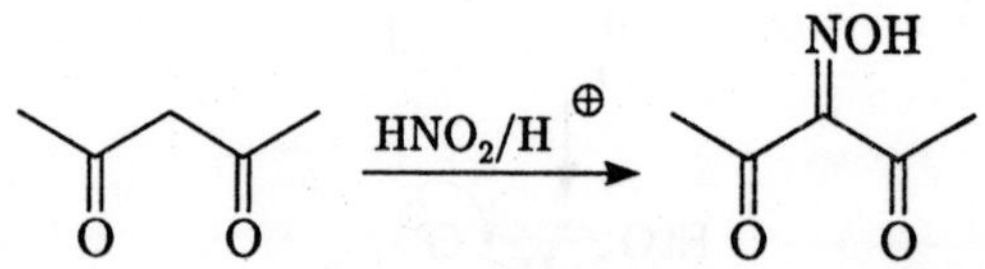

(d) 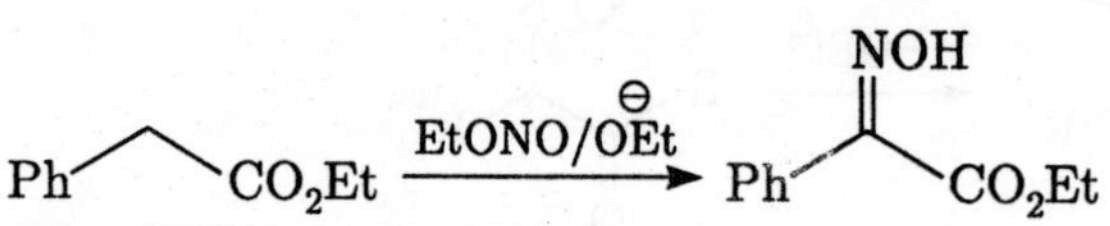

The products of nitrosations have two main synthetic uses. First, reduction leads to amino derivatives. These derived from ketones are unstable because

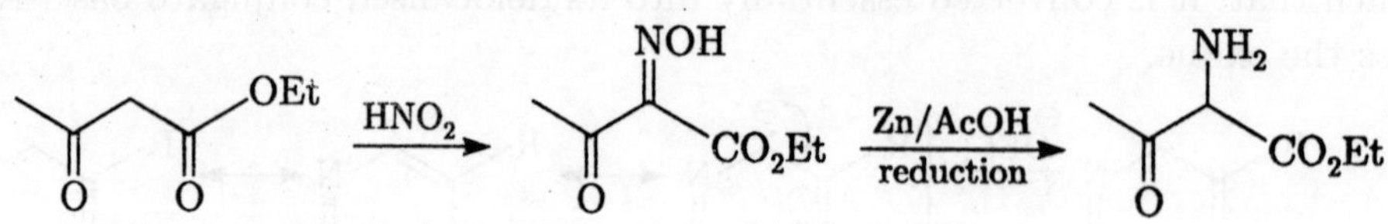

(EAA)

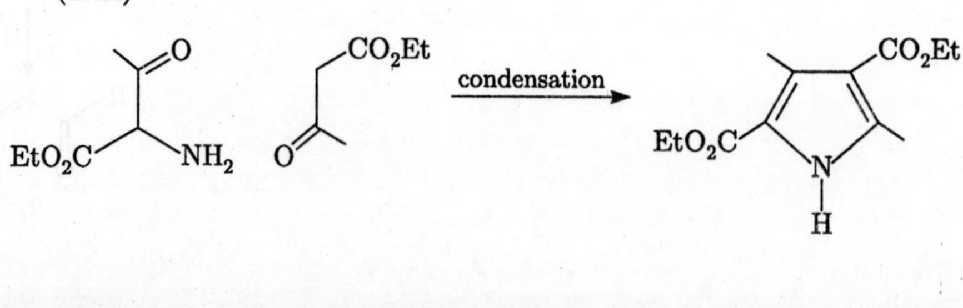

they readily undergo self-condensation, but several heterocyclic syntheses are successfully carried out by reducing β–ketooximes in the presence of compounds with which the products react to form ring systems such as pyrroles.

Second, hydrolysis converts the oxime into a carbonyl group, *e.g.*

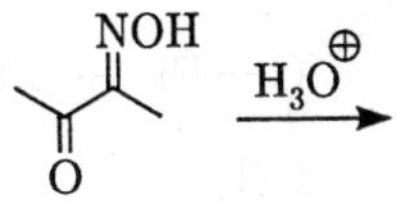

, so that the overall process can be used for the transformation, $-COCH_2-$ to $-\underset{\text{O}}{\underset{\|}{\text{C}}}-\underset{\text{O}}{\underset{\|}{\text{C}}}-$

Substitution at α–Position of Carbonyl Compound by Nitration Reaction

The nitronium ion is generated (NO_2^+ ion) analogously to the nitrosonium ion by treating concentrated nitric acid with a powerful acid such as sulphuric acid. This method is widely used for bonding aromatic carbon to the nitro group, but it is not suitable for the nitration of aliphatic systems because of oxidations and degradations which tend to occur in these rigorous conditions. However, a base catalysed procedure analogous to nitrosation may be used; an enolate forming compound is treated with base in the presence of an organic nitrate. For example, benzyl cyanide and methoxy nitrate (methoxy nitrate is prepared from methyl alcohol and nitric acid in the presence of concentrated H_2SO_4; CH_3ONO_2 is not very stable and is used immediately.) react in the presence of ethoxide ion ($\overset{\ominus}{\text{O}}$Et) ion to give a nitro compound, which on alkaline hydrolysis followed by acidification gives phenylnitromethane.

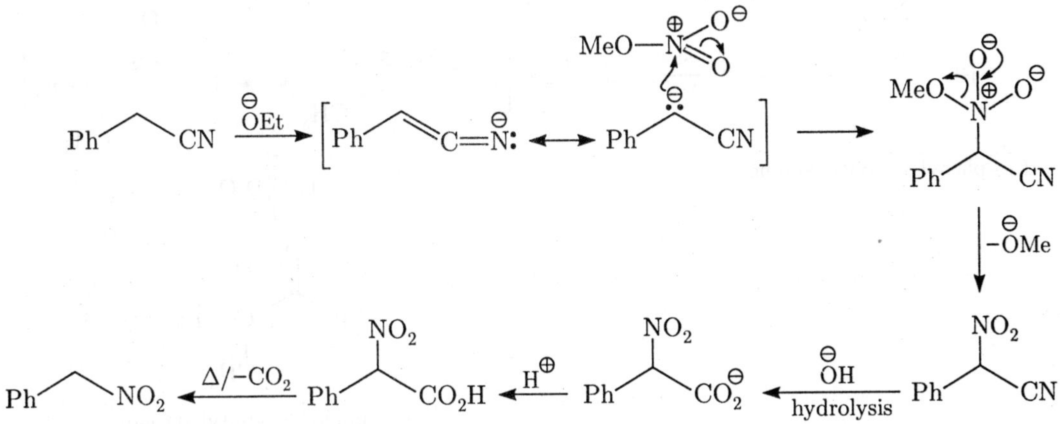

Electrophilic Substitution at α–Position of Carbonyl Compounds

Deuterium exchange : Ketones containing at least one α–hydrogen atom is found to undergo exchange of its α–hydrogen atom for deuterium when treated with base ($OD^{\ominus}$) in solution in D_2O.

When the reaction is carried out on an optically active ketone containing α–H, it undergoes loss of optical activity at the same rate as deuterium exchange. In other words, racemisation occurs at the same rate as deuterium exchange.

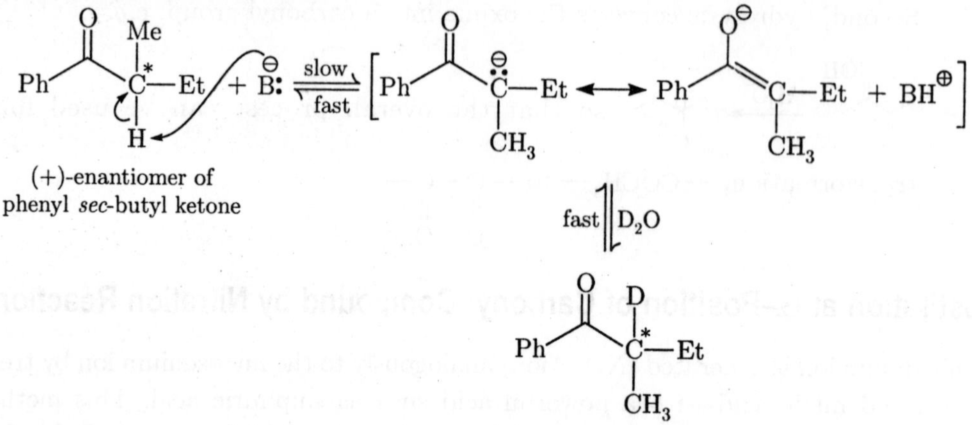

(+)-enantiomer of phenyl *sec*-butyl ketone

(Deuteriated compound)
(±) phenyl *sec*-butyl ketone

Base employed here, generally is NaOD in dioxane/D_2O system. When analogous compound containing D in place of H underwent exchange in H_2O, there was found to be a kinetic isotope effect (k_H/k_D) on comparing the rates of exchange for the two compounds.

All these suggests slow, rate limiting breaking of the C—H bond to form the stabilised carbanion intermediate, followed by fast uptake of $D^{\oplus}$ from the solvent D_2O.

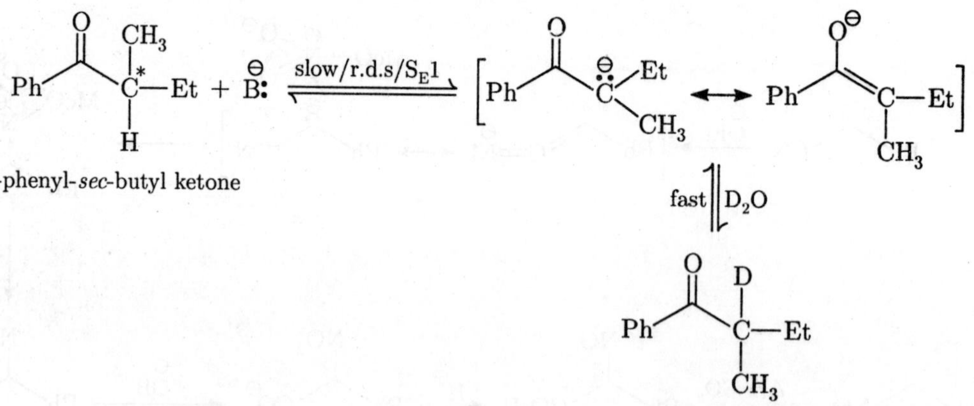

(+)-phenyl-*sec*-butyl ketone

(±) phenyl-*sec*-butyl ketone)
(deuteriated)

Rate = k 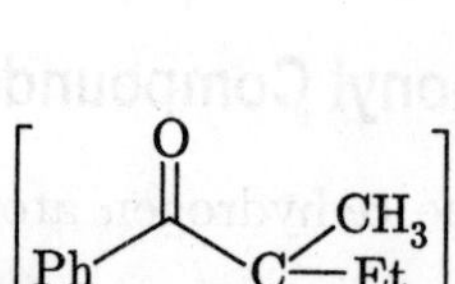 or Rate=k[substrate, *i.e.* ketone]

Although carbanion is pyramidal in geometry, the bonds to the carbanion carbon atom will need to assume a planar configuration if stabilisation by delocalisation over the adjacent C=O is to occur. Subsequent addition of $D^{\oplus}$ is then statistically equally likely to occur from either side to this planar carbanion moiety. This slow, rate determing formation of a carbanion intermediate followed by rapid electrophilic attack to complete the overall substitution is similar to rate limiting carbocation formation in S_N1 pathway. It is therefore referred to as the S_E1 pathway.

Halogenation and Haloform Reaction

α–Hydrogen atoms of a carbonyl compound are active because of the (–I) effect of the carbonyl group. Active α–hydrogen atoms may be replaced by halogen atoms and the process is known as *halogenation reaction.*

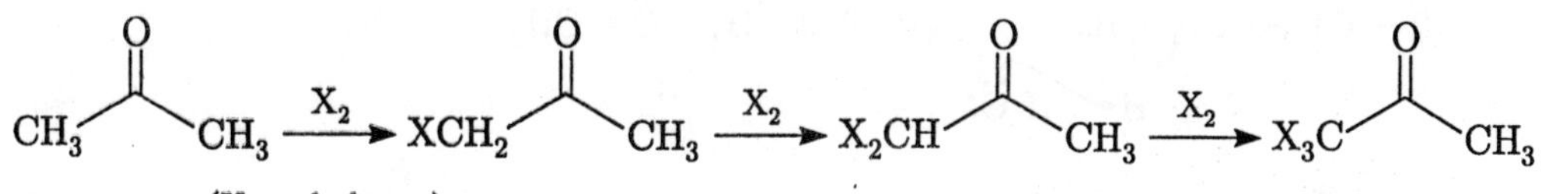

(X = halogen)

Bases promote the halogenation reaction whereas acids catalyse the reaction. The acid catalysed reaction may be stopped at a monohalogenation step and thus, has a preparative value.

(a) 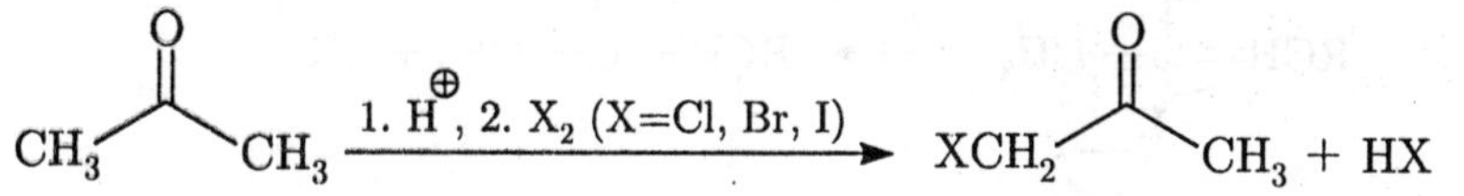

(b) 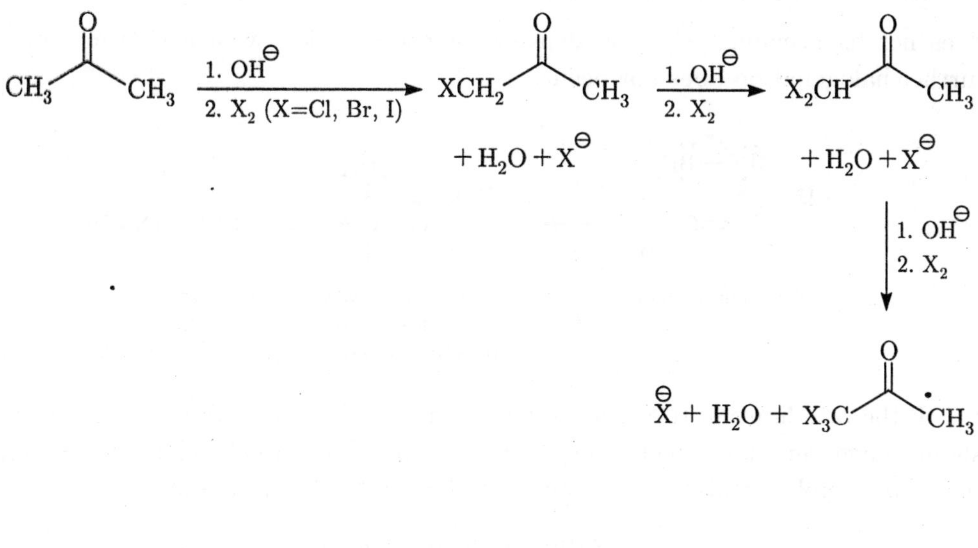

Mechanism of acid–catalysed halogenation reaction :

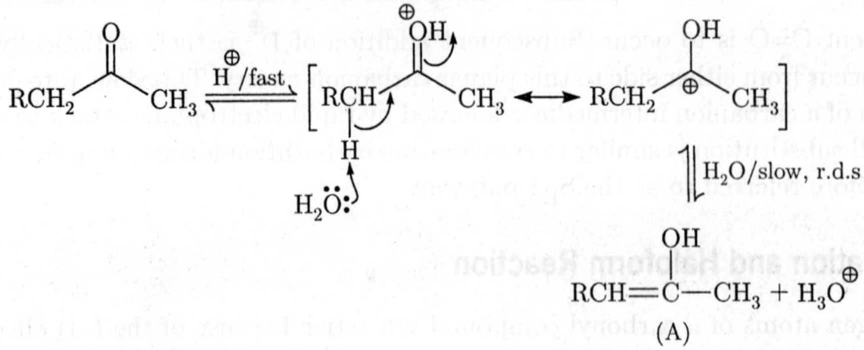

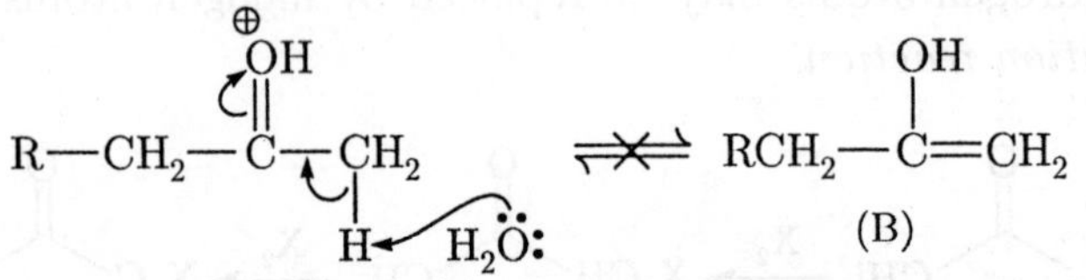

Compound (A) is formed preferentially since the hyperconjugative effects of the H atoms of CH_3 group and R group stabilise (A) more than compound (B) by (+I) effect. Compound (B) has only two H atoms in $—CH_2—$ for hyperconjugation.

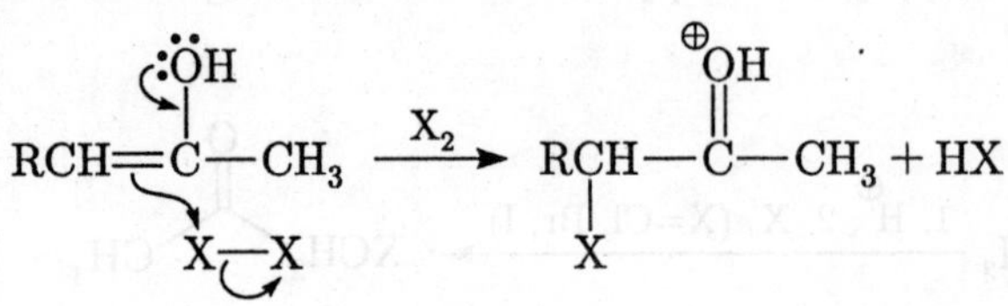

As X of RCH(X) moiety has an –I effect, the oxygen atom of the carbonyl group does not have enough electron density for coordination with a proton and therefore further halogenation does not occur.

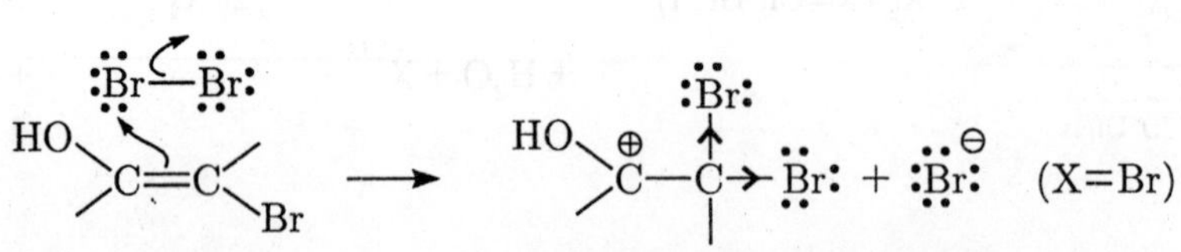

(Halogenated enol)

Carbocation intermediate destabilised by polar effect (electron withdrawing) of two bromines

If the rate limiting transition state resemble this carbocation, then transition state should have very high energy and the rate would be small. The slowest step of the reaction is enol formation and it involves the substrate and the acid only.

$$\text{Rate} = k.\ [\text{substrate}]\ [H^{\oplus}]$$

The reaction is an example of S_E1 reaction. The evidences in favour of the mechanism are as follows.

1. The rates of acid catalysed chlorination, bromination and iodination of acetone are the same, *i.e.*, the rate is independent of the concentration of halogen. In other words, the rate is zero order with respect to halogen.
2. The rate of deuteriation in the presence of heavy water and the rate of acid–catalysed halogenation are the same.
3. The acid catalysed racemesation of an optically active phenyl secondarybutyl ketone and acid catalysed halogenation follow the same rate equation.

   These observations tell us that the enolisation step, *i.e.*, step 1 is the rate–determining step.

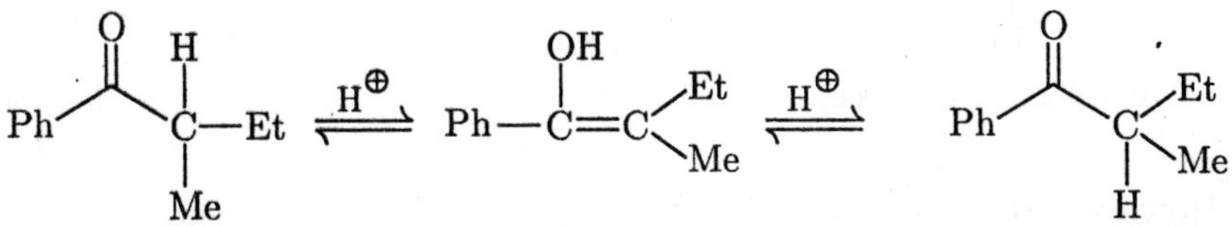

(+)-form (enol form) (±) forms of phenyl secondarybutyl ketone (racemic mixture)

Mechanism of Base–promoted Halogenation Reaction :

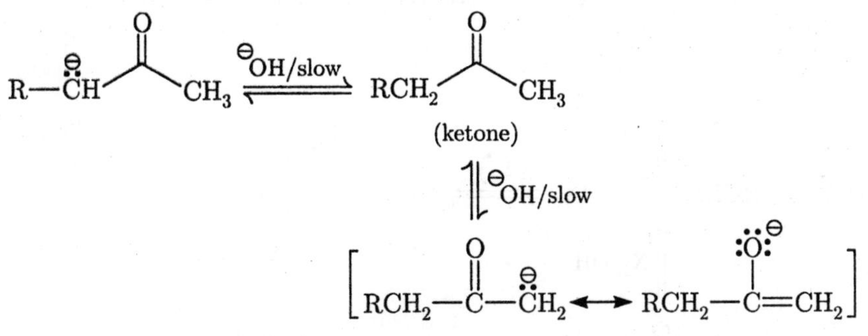

H atom of RCH_2– group is less acidic than hydrogen of CH_3 group. (+I) effect of R group decreases the acidity of RCH_2 moiety.

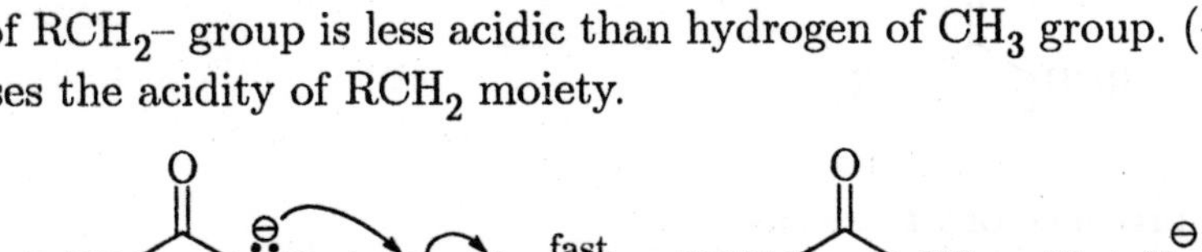

The formation of monohaloderivative follows second order kinetics.

$$\text{Rate} = k[\text{substrate}]\,[\overset{\ominus}{\text{OH}}]$$

Evidences in favour of the mechanism :

1. Reversible formation of the carbanion is supported by the fact that, when the reaction is carried out with $\overset{\ominus}{\text{OD}}/D_2O$, exchange of deuterium occurs.

2. The kinetic studies show that the rate of the reaction is independent of concentration of the halogen but it depends on the concentrations of the substrate and the base.
3. Base promoted halogenation of acetone shows that the rates of bromination and iodination of acetone are the same. It indicates that the rate does not depend on the concentration of halogen taken.
4. The rate of base promoted racemisation of optically active phenyl sec-butyl ketone is the same as that of halogenation.

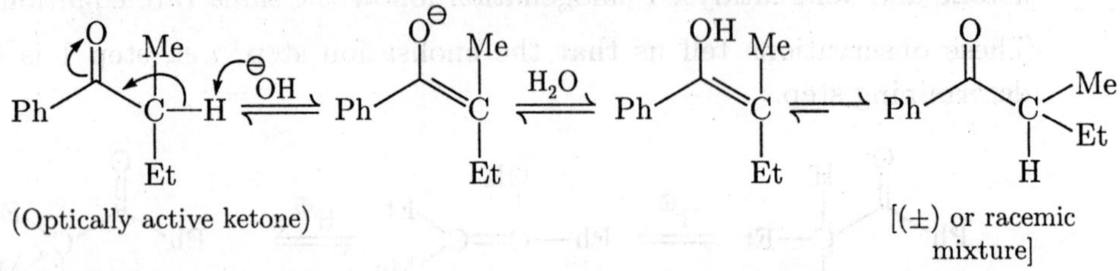

However, the reaction does not stop at the monohalogenated stage, usually a trihalogenated product is formed.

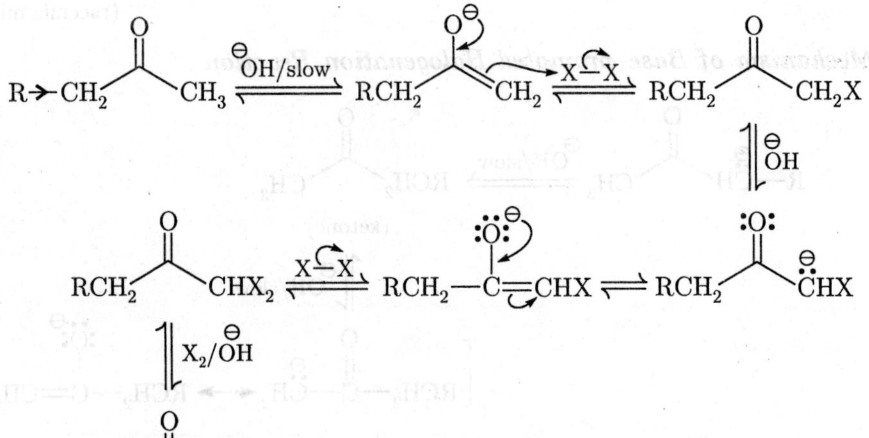

In the presence of *excess* base,

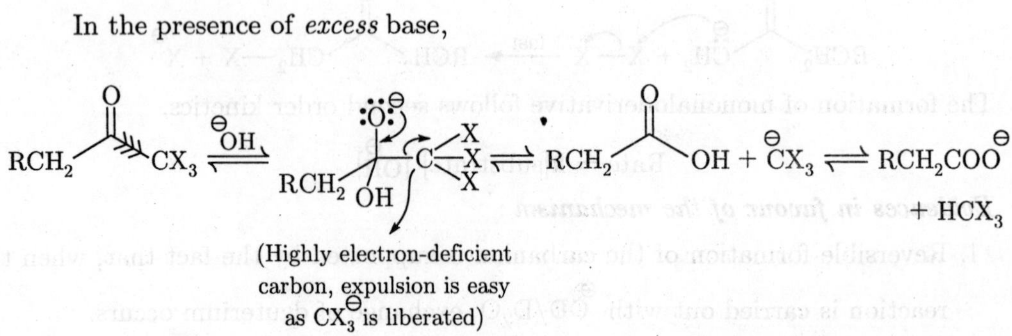

The term "*haloform reaction*" is given to all these reactions which give haloform by the reaction between an organic compound and a halogen atom in alkaline solution. This is a characteristic reaction of a *ketomethyl* or acetyl ($-\overset{O}{\overset{\|}{C}}-CH_3$) group.

For example :

$$\text{(a)}\ R-\overset{O}{\overset{\|}{C}}-CH_3 + \overset{\ominus}{O}H + X_2 \longrightarrow RCO\overset{\ominus}{O} + CHX_3 + 3X^{\ominus} + 3H_2O$$

$$\text{(b)}\ CH_3CHO + \overset{\ominus}{O}H + 3I_2 \longrightarrow HCO\overset{\ominus}{O} + CHI_3 + 3I^{\ominus}$$

$$\text{(c)}\ CH_3CH_2OH + 2NaOX \longrightarrow CH_3CHO + 2NaX + H_2O$$

$$CH_3CHO + NaOX \longrightarrow CHX_3 + HCOONa$$

$$\text{(d)}\ RCH_2CH(OH)CH_3 + NaOX \longrightarrow RCH_2COCH_3 + NaX + H_2O$$

$$RCH_2COCH_3 + \overset{\ominus}{O}H + 3X_2 \longrightarrow RCH_2CO\overset{\ominus}{O} + CHX_3 + 3X^{\ominus} + 3H_2O$$

There are molecules which give haloform reaction beyond our expectation. Isopropyl amine and compounds of the type $RCOCH_2COR$, $RCH(OH)CH_2CH(OH)R$, $CH_3CH(NHCOR)COR$ etc. form haloform on treatment with alkaline halogen solutions. On the other hand, though acetic acid and acetoacetic ester possess ketomethyl group, they do not respond to haloform reaction. However, the reaction takes place merely on mixing a methyl ketone with an alkaline solution of hypohalite. Haloform reaction is an *oxidative degradation* reaction. By this reaction, one can determine whether a compound contains a ketomethyl group or not. In practice, iodoform test is performed instead of chloroform or bromoform tests since iodoform is a *yellow crystalline solid* insoluble in water and can be identified by its melting point. The iodoform reaction is carried out by taking the substance in water and can be identified by its melting point. The iodoform reaction is carried out also by taking the substance in dioxan and treating it first with dilute sodium hydroxide and then with a slight excess of iodine in potassium iodide solution, warming the mixture and finally adding water to it. If the compound contains $-COCH_3$, $CH_3\underset{|}{C}H(OH)$ or it is CH_3CHO or CH_3CH_2OH, yellow precipitate of iodoform (CHI_3) will be obtained.

Besides structure determination, the reaction may be used to prepare aromatic acids where other oxidising agents can not be used. 2-Methylnaphthalene and 2-acetylnaphthalene are succeptible towards oxidation when they are treated with strong oxidising agents. But, 2-napthoic acid is obtained when 2-acetylnaphthalene is treated with alkali and halogen ($NaOH + X_2 \longrightarrow NaOX$, a mild oxidising agent). Sodium hypohalite (NaOX) converts $-COCH_3$ group to carboxylate anion (COO^-) without destroying the aromatic ring.

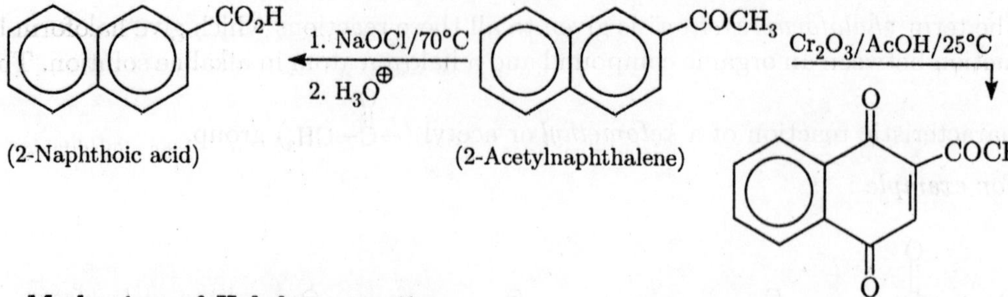

Mechanism of Haloform reaction :

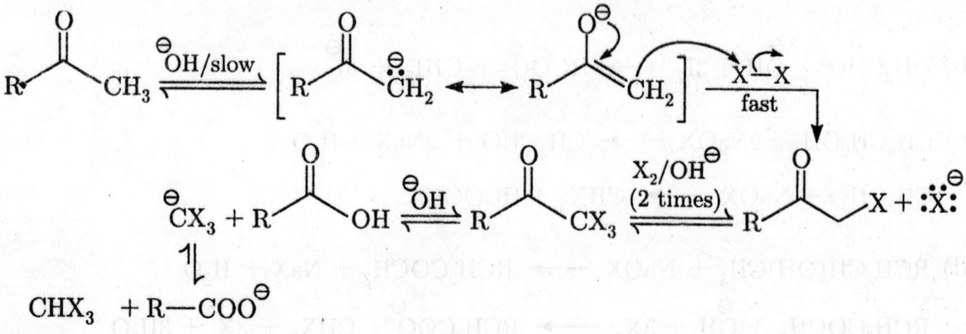

Applications of Haloform reaction :

1. Me_2CHNH_2 responses iodoform test.

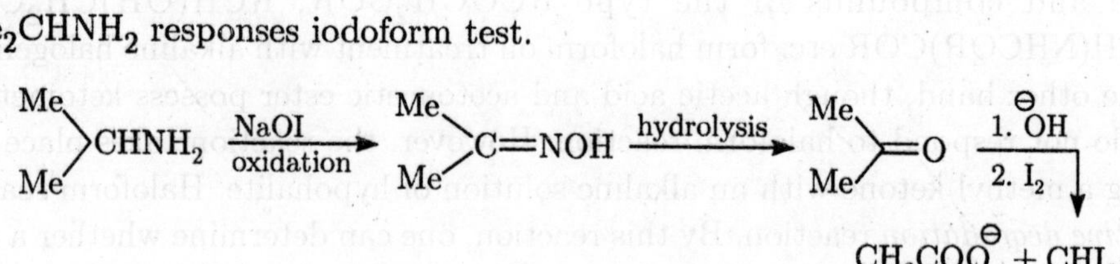

2.

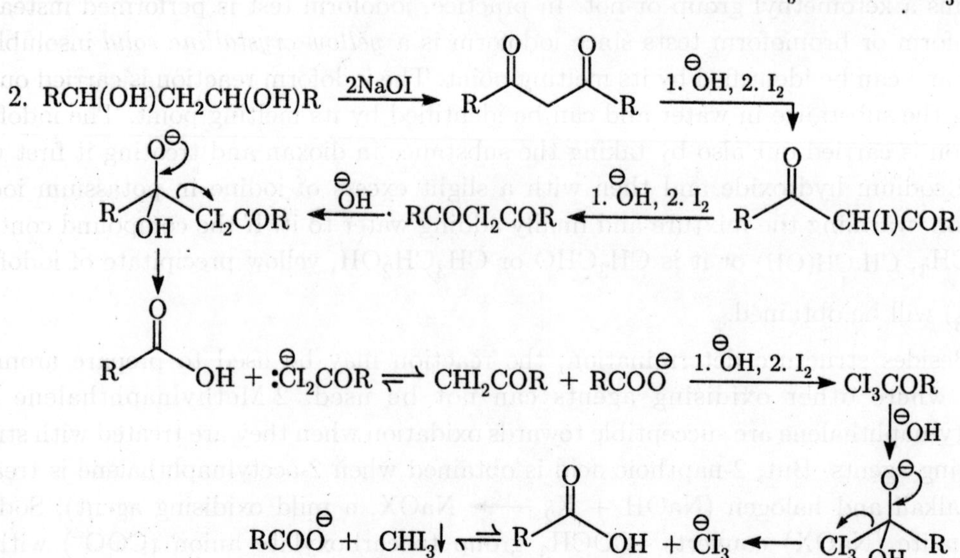

3. Acetoacetic ester and acetic acid do not respond to iodoform test though they contain $CH_3-\overset{\overset{\large O}{||}}{C}-$ group.

(a) $CH_3COOH \xrightarrow{\text{base}} CH_3CO\overset{\ominus}{O}$; $CO\overset{\ominus}{O}$ group has no tendency to withdraw electron from $CH_3-CO\overset{\ominus}{O}$ bond. Thus, the hydrogens of methyl (CH_3) group are no longer acidic. For this reason, acetic acid CH_3COOH does not respond to iodoform test.

(b) 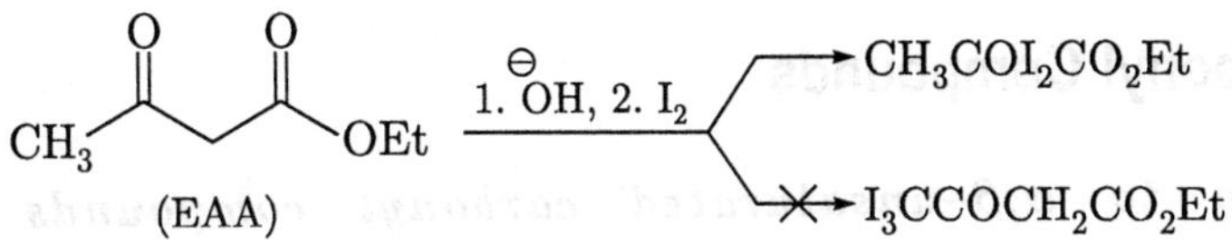

The $-CH_2-$ hydrogens of ethyl acetoacetate (EAA) is more acidic than the end methyl group as the former is flanked by a carbethoxy and a carbonyl group. So when ethyl acetoacetate (CH_3COCH_2COOEt) is treated with an aqueous solution of I_2/KI and aqueous alkali, $CH_3COCI_2CO_2Et$ is formed preferentially.

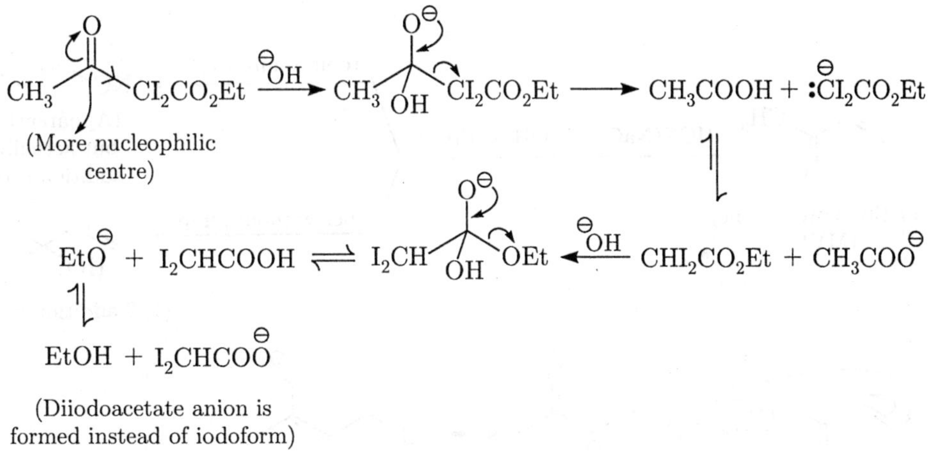

4. Acetone gives iodoform with NH_4OH/I_2 (weaker base) but ethyl alcohol does not. ethyl alcohol (EtOH) forms iodoform (CHI_3) when it is allowed to react with an aqueous solution of NaOH and I_2. Explain.

When ethanol gives iodoform, it first gets converted to CH_3CHO by NaOI (sodium hypoiodite), the latter being an oxidising agent.

$$2NaOH + I_2 \longrightarrow NaI + NaOI + H_2O$$

$$CH_3CH_2OH + NaOI \longrightarrow CH_3CHO$$

and then iodoform reaction proceeds well with CH_3CHO. But with NH_4OH/I_2 we do not get any NH_4OI which can oxidise CH_3CH_2OH to CH_3CHO. CH_3COCH_3

possesses the required $-\underset{\underset{O}{\|}}{C}-CH_3$ group and thus responses even in weaker alkali (NH_4OH and I_2) as no further oxidation is needed here.

$$NH_4OH + I_2 \not\rightleftharpoons NH_4OI + NH_4I + H_2O$$

$$CH_3CH_2OH + NH_4OI \not\rightleftharpoons CH_3CHO$$

(No further reaction is possible to form iodoform)

α, β–Unsaturated Carbonyl Compounds

Nucleophilic addition to α,β–unsaturated carbonyl compounds : An α,β–unsaturated carbonyl system and many other similar systems may be looked upon a single functional group consisting of two parts, a carbonyl and a C=C part. When one specific part undergoes the reaction of a single functional group and not the other, the reaction may be called a regioselective one. For example, hydrocyanic acid (HCN) adds to methyl vinyl ketone in two ways.

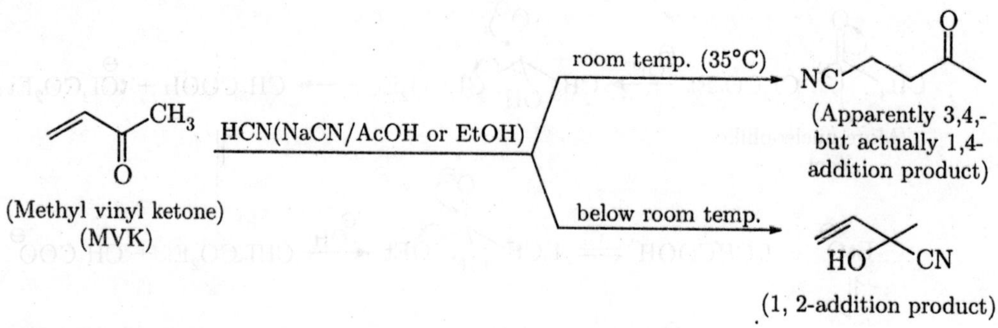

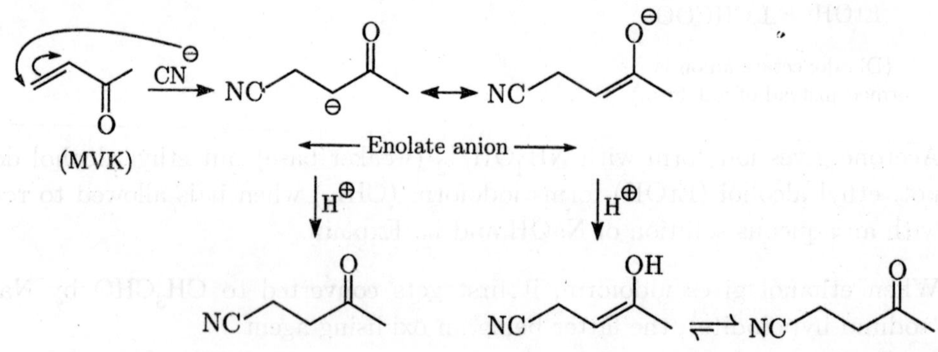

The enolate anion is resonance stabilised. This enolate anion can protonate either on oxygen or on carbon as shown above. In either case, the carbonyl group is generated. With normal double bond, hydrocyanic acid (HCN) does not add to it. (⁀⁀ + HCN $\xrightarrow{r.t}$ no reaction); hydrocyanic acid (HCN) being a very weak acid as H–CN bond is mostly *covalent*, does not form enough proton to form the protonium ion complex with an alkene). So the electrophilic addition does not occur.

Why the same reactant (HCN) under two reaction conditions give two addition reactions (both are regioselective) with the same substrate, follow some *general principles.*

1. Carbon oxygen double bond (C=O) is more stable than carbon carbon double bond (C=C) under the same environment. So 1,4– or conjugate addition product is the thermodynamically controlled product where C=O is retained and C=C bond is destroyed. (carbon–carbon π–bond dissociation energy is 264 kJ/mol and carbon–oxygen π–bond dissociation energy is 390 kJ/mol).

2. Kinetically, C–4 atom $(\underset{4}{CH_2}=\underset{3}{CH}-\underset{2}{\overset{\overset{1}{O}}{\overset{\|}{C}}}-CH_3)$ is a soft acid whereas carbonyl carbon is a hard acid. So, a strong base or hard nucleophile tends to undergo 1, 2–addition (SHAB PRINCIPLE) through *hard-hard* interaction, while a weak base or soft nucleophile tends to undergo 1,4–addition, through *soft–soft* interaction.

3. The 1,4–addition is more easily reversed than 1,2–addition. With softer nucleophiles, the reaction becomes more reversible, *i.e.*, conjugate or 1,4–addition is favoured. In general, RLi, $:\overset{\ominus}{N}H_2$, $R\ddot{\underset{..}{O}}:^{\ominus}$ and $H:^{\ominus}$ are hard nucleophiles which undergo 1,2–addition and $R\ddot{\underset{..}{S}}:^{\ominus}$, neutral amines, RMgX (R=alkyl) and stable carbanions are soft nucleophiles which undergo 1,4–additions.

***Examples* :**

1. 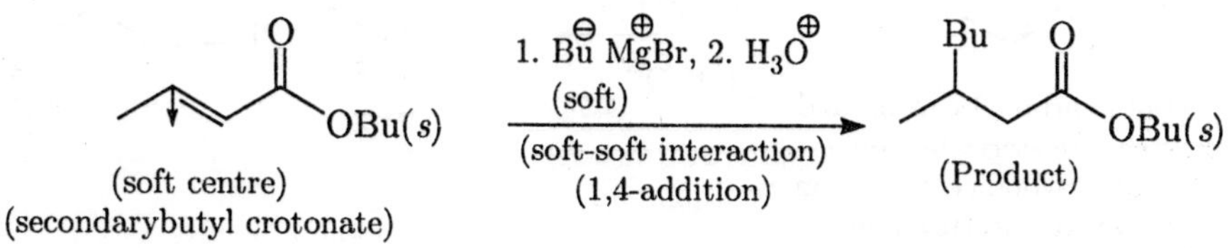

2. 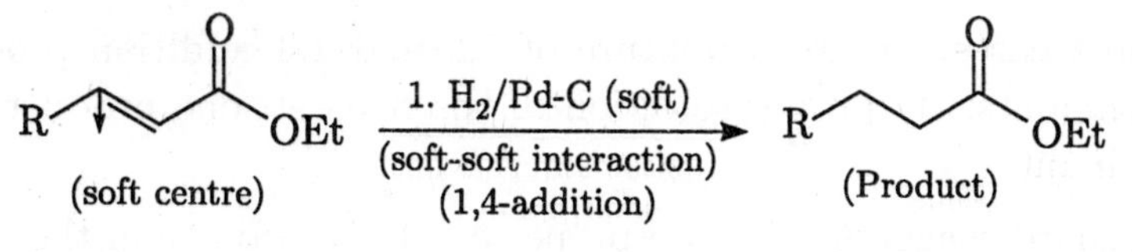

3. 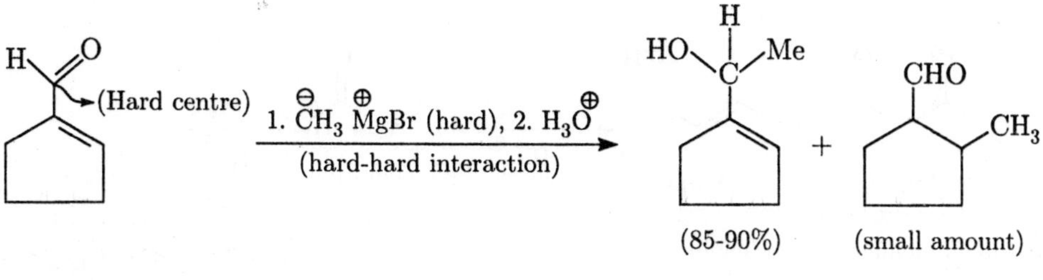

What is conjugate addition?

An addition to the double bond of an α, β–unsaturated carbonyl compound is called a *conjugate addition.* The nucleophilic conjugate addition, such as the addition of cyanide to ethyl crotonate $CH_3CH{=}CHCO_2Et$ has no parallel reactions of butadiene. Such reactions are in general known as **Michael additions.**

Whether direct addition or conjugate addition will predominate, depends on steric and electronic factors. If the carbonyl carbon is sterically congested, then conjugate addition will occur more readily than the direct addition. On the other hand, if β–carbon is more congested, direct addition will take place.

Examples :

1. 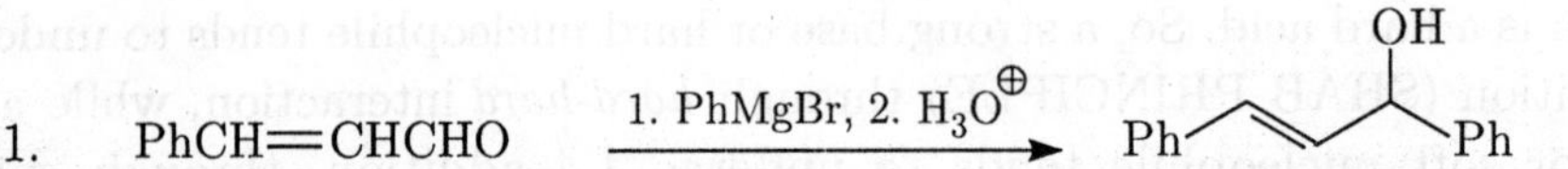

(Carbonyl carbon has no steric congestion whereas β-carbon contains bulky phenyl group)

(1,2-addition product) (100%)

2. 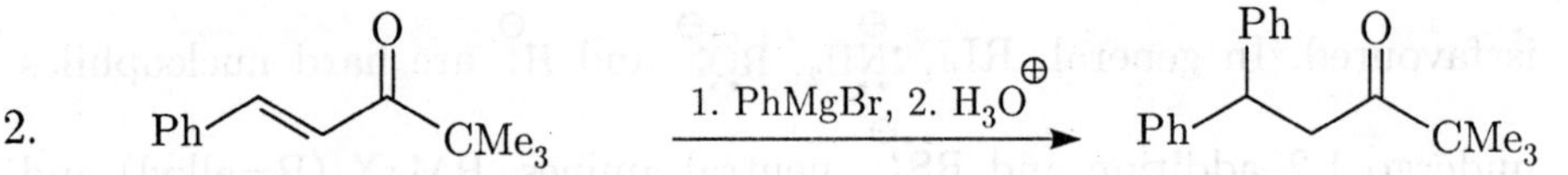

(Carbonyl carbon is sterically congested to compared β-carbon)

(1,4-addition product) (100%)

3. 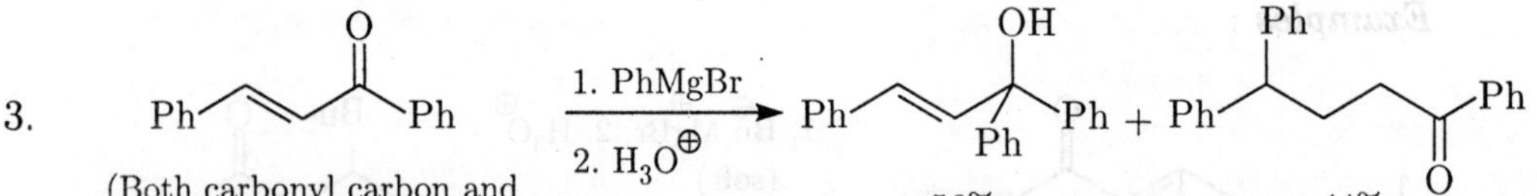

(Both carbonyl carbon and β-carbon are sterically congested. Carbonyl carbon centre becomes weakly electrophilic due to congestion)

In fact, in most cases, we get a mixture of 1,2–and 1,4–addition products in comparable amounts. By proper selection of the reagent, one product may be made predominant.

4. Aliphatic Grignard reagents are more prone to 1,4–addition than the aromatic ones.

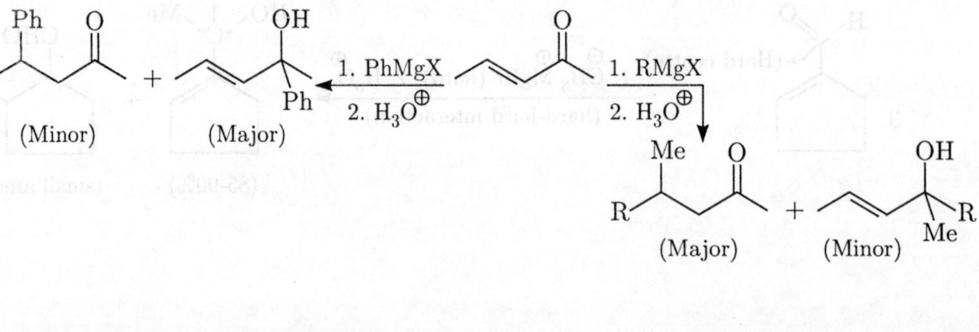

5. Organolithiums undergo 1,2–addition in better yield than the corresponding Grignard reagents.

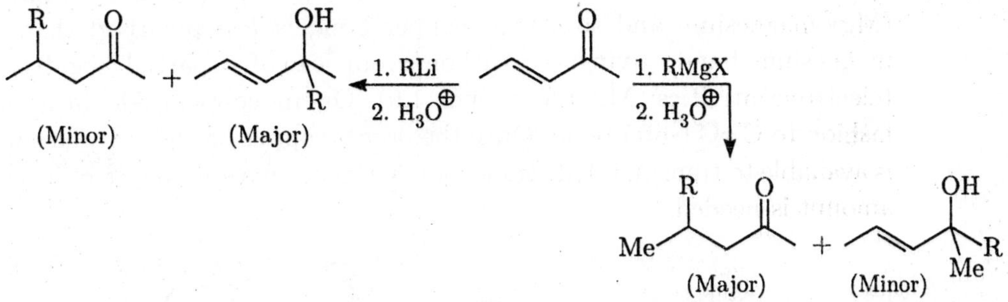

6. The inclusion of a copper (I or II) salt in the addition reactions of organo–lithiums and Grignard reagents to an α, β–unsaturated system promotes 1,4– or conjugate addition.

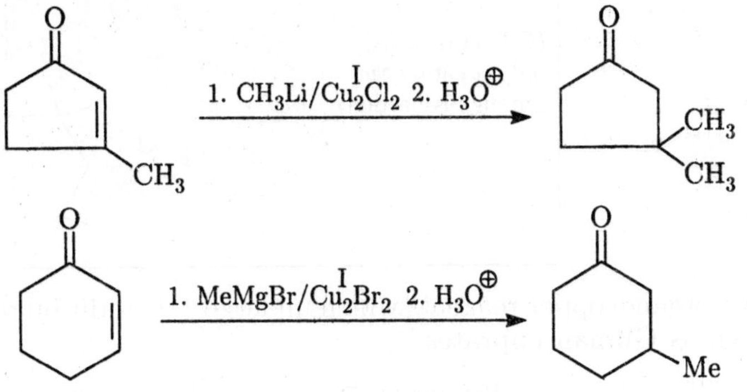

Explanation :

Copper (I) salts have a remarkable effect on oganometallic reagents.

'Hard' Grignard reagents prefer to add 'hard' C=O electrophilic centre rater than to 'soft' C=C centre.

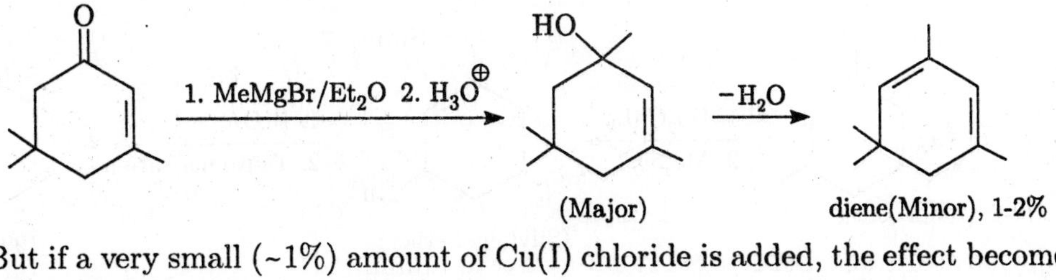

But if a very small (~1%) amount of Cu(I) chloride is added, the effect becomes dramatic. It makes the Grignard reagent undergo conjugate addition, practically no diene is formed.

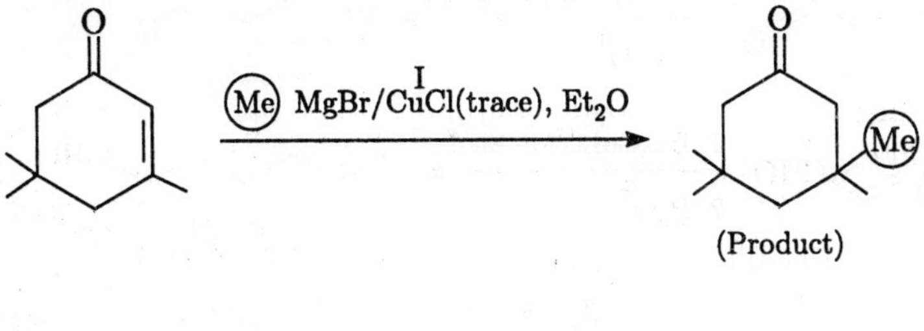

Organocopper reagents undergo conjugate addition : The copper works by transmetallating Grignard reagent to give an organocopper reagent. Organocoppers are *softer* than Grignard reagents because copper is less electropositive than (Mg) magnesium and so carbon-copper bond is *less* polarised than carbon–magnesium bond, giving the carbon atom less of a partial negative charge. (electronegativities: Mg 1.3, copper 1.9). Organocoppers add in a conjugate fashion to C=C (soft) bond. Once the organocopper has added, the copper salt is available to transmetallate some more Grignard reagent and so only a catalytic amount is needed.

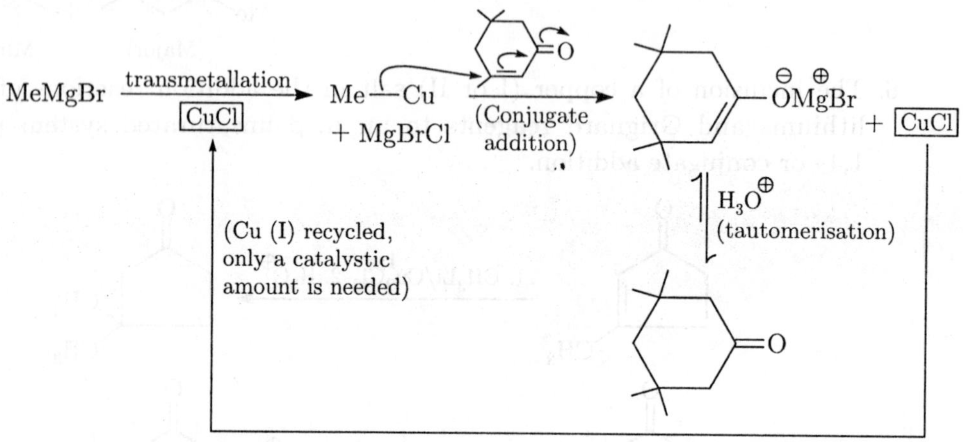

Other organocopper reagents which undergo 1,4–addition reactions are $R_2Cu^{\ominus}Li^{\oplus}$, known as **Gilman cuprates**.

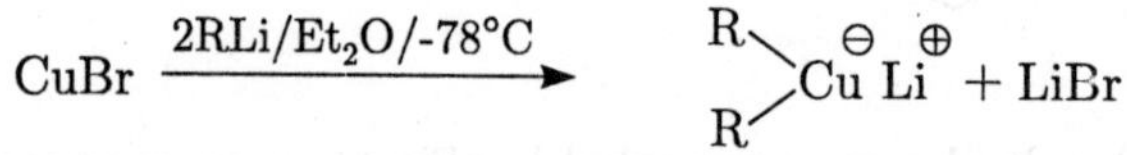

(Lithium cuprate)
(not stable, may form tetramer; to be used immediately)

7. (a)

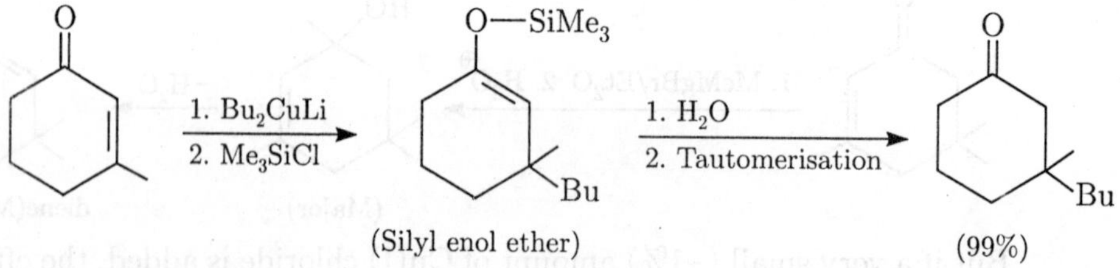

(b)

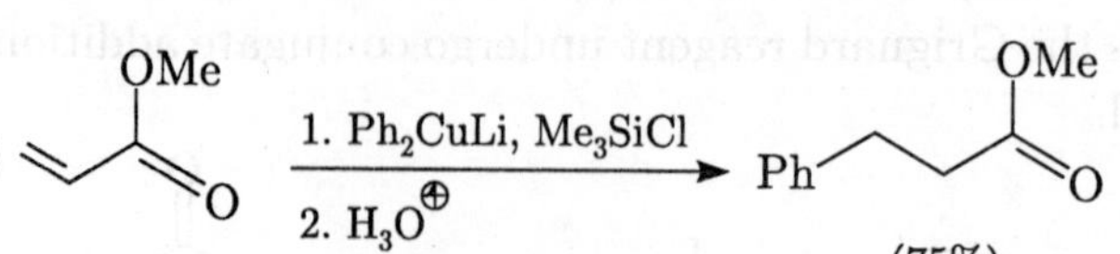

(c)

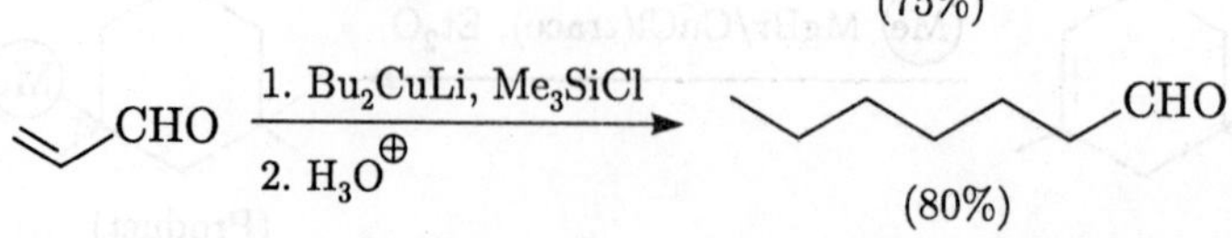

Summary

Conjugate or 1,4–addition is favoured by,

1. Thermodynamic control like high temperature, long reaction hour etc.
2. Unreactive C=O group (amide, ester etc.)
3. Unhindered β–carbon.
4. Soft nucleophiles.
5. Organocopper or catalytic Cu(I).

Direct or 1,2-addition is favoured by,

1. Kinetic control like low temperature, short reaction hour etc.
2. Reactive C=O group (aldehyde, acyl chloride)
3. Hindered β-carbon.
4. Hard nucleophiles.
5. Organolithium, Grignard reagents etc.

Applications :

1. 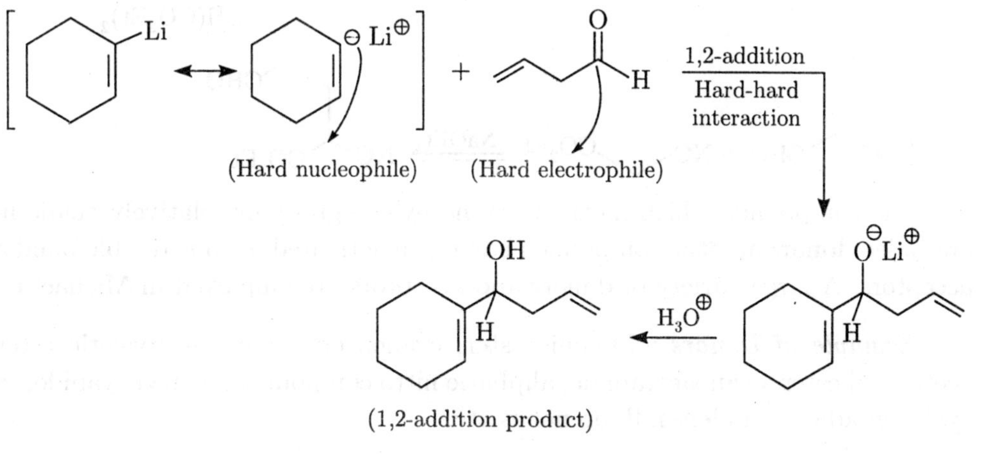

2. 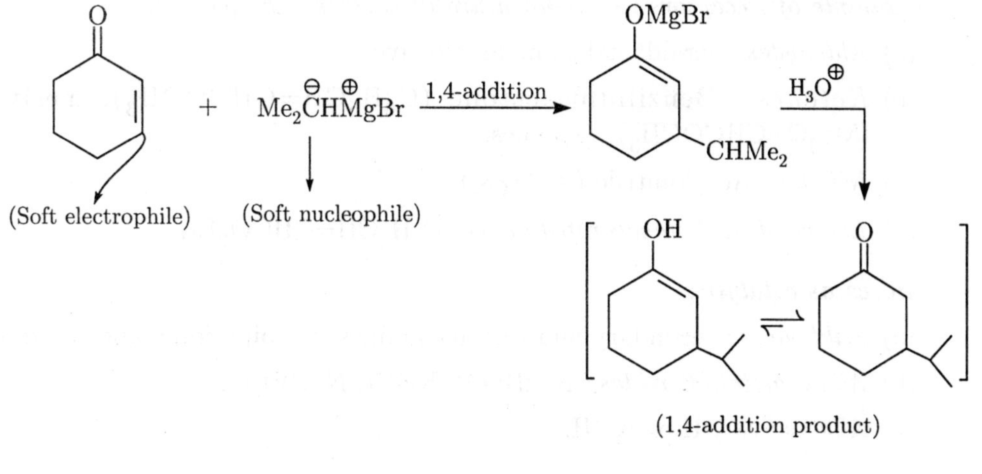

3. 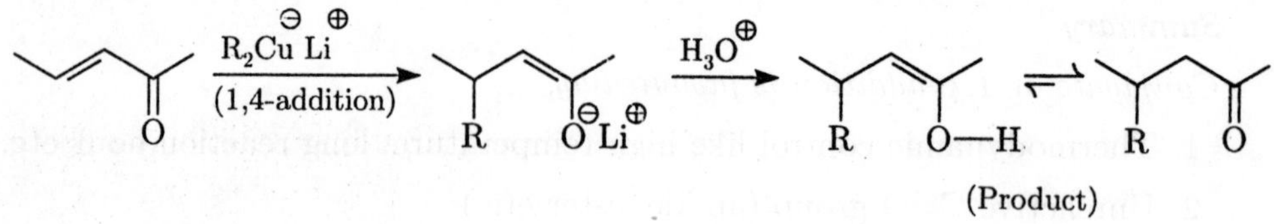

The Michael Reaction

The base-catalysed addition of compounds having active methylene group (or relatively acidic hydrogens) to an activated olefinic bond of the type –C=C–Z (Z=electron withdrawing) is classified as **Michael reaction**. The bases commonly used are alkali, alkoxides, secondary amines etc.

Examples :

(a) 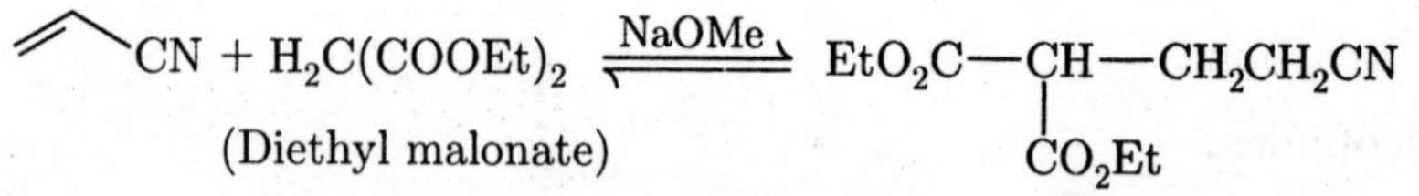

(b) 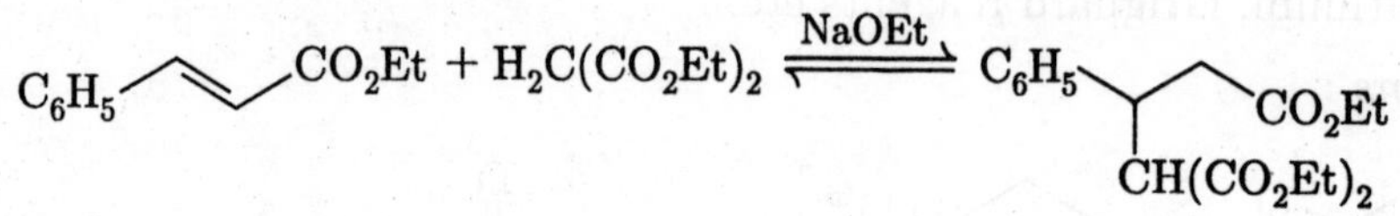

(c) 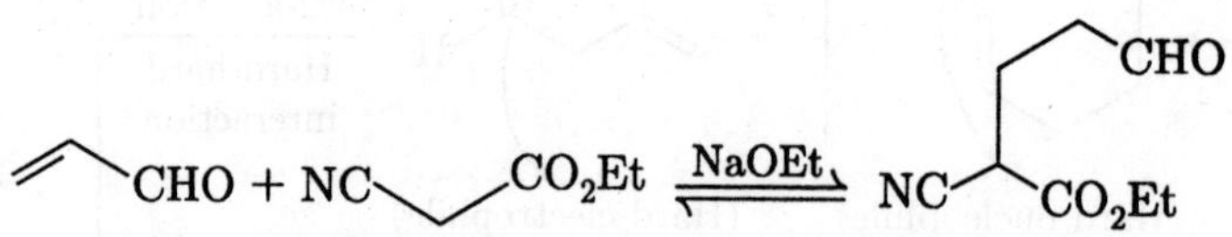

The compounds which have active methylene group or relatively acidic hydrogens are called **donors** and the compounds having an activated olefinic double bond are called **acceptors**. A large variety of donors and acceptors are employed in Michael reaction.

Example of Donors : Malonic ester, cyanoacetic ester, acetoacetic ester, phenyl acetic acid ester, cyanoacetamide, aliphatic nitro compounds, benzyl cyanide, sulphones, cyclopentadienes, indenes, fluorenones etc.

Example of Acceptors : *α, β–unsaturated carbonyl compounds:*

(a) *Aldehydes* : acraldehyde, cinnamaldehyde

(b) *Ketones* : Benzilidineacetone ($C_6H_5CH{=}CHCOCH_3$), mesityl oxide ($Me_2C{=}CHCOCH_3$), quinones.

(c) *Nitriles* : Acrylonitrile (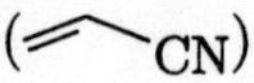)

(d) *Esters of α, β–unsaturated acids* : $C_6H_5CH{=}CHCO_2Et$.

Bases as catalyst :

(a) *Mild bases* : secondary and tertiary amines like piperidine and pyridine.

(b) *Alkali metal alkoxides* : $K^+ tBuO^-$, KOEt, NaOEt etc.

(c) *Alkalis* : NaOH or KOH.

Mechanism of Michael reaction :

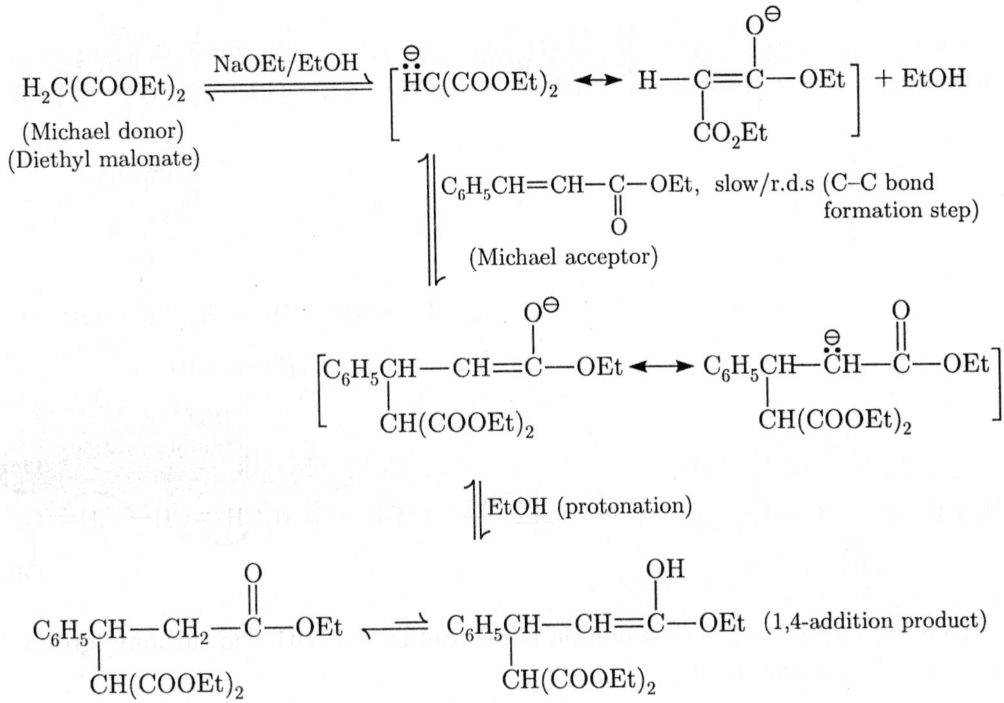

Although 1,4–addition occurs initially, the final product is 3,4–addition leading to more stable ketone. In the presence of strong bases, cyclisation may occur, which can be avoided by using mild bases like secondary or tertiary amines like piperidine.

Compounds with two double bonds in conjugation with the electron withdrawing group may undergo nucleophilic attack at *β–carbon* or *δ–carbon* to give a total of *three products.*

(a) ***Attack at β–carbon*** :

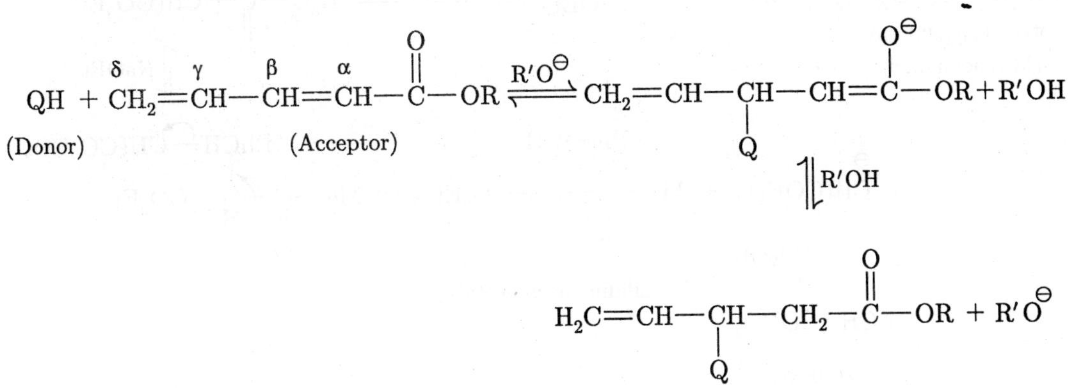

(Product I)

(b) ***Attack at δ–carbon*** :

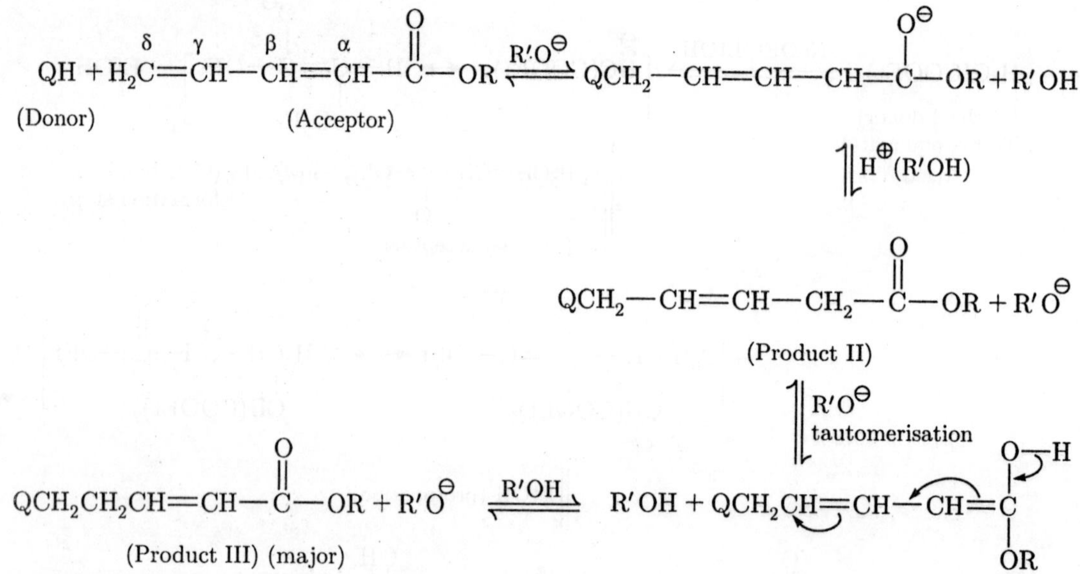

Since product III contains a double bond conjugated with the carbonyl group, this product will be predominant.

Michael addition reaction is *reversible.* Michael 3,4–addition products (*i.e.*, addition products across the double bond) may often be decomposed by heating with or without alkali, to produce products different from the starting substrate. This is known as Michael retrogression or reversal.

Example :

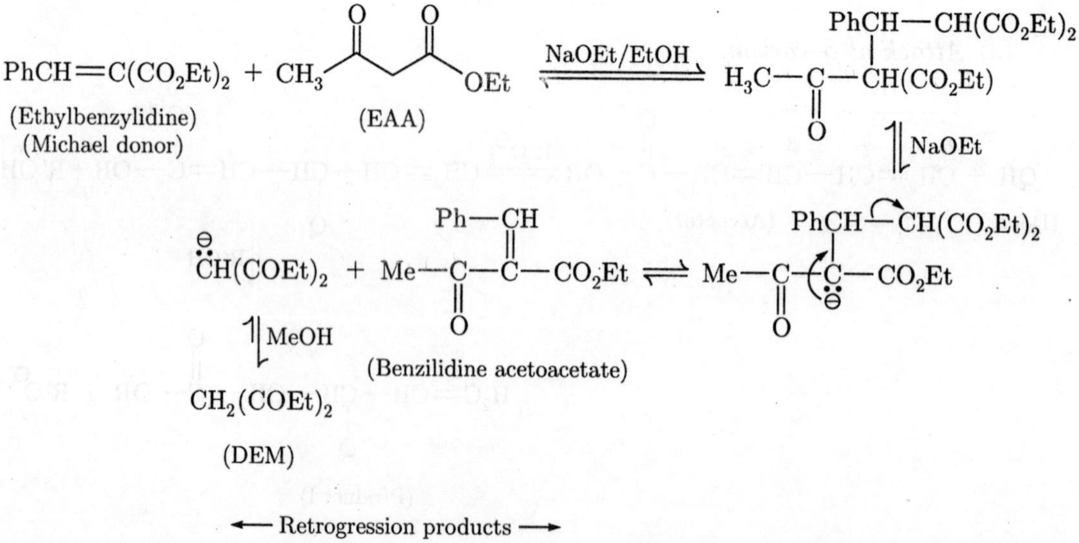

← Retrogression products →

***Examples of Michael reaction* :**

1. 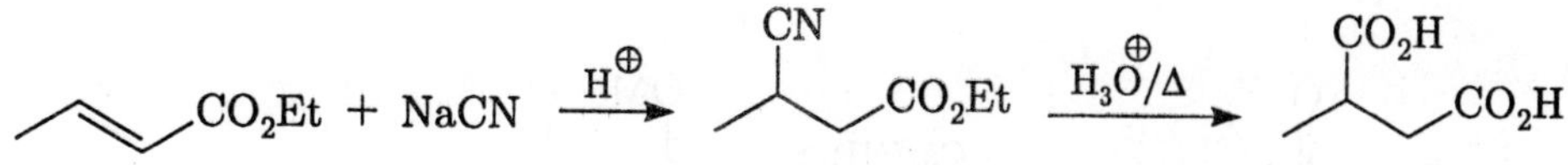

2. 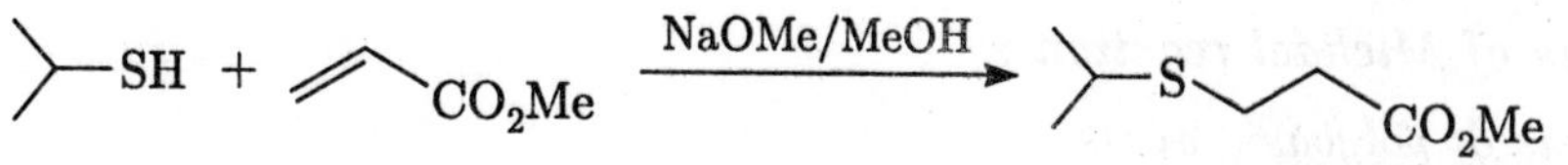

3. 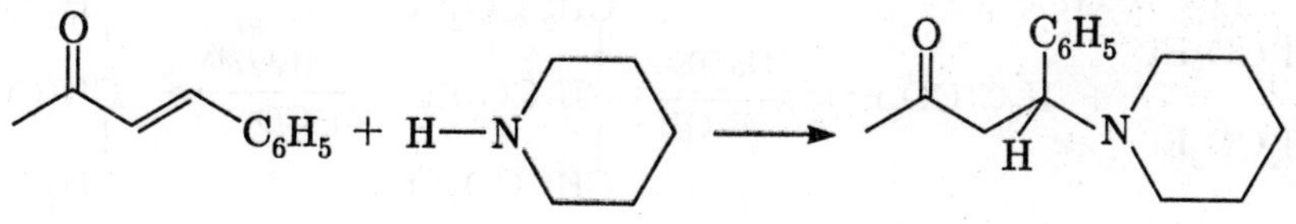

4. 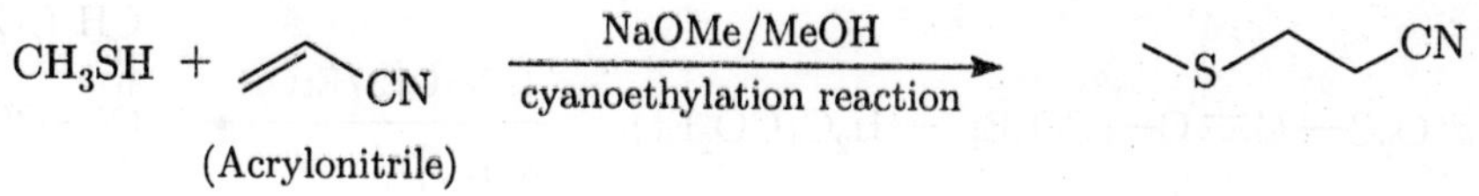

5. 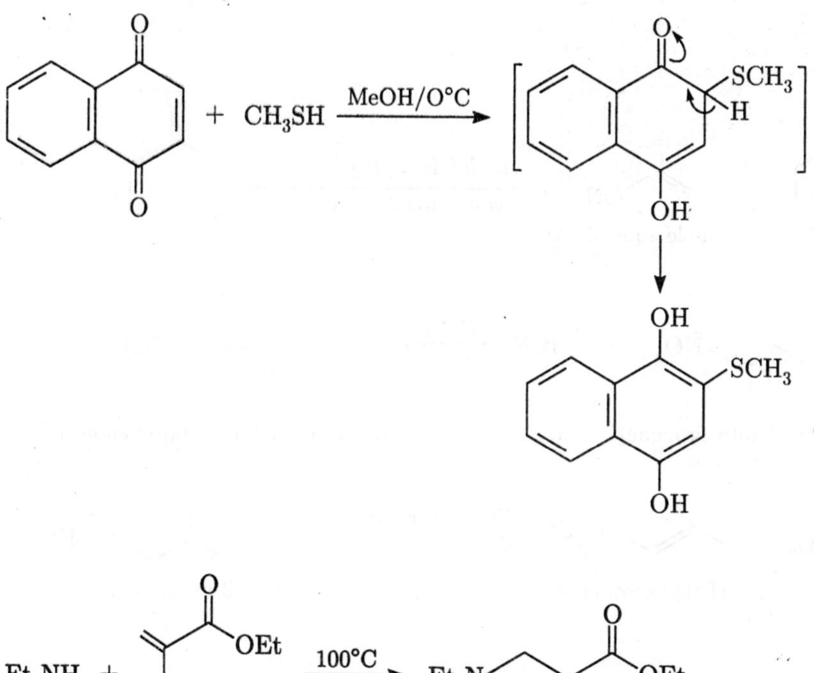

6. 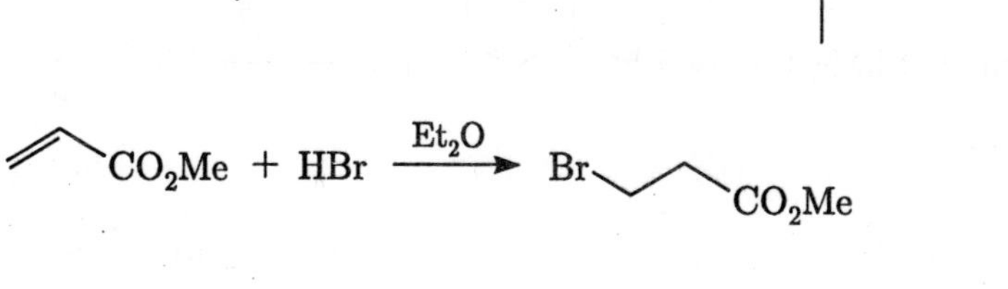

7.

8. 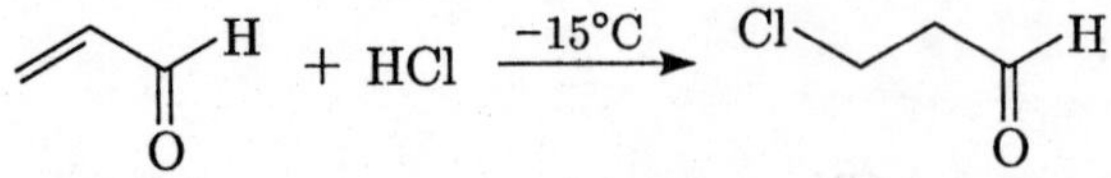

9. 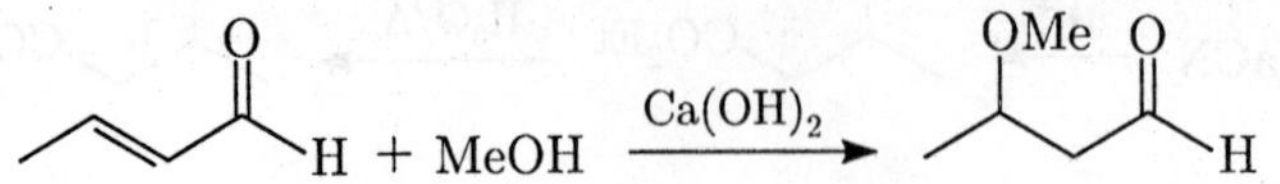

Applications of Michael reaction :

1. *Synthesis of polybasic acids*

$$\text{(a)}\ \begin{matrix}\text{CH CO}_2\text{Et}\\ \|\\ \text{CH CO}_2\text{Et}\end{matrix} + \text{H}_2\text{C(CO}_2\text{Et)}_2 \xrightleftharpoons[\text{EtOH}]{\text{NaOEt}} \begin{matrix}\text{CH}_2\ \text{CO}_2\text{Et}\\ |\\ \text{CH CO}_2\text{Et}\\ |\\ \text{CH (CO}_2\text{Et)}_2\end{matrix} \xrightarrow[-\text{CO}_2]{\text{H}_3\overset{\oplus}{\text{O}}/\Delta} \begin{matrix}\text{CH}_2\ \text{COOH}\\ |\\ \text{CH(COOH)}\\ |\\ \text{CH}_2\ \text{COOH}\end{matrix}$$

$$\text{(b)}\ \text{EtO}_2\text{C—C}\equiv\text{C—CO}_2\text{Et} + \text{H}_2\text{C(CO}_2\text{Et)}_2 \xrightarrow[\text{2. H}_3\overset{\oplus}{\text{O}}/\Delta]{\text{1. NaOEt/EtOH}} \begin{matrix}\text{CH COOH}\\ \|\\ \text{C—COOH}\\ |\\ \text{CH}_2\ \text{COOH}\end{matrix}$$

(Activated triple bond) (Aconitic acid)

2. 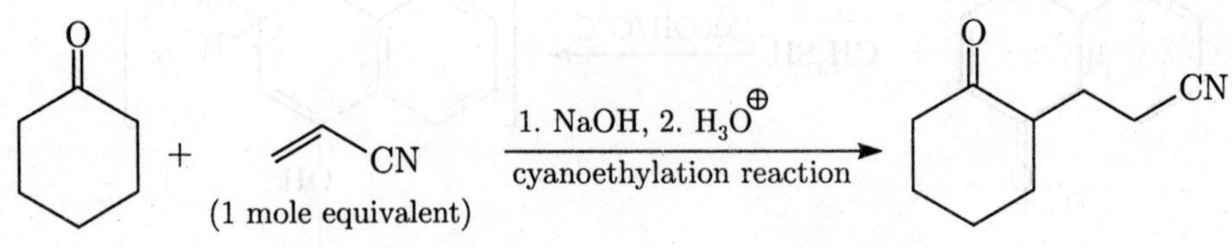

3. 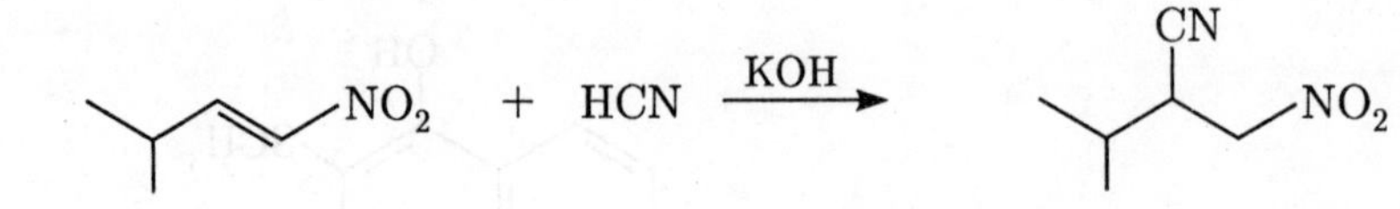

(2-methyl-1-nitropropene) (2,2-dimethyl-3-nitropropanonitrile)

4. 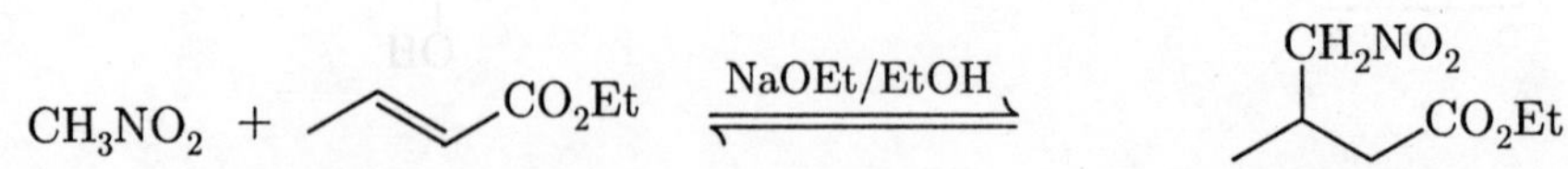

(Ethyl crotonate) (Ethyl-3-methyl-4-nitrobenzoate)

5. 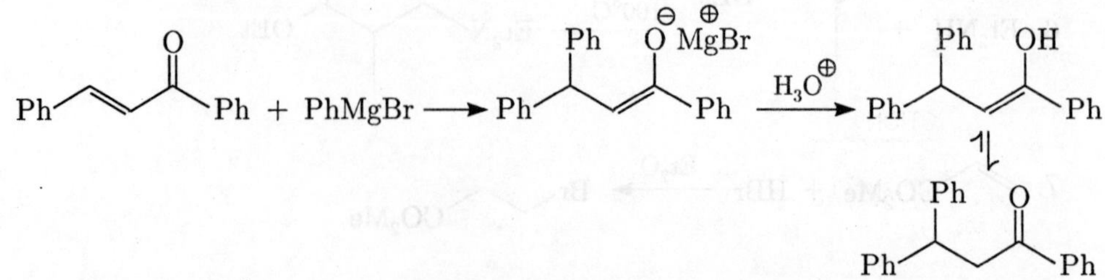

6. *Building of Ring System (Double Michael Addition)*

(a)

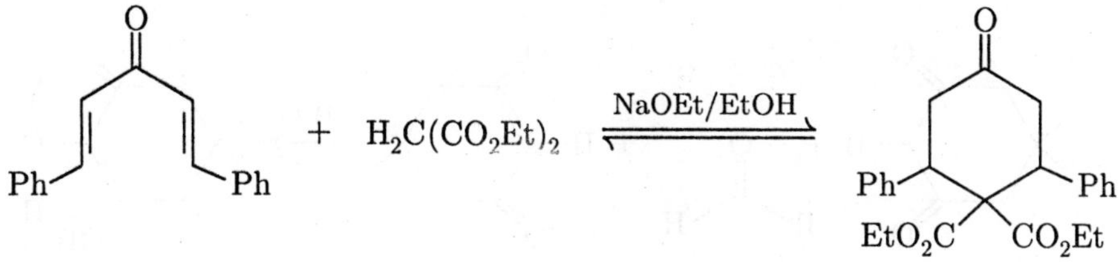

(b)

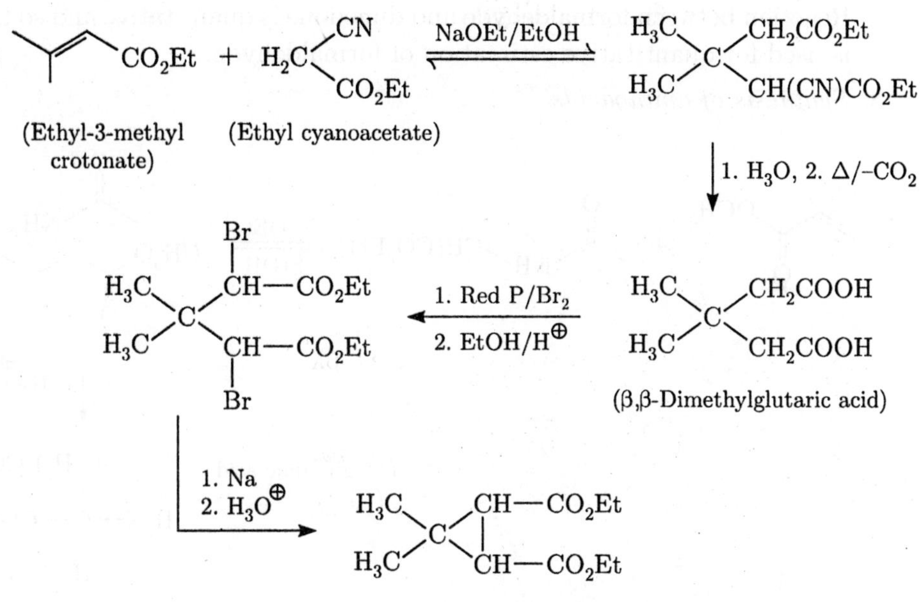

(Caronic acid)

7. *Synthesis of Dimedone* : Dimedone is a reagent for the identification of aldehydes in the presence of ketones.

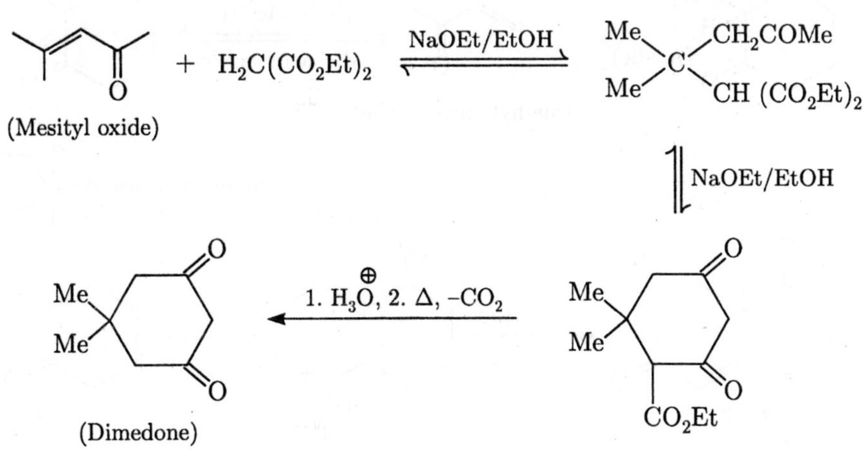

Dimedone reacts with aldehydes, but not with ketones and this reaction is taken as a distinction test to separate them from a mixture containing both.

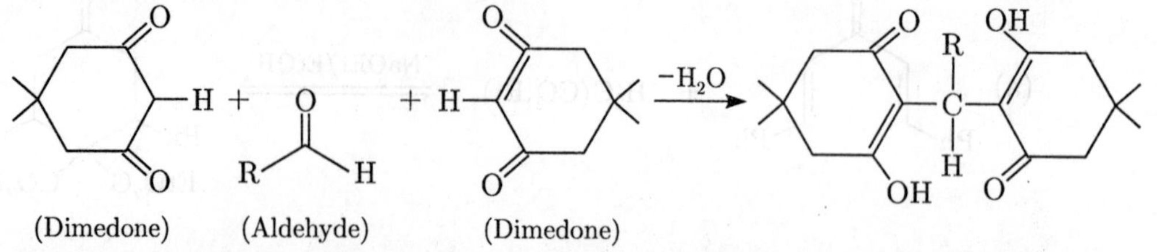

Reaction between formaldehyde and dimedone is quantitative and so this reagent is used for quantitative estimation of formaldehyde.

8. *Synthesis of aminoacids*

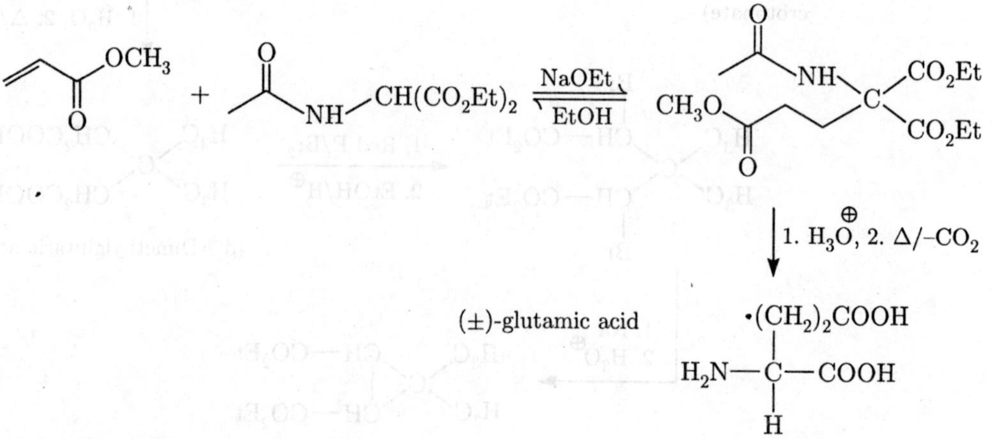

9. *Robinson's annulation reaction*

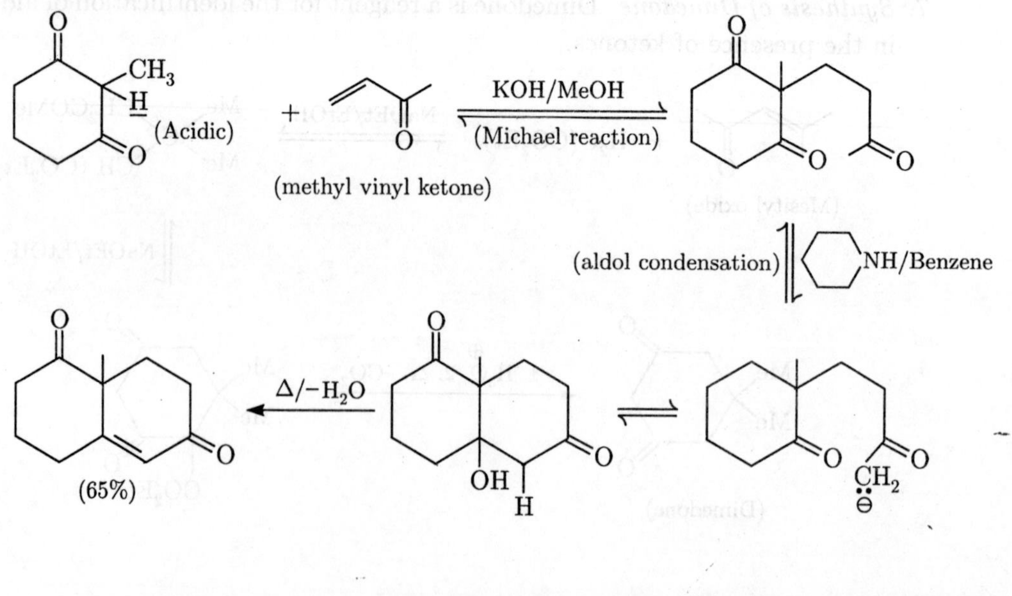

Reduction of α, β-unsaturated carbonyl compounds

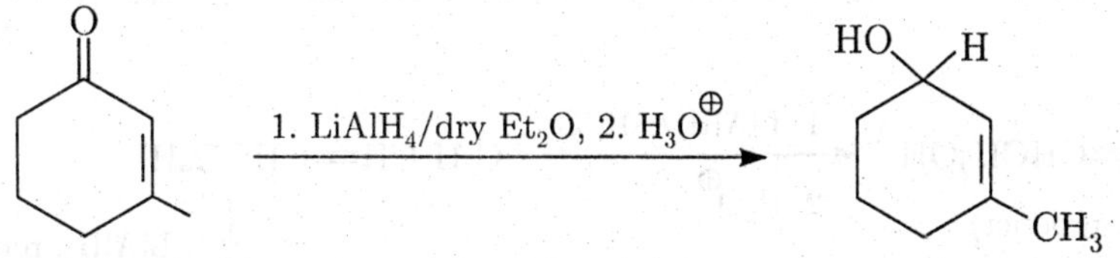

The reaction like other lithium aluminium hydride ($LiAlH_4$) reductions, involve the attack of hydride ion ($\overset{\ominus}{H}$: ion) at the carbonyl carbon and is therefore a carbonyl addition, not a conjugate addition. Carbonyl addition is not only faster than conjugate addition, but in this case, also *irreversible*, as hydride is a poor leaving group. Because addition of $LiAlH_4$ is irreversible, conjugate addition never has a chance to occur and is therefore not observed.

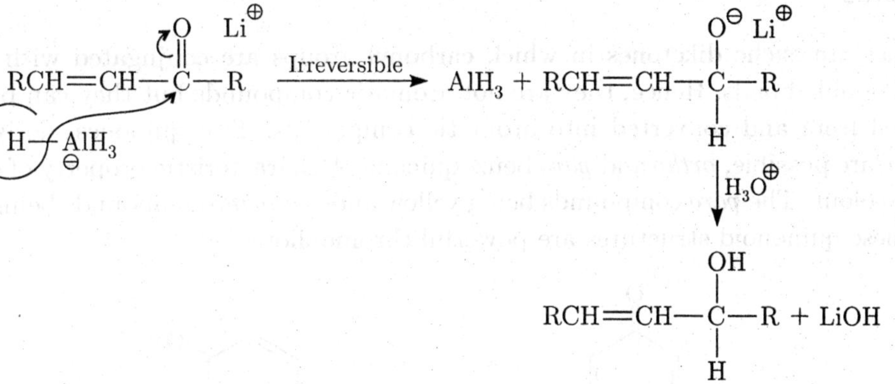

In other words, reduction of the carbonyl group with $LiAlH_4$ is a kinetically controlled reaction. Many α, β–unsaturated carbonyl compounds are reduced by $NaBH_4$ to give mixtures of both carbonyl addition products and conjugate addition products. Because mixtures are obtained, sodium borohydride ($NaBH_4$) reduction of α, β-unsaturated carbonyl compounds are not useful. So $LiAlH_4$ can reduce the carbonyl group of an α, β-unsaturated carbonyl compound without affecting the double bond. The carbon–carbon double bond of an α, β-unsaturated carbonyl compound can in most cases be reduced selectively by catalytic hydrogenation.

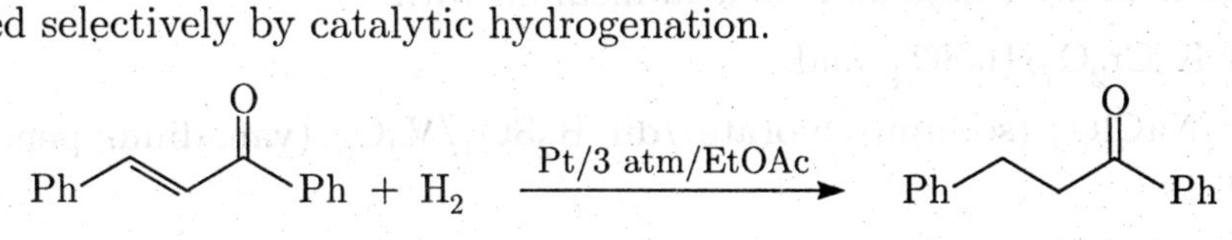

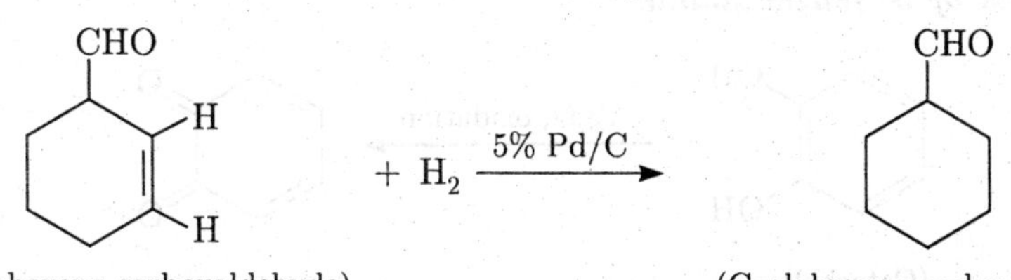

(2-Cyclohexene carboxaldehyde) (Cyclohexane carboxaldehyde)

When a phenyl group is attached to the β–carbon atom of an α, β-unsaturated carbonyl compound, both the double bond and the carbonyl group are reduced by $LiAlH_4$.

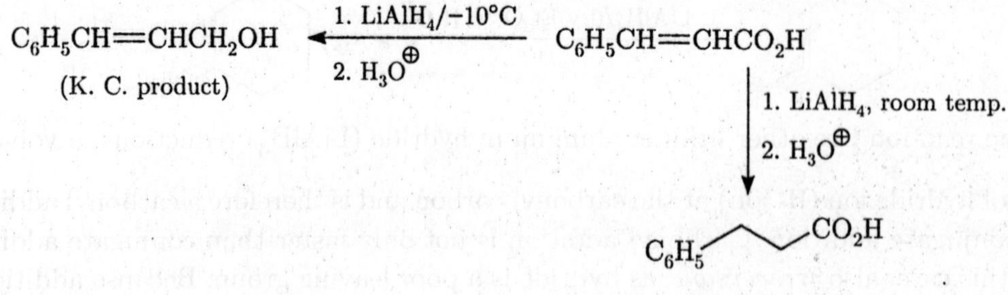

Quinones

Quinones are cyclic diketones in which carbonyl groups are conjugated with carbon–carbon double bonds. Hence, they are not aromatic compounds but they can be readily prepared from and converted into aromatic compounds. Two quinones, derived from benzene are possible, *ortho* and *para* benzoquinone. A characteristic property of quinones is their colour. The *para* compounds being yellow and the *ortho* compounds being usually red. These quinonoid structures are powerful chromophores.

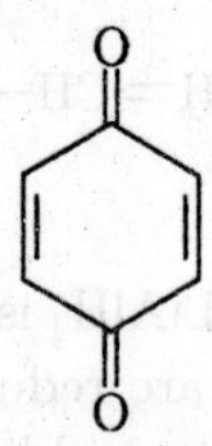

(*p*-Benzoquinone)

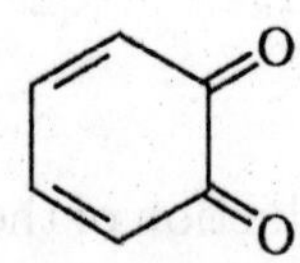

(*o*-Benzoquinone)

Preparation of quinones **:**

Quninones are usually prepared by the oxidation of the corresponding dihydroxy, diamino and aminohydroxy compounds in acid medium with,

(a) MnO_2 or $K_2Cr_2O_7/H_2SO_4$, and

(b) $FeCl_3$ or $NaClO_3$ (sodium chlorate)/dil H_2SO_4/V_2O_5 (vanadium pentoxide catalyst)

1. ***Synthesis of o-Benzoquinone***

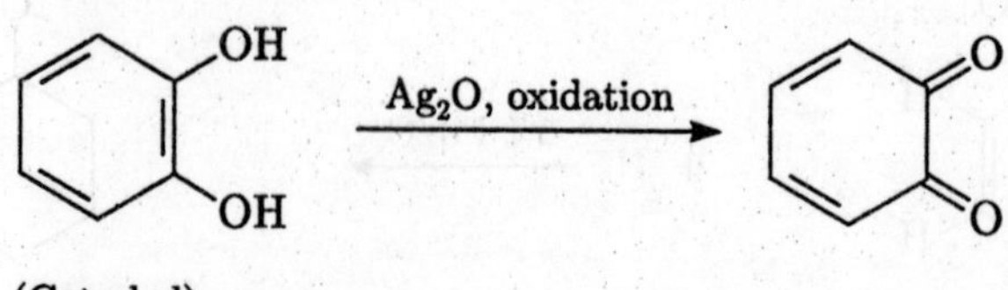

(Catechol)

2. *Synthesis of p-Benzoquinone*

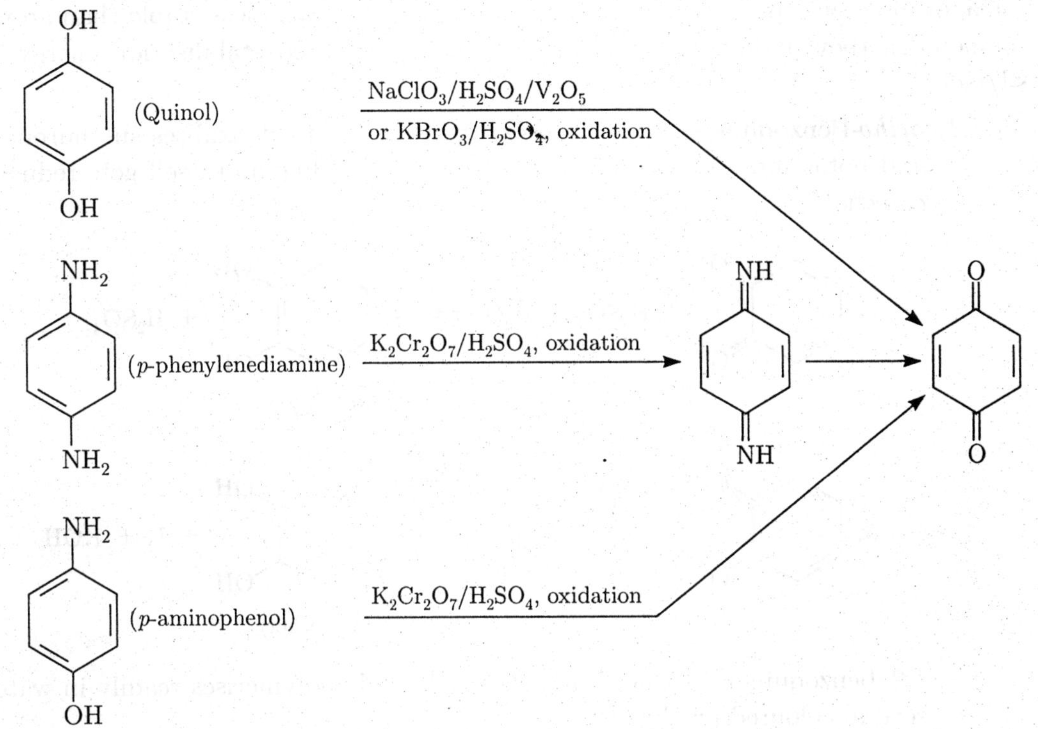

Some intermediate products like HN=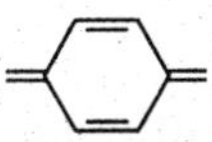=NH and O=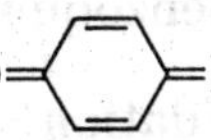=NH have been isolated.

Structure and Physical Properties of Quinones : Benzoquinones do not have aromatic rings and these rings are said to be quinonoid rings. Therefore, quinones are less stable than the corresponding aromatic compounds. On the other hand, the π-orbitals involved in the quinonoid system embrace π–bonded carbon and oxygen atoms, so they are not very unstable. In all quinones (except in 1,2–quinones), one of the two C=C double bonds is cross-conjugated. However, owing to conjugation between carbonyl groups and C=C bonds, quinones are good chromophores and they bear colour. The colour is attributed to n–π^* transition. They can form weak hydrogen bond with water and alcohol; this makes them slightly soluble in water, but readily soluble in alcohol.

Name	m.p.	Colour and Odour	Solubility	Steam–volatility
1. 1,2–Benzoquinone	60°–70°C	Red palate (Odourless)	Alcohol	Hot, steam-volatile
(*ortho*-benzoquinone)		Green needles (Odourless)	Alcohol	unstable
2. 1,4–Benzoquinone (*para*-benzoquinone)	116°C	Yellow prisms, sharp smell, sublimes	Slightly soluble in water, alcohol	steam-volatile

Chemical reactions : Since, carbon–carbon double bonds are conjugated with the carbonyl groups in quinone, they behave as α, β-unsaturated ketones and undergo 1,4–addition reactions. Since, the addition products are much less stable than aromatic compounds, they undergo aromatisation readily (increased stabilisation energy:125.5 kJ/mol).

1. ***ortho*-Benzoquinone** : It is a good oxidising agent; it oxidises sulphurous acid and potassium iodide solution to H_2SO_4 and iodine and itself gets reduced to catechol.

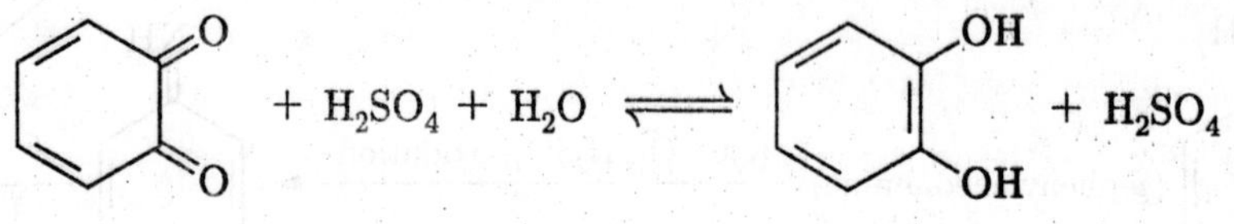

(Catechol)

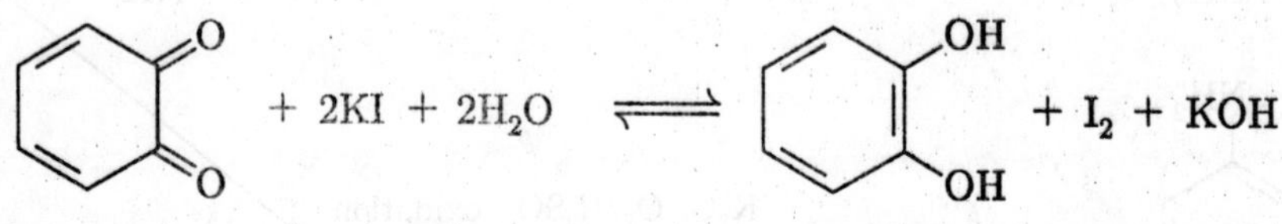

(Catechol)

1,2–benzoquinone is very unstable in water. It polymerises readily in water to several coloured products.

2. ***para*-Benzoquinone** :

A. **Oxidation of *p*-benzoquinone**

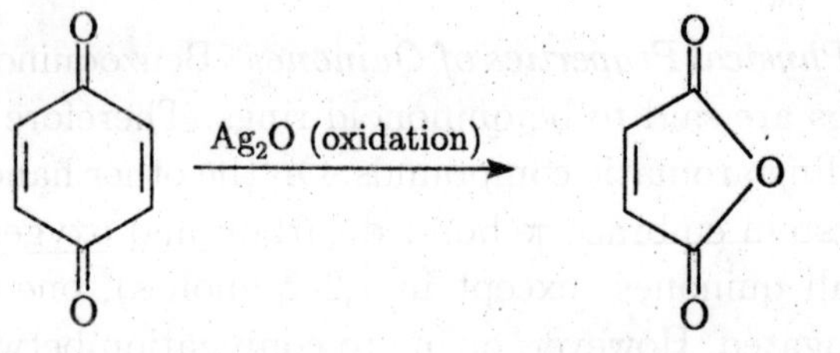

(Maleic anhydride)

B. ***Reduction***

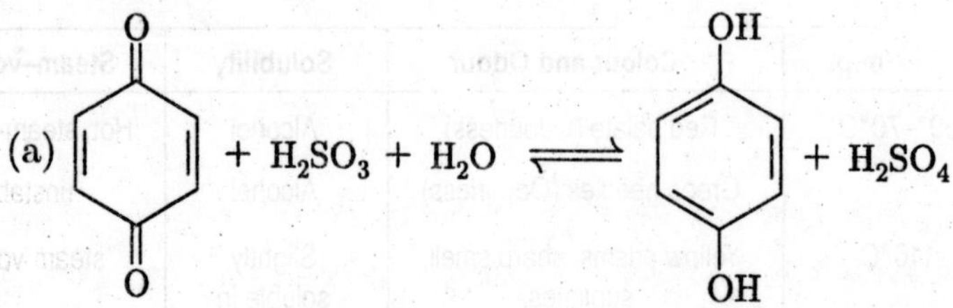

(Quinol)

(b) 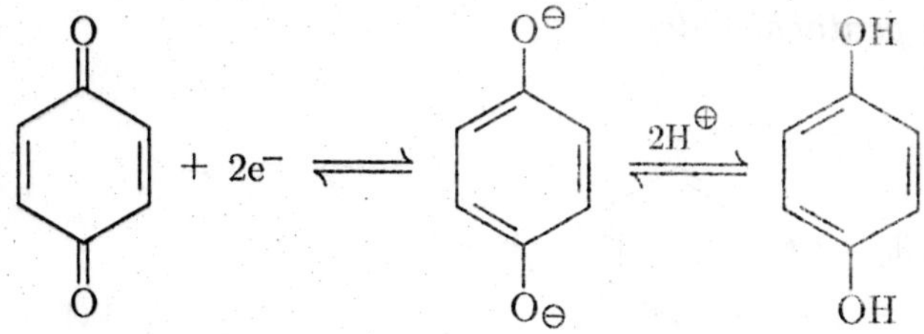 Δ R.E = (20.9–125.5)kJ/mol

R.E. ≅ 20.9 kJ/mol

(c) $2I^{\ominus} \longrightarrow I_2 + 2e^-$; $2I \longrightarrow I_2$

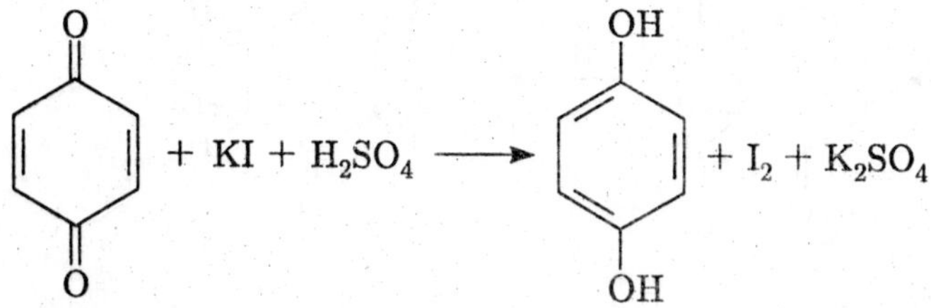

The oxidising power of the quinones is attributed to the fact that, by accepting two electrons a quinone gets aromatised with a large resonance energy.

The redox potential of quinol/*p*–benzoquinone system is appreciably high and it is 0.70 volt and that of catechol/*o*–benzoquinone system is 0.79 volt. It has been found that, (–I) substituents and (+I) substituents in a quinone respectively increase and decrease oxidation/reduction potential of the system. In chloranil, four Cl atoms are present and they exert strong (–I) effect. This raises the oxidation–reduction potential of the chloranil–tetrachloroquinol system and hence chloranil is used as a strong oxidising agent.

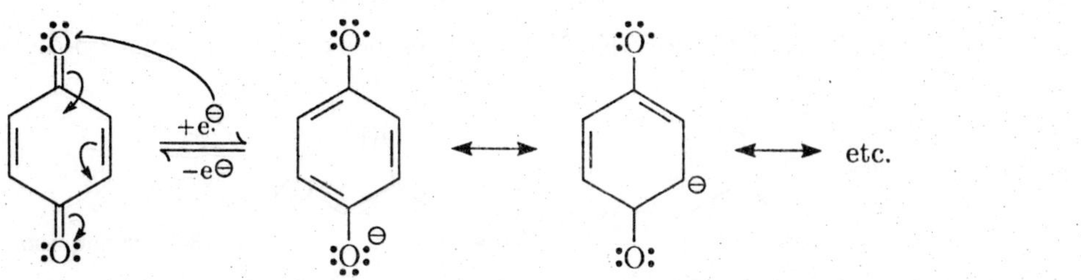

← Resonance-atabilised anionic free radical on electrolytic reduction →

3. ***Oxime Formation***

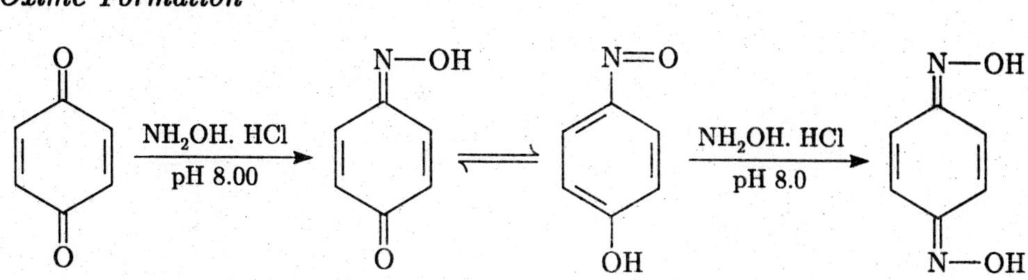

4. ***With phosphorus pentachloride*** :

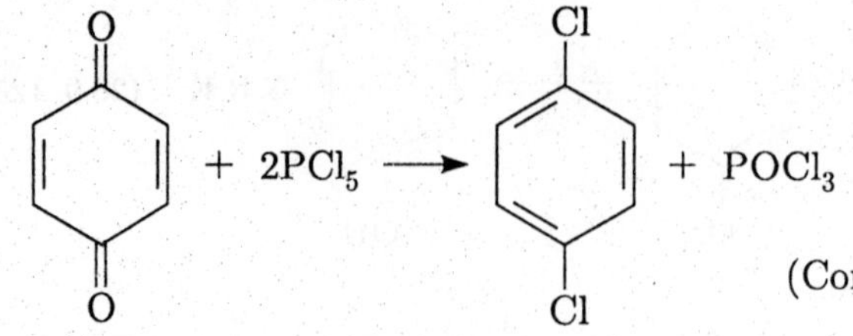

(Compare RCOR $\xrightarrow{PCl_5}$ $RCCl_2R$)

5.

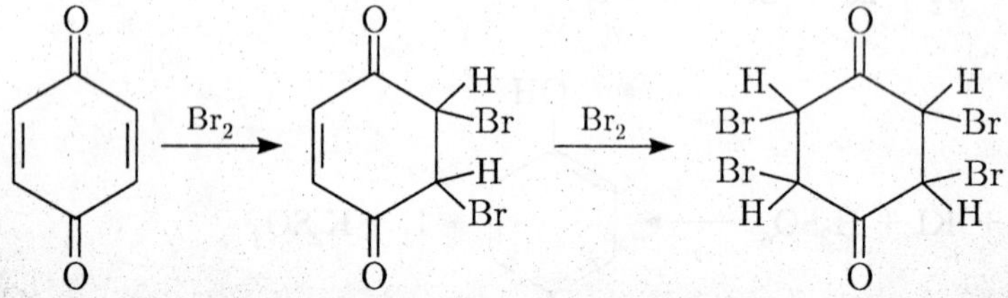

6. ***1,4–Addition reactions*** :

(a) *With HCl* : HCl adds to *p*–benzoquinone to form 2-chloroquinol.

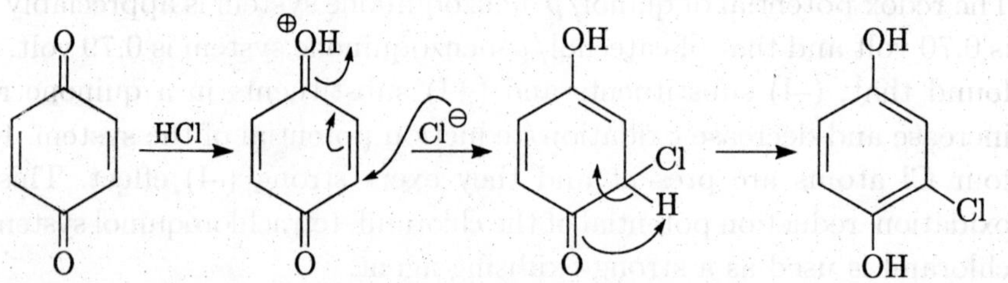

(b) *With KCN*: Ethanolic KCN in the presence of H_2SO_4 forms 2,3-dicyanoquinol.

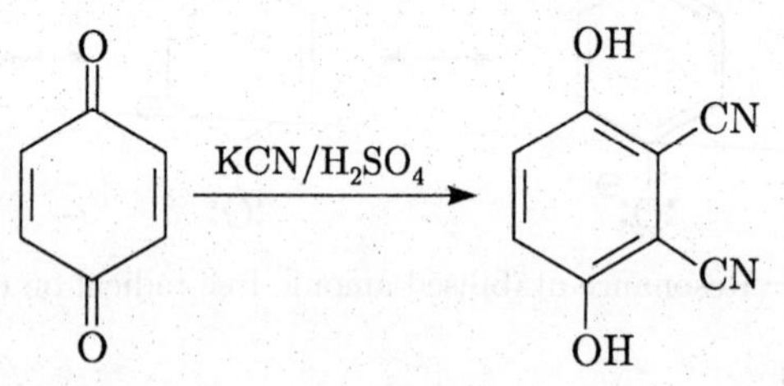

(2,3-Dicyanoquinol)

(c) *With primary and secondary amines* :

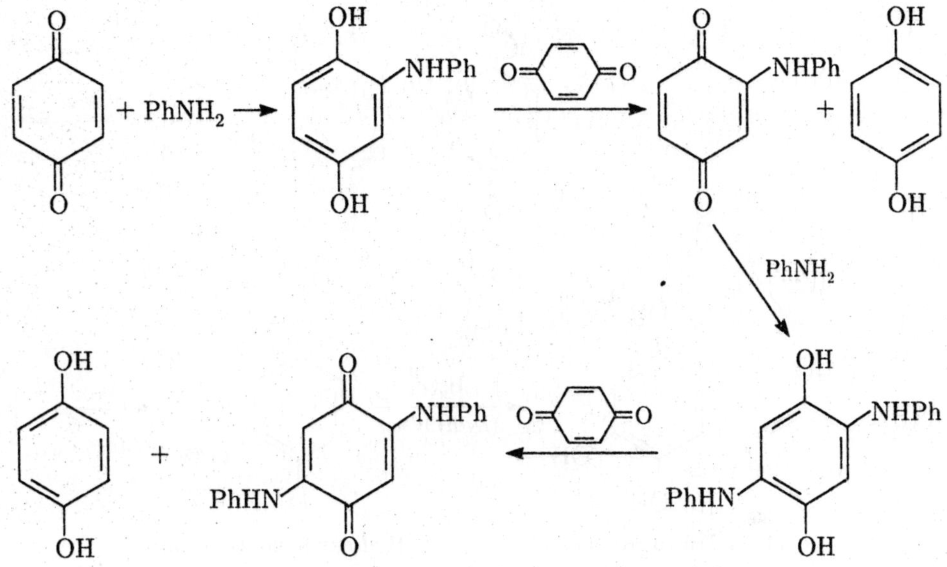

(2,5-Diamino- *p*-benzoquinone)

(d) *With primary alcohols* :

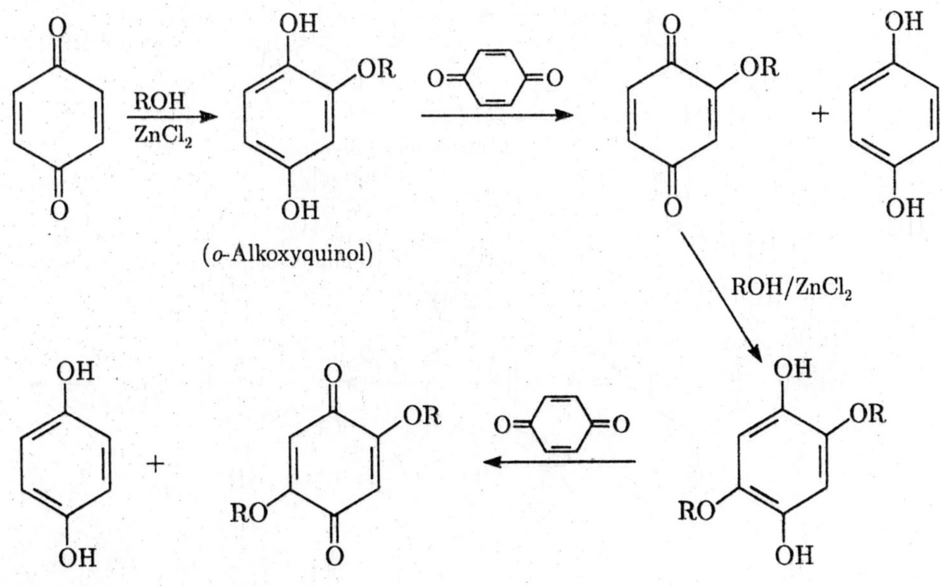

(Quinol) (2,5-Dialkoxy- *p*-benzoquinone)

(e) **Thiele's acetylation** : In the presence of H_2SO_4, acetic anhydride (Ac_2O) adds to *p*–benzoquinone to form hydroxyquinol triacetate.

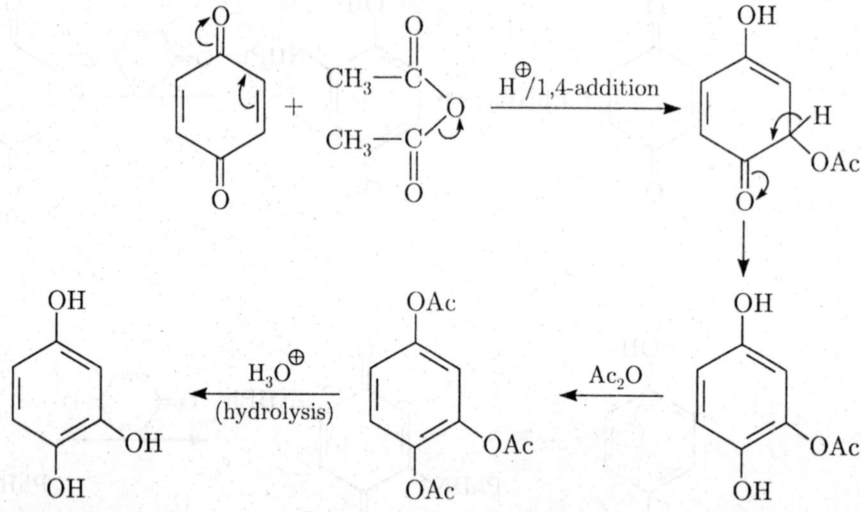

(1,3,4-Trihydroxyphenol) (Hydroxyquinol triacetate)

(f) *Reaction with chlorine*

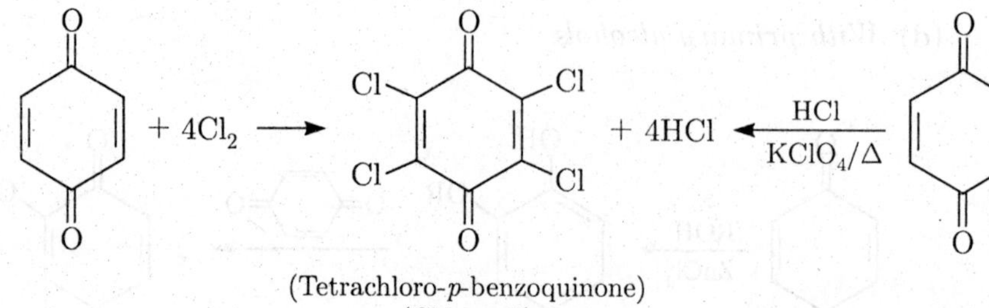

(Tetrachloro-*p*-benzoquinone)
(Chloranil)

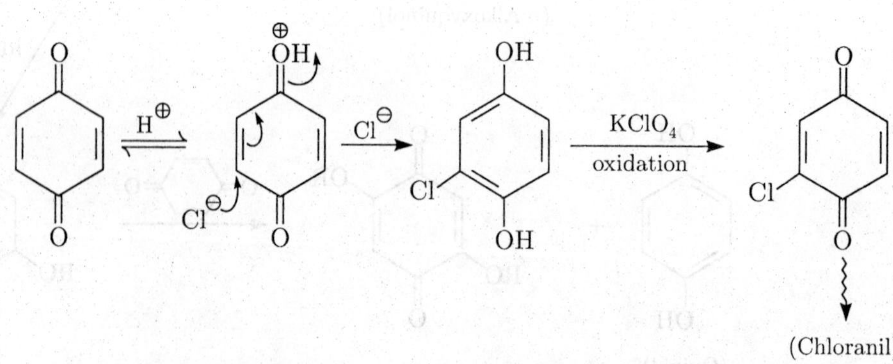

(Chloranil)

Chloranil is a good fungicide, it is also a good oxidising agent and so is used as an aromatising agent.

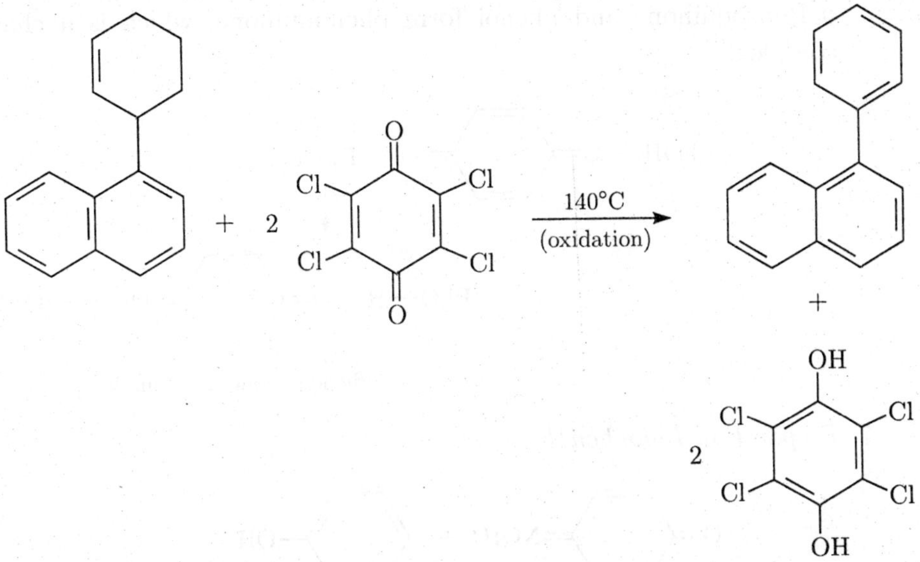

(g) *Addition* of *conjugated dienes*: *p*-Benzoquinone undergoes the Diels–Alder reaction with conjugated dienes.

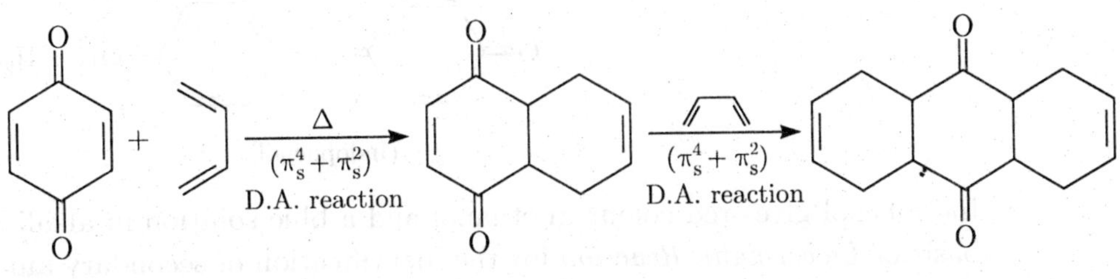

(Dienophile) (Diene)

(h) *Formation* of *quinhydrone* : When a concentrated alcoholic solution of quinone is added to a concentrated alcoholic solution of hydroquinone (quinol), crystals of quinhydrone are obtained; quinhydrone is a dark green solid with metallic lusture (m.p. 121°C). They are believed to be charge transfer molecular complex having colour and formed from quinones and phenols.

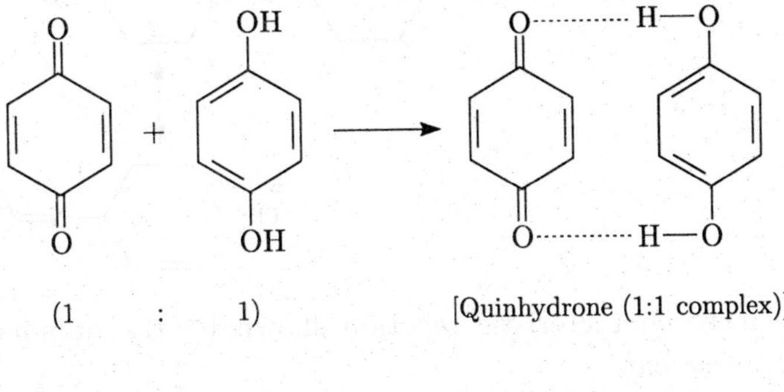

(1 : 1) [Quinhydrone (1:1 complex)]

p–Benzoquinone and phenol form phenoquinone, which is a charge transfer complex.

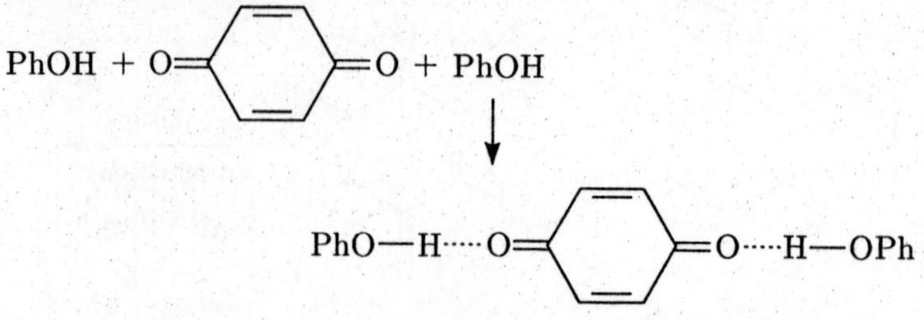

[Phenoquinone (2:1 complex)]

7. *Preparation Indophenol* :

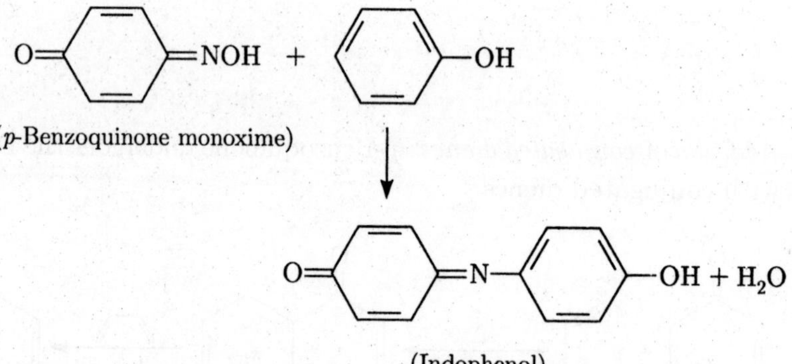

Indophenol gives red colour in ethanol and a blue solution in alkali; this is the basis of *Liebermann Reaction* for the identification of secondary amines.

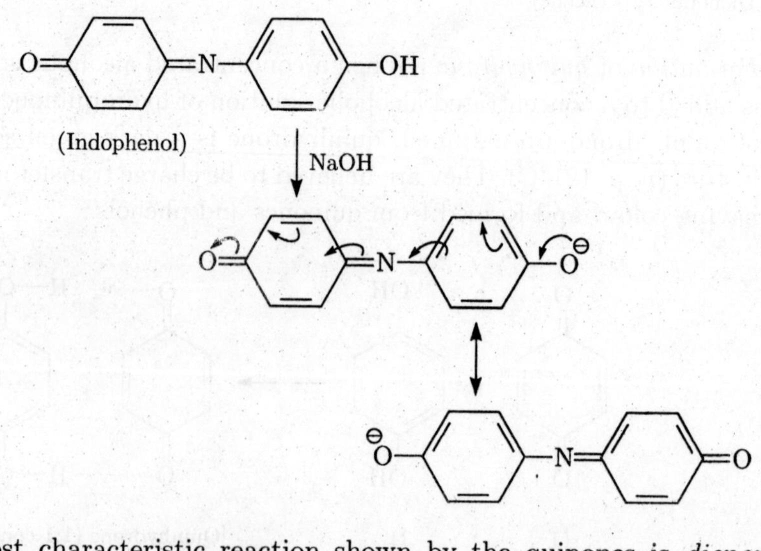

8. The most characteristic reaction shown by the quinones is *dienone–phenol rearrangement.*

THE DIENONE–PHENOL REARRANGEMENT

When 4,4–dialkylcyclohexadienone is treated with acid, it is converted to phenol with migration of one of the alkyl groups to the adjacent carbon. This is known as *dienone – phenol rearrangement.*

The dienone is dissolved in acetic anhydride and treated with catalytic amount of sulphuric acid. The product on hydrolysis gives phenol.

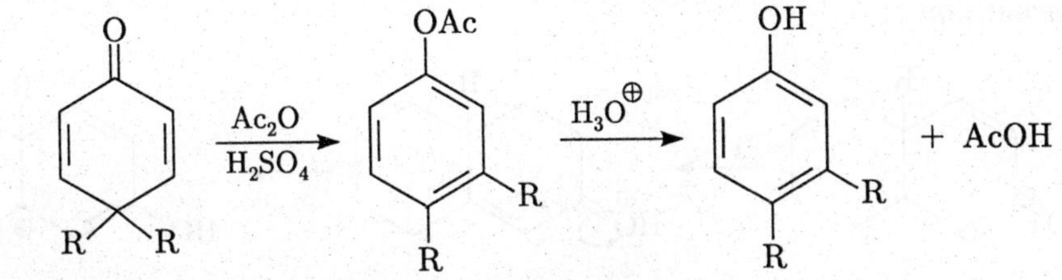

Mechanism of dienone–phenol rearrangement :

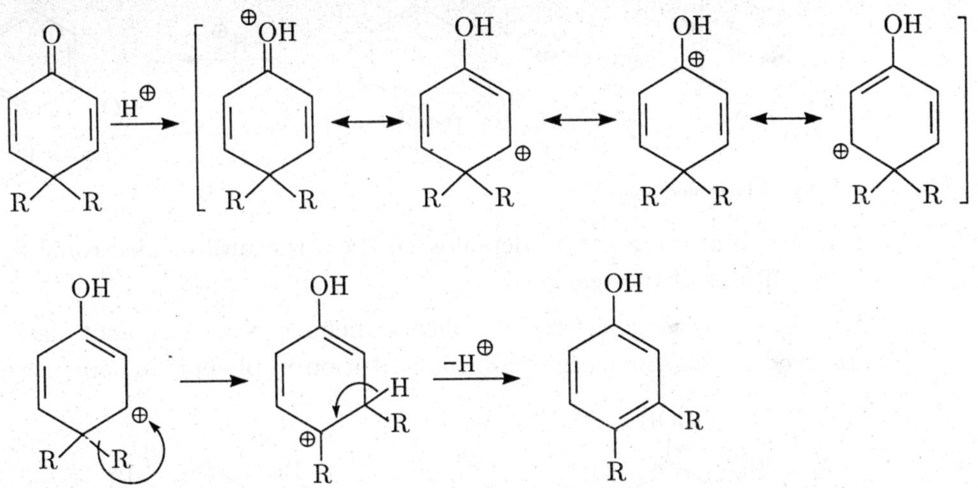

(Carbocation rearrangement) (3,4-Disubstituted phenol)

The ease of dienone–phenol rearrangement is due to the creation of a stable aromatic system. When one of the alkyl groups is an integral part of the cyclic system, either the other alkyl group or methylene group may migrate.

(a) *Alkyl Migration*

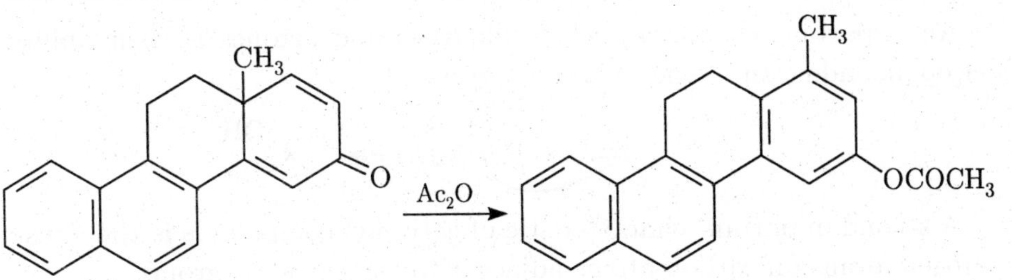

(b) *Migration of Ring-methylene group*

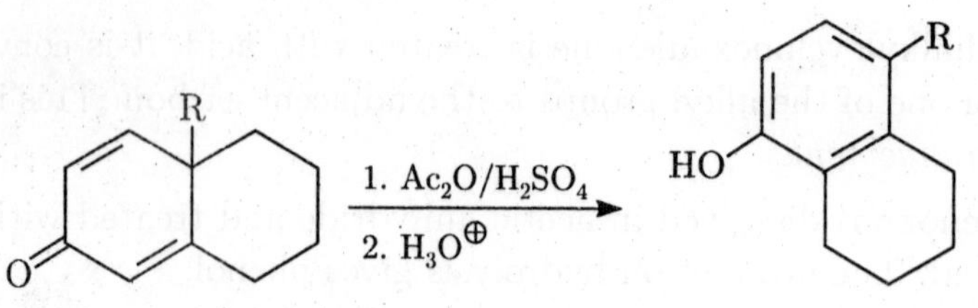

Mechanism :

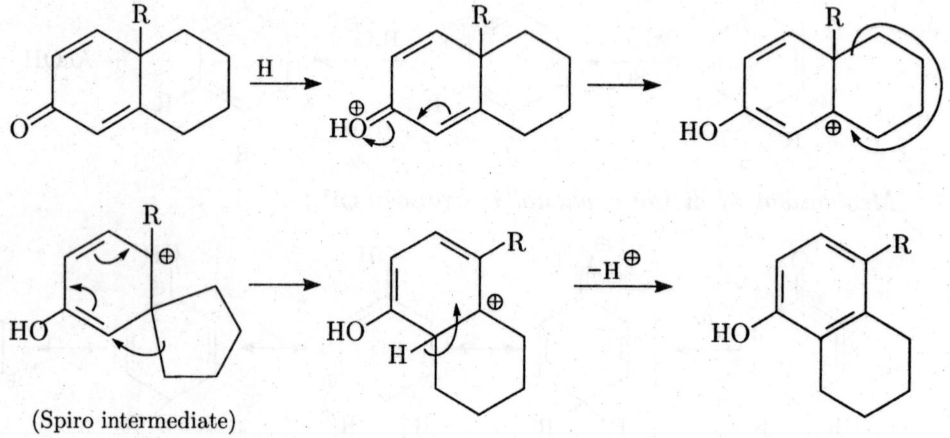

The course of the reaction depends on the structural or electronic factors and on conditions of the reaction.

A reverse rearrangement, *i.e.*, phenol–dienone rearrangement has also been observed during the electrophilic substitution in phenols in some cases.

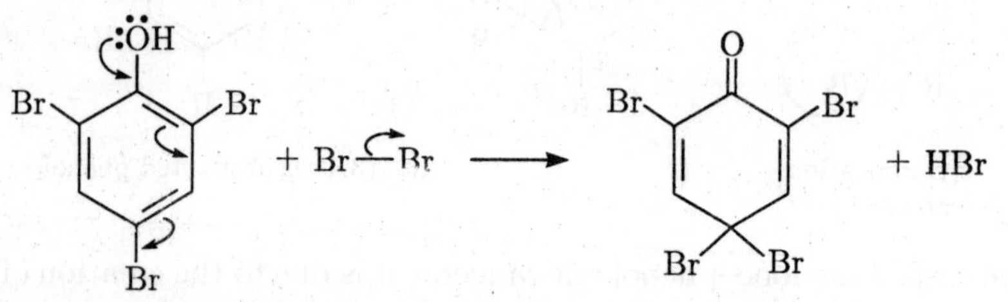

THE ENOLATES AND ENAMINES

The acidity of the α–hydrogens of carbonyl compounds : Enolate anions

An important characteristic of aldehydes and ketones is their ability to undergo nucleophilic addition at their carbonyl groups.

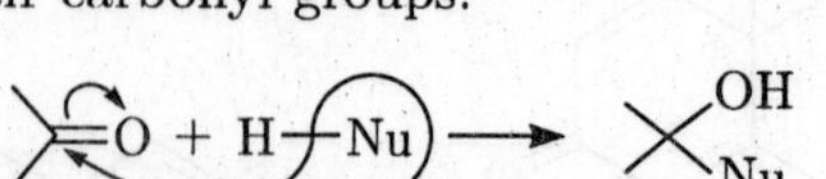

A second important characteristic of carbonyl compounds is the unusual acidity of hydrogen atoms on carbon atoms adjacent to the carbonyl group.

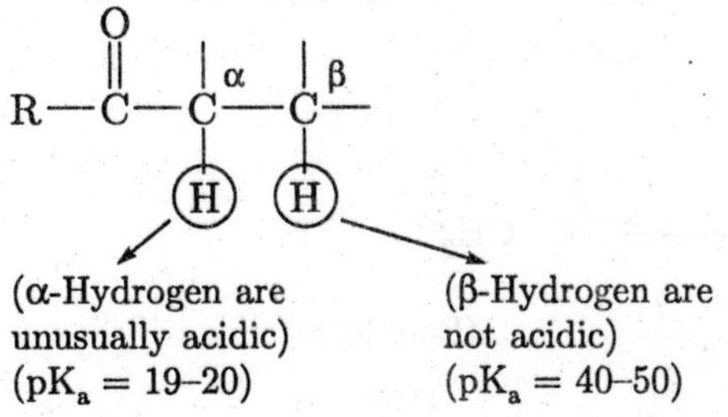

These α–hydrogens are more acidic than acetylenic hydrogens (pK_a=25) and far more acidic ethylenic hydrogens (pK_a=40) or of ethane (pK_a=50).

Carbonyl group is electron withdrawing and when a carbonyl compound loses an α–proton, the anion that is produced is *stabilised by resonance.* The negative charge of the anion is *delocalised.*

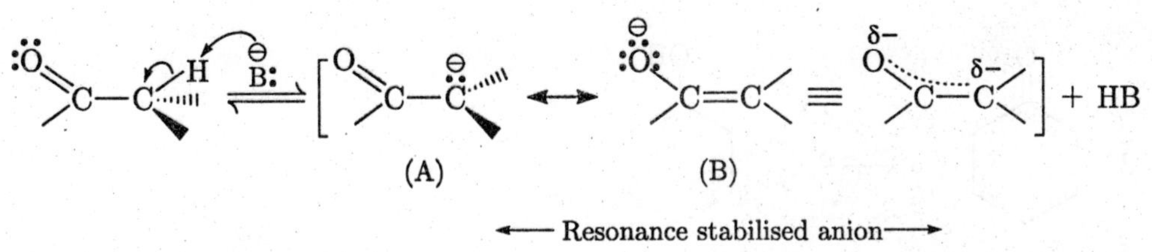

Although structure (A) contains more stable π-bond between carbon and oxygen than carbon–carbon π bond in structure (B), structure (B) has got more contribution over (A) to the resonance hybrid. Oxygen being more electronegative, is better able to accomodate the negative charge.

When this resonance stabilised anion accepts a proton, it can do so in either of the two ways. It can accept the proton at carbon to form the original carbonyl compound known as the *keto form* or it may accept the proton at oxygen to form an *enol.*

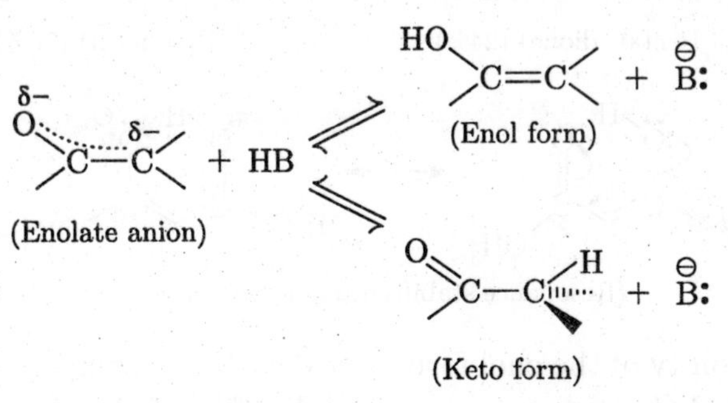

Both of these reactions are reversible. Because of its relation to the enol, the resonance–stabilised anion is called an *enolate anion.*

Keto–and Enol–tautomers : Keto– and enol forms of carbonyl compounds are constitutional isomers and they can be interconverted easily in the presence of traces of acids and bases. These are also known as tautomers and the process is known as *tautomerisation.* Generally the keto form of mono carbonyl compounds is more stable due to the greater stability of C=O π bond.

1. 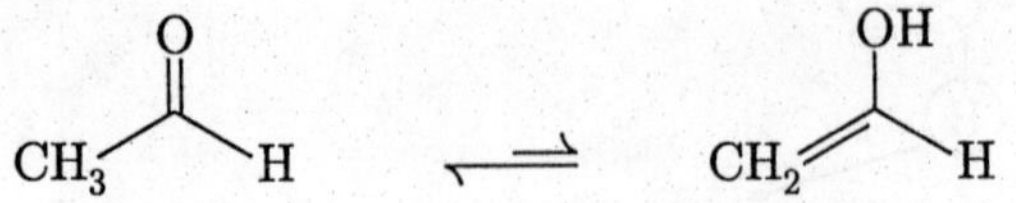

(Keto form) (100%) — (Enol form) (trace)

2. 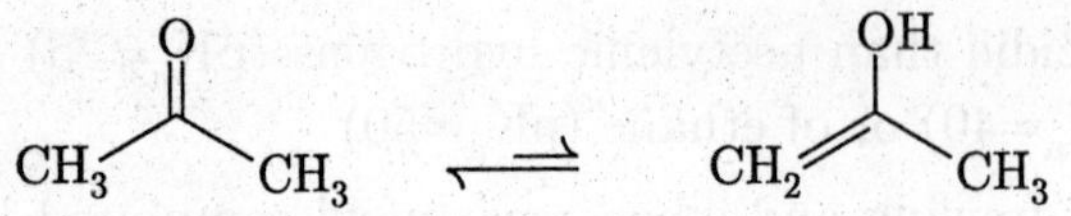

(Keto form) (> 99%) — (Enol form) (1.5×10^{-4}%)

3. 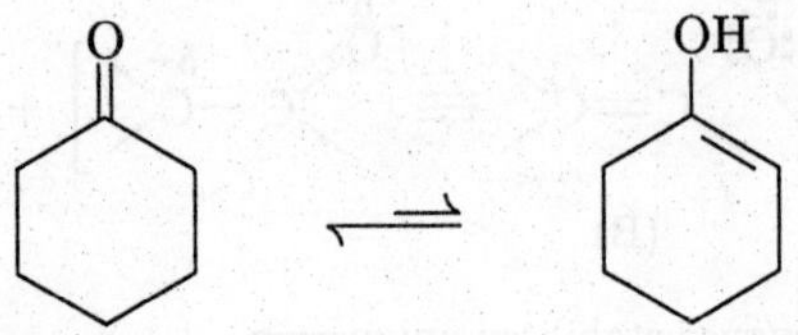

(Keto form) (98.8%) — (Enol form) (1.2%)

β–Dicarbonyl compounds contain much higher enol percentage in the equilibrium.

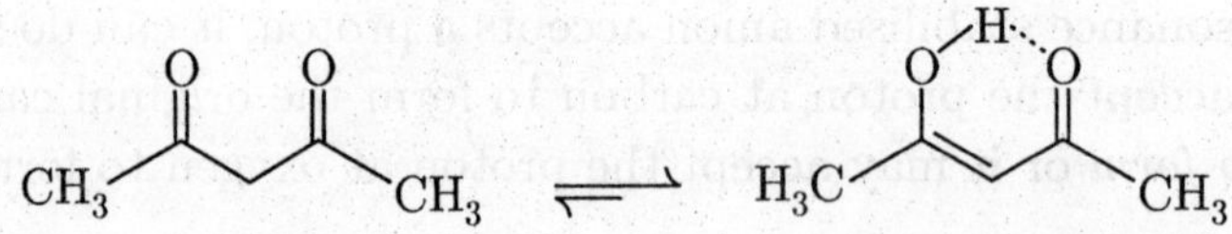

(2,4-Pentanedione) (24%) — (Enol form) (76%)

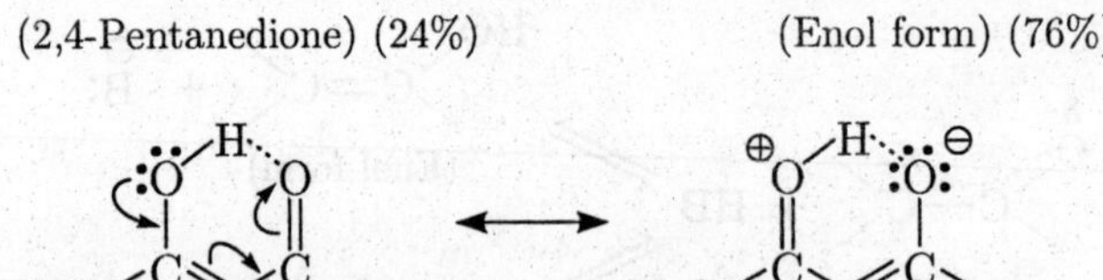

(Resonance stabilisation of enol form)

The greater stability of the enol form of β–dicarbonyl compounds can be attributed to the stability gained through resonance stabilisation of the conjugated double bonds and though hydrogen bonding in a cyclic form.

Reactions via enols and enolate anions

1. ***Racemisation*** : When a solution of (+)–*sec*-butyl phenyl ketone in aqueous ethanol is treated with either acid or base, the solution gradually loses its optical activity. After a time, isolation of the ketone shows that it has been racemised.

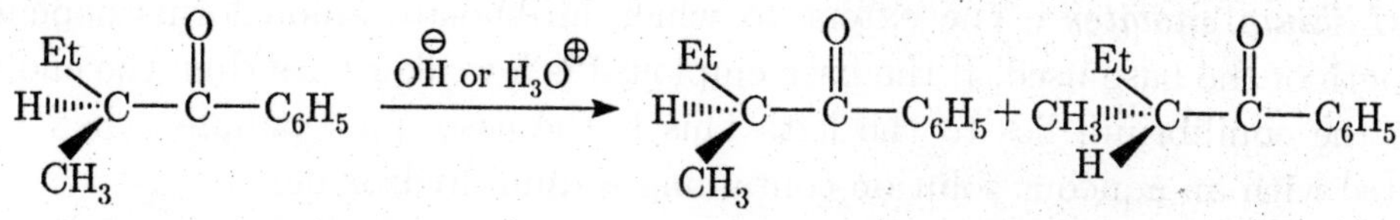

(+)–*Sec*-butyl phenyl ketone (±) *Sec*-butyl phenyl ketone (racemic mixture)

Racemisation occurs because the ketone slowly but reversibly changes to enol either in the presence of acid or base and the *enol is achiral.* When the enol reverts to the ketoform, it produces equal amounts of two enantiomers.

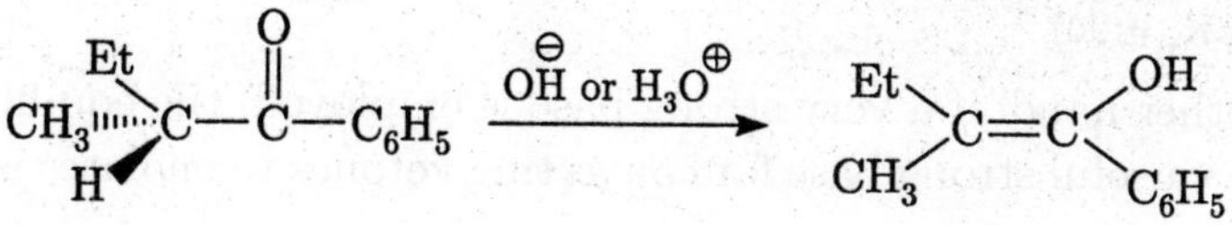

(Chiral) Enol (achiral)

Mechanism of the reaction :

(a) ***Base–catalysed enolisation*** :

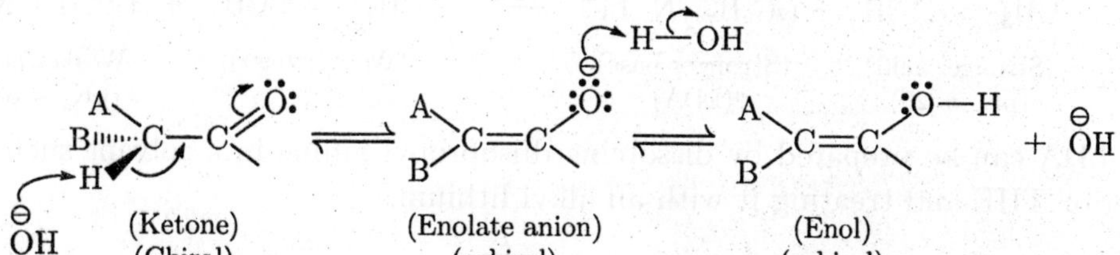

(b) ***Acid–catalysed enolisation*** :

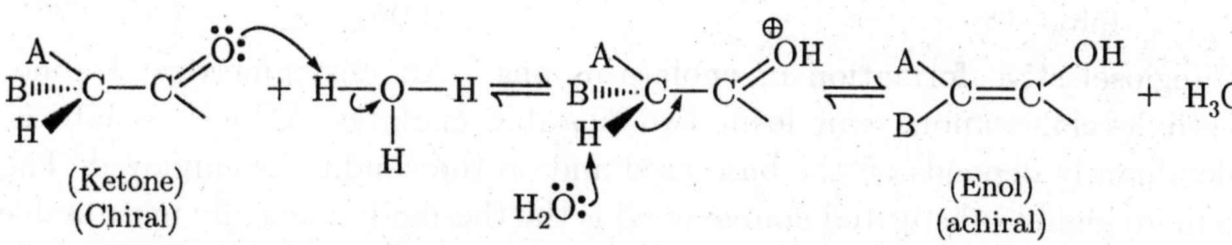

In cyclic ketones, the enol or enolate anion formed can be (E) or (Z). Protonation on one face of (E)–isomer and protonation on the same face of (Z)–isomer produces enantiomers.

Keto–enol tautomerism can sometimes be used to convert a less stable epimer. This equilibriation process is known as epimerisation.

Example :

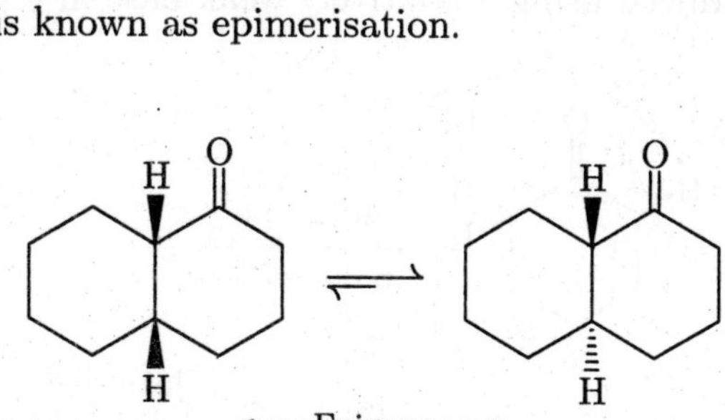

← Epimers →

N.B.: Epimers are diastereoisomers which differ in cnfiguration at *only one* stereocentre.

Lithium enolates : The extent to which an enolate anion forms depends on the strength of the base used. If the base employed is a weaker base than the enolate anion, then the equilibrium lies to the left. This is the case, for example, when a ketone is treated with an aqueous solution containing sodium hydroxide.

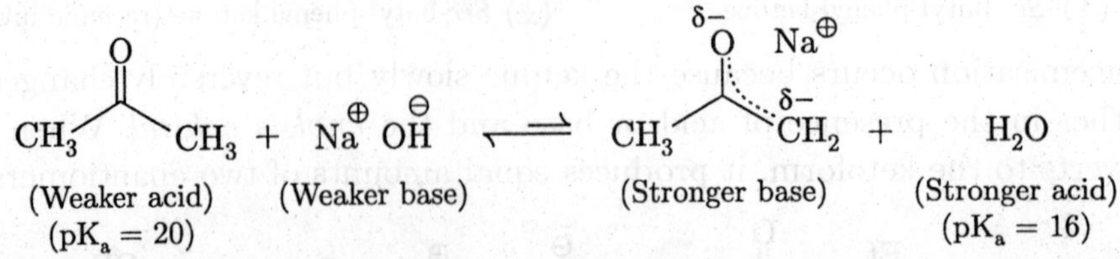

On the other hand, if a very strong base is employed, the equilibrium lies far to the right. One very useful strong base for converting ketones to enolates is *lithium diisopropyl amide* (LDA), $(iC_3H_7)_2\overset{\ominus}{N}\!:\,Li^{\oplus}$.

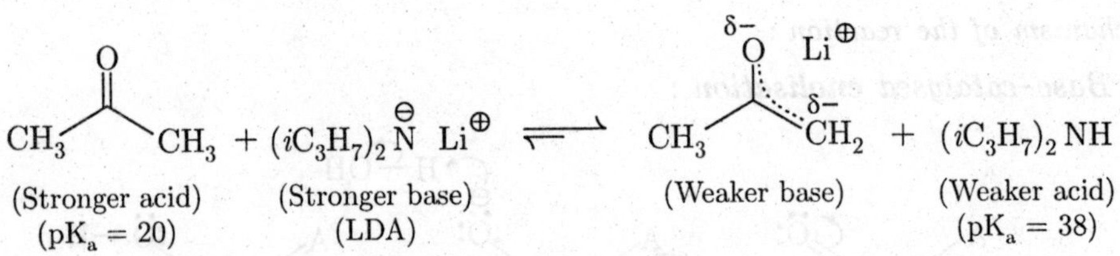

LDA can be prepared by dissolving diisopropyl amine in a solvent such as diethyl ether or THF and treating it with an alkyl lithium.

$$\underset{\substack{\text{(Stronger acid)}\\(pK_a = 38)}}{(iC_3H_7)_2NH} + \underset{\text{(Stronger base)}}{C_4H_9Li} \rightleftharpoons \underset{\substack{\text{(Weaker base)}\\\text{(LDA)}}}{(iC_3H_7)_2\overset{\ominus}{N}\;Li^{\oplus}} + \underset{\substack{\text{(Weaker acid)}\\(pK_a = 50)}}{C_4H_{10}}$$

Regioselective formation of enolate anions : An unsymmetrical ketone such as 2–methylcyclohexanone can form two possible enolates. Which enolate is formed predominantly depends on the base used and on the conditions employed. The enolate with more highly substituted double bond is the thermodynamically more stable enolate in the same way that an alkene with the more substituted double bond is the more stable alkene. This enolate, called the *thermodynamic enolate,* is formed predominantly under conditions that permit the establishment of an equilibrium. This will generally be the case if the enolate is produced using a relatively weak base in a protic solvent.

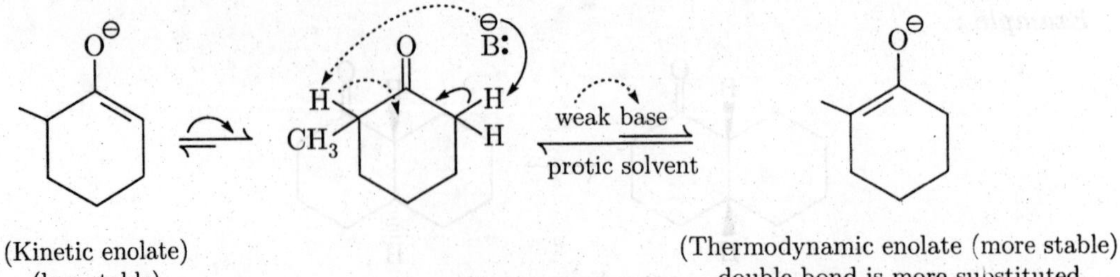

(Kinetic enolate)
(less stable)

(Thermodynamic enolate (more stable)
double bond is more substituted
and is the predominant
enolate present in the equilibrium)

On the other hand, the enolate with the less substituted double bond is usually formed faster, because removal of the hydrogen necessary to produce this enolate is *less* sterically hindered. This enolate, called the kinetic enolate is formed predominantly when the reaction is kinetically controlled or rate controlled.

The kinetically favoured enolate can be formed through the use of LDA. This strong sterically hindered base rapidly removes the proton from the less substituted α–carbon of the ketone.

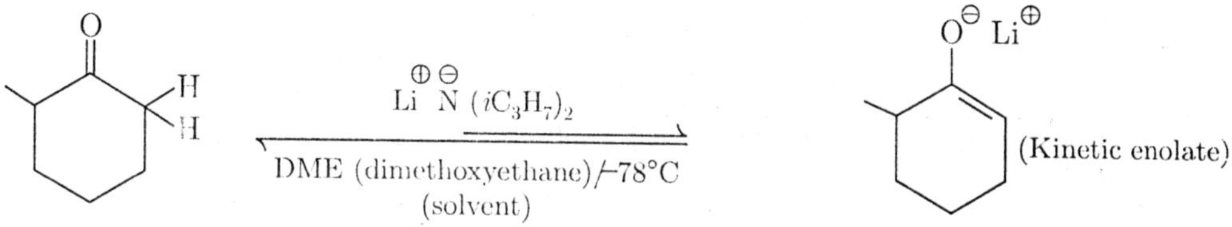

(2-methylcyclohexanone)

(This enolate is formed faster because the hindered strong base (LDA) removes the less hindered proton faster)

Lithium enolates in directed aldol condensation : One of the most effective and versatile ways to bring about a crossed aldol reaction is to use a lithium enolate obtained from a ketone as one component and an aldehyde or ketone as the other. An example of that is called a directed aldol condensation.

Regioselectivity can be achieved when unsymmetrical ketones are used in directed aldol reacvtions by generating the kinetic enolate anion using LDA. This ensures production of the enolate in which the **proton has been removed from the less substituted α–carbon.**

Examples :

An aldol reaction via the kinetic enolate with LDA

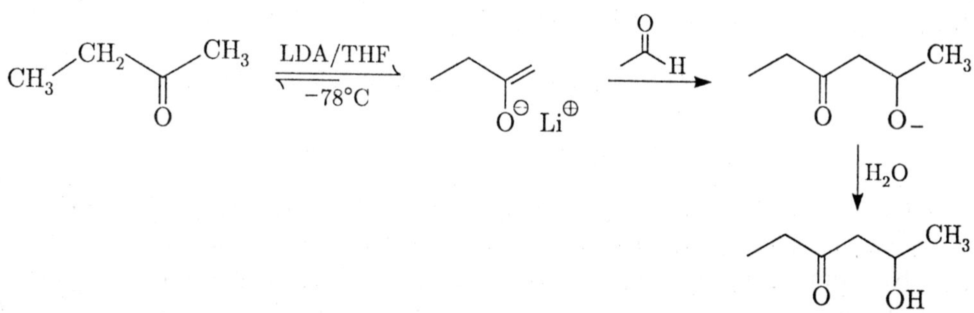

(A single crossed aldol product results (75%))

If this aldol reaction (Claisen Schmidt reaction) had been carried out in the classical way using hydroxide ion as the base, then at least two products would have been formed in significant amounts. Both the kinetic and thermodynamic enolates would have been formed from the ketone, and each of these would have added to the carbonyl carbon of the aldehyde.

Direct alkylation of ketones via Lithium enolates : The formation of lithium enolates using LDA furnishes a useful way of alkylating ketones in a regioselective way. For example, the lithium enolate formed from 2–methylcyclohexanone can be methylated or benzylated by allowing it to react with methyl iodide or benzyl bromide respectively.

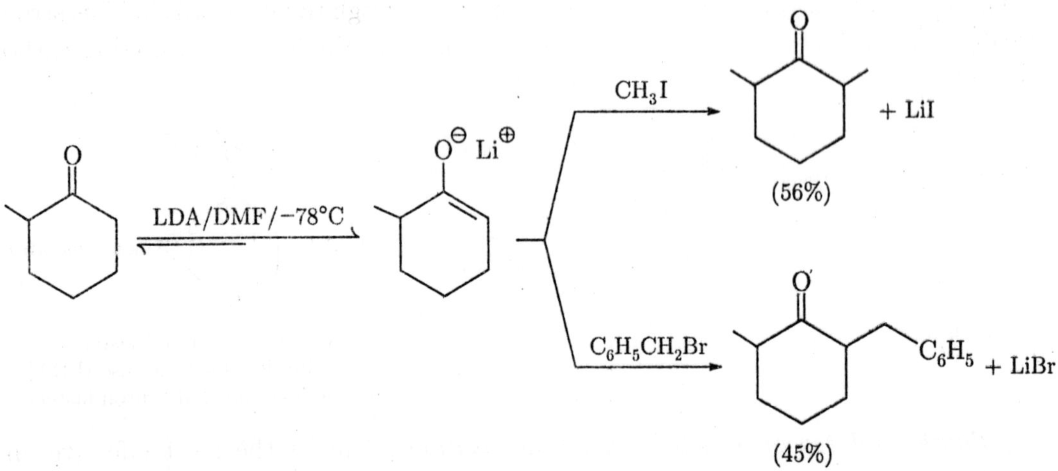

These alkylation reactions have one serious limitation. because the reactions are of S_N2 nature and enolate anions are strong bases, successful alkylations occur only when primary alkyl, primary benzylic and primary allylic halides are used. With secondary and tertiary halides, elimination becomes the main course of the reaction.

Some salient features of enolate anions : Enolate anions bear a partial negative charge on an oxygen atom and they can react in nucleophilic substitution reactions as if they are alkoxide anions. because they have a partial negative charge on a carbon atom, they can also react as carbanions. Nucleophiles like this, these that are capable of reacting at two sites, are called *ambident* nucleophiles.

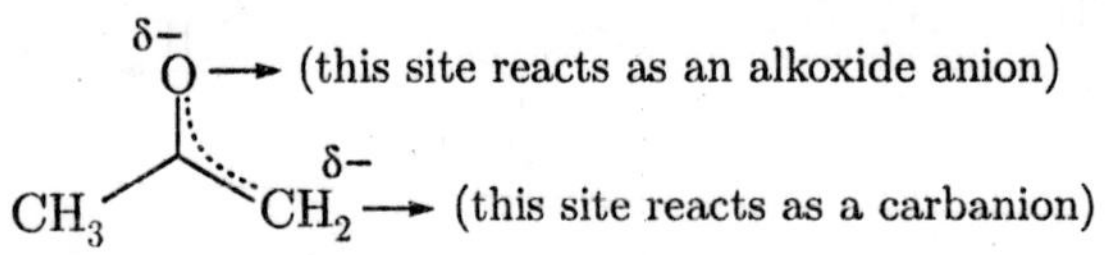

Just how an enolate anion reacts depends in part, on the substrate with which it reacts. Chloroalkylsilances tend to react almost exclusively at the oxygen atom of an enolate. Reagents include chloromethylsilane, tertiarybutylchlorodimethylsilane (TBDMSCl) and tertiarybutylchlorodiphenylsilane (TBDPSCl).

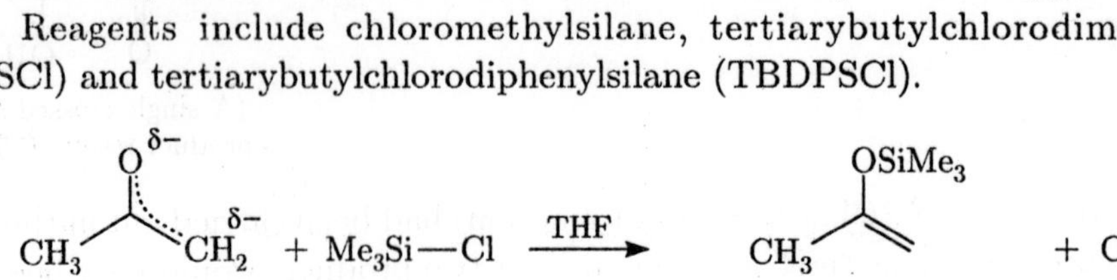

(Trimethylsilyl enol ether)

This reaction called silylation is a nucleophilic substitution at the silicon atom by the oxygen atom of the enolate and it takes place as it does because the O–Si bond that forms in the trimethylsilyl enol ether is very strong (much stronger than C–Si bond). This factor makes formation of the trimethylsilyl enol ether highly exothermic, and, consequently, the free energy of activation for reaction at O atom is lower than that for reaction at the α–carbon.

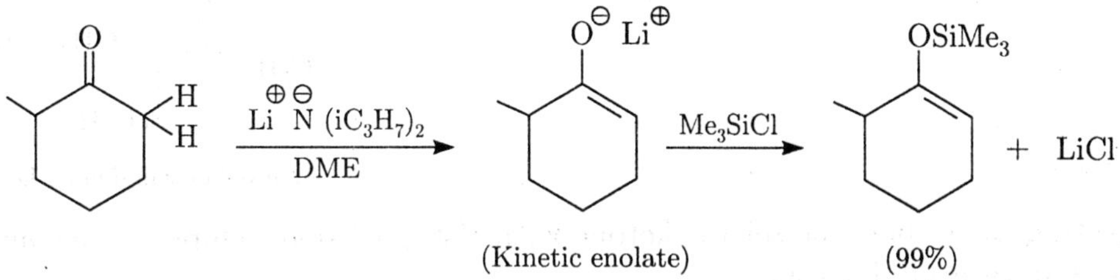

This example shows how the enolate anion can be trapped by converting it to the trimethylsilyl enol ether. This procedure is particularly useful, because the trimethylsilyl enol ether can be purified, if necessary, and then converted back to an enolate. One way of achieving this conversion is by treating the trimethylsilyl enol ether with as aprotic solution containing fluoride ($F^{\ominus}$) ions. The source of $F^{\ominus}$ ions is $Bu_4\overset{\oplus}{N}F^{\ominus}$(TBAF).

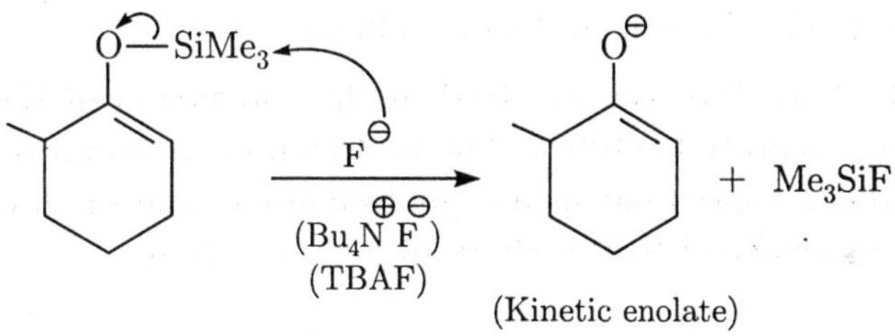

This reaction is a nucleophilic substitution at the Si atom brought about by a $F^{\ominus}$ ion. Fluoride ions have an extremely high affinity for silicon atoms because Si–F bonds are very strong. Another way to convert a trimethylsilyl enol ether back to enolate anion is to treat it with methyllithium.

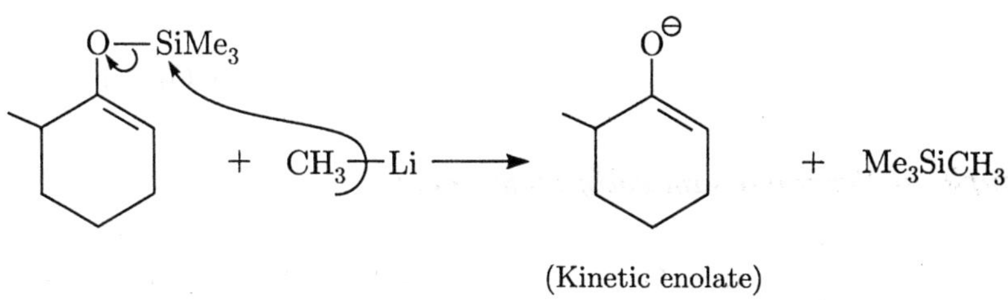

α–Selenation : A synthesis of α, β–unsaturated carbon compounds

Lithium enolates react with benzeneselenyl bromide (C_6H_5SeBr) or with C_6H_5SeCl to yield products containing a C_6H_5Se group at the α position.

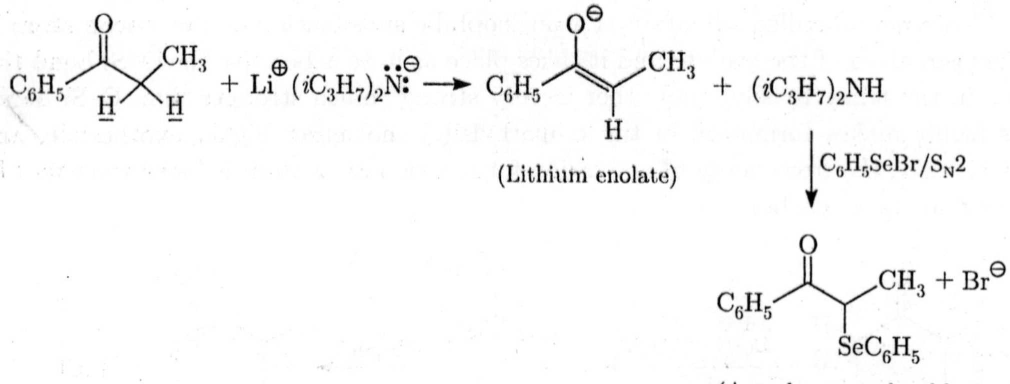

(Lithium enolate)

(An α-benzeneselenyl ketone)

Treating the α–benzene selenyl ketone with H_2O_2 at room temperature converts it to an α, β–unsaturated ketone.

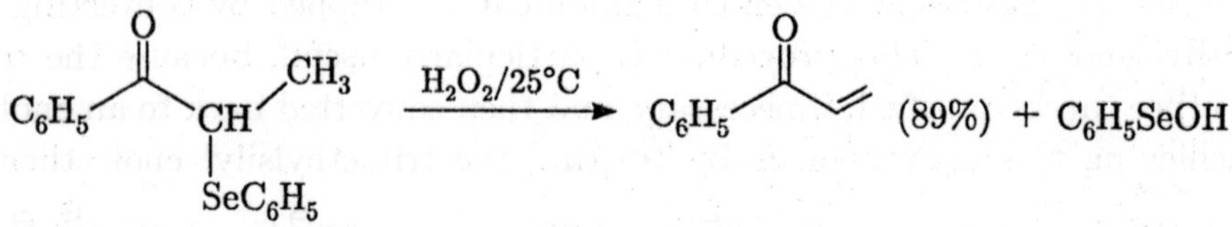

These are very mild conditions for the introduction of a double bond (room temperature and neutral solution) and so is valuable.

Mathematically, two steps are involved in the conversion of the α–benzeneselenyl ketone to the α, β–unsaturated ketones. The first step is an oxidation brought about by H_2O_2. The second step is a spontaneous intramolecular elimination in which the negatively charged oxygen atom attached to the Se atom acts as a base.

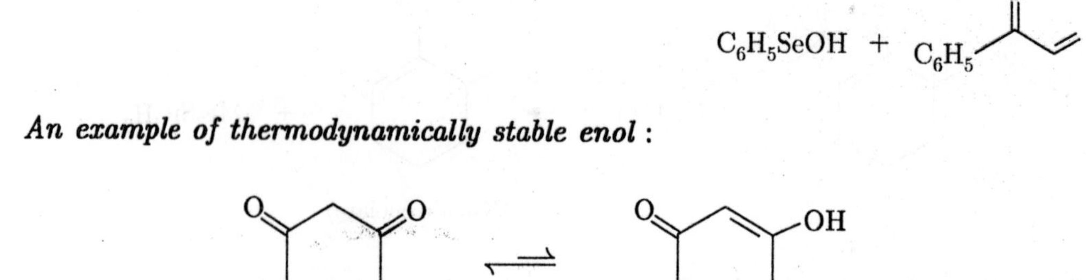

An example of thermodynamically stable enol :

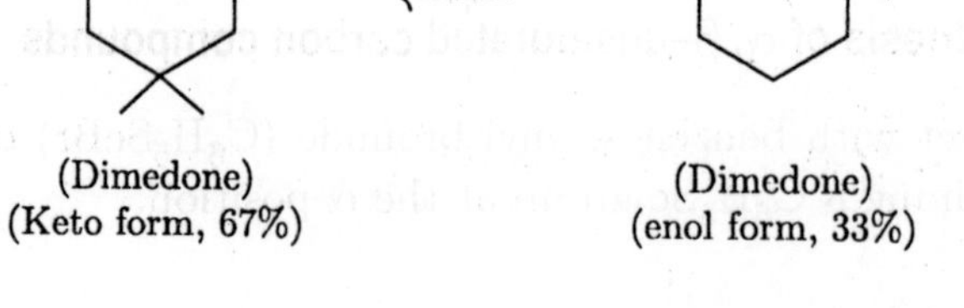

(Dimedone)
(Keto form, 67%)

(Dimedone)
(enol form, 33%)

The normal stability of this enol is due to the unique arrangement of two functional groups lead to enols that are conjugated rather like a carboxylic acid.

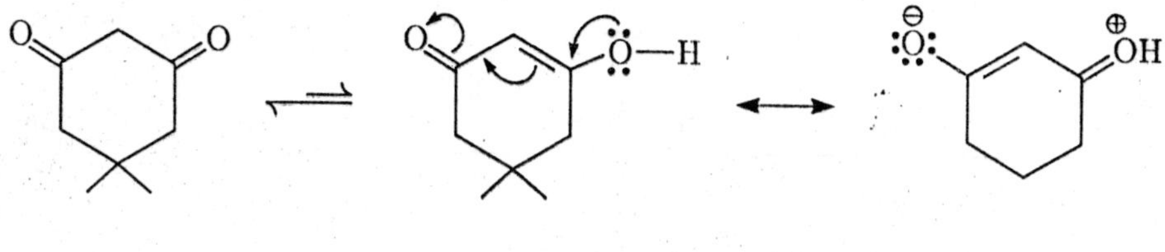

(Equilibration of enol form of dimedone)

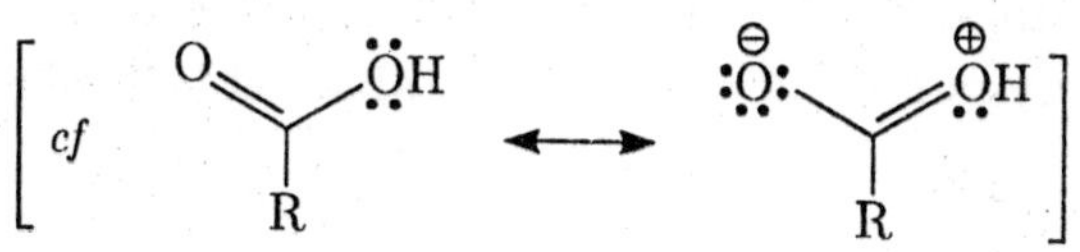

Deuterium exchange and nitrosation reaction at the α–carbon to a carbonyl group containing at least one α–H atom are examples of electrophilic substitution reaction which proceed via an *enolate anion.*

Enamines

Synthesis of enamines : Stork enamine synthesis

Aldehydes and ketones with at least one α–H atom react with secondary amines to form compounds called *enamines.* The general reaction for the formation of enamines can be written as follows.

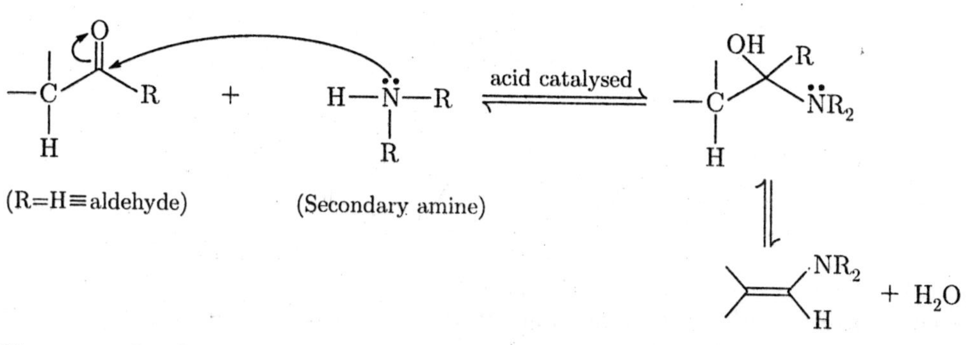

Since enamine formation requires the loss of a molecule of water, enamine preparations are usually carried out in a way that allows water to be removed as an azeotrope or by a drying agent. This removal of water drives the reversible reaction to completion. Enamine formation is also catalysed by the presence of a trace amount of acid. The secondary amines most commonly used to prepare enanmines are cyclic amines such as

pyrrolidine 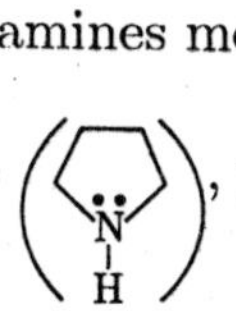, piperidine 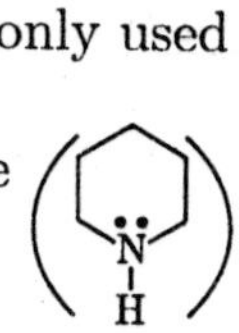 and morpholine 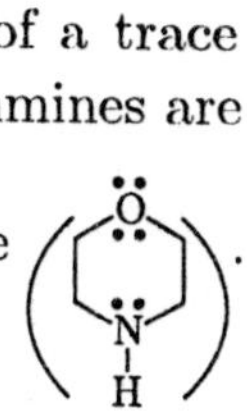.

The choice of morpholine, pyrrolidine and piperidine are taken as both the starting amines and the enamines are more nucleophilic (the alkyl groups are tied back and can not get in the way of reaction).

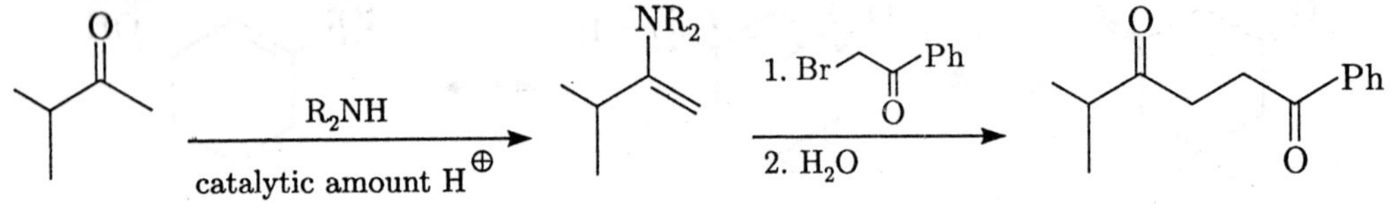

As the original ketone is unsymmetrical, two enamines are possible. Less substituted enamine is predominant. For the more substituted enamines, steric hindrance forces the enamines to lose the planarity and destabilises it. Thus the less substituted enamine is more stable. (Compare the opposites– *more* substituted *enols* are stable but *less* substituted *enamines* are stable.)

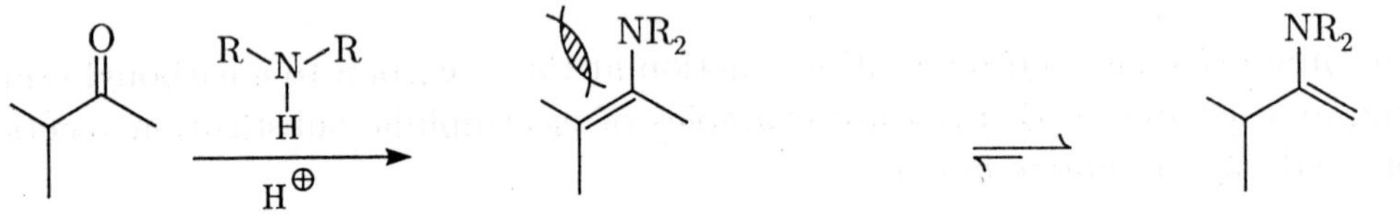

(More hindered enamine)
(Steric hindrance prevents complete planarity of conjugated enamine)

(Less hindered enamine)

Example :

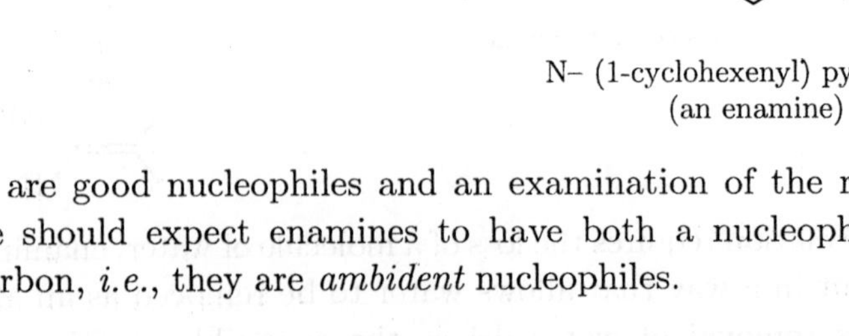

(Cyclohexanone)

N– (1-cyclohexenyl) pyrrolidine
(an enamine)

Enamines are good nucleophiles and an examination of the resonance structures that follow we should expect enamines to have both a nucleophilic nitrogen and a nucleophilic carbon, *i.e.*, they are *ambident* nucleophiles.

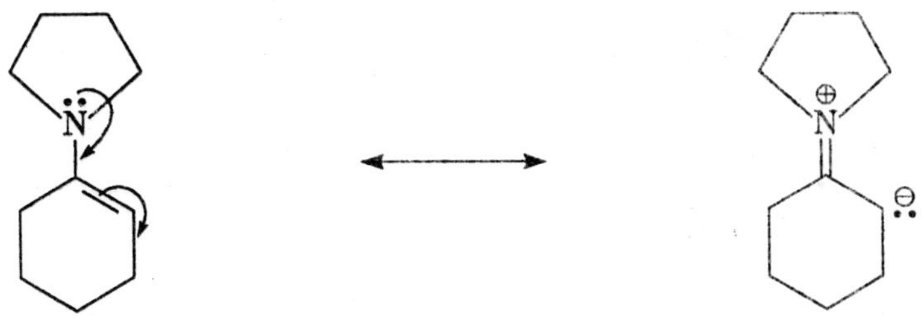

(Contribution to the hybrid made by this structure confers nucleophilicity on nitrogen)

(Contribution to the hybrid made by this structure confers nucleophilicity on C and decreases nucleophilicity on N)

The nucleophilicity of the carbon of enamines makes them particularly useful reagents in organic synthesis because they can be acylated, alkylated, and used in Michael additions. Thus reactions as a whole is known as *Stork enamine reactions* (Inventor : Gilbert Stork). When an enamine reacts with an acyl halide or an acid anhydride, the product is the C–acylated compound. The imminium ion that forms hydrolyses when water is added, and the overall reaction provides a synthesis for β–diketones.

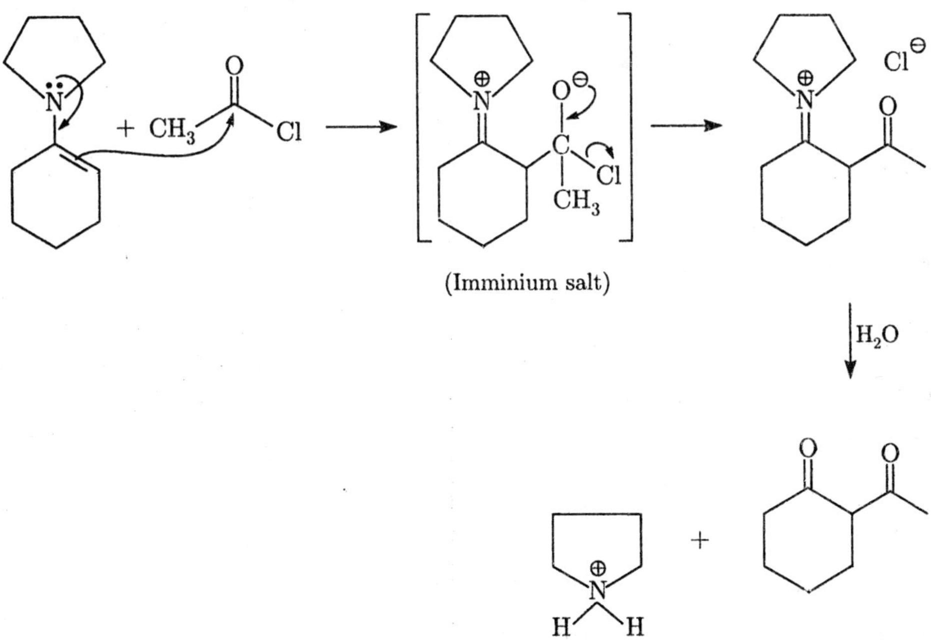

(2-Acetylcyclohexanone)
(α β-diketone)

Although N–acylation may occur in this synthesis, the N–acyl product is unstable and can act as an acylating agent itself.

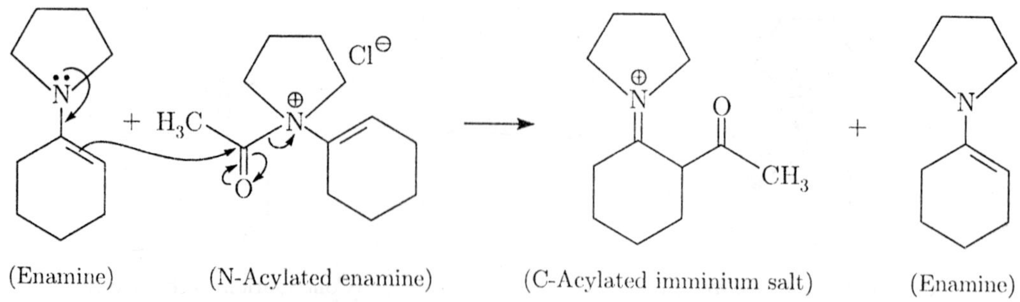

As a consequence, the yields of C–acylated products are generally high.

Enamines can be alkylated as well as acylated. Although alkylation may lead to the formation of a considerable amount of N–alkylated product, heating the N–alkylated product often converts it to a C–alkyl compound. This rearrangement is particularly favoured when the alkyl halide is an allylic halide, benzylic halide or an α–haloacetic ester.

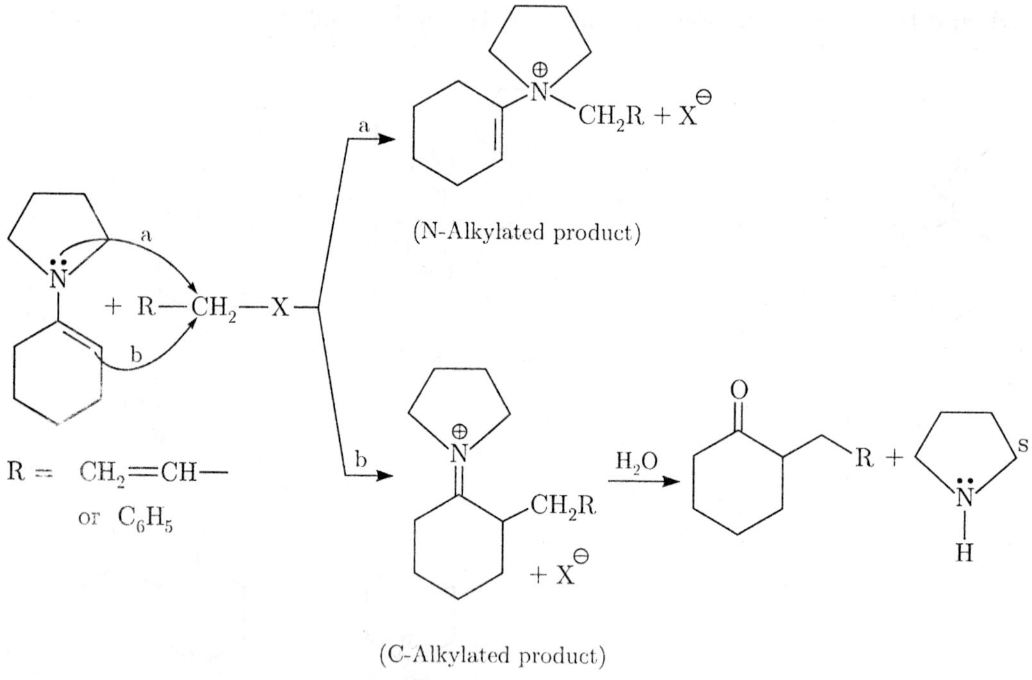

Enamine alkylation reactions are S_N2 reactions, therefore, when we choose our alkylating agents, we are usually restricted to the use of methyl, primary, allylic and benzylic halides. α–Haloesters can also be used as alkylating agents, and this reaction provides a convenent synthesis of γ–keto esters.

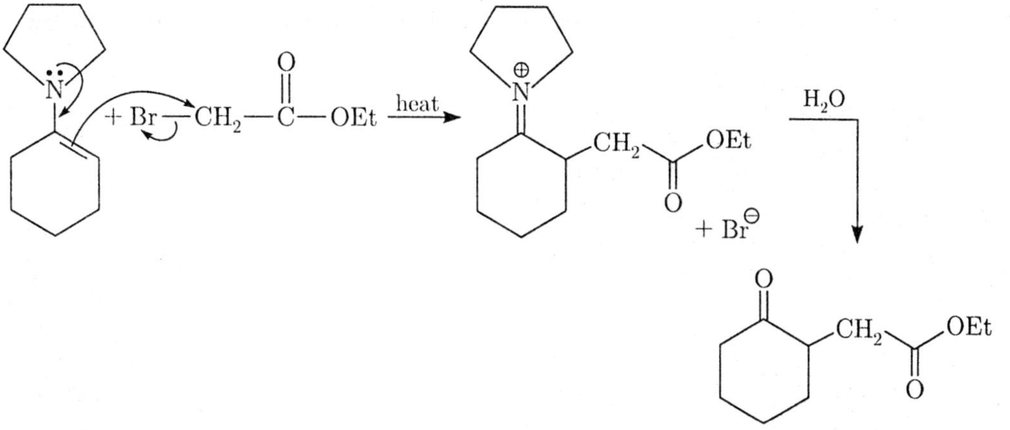

(a γ-Ketoester) (75%)

An especially interesting set of enamine alkylations is shown in the following reactions (Developed by J.K. Whitesell). The enamine (prepared from a single enantiomer of a secondary amine) is chiral. Alkylation from the bottom of the enamine is *severely hindered* by the methyl group. This hindrance exists even if rotation of the group takes place about the bond connecting the two rings. Consequently, alkylation takes place much more rapidly from the **top side**. This reaction yields (after hydrolysis) 2–substituted cyclohexanones consisting almost entirely of a *single enantiomer*.

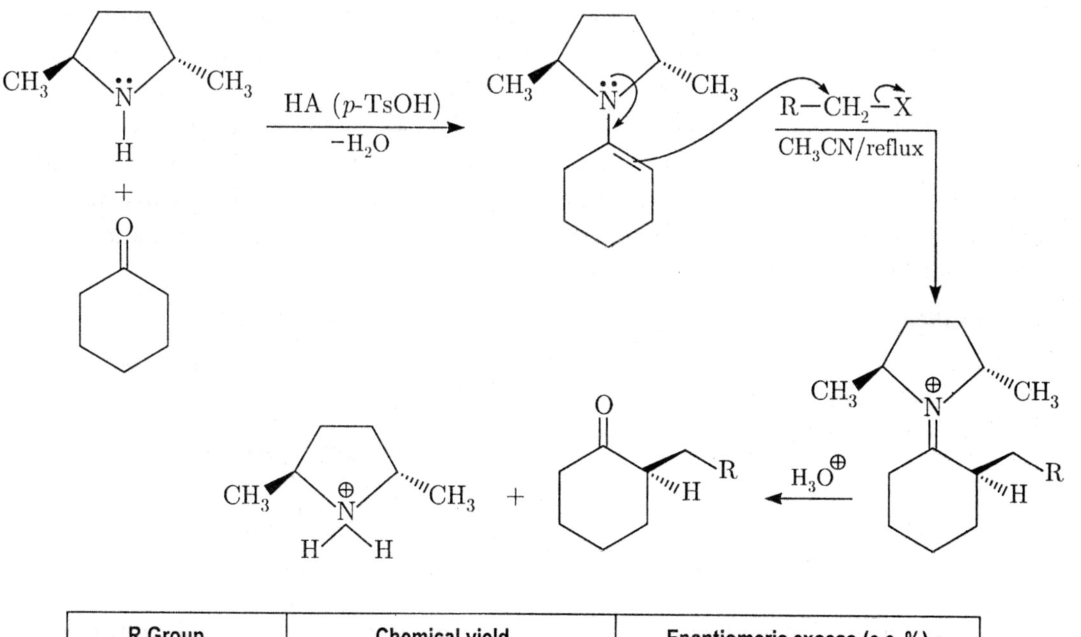

R Group	Chemical yield	Enantiomeric excess (e.e. %)
H	50	83
CH_3CH_2—	57	93
CH_2=CH—	80	82

Enamines can also be used in *Michael additions.* One example is given below.

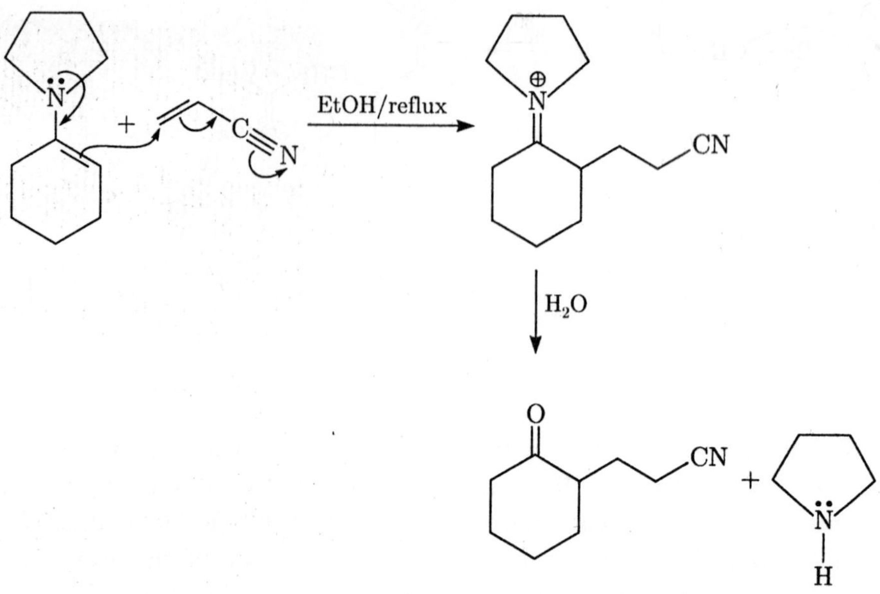

Tautomerism

There are many constitutional isomers which are interconvertible by a low energy barrier and the isomerisation involves migration of an atom or group from one position to another. Sometimes these isomers are interconvertible by electron distribution along with migration of atomic nuclei and the phenomenon is known as *tautomerism* and the isomers as *tautomers.* Tautomerism is an equilibrium controlled phenomenon and so different tautomers can exist under different thermodynamic conditions like pressure, temperature, solvent, pH, etc. Tautomerism is generally exhibited in liquid and gaseous forms of molecules, not in their solid forms.

Examples :

1. Ethyl acetoacetate can remain in two isomeric forms in a dynamic equilibrium under normal conditions.

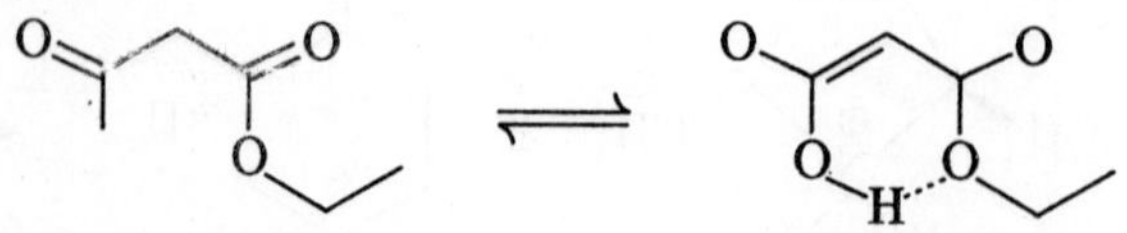

(Keto form) (Enol form)

Ethyl acetoacetate has two tautomeric forms like keto- and enol tautomers.

Due to the presence of above two isomeric (tautomeric) structures, ethyl acetoacetate shows the presence of functional groups like (a) keto group, (b) ester group, (c) ethylenic unsaturation and (d) hydroxyl group.

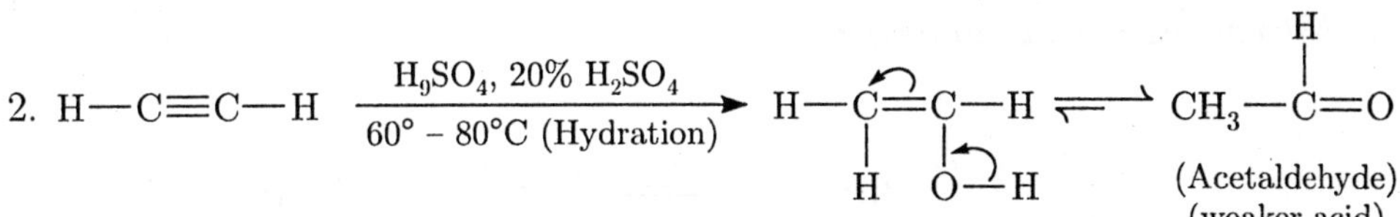

(Vinyl alcohol) (stronger acid) (Enol form) — (Acetaldehyde) (weaker acid) (Keto form)

Tautomerism can be divided into *three* categories : 1. **Cationotropy**, 2. **Anionotropy, and** 3. **Valence tautomerism**

1. ***Cationotropy*** : When a proton (H^+) changes its position as a cation, the tautomerism is known as *prototropy.* Thus, prototropy is a special class of cationotropy.

Some examples of prototropy :

1. ***Keto-enol tautomerism*** :

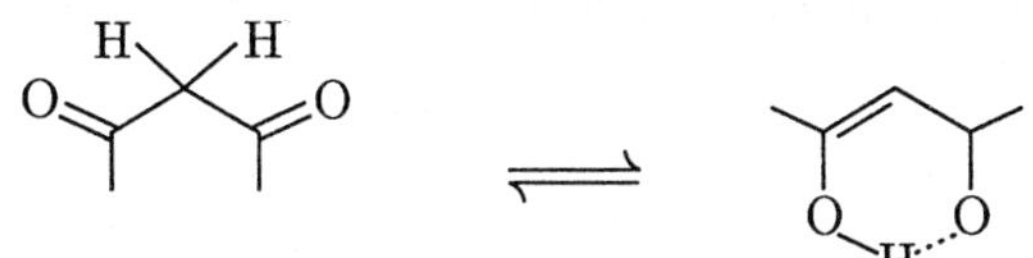

(Acetylacetone) (Keto form) — (Enol form)

2. ***Phenol–keto tautomerism*** :

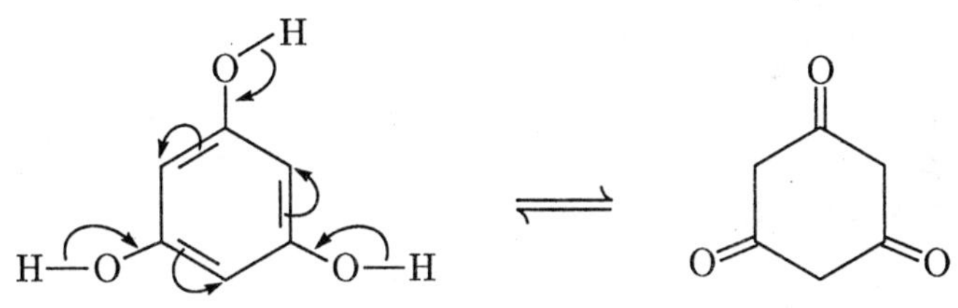

(Phloroglucinol) (Phenol form) — (Keto form)

3. ***Amido–imidol tautomerism*** :

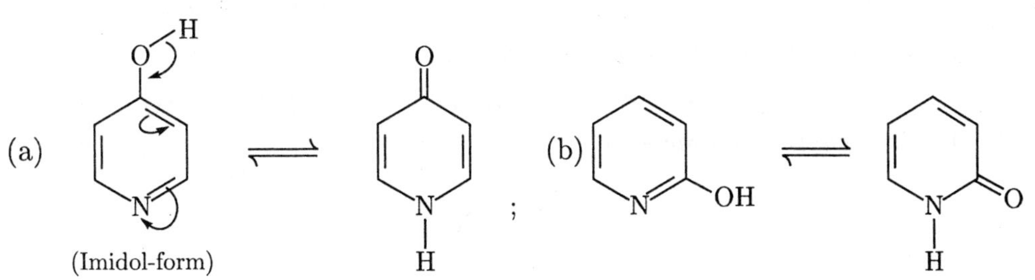

(Imidol-form) — (Amide form)

4. *Nitroso–oxime tautomerism* :

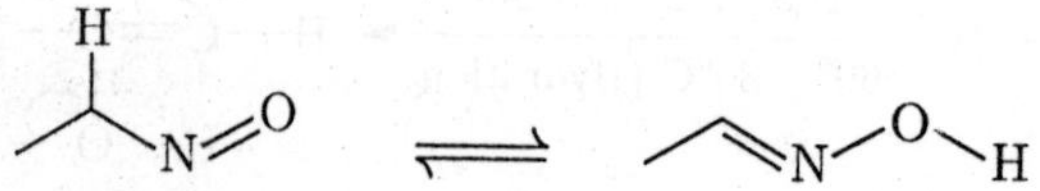

(Nitroso form) (Oxime form)

Nitrosoform is only stable when there is no α–H, otherwise oxime form predominates in the equilibrium.

5. *Nitro–and acinitro tautomerism* :

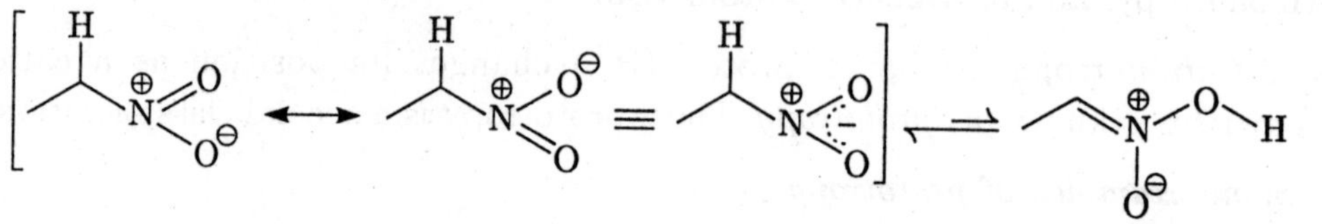

(Resonance stabilised nitro form) **(Acinitro form) (less stable)**

6. *Imine–enamine tautomerism* :

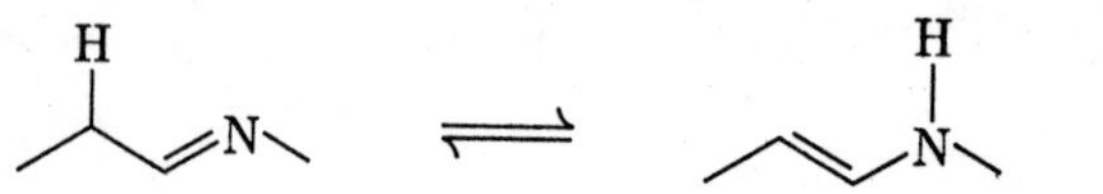

(Imine) (more stable) **(Enamine) (less stable)**

Enamine formation is possible only when there is *an α–H* atom and is stable when *no hydrogen* is attached to nitrogen.

7. *Amidine-Imidine tautomerism* :

$$-NH-\overset{|}{C}=N \rightleftharpoons -N=\overset{|}{C}-NH-$$

8. *Azo–hydrazone tautomerism* :

$$-N=N-\underset{|}{\overset{|}{C}}-H \rightleftharpoons -HN-N=C\langle$$

9. *Diazo–amino tautomerism* :

$$-N=N-\overset{|}{N}-H \rightleftharpoons -NH-N=N-$$

10. *Diazo–nitrosoamine tautomerism* :

$$Ar-N=N-OH \rightleftharpoons Ar-NH-N=O$$

11. *Ring–chain tautomerism* :

(a) 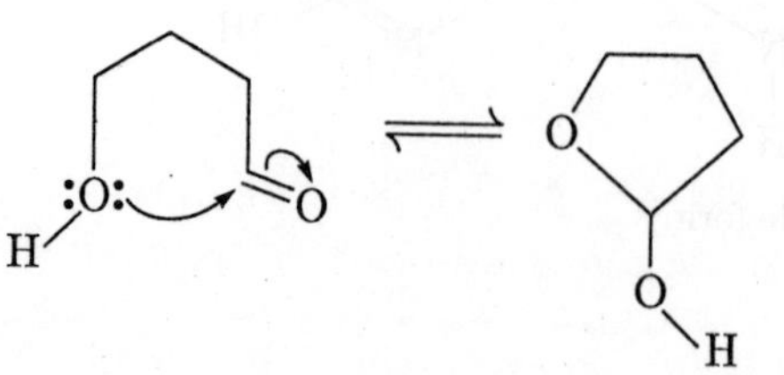

(b) 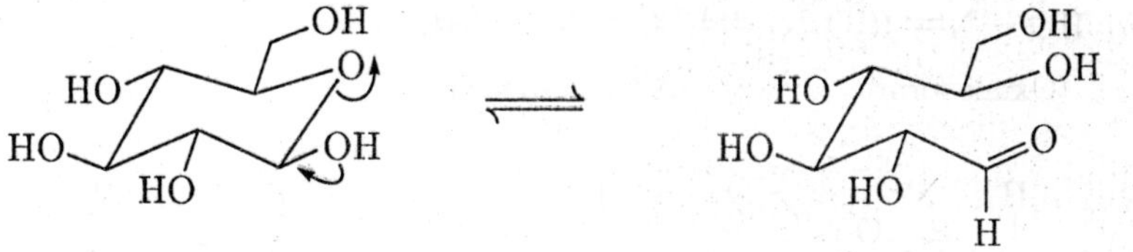

(Ring structure of β-D-glucopyranose) (Open chain form of D-glucose)

Equlibrium in prototropy : The characteristics of equilibrium between the tautomers involving prototropy are as follows.

(a) 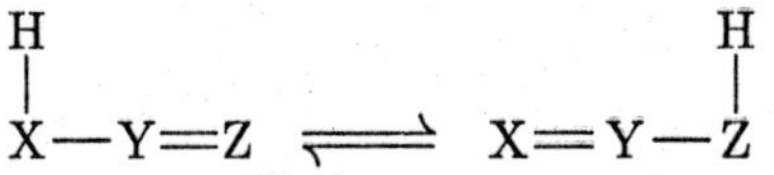

(b) 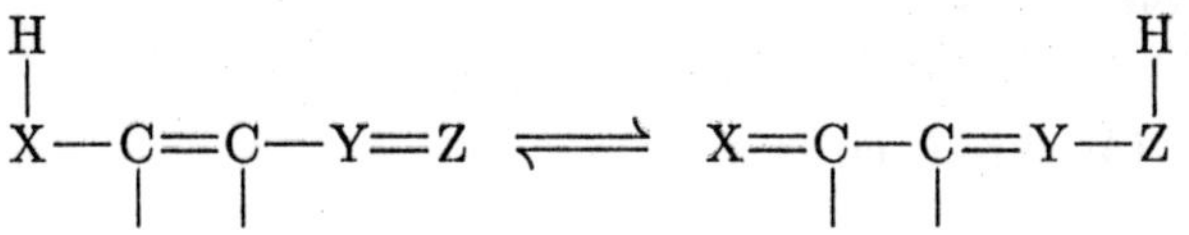

(c) 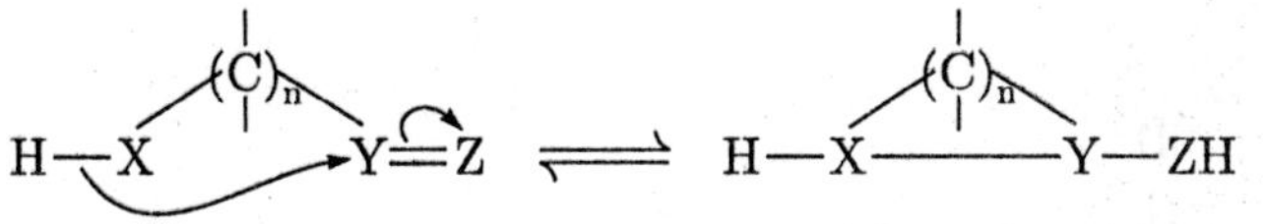

Let the two tautomers be in equilibrium as $A \rightleftharpoons B$

So, at a certain temperature, $K_e = \frac{[B]_e}{[A]_e}$ where $[A]_e$ and $[B]_e$ are the equilibrium concentrations of A and B.

$$\therefore \ln K_e = \frac{-\Delta G^\circ}{RT} = \frac{-(\Delta H^\circ - T\Delta S^\circ)}{RT}$$

When carbon is attached to a heteroatom like N, O or S, (C=N, C=O or C=S), the bond energy is more and it is more than twice of C–X(X=heteroatom) single bond energy. It follows then,

B. E. of C=X(X=N, O, S etc.)>B. E of 2×[C–X] (X=N, O, S) and the B. E. of C=C <B. E. of 2×(C–C). (where B.E stands for bond energy)

(a) For the following transformation, $\Delta H^\circ > O$ and the equilibrium is shifted to the left.

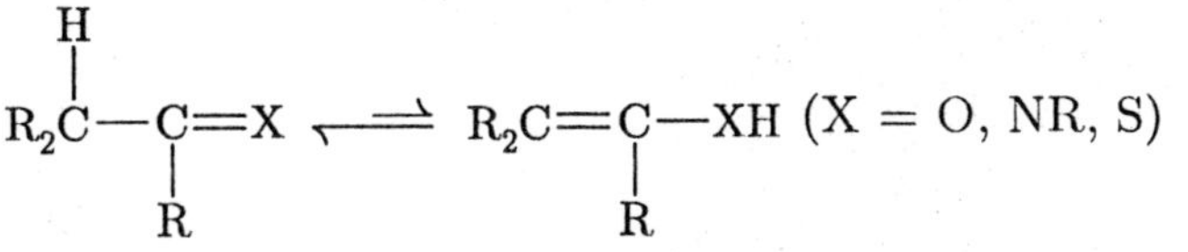

For this reason, acetone has a poor enol content (~0.01%) and the keto content is ~ 99.09%.

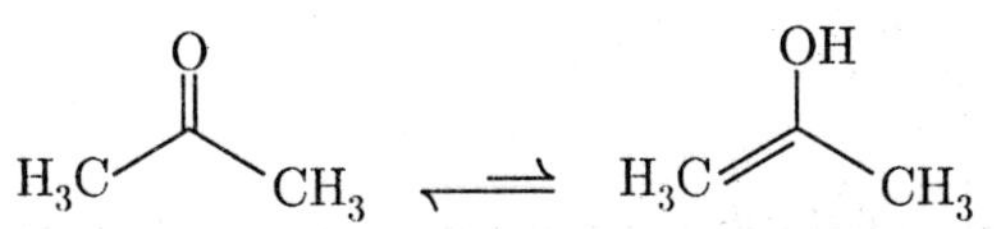

~99.09% (keto form) ~0.01% (enol form)

(b) $HO—N=R_2C \rightleftharpoons O=N—CHR_2$

(Oxime form) (Nitroso form)

(c) 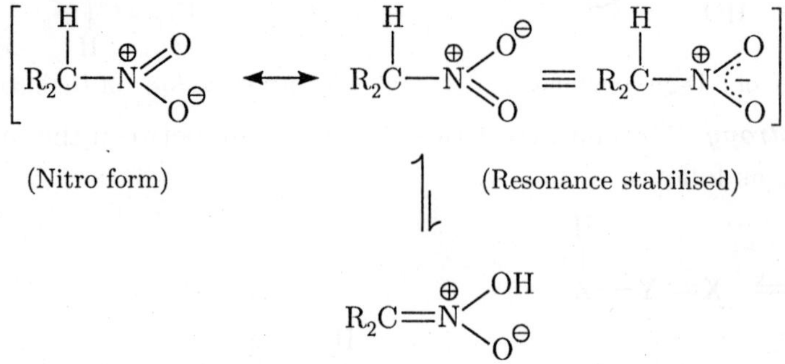

(Nitro form) (Resonance stabilised)

(Acinitro form)

Keto–enol tautomerism :

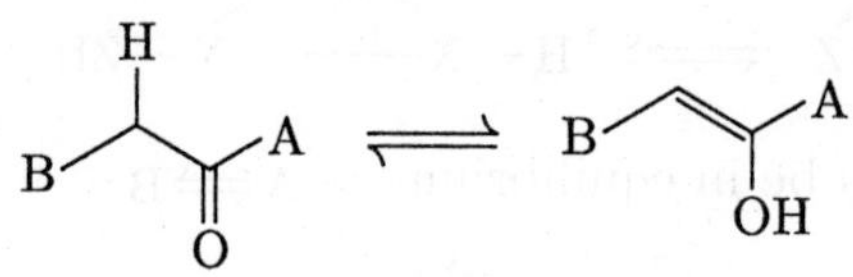

(Keto-form) (Enol-form)

The ratio of keto– and enol forms depends on the nature of A and B.

1. If B is an alkyl group, the enol form gets hyperconjugative stability although the extent of stabilisation is not much.
2. If B is an unsaturated or aryl group, the enol conformer gets resonance stabilisation. The enol content of $C_6H_5CH_2COCH_3$ is more than that of $CH_3CH_2COCH_3$.

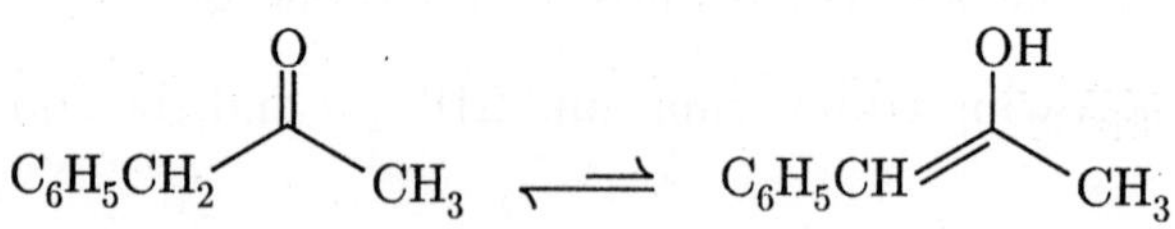

(I)

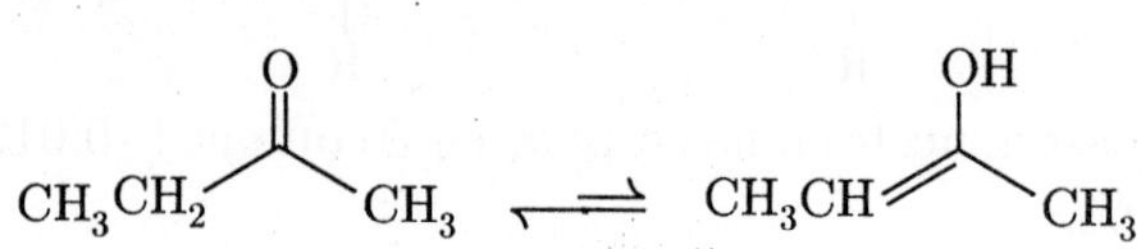

(II)

Enol content of (I) in equilibrium is more than that of (II).

If B is vinyl, then by two consecutive keto–enol and enol– keto tautomerism, an α,β–unsaturated compounds are formed during any preparation of β–γ–unsaturated compounds.

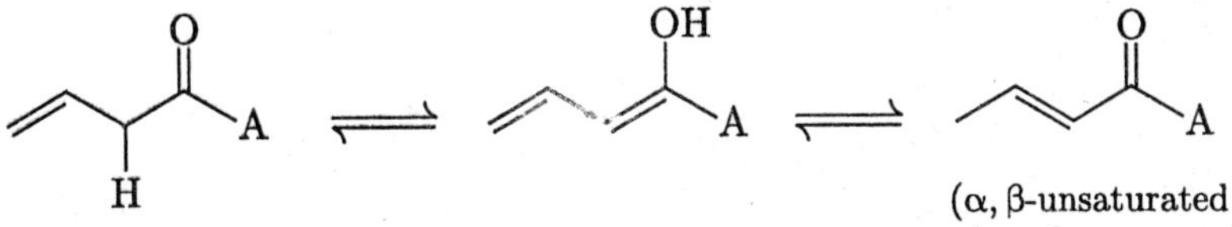

(β-γ-unsaturated carbonyl compound) (α, β-unsaturated carbonyl compound)

3. If B contains any electronegative element, the enol form is stabilised by intramolecular hydrogen bonding. This intramolecular hydrogen bonding becomes less important if the solvent molecules form hydrogen bonding with the molecule concerned.

In gaseous state, or in apolar solvents, $CF_3CH_2\overset{O}{\overset{\|}{C}}-CH_3$ has get more enol content than $CH_3CH_2\overset{O}{\overset{\|}{C}}-CH_3$ as the former molecule is stabilised by intramolecular hydrogen bonding.

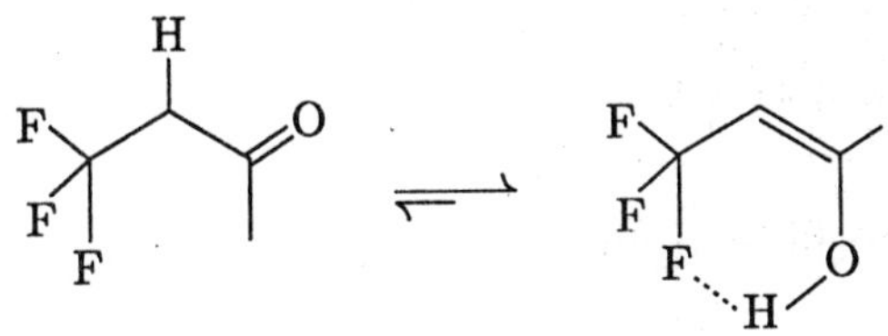

Highly fluorinated ketones like $CF_2H-\overset{O}{\overset{\|}{C}}-CF_3$ is stable in its keto form, not in the enol form. The enol form gets converted to the keto form upon prolonged heating, as the tautomerisation reaction is very slow due to electron withdrawing power of fluorine atoms.

$$F_2C{=}\underset{\displaystyle OH}{\underset{|}{C}}-CF_3 \xrightleftharpoons{200°C/3h} CF_2H-\underset{\displaystyle O}{\underset{\|}{C}}-CF_3$$

4. If B is C=O, N=O etc. (where double bond is joined to an electronegative atom) then the enol form is stabilised by both intramolecular hydrogen bonding and resonance. The extent of resonance stabilisation depends on the nature of the group. If it is –COOR, –COOH, –$CONH_2$ etc. then enol form attains no extra stability out of resonance. In those cases, groups with + R effect (*e.g.*, OH, OR, NH_2 etc.) are attached to the carbonyl carbon and C=C bond remains in *cross conjugation* with the C=O group. As a result, resonance between C=C and C=O becomes less important. But, if B is either aldehyde or keto carbonyl,

then the enol form gets considerable resonance stabilisation. This resonance stabilisation is the reason for the higher enol content of acetylacetone than that of ethyl acetoacetate.

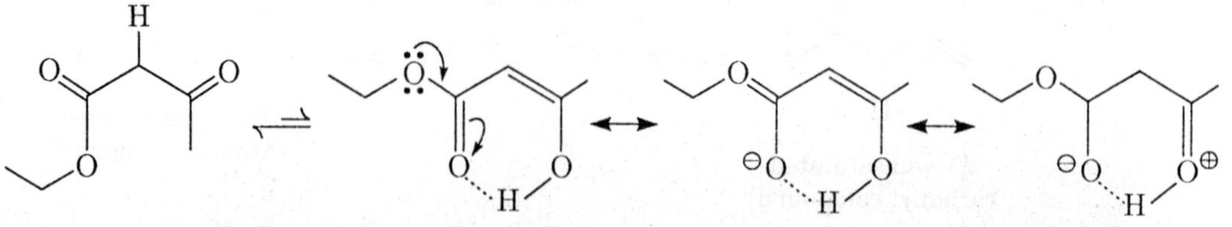

EAA (92%) (Enol form) (8%)

Another reason for the high keto content of ethyl acetoacetate is that free rotation around the bonds is more probable which makes the entropy of the system more positive for the keto form compared to the enol form where the entropy change is negative due to ring formation. As a result, free energy of the keto form becomes less.

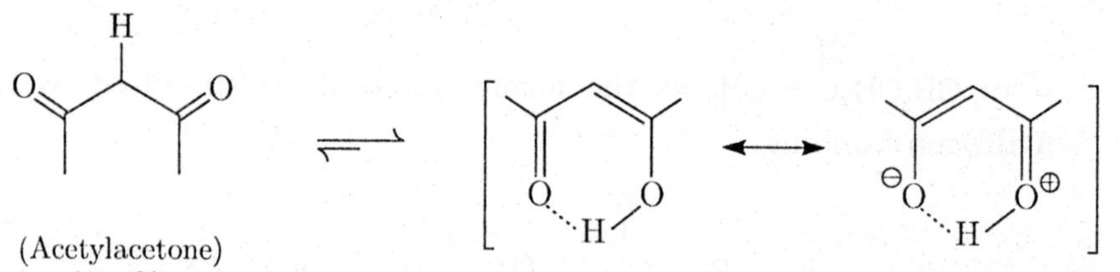

(Acetylacetone) (23.6%) (76.4%)

5. If any enol form is aromatic, it becomes stable and hence predominates in the equilibrium.

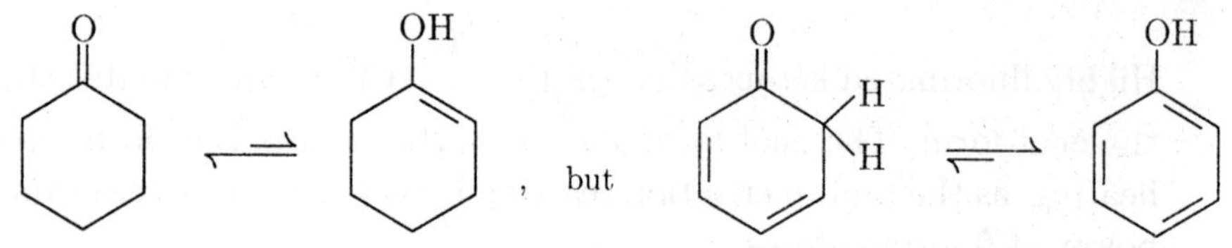

(Keto form) (99.98%) (Enol form) (0.02%) (0%) (~100%) (Aromatic)

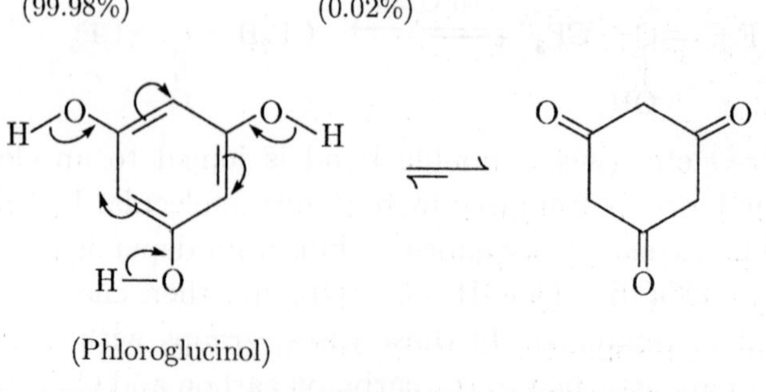

(Phloroglucinol)

A great stability is achieved by three C=O bonds as C=O double bond has bond energy more than twice that of C–O single bond energy and even exceeds the aromatic stability present in 1,3,5-trihydroxyphenol (phloroglucinol). For this reason, triketo form of phloroglucinol predominates in the equilibrium.

6. The carbon atoms which are joined to ethylenic double bond should lie in the same plane in order to have the enol form. If by configurational or due to steric reasons, the ethylenic part of the enol form can not form a planar geometry, then keto to enol conversion gets inhibited.

Examples :

(a) 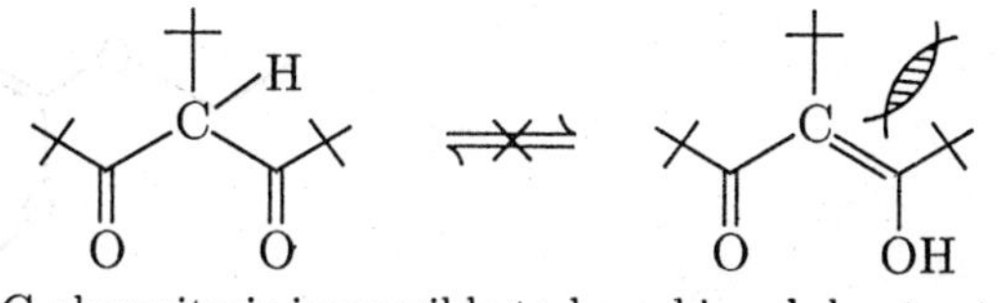

(C=C planarity is impossible to be achieved due to strong steric repulsion exerted by bulky tertiarybutyl groups)

(b) 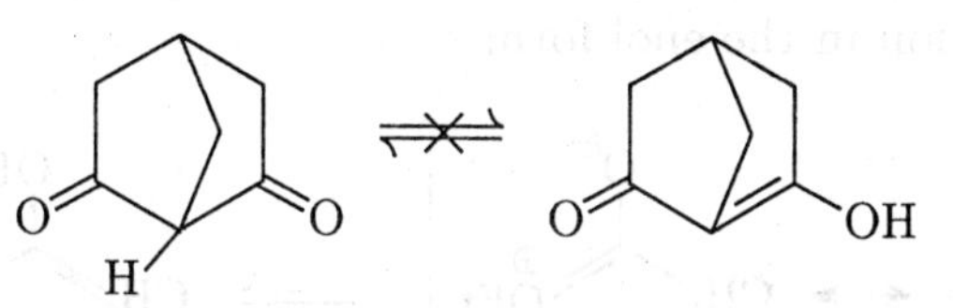

(Bicyclo [2.2.1] heptane-2,6-dione)
(By Bredt's rule, the bridge head carbon cannot attain a planar geometry on enolisation because of rigid bicyclic structure of the molecule)

(c) 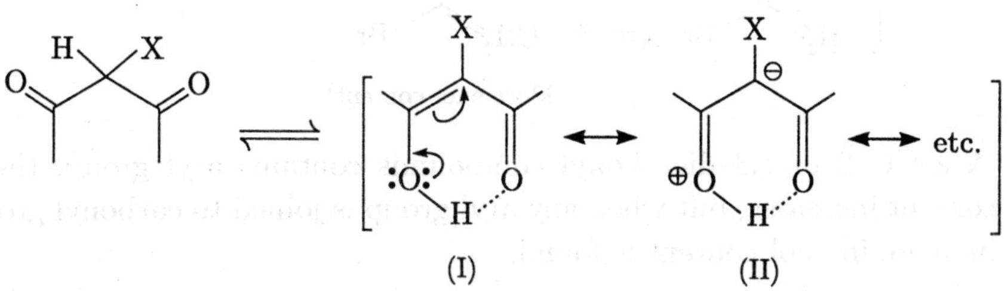

If X has (–I) or (–R) effect, the negative charge in structure (II) gets delocalised and the enol form gets stabilised. If X is phenyl (–R effect), resonance stability is more and the extent of enol form in equilibrium increases and if X=CH_3 (+R effect), the resonance stability of enol form decreases.

7. Acids, esters, amides etc. have negligible enol content as the resonance stability is lost in the enol form.

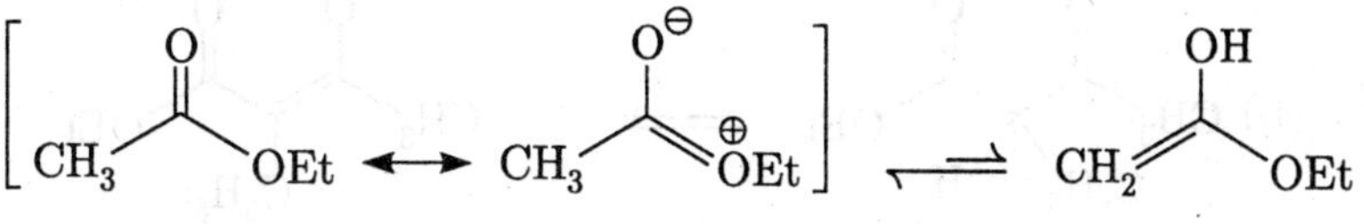

Diethyl malonate *has even lower enol content than* ethyl acetoacetate; the enol form of diethyl malonate loses its resonance stability.

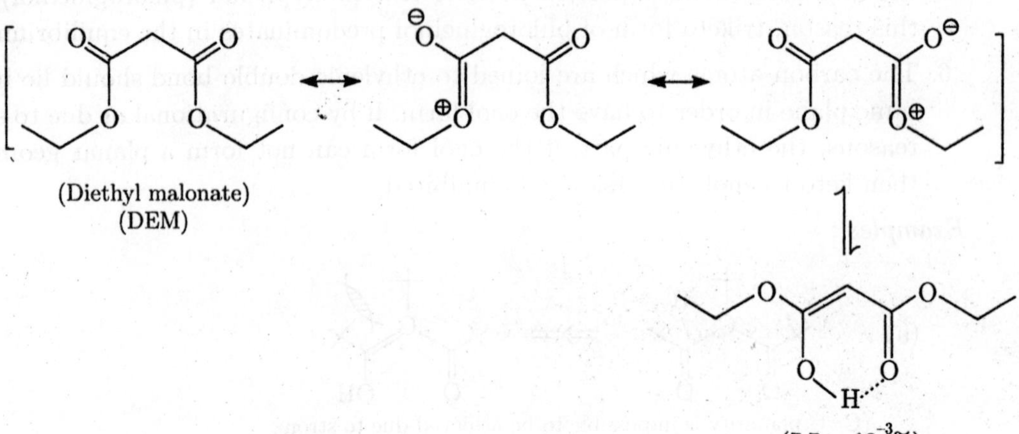

(Diethyl malonate)
(DEM)

(7.7×10^{-3}%)

Acetyl bromide has more enol content than ethyl acetate; the *ester group* loses its resonance stabilisation in the enol form.

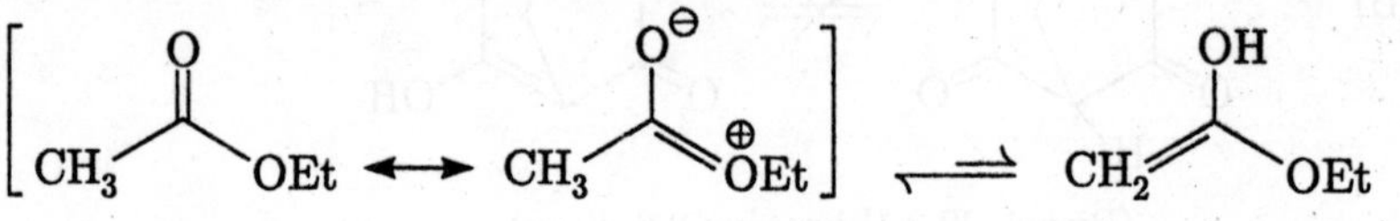

(Less enol content)

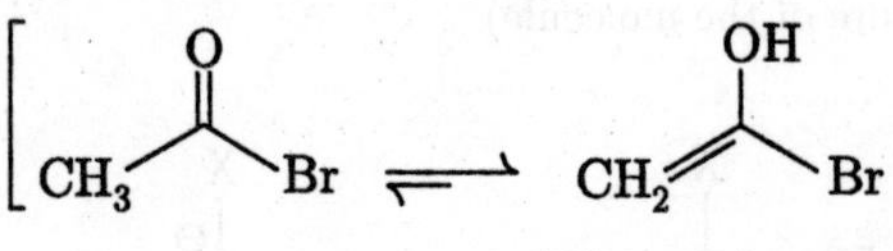

(More enol content)

8. When C–2 of 1,3–dicarbonyl compounds contains aryl group, the % of enol content increases; but when any aryl group is joined to carbonyl group, no such increase in enol content is found.

I. (a)

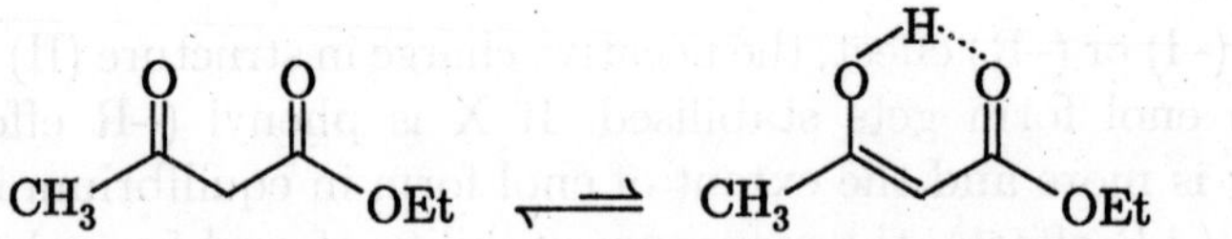

(92%) (8%)

(b)

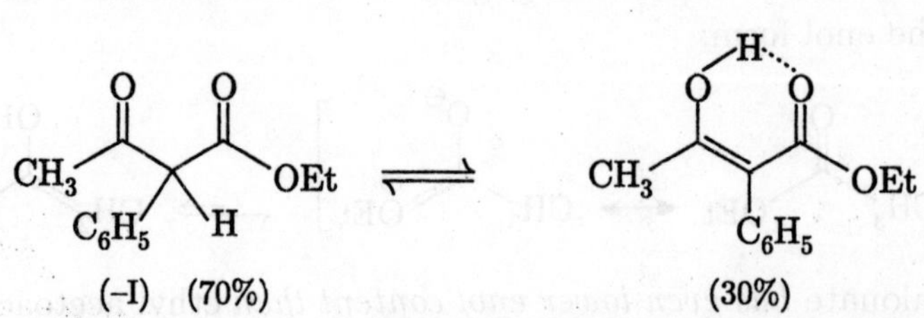

(–I) (70%) (30%)

(Resonance stabilisation increases)

II. (a) 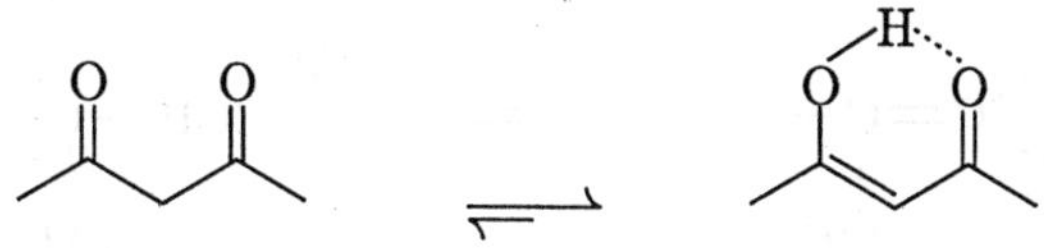

(24%) (76%)

(b) 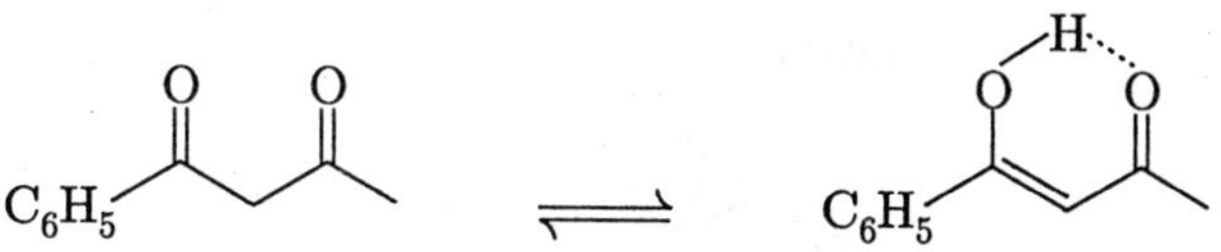

(11%) (89%)

(Increment in enol content is not that dramatic as no resonance stabilisation of enol occurs)

9. Open–chain 1,2–dicarbonyl compounds remain in anti position to avoid dipole–dipole interaction, and their enol content is also less compared to ordinary ketones.

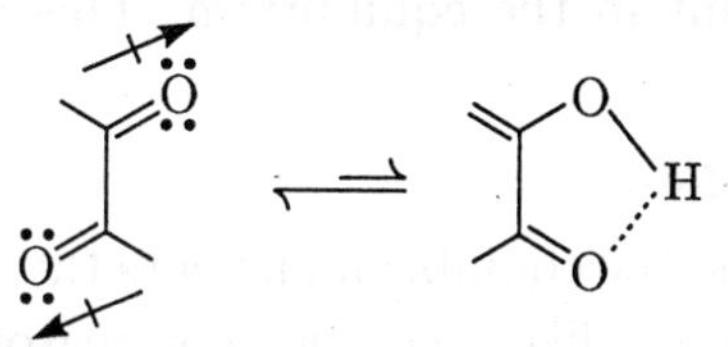

But in small membered cyclic 1,2–diones, like cyclobutane–1,2–dione or cyclopentane– 1,2–dione, the two carbonyl groups are compelled to attain *cis*–configuration whereby a strong dipole-dipole interaction is generated and the diketo form loses its stability. On the other hand, enol form is stabilised by intramolecular hydrogen bonding and the extent of dipole-dipole interaction gets minimised. So these compounds remain almost 100% in the enol form in the equilibrium.

(a) 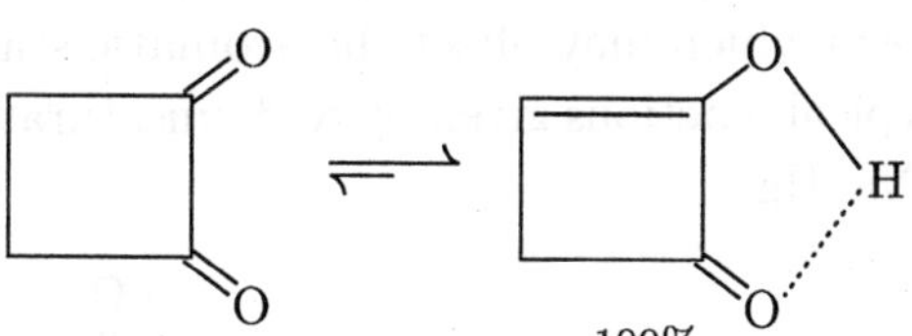

~100%

(b) 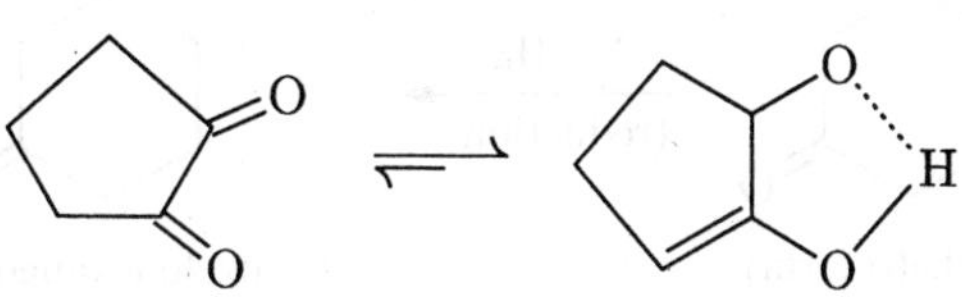

~100%

N.B. : In any dicarbonyl compound, maximum distance is maintained between two oxygen atoms to avoid dipole-dipole interaction which becomes the preferred conformer.

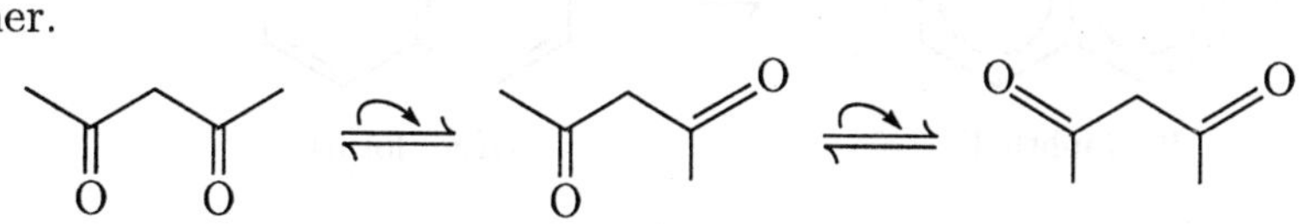

10.

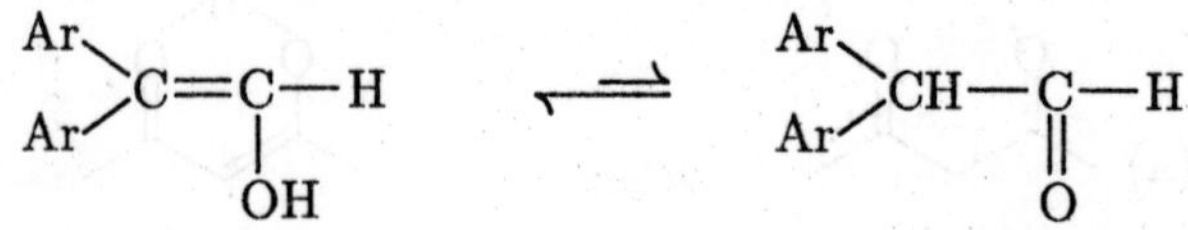

(2,2-dimesityl alcohol) (5%)

(95%)

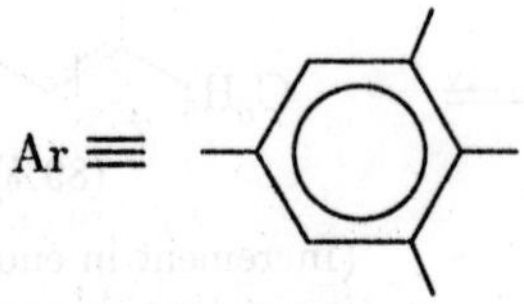

The destabilisation of keto form is due to steric hindrance. In enol form, two aryl groups are about 120° apart (carbon is sp^2 hybridised), but in the enol form, they move to 109°28′ (carbon becomes sp^3 hybridised). So the latter form suffers more steric hindrance and remains in less amount in the equilibrium. These enols are known as *fusion type* enols.

Other prototropic shifts :

1. For simple phenols, the equilibrium favours the enol form and there is no evidence where phenol behaves like a ketone. The reason is obviously **aromaticity** which is present in the enol form but not in the keto form, the stabilisation energy is lost.

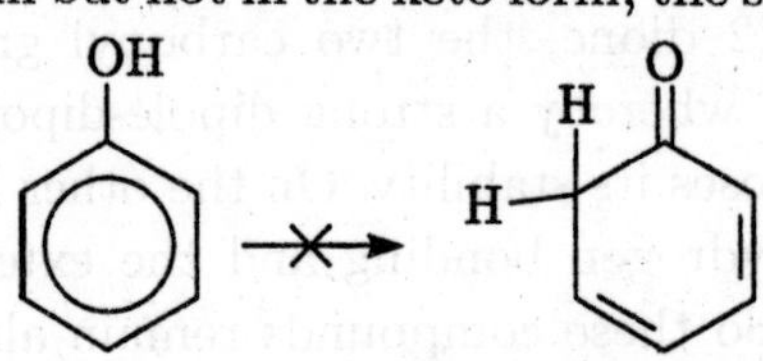

However in resorcinol, where two –OH groups are present, two C=O double bonds are formed in the keto form which may offset the aromatic stability. Keto form of resorcinol shows some typical reactions given by α, β–unsaturated carbonyl compounds like reduction by Na/Hg.

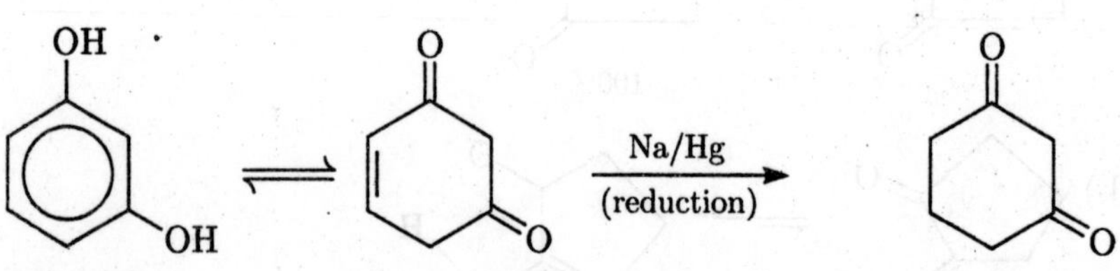

(Resorcinol) (Diketo form) (1,3-cyclohexanedione)

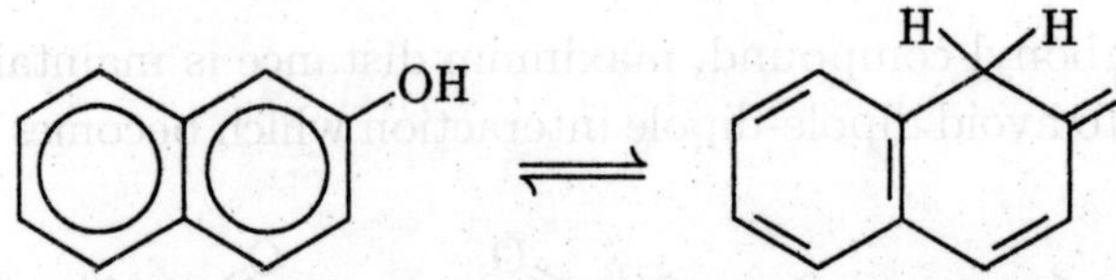

(β-Naphthol) (Keto form)

Upon tautomerisation, β-naphthol does not lose all of its aromatic stability like phenol (as one benzene ring remains intact) and so it shows some percentage of keto form in the equilibrium.

2. ***Heterocyclic compounds*** : Keto form of 4–hydroxy– and 2–hydroxypyridine is more stable in liquid or in solution phase whereas the enol form is only detectable in vapour phase.

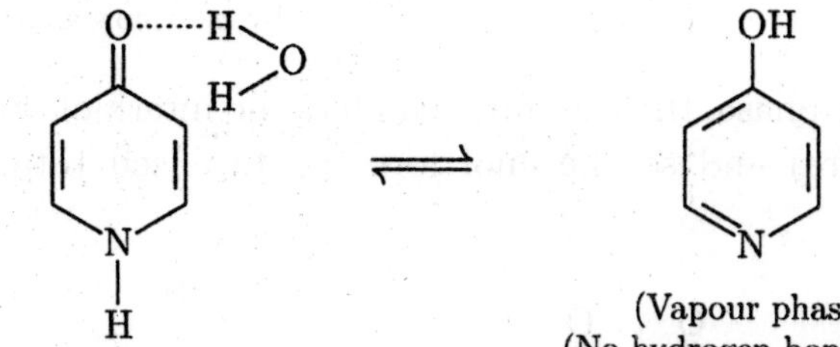

(Solution in water)

(Vapour phase)
(No hydrogen bonding is possible as there is no solvent)

A strong C=O bond is formed which offsets the aromatic stability and C=O bond is stabilised through intermolecular hydrogen bonding with the solvent molecules if the solvent be polar and protic. The same reason is applicable to 2–hydroxypyridine.

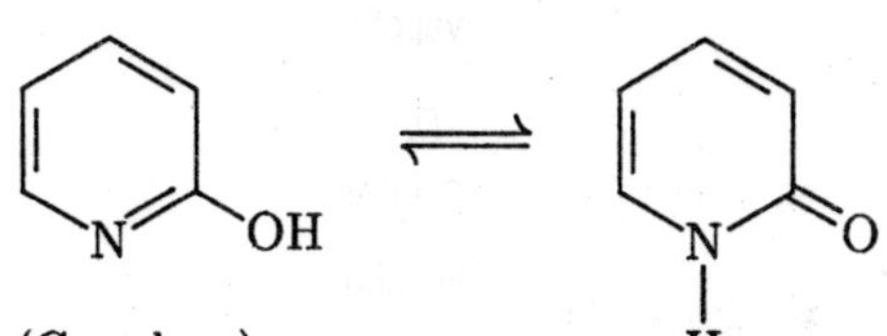

(Gas phase)

(Liquid phase)

Effect of solvent on keto–enol tautomerism : The σ–moment and π–moment of keto C=O group operate in the same direction in keto carbonyl compounds which make C=O a very strong dipole; whereas in enol form, the direction of σ–and π–moments operate opposite to each other, making the enol form a weaker dipole.

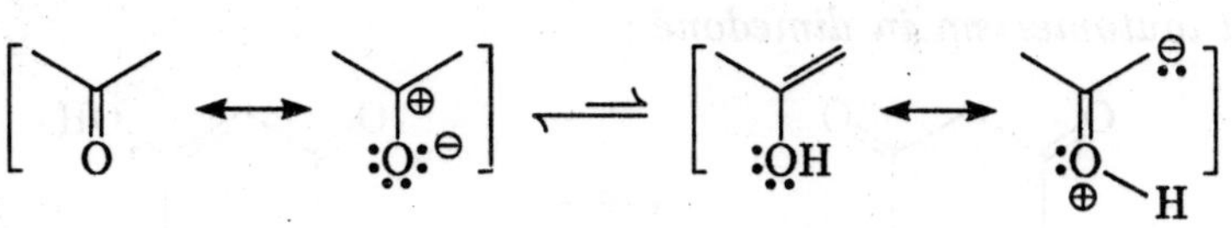

Polar solvents form intermolecular hydrogen bonding with C=O bond and thus, solvation stability is attained. On the other hand, if the polarity of the solvent is less, the enol form becomes predominant. So the magnitude of $\Delta H°$ for *keto* $\rightleftharpoons$ *enol* conversion is less in non polar solvents compared to polar solvents. Again, in the liquid form, the keto form can behave as an autosolvent, which is absent in the vapour phase. The enols which undergo intramolecular hydrogen bonding change their extent of enol content drastically on changing the conditions or solvent.

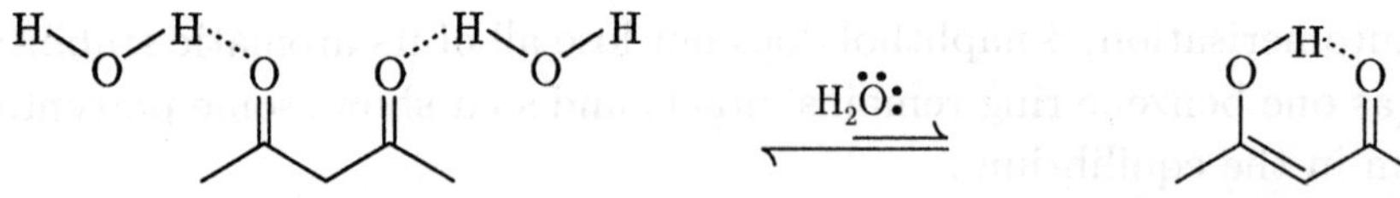

(Keto form of 2,4-pentanedione is stabilised by intermolecular hydrogen bonding with solvent (H_2O) molecules)

(Enol form of 2,4-pentanedione is stabilised by intramolecular hydrogen bonding which becomes less important in polar protic solvent as the keto form is stabilised more by intermolecular hydrogen bonding)

But in the vapour phase, the keto form can have no intermolecular hydrogen bonding (as no solvent is there) and so the enol form is stabilised totally by intramolecular hydrogen bonding.

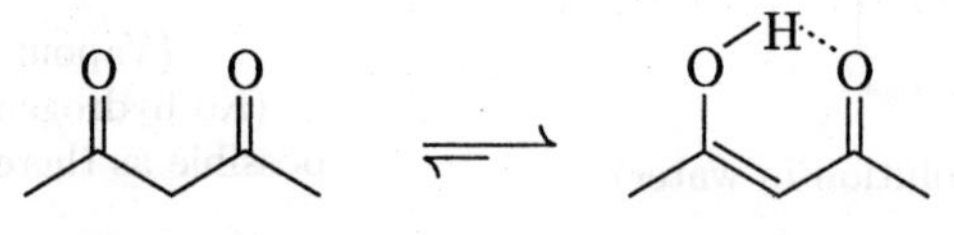

(Vapour phase) (2,4-pentanedione)

(Enol form) (more stable)

Compound	Condition/solvent	% Enol content
1. Pentane–2, 4–dione	liquid	76.4
	vapour	92.0
	H_2O	15.0
	CH_3CN	58.0
	hexane	92.0
2. Ethyl acetoacetate	liquid	8.0
	vapour	50.0
	H_2O	0.4
	hexane	46.0

The percentage of enol present also depend on the *temperature.*

***Keto–enol tautomerism in dimedone* :**

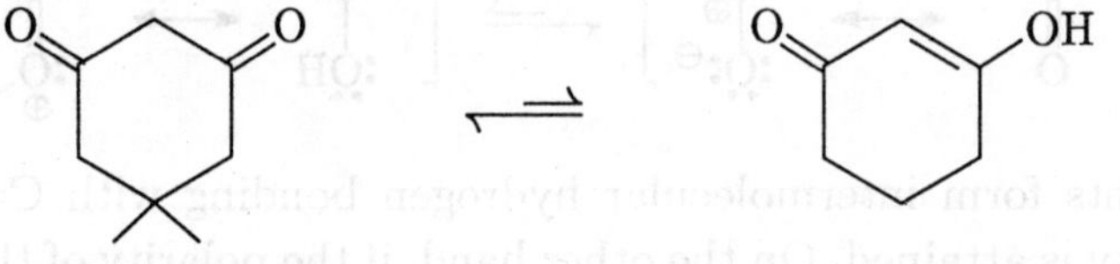

(Keto form of dimedone) (67% in $CDCl_3$)

(Enol form of dimedone) (33% in $CDCl_3$)

We need to examine why these enols are so stable. The main reason is that this unique (1,3) arrangement of the two functional groups leads to enols that are conjugated like a carboxylic acid.

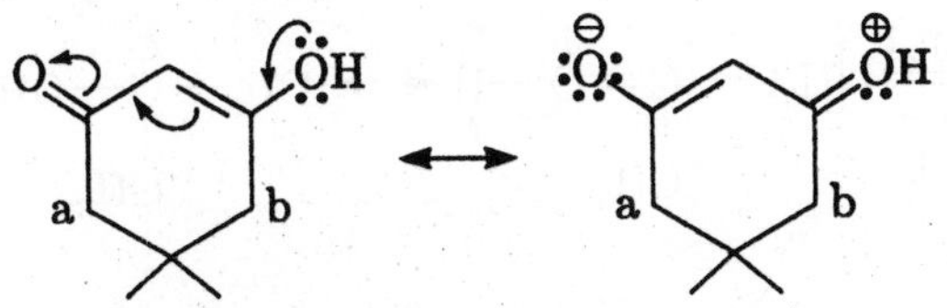

(Delocalisation in the enol form of dimedone)

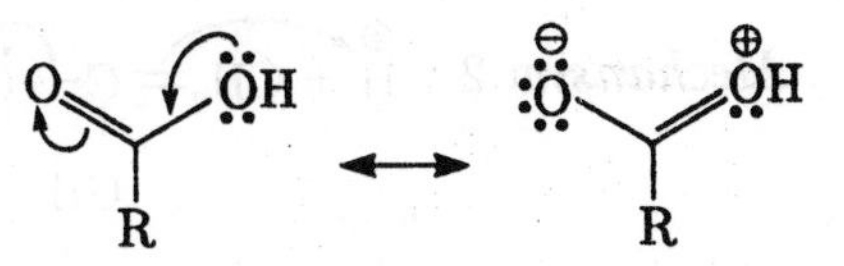

(Delocalisation in a carboxylic acid)

The two $-CH_2$ groups (a and b as shown above) seems to be the same (also in ^1H–NMR spectrum) and the delocalisation due to tautomerism made them same.

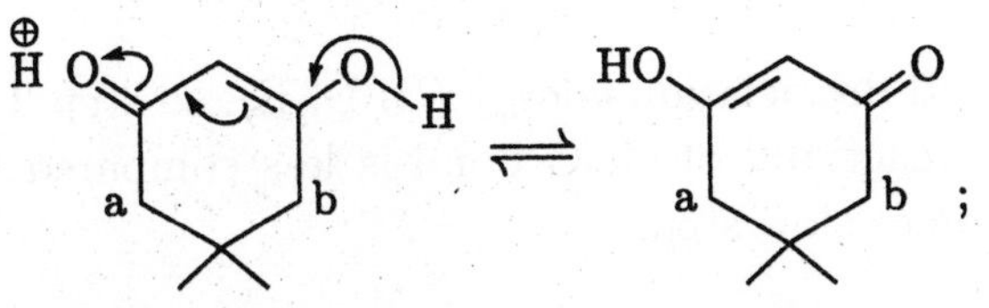

(Equilibration of the enol form of dimedone)

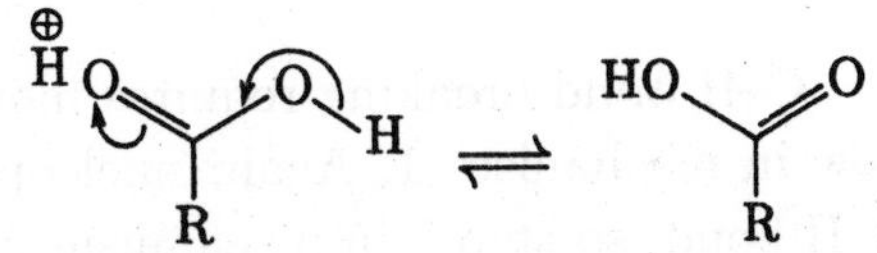

(Equilibration of a carboxylic acid)

Effect of entropy on keto–enol tautomerism : For acyclic ketones, free rotation around the single bonds is possible which makes the conformational randomness more. But in the enol form, the rotation around the rigid double bond is not possible. As a result, the enol form has less number of conformers. So when a keto form transforms into an enol form, the randomness decreases, *i.e.*, $\Delta S° < O$. This is one of the reasons for the poor enol content of acyclic ketones. In cyclic ketones, the conformational randomness is less due to their rigid structure. So, when a cyclic ketone transforms to an enol form, the decrease in randomness is comparatively less and thus the enol content becomes more compared to acyclic ketones. Other reason of enol stabilisation is intramolecular hydrogen bonding.

Mechanism of interconversion of tautomers : In case of prototropy, it appears that, one proton (H^+) gets transferred from one tautomer to another and no internal exchange of proton (H^+) takes place. Prototropy is assisted only in the presence of acid, alkali, wall of reaction vessel (carrier). Sometimes tautomers themselves act as autocarriers.

Example 1 : Acid catalysed conversion of CH_3COCH_3 to $CH_2{=}\overset{\displaystyle OH}{\overset{|}{C}}{-}CH_3$ and *vice–versa.*

Mechansim 1 :

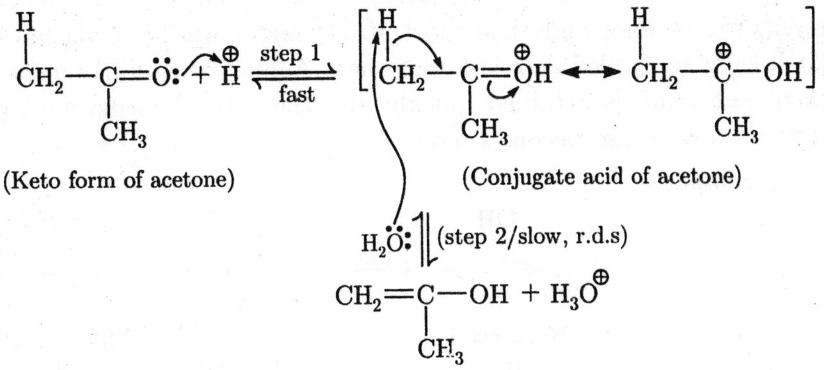

(Keto form of acetone) (Conjugate acid of acetone)

***Mechansim* 2 :**

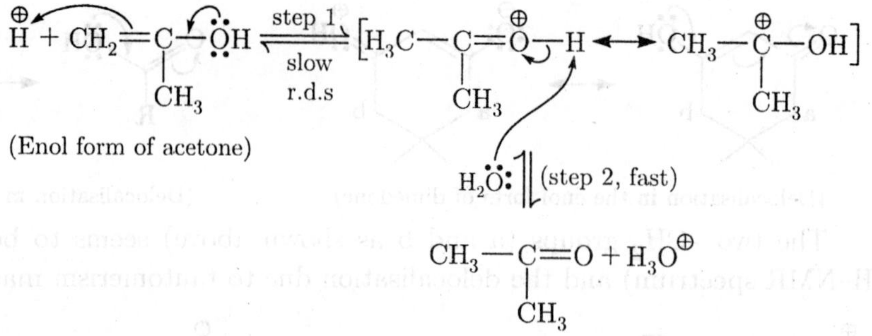

C–H bond breaking requires more bond dissociation energy (B. D. E), so step 2 is slow in mechanism 1. Again nucleophilic reactivity of C=C bond is less compared to O–H bond, so step 1 in mechanism 2 becomes slow step.

Energy profile diagram of $CH_3COCH_3 \rightleftharpoons CH_2{=}C(OH)CH_3$ ***conversion***

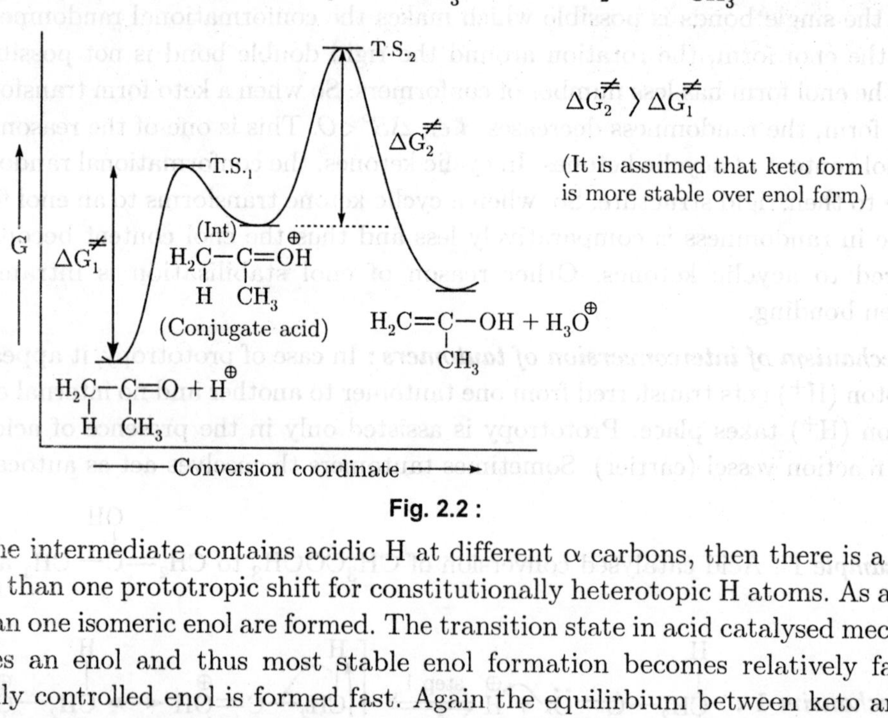

Fig. 2.2 :

If the intermediate contains acidic H at different α carbons, then there is a chance for more than one prototropic shift for constitutionally heterotopic H atoms. As a result, more than one isomeric enol are formed. The transition state in acid catalysed mechanism resembles an enol and thus most stable enol formation becomes relatively fast and kinetically controlled enol is formed fast. Again the equilirbium between keto and enol (*keto* ⇌ *enol*) is attained quickly and the rate of formation of thermodynamically controlled enol also becomes more.

***Example* :**

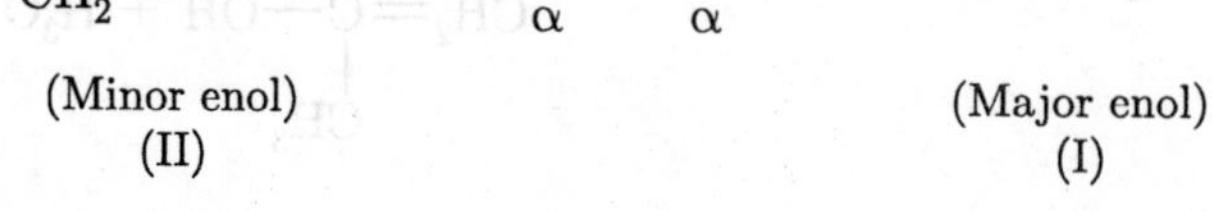

(Minor enol) (II) (Major enol) (I)

But-2-en-2-ol, is the major enol (I) as it contains six hyperconjugative structures whereas only *two* are there for but-1-en-2-ol (II). So in the presence of acid catalyst, the rate of formation of but-2-en-2-ol is more than but 1-en-2-ol.

2. ***Base catalysed mechanism of prototropy*** :

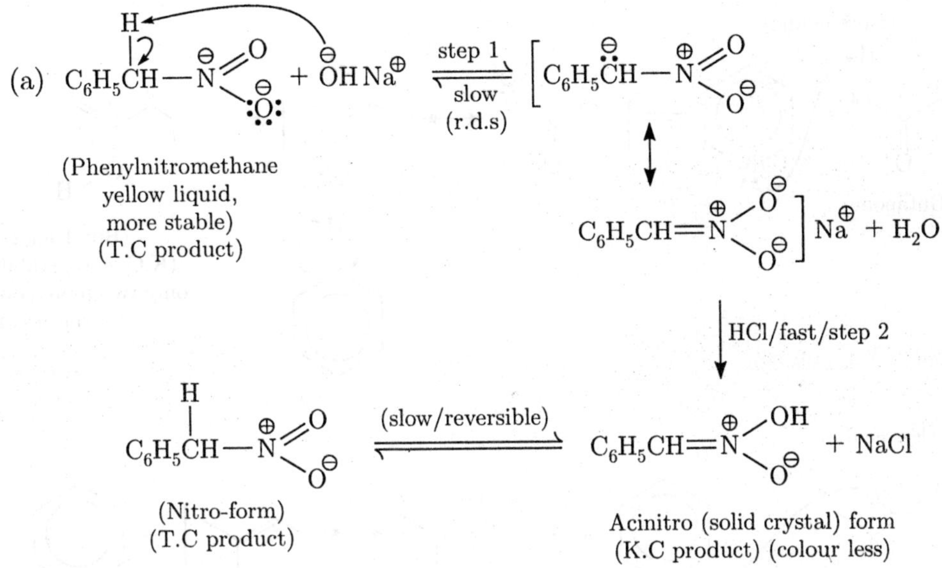

Step 1 is *slow* as it requires more activation energy because bond dissociation energy of C–H bond is more. *Step 2* is fast, as quick protonation occurs on the electron rich oxygen atom of conjugate base of nitro form which needs less activation energy to form the less stable K. C product acinitro form. Reversible formation of acinitro to nitro form (T. C. product) is attained quickly as bond dissociation energy of O–H bond is comparatively less.

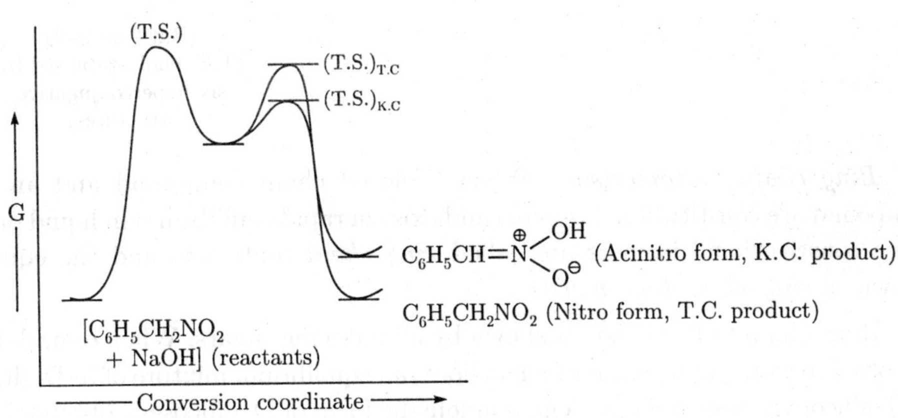

Fig. 2.3 :

(b) In the presence of pyridine, 2–butanone undergoes prototropic shift to produce but-1-en-2-ol and but-2-en-2ol, of which but-1-en-2-ol is formed at a faster rate. The acidity of C_3–H is less due to the methyl group (+I effect) attached to it and pyridine experiences a steric repulsion due to CH_3 group when it abstracts C_3–H. So, the rate of prototropic shift of C_1–H is more in the presence of pyridine.

(more acidic)

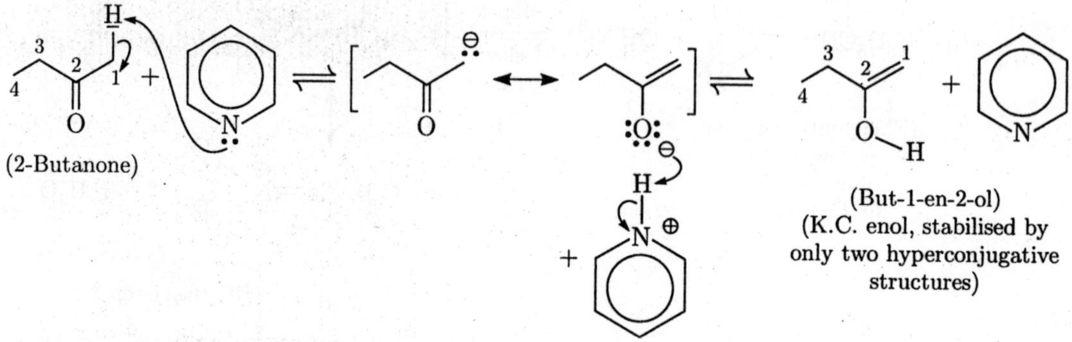

(2-Butanone)

(But-1-en-2-ol)
(K.C. enol, stabilised by only two hyperconjugative structures)

(less acidic)

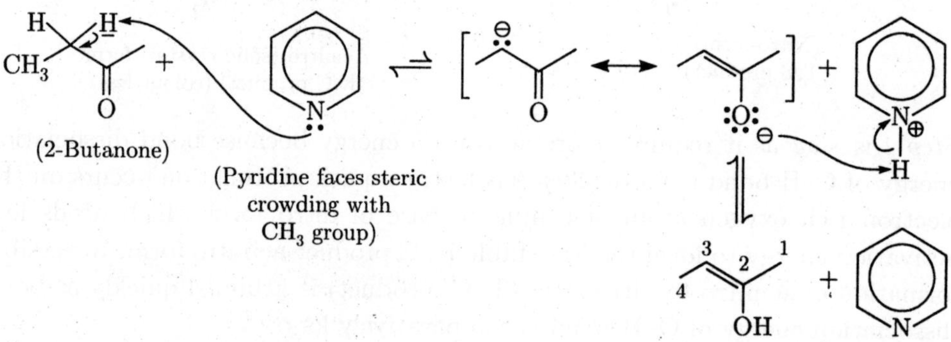

(2-Butanone)

(Pyridine faces steric crowding with CH_3 group)

(But-2-en-2-ol)
(T.C. enol, stabilised by six hyperconjugative structures)

Ring–chain tautomerism : When a closed chain compound and an open chain compound are constitutional isomers and exist in rapid equilibrium in liquid or in solution, these constitutional isomers are called *ring–chain tautomers* and the equilibration is known as *ring–chain tautomerism.*

Ring–chain tautomerism is shown by all reducing sugars. When α–or β–D-glucose is dissolved in water, and kept for half an hour, an equilibrium mixture of α–D-glucopyranose, β–D–glucopyranose and open chain aldehydic form of D–glucose is obtained. in fact due to *ring chain tautomerism*, reducing sugars show *mutarotation.*

(a) 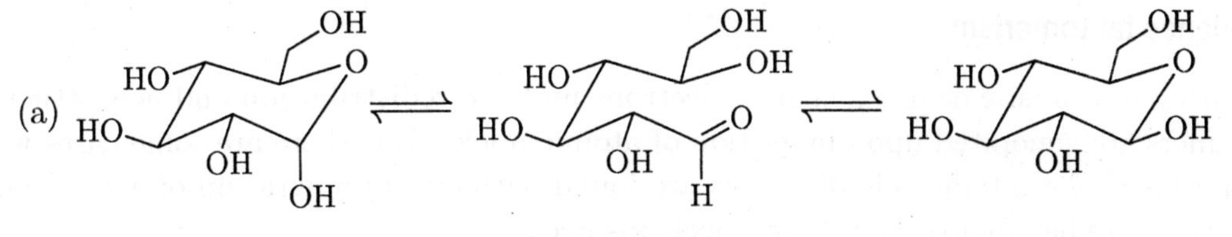

(α-D-glucopyranose) (~38%) (Open chain aldehyde form) (~0.02%) (β-D-glucose) (~62%)

(b) Ring–chain tautomerism is usually exhibited by compounds having two functionalities.

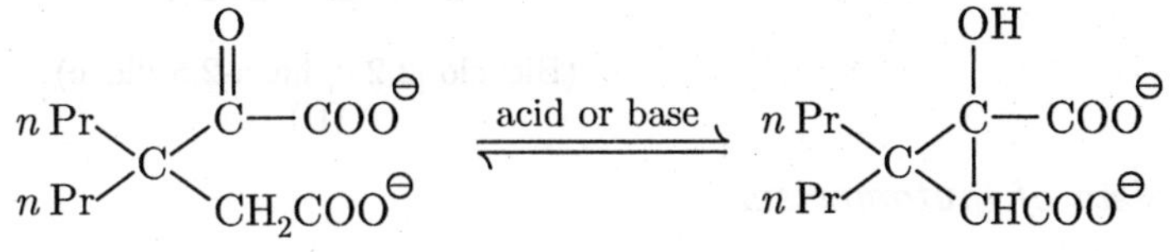

(c) 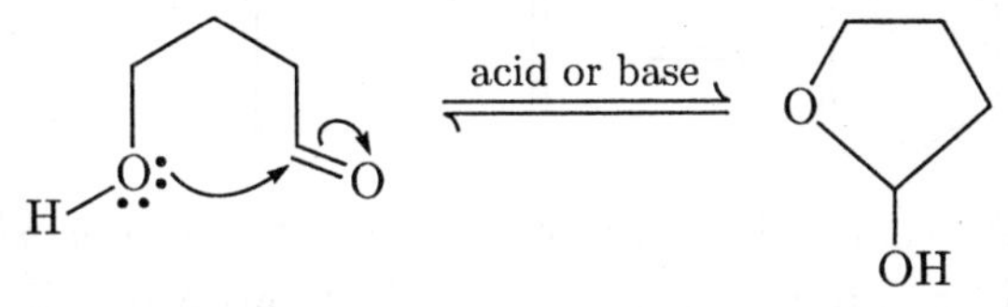

The interconversion of ring–chain tautomers may be either by *cationotropy* or by *anionotropy*.

Example of cationotropy : Interconversion of *α–D– and β–D–glucopyranose* to the open chain aldehyde form.

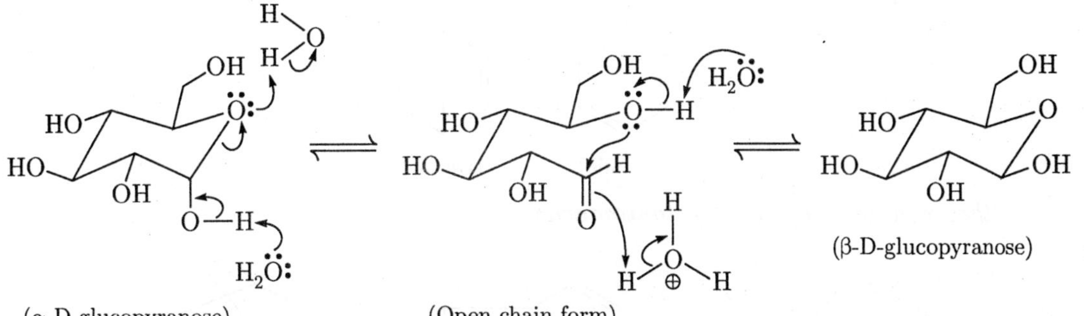

(α-D-glucopyranose) (Open chain form) (β-D-glucopyranose)

Example of anionotropy :

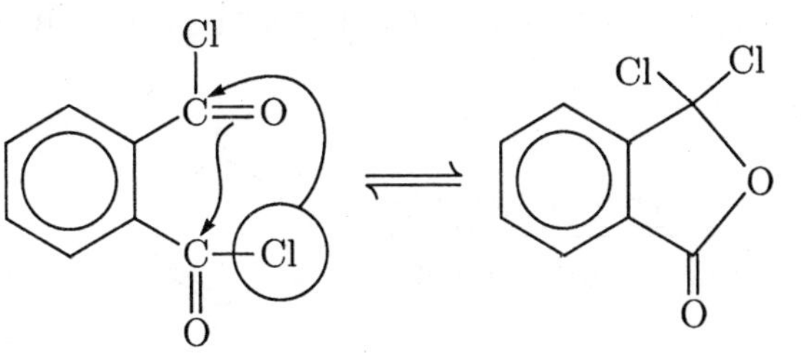

Valence tautomerism

During tautomeric change, valence electrons undergo redistribution and new structural isomers are generated upon migration of atomic nuclei. But there are some cases where changes in the interatomic distances are found without any migration of atomic nuclei although redistribution of valence electrons occurs.

Example :

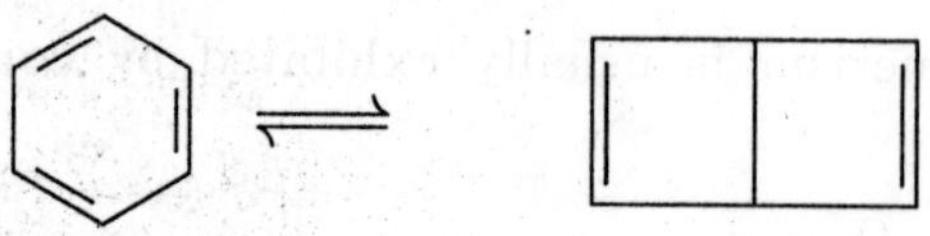

(I) (Bicyclo [2.2.0] hexa-2,5-diene) (II)

Mechanism of tautomerism :

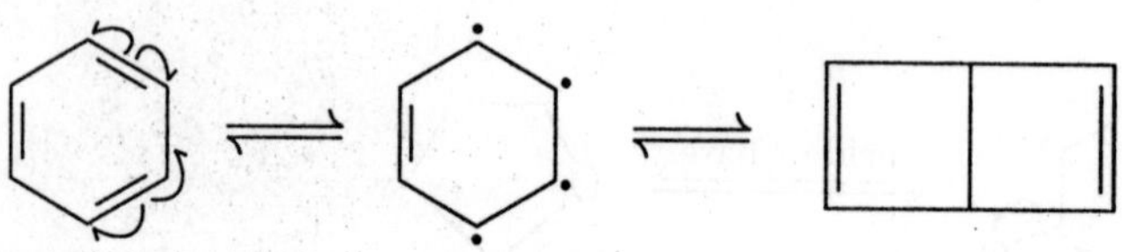

(I) and (II) represent different structures because of different *σ–frame work* and no shift of atomic nucleus takes place. In resonance, the valence electrons are redistributed in the same *σ–framework* to form different structures. But in valence tautomerism, shift of valence electrons is accompanied with the change in basic structure but not involving change in the positions of atomic nuclei.

N. B : Kekule's benzene and Dewar's benzene are *examples of resonance, not valence tautomerism* as the basic cyclic structure is not disturbed.

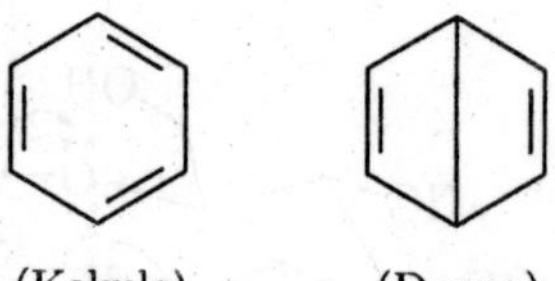

(Kekule) (Dewar)

Other examples of valence tautomerism :

1. 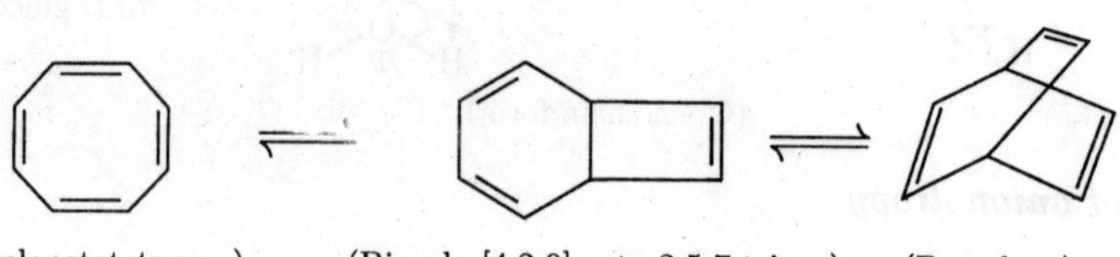

(Cyclooctatetraene) (COT) (Bicyclo [4.2.0] octa-2.5,7-triene) (Barrelene)

2. 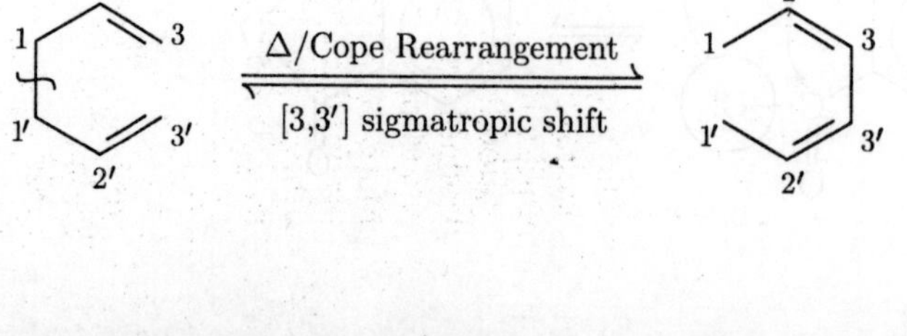

3. 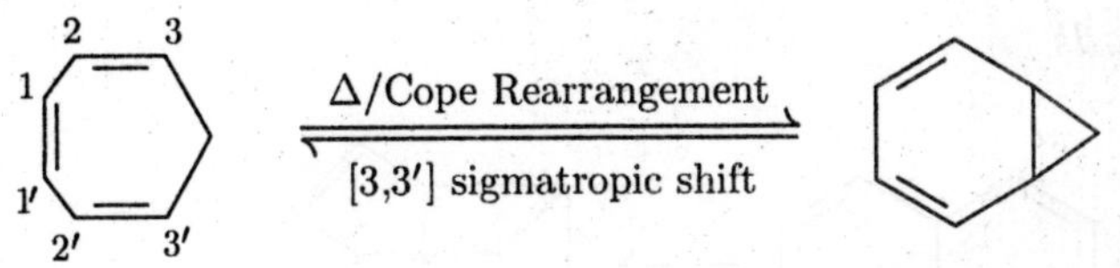

At 180°C, the ^{1}H–NMR spectra of compounds formed on Cope rearrangement (examples 2 and 3) show that the above two structures remain in equilibrium and they are called *fluxional* structures.

4. 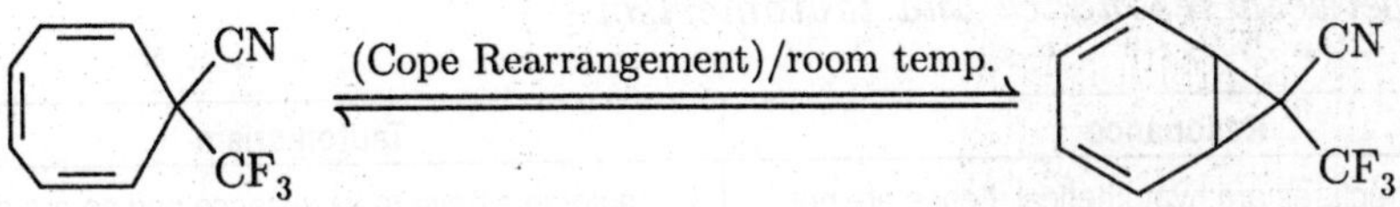

5. 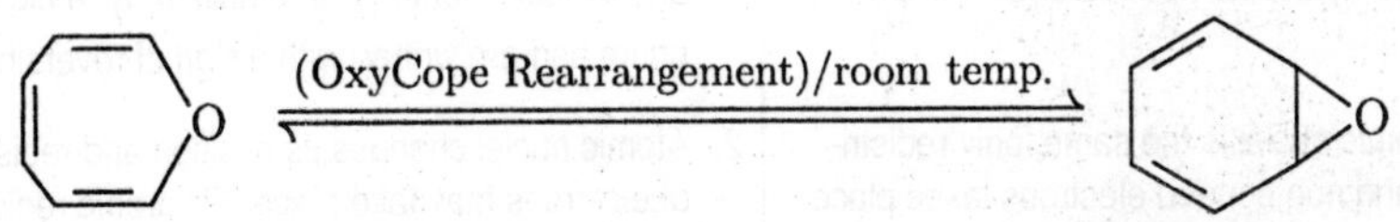

(Oxepin) (Benzene oxide)

6. 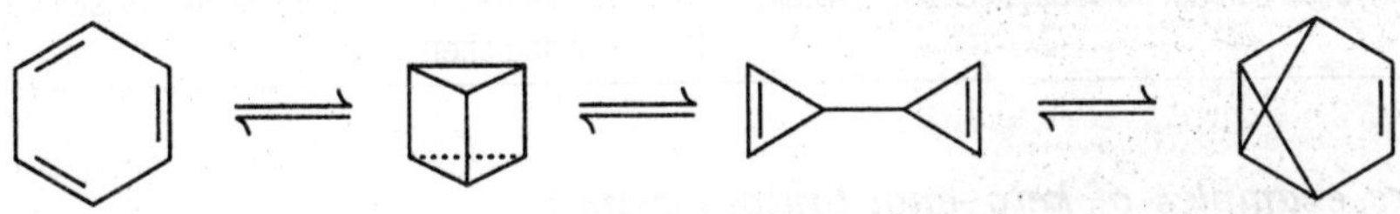

(Benzene) (Prismane) (Bicyclopropenyl) (Benzvalene)

7. 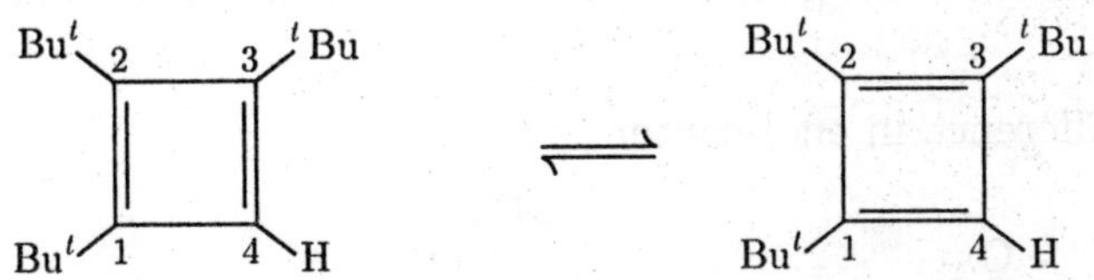

(1,2,3-Tritertiarybutylcyclobutane)

The compounds remain in dynamic equilibrium even at –185°C.

8. 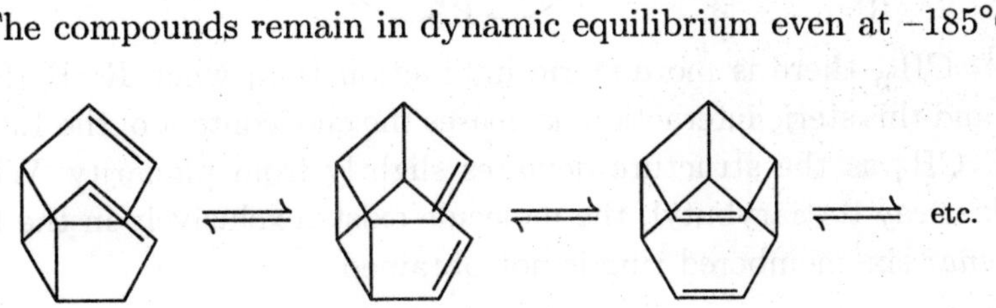

(Hypostrophene)

This is an example of *infinite degenerate Cope Rearrangement.*

9. *$(CH)_{10}$ type compounds*

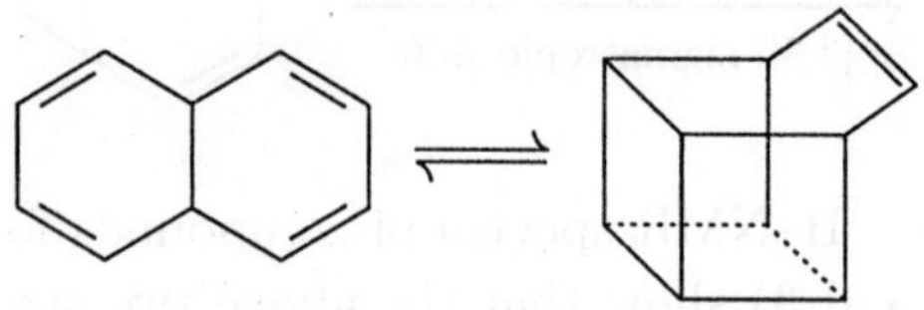

(Dihydronaphthalene) (Basketene)

Difference between resonance and tautomerism

Resonance	Tautomerism
1. Resonating structures are hyptothetical, hence are not isolable, designated by double headed arrow (⟷) among them.	1. Tautomers have real existence and so are detectable and isolable. Tautomers remain in dynamic equilibrium and are written with a sign of reversibility (⇌).
2. The position of atomic nuclei is the same, only redistribution of bonded and non bonded electrons takes place.	2. Atomic nuclei changes its position and redistribution of electrons may take place. Electronic redistribution with no change in position of atomic nuclei applies to valence tautomerism.
3. Resonance hybrids can not be separated or chemically detected.	3. Tautomers are isolable and their existence can be detected chemically.

Some more examples of keto–enol tautomersim :

1. 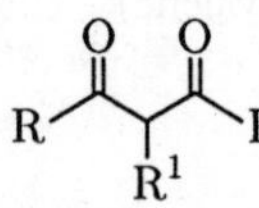, when R^1=CH_3, enol% =44 and R^1=H (acetylacetone), enol % =76.

Explain the difference in enol content.

Ans. : 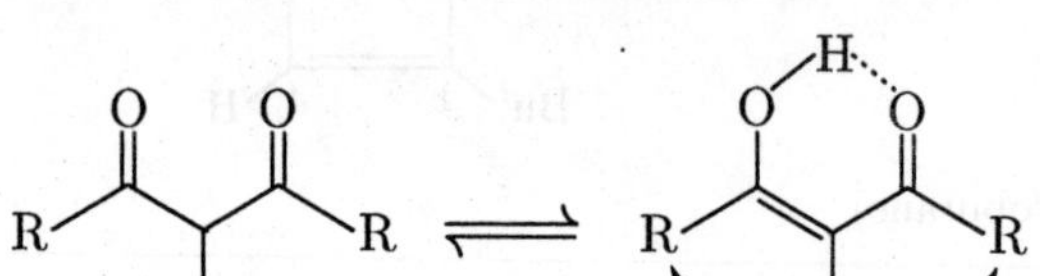

When R^1=CH_3, there is more steric interaction than when R=H (for acetylacetone) and this steric interaction decreases the enol content of the 1,3–diketone when R^1=CH_3 as the structure deviates slightly from planarity. When R^1 is even bulkier say tertiarybutyl, the molecule exists exclusively in the keto form as the *planar* six–membered ring is not obtained.

2. The percentage enol form of 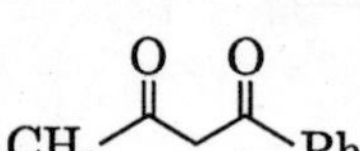 is more than the most percent present in 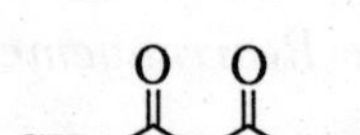

Ans. :

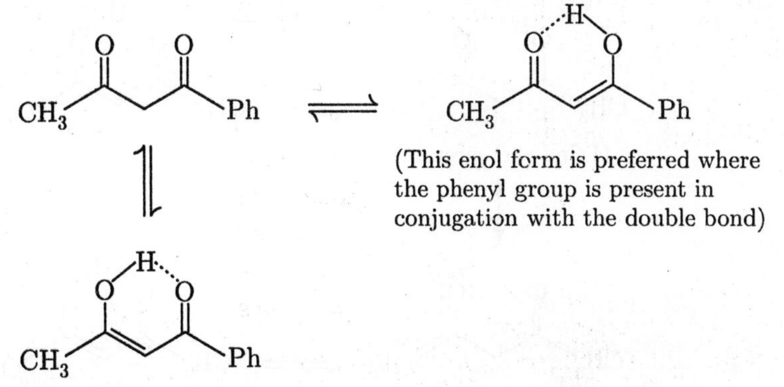

(This enol form is preferred where the phenyl group is present in conjugation with the double bond)

(This enol form is less preferred as the phenyl is in cross conjugation)

The phenyl ring which is in conjugation with the double bond is reponsible for the molecule's higher enol content.

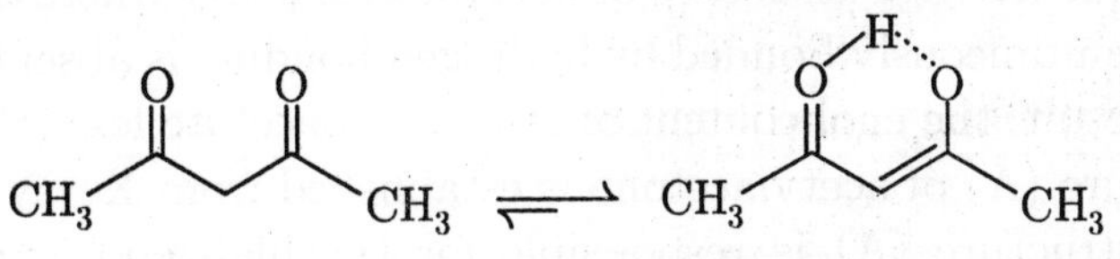

In acetylacetone, no phenyl group is present which may contribute to its extended conjugation in the enol form, so this molecule has lower enol content compared to the former molecule.

3. Neat (devoid of any solvent) ethyl acetoacetate has 8% enol content whereas acetylacetone has 76% and $PhCOCH_2COCH_3$ has 89% enol content. Explain.

Ans. :

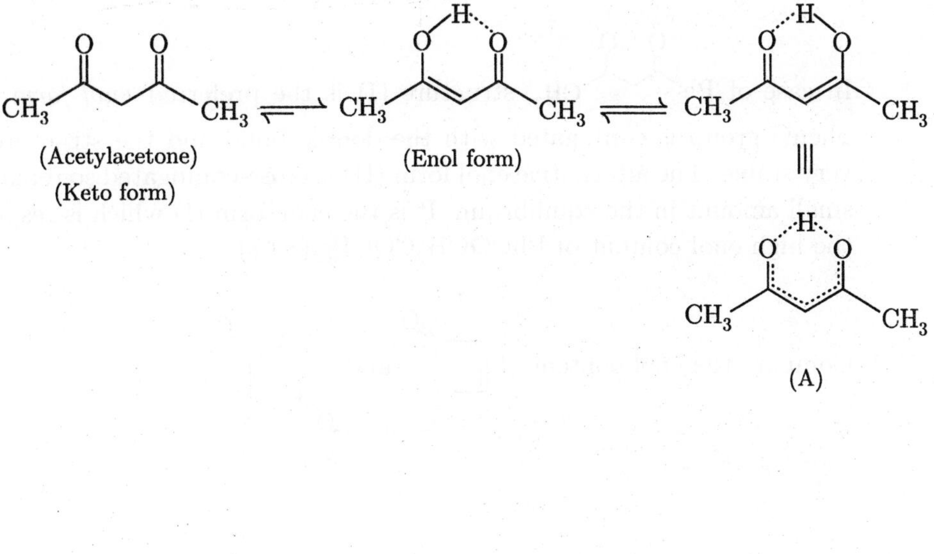

(Acetylacetone) (Keto form) (Enol form)

(A)

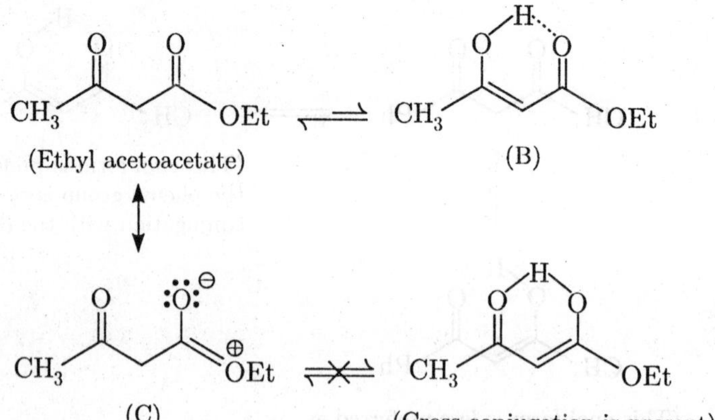

(Ethyl acetoacetate) (B)

(C) (Cross conjugation is present)

(C) is the most important resonating structure of ethyl acetoacetae. Samples are taken neat so that solvents can not interfere in the keto–enol tautomerism.

The time average structure of acetylacetone (A) where both the oxygen atoms are simultaneously bonded by hydrogen bonding is absent in ethyl acetoacetate. As a result, the enol content of ethyl acetoacetate less (8%). The time averaged structure (A) of acetylacetone is established from X–ray crystallographic data. This structure (A) is responsible for the high enol content of acetylacetone (76%).

$PhCOCH_2COCH_3$ has 89% enol content. The reason for the molecule's high enol content is as follow.

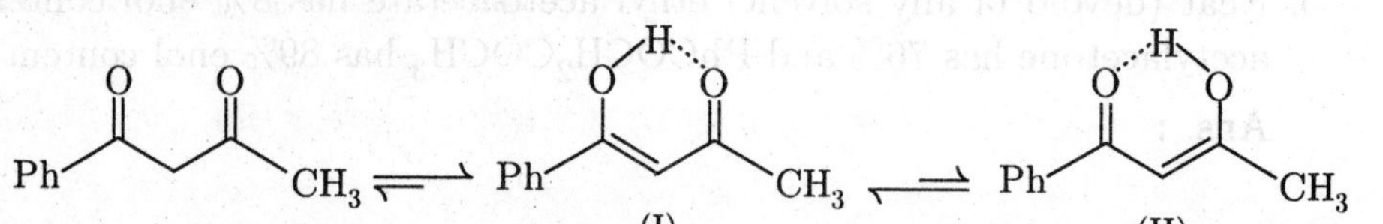

(I) (II)

In case of 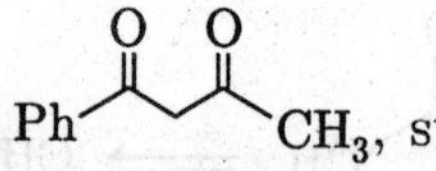, structure (I) is the preferred *enol form* where the phenyl group is conjugated with the double bond and the structure becomes very stable. The alternative enol form (II) is cross-conjugated so remains in very small amount in the equilibrium. It is the enol form (I) which is responsible for the high enol content of $PhCOCH_2COCH_3$ (89%).

4. Compare the enol content of 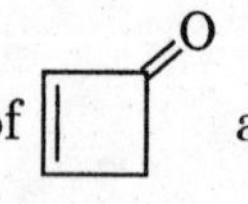 and 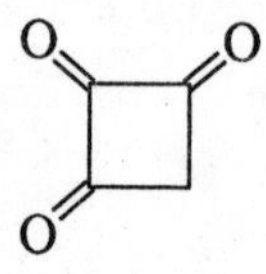.

Ans. : 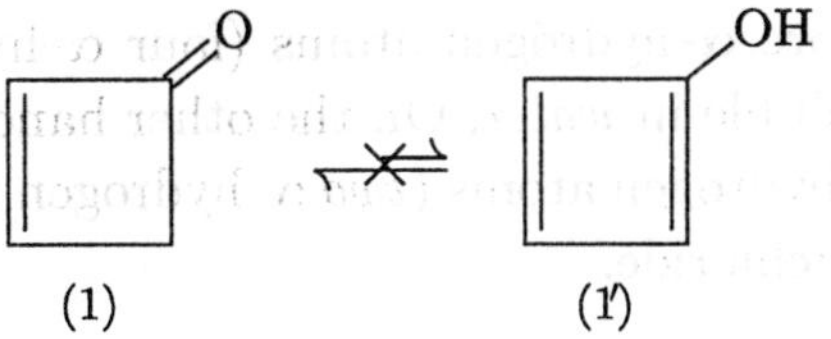 (Antiaromatic)

(1) (1′)

The enol form of (1) *i.e.*, (1′) is *antiaromatic*, which is very unstable and so is non existant in the equilibrium. We get *only* the *keto form* (1), in the equilibrium.

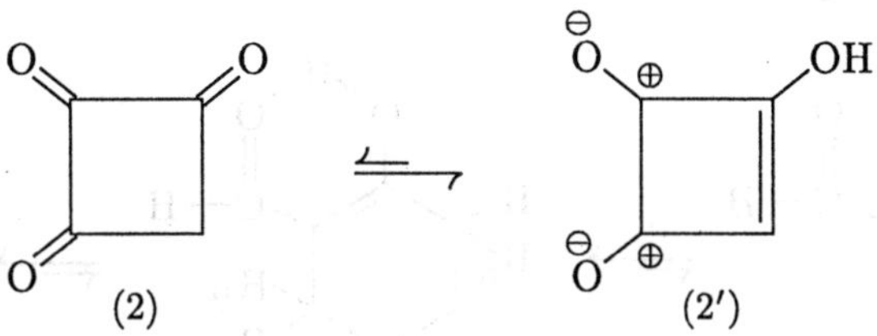 (Aromatic)

(2) (2′)

The enol form of (2) is (2′), which is aromatic and thus has a high stability. So in the equilibrium (2) remains exclusively as (2′).

So the enol form of (2) is more than the enol form of (1) in the equilibrium.

5. The following bicyclo heptane– 1,3–dione is not soluble in alkali.

Ans. : 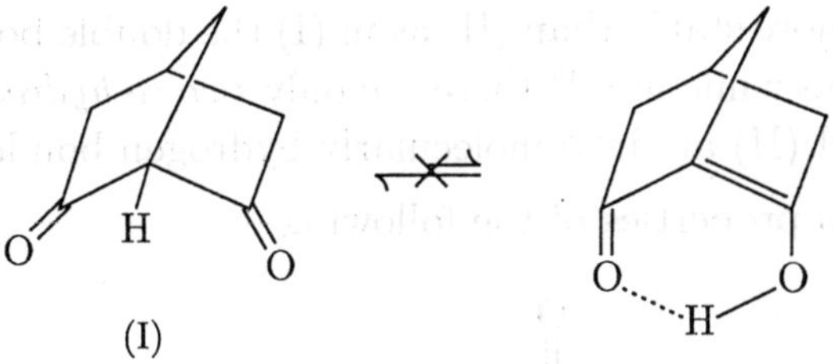

(I) (I′)

The enol form of (I) is not permissible by *Bredt's rule* where a double bond is formed at the *bridge–head* position. As the abstraction of bridge–head hydrogen is not possible, the compound is not soluble in alkali.

6. For the molecule $CH_3-\overset{\overset{\large O}{||}}{C}-CH_2CHO$.

(a) Write down the enol form of this dicarbonyl.

(b) If it at all exists in the enol form, one structure will be soluble in water and another will be soluble in carbon tetrachloride. *Explain the observation.*

Ans. : 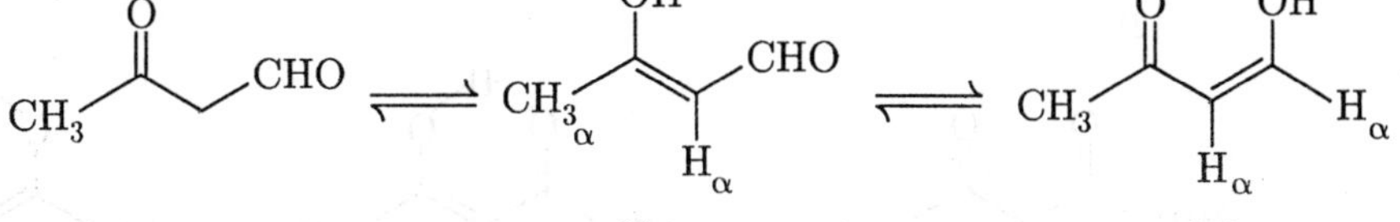

(I) (II)

The enol form (I) contains more α–hydrogen atoms (four α–hydrogen atoms) thus more polar and so it is soluble in *water.* On the other hand, the enol form (II) contains less number of α-hydrogen atoms (*two* α–hydrogen atoms) and this form in soluble in carbon tetrachloride.

7. The molecules 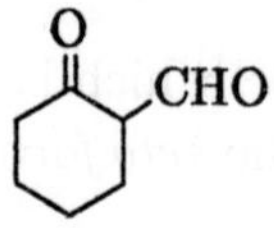 enolises to the extent of 100%.

Ans. : 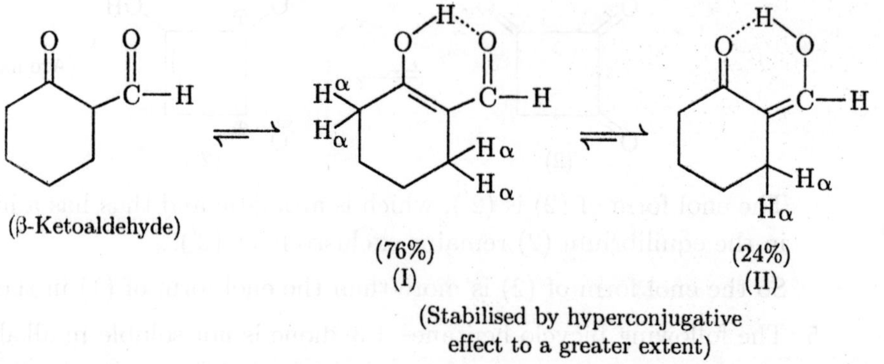

The enol form (I) is more stable than (II) as in (I) the double bond is flanked by *four α–hydrogen atoms* while in (II) there are only *two α–hydrogen atoms.* Both the structures (I) and (II) are intramolecularly hydrogen bonded.

8. Compare the physical properties of the following—

Ans. : The molecules (2) and (3) are soluble in alkali but (1) is not.

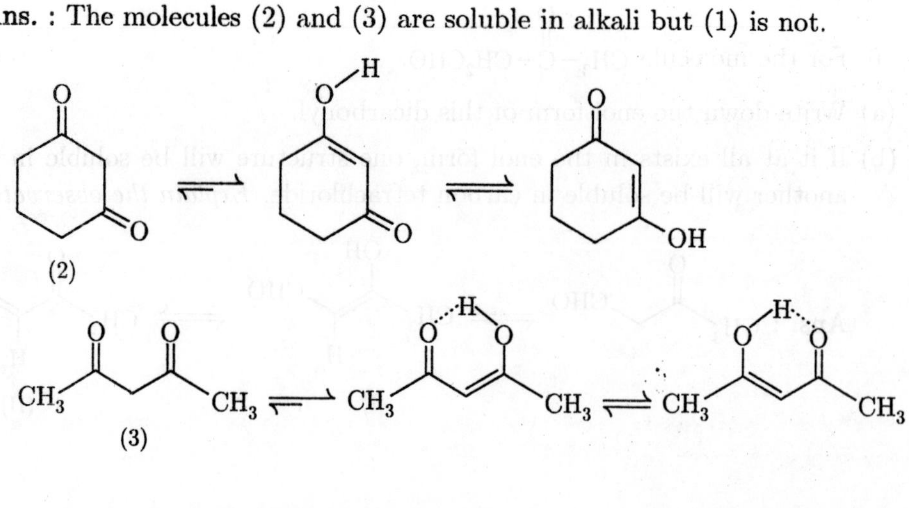

Both (2) and (3) can enolise to a great extent and so are soluble in alkali, but (3) has higher enol content as the enol forms are stabilised through intramolecular hydrogen bonding.

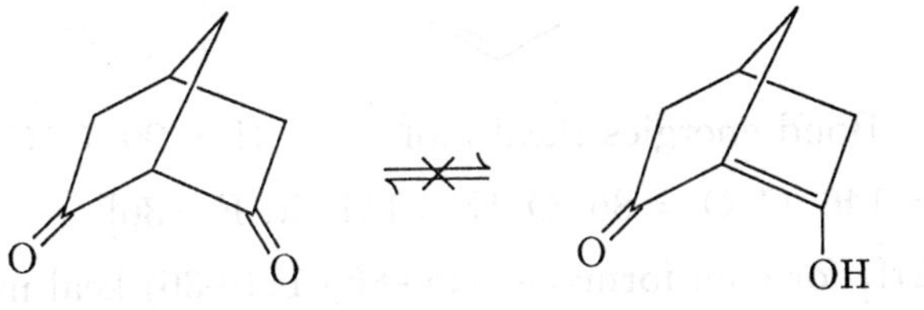

(1)

In structure (1), the double bond is generated at the bridge–head position which is not permissible by Bredt's rule. As a result, molecule (1) can not enolise and does *not* dissolve in alkali.

1. ***Instability of enol form where hydrogen bonding is absent*** : (*From thermodynamic considerations*).

The non–spontenity of the equilibrium keto ⇌ enol can be easily understood from bond energy data for acetone:

$$CH_3-\underset{\underset{O}{\|}}{C}-CH_3 \rightleftharpoons H_2C=\underset{\underset{OH}{|}}{C}-CH_3$$

[No H–bonding possible]

[Given the bond energies in kcal/mol:

C–H=99; C–C=83, C=O=179; C=C = 146, O–H = 111; C–O=86]

In the above equilibrium Enthalpy of LHS (keto form)

ΔH_1=–(99+83+179)kcal mol^{-1} =361 kcal mol^{-1}

and Enthalpy of RHS (enol form) ΔH_2=–(146+86+111)kcal =–343 kcal mol^{-1}

Hence $\Delta H_{keto \to enol} = \Delta H_2 - \Delta H_1$ =–343–(–361) kcal mol^{-1} =+18 kcal mol^{-1}

Here ΔS=O as number of moles are same in equilibrium.

So, ΔG=ΔH–TΔS=ΔH–T×O=ΔH=+18 kcal=non spontaneous process

Hence acetone exists absolutely in keto form; the enol content is only about 0.004%

2. ***Ease of aromatic characters*** : **Stability of enols**

(a) ***Phenol*** : Phenol exists entirely in enol form; this is because on passing to keto form which is a dienone but not aromatic, about 150 kJ mol^{-1} (36 kcal mol^{-1}) "Resonance energy" has to be sacrified which tends the equilibrium towards the enol form. This can easily be predicted, considering the bond energy changes during enol to keto equilibrium :

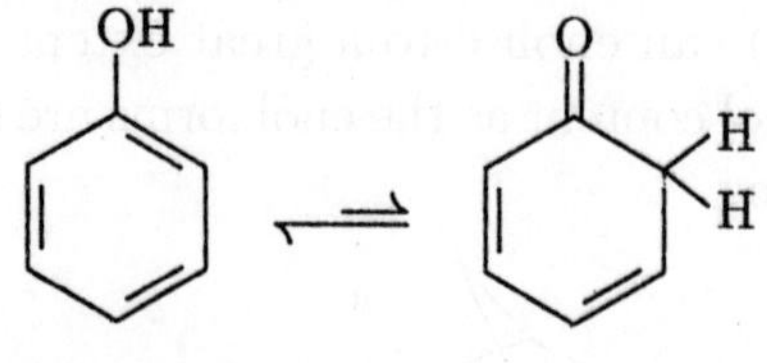

[*Given* : Bond energies (kcal mol^{-1}): C–H = 99; C–C = 83; C=O = 179; C=C = 146; C–O = 86; O–H = 111; R. E =36]

Here ΔH_1 for enol form= –(146+86+111+36) kcal mol^{-1}=–379 kcal mol^{-1}

& ΔH_2 for keto form=–(99+83+179) kcal=–361 kcal mol^{-1}.

So, $\Delta H_{keto \rightarrow enol} = \Delta H_1 - \Delta H_2$

$= -379-(-361) = -18$ kcal mol^{-1}

Hence as here, ΔS=0 (number of moles remaining same and other entropy factors like conformational entropy factors unchanged).

$\Delta G_{keto \rightarrow enol} = \Delta H_{keto \rightarrow enol} = -18$ kcal=a spontaneous process.

(b) ***Resorcinol*** : *m*–Dihydroxybenzene or resorcinol exists both in keto and enol form because the aromatic stabilization in the enol form is almost compensated by two strong carbonyl bonds in the keto form; supported by bond energy data as follows.

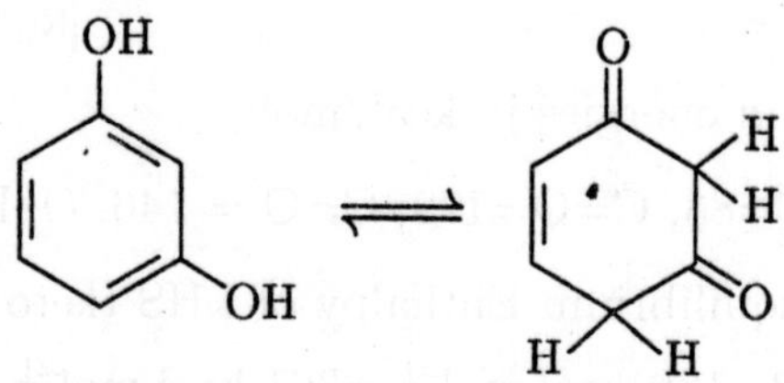

(I) (II)

Hence, $\Delta H_1 = -(2\times146+2\times86+2\times111+36) = -722$ kcal mol^{-1}

$\Delta H_2 = -(2\times99+2\times83+2\times179) = -722$ kcal mol^{-1}

Hence $\Delta H_{enol \rightleftharpoons keto} = \Delta H_1 - \Delta H_2 = 0 = \Delta G$

So both the forms exist equally in the equilibrium.

Carboxylic Acids And Their Derivatives

Carboxylic acid derivatives (General formula $R-\overset{O}{\overset{\|}{C}}-X$)

1. Acid Chlorides ($R-\overset{O}{\overset{\|}{C}}-Cl$, X=Cl)
2. Acid Anchydrides ($R-\overset{O}{\overset{\|}{C}}-O-\overset{O}{\overset{\|}{C}}-R'$, X= $-O-\overset{O}{\overset{\|}{C}}-R'$)
3. Carboxylic acid esters ($R-\overset{O}{\overset{\|}{C}}-OR'$, X= -OR′)
4. Carboxylic acid amides ($R-\overset{O}{\overset{\|}{C}}-NH_2$, X= $-NH_2$)

   All of them contain acyl ($R-\overset{O}{\overset{\|}{C}}-$) ***group***
5. Cyanides or nitriles ($R-C\equiv N$)

Structure of Carboxylic acid Derivatives

The structures of carboxylic acid derivatives have resemblence with their carbonyl compounds. C=O bond length is about 1.21Å and the carbonyl group and its two attached atoms are planar. The nitrile $C\equiv N$ bond length, 1.16Å is significantly shorter than the acetylenic $C\equiv C$ bond length (1.20Å). In an amide, both carbonyl carbon and the amide nitrogen have essentially trigonal planar bonding patterns, which may be understood from the following resonating structures, which show that the bond between the nitrogen and the carbonyl carbon has considerable double bond character.

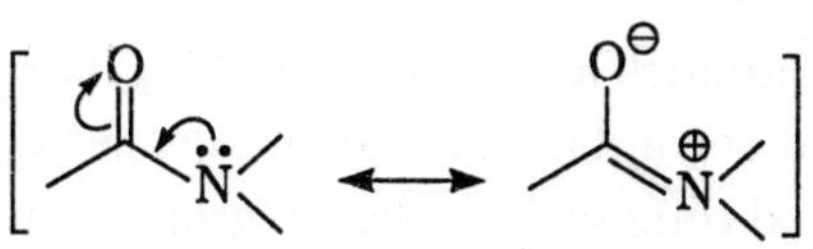

(Amide resonance structures)

Because of the trigonal planar geometry at nitrogen, secondary and tertiary amides can exist in both E- and Z- configurations about the carbonyl-nitrogen bond. Z-configuration predominates generally as in this form, van der Waals repulsion between the largest groups is avoided.

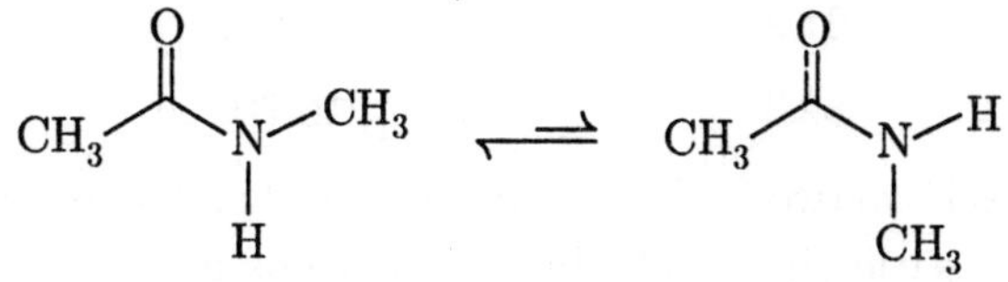

Z– E–

The interconversion of E- and Z- forms of amides is too rapid at room temperature to permit their separation, but comparatively slow if compared with rotation around carbon-carbon single bond. The typical energy barrier for rotation about the carbonyl-nitrogen bond of an amide is 71 kJ/mol (17 kcal/mol) [corresponds to internal rotation rate of about *10 times per second*]. In contrast, internal rotation in butane occurs about 10^{11} times per second. The relatively low rate of internal rotation is caused by the significant double bond character in the carbonyl carbon-nitrogen bond.

Physical Properties of Carboxylic Acid Derivatives

1. **Esters :** Esters are polar molecules but cannot undergo hydrogen bonding as the carboxylic acids do. Lower esters are volatile, fragrant and have densities lower than water. Most esters are insoluble in water.

	CH_3CH_2COOH	$CH_3CH_2-C(=O)-OCH_3$	$CH_3-C(=O)-OCH_3$	$CH_3-C(=O)-CH_2CH_3$
b.p.	114°C	80°C	57°C	31.2°C

2. **Anhydrides and Acid chlorides :** Most lower anhydrides and acid chlorides are dense water-insoluble liquids with acrid piercing odours. Their boiling points are not very different from other polar molecules with same mass (molecular) and shape. The simplest acid chloride and acid anhydride (formyl chloride and formic anhydride) are unstable and can not be isolated under ordinary conditions.
3. **Nitriles :** Nitriles are among the most polar organic compounds. Acetonitrile, *e.g.*, has a dipole moment of 3.4 D. The polarity of nitrile is reflected in their boiling points which are rather high despite absence of hydrogen bonding.

	$CH_3-C\equiv N$	$CH_3CH_2-C\equiv N$	$CH_3C\equiv C-H$
b.p.	81.6°C	97.4°C	-23.3°C

4. **Amides :** The lower amides are water soluble, polar molecules with high boiling points. Primary and secondary amides like carboxylic acids, tend to associate into hydrogen bonded dimers or higher aggregates in the solid state, in the pure liquid state or in solvents that do not form hydrogen bonds. So simple amides may have very high boiling points, many are solids.

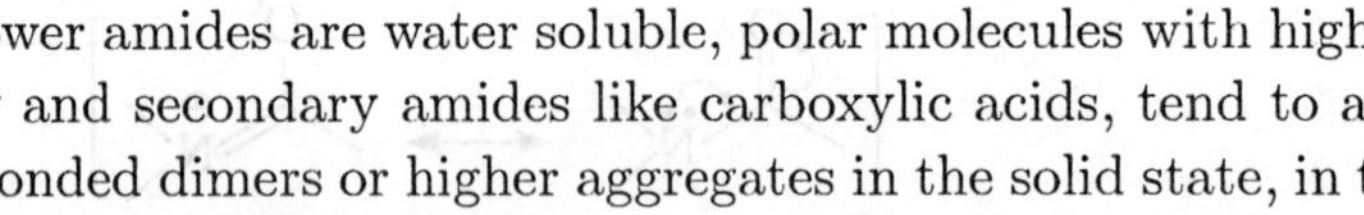

b.p.	221.2°C	117.9°C	56.5°C
m.p.	82.3°C	16.7°C	-94°C

Primary amides have two hydrogens on the amide nitrogen that can form hydrogen bonds. Along a series in which these hydrogens are replaced by methyl groups, the capacity for hydrogen bonding is reduced, and boiling points decrease in spite of the increase in the molecular mass.

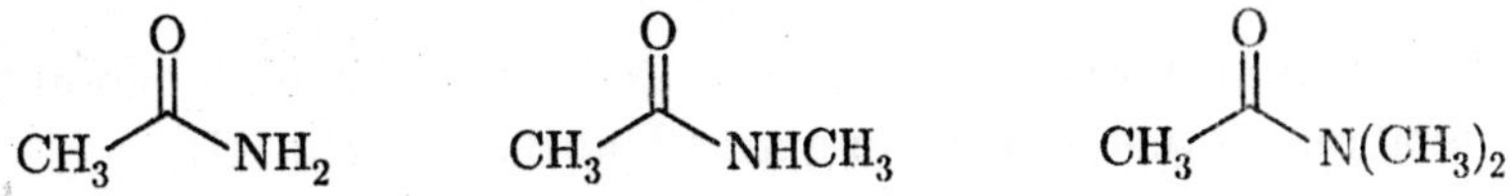

b.p.	221.2°C	204–206°C	166.1°C
m.p.	82.3°C	28°C	–20°C

A number of amides have high dielectric constants. N-N-Dimethylformamide (DMF) which has a dielectric constant (ε) of 37, for example dissolves a number of inorganic salts and is widely used as a polar aprotic solvent, despite of its high boiling point.

Basicity of Carboxylic Acid Derivatives

Like carboxylic acids, carboxylic acid derivatives are weakly basic as the carboxyl oxygen can be protonated by strong acids. Similarly, cyanides are very weakly basic at its nitrogen. The basicity of an ester is about the same as that of corresponding carboxylic acid.

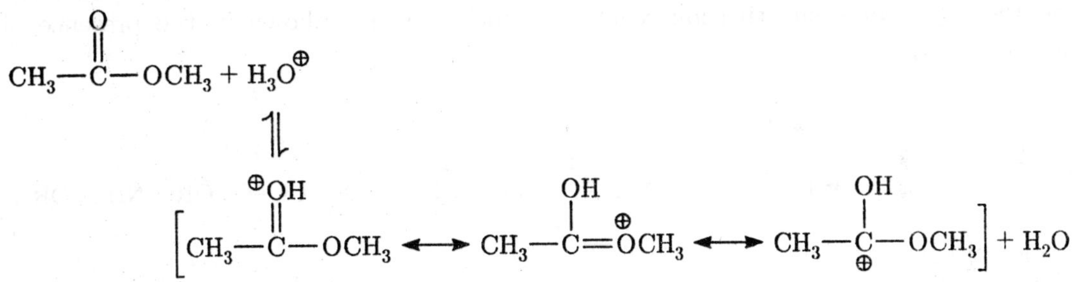

Protonated ester, pK_a=–6

Amides are considerably more basic than other carboxylic acid derivatives. This is a reflection of reduced electronegativity of nitrogen relative to oxygen.

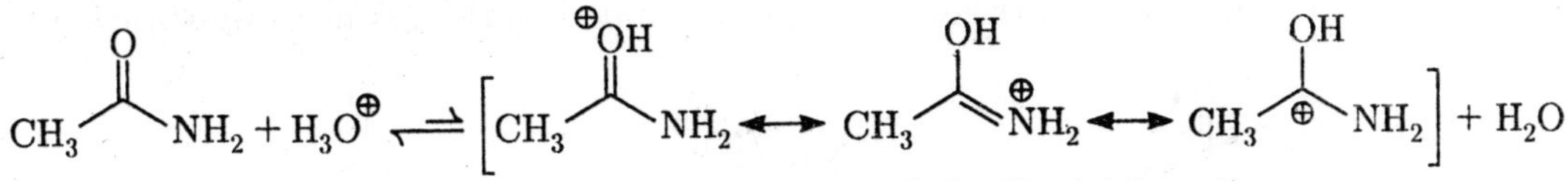

Protonated amide, pK_a=(–0.5 to –1)

Both esters and amides protonate or carbonyl oxygen, if esters protonate on oxygen atom of $R-C(=O)-\underline{O}R'$ or amide on nitrogen atom ($R-C(=O)-\underline{N}H_2$), then the cation generated would not be resonance stabilised, and moreover will be destabilised by electron-withdrawing carbonyl group. The nitrogen protonation on amide is less favourable than carbonyl protonation by about 8 pK_a units.

Nitriles are very weak bases, protonated nitriles have pK_a about –10 and a protonated nitrile is about as acidic as strong acid hydroiodic acid (HI).

$$H_3C{-}C{\equiv}N\!: + H_3O^{\oplus} \rightleftharpoons \left[CH_3{-}C{\equiv}\overset{\oplus}{N}H \longleftrightarrow CH_3{-}\overset{\oplus}{C}{=}NH\right] + H_2O$$

(Lone pair of electrons resides in sp hybrid orbital)   Protonated nitrile $pK_a \cong -10$

Nucleophilic Substitution at the Acyl Carbon—Role of the Carbonyl Group

The derivatives of carboxylic acid like the carboxylic acids contain the carbonyl group C=O and this group is retained in the most of the reactions undergone by these compounds. This carbonyl group performs two functions:

(a) It provides a site for nucleophilic substitution.

(b) It increases the acidity of hydrogen(s) attached to the α-carbon.

Carboxylic acid derivatives undergo nucleophilic substitution in which –OH, Cl, –OCOR, –NH_2 or OR′ etc. are replaced by some other basic groups. Substitution occurs much more readily compared to nucleophilic substitution at a saturated carbon atom and there are some substitution reactions which are only shown in the presence of carbonyl group.

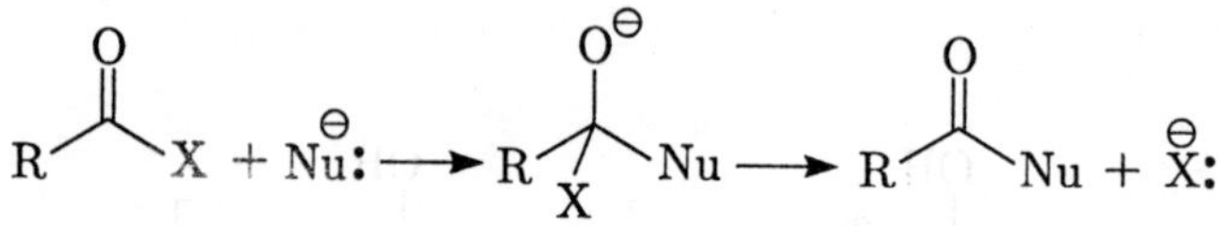

(X=OH, Cl, –OCOR, –NH_2, –OR′)

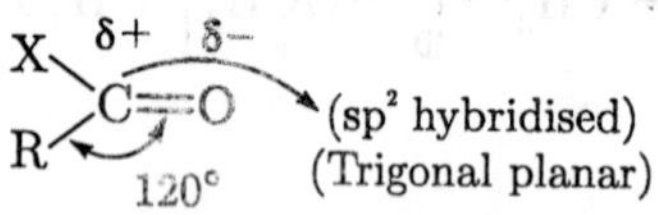

Both steric and electronic factors make the carbonyl group susceptible to nucleophilic attack at the carbonyl carbon. The tetrahedral intermediate from an acyl compound ejects X: group returning to a trigonal compound and thus the result is *substitution.*

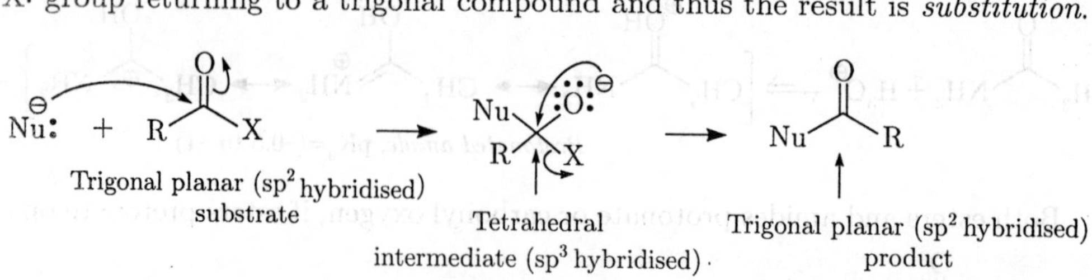

The tetrahedral intermediate formed is unstable because the trigonal planar carbon atom (sp^2 hybridised) becomes tetrahedral (sp^3 hybridised).

Evidences in favour of formation of tetrahedral intermediate :

Bender (1951) reacted water with carboxylic acid derivatives RCOX that had been labelled with ^{18}O.

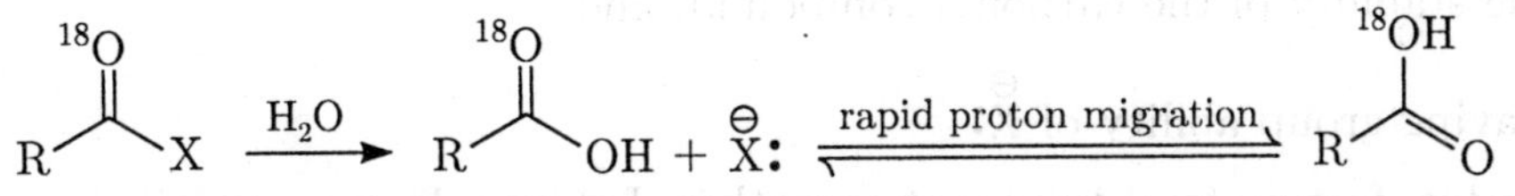

The population of labelled molecules in the remaining starting material had decreased significantly (*i.e.*, the substrate contains normal ^{16}O also) which indicates the formation of an intermediate where ^{16}O and labelled ^{18}O can change places.

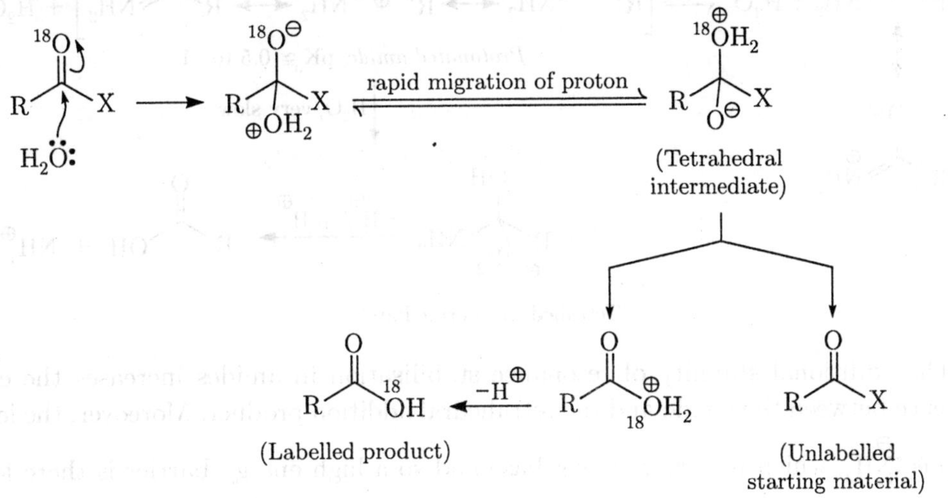

Why is X: always ejected from the tetrahedral intermediate?

The answer lies in the leaving group ability.

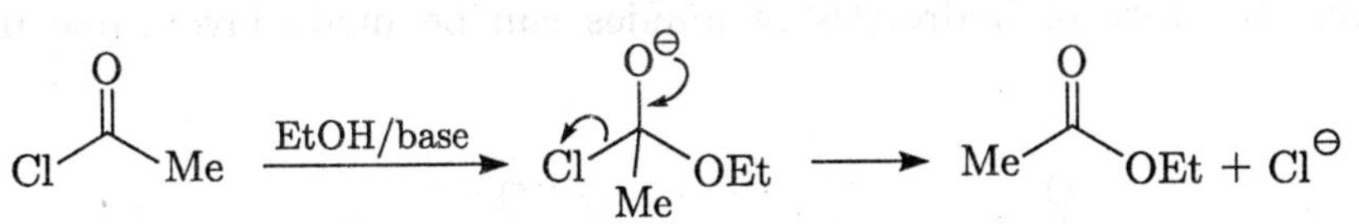

Now $\overset{\ominus}{Me}$ and $\overset{\ominus}{O}Et$ are *bad leaving groups* as these are *strong bases* where Cl^- is quite a good leaving group as it is stable, less basic and quite unreactive. [pK_{aH} for $Me^{\ominus}$ = 50, for $EtO^{\ominus}$ = 16 and for $Cl^{\ominus}$ = 7). This is the leaving group ability by which acyl compounds differ from aldehydes and ketones in reactions. With aldehydes and ketones the product formed is an *addition product* not a substitution one, as to undergo a substitution reaction, the leaving group would have to be $\overset{\ominus}{H}$: ion (in case of aldehydes) or alkide ($\overset{\ominus}{R}$:) in case of ketones from the tetrahedral intermediate. Both $\overset{\ominus}{H}$: and $\overset{\ominus}{R}$: being strong bases are poor leaving groups. So in case of acyl compounds, $\overset{\ominus}{X}$: is ejected from the tetrahedral intermediate to lead to a substitution product, aldehydes and ketones give rise to addition products.

The rate of carbonyl substitution reaction depends on—

1. The stability of the carbonyl compound, and

2. Leaving group ability of $\overset{\ominus}{X}$:

These two factors tend to operate together. Let us take two extreme cases.

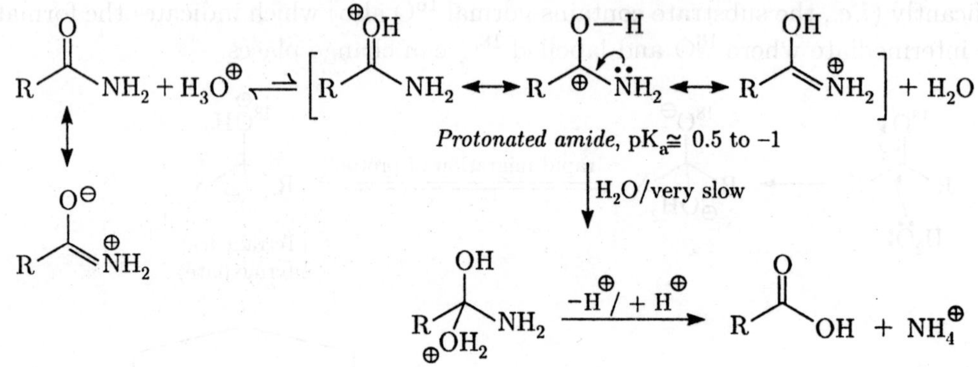

(Tetrahedral intermediate)

The additional stability of resonance stabilisation in amides increases the energy difference between the amide and the tetrahedral addition product. Moreover, the leaving group is $:\overset{\ominus}{N}H_2$, which is a very strong base and so a high energy barrier is there for the second step (ejection of $:\overset{\ominus}{N}H_2$ from the tetrahedral intermediate). As a result, the second step becomes rate limiting. So amide hydrolysis under acidic condition is a particularly slow reaction and requires harsh conditions to proceed at a reasonable rate.

However, the rate of hydrolysis of amides can be made favourable under basic conditions.

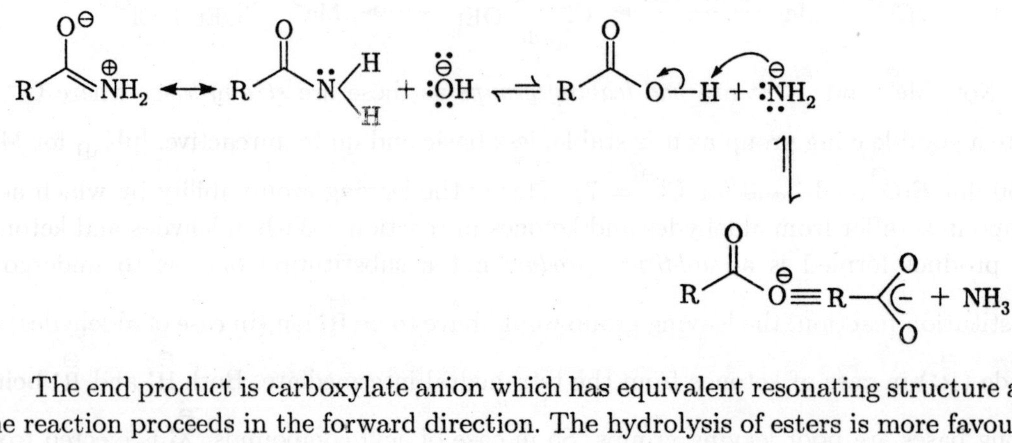

The end product is carboxylate anion which has equivalent resonating structure and the reaction proceeds in the forward direction. The hydrolysis of esters is more favoured under basic conditions. An ester molecule is also resonance stabilised but the extent of resonance stabilisation is less compared to an amide. Moreover, an alkoxide ion is a better leaving group compared to $:\ddot{N}H_2^{\ominus}$ as the basicity of the former is less. As a result, the esters become more reactive towards hydrolysis.

For the hydrolysis of acid chlorides, we see that the acid chlorides are much less resonance stabilised (ineffective overlap between chlorine 3p orbital and carbon 2p orbital) and also the polar effect (–I) of Cl atom destabilises the carbonyl compound, through an unfavourable interaction of the carbon chlorine bond dipole with the partial positive charge on the carbonyl carbon.

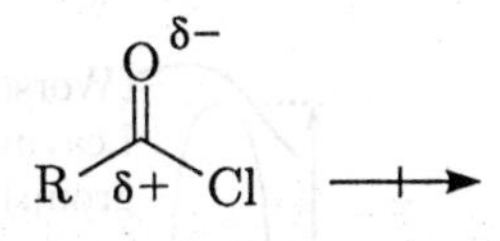

Partial positive charge on the carbonyl carbon interacts unfavourably with the positive end of the C—Cl bond dipole.

So, an acid chloride is comparatively destabilised compared to amides and esters in the ground state and this destabilisation reduces the standard free energy difference between the acid chloride and the transition state Moreover, $Cl^{\ominus}$ being a good leaving group, the tetrahedral intermediate breaks down quickly to afford the product. Even the first step (attack of a nucleophile) becomes rate limiting, so the hydrolysis of an acid chloride occurs at a much faster rate compared to those of esters and amides.

An acid anhydride is more resonance stabilised than an acid chloride but less than an ester because of the positive charge on the carboxylate oxygen and partial positive charge on the carbonyl carbon.

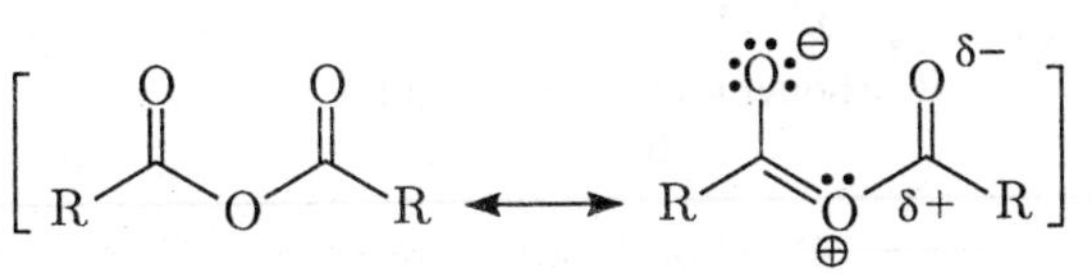

(Repulsion between like charges)

The leaving group in case of acid anhydride is a carboxylate anion which is undoubtedly more basic than chloride ion ($Cl^{\ominus}$) but less basic than alkoxide anion so the reactivity of acid anhydrides is in between acid chlorides and esters. So we may conclude that, (a) stabilisation of a carbonyl compound decreases its reactivity and destabilisation of the carbonyl compound increases its reactivity; (b) Higher basicity of the leaving group decreases reactivity and lower basicity increases reactivity.

So the reactivity order of acyl compounds is as follows.

Acid chlorides > acid anhydrides > esters > carboxylic acids > amides

— Reactivity decreases →

This is a conclusion derived from negatively charged nucleophiles, but same conclusions are obtained from acid catalysed reactions also.

Reactions of nitriles in bases are slower than these of other acid derivatives because nitrogen is less electronegative than oxygen and accepts additional electrons less readily. Reactions of nitriles are slow in acid medium due to their extremely low basicities. It is the protonated form of a nitrile that reacts with nucleophiles in acid solution; but so little of this form is present that the rate of the reaction is very small.

$$R-C\equiv N + H_3O^{\oplus} \rightleftharpoons \left[R-C\equiv \overset{\oplus}{N}H \longleftrightarrow R-\overset{\oplus}{C}=NH \right] + H_2O$$

Protonated nitrile, $pK_a \cong 10$

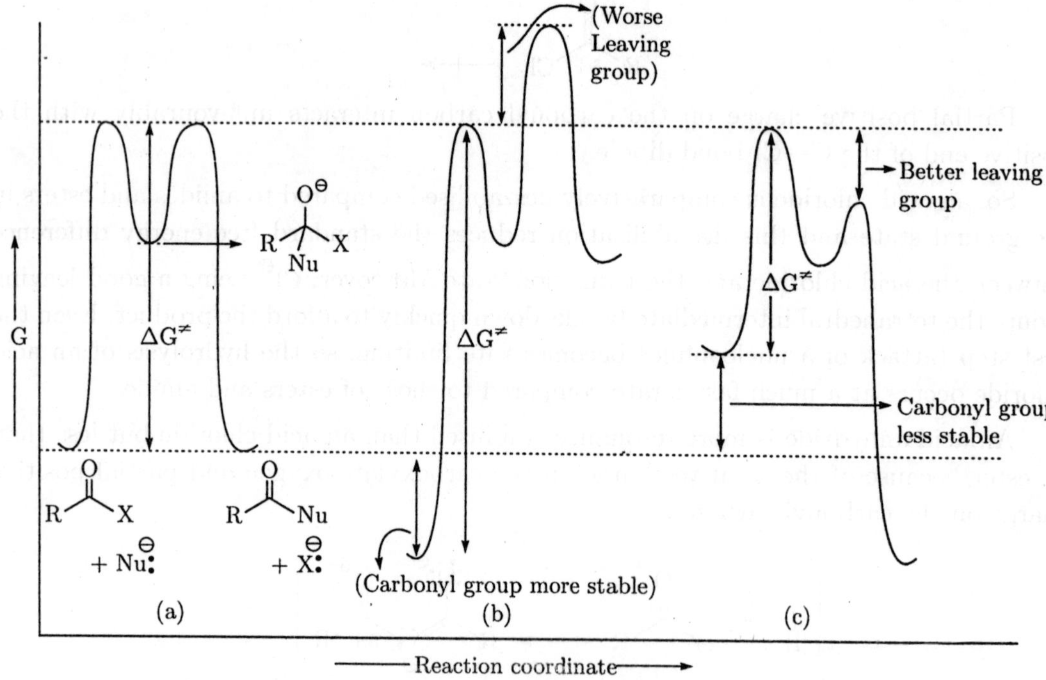

Fig. 2.4 :

(a) A free energy diagram for a generalised reaction in which the reactants and the products have the same standard free energy and the transition state for the two steps also have same standard free energy.

(b) When a carbonyl compound (*e.g.*, an amide) is stabilised by resonance and it contains a poor leaving group the rates of formation and breaking of tetrahedral intermediate both decrease and the rate of nucleophilic substitution gets slower. An increase in the $\Delta G^{\neq}$ between the reactant and the transition state is increased.

(c) When a carbonyl compound (*e.g.*, an acid chloride) is destabilised and it contains an excellent leaving group, the rates of formation and breaking down of the intermediate (tetrahedral) both increase and the rate of nucleophilic substitution becomes faster.

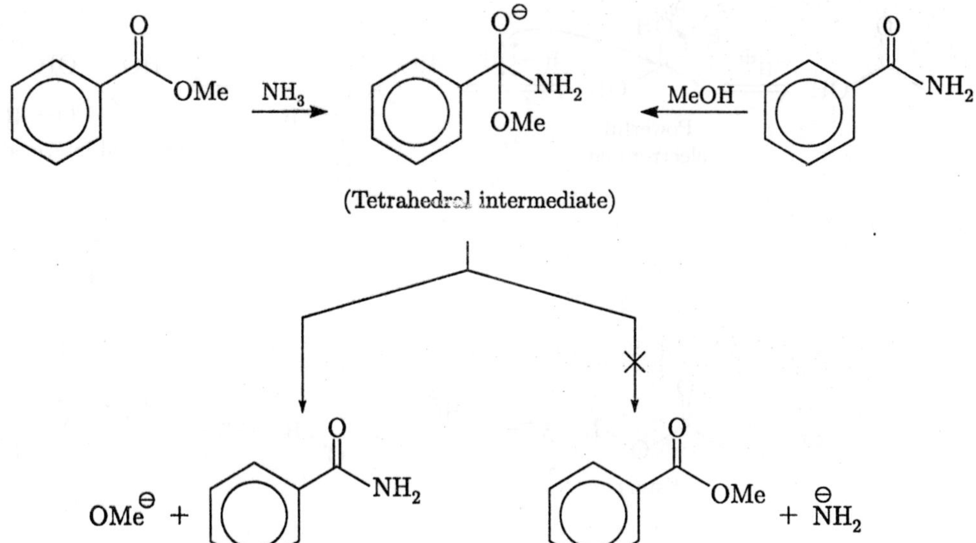

As the basicity of $:\ddot{N}H_2^{\ominus}$ is much more (therefore a bad leaving group) than $OMe^{\ominus}$ (evident from pK_a values), amide is formed readily but not the ester.

Carboxylic acids do not undergo substitution reactions under basic conditions

When carboxylic acids are reacted with alcohols in the presence of base, the product is only carboxylate anion by deprotonation of acid. Similarly, carboxylic acids *do not* react with amines to give amides but gives ammonium carboxylate anion.

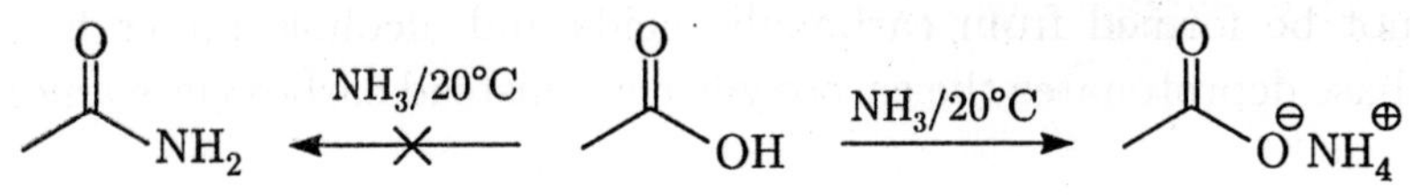

Once the carboxylate anion is formed, no further nucleophilic attack at the carbonyl centre is possible because of the following resonating structure of carboxylate anion.

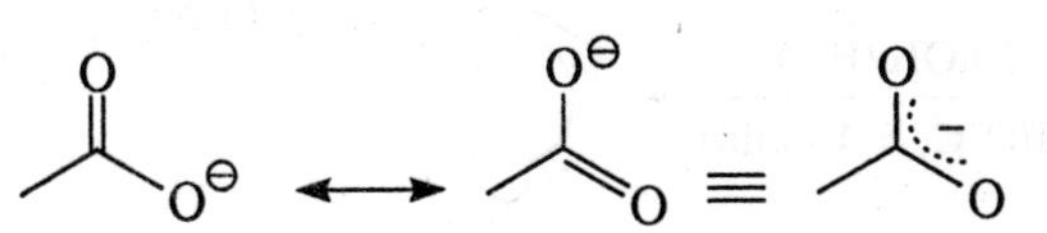

A double bond is generated which prevents the nucleophilic attack at the carbonyl carbon.

Under neutral conditions, alcohols are not reactive enough to add to carboxylic acids, but in the presence of *acids*, esters can be formed from alcohols and carboxylic acids. Carbonyl groups on protonation become extremely powerful electrophilies. For this reason, alcohols react with carboxylic acids under acid catalysis (HCl or H_2SO_4), although they (alcohols) are weak nucleophiles.

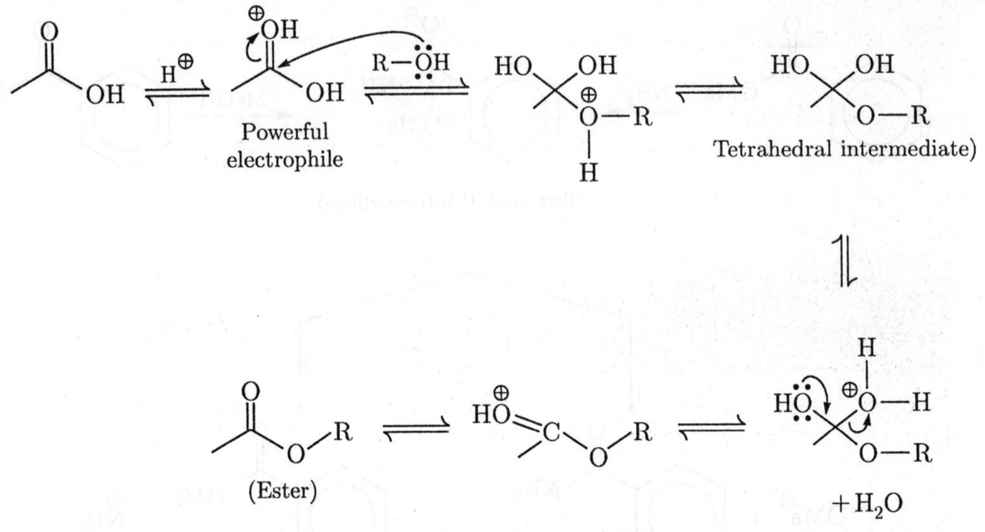

(pK_{aH} of $\overset{\ominus}{O}H$ is 15 and that of H_2O is –2)

Tetrahedral intermediates are unstable as the energy gained to reform a C=O bond is greater than the energy consumed to break two C—O bonds. On protonation bad leaving groups like $OH^{\ominus}$ or $OR^{\ominus}$ become good leaving groups as they form H_2O or ROH molecules. Loss of ROH from the tetrahedral intermediate gives back to starting material whereas loss of water gives the desired product; *i.e.*, ester.

Base-catalysed hydrolysis of esters is irreversible

Esters can not be formed from carboxylic acids and alcohols under basic conditions because the base deprotonates the carboxylic acid, instead carboxylate anion and alcohol are formed.

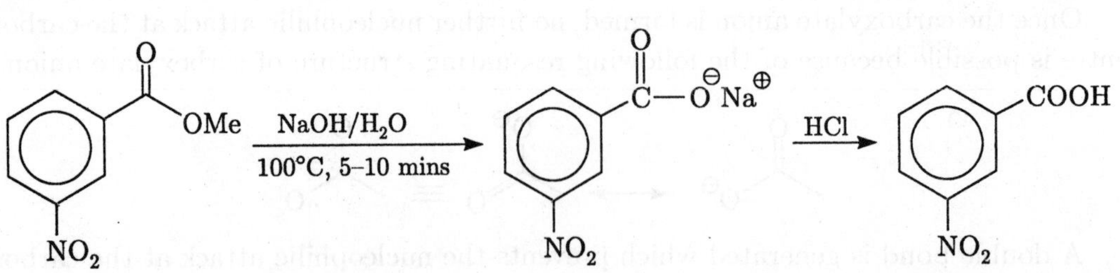

In acid-catalysed ester hydrolysis, the ester carbonyl oxygen gets protonated. In base-catalysed ester hydrolysis, this is not possible. But, however, unprotonated ester is good enough electrophile because $OH^{\ominus}$, not the neutral H_2O is the nucleophile. The tetrahedral intermediate may collapse to give back the tarting material (ester) or may proceed forward to produce acid and water.

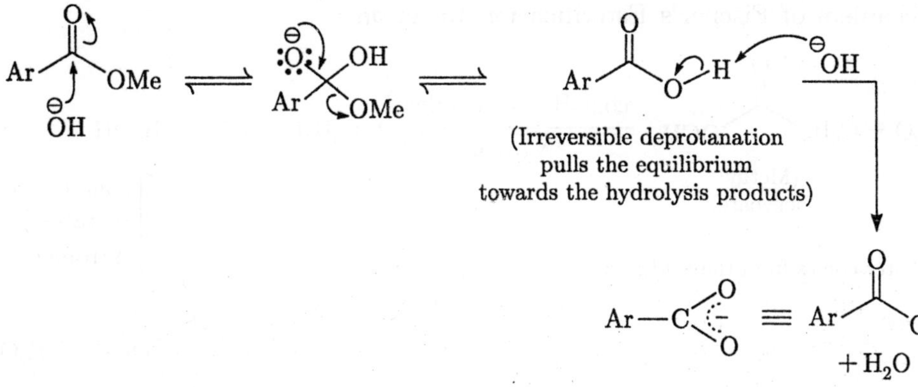

Esterification of Carboxylic Acids

1. Fischer's method of esterification : Carboxylic acids and *excess* alcohol are heated in the presence of concentrated sulphuric acid (H_2SO_4) as a catalyst. The reaction is fully *reversible* in nature.

(a) 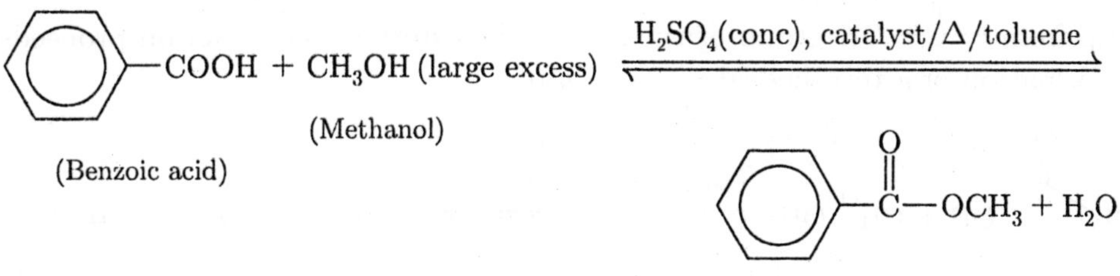

(b) $$HO_2C(CH_2)_4COOH + C_2H_5OH\text{(excess)} \xrightleftharpoons{\text{conc.}H_2SO_4\text{ (catalyst)}/\Delta/\text{toluene}} EtO{-}\overset{O}{\overset{\|}{C}}{-}(CH_2)_4{-}\overset{O}{\overset{\|}{C}}{-}OEt + H_2O$$

(Adipic acid) (Ethanol) (Diethyl adipate)

These reactions are run to *completion* using large excess of alcohol acting both as a reactant and a solvent. Concentrated sulphuric acid (H_2SO_4) also plays a double role – a catalyst and a dehydrating agent to remove water formed in the reaction mixture. Water is also removed from the equilibrium as an azeotrope by adding toluene in the reaction mixture and distilling it off. Fischer's esterification reaction is not suitable for esterification of phenols and tertiary alcohols.

Mechanism of Fischer's Esterification Reaction :

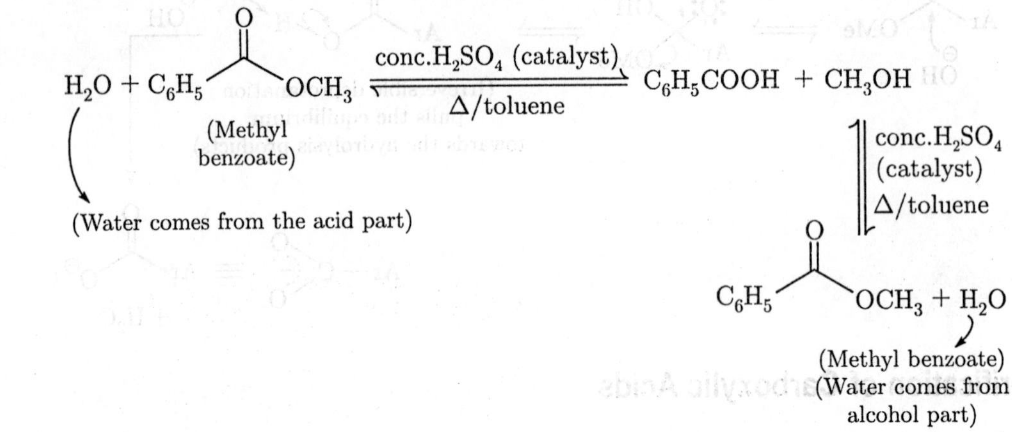

The water librerated in the reaction may come either from the acid or from the alcohol part. When ^{18}O labelled methanol ($CH_3{}^{18}OH$) is used, it is found that the *water* comes exclusively from *carboxylic acid.* The reaction is therfore, displacement of –OH group from $-\overset{\overset{\displaystyle O}{\|}}{C}-OH$ group of the acids. The esterification reaction proceeds through the formation of a tetrahedral intermediate.

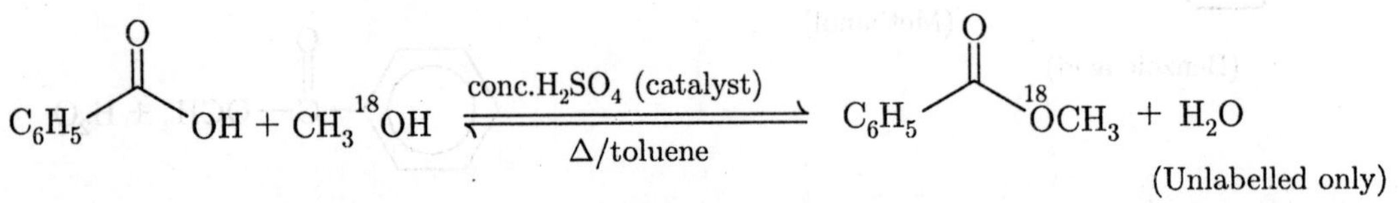

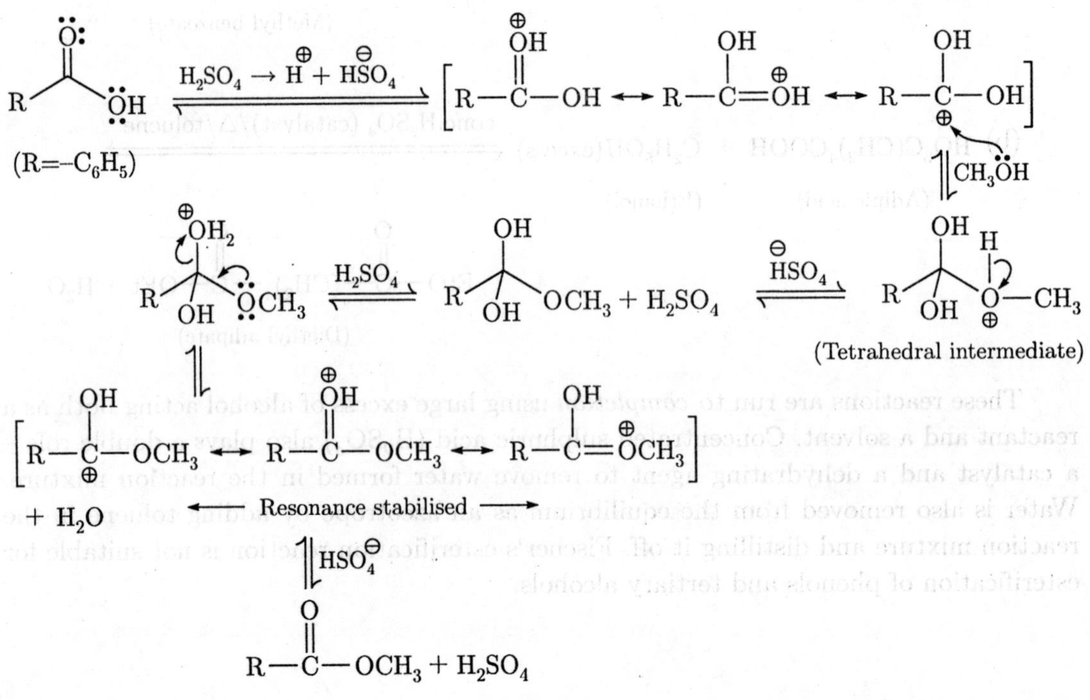

The evidence for the formation of tetrahedral intermediate comes from the isotope labelled experiment with ^{18}O labelled atoms. If any tetrahedral intermediate be formed, then the two –OH groups attached to it must be in identical environemt and water may be eliminated from any of the two –OH groups. To prove the formation of tetrahedral intermediate, the reverse reaction, *i.e.*, hydrolysis of ester is taken into consideration, which is logical as esterification and ester hydrolysis reactions are microscopically reversible.

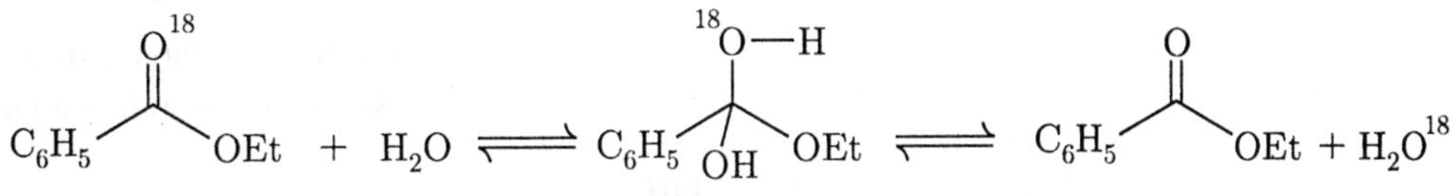

(^{18}O labelled ester) (Tetrahedral intermediate)

The reaction is reversible in nature and the unconverted ester recovered from the reaction mixture contains a mixture of labelled ester and unlabelled ester. The formation of unlabelled ester proves the formation of tetrahedral intermediate, where the two –OH groups are identical.

The esterification reaction may be called a nucleophilic displacement or nucleophilic substitution reaction at the carbonyl group where –OH group attached to C=O group of carboxylic acid is being substituted by a nucleophile. For acid derivatives, further addition to >C=O moiety is not favourable as we get for aldehydes and ketones (formation of acetals and ketals).

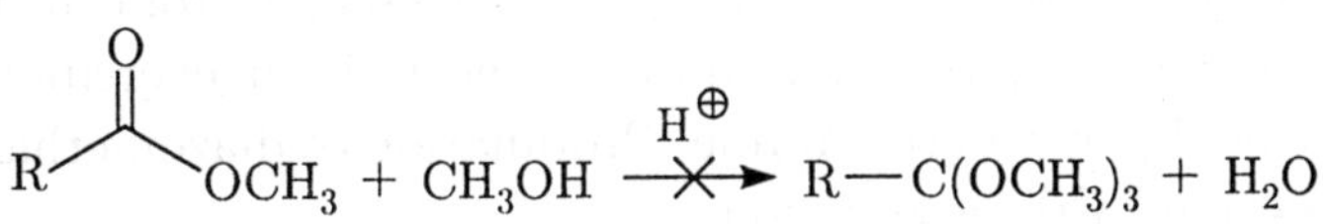

(*Ortho* ester)

Although *ortho* esters are known, they are not formed by this mechanism. The unreactivity of ester carbonyl group is due to the resonance stabilised structure of an ester molecule.

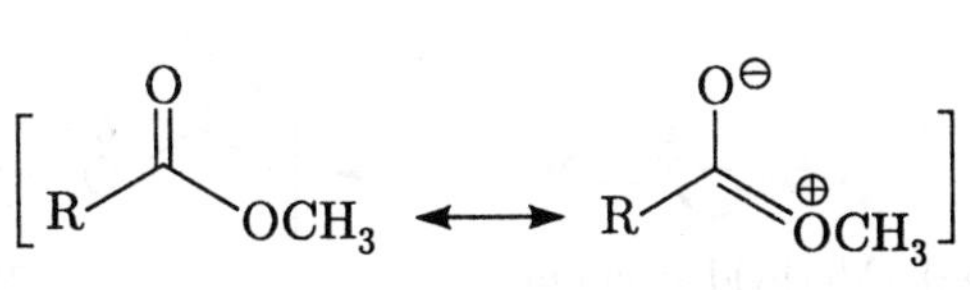

Partial double bond character makes the carbonyl carbon less electrophilic and unreactive towards nucleophiles.

The equilibrium constants for the addition to the >C=O group of acid derivatives are *10^8 times smaller* than those for formation of aldehyde addition compounds. Most carbonyl displacement reactions of esters and acids are much slower than the *analogous* reactions of *aldehydes and ketones.* Carboxylic esters are less reactive as they have resonance stabilised structures compared to aldehydes and ketones. This resonance stabilisation is absent in the tetrahedral intermediate and so the formation of tetrahedral intermediate proceeds at a sluggish rate for acids or esters compared to those for aldehydes and ketones.

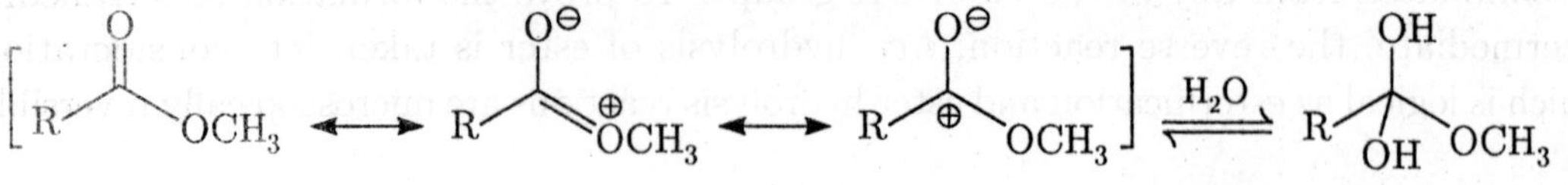

(Tetrahedral intermediate)
(No resonance stabilisation)

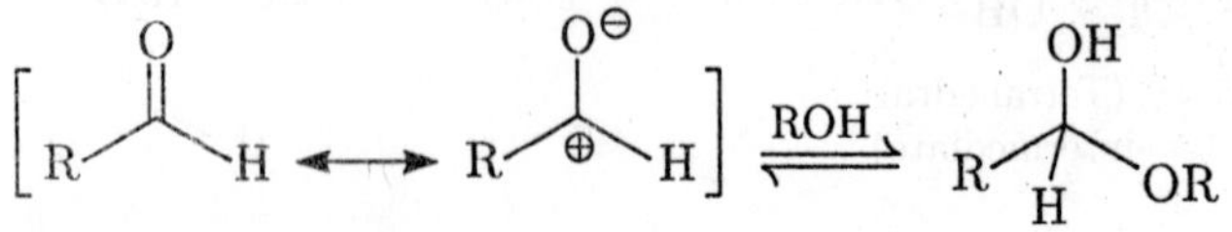

(Less stabilised by resonance) (Tetrahedral intermediate)
(No resonance stabilisation is present)

2. Esterification by Alkylation Reaction

(a) $CH_3(CH_2)_4CH{=}CHCOOH + CH_2N_2$ (diazomethane) $\xrightarrow{\text{ether}}$ $CH_3(CH_2)_4CH{=}CH{-}\overset{O}{\overset{\|}{C}}{-}OCH_3 + N_2\uparrow$

The reaction is almost irreversible as nitrogen escapes from the reaction mixture as a gas, and the equilibrium shifts to the right irreversibly. The acidity of carboxylic acid plays a critical role. Protanation of diazomethane by carboxylic acid gives a methyldiazonium ion.

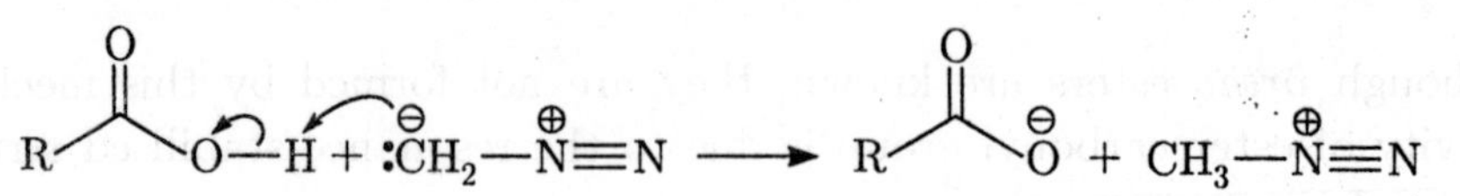

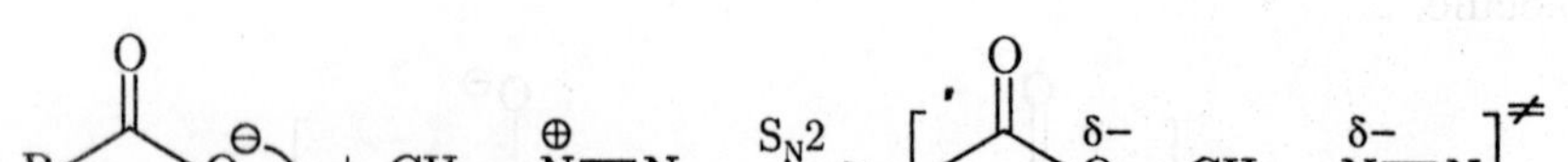

(Carboxylate anion) (Methyldiazonium cation) T.S

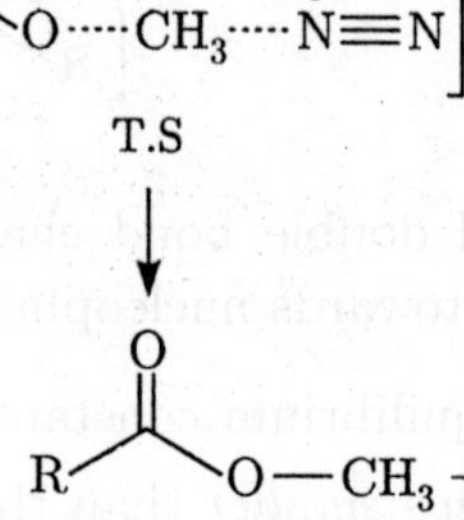

(Good leaving group)

(b) 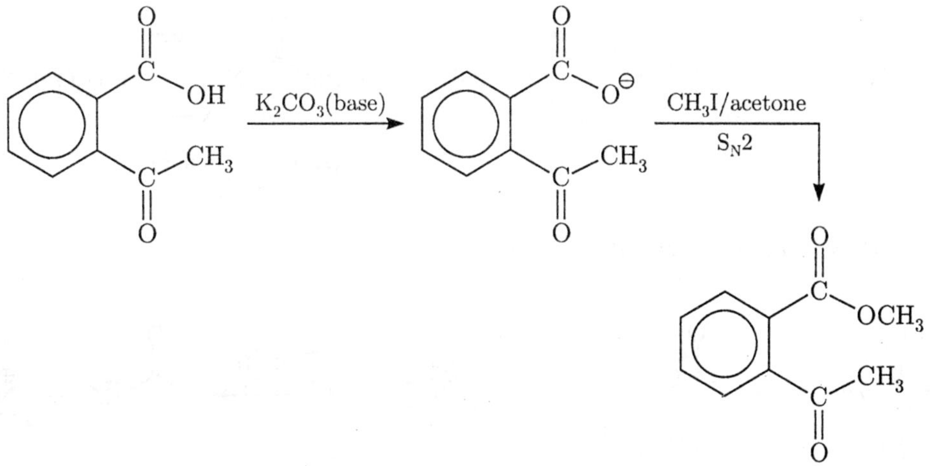

3. Formation esters of tertiary alcohols with alkenes and acids in the presence of concentrated sulphuric acid (H_2SO_4) as a catalyst.

$$CH_3-\overset{\displaystyle CH_3}{\overset{|}{C}}=CH_2 + CH_3COO^{\ominus}\,H^{\oplus} \xrightarrow[\text{pressure}]{H_2SO_4\text{(conc.), (catalyst)}} Me_3C-OCOCH_3$$

(Tertiarybutyl acetate)
(Markownikoff addition product)

Reactions of Carboxylic Acid Derivatives With Nucleophiles

1. ***Reactions*** of ***acid chlorides with ammonia and amines*** :

(a) $CH_3(CH_2)_8COCl + 2\ddot{N}H_3\,\text{(conc. } NH_4OH) \xrightarrow{\text{rapid and irreversible}} CH_3(CH_2)_8-\overset{O}{\overset{\|}{C}}-NH_2 + NH_4Cl$

(Dedecanoyl chloride) → (Dodecanamide)(73%)

(b) 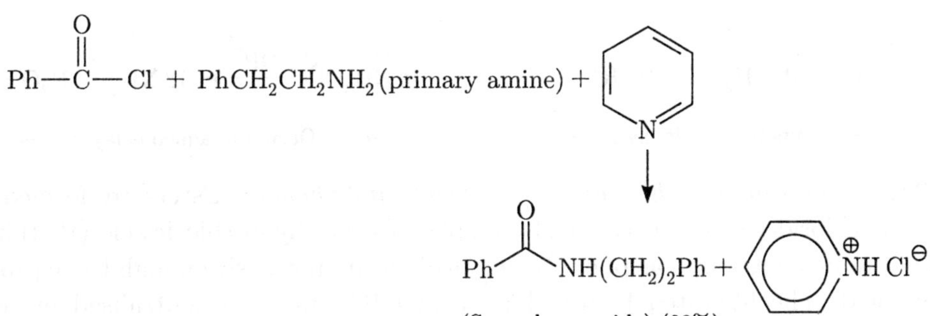

(Secondary amide) (98%)

(c) 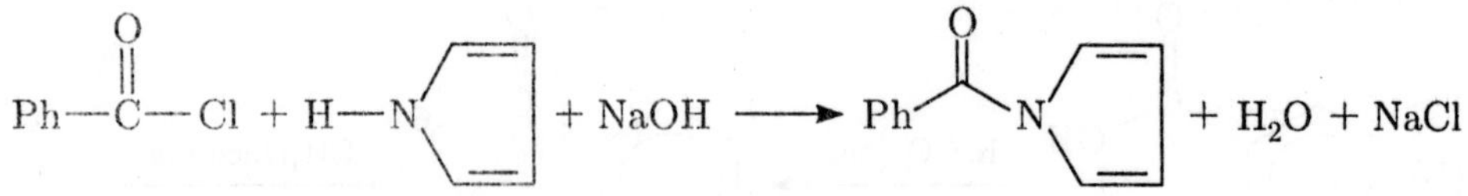

(A secondary amine) (A tertiary amide) (81%)

Mechanism of the reaction :

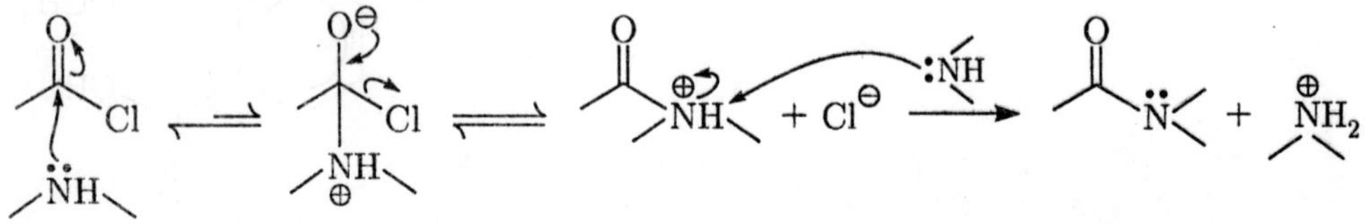

The proton is removed from the amide nitrogen in the last step of the mechanism. Unless additional base is added, the starting amine acts as a base in this step. Hence, for each equivalent of amide that is formed, an equivalent of amine is protonated, *i.e.*, the amine is no longer nucleophile. So we can conclude that, $R_2\ddot{N}H$ (strong base) is a good nucleophile but $R_2\overset{\oplus}{N}H_2$ (protonated amine) is not a nuclephile.

Hence if only the base present is the amine nucleophile, then **at least two equivalents** must be added; one equivalent is used as the nucleophile and another equivalent is used in the final proton transfer step. The use of excess amine is practical when it is cheap, otherwise tertiaryamines like triethylamine (Et_3N) or pyridine are used as bases. Presence of tertiary amines does not interfere with the amide formation reaction as it can not form an amide.

Schotten Baumann Techniqne : The reaction is run with an acid chloride in a separate layer (either alone or in a solvent) over an aqueous solution of sodium hydrioxide. Hydrolysis of the acid chloride by sodium hydrioxide is avoided as acid chlorides are typically insoluble in water and therefore can not come in direct contact with the water soluble hydroxide ions. The amine reacts with acid chloride to yield the amide and aqueous NaOH solution neutralises the protanated amine that is formed.

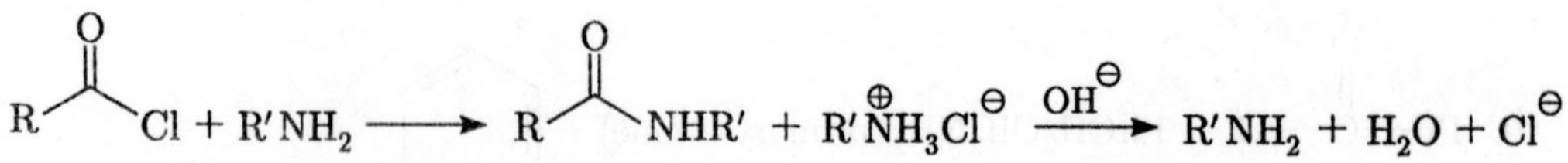

← Occurs in organic layer → ← Occurs in aqueous layer →

2. *Reactions of acid chlorides with alcohols and phenols* : Esters are formed rapidly when acid chlorides react with alcohols and phenols. The hydrochloric acid (HCl) liberated need not to be neutralised as phenols and alcohols are not basic enough to be protonated by the acid. The liberated hydrochloric acid (HCl) may be neutralised by adding a tertiary amine like pyridine. Pyridine may be used as a solvent also.

(a) 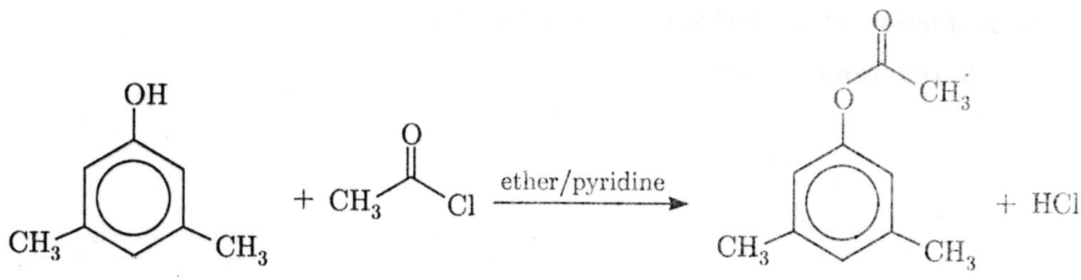

(3,5-dimethylphenol) (3,5-dimethylphenyl acetate)

(b) 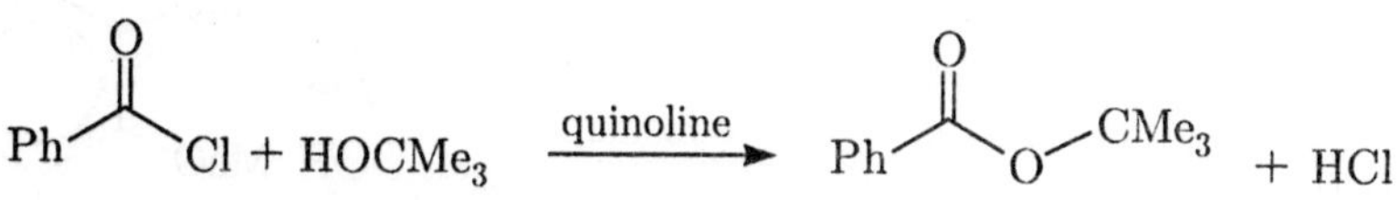

(Tertiarybutanol)

Esters of tertiary alcohols and phenols which can not be prepared by acid-catalysed esterification can be prepared by this method.

(c) 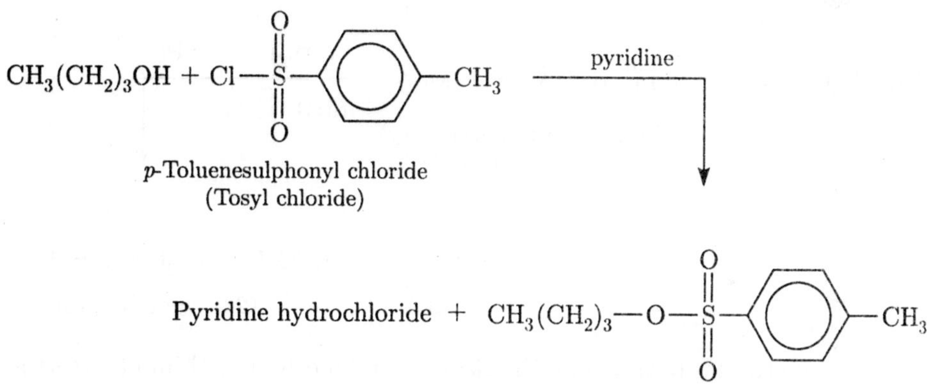

p-Toluenesulphonyl chloride (Tosyl chloride)

Butyl tosylate

3. ***Reaction of acid chlorides with carboxylate salt***

$$CH_3CH_2-\overset{O}{\overset{\|}{C}}-Cl + Na^{\oplus}\ \overset{\ominus}{O}-\overset{O}{\overset{\|}{C}}-CH_3 \xrightarrow{\text{ether}} CH_3CH_2-\overset{O}{\overset{\|}{C}}-O-\overset{O}{\overset{\|}{C}}-CH_3 + Na^{\oplus}Cl^{\ominus}$$

(Propanoyl chloride) (Sodium acetate) (weak nucleophile)

The method is also useful to prepare *mixed anhydrides.*

4. 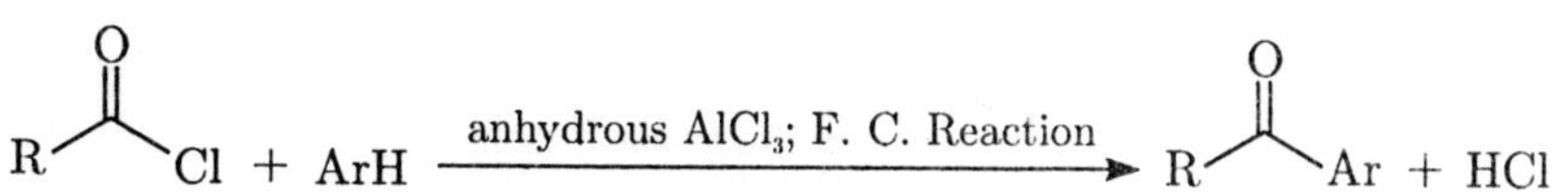

(a ketone)

5. ***Reduction of acid chlorides to aldehydes***

(a) ***Rosenmund Reduction***

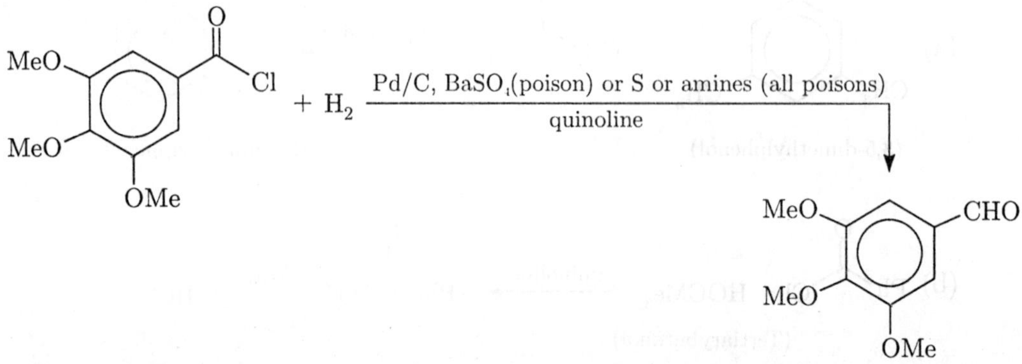

The catalyst (Pd/C) is deactivated or poisoned to prevent further reduction of the aldehyde formed.

(b)
$$Me_3C-\overset{O}{\overset{\|}{C}}-Cl + \overset{\oplus}{Li}\ H-Al\text{+}OCMe_3)_3 \xrightarrow[\text{(ii) } H_3\overset{\oplus}{O}]{\text{(i) Diglyme/}-78^\circ C} Al^{3+} + LiCl + 3Me_3COH + Me_3C-\overset{O}{\overset{\|}{C}}-H$$

Lithium tri(tertiarybutoxy) aluminium hydride; (Salt); (2,2-Dimethylpropanal)

This method is better than the Rosenmund method. Lithium tri (tertiarybutoxy) aluminium chloride is far less reactive than $LiAlH_4$ as the former contains only one hydride ion to be used for reduction. This hydride ion reduces only the most reactive functional group. Acid chlorides are more reactive than the aldehydes towards nucleophiles. So the reagent preferentially attacks only the acid chloride and reduces it to aldehydes but does not attack the product aldehyde. In contrast, $LiAlH_4$ can not discriminate between aldehyde and acid chloride and thus, acid chlorides are reduced to primary alcohols.

Preparation of tri(tertiary butoxy)aluminium hydride :

$$\overset{\oplus}{Li}\ \overset{\ominus}{AlH_4} + 3Me_3COH \longrightarrow \overset{\oplus}{Li}\ H-\overset{\ominus}{Al}[OCMe_3]_3 + 3H_2$$

In other words, with lithium tri (tertiarybutoxy) aluminium hydride, the reduction of acid chlorides stops at the aldehyde stage.

6. ***Reaction of acid chlorides with organometallics*** : Because acid chlorides are more reactive than ketones, they (acid chlorides) form ketones with Grignard reagent. But Grignard reagents are very reactive to stop the reaction at the ketone stage and the product ketone reacts further with Grignard reagent to form an alcohol. Another type of organometallic reagent called lithium dialkylcuprate ($Li^{\oplus}\, R_2Cu^{\ominus}$) can be used to effect this transformation cleanly. These are commonly known as Gilman cuprates.

Preparation of $Li^{\oplus}\, R_2Cu^{\ominus}$: Two equivalents of an organolithium reagent is used with one equivalent of cuprous chloride (CuCl).

$R—Li + CuCl \longrightarrow RCu + Li^{\oplus}\, Cl^{\ominus}$, the equilibrium is shifted towards right as Li, a very electropositive metal forms the ionic compound Li^+Cl^-.

$$\overset{\oplus}{Li}\ \overset{\ominus}{R}\!: + Cu—R \longrightarrow R—\overset{\ominus}{Cu}—RLi^{\oplus}$$

(Lewis acid) (Lithium dialkylcuprate)

Although copper bears negative charge, it is more electropositive relative to carbon and the reagent is conceptualised as an alkyl anion complexed to copper.

$$R—Cu\cdots\cdots:\overset{\ominus}{R}Li^{\oplus}$$

Lithium dialkylcuprates react in some ways like Grignard reagent or lithium reagent, however, as the alkyl anion is complexed with copper (less electroposotive than Li), alkyl-copper bond has more covalent character and these reagents are *less reactive.* They typically react with acid chlorides and aldehydes, very slowly with ketones and not at all with esters. The reaction of lithium dialkylcuprate with acid chlorides gives *ketones* in excellent yield.

$$CH_3(CH_2)_4COCl + Me_2Cu^{\ominus}\, Li^{\oplus} \xrightarrow[THF]{-78°C/15\ min} \xrightarrow{H_2O} Li^{\oplus}\, Cl^{\ominus} + CH_3Cu + CH_3(CH_2)_4COCH_3$$

(Lithium dimethylcuprate)

CH_3Cu: (Reacts with water)

$CH_3(CH_2)_4COCH_3$: (2-heptanone) 81%

Ketones being much less reactive than acid chlorides towards lithium dialkylcuprate, they do not react further.

Carboxylic Acids

General formula C_nH_{2n+1} COOH, also known as fatty acids; some higher members like stearic and palmitic acids occur in natural fats.

Synthesis of Carboxylic Acids

1. (a) $$RCH_2OH/(ArCH_2OH) \xrightarrow[\text{or } KMnO_4/\text{conc. } H_2SO_4 \text{ (oxidation)}]{K_2Cr_2O_7/\text{conc. } H_2SO_4} RCHO/(ArCHO) \xrightarrow[\text{(oxidation)}]{K_2Cr_2O_7/H^{\oplus} \text{ or } KMnO_4/H^{\oplus}} RCOOH/ArCOOH$$

(b) $$RCHO/(ArCHO) \xrightarrow[\text{or } KMnO_4/\text{conc. } H_2SO_4 \text{ (oxidation)}]{K_2Cr_2O_7/\text{conc. } H_2SO_4} RCOOH/(ArCOOH)$$

(c) $$R_2CHOH \xrightarrow[\text{Drastic Oxidation}]{K_2Cr_2O_7/H^{\oplus}} R_2CO \xrightarrow[\text{Drastic Oxidation}]{K_2Cr_2O_7/H^{\oplus}} 2RCOOH$$

2. $$RCOCH_3/(ArCOCH_3) \xrightarrow[\text{(ii) } H_3O^{\oplus}]{\text{(i) } NaOH/I_2 \text{ (oxidation by haloform reaction)}} RCOOH/(ArCOOH)$$

3. $$\underset{\text{(Symmetric alkene)}}{RCH{=}CHR} \xrightarrow[\text{Oxidation}]{KMnO_4/H^{\oplus}} 2RCOOH$$

4. $$RCN/(ArCN) \xrightarrow[\text{or by dilute alkali followed by } H_3O^{\oplus}]{\text{Hydrolysis by dilute acid}} RCOOH/(ArCOOH)$$

5. $$RCONH_2/(ArCONH_2) \xrightarrow[\text{(ii) } H_3O^{\oplus}]{\text{(i) Hydrolysis by } \overset{\ominus}{O}H \text{(alkali)}} RCOOH/(ArCOOH)$$

6. $$RCOCl/(ArCOCl) \xrightarrow{H_3O^{\oplus}} RCOOH/(ArCOOH)$$

7. $$RCOOR'/(ArCOOR') \xrightarrow[\text{reflux}]{\overset{\ominus}{O}H \text{ or } H_3O^{\oplus} \text{ (hydrolysis of esters)}} RCOOH/(ArCOOH)$$

8. (a) $$RMgX/(ArMgX) \xrightarrow[\text{(ii) } H_3O^{\oplus}]{\text{(i) } CO_2/-78°C} RCOOH/(ArCOOH)$$

(b) $RLi/(ArLi) \xrightarrow[\text{(ii) } H_3O^{\oplus}]{\text{(i) } CO_2/-78^\circ C} RCOOH/(ArCOOH)$

9. $RCH{=}CH_2 \xrightarrow[\text{(iii) } H_3O^{\oplus}]{\text{(i) conc. } H_2SO_4 \text{ (ii) CO (carbon monoxide)}} RCH(CH_3)COOH$

10. 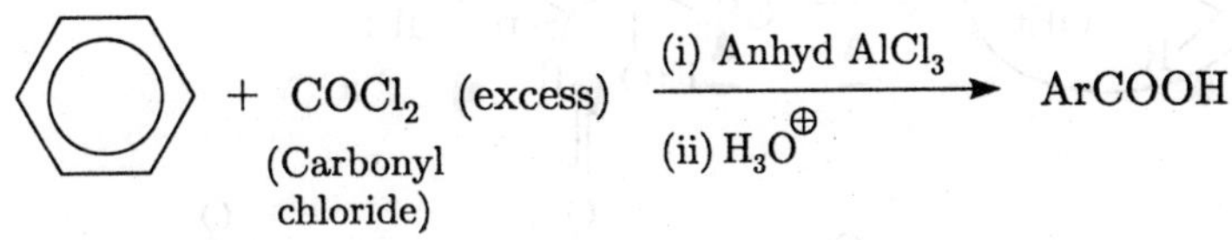

Excess $COCl_2$ should be used otherwise benzophenone will be the major product.

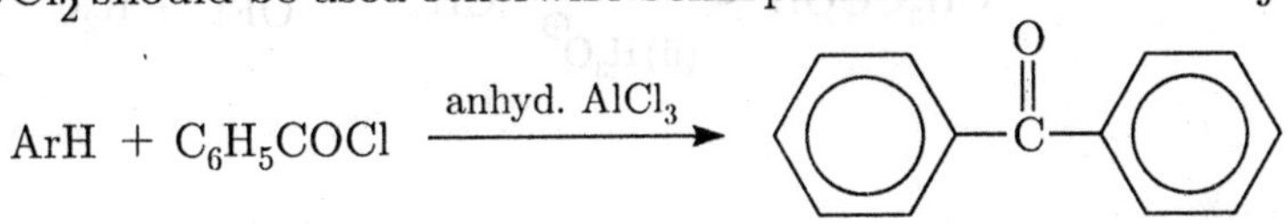

11. $ArCHO + (CH_3CO)_2O \xrightarrow[\text{Perkin's Reaction}]{\text{(i) NaOAc, (ii) } H_3O^{\oplus}} ArCH{=}CHCOOH$

12. 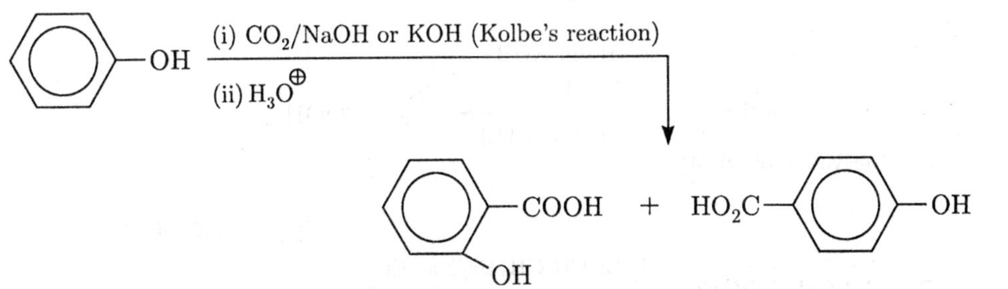

[*o*-hydroxybenzoic acid (major), when NaOH is used as a base]   [*p*-hydroxybenzoic acid (mijor), acid (major), when KOH is used as a base]

13. 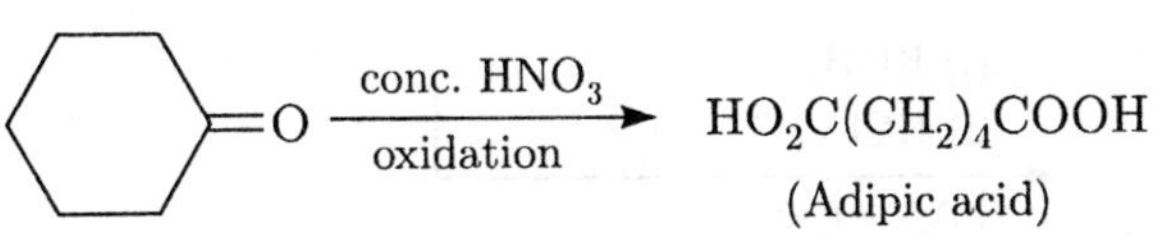

14. $Br(CH_2)_nBr \xrightarrow{\text{KCN(alcoholic)}} NC(CH_2)_nCN \xrightarrow{\overset{\oplus}{H_3O}\text{(hydrolysis)}} HO_2C(CH_2)_nCOOH$

15. (a) 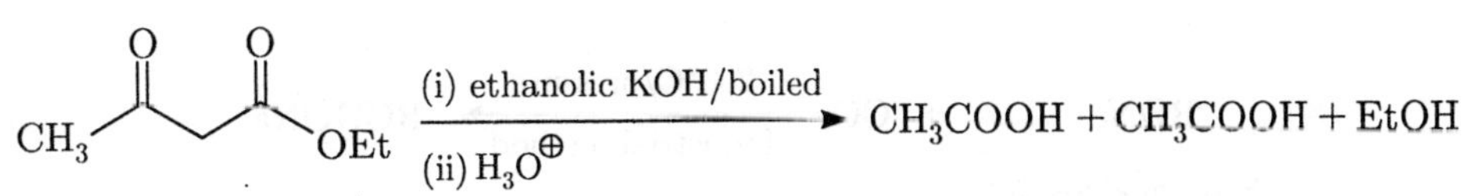

(Ethyl acetoacetate)

(b) 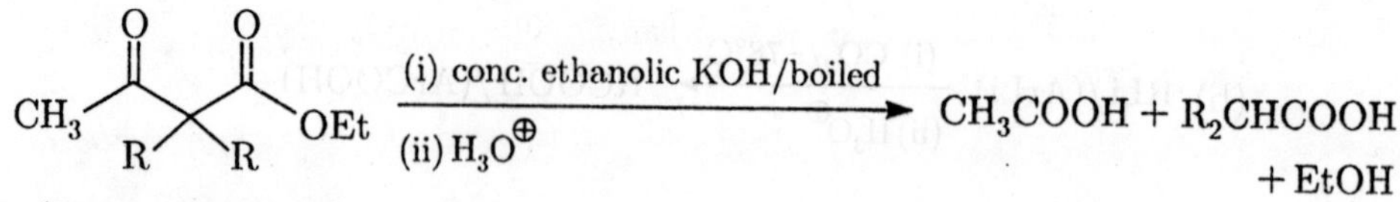

(Derivative of EAA)

Mechanism :

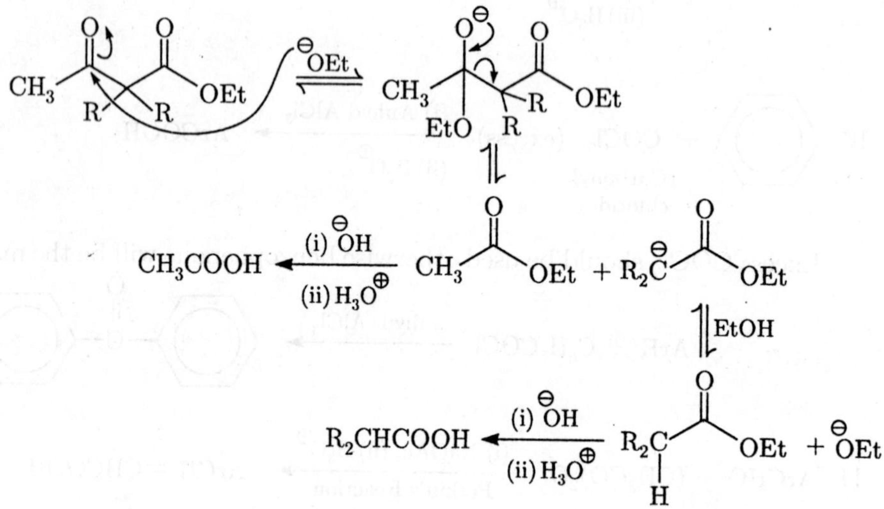

16. $R_2C(COOEt)_2 \xrightarrow[\text{(iii)}\Delta/(-CO_2)]{\text{(i) dil. KOH, (ii) HCl}} R_2CHCOOH$

(Derivative of DEM)

17. $2NC\ CH_2\ COOEt \xrightarrow[\text{EtOH}]{\text{(i) Br } CH_2CH_2 \text{ Br/NaOEt}}$ $NC—CHCOOEt$ | CH_2 | CH_2 | $NC—CHCO_2Et$

$\xrightarrow[\text{(iii)}\Delta(-CO_2)]{\text{(i) KOH, (ii) HCl}}$ CH_2COOH | CH_2 | CH_2 | CH_2COOH

18. $RONa + CO \xrightarrow[\text{Industrial method}]{200°C/\text{pressure}} RCOONa$

(Sodium alkoxide)

19. $$C_6H_5CHO + CH_3COOEt \xrightarrow[\text{(ii) } H_3O^{\oplus}]{\text{(i) NaOEt/EtOH(Claisen Reaction)}} C_6H_5CH{=}CHCOOH + EtOH$$

(Cinnamic acid)

20. $$C_6H_5CHO + CH_2(COOEt)_2 \xrightarrow[\text{Knoevenagel reaction}]{\text{pyridine}} C_6H_5CH{=}C(COOEt)_2 \xrightarrow{\text{(i) KOH; (ii) } H_3O^{\oplus}\text{; (iii) }\Delta(-CO_2)} C_6H_5CH{=}CHCOOH$$

21. $$2CH_2(COOEt)_2 \xrightarrow[\text{(ii) } OH^{\ominus} \text{ (iii) } H_3O^{\oplus} \text{ (iv) } \Delta/(-CO_2)]{\text{(i) Br } CH_2CH_2 \text{ Br/NaOEt/EtOH}} HOOC(CH_2)_4COOH$$

Physical Properties of Carboxylic acids

Carboxylic acids usually remain in dimeric form, either in solid, liquid or gaseous state or even in solution through hydrogen bonding between the hydroxyl hydrogen and carbonyl oxygen as shown below.

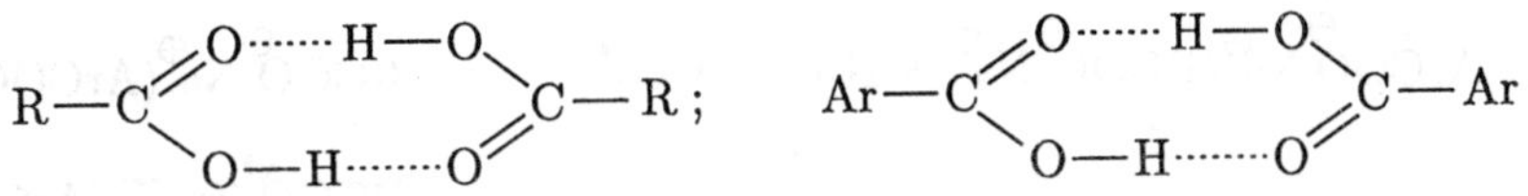

The dimeric state of a carboxylic acid has been determined by the M.W. determination of acetic acid and benzoic acid by vapour density method, in which the respective molecular weights are found to be 120 and 344 (instead of 60 and 172). Owing to this dimerisation, the vapour pressure of carboxylic acids gets reduced and therefore they boil at higher temperatures than the corresponding alcohols.

	Acetic acid	Acetaldehyde	*n*-propylalcohol	*n*-butane	(All have comparable molecular weights)
b.p.	118°C	20°C	98°C	–55°C	

The b.p of a molecule increases with increasing M.W, since the London force increases (increase in b.p is 18°C/carbon atom). The carboxylic acids with even number of carbon atoms is more symmetrical than those with odd number of carbon atoms. So carboxylic acids with even number of carbon atoms boil at a higher temperature compared to acids having odd number of carbon atoms. Carboxylic acids ionise partly in water, and the carboxylate anion is better hydrated. So the parent acid is more soluble in alcohols than in water. Benzoic acid is soluble in hot water but other aromatic acids are slightly soluble in water.

First four members of aliphatic monocarboxylic acids are colourless pungent smelling, corresive liquids, miscible in all part of water. C_5–C_{10} numbers are sharp smelling colourless liquids. Above C_{10}, the acids are odourless solids (odourless due to low volatility).

Reactions given by carboxylic acids

The sole reactivity of a carboxylic acid depends upon $-CO_2H$ functionality. It may be divided into *five groups.*

(a) Substitution of ionisable H of $-CO_2H$ group.

(b) Reactions involving C=O functionality

(c) Reactions involving the α-carbon with respect to $-CO_2H$ group.

(d) Decarboxylation of $-CO_2H$ group

(e) Nucleophilic substitution at the acyl carbon of carboxylic acids.

(a) Substitution of ionisable hydrogen of $-CO_2H$ group

(i) 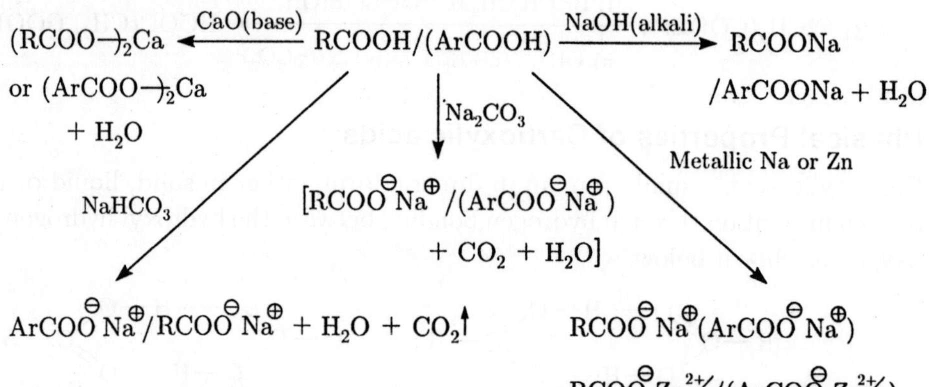

(ii) $RCOOH/(ArCOOH) \xrightarrow{CH_2N_2} RCOOCH_3/(ArCOOCH_3)$

(iii) $RCOOH/(ArCOOH) \xrightarrow{\text{(i) } NH_3, \text{ (ii) } \Delta} RCO\overset{\ominus}{O}\ \overset{\oplus}{NH_4}/(ArCO\overset{\ominus}{O}\overset{\oplus}{NH_4})$

(b) Reaction involving C=O functionality of carboxylic (–COOH) group

(i) $RCOOH/(ArCOOH) \xrightarrow{LiAlH_4/\text{ether}} RCH_2OH/(ArCH_2OH)$

This is an important method for the preparation of primary alcohols.

Mechanism of reduction :

$LiAlH_4$, a source of strongly basic ($\overset{\ominus}{H}$:) ion reacts with acidic hydrogen of the hydride carboxylic acid as shown below.

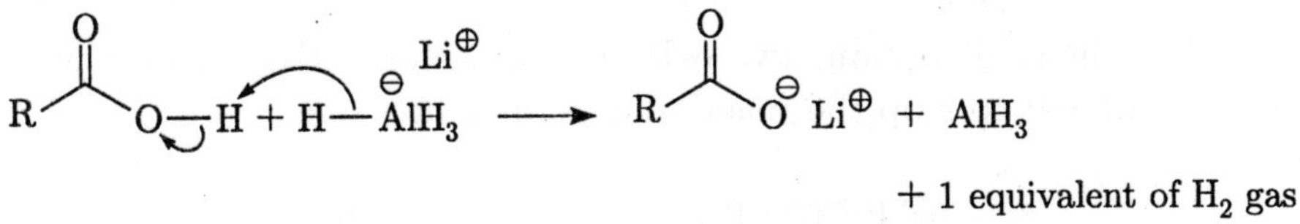

The lithium salt of the carboxylic acid is the actual species which is reduced.

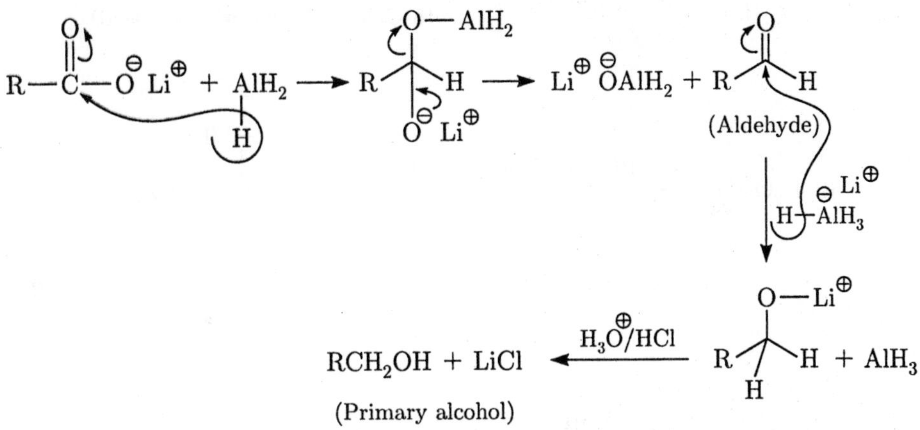

Aldehydes being more reactive than carboxylic acids, can not be isolated, and so reacts with another molecule of $LiAlH_4$ to form primary alcohol followed by acidification. So we see that, $LiAlH_4$ reduction of a carboxylic acid incorporates two types of carbonyl reaction. The first is a net substitution at the carbonyl carbon to give the aldehyde intermediate. The second is an *addition* to the aldehyde to form the primary alcohol. $NaBH_4$, another important hydride reducing agent *does not* reduce carboxylic acids. $LiAlH_4$ reduction of carboxylic acids can be combined with Grignard synthesis of carboxylic acids (alkyl magnisium halide + CO_2, followed by acidification) to provide a one-carbon chain extension of carboxylic acids.

(ii) $RCOOH \xrightarrow[\text{or } H_2/\text{Raney Ni}]{\text{HI/red P/pressure}} RCH_3 + H_2O$

(c) Reaction involving the α-carbon to the –CO_2H group of carboxylic acids :

Hell-Volhard-Zelinsky Reaction (H.V.Z. Reaction)

Aliphatic carboxylic acids containing α-H atoms can easily be converted to its halo-derivative by the action of chlorine or bromine in the presence of *catalytic amount* of red phosphorus and the reaction is known as Hell-Volhard-Zelinsky (HVZ) reaction. This reaction does not occur with fluorine or iodine.

The halogenation of carboxylic acids by HVZ reaction takes place very readily and exclusively at α-position. The readiness and exclusive halogenation at α-position give the reaction a great value in synthesis. α-Haloacids can easily be converted to α-hydroxy acids, α-amino acids and α-cyano acids. The α-cyano acids in their turn may be converted to compounds having synthetic importance such as malonic acid and its derivatives.

When the acid contains two α-H atoms, one or both may be replaced by halogens, but it is difficult to stop the reaction at monohalo stage.

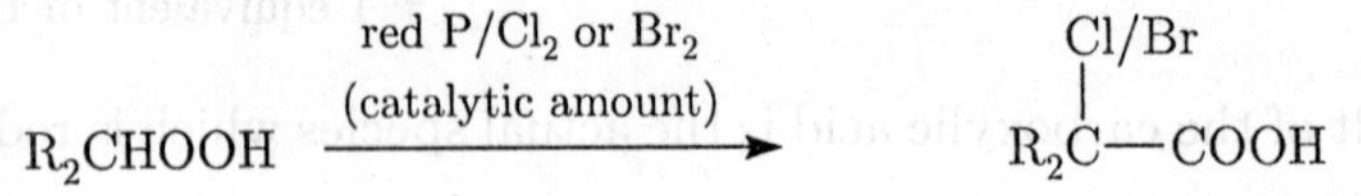

(α-Chloro/Bromocarboxylic acid)

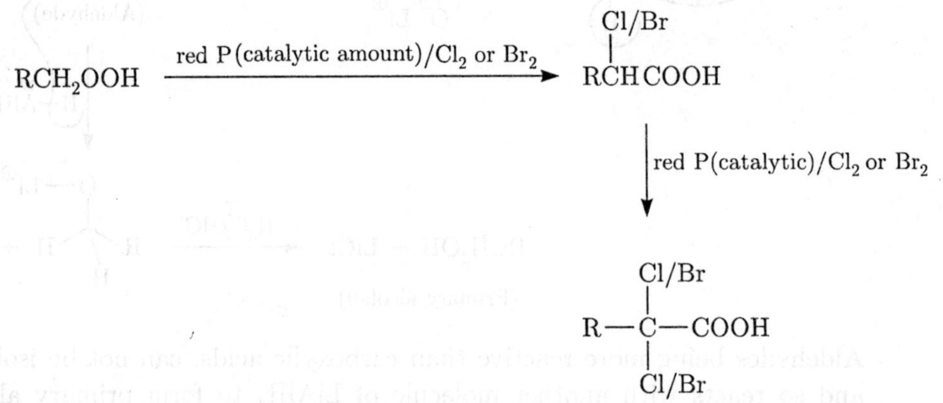

Chlorine is less specific compared to bromine towards the halogenation at α-position. This may be due to the presence of some free radical chlorine ($\dot{C}l$).

$$RCH_2CH_2COOH \xrightarrow{\text{red P(catalytic)}/Cl_2} RCH_2CH(Cl)COOH + RCH(Cl)CH_2COOH$$

However, bromine (Br_2), is specific to halogenate a carboxylic acid at α-position and the reaction can be stopped at monohalo stage.

Mechanism of Hell-Volhard-Zelinsky reaction :

$$2P + 3Br_2 \longrightarrow 2PBr_3$$

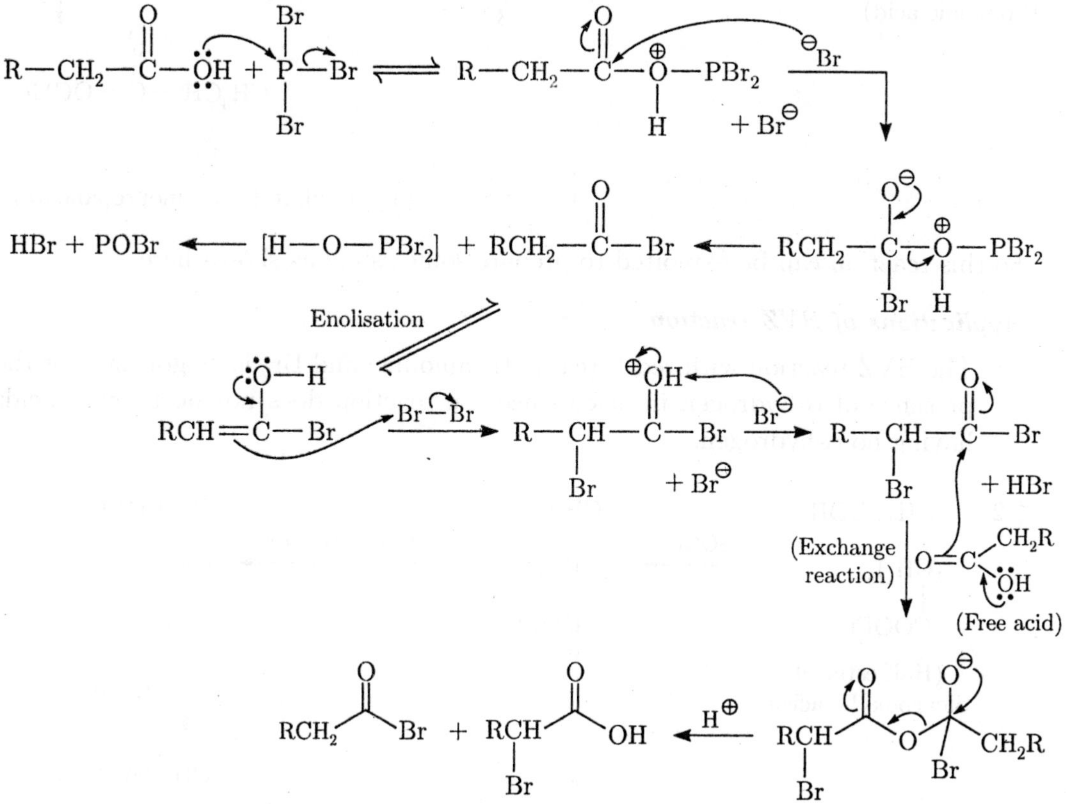

Since RCH_2COBr is generated at the last step, the reaction can run smoothly without catalyst. The catalyst is required only to initiate the reaction. It has been found that, when a carboxylic acid is chlorinated, in the presence of PBr_3 as a catalyst, only α-chloro acid *and no α-bromo acid* is obtained.

$$RCH_2COOH + Cl_2 \xrightarrow{PBr_3} \underset{}{R\overset{Cl}{\overset{|}{C}}HCOOH} \text{ but no } R\overset{Br}{\overset{|}{C}}HCOOH$$

HVZ reaction is applicable to di- and polycarboxylic acids where all the α-positions get substituted if sufficient bromine is used.

When a *small amount of PBr_3* catalyst is used, the α-bromo acid bromide formed reacts with the carboxylic acid to form more acid bromide, which is then brominated as usual.

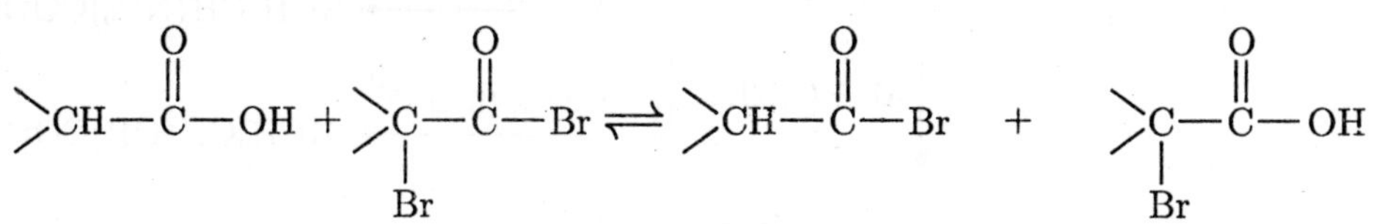

(When catalytic amount of PBr_3 is used)

If one equivalent of PBr_3 is used, the α-bromo acid bromide is the reaction product.

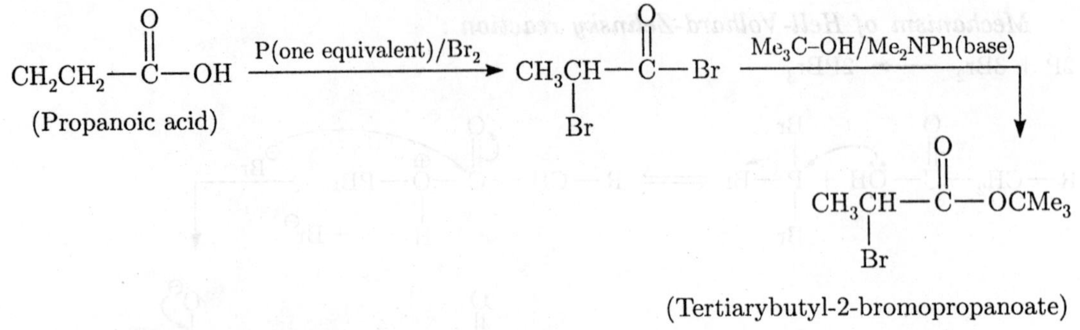

So this reaction can be exploited to prepare some esters as shown here.

Applications of HVZ reaction

1. The HVZ reaction with red P (catalytic amount) and Br_2 is diagonostic for the presence of α-hydrogen in acids since the reaction does not occur with acids having no α-hydrogen.

2. 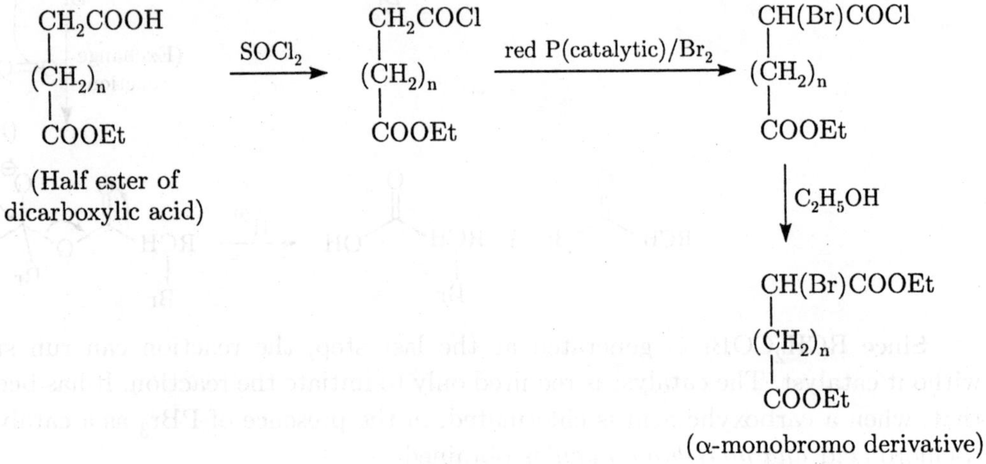

3. *Nucleophilic displacement and elimination* of *halogen from α-haloacids*

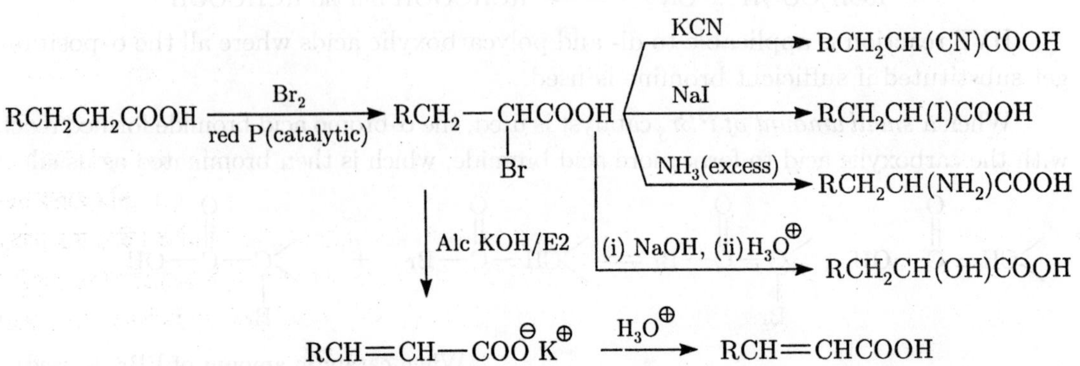

(d) Decarboxylation of –COOH group

(i) $RCOONa(anhydrous) + NaOH(CaO) \xrightarrow{\Delta} R{-}H + Na_2CO_3$

(Sodalime)

(ii) $2RCOO^{\ominus}K^{\oplus} + 2H_2O \xrightarrow[\text{Kolbe's electrolytic method}]{\text{electrolysis}} R{-}R + 2CO_2 + 2KOH + H_2$

(Potassio salt of carboxylic acid) (Alkane)

(iii) ***Hunsdiecker Reaction***

Silver salt of carboxylic acids in dry carbon tetrachloride solution are decomposed by chlorine or bromine to form alkyl halides.

$$RCOOAg + Br_2 \longrightarrow RBr + CO_2\uparrow + AgBr\downarrow$$

The yield of alkyl halides formed follows the order :

Primary halide > secondary halide > tertiary halide

— yield decreases →

The use of bromine is advantageous as the yield of alkyl halide is poor if chlorine is used instead.

Mechanism of Hunsdiecker reaction :

Mechanistic pathway is not certain; one proposed is the formation of free radical as follows.

$$RCOOAg + Br_2 \longrightarrow RCOOBr(\text{hypohalite}) + AgBr\downarrow$$

$$RCOOBr \longrightarrow RCO\dot{O} + \dot{Br}$$

$$RCO\dot{O} \longrightarrow \dot{R} + CO_2\uparrow$$

$$\dot{R} + Br{-}Br \longrightarrow RBr + \dot{Br}$$

$$\dot{R} + RCOOBr \longrightarrow RBr + RCO\dot{O}$$

$$RCO\dot{O} \longrightarrow \dot{R} + CO_2$$

Iodine does not form RI with RCOOAg instead forms an ester and silver iodide.

$$2RCOOAg + I_2 \longrightarrow RCOOR + CO_2\uparrow + 2AgI\downarrow$$

Decarboxylation of Carboxylic Acids and Its Derivatives

1. Decarboxylation of Carboxylic acids : The loss of CO_2 from a carboxylic acid is called decarboxylation.

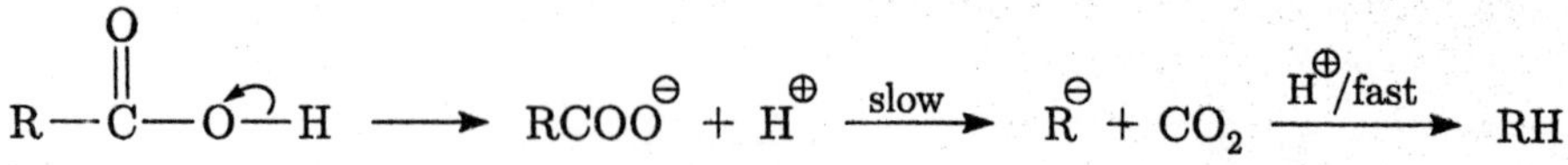

$$\text{Rate of the reaction} = k[RCOO^-]$$

Decarboxylation reaction is promoted by electron withdrawing substituents in R that could stabilise the carbanion intermediate ($R-\overset{O}{\overset{\|}{C}}-O^{\ominus} \xrightarrow{slow} :R^{\ominus} + CO_2 \xrightarrow[fast]{H^{\oplus}} RH$) by delocalisation of its negative charge. This is borne out by very much readier decarboxylation of the nitro substituted carboxylate anion than of $Me_2CHCOO^{\ominus}$ itself.

Carboxylic acids have inherent tendency to undergo decarboxylation, as –

(i) CO_2 is a highly stable molecule ($\Delta H < 0$)

(ii) The system becomes disordered ($\Delta S > 0$)

Example : Decarboxylation of $Me_2C(NO_2)COO^{\ominus}\ Na^{\oplus}$ in the presence of Br_2.

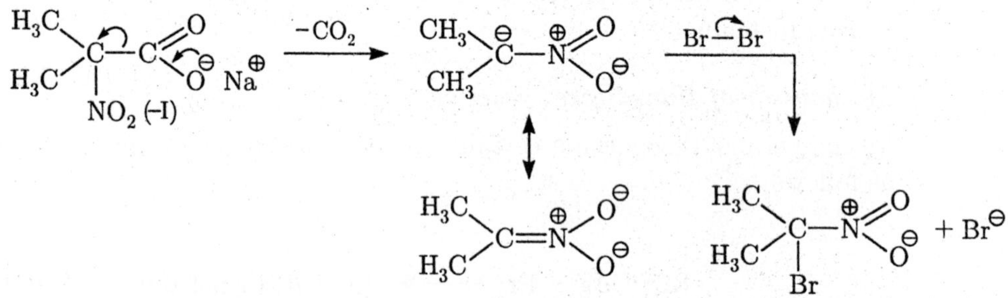

When sodio salts of carboxylic acids are heated with sodalime, we get an alkane.

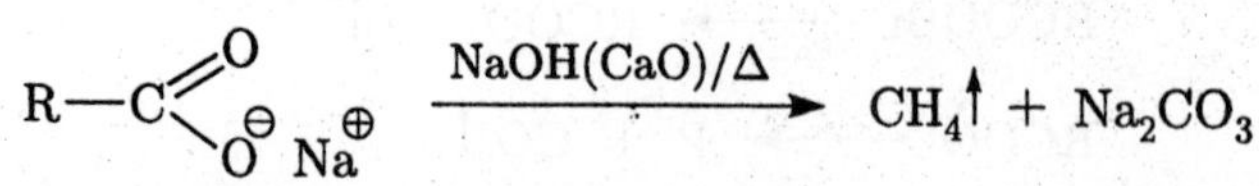

2. Hundsdiecker Reaction : Silver salts of carboxylic acids in dry carbon tetrachloride (CCl_4) solution are decomposed by Br_2 (preferably) or chlorine to form alkyl halide alongwith decarboxylation.

$$RCOOAg + Br_2 \longrightarrow RBr + CO_2 + AgBr\downarrow$$

There are certain types of carboxylic acids which are readily decarboxylated. Among these are,

(i) β-keto acids.

(ii) Malonic acid derivatives

(iii) Carbonic acid derivatives.

3. a. Decarboxylation of β-keto acids : β-keto acids decarboxylate readily at room temperature in acidic medium. The rate being 50 times more compared to that in basic medium.

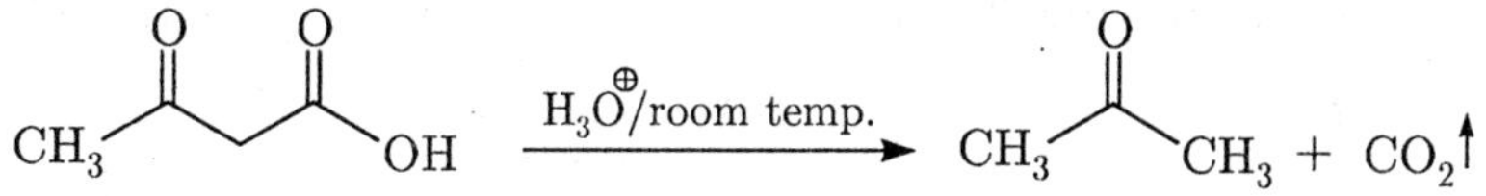

Decarboxylation of a β-keto acid involves an enol intermediate that is formed by an internal proton (H^+) transfer from the carboxylic acid group to the carbonyl oxygen atom of the ketone. The enol is transferred spontaneously to the corresponding ketone. The reaction is believed to proceed through a six-membered cyclic transition state.

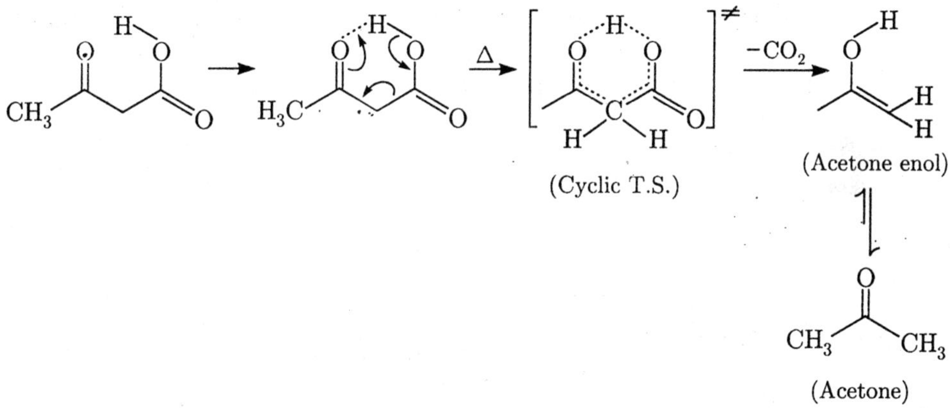

b. ***Decarboxylation of malonic acids*** :

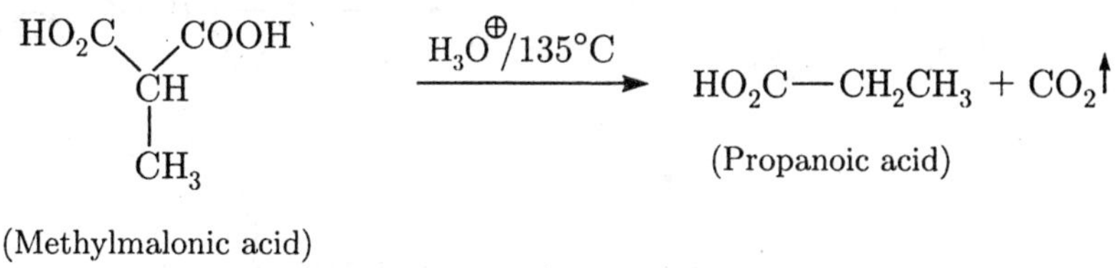

Decarboxylation of malonic acid or its derivatives do not occur in bases and proceeds through a similar six-centred cyclic transition state as we find in case of β-keto acids. Malonic acid contains its carboxyl C=O group β to $-CO_2H$ group and carbonyl group is present β to $-CO_2H$ group in case of β-keto acids.

$$HO-\underset{\beta}{\overset{\overset{\displaystyle O}{\|}}{C}}-CH_2COOH \qquad\qquad R-\underset{\beta}{\overset{\overset{\displaystyle O}{\|}}{C}}-CH_2COOH$$

(Malonic acid) (β-Keto acid)

Decarboxylation of malonic acid and its derivatives require heating and so the acids themselves can be isolated at room temperature.

4. Glycidic acid undergoes decarboxylation when warmed with dilute acid.

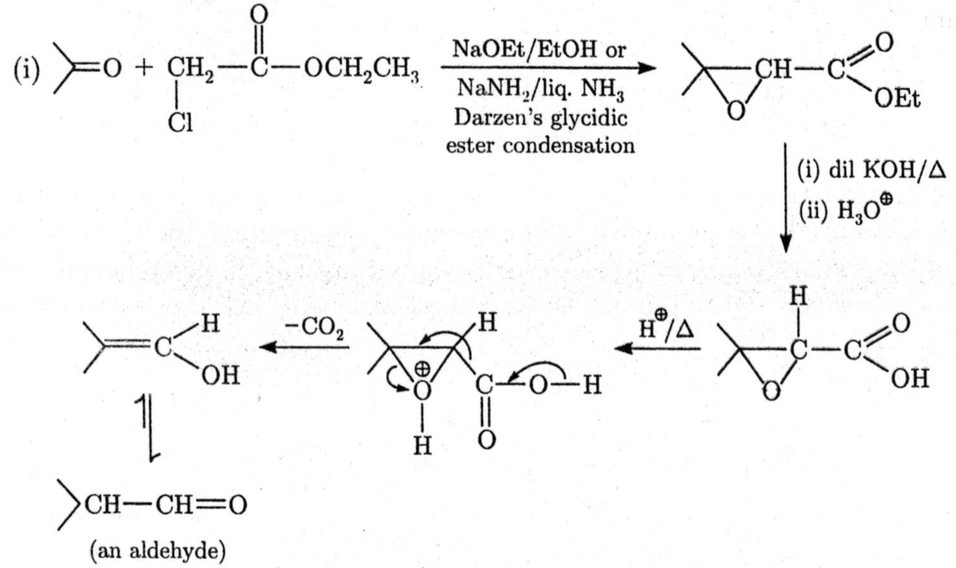

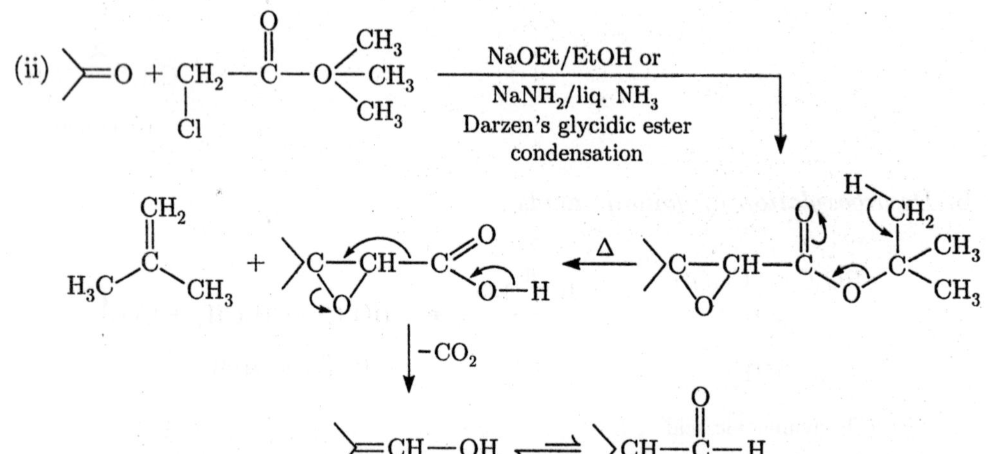

5. Kolbe's electrolytic method for decarboxylation of carboxylic acids

$$2RCOOK + 2H_2O \xrightarrow{\text{electrolysis}} R{-}R + 2CO_2\uparrow + 2KOH + H_2\uparrow$$

6. Carbonic acid is unstable and decarboxylates spontaneously in acidic solution to CO_2 and H_2O.

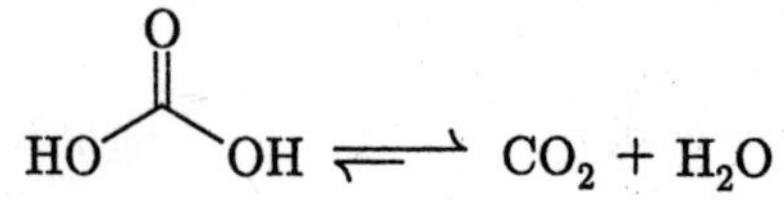

Similarly, any carbonic acid derivative with a free carboxylic acid group will also decarboxylate under acidic conditions.

(i) 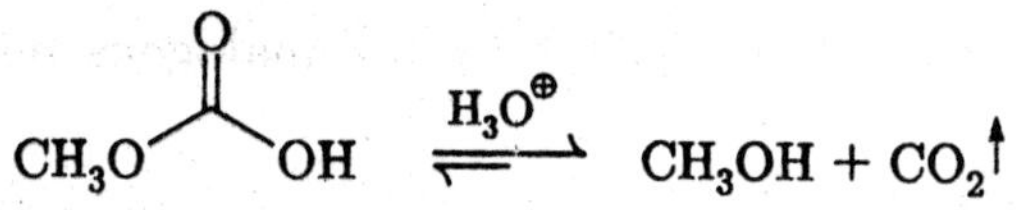

(Methyl carbonate)

(ii) 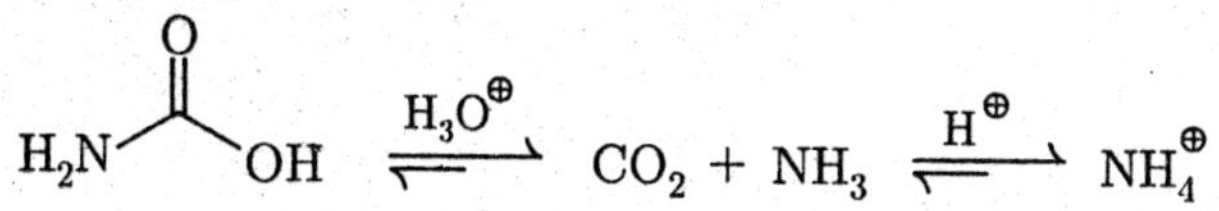

(Carbamic acid)

Under basic conditions carbonic acid and its derivatives exist as carboxylate salts and do not decarboxylate. For example, sodium salts of carbonic acids such as $NaHCO_3$ or Na_2CO_3 are familiar stable compounds.

Carbonic acid diesters and diamides are stable. Dimethyl carbonate (a diester of carbonic acid) and urea (diamide of carbonic acid) are examples of such stable compounds.

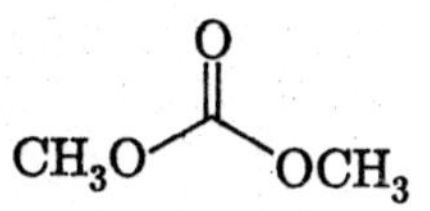

(Dimethyl carbonate)

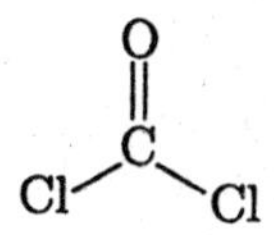

(Phosgene)

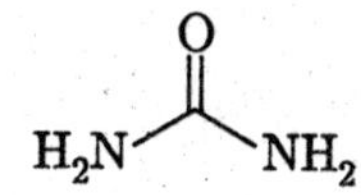

(Urea)

Decarboxylation of carbonic acids proceeds via a carbanion intermediate.

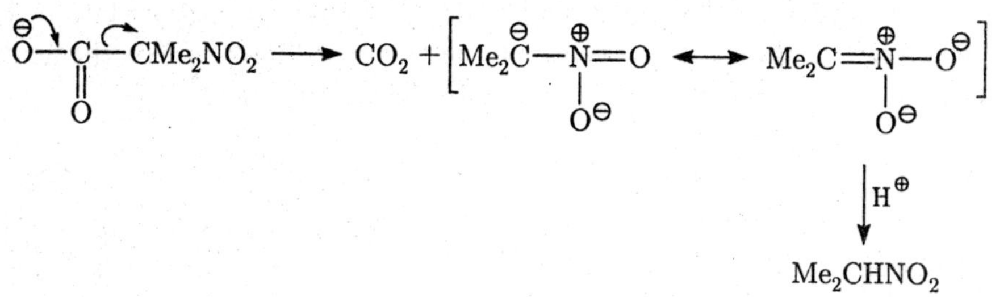

Evidence that carbanion intermediates are involved are provided by carrying out the decarboxylation in the presence of bromine. This is without effect on the overall rate of the reaction but the end product is now $Me_2C(Br)NO_2$ rather than Me_2CHNO_2— under the conditions where neither $Me_2C(NO_2)COO^{\ominus}$ nor Me_2CHNO_2 undergoes bromination. The bromo product arises from rapid attack of Br_2 on the carbanion intermediate which is thereby trapped.

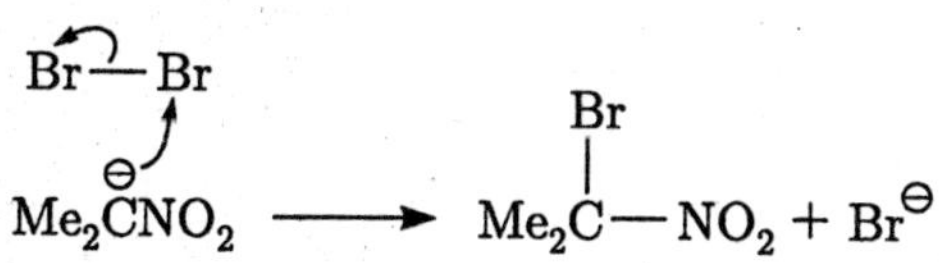

β,γ unsaturated acids probably also decarboxylates by an analogous pathway as shown for β-keto acids.

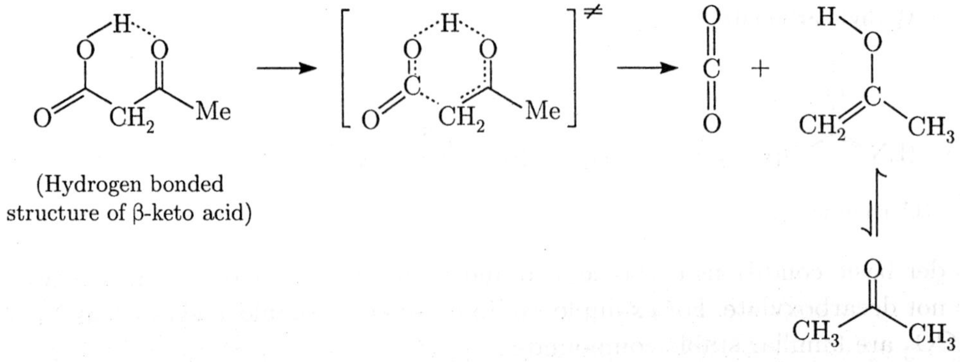

(Hydrogen bonded structure of β-keto acid)

Rate=k[keto acid]

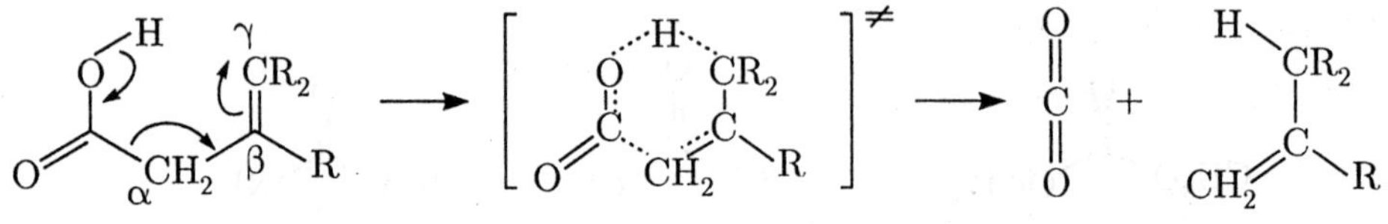

α, β-Unsaturated acids $R_2CH(R){=}CHCO_2H$ probably decarboxylates by this pathway also, as it has been shown that they isomerise to coresponding β,γ-unsaturated acid prior to decarboxylation.

7. Another example in which free acid undergoes ready decarboxylation, but this time via a carbanion intermediate (actually an ylid) is pyridine-2-carboxylic acid, which is decarboxylated very much more readily than its 3- or 4-isomers.

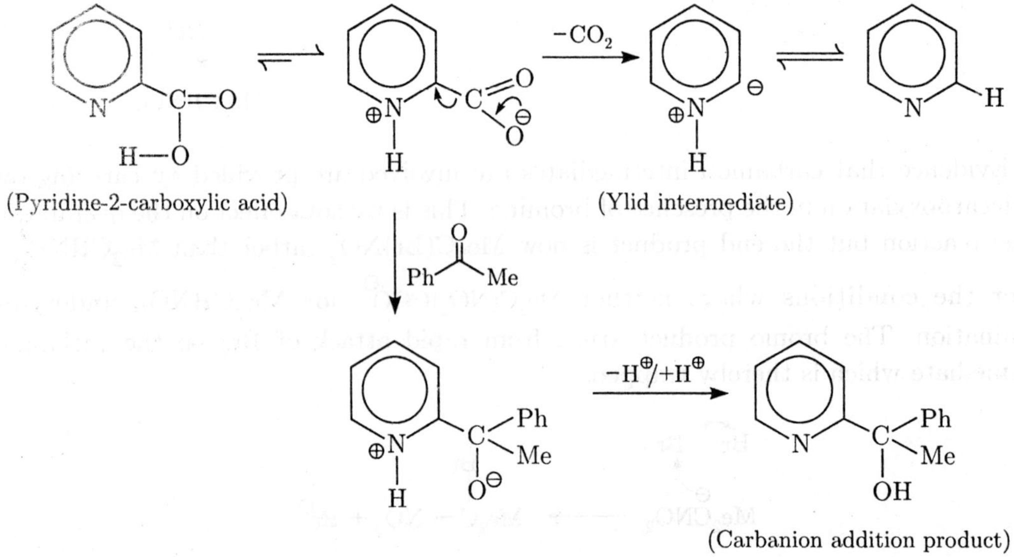

(Pyridine-2-carboxylic acid) (Ylid intermediate)

(Carbanion addition product)

The ylid intermediate can be trapped by carrying out decarboxylation in the presence of carbonyl compounds, *e.g.*, PhCOMe, to yield the carbanion addition product. The reason for the much easier decarboxylation of pyridine-2-carboxylic acid than of its 3-and 4- isomers, is the stabilisation that the positively charged nitrogen ($\overset{\oplus}{N}$) can effect on the adjacent carbanion carbon atom in the intermediate ylid.

8. Aromatic carboxylic acids can be decarboxylated by converting them to a cuprous salt and then heating the salt with quinoline in an inert atmosphere in the presence of cuprous oxide.

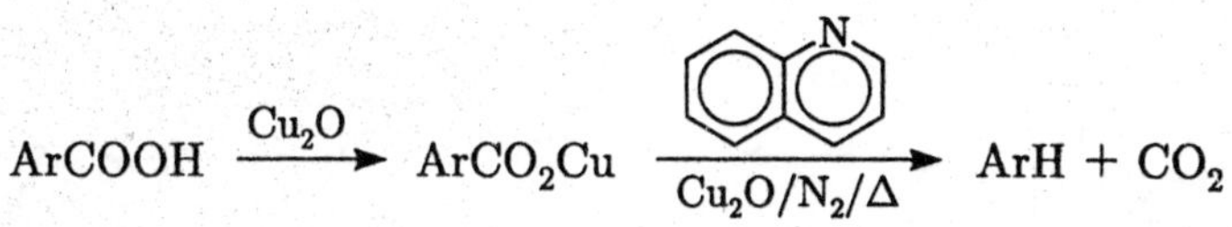

9. ***Decarboxylation of carboxyl radicals*** : Although the carboxylate ions ($RCOO^{\ominus}$) of simple aliphatic acids do not decarboxylate readily, carboxyl radicals ($RCOO^{\bullet}$) do. They decarboxylate by losing CO_2 and producing alkyl radicals.

$$RCO\dot{O} \longrightarrow \dot{R} + CO_2\uparrow$$

Examples :

1. ***Amine catalysed decarboxylation***

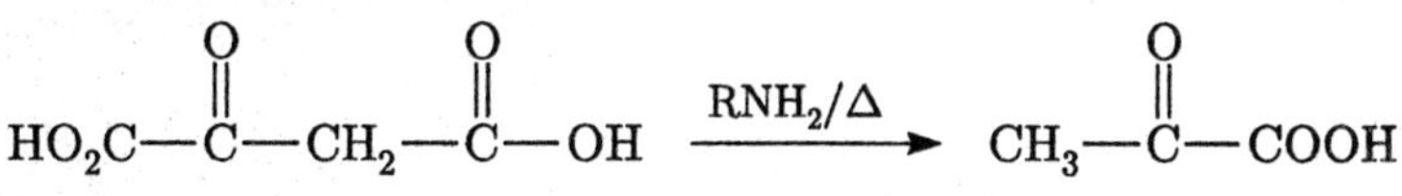

(Oxalacetic acid)

Mechanism :

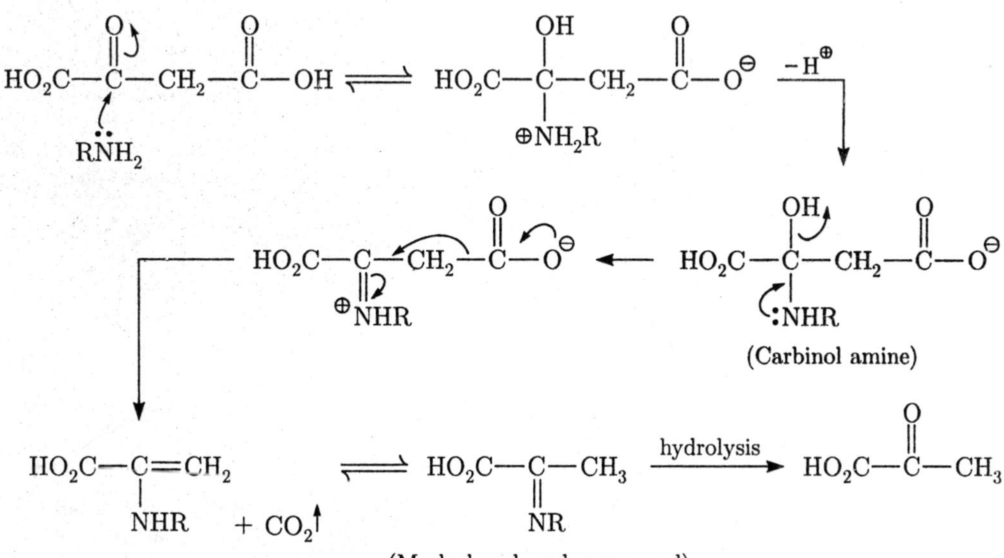

2. ***Decarboxylation under non-hydrolytic conditions***

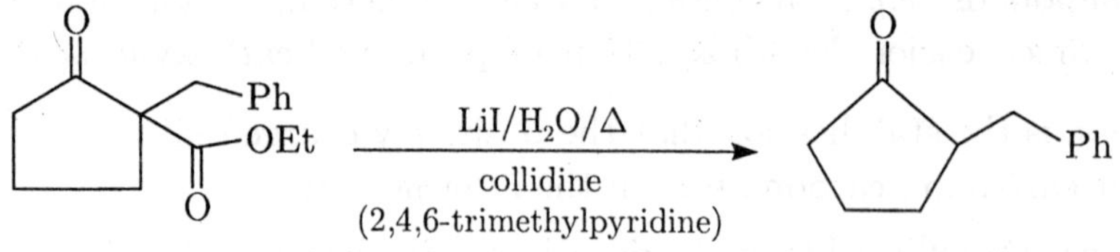

Mechanism :

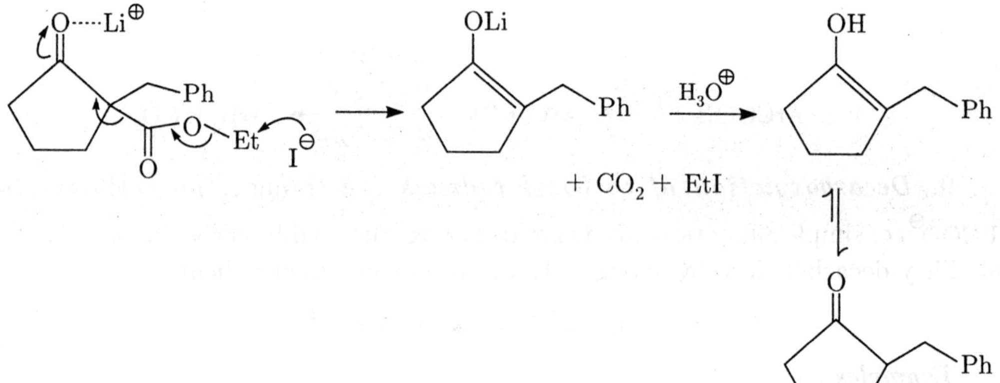

3. The following undergoes decarboxylation with extreme difficulty.

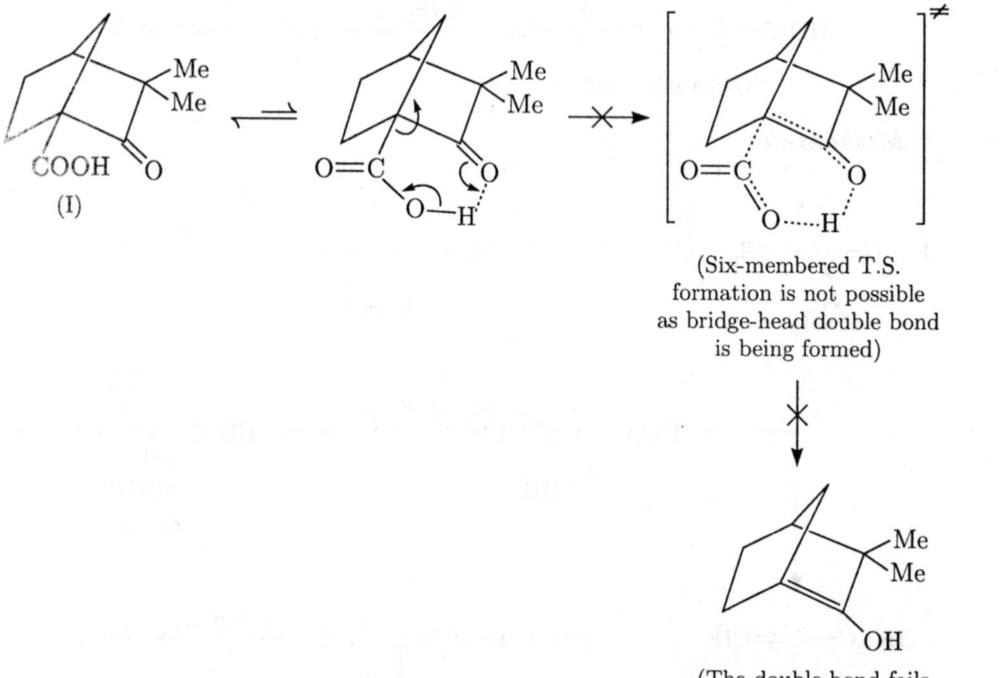

(Six-membered T.S. formation is not possible as bridge-head double bond is being formed)

(The double bond fails to attain coplanarity with the ring)

But the following silver salts (II and III) having bridge-head carboxylate groups readily undergo Hunsdiecker reaction (*i.e.*, decarboxylation reaction)

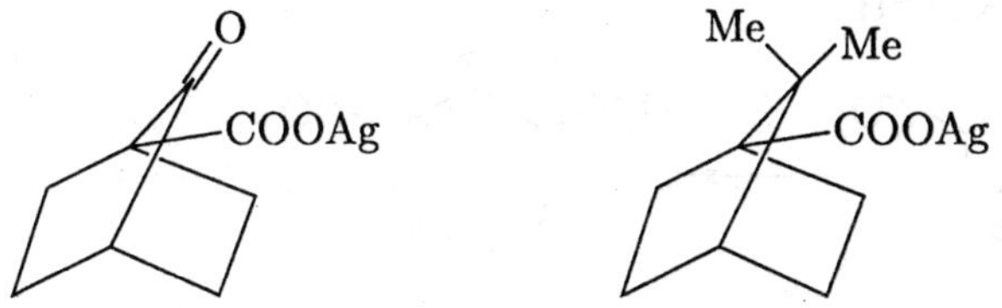

(II) (III)

From the mechanism of Hunsdiecker reaction, an intermediate 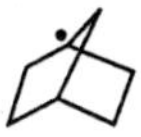 is formed where the single electron resides at the bridge-head carbon. So we may conclude that coplanarity of the bonds to a *tervalent carbon atom* is a far less compelling requirement for free radicals than for carbonium ions.

4. 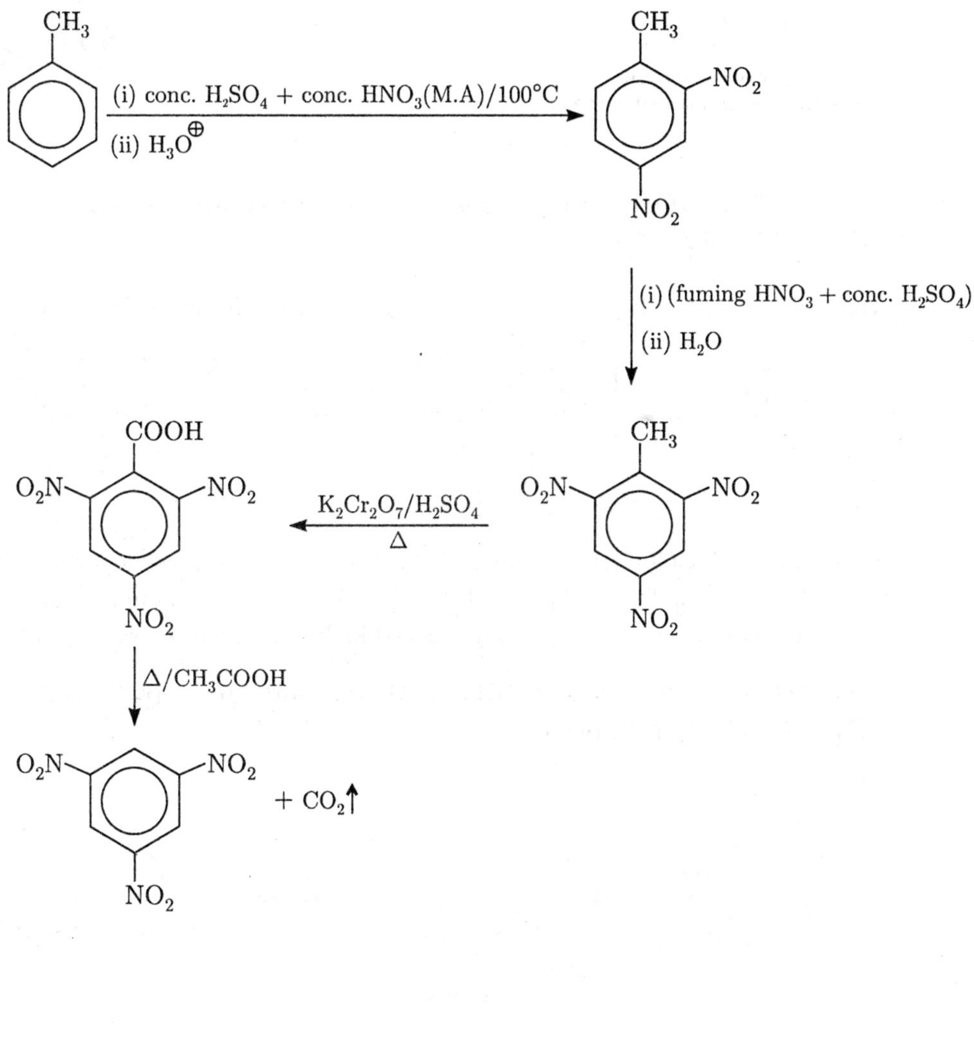

Mechanism of decarboxylation

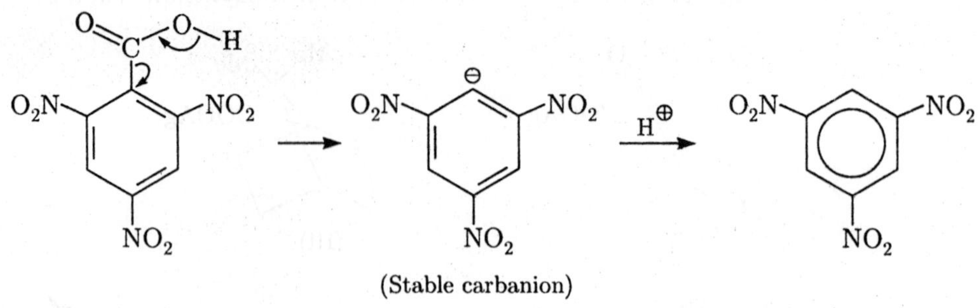

5. 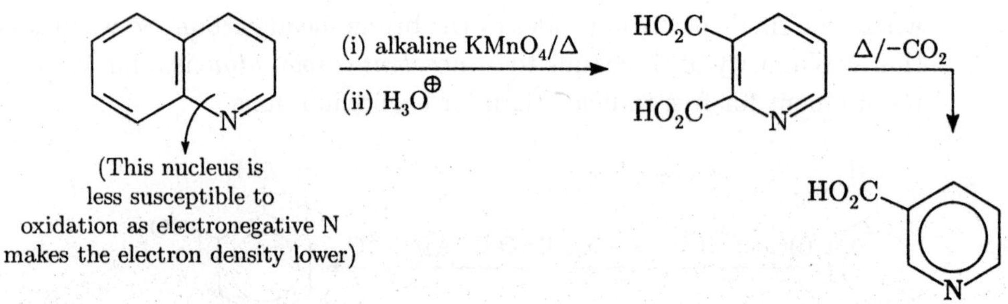

6. CH_3COCH_2COOH undergoes decarboxylation easily but not $CH_3COCH_2CH_2COOH$.

Ans. : A β-keto acid undergoes decarboxylation in the following way.

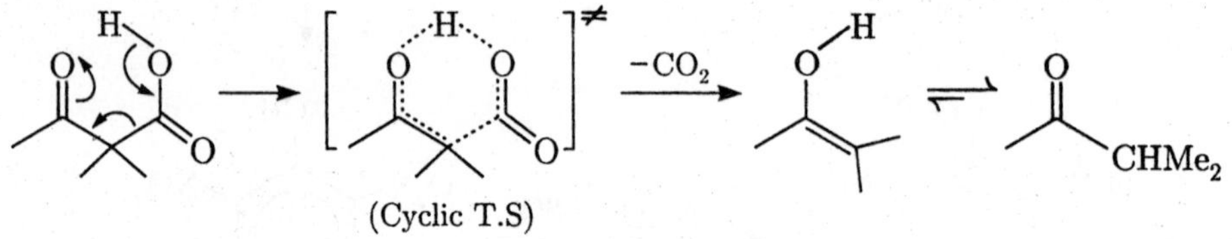

Now CH_3COCH_2COOH is a β-keto acid and so it undergoes decarboxylation to yield CH_3COCH_3. But $CH_3COCH_2CH_2COOH$ is a γ-keto acid, where the above mechanism of decarboxylation is not possible due to one intervening $-CH_2$-group.

7. CF_3COCH_2COOH can be distilled without decomposition but not CH_3COCH_2COOH. Explain.

Ans. :

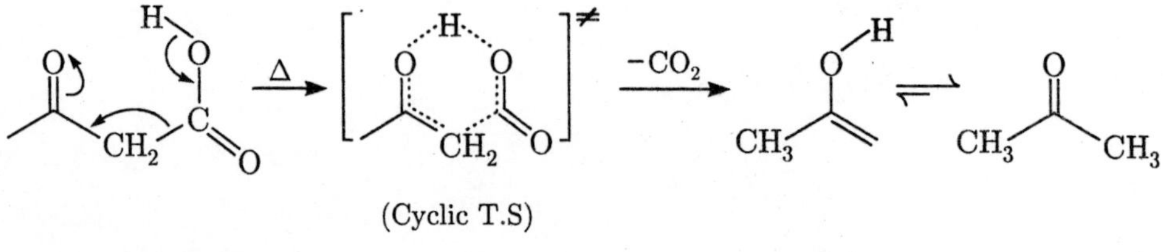

But when CH_3 is replaced by CF_3 group, the normal polarisation of $>$=O group (*i.e.* $>$=O) is not possible as $-CF_3$ group has strong –I effect. So CF_3COCH_2COOH doen not undergo decarboxylation during distillation.

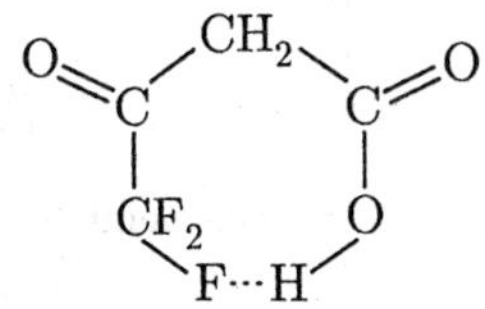

(Very strong hydrogen bonding inhibits decarboxylation)

8. 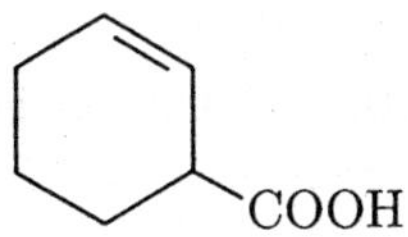 does not decarboxylate but 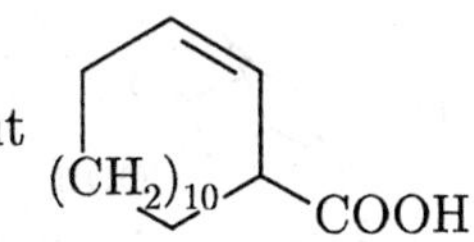 does.

Ans. : The mechanism of β,γ-unsaturated acid is as follows.

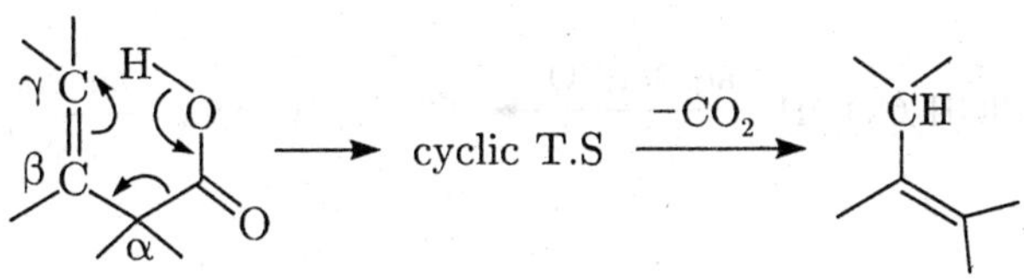

α,β,γ carbons are the units of a ring for the formation of six membered cyclic transition state which is not attainable by a smaller ring but can be easily attained by a larger ring. Thus, 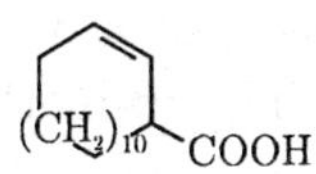 undergoes easy decarboxylation but 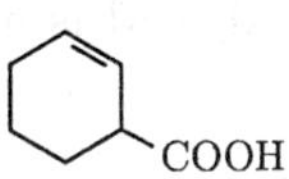 can not.

9. Of the following two compounds 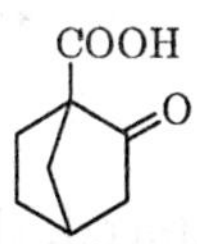 (A) and 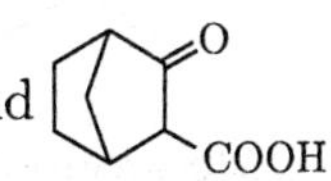 (B); (B) undergoes decarboxylation easily but not (A). Why?

Ans.:

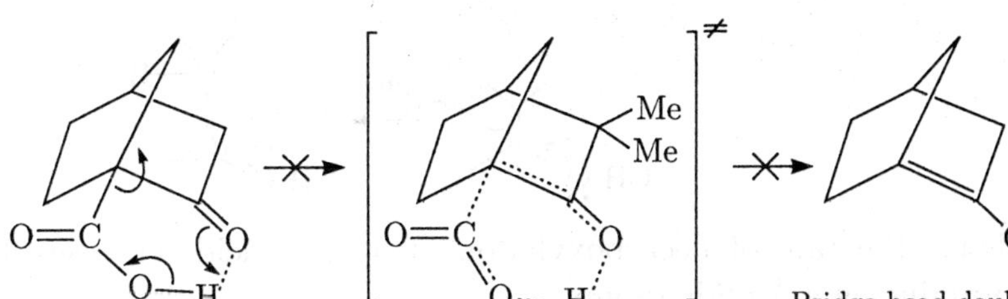

(A)

Bridge head double bond (nceds planarity at the bridge head which violates Bredt's rule)

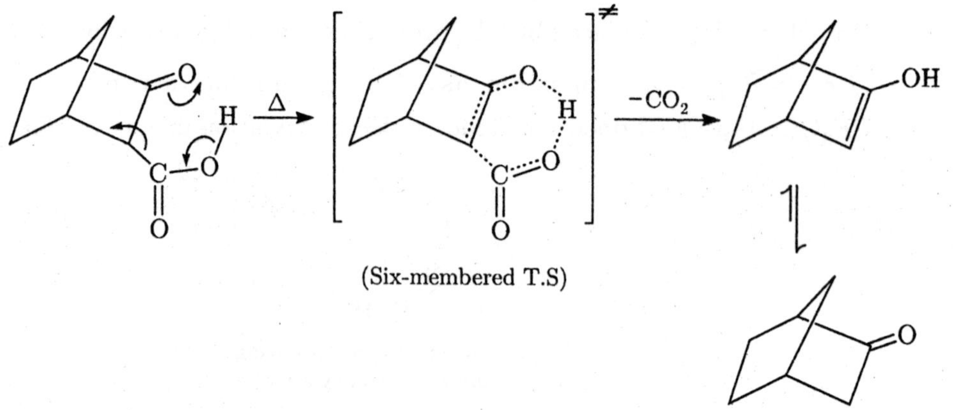

(Six-membered T.S)

Molecule (B), 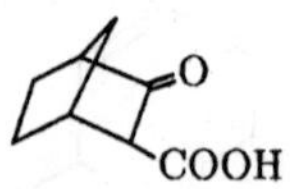 does not involve any double bond at the bridge head position, so it can undergo decarboxylation smoothly.

10. Conversion of $ClCH_2COOH$ to CH_3NO_2.

Ans. : $ClCH_2COOH \xrightarrow{\text{aq. } Na_2CO_3} ClCH_2COONa \xrightarrow[S_N2]{\text{aq. } NaNO_2} O_2NCH_2COONa \xrightarrow{H_3O^{\oplus}} [O_2N—CH_2COOH] \xrightarrow{-CO_2} CH_3NO_2$

11. The rate of decarboxylation of a β, γ-unsaturated acid was increased about 10^5–10^6 times by introducing a β-methoxy group. Explain

Ans. : Mechanism of decarboxylation of β,γ– unsaturated acid is as follows.

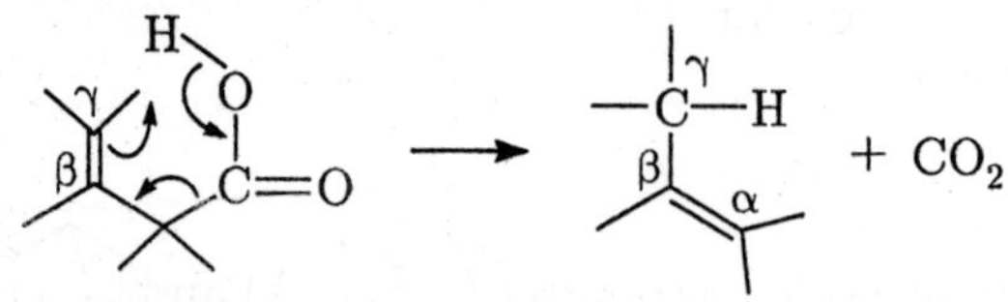

When the β-OMe group is introduced, the unsaturated part behaves like a vinyl ether which is succeptible to be attacked by a proton.

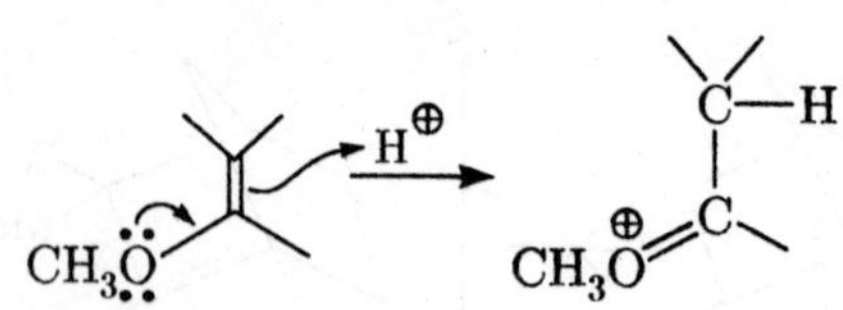

Thus, the rate of decarboxylation of a β,γ– acid increases 10^5–10^6 fold by introducing a β–OMe group.

12. $RCH_2CH{=}CHCOOH$ undergoes decarboxylation on heating but not $R_3CH{=}CHCOOH$. Why?

Ans. : An α, β-unsaturated acid undergoes decarboxylation *via* an intermediate which isomerises to β,γ– unsaturated acid.

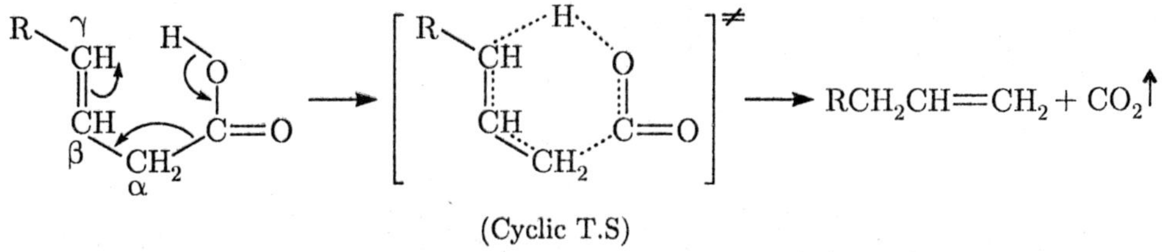

With acids like $R_3CH{=}CHCOOH$, the isomerisation to a β,γ-unsaturated acid system is not possible and thus, it does not undergo decarboxylation.

13. Complete and explain.

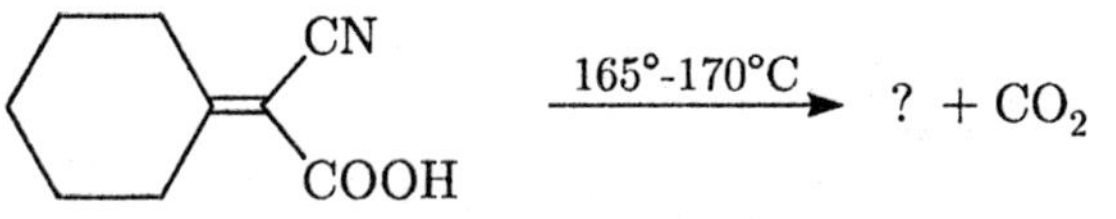

Ans. :

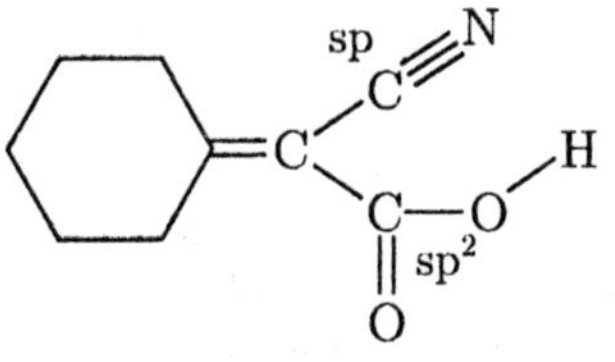

Carbon of C≡N group is sp hybridised and that of C=O is sp^2 hybridised. Thus, decarboxylation via six membered cyclic transition state becomes difficult with the involvement of CN group. So the molecule undergoes decarboxylation through a β,γ-unsatured acid.

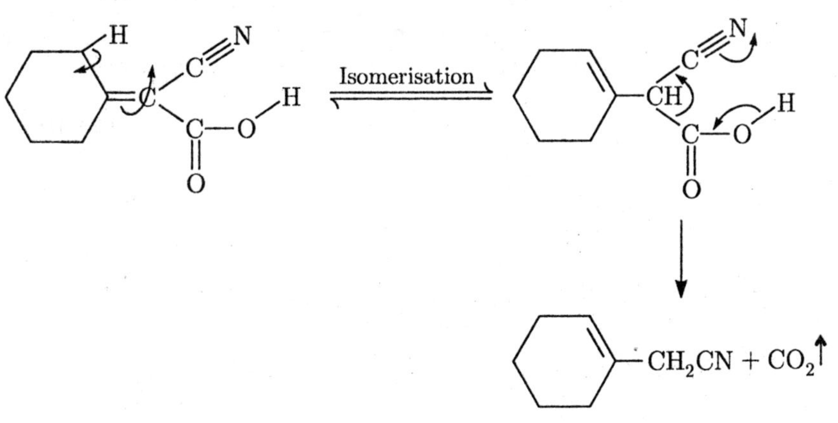

14. Explain the following observation.

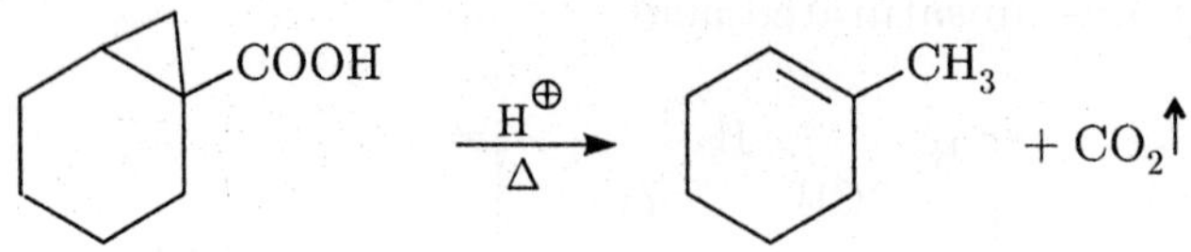

Ans. :

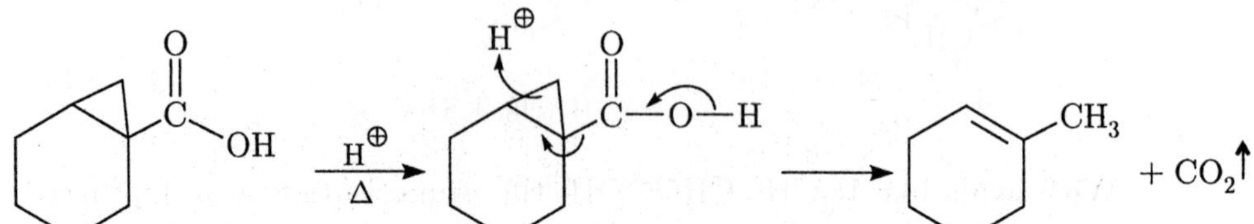

C—C bond of cyclopropane ring has some π-character and so it is protonated and we get the product.

5.

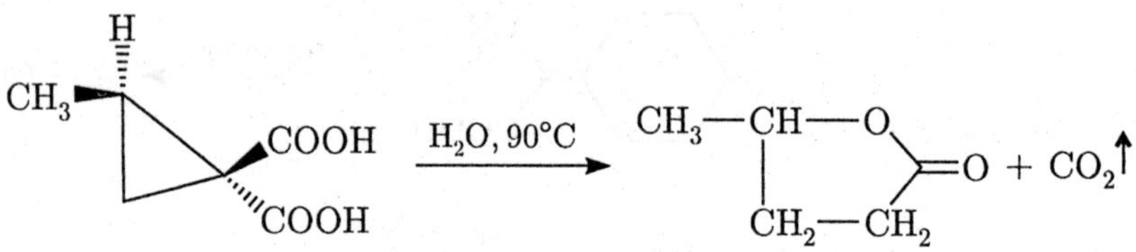

Ans. :

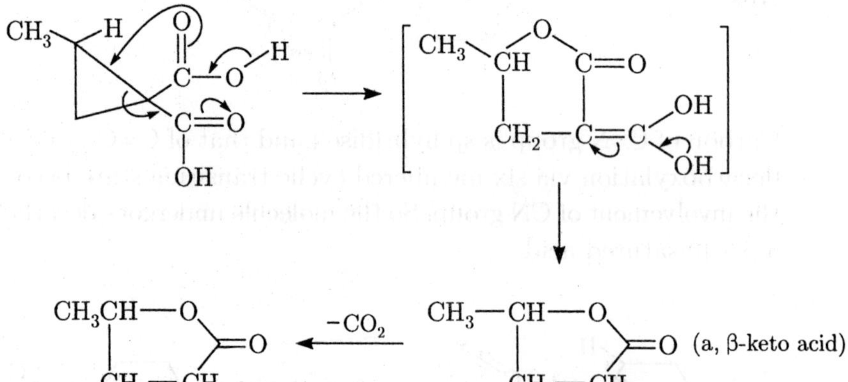

16.

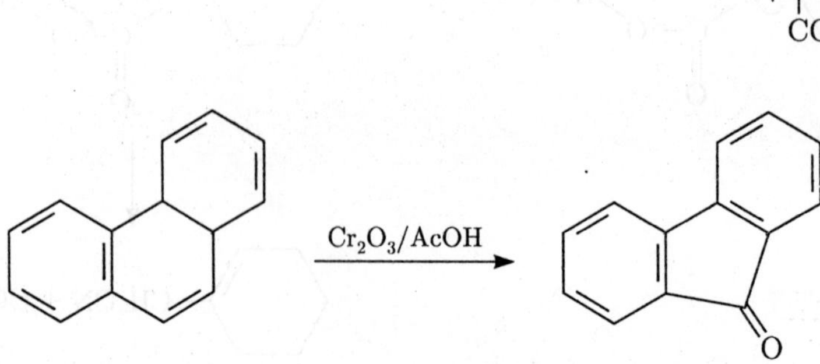

(Phenanthrene) (Fluorenone)

Ans. :

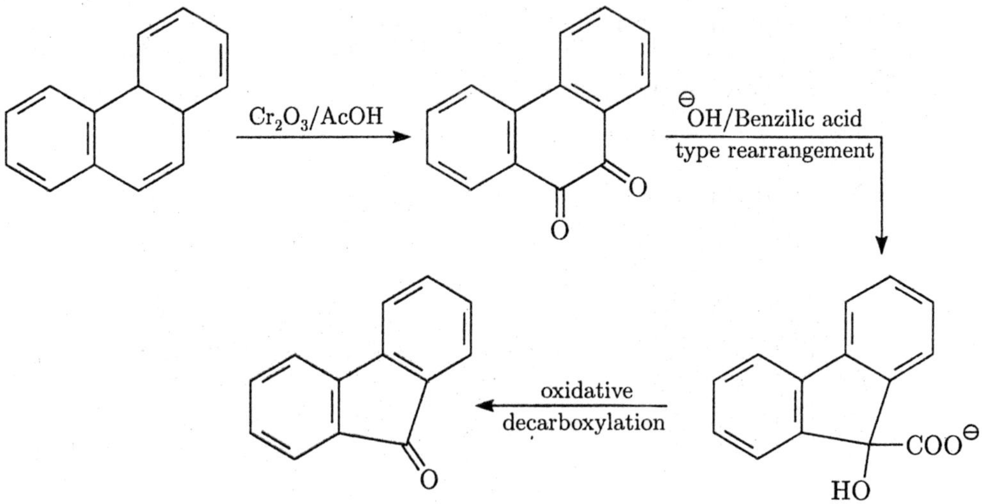

(Fluorenone)

17. Explain mechanistically the following reaction.

Ans. :

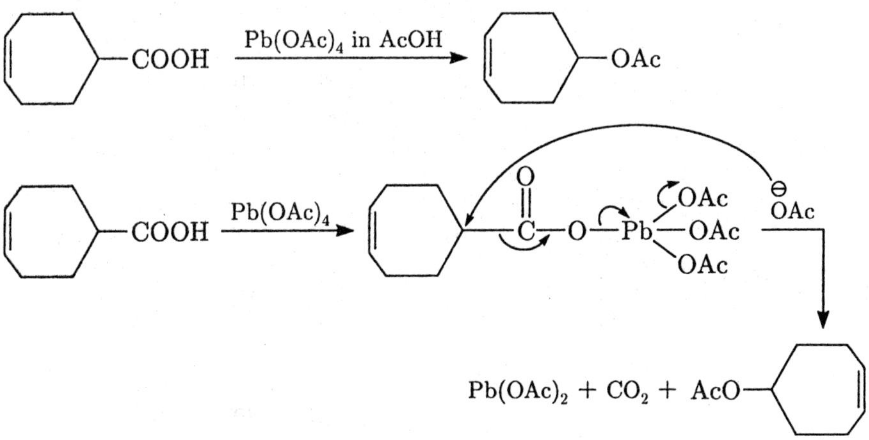

Such decarboxylation is retarded by oxygen and catalysed by Cu(II) salts. Thus, the mechanism of the reaction is believed to proceed as follows.

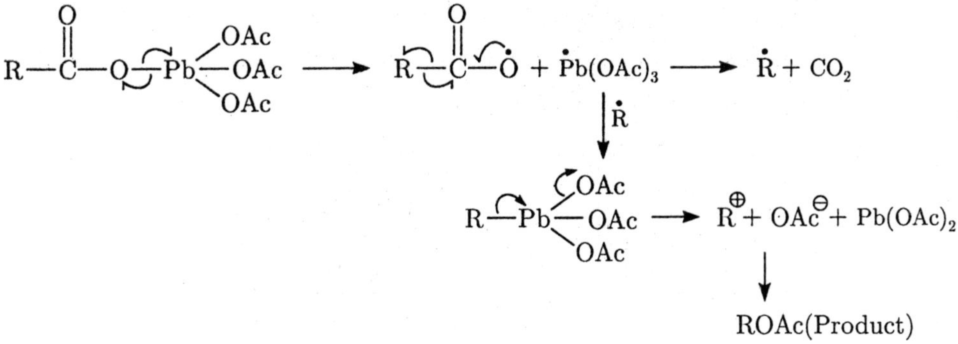

18. 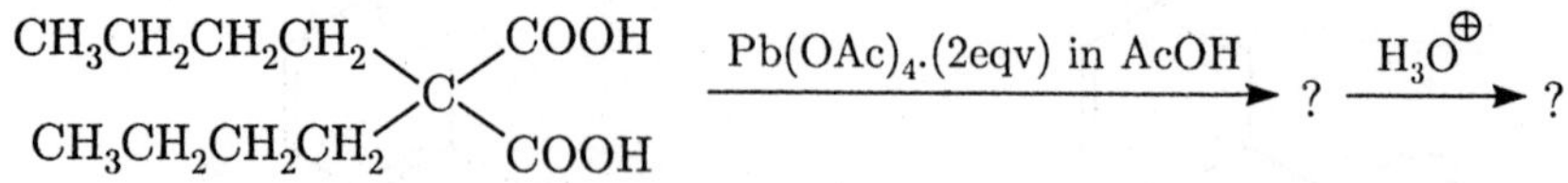

Ans. : 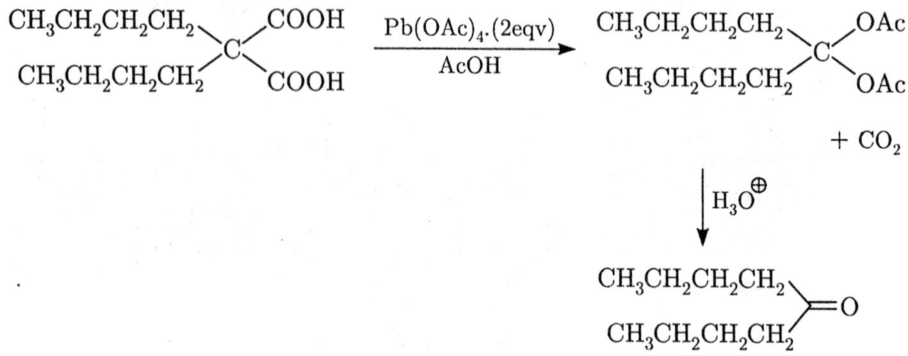

19. Complete the following reaction.

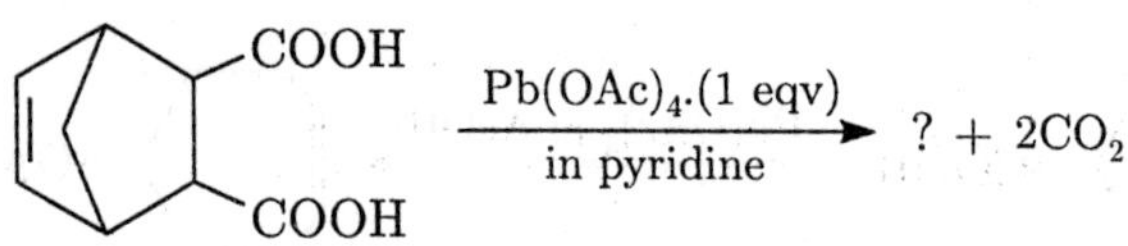

Ans. : 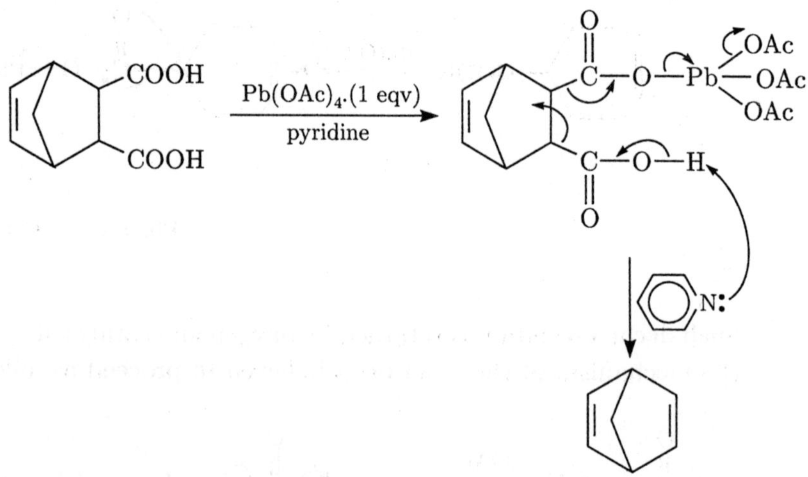

(Product)

20. Explain mechanistically the following reaction.

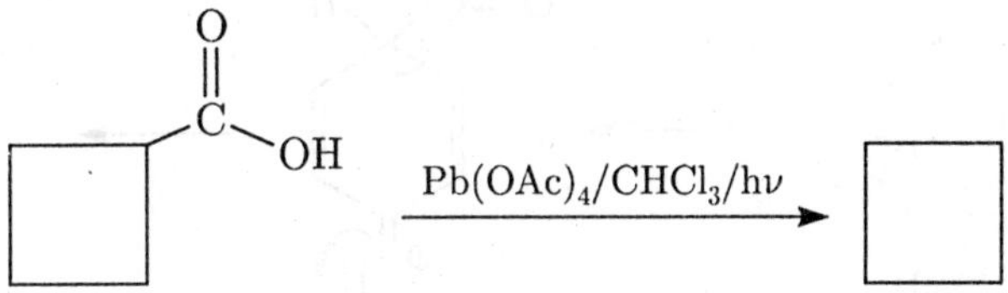

Ans.:

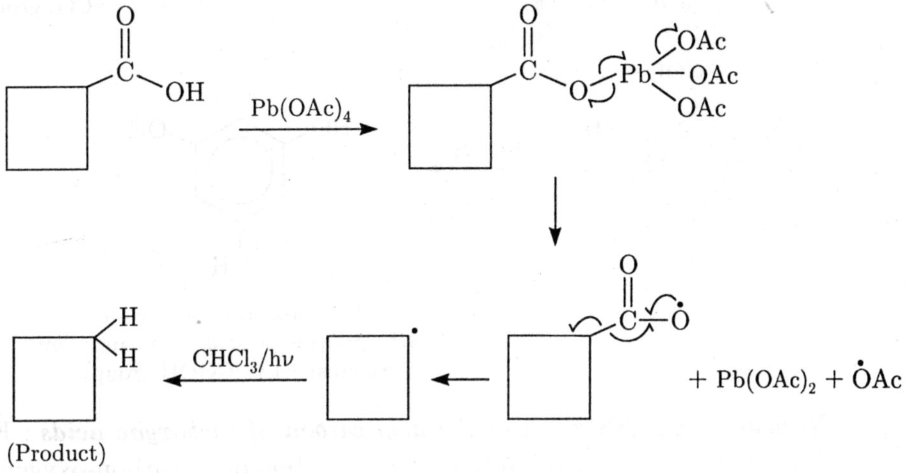

21. 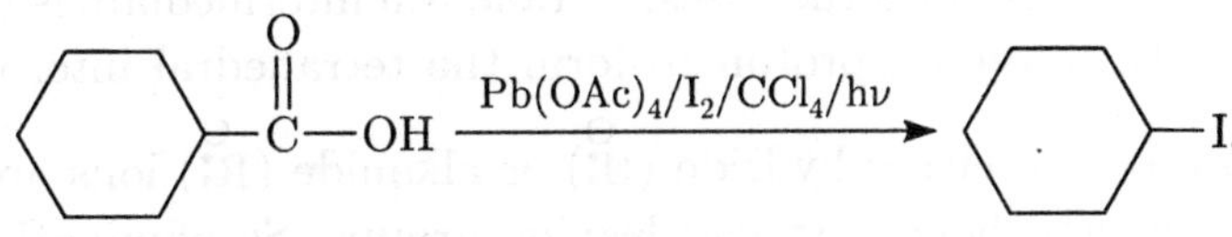 Explain with mechanism.

Ans. :

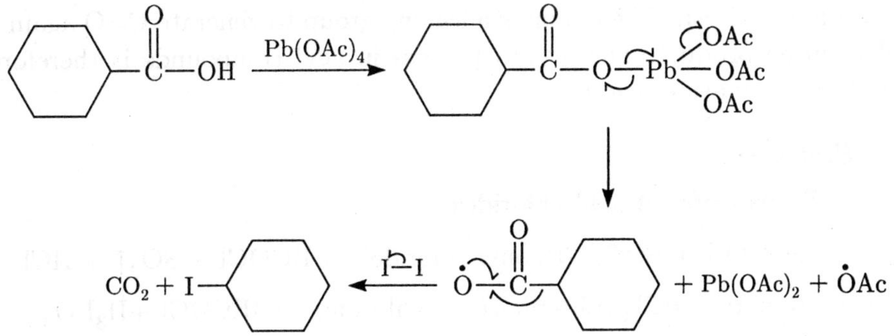

22. 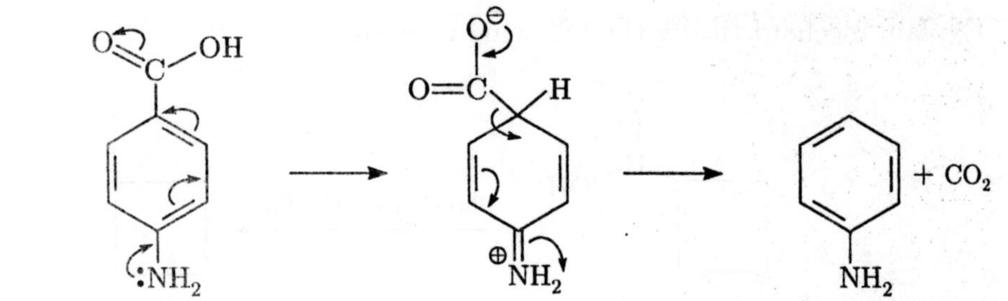

(–NH_2 may be replaced by –OH group which also activates the benzene ring)

(–NH_2 or –OH should be present *ortho* or *para* with respect to –CO_2 group)

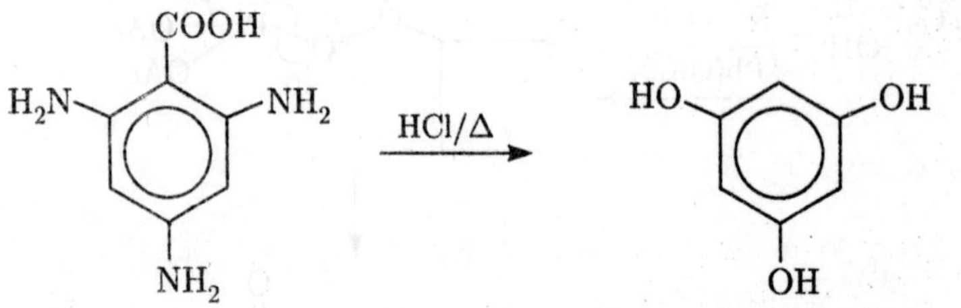

(Decarboxylation occurs as –NH_2 group is present *ortho* and *para* withrespect to COOH group)

e. ***Nucleophilic substitution at the acyl carbon of carboxylic acids*** : For aldehydes and ketones, nucleophilic addition to carbonyl carbon or to carbon-oxygen double bond is a characteristic reaction. For carboxylic acids, a nucleophilic addition elimination reaction is done at the acyl carbon. In both the cases, tetrahedral intermediate is formed. Aldehydes and ketones usually accepts a proton to form the tetrahedral intermediate and for elimination step to proceed, either hydride ($\overset{\ominus}{H:}$) or alkanide ($\overset{\ominus}{R:}$) ions are to be ejected which are strong bases and hence are bad leaving groups. So elimination step does not occur with aldehydes and ketones. In contrast, the intermediate formed from an acyl compound usually eliminates a leaving group to generate C=O again and leads to a substitution product. The overall process in acyl compounds is therefore nucleophilic addition-elimination reaction.

Examples :

1. Preparation of acid chlorides

(a) $RCOOH + SOCl_2$ (thionyl chloride) $\rightarrow RCOCl + SO_2\uparrow + HCl$

(b) $ROOH + PCl_3$ (phosphorus trichloride) $\rightarrow 3RCOCl + H_3PO_3$

(c) $RCOOH + PCl_5$ (phosphorus pentachloride) $\rightarrow RCOCl + POCl_3 + HCl$

Mechanism of acid chloride formation using thionyl chloride ($SOCl_2$) :

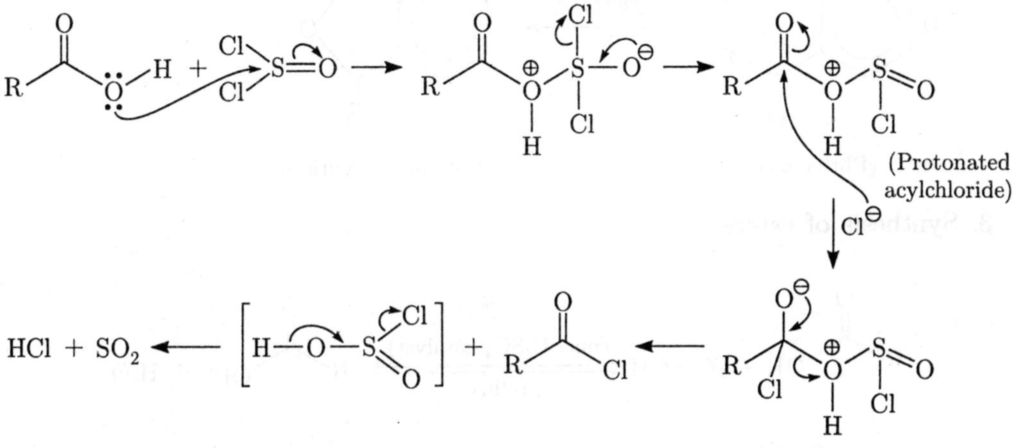

(Tetrahedral intermediate)

2. (a) 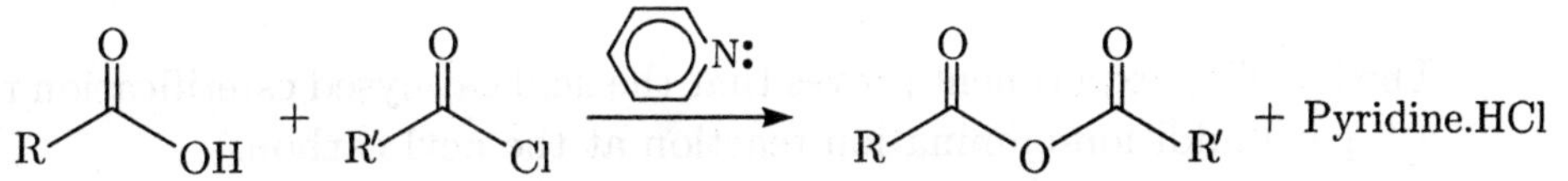

(R=R′ =simple anhydrides,
R≠R′=Mixed anhydride)

(b) 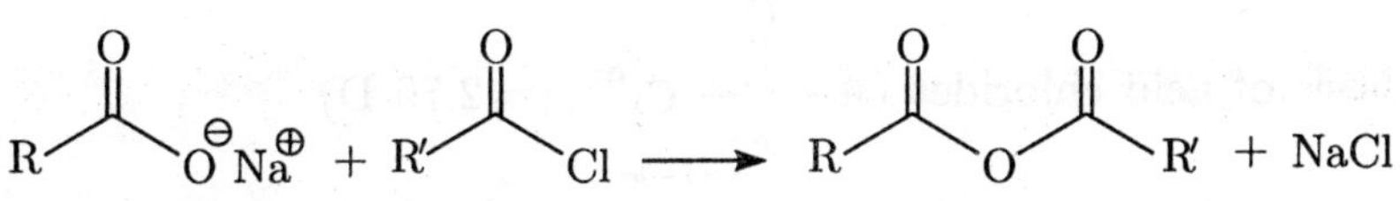

(Sodio salt of carboxylic acid) (Anhydride)

(c) 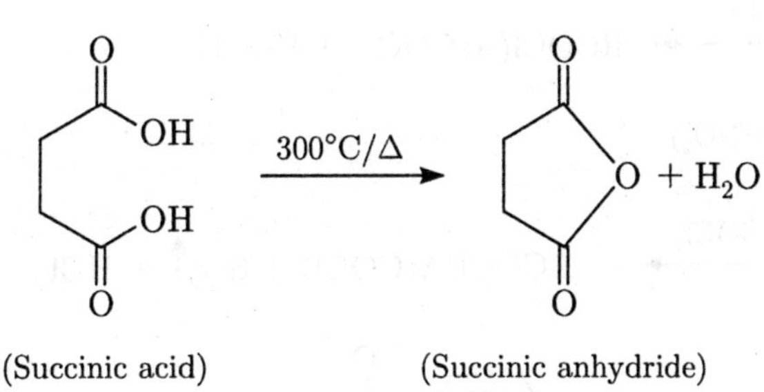

(Succinic acid) (Succinic anhydride)

(d) 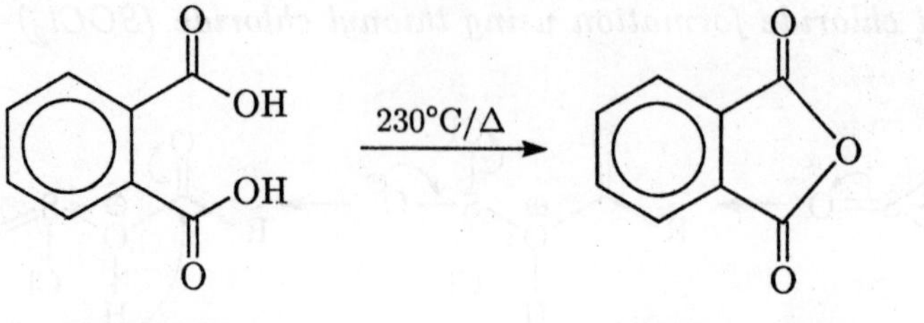

(Phthalic acid) (Phthalic anhydride)

3. Synthesis of esters

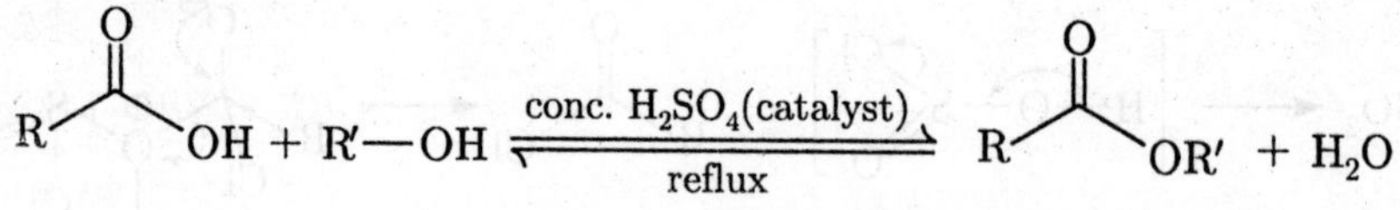

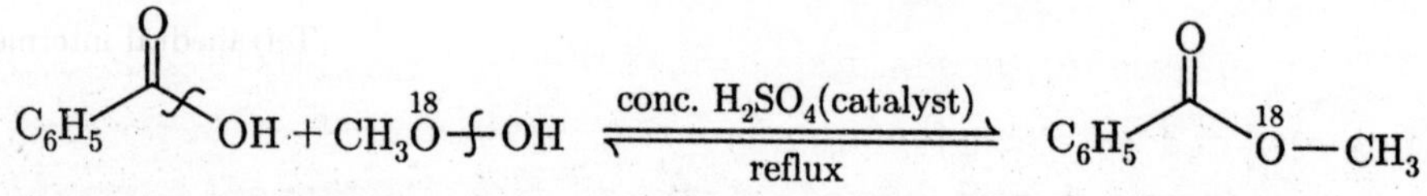

The labelling experiment proves that the acid catalysed esterification reaction is a typical addition-elimination reaction at the acyl carbon.

Synthesis of Carboxylic Acid Derivatives

1. Synthesis of acid chlorides $(R-\underset{\delta+}{\overset{O^{\delta-}}{\overset{\|}{C}}}-Cl^{\delta-}, \mu = 2.70\ D)$

(a) $RCOOH(ArCOOH) \xrightarrow{PCl_3} RCOCl(ArCOCl) + H_3PO_3$

(b) $RCOOH(ArCOOH) \xrightarrow{PCl_5} RCOCl(ArCOCl) + POCl_3$

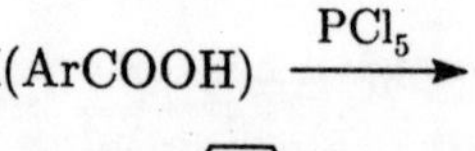

(c) $RCOOH(ArCOOH) \xrightarrow{SOCl_2} RCOCl(ArCOCl) + SO_2\uparrow + HCl$

(d) 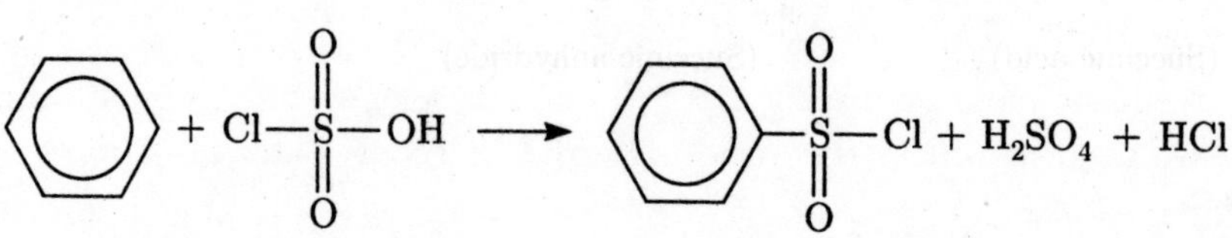

(Chlorosulphonic acid) (Benzenesulphonyl chloride)

Formation :

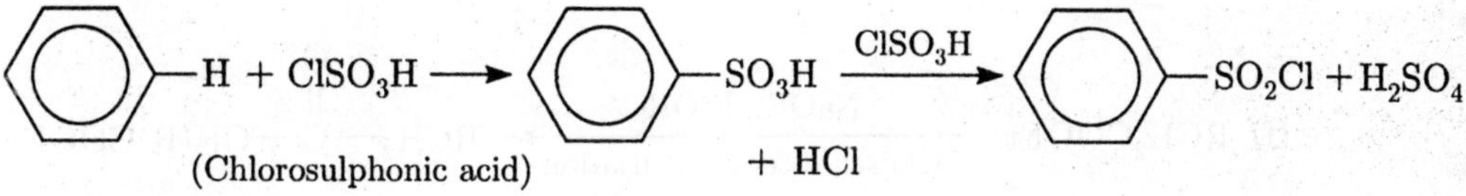

2. **Synthesis of esters**

(a) $RCOOH(ArCOOH) + R'OH \xrightleftharpoons{\text{conc. } H_2SO_4\text{(catalyst)}} R'COOR(ArCOOR') + H_2O$

Mechanism of acid catalysed esterification reaction :

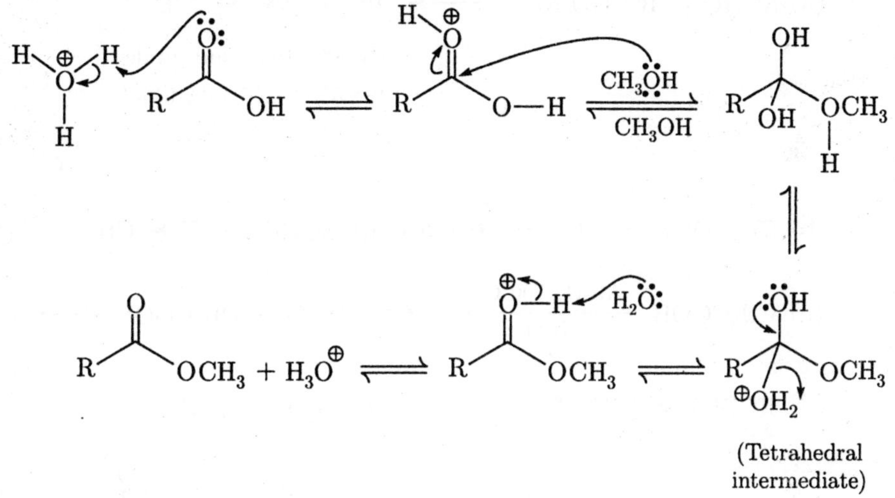

Acid catalysed esterification and hydrolysis of esters are *microscopically reversible* processes.

(b) $RCOCl(ArCOCl) + R'OH \longrightarrow RCOOR'(ArCOOR') + HCl$

(c) $(RCO_2)O + R'OH \longrightarrow RCOOR' + RCOOH$

(d) $RCOOAg(ArCOOAg) + R'Br \longrightarrow RCOOR'(ArCOOR') + AgBr\downarrow$

(e) $RCOOH(ArCOOH) \xrightarrow{CH_2N_2} RCOOCH_3(ArCOOCH_3) + N_2\uparrow$

(f) $R_2O + CO \xrightarrow{BF_3/Et_2O,\ 125°\text{–}180°C/500\ atm} RCOOR$

(g) $RCHO + Al(OEt)_3 \xrightarrow{\text{Tischenko reaction}} RCOOCH_2R$

(h) $RCOR \xrightarrow[\text{Bayer-Villiger oxidation}]{RCO_3H,\ \text{oxidation}} RCOOR$

(i) $RCH_2COOEt \xrightarrow[\text{Claisen ester condensation}]{NaOEt/EtOH} RCH_2-\overset{O}{\overset{\|}{C}}-CH(R)COOEt$

(j) $H_2C{=}C{=}O \xrightarrow{ROH} CH_3COOR$

Synthesis of anhydrides

1. (a) $RCOCl + R'COO^{\ominus}Na^{\oplus} \longrightarrow$ 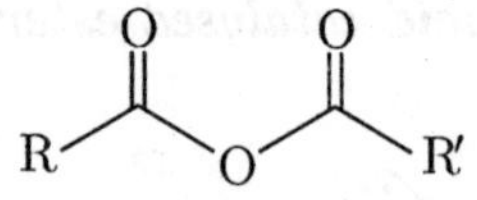

(R=R′ ≡simple anhydrides,
R≠R′ ≡Mixed anhydride)

(b) $CH_3COOH + C_2H_2 \xrightarrow{Hg^{2+}} CH_3CH(OCOCH_3)_2 \xrightarrow{\Delta}$ 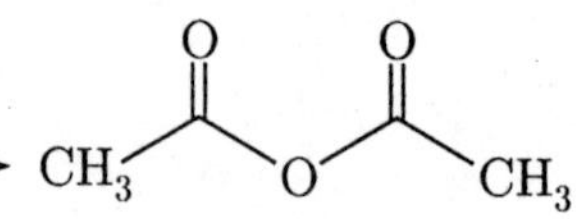

(c) $CH_3COOH \xrightarrow[-H_2O]{AlPO_4/700°C} H_2C{=}C{=}O + CH_3COOH \longrightarrow (CH_3CO)_2O$

(d) $RCOOH + (CH_3CO)_2O \longrightarrow (RCO)_2O + AcOH$

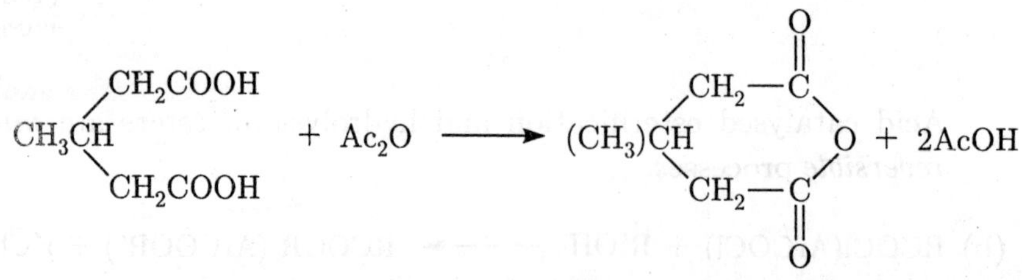

(β-Methylglutanic anhydride)

(e) $RCOCl + RCOOH \xrightarrow{\text{Pyridine}} (RCO)_2O + Py.HCl$

(f) (i) 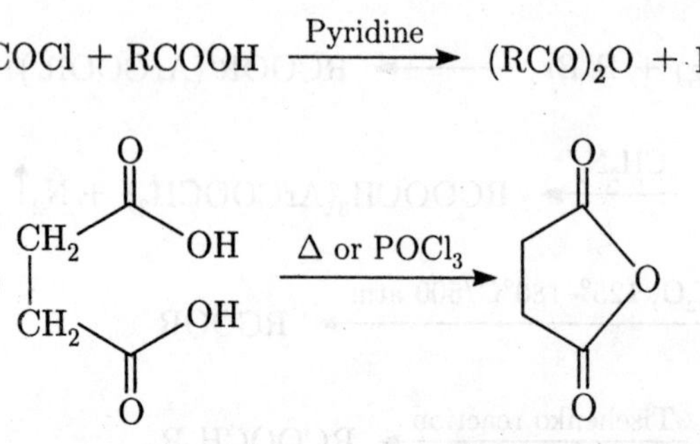

(Succinic anhydride)

(ii) 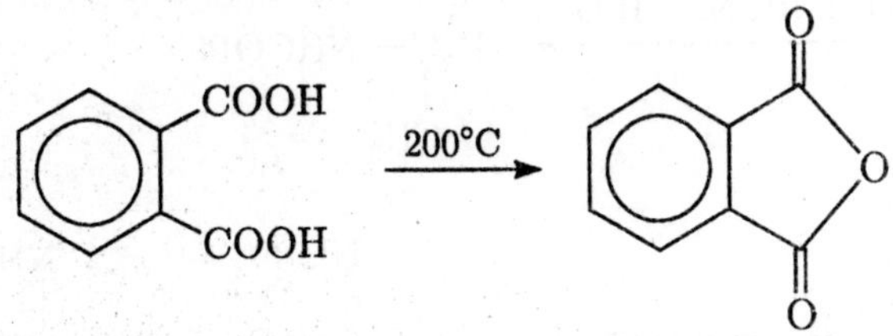

(Phthalic anhydride)

Ring size is crucial with adipic acid; no seven-membered ring is formed on anhydride formation, instead CO_2 is lost and a five-membered ring ketone is product.

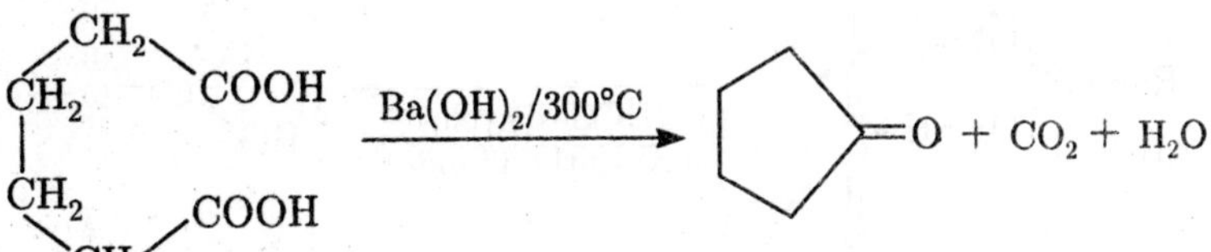

(Cyclopentanone)

(g) 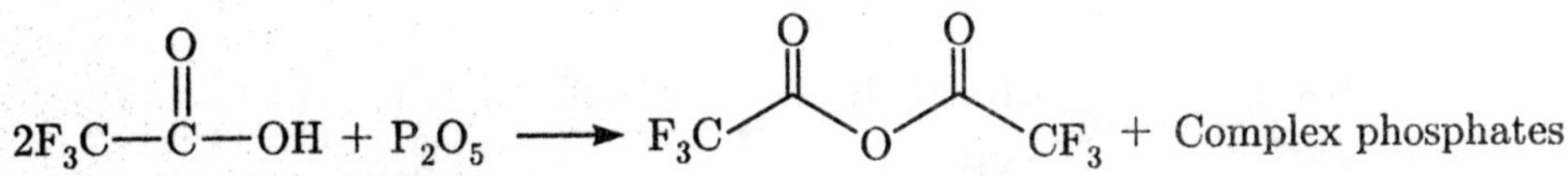

(Strong dehydrating agent)

Synthesis of Amides

1. (a) $RCOONH_4(ArCOONH_4) \xrightarrow{\Delta} RCONH_2(ArCONH_2) + NH_3$

(b) $RCOOR' \xrightarrow{NH_3} RCONH_2(ArCONH_2) + R'OH$

(c) $RCOCl(ArCOCl) \xrightarrow{NH_3} RCONH_2(ArCONH_2) + NH_4Cl$

(d) $(RCO)_2O/(ArCO)_2O \xrightarrow{NH_3} RCONH_2(ArCONH_2) + RCOOH(ArCOOH)$

(e) $RCN \xrightarrow{HCl/H_2O \text{ (controlled hydrolysis)}} RCONH_2$

(f) $RCOOH(ArCOOH) + O{=}C(NH_2)_2 \xrightarrow{\Delta} RCONH_2(ArCONH_2)$

(Urea)

(g) $R_2C{=}CH_2 \xrightarrow{1.\ H_2SO_4\ 2.\ R'CN,\ 3.\ H_2O} R_2C(CH_3){-}NHCOR'$

(h) $R_2C{=}CH_2 \xrightarrow[2.\ CO,\ 3.\ R'NH_2(NH_3)]{1.\ H_2SO_4} R{-}CH(CH_3){-}C(NHR'){=}O\ /\ (RCH(CH_3){-}C(NH_2){=}O)$

(i) ***Dicyclohexylcarbodiimide (DCC)- promoted Amide synthesis***

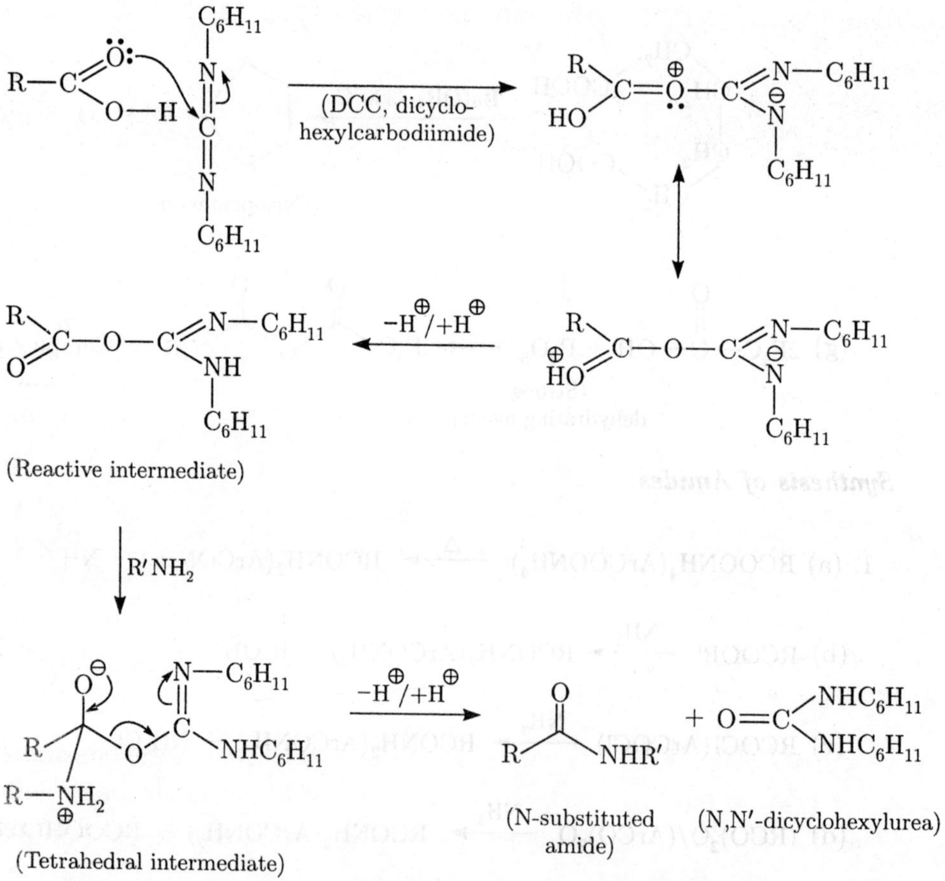

Synthesis of Imides :

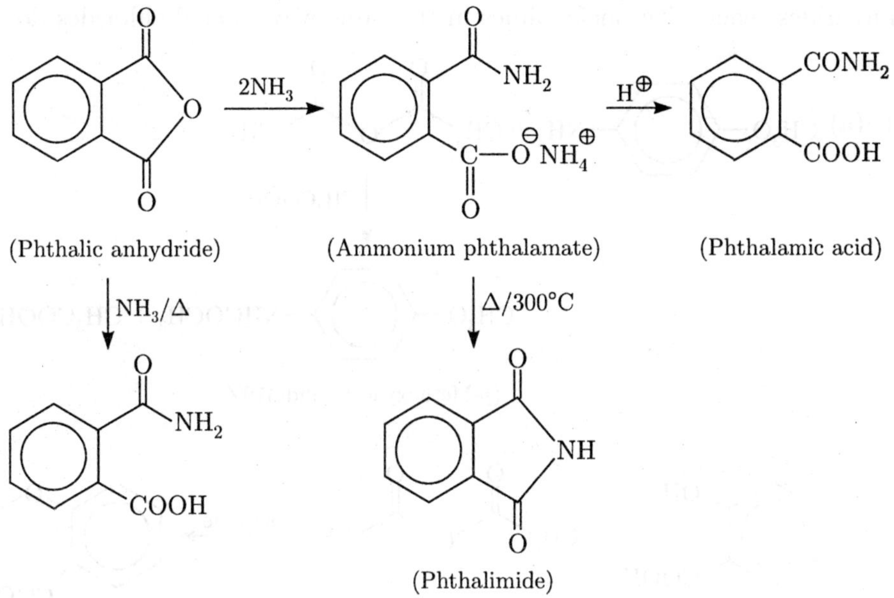

Synthesis of nitriles

1. (a) $RCONH_2 + (ArCONH_2) \xrightarrow{P_2O_5/\Delta/-H_2O} RCN(ArCN)$

(b) $RCOOH(ArCOOH) + NH_3 \xrightarrow[\text{Industrial method}]{Al_2O_3/500°C} RCN(ArCN)$

(c) $RCOOH(ArCOOH) \xrightarrow[\text{Industrial method}]{O_2/\text{catalyst}/500°C} RCN(ArCN)$

(d) $RCH{=}NOH(ArCH{=}NOH) \xrightarrow[-H_2O]{P_2O_5 \text{ or } Ac_2O} RCN(ArCN)$

(e) $R{-}X + KCN \xrightarrow[S_N2]{\text{aqueous ethanolic medium}} \underset{\text{(Major)}}{RCN} + \underset{\text{(Trace)}}{RNC}$

(f) $ROSO_2K + KCN \xrightarrow{\text{warmed}} \underset{\text{(Major)}}{RCN} + \underset{\text{(Trace)}}{RNC}$

(g) $CH_3{-}C_6H_4{-}SO_3R + KCN \xrightarrow{\Delta} RCN$

(h) $RMgCl(ArMgBr) + ClCN \longrightarrow RCN(ArCN)$

(i) $RNC \xrightarrow{\text{prolonged heating}} RNC$

Reactions of anhydrides with nucleophiles :

Anhydrides react with nucleophiles in the same way as acid chlorides do.

1. (a)

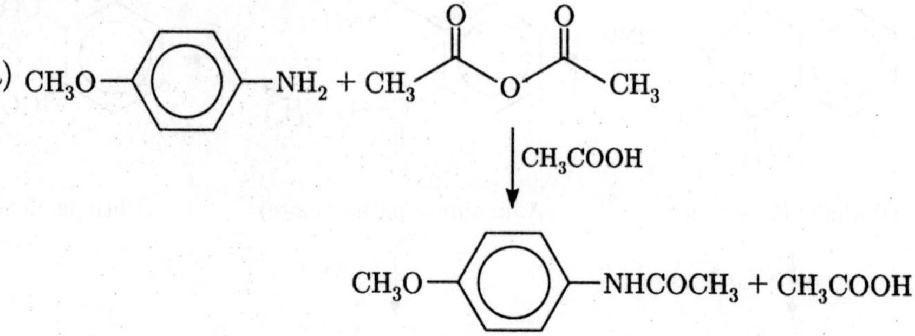

(p-Methoxyacetanilide)79%

(b)

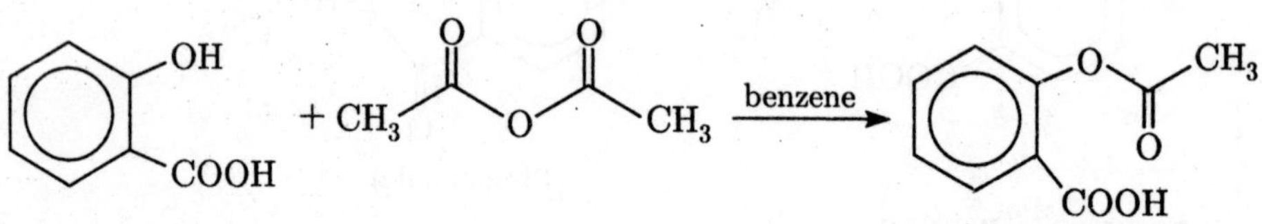

(Salicylic acid) (Acetylsalicylic acid) (aspirin), 90%

+ CH_3COOH

Most anhydries are formed from the corresponding acids. So when anhydrides are used to prepare esters or amides, one mole of acid is liberated as the leaving group. This is only possible in practice when the acid is not expensive.

(c) *Formation* of *half esters and half amides*

i.

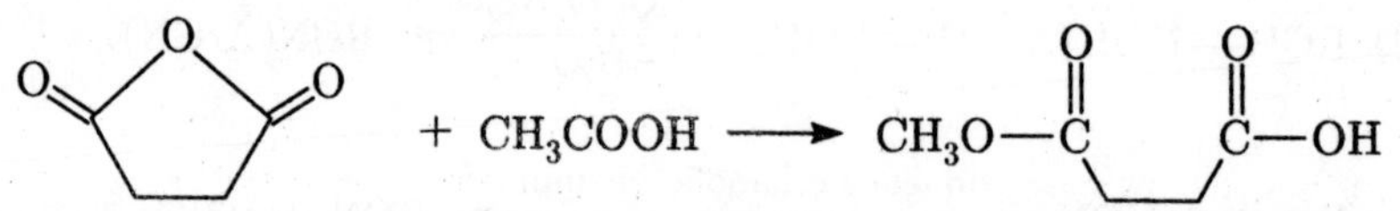

(Succinic anhydride) (Methyl hydrogen succinate) (half ester)

ii.

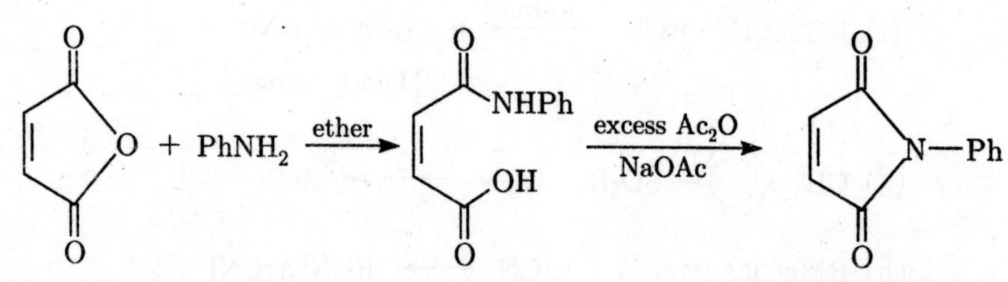

(Maleic anhydride) (Half amide) (N-phenylmaleimide)

(d) i.

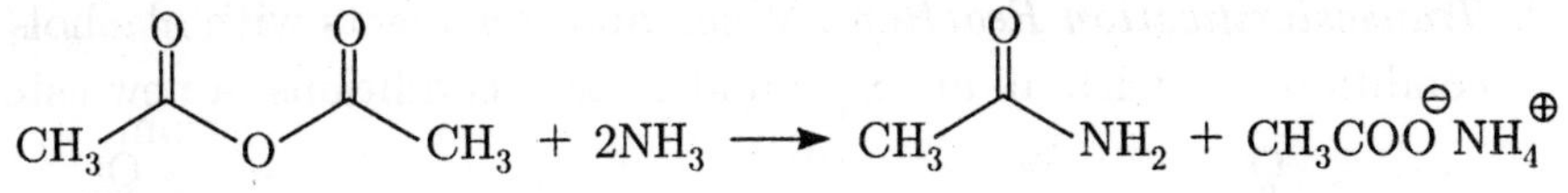

(Acetic anhydride) (Acetamide) (Ammonium acetate)

ii.

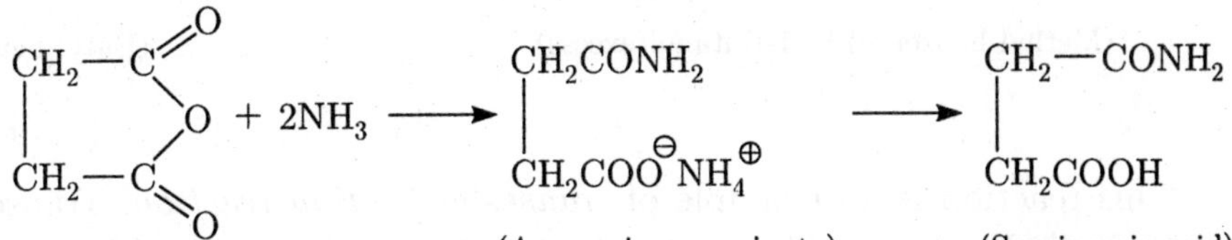

(Ammonium succinate) (Succinamic acid)

2.

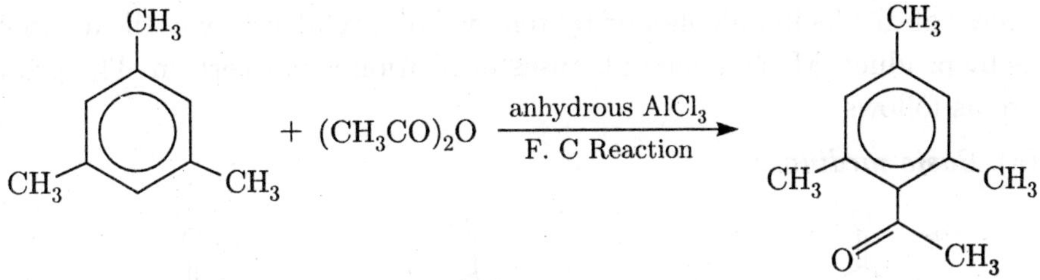

3. $(RCO)_2O \xrightarrow{HCl} RCOCl + RCOOH$

4. $(CH_3CO)_2O + CH_3CHO \longrightarrow CH_3CH(OCOCH_3)_2$

5. $(CH_3CO)_2O + N_2O_5 \longrightarrow CH_3COONO_2$

(Acetyl nitrate)

Reactions of esters with nucleophiles

1. (a)

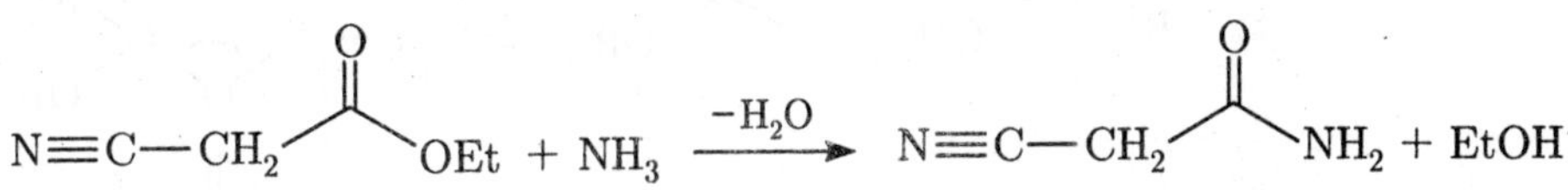

(86%)

(b)

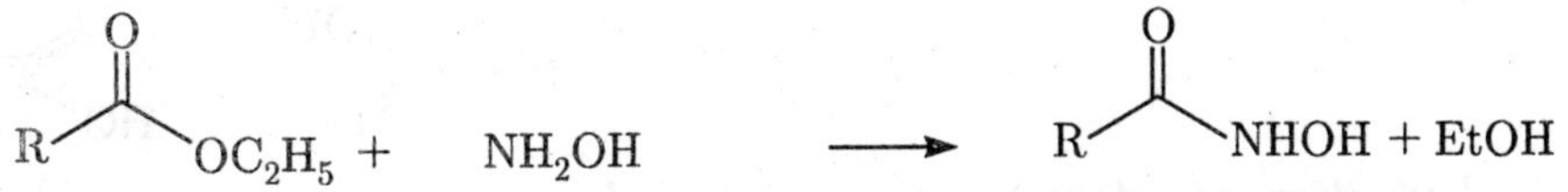

(Hydroxylamine) (Hydroxamic acid)

This test is the identification test for esters (hydroxamate test) in the laboratory, as hydroxamic acid products form highly coloured complexes with ferric iron. Acid chlorides and anhydrides also produce hydroxamic acids with hydroxylamine.

(c)

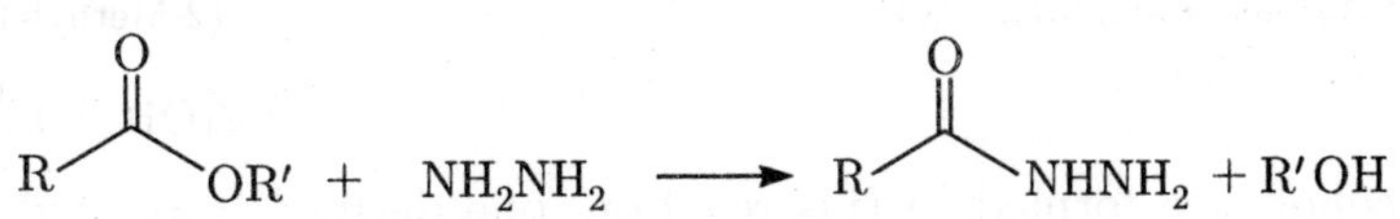

(Hydrazine)

2. ***Transesterification Reaction*** : When an ester reacts with alcohols under acidic conditions, or with an alkoxide under basic conditions, a new ester is formed.

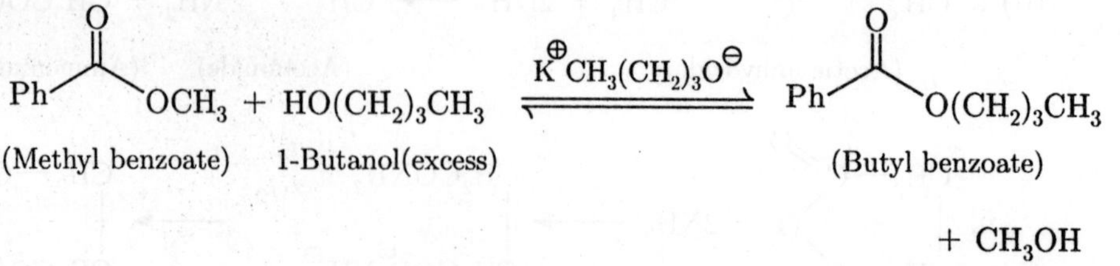

(Methyl benzoate) 1-Butanol(excess) (Butyl benzoate)

This reaction is an example of *transesterification reaction.* Transesterification typically has an *equilibrium constant* near *unity*, because neither ester is strongly favoured at equilibrium. The reaction is driven to completion by the use of an excess of displacing alcohol or by removal of a relatively volatile alcohol formed as by product. Mechanism of transesterification is not certain. The probabilities are as follows :

(a) ***Basic medium*** :

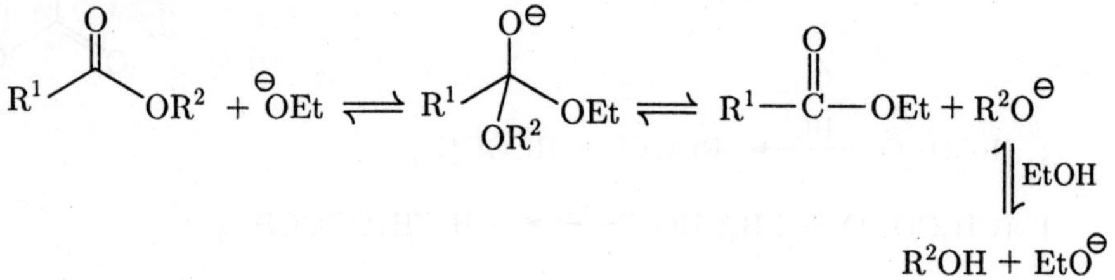

(b) ***Acid medium*** :

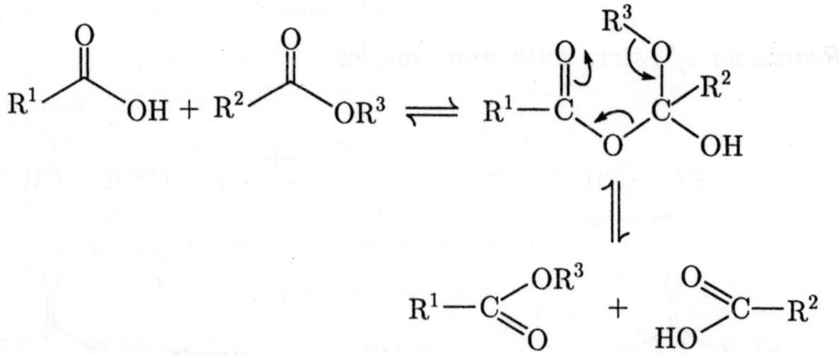

3. ***Reduction of esters to primary alcohols***

(a) 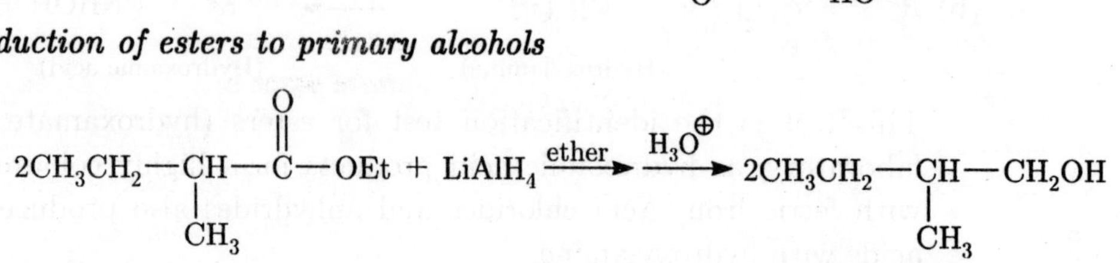

(Ethyl 2-methylbutanoate) (2-Methyl-1-butanol)

Two alcohols are formed in this reaction, one derived from acyl group of the ester and another derived from alkoxy group. In most cases, methyl or ethyl esters are used and the by product — methanol or ethanol is discarded. The active nucleophile in $LiAlH_4$ reductions is the hydride ($\overset{\ominus}{H}:$) ion from $\overset{\ominus}{Al}H_4$.

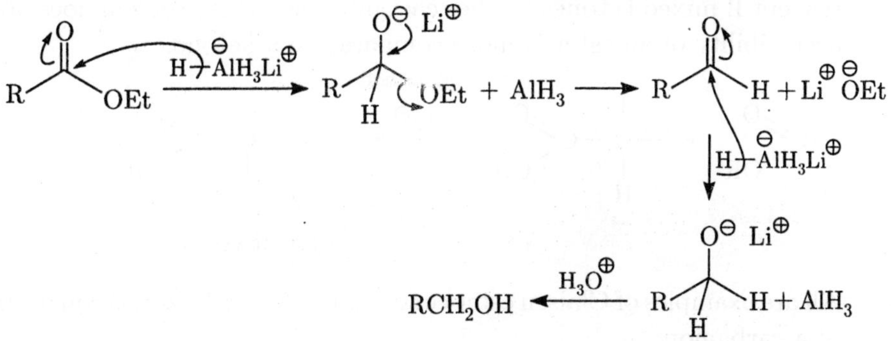

Sodium borohydride ($NaBH_4$), is another useful hydride reducing agent. $NaBH_4$ can reduce aldehydes and ketones but cannot reduce ester functionality. So $NaBH_4$ can be used to reduce aldehydes and ketones selectively in the presence of esters. $LiAlH_4$ can reduce acid chlorides and anhydrides to primary alcohols, but is seldom used.

(b) ***Catalytic hydrogenation*** : ***Hydrogenolysis*** : Hydrogenolysis of an ester requires more severe conditions than simple hydrogenation of carbon-carbon double bond.

$$CH_3(CH_2)_{10}COOCH_3 \xrightarrow[150°C,\ 5000\ lb/cm^3]{H_2/CuO.CuCr_2O_4} CH_3(CH_2)_{10}CH_2OH + CH_3OH$$

(hydrogenolysis) (1-Dodecanol)

4. ***Reaction with Grignard reagents***

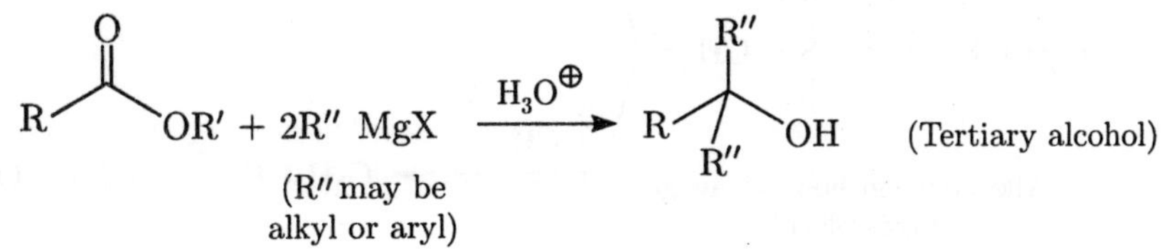

This is an excellent method to prepare tertiary alcohols.

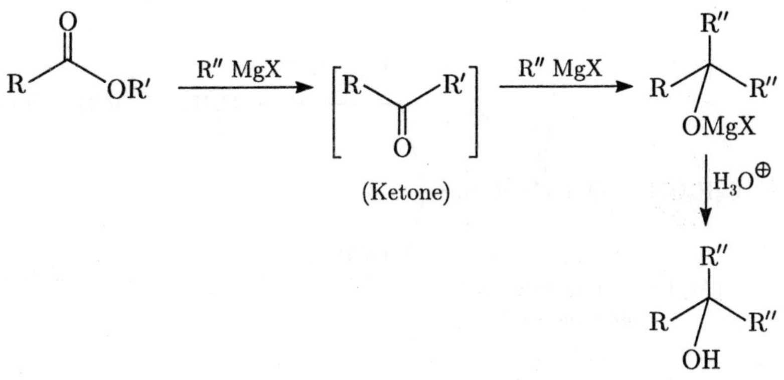

In some cases, ketones are also isolated. Two of the three groups attached to the carbon bearing –OH comes from Grignard reagent and hence must be identical. This is one drawback to prepare tertiary alcohol from esters with Grignard reagent If mixed ketones be the reactants, then this problem does not arise. But accessibility of an ester is more compared to a ketone.

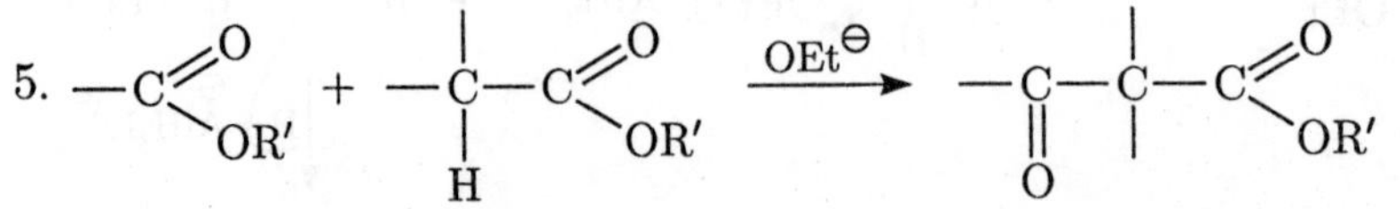

(β-Keto ester)

All are examples of Claisen ester condensation which passes through the formation of a carbanion.

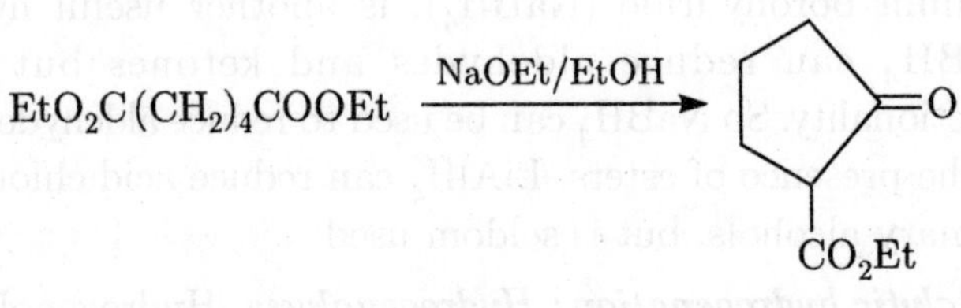

Comparison of reactivity of carboxylate and sulphonate esters : Althouh sulphonate and carboxylate esters are synthesised in similar ways, their reactions with nucleophiles are different.

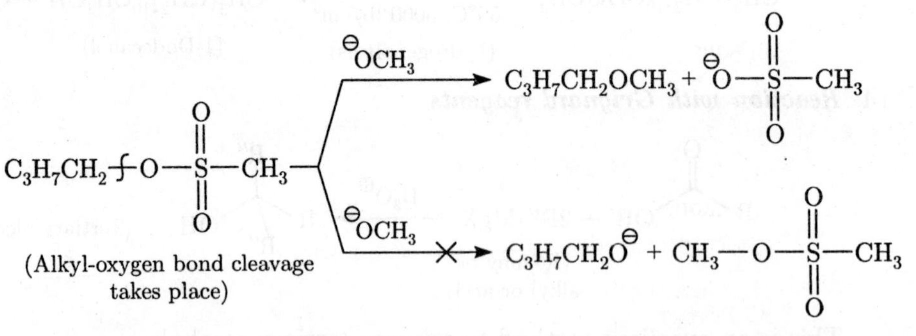

(Alkyl-oxygen bond cleavage takes place)

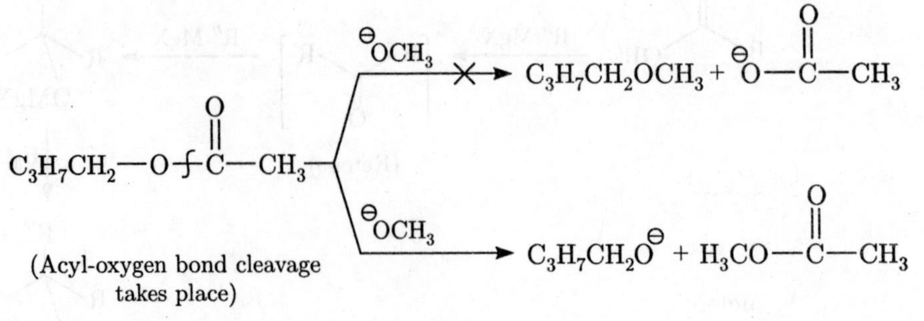

(Acyl-oxygen bond cleavage takes place)

Sulphonate group is a weaker base and hence a good leaving group compared to carboxylate group. –OH group of an alcohol is a poor leaving group, but when converted to a sulphonate ester group it becomes a good leaving group.

Reactions of Amides :

1. Reduction of amides to amines

(a) 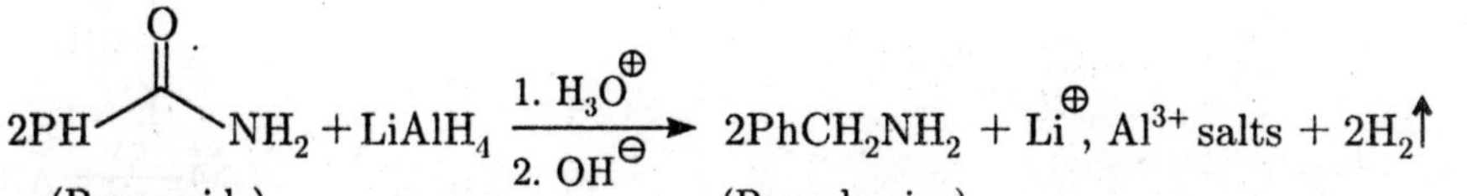

(Benzamide) (Benzylamine)

$^{\ominus}$OH ion (base) is required for work up, as the amine formed remains protonated (the corresponding conjugate acid) and become neutralised to form the free amine.

(b) 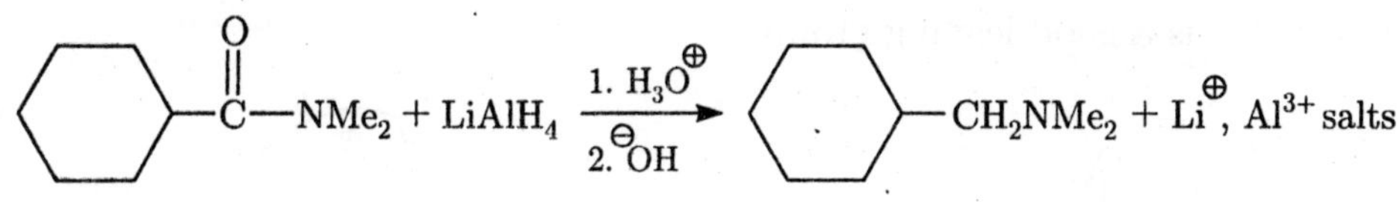

(Tertiary amide) (88%)

The reduction of an amide with $LiAlH_4$ differs from reduction of esters to primary alcohols. During the reduction of esters, carboxylate oxygen is lost as a leaving group but in amide, nitrogen is *not* lost as if it is lost then amide reduction by $LiAlH_4$ would also produce a primary alcohol.

Ester Reduction :

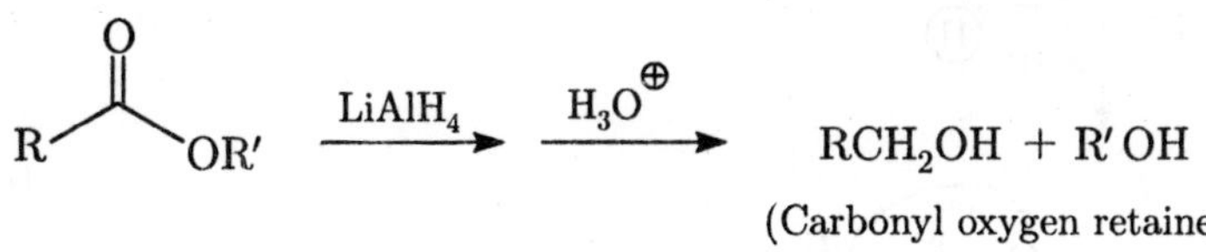

(Carbonyl oxygen retained)

Amide Reduction

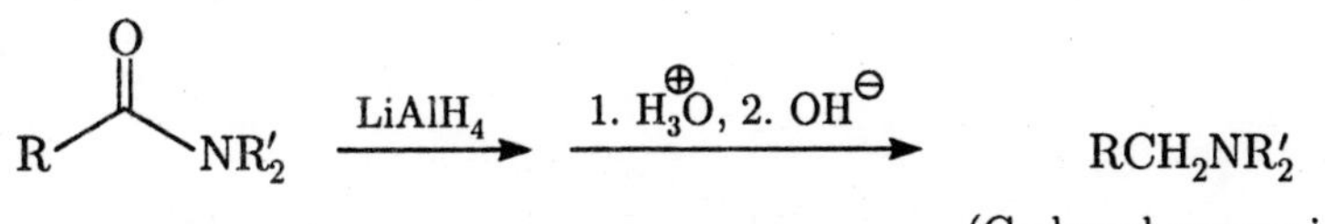

(Carbonyl oxygen is lost)

Mechanism of the reduction :

(a) 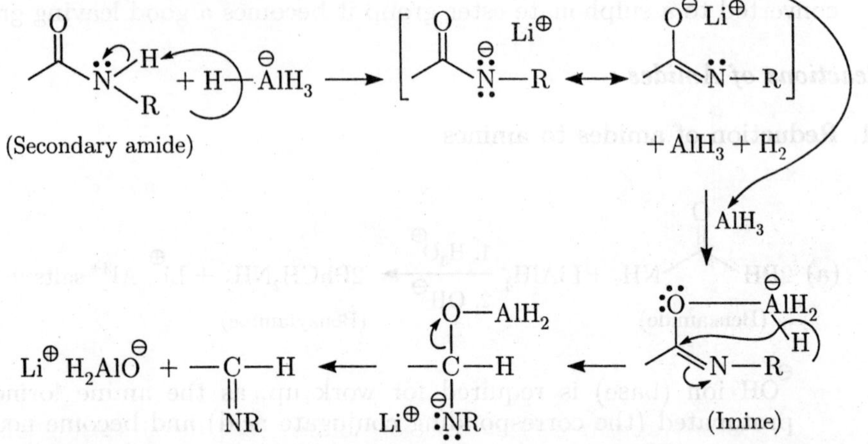

Oxygen is lost rather than nitrogen because $-OAlH_2$ is a weak base and so is a good leaving group.

(b) 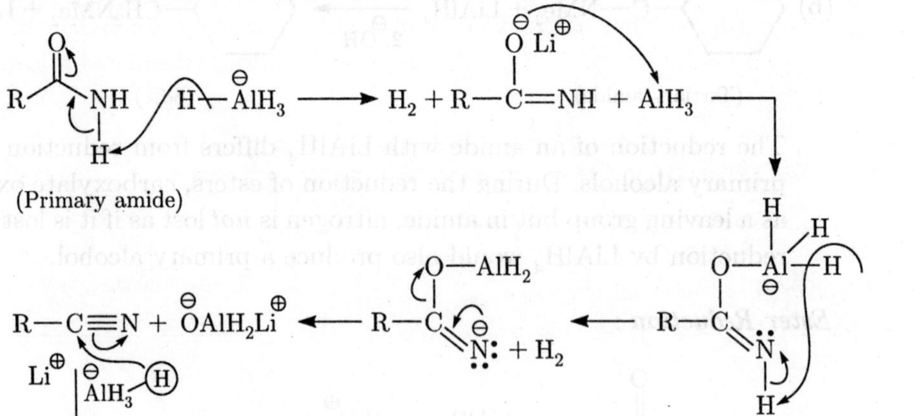

2. (a) $HCONMe_2 \xrightarrow[2.\ H_3O^{\oplus}]{1.\ R^1MgX \text{ or } R^1Li} R^1CHO$ (Aldehyde)

(b) $RCONMe_2 \xrightarrow[2.\ H_3O^{\oplus}]{1.\ R^1MgX \text{ or } R^1Li} RCOR^1$ (Ketone)

3. $RCONH_2 \xrightarrow{HNO_2} RCOOH + N_2 + H_2O$

4. $RCONH_2 \xrightarrow{H^{\oplus}/\text{acidic}} \left[R{-}\overset{\overset{\oplus}{O}H}{\overset{\|}{C}}{-}NH_2 \longleftrightarrow R{-}\overset{OH}{\overset{|}{C}}{=}\overset{\oplus}{N}H_2 \longleftrightarrow R{-}\overset{OH}{\overset{|}{\underset{\oplus}{C}}}{-}NH_2\right]$

5. $RCONH_2 \xrightarrow{NaNH_2/\text{basic}} \left[RCO\overset{\ominus}{\ddot{N}}H \longleftrightarrow R{-}\overset{O^{\ominus}}{\overset{|}{C}}{=}NH\right]$

6. An unique reaction given by primary amide is the dehydration of primary amides to nitriles.

(a) 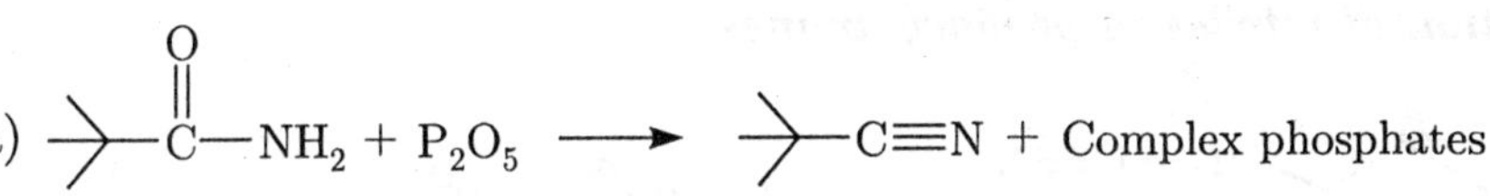

(b) $CH_3(CH_2)_3\underset{Et}{\underset{|}{C}H}{-}\overset{O}{\overset{\|}{C}}{-}NH_2 + SOCl_2 \longrightarrow CH_3(CH_2)_3{-}\underset{Et}{\underset{|}{C}H}{-}C{\equiv}N + SO_2 + HCl$

Mechanism of the reaction :

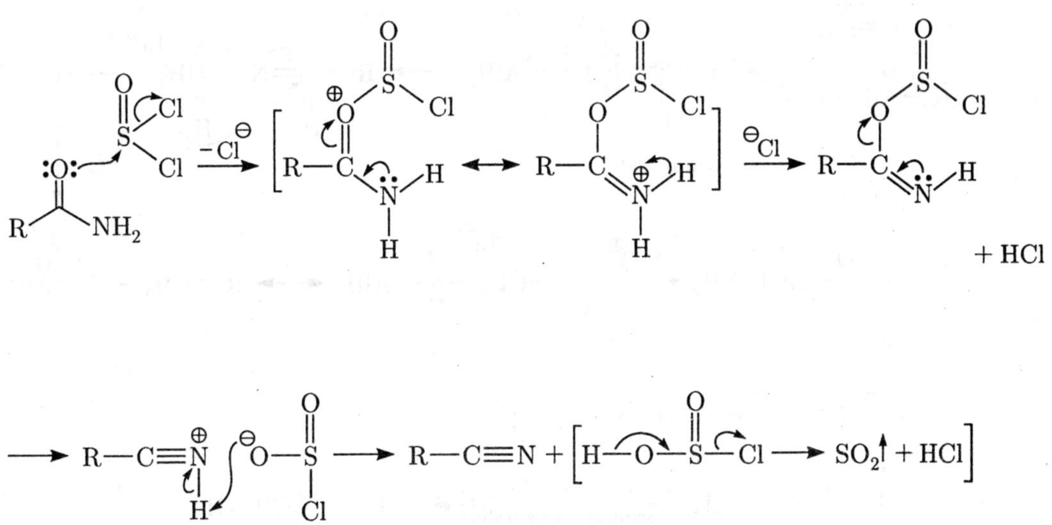

Lactams

Cyclic amides are called lactams.

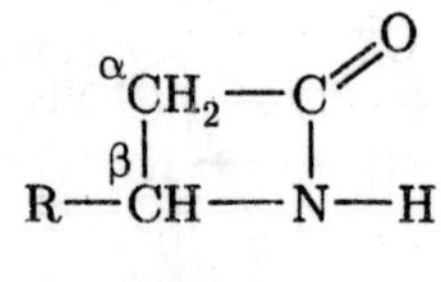

(β-Lactam)

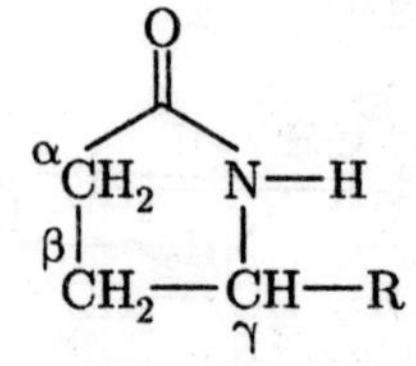

(γ-Lactam)

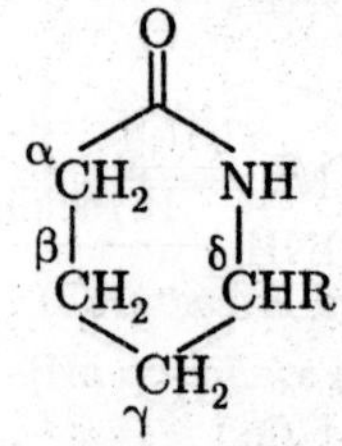

(δ-Lactam)

γ-and δ- Lactams are formed spontaneously from γ- and δ- amino acids. β- Lactams are highly reactive as their strained four-membered rings open easily in the presence of nucleophilic reagents.

Reduction of nitriles to primary amines

1. 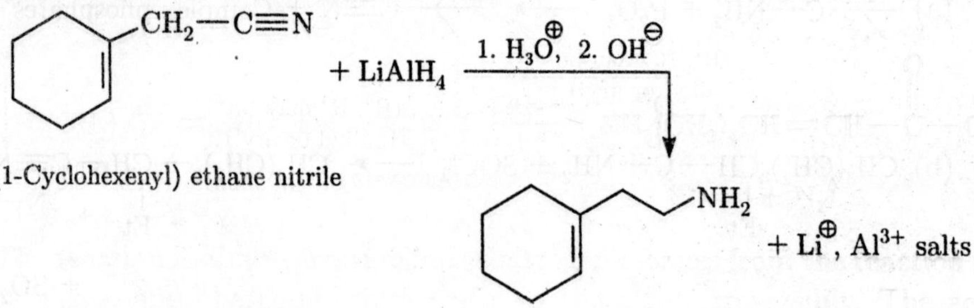

2(1-Cyclohexenyl) ethane nitrile

Mechanism of the reaction :

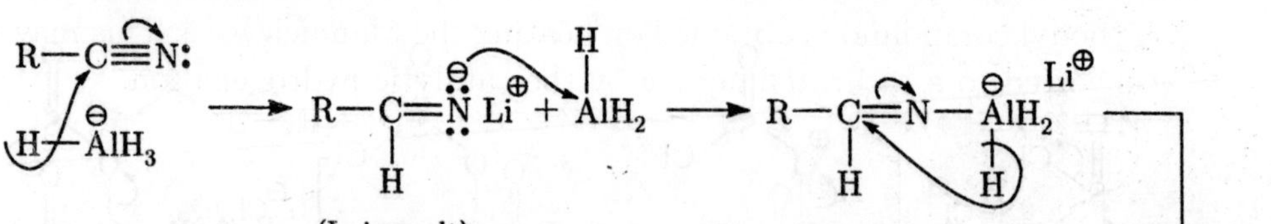

(Imine salt)

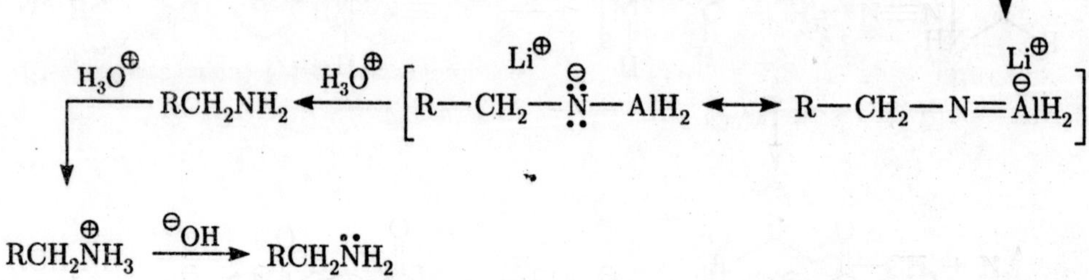

2. $CH_3(CH_2)_4C{\equiv}N + 2H_2 \xrightarrow[\text{2000 psi, 120–130°C}]{\text{Raney Ni}} CH_3(CH_2)_4CH_2NH_2$

Imine is formed as an intermediate, which is not isolated and is hydrogenated to the amine product.

$$R{-}C{\equiv}N \xrightarrow{H_2/\text{catalyst}} \underset{\text{(Imine)}}{[R{-}CH{=}NH]} \xrightarrow{H_2/\text{catalyst}} RCH_2NH_2$$

Hydrolysis of Carboxylic Acid Derivatives

1. Hydrolysis and formation of lactones

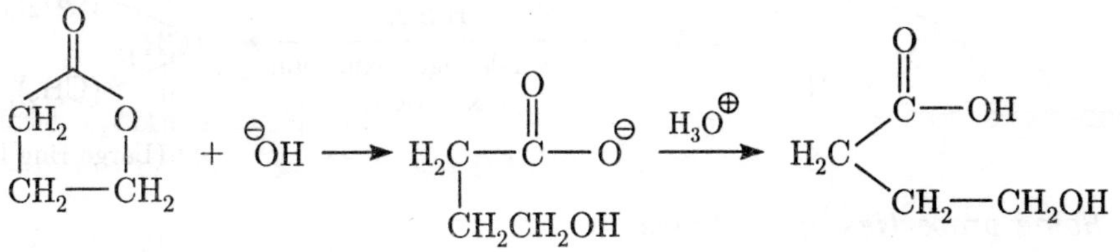

(γ-Butyrolactone) (A cyclic ester) (γ-Hydroxybutyrate) (γ-Hydroxy acid)

If a hydroxy acid is allowed to stand in acidic solution it comes to equilibrium with the corresponding lactone and thus, lactone formation reaction is acid catalysed intramolecular esterfication reaction.

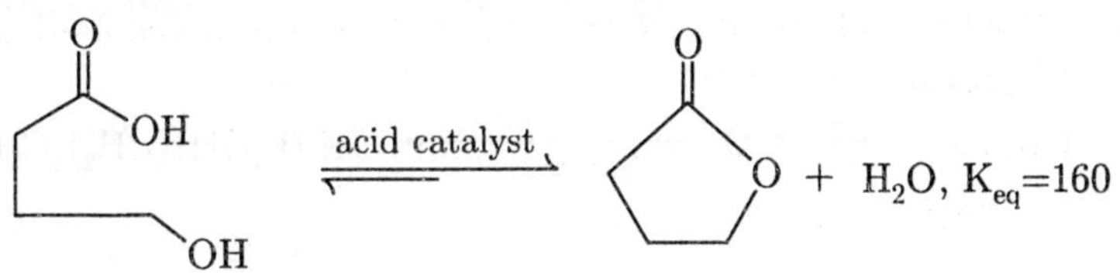

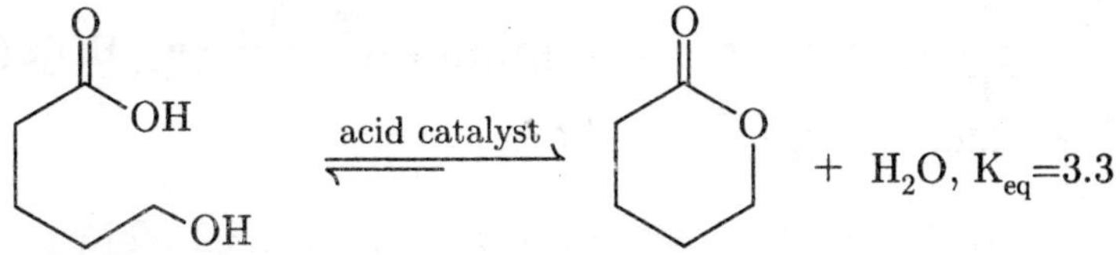

Lactones containing five- and six-membered rings are favoured at equilibrium over their corresponding hydroxy acids. Lactones containing smaller or larger rings are less stable than their corresponding hydroxy acids.

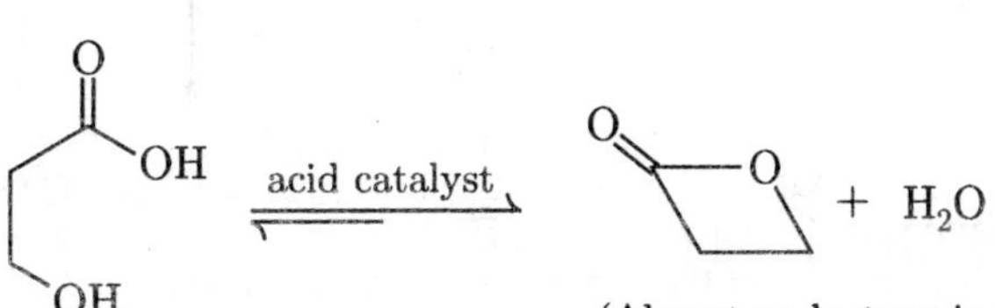

(Almost no lactone is present at equilibrium)

By using high dilution principle, large ring lactones have been prepared from hydroxyacids in which hydroxyl group is far away from $-CO_2H$ group. A sufficiently dilute solution is taken where the distance between –OH and $-CO_2H$ groups of different molecules are greater than the distance between –OH and $-CO_2H$ groups of the same molecule. Then only a cyclic ester (lactone) is formed instead of linear ω-Hydroxypentadecanoic acid and gives a high yield of lactone on heating in a very dilute solution.

2. Large ring lactones (14–18 membered rings) have been prepared by the oxidation of cyclic ketones with peracid or Caro's acid.

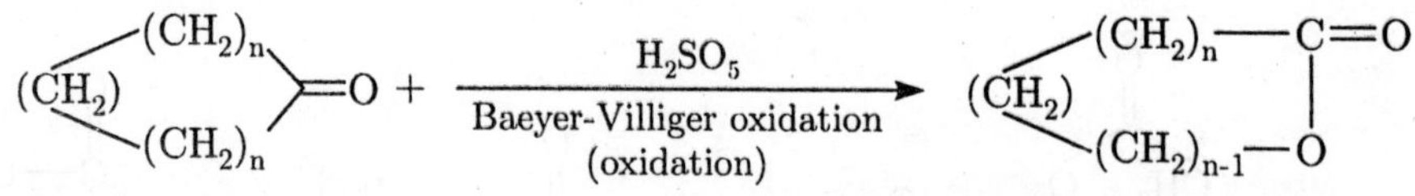

(Large ring lactone)

Some properties of Lactones

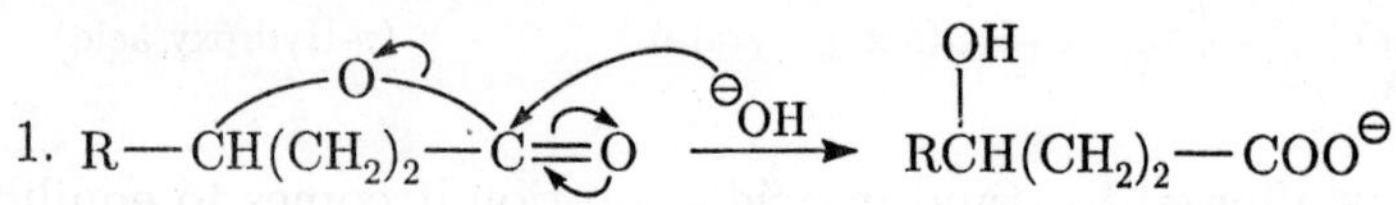

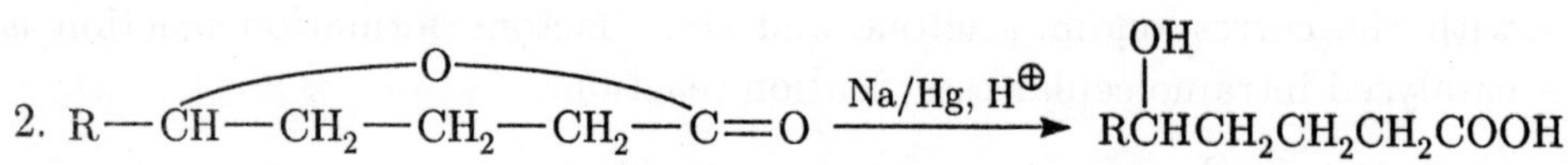

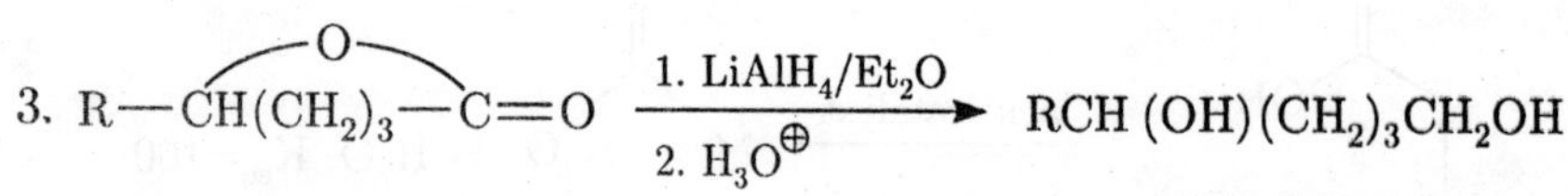

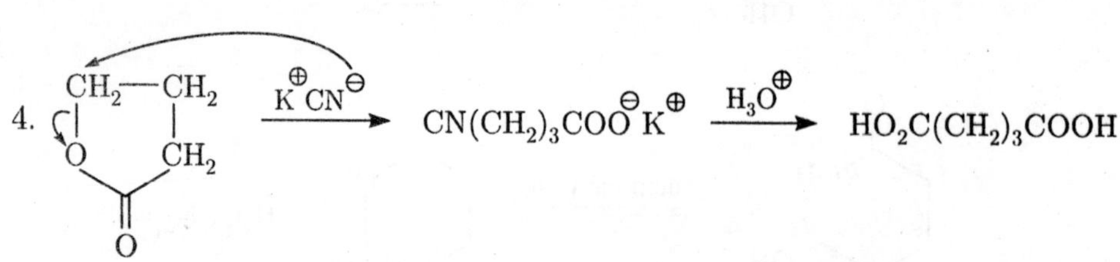

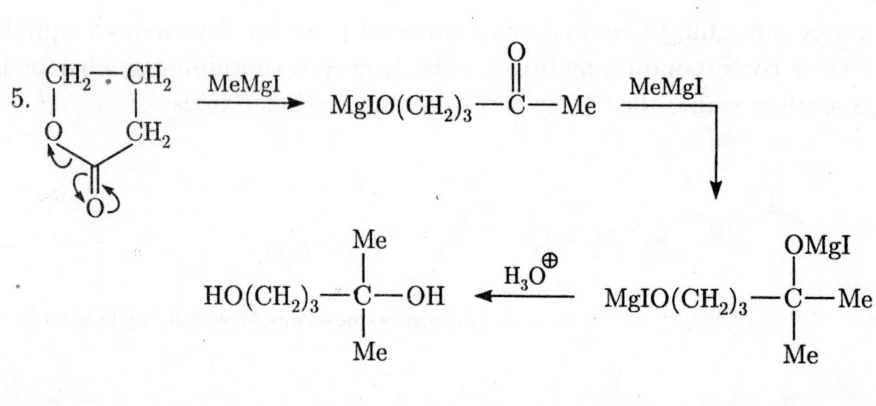

Hydrolysis of Amides

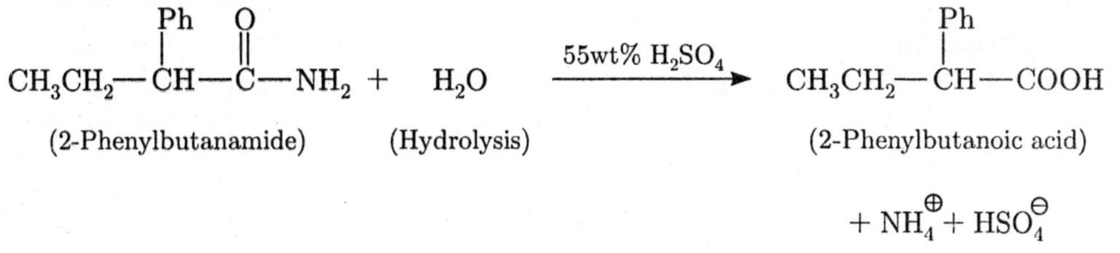

Protonation of NH_3 or amine by product drives the hydrolysis equilibrium to completion. The amine is isolated as follows.

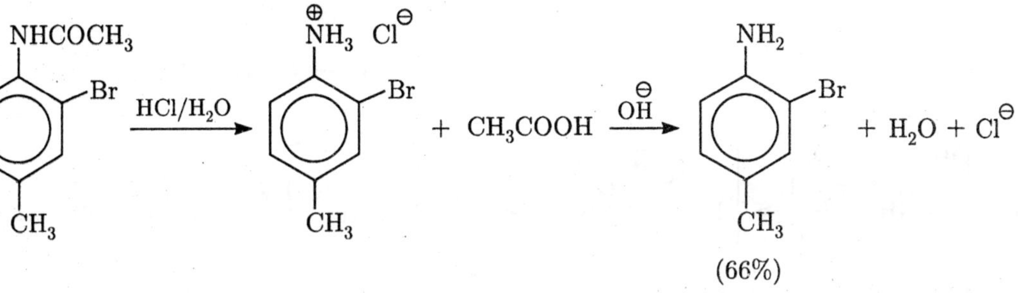

Hydrolysis of amides in bases is analogous to saponification of esters. In bases the reaction is driven to completion by the formation of carboxylate anion.

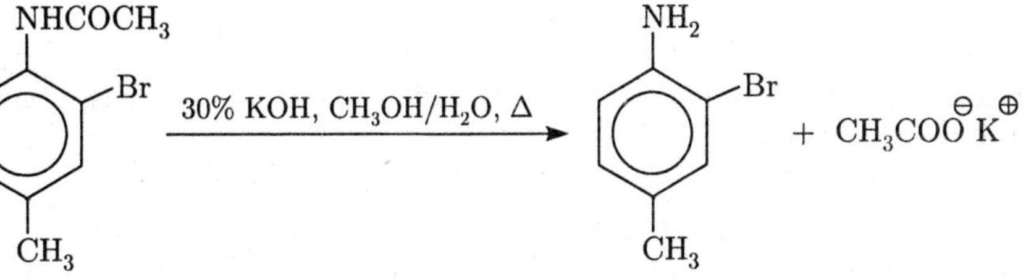

Amides are less succeptible to hydrolysis compared to that of esters.

Hydrolysis of Nitriles

$$\underset{\text{(Phenylacetonitrile)}}{PhCH_2C{\equiv}N} + 2H_2O + H_2SO_4\,(57\text{ wt\%}) \xrightarrow{\Delta/3h} \underset{\text{(Phenylacetic acid)}}{PhCH_2COOH} + \overset{\oplus}{N}H_4 + HSO_4^{\ominus}$$

Nitriles hydrolyse slower than esters and amides, so they require more harsh conditions.

Mechanism of hydrolysis of nitriles :

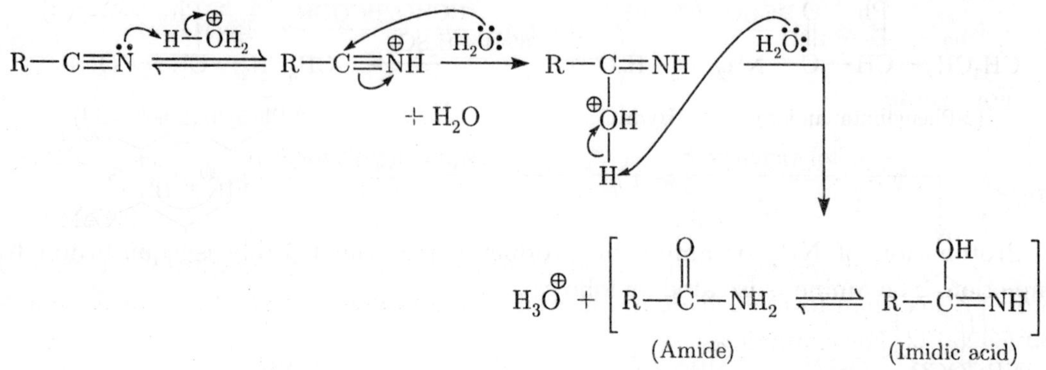

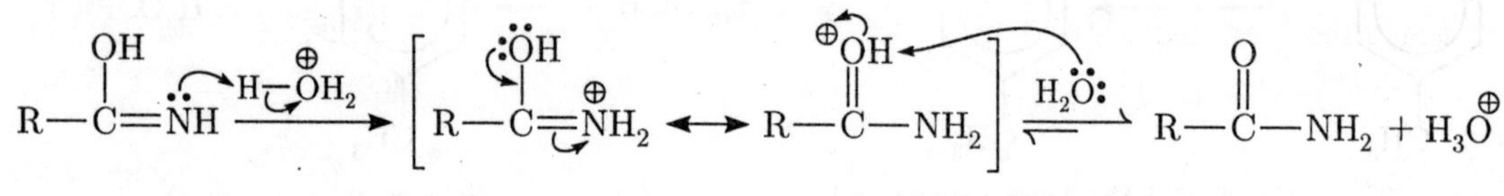

Amide hydrolysis is faster than nitrile hydrolysis, so under the harsh conditions of nitrile hydrolysis, amides do not survive, they form carboxylic acids.

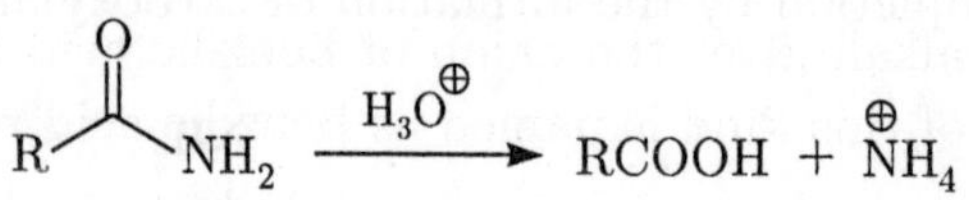

Nitriles behave like carbonyl compounds which is evident from the base catalysed hydrolysis of them (nitriles).

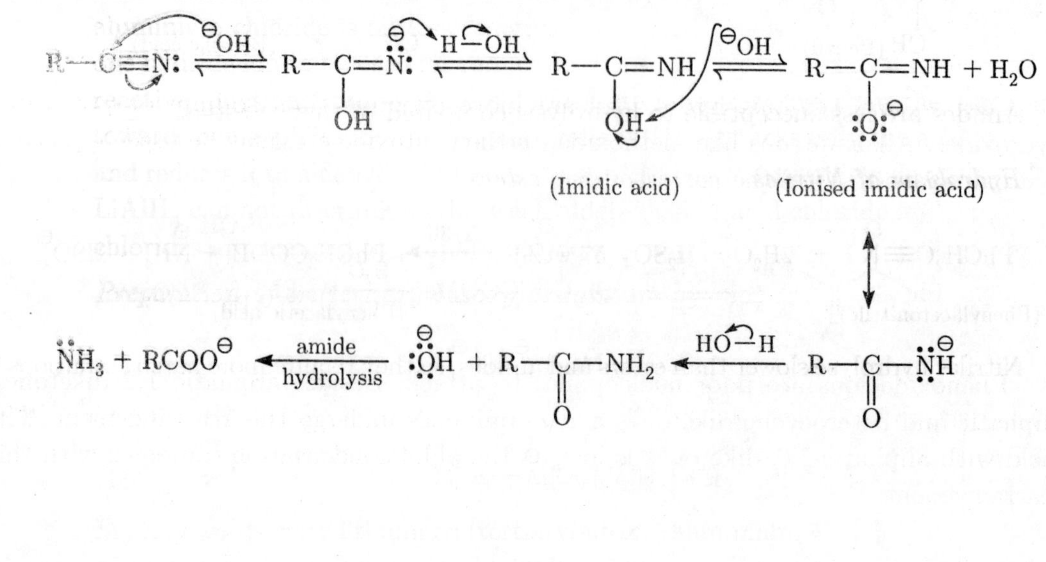

Hydrolysis of acid chlorides and anhydrides

Acid chlorides and anhydrides react rapidly with water even in the absence of acids and bases.

1. 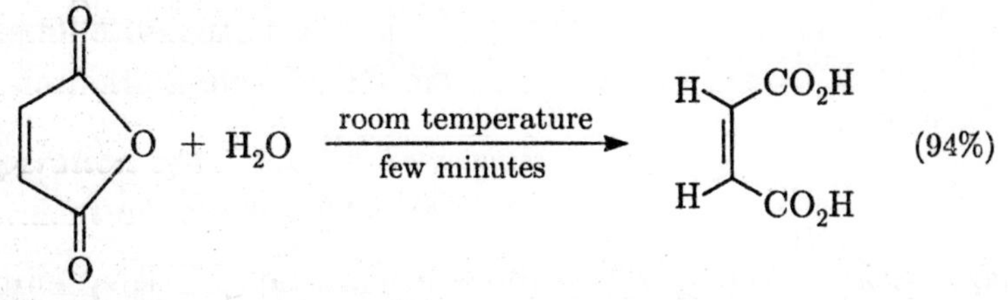

2. 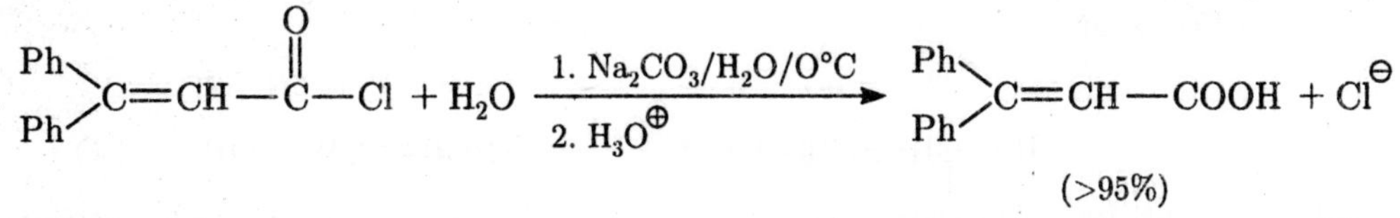

However, carboxylic acids are not generally prepared from the acid chlorides or acid anhydrides. In the presence of little moisture, acid chlorides and acid anhydrides form their corresponding acids.

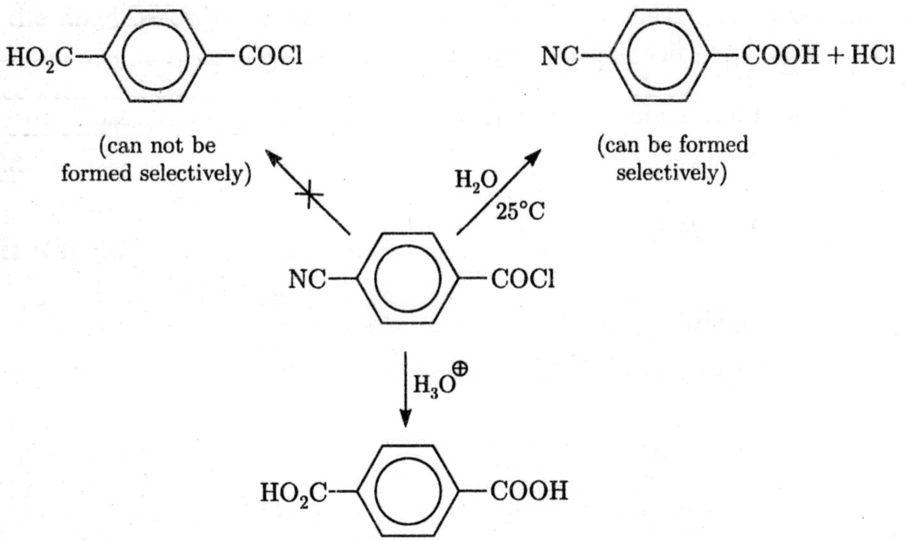

Action of Heat on Hydroxyacids

When hydroxyacids are heated, the product formed depends on the relative positions of –OH and –CO_2H groups.

1. **With α-hydroxy acids :**

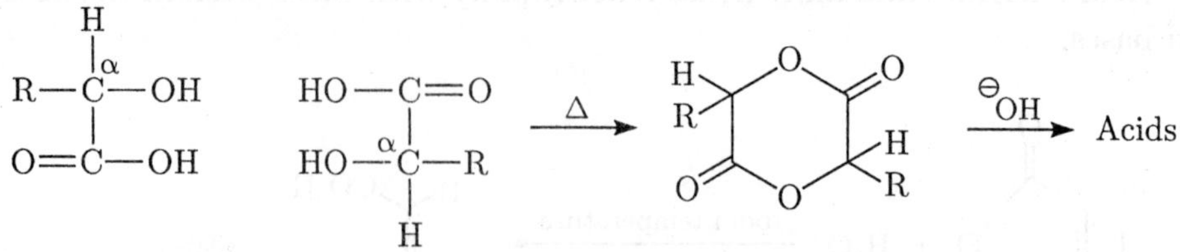

(α-Hydroxy acid) (3,6-Dialkyl-1,4-dioxan-2,5-dione)

2. **With β-hydroxy acids :** When β-hydroxy acids are heated, they eliminate a molecule of water to form mainly α, β-unsaturated acid and a very small amount of β, γ-unsaturated acid.

$$R-\underset{OH}{\underset{|}{\overset{\beta}{C}H}}-\overset{\alpha}{C}H_2COOH \xrightarrow{\Delta} RCH{=}CHCOOH + H_2O$$

(β-Hydroxy acid)

3. **With γ-hydroxy acids :**

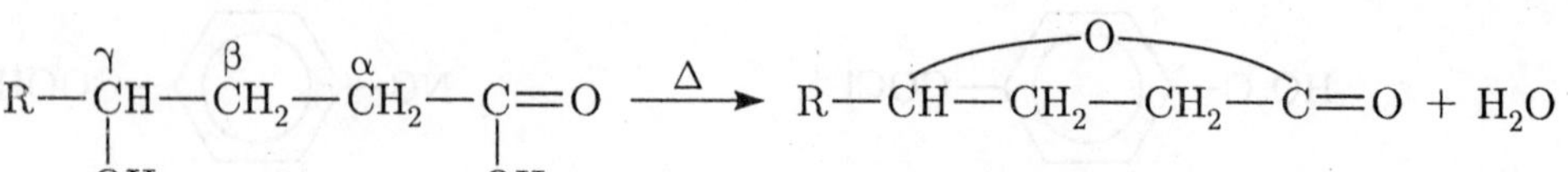

(γ-Hydroxy acid) (γ-Lactone)

4. **With δ-hydroxy acids :**

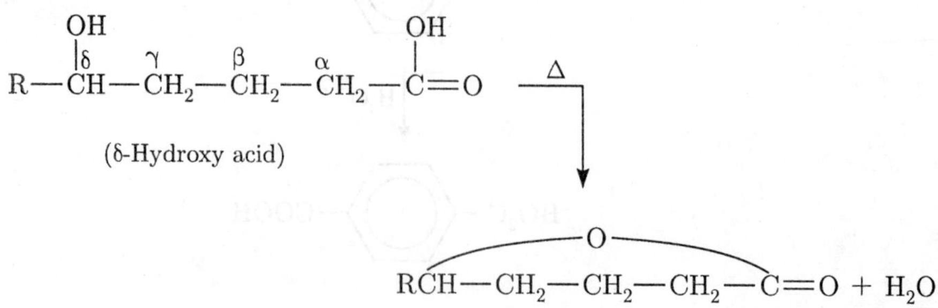

(δ-Hydroxy acid)

(δ-Lactone)

Hydrolysis of Carboxylic Acid Esters

Hydrolysis of esters may be carried out by refluxing them either with dilute acid or with dilute alkali.

$$R'OH + RCOO^{\ominus} \xleftarrow{\ ^{\ominus}OH/H_2O\ } R-\overset{\overset{\large O}{\|}}{C}-OR' \xrightleftharpoons{H^{\oplus}/H_2O} RCOOH + R'OH$$

OR′ is a poor leaving group compared to anhydrides (OCOR) or halide, and thus, water can not alone hydrolyse most esters. When bases catalyse the reaction, the attacking species is $^{\ominus}OH$, a more powerful nucleophile than water. This reaction is called *saponification* and gives salts of acids. Acid catalyses the reaction by making the carbonyl carbon more positive and therefore more succeptible to attack by the nucleophile. Acid catalysed reactions are reversible or equilibrium reactions and are practicable only when the equilibrium shifts to the right. Ester hydrolysis can also be catalysed by metal ions, cyclodextrins, enzymes, methanesulphonic acid or guanidine. Phenolic esters are cleaved easily and rapidly; lactones also undergo hydrolysis (if the lactone is five or six-membered, spontaneous lactonisation takes place). Hinderd esters are hydrolysed with difficulty, *n*-propyllithium being a good cleaving agent. For insoluble esters, the rate of two phase ester saponification is increased by the application of ultrasound.

Ingold classified the acid- and base- catalysed hydrolysis of esters into **eight** possible mechanisms depending on the following criteria.

1. Acid- or base- catalysed. 2. Unimolecular or bimolecular, and 3. Acyl cleavage or alkyl cleavage

All the eight of these are S_N1 or S_N2 or tetrahedral mechanisms. The acid catalysed mechanisms are reversible as well as symmetrical, *i.e.*, the mechanisms for the ester formations are exactly the same as for the hydrolysis, only H replaces R.

Mechanisms for Esterification and Ester Hydrolysis

Type	Remarks
$B_{Ac}2$	Very common; includes all basic ester hydrolyses (saponification)
$A_{Ac}2$	Very common; includes acid hydrolysis of esters of primary and most secondary alcohols, and most ordinary esterification reactions.
$B_{Ac}1$	Not observed to date.
$A_{Ac}1$	Rare. Some esterifications and hydrolysis in concentrated solutions of very strong acids are of this type.
$B_{AL}2$	Extremely rare. Observed only for hydrolysis of β-lactones in the absence of both strong acid and strong base.
$A_{AL}2$	Very rare; requires water as a nucleophile in an S_N2 process.
$B_{AL}1$	Apparently quite general for the hydrolysis of tertiary alcohols and those secondary alcohols that yield the most stable carbonium ions (for example benzhydrol and α-methylallyl alcohol). Not generally observed for hydrolysis in concentrated bases.
$A_{AL}1$	Generally observed for tertiary alcohol, secondary alcohol and benzyl esters where the alcohol-alkyl groups can generate stable carbocations.

B stands for base catalysed hydrolysis while A stands for acid catalysed hydrolysis.

Ac stands for acyl-oxygen ($R—\overset{O}{\overset{\|}{C}}—OR'$) bond fission and AL stands for oxygen-alkyl ($R—\overset{O}{\overset{\|}{C}}—O—R'$) bond fission. The 1 and 2 indicate respectively unimolecularity and bimoleculartiy of the reactions. $B_{Ac}2$ and $A_{Ac}2$ are the most commonly found mode of hydrolysis of ester.

Both $B_{Ac}2$ and $A_{Ac}2$ have tetrahedral mechanisms and involve acyl-oxygen cleavage. The evidences are as follows.

1. Hydrolysis with H_2O^{18} results in the O^{18} appearing in the acid and not in the alcohol.
2. Esters with chiral R′ groups give alcohols with retention of configuration.
3. Allylic R′ gives no allylic rearrangement.
4. Neopentyl R′ gives no neopentyl rearrangement.

All these facts indicate that O—R′ bond is *not broken* (*i.e.*, oxygen-alkyl bond) in $A_{Ac}2$ and $B_{Ac}2$ mechanisms.

A carboxylic acid in a basic medium is converted to a carboxylate anion, $RCOO^{\ominus}$, which because of its negative charge, is *not* subjected to nucleophilic attack by alcohols or their conjugate bases. *Esterifications in basic media are therefore not observed.*

1. **$B_{Ac}2$ *Mechanism*** (Base-catalysed acyl oxygen fission, bimolecular) :

$B_{Ac}2$ follows tetrahedral mechanism.

Step 1 : Nucleophilic attack by the base on the carbonyl carbon of the ester. This step is slow and hence is rate determining.

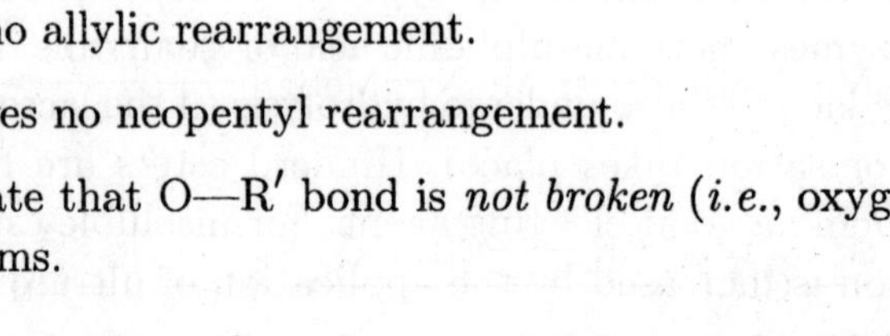

(Tetrahedral intermediate)

Step 2 : Cleavage of acyl-oxygen bond. This is a fast step.

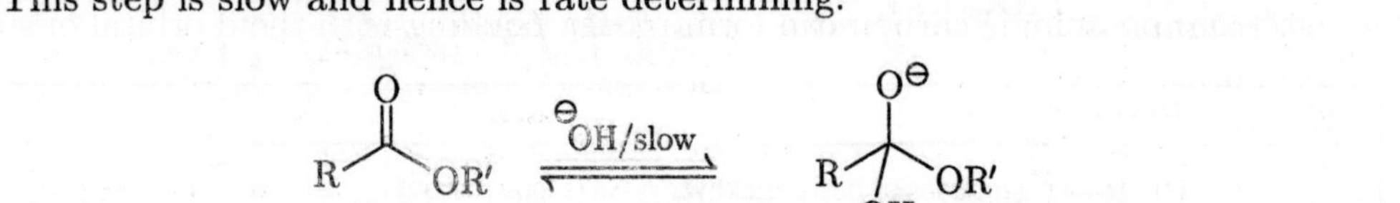

The reaction follows a second order kinetics. Rate = k[ester] $[OH^{\ominus}]$ when an ester with a chiral R′ group is hydrolysed, an optically active alcohol is obtained. If alkyl-oxygen bond be cleaved then a racemised alcohol would have been obtained, because $R'^{\oplus}$, the carbocation would be free then. An optically active alcohol can form only when acyl-oxygen bond is cleaved. Furthermore, when the hydrolysis is carried out in presence of H_2O^{18}, the alcohol formed does not contain O^{18}, which indicates that acyl-oxygen fission takes place.

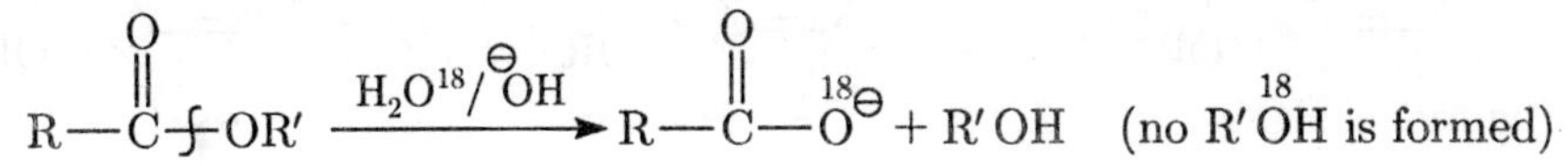

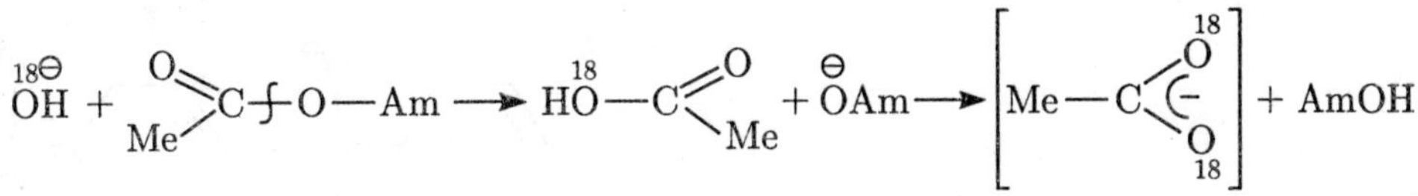

($Am \equiv C_5H_{11}$)

$B_{Ac}2$ is the most common type of mechanism of ester hydrolysis. If R group of the ester contains an electron withdrawing group, the rate of the reaction increases. (electron withdrawing group at R makes C=O centre more electropositive and the attack of $\overset{\ominus}{O}H$ to that centre becomes more facile). If R′ is bulky, the rate of hydrolysis decreases owing to steric effect.

The overall reaction is essentially *irreversible* as $\overset{\ominus}{O}R'$ should remove proton from RCOOH rather than attack its carbonyl carbon atom while $RCOO^{\ominus}$ will be insucceptible to nucleophilic attack by R′OH or $R'O^{\ominus}$. Carbonyl carbon of $RCOO^{\ominus}$ bears partial double bond character and so becomes less electrophilic to be attacked by a nucleophile.

$\frac{K}{K_{MeOAc}}$	CH_3COOMe	$CH_2ClCOOMe$	$CHCl_2COOMe$
	1	761	16,000

$\frac{K}{K_{MeOAc}}$	$(COOMe)_2$	CH_3COOEt	CH_3—C(=O)—CO_2Et
	170,000	0.60	10,000

Groups with (–1) effect accelerate the rate of $B_{Ac}2$ hydrolysis

$\frac{K}{K_{EtOAc}}$	CH_3COOEt	C_2H_5COOEt	Me_2CHCO_2Et	Me_3CCO_2Et
	1	0.47	0.10	0.011

Steric crowding retards the formation of tetrahedral intermediate which is reflected in the sluggish rate of $B_{Ac}2$ hydrolysis of the esters depicted in the above series. Benzoate esters undergo $B_{Ac}2$ hydrolysis at a comparatively slower rate. The π-electrons of the benzene ring undergo conjugation with the carbonyl group of the ester thereby lowering its electrophilicity, as a partial double bond develops there.

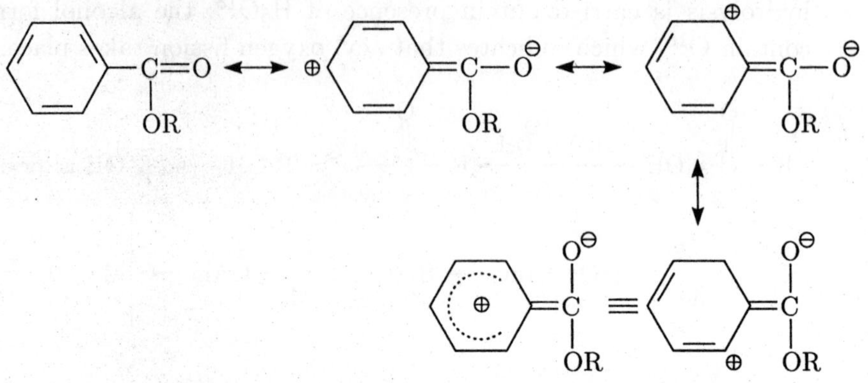

The effect of substituent at *meta* or *para* positions on $B_{Ac}2$ hydrolysis of aromatic esters depend on the step of nucleophilic attack of $H\overset{\ominus}{O}$ which is the rate determining step. The presence of electron withdrawing substituents like $-NO_2$, $-Cl$, $-COCH_3$ etc. accelerate the rate of hydrolysis by increasing the electrophilicity of the ester carbonyl carbon, whereas electron donor groups like $-OCH_3$, $-NMe_2$ etc. at same position retard the rate. For example, rate of alkaline hydrolysis of methyl 4-nitrobenzoate is much faster than methyl benzoate.

2. $A_{Ac}2$ ***Mechanism*** (acid catalysed acyl oxygen fission bimolecular) :

$A_{Ac}2$ mechanism follows tetrahedral mechanism. Like $B_{Ac}2$, $A_{Ac}2$ mechanism is also very common regarding the hydrolysis of esters.

The most obvious difference between the basic hydrolysis of esters and their acid-catalysed hydrolysis is that the latter is *experimentally reversible*, its reversal being the acid catalysed esterification reaction. $A_{Ac}2$ mechanism in fact follows the principle of **microscopic reversibility**, *i.e.*, given sequence of steps constitutes the favoured mechanism for the forward reaction, the reverse sequence of these steps constitutes the favoured mechanism for the reverse reaction.

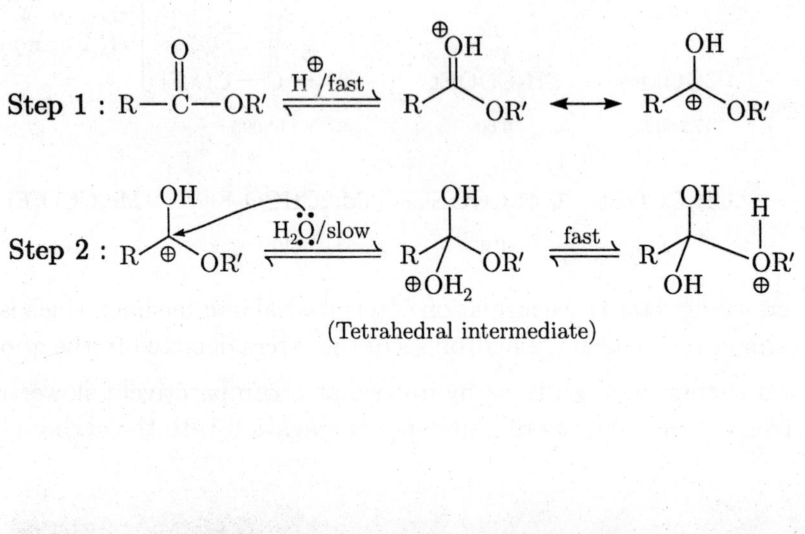

(Tetrahedral intermediate)

Step 3 : 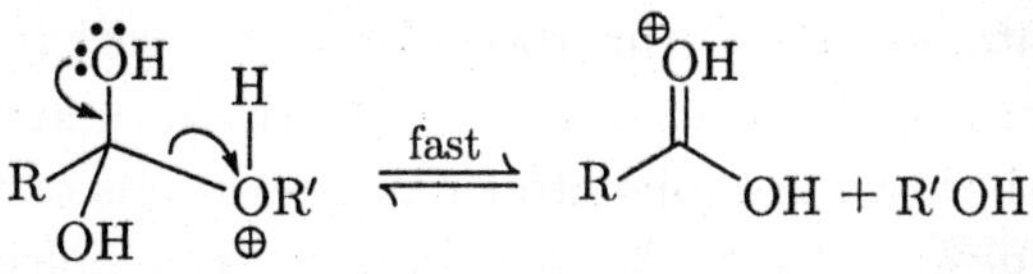

Step 4 : 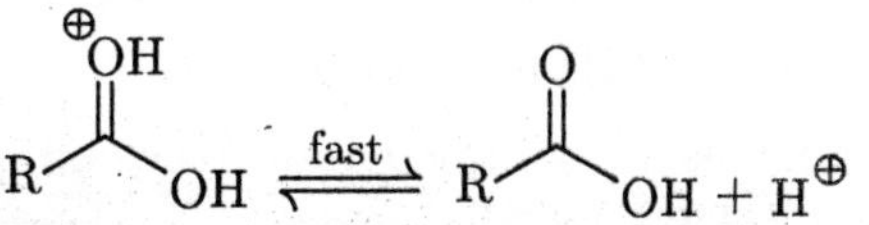

Rate = k[ester] $[H_2O]$ $[H^+]$, when the solvent is not water

Rate = k[ester] $[H^+]$, when the solvent is water. Water is taken in **excess** when used as solvent and hence the rate of the reaction becomes zero order with respect to water then.

Examples :

(a) 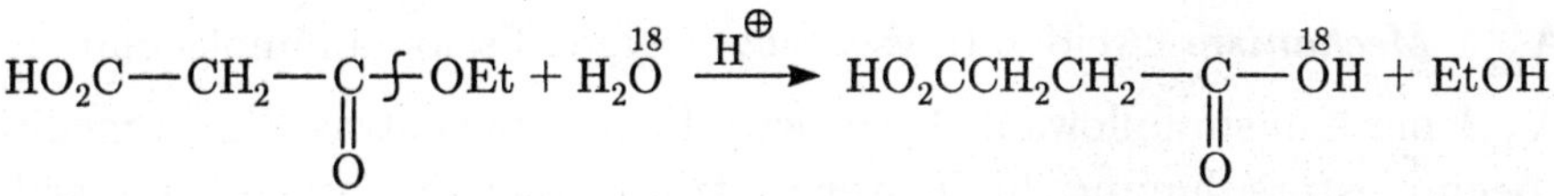

(b) 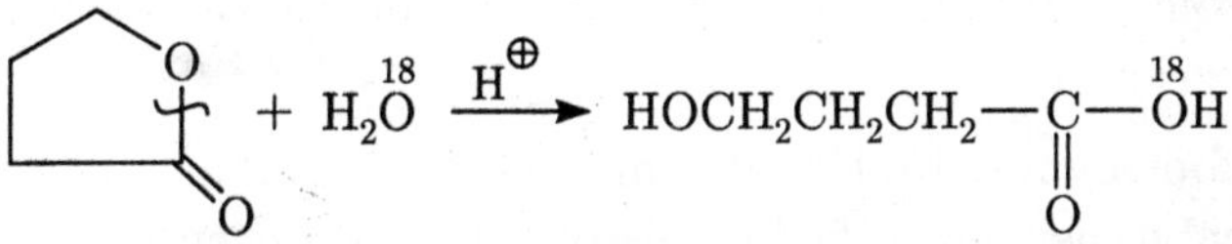

The product profile and the scrambling of ^{18}O suggest that hydrolysis proceeds *via* $A_{Ac}2$ pathway. The formation of optically active R′OH where R′ is asymmetric with *full retention of configuration* suggests that alkyl oxygen bond is not cleaved, as there would have been racemisation of $R'^{\oplus}$. Also, when H_2O^{18} is used as a solvent, unlabelled R′OH is formed not $R'O^{18}H$ which also supports acyl-oxygen cleavage, not alkyl-oxygen one. The formation of tetrahedral intermediate in the rate determining step can be proved by the following experiment.

$\frac{K}{K_{HOAc}}$	CH_3COOH	nC_3H_7COOH	Me_3COOMe	Me_3CCOOH	$Me_3C—CH(CH_3)COOH$
	1	0.51	0.037	0.023	0.00062

$\frac{K}{K_{HOAc}}$	$Me_3C—CMe_2COOH$	Et_3CCOOH	$(iPr)_2CHCOOH$	$Me_3C—CH(CH_3)COOH$
	0.00013	0.00016	$<10^{-4}$	$<10^{-4}$

With increase in steric crowding, the rate of formation of tetradedral intermediate decreases as the intermediate faces severe steric repulsion with the bulky substituents with tetrahedral bond angle.

2,4,6-tribromobenzoate and 2,4,6-trinitrobenzoates are resistant to $A_{Ac}2$ mode of hydrolysis. A severe steric repulsion arises on the formation of tetrahedral intermediate with either two bromine atoms at *o*-positions or two $-NO_2$ groups at the *o*-positions (*ortho* effect). As acid catalysed bimolecular pathway of hydrolysis follows microscopic reversibility, the above observations hold good for the reverse reaction, *i.e.*, esterification reaction also.

As in $A_{Ac}2$ mechanism, there is a competition between protonation and nucleophilic attack of water (H_2O) to the cationic carbonyl carbon of the protonated ester which is the rate determining step, the overall rate must depend upon the resultant effect of these two steps. The protonation will be retarded if an electron withdrawing group like $-NO_2$ is present at *para* or *meta* positions whereas the step of nucleophilic attack by water will be facilitated. As a result of competition, practically, aromatic esters have no/little effect toward $A_{Ac}2$ hydrolysis if electron withdrawing/donor groups are attached to *m*- or *p*- positions.

3. $A_{Ac}1$ ***Mechanism*** (Acid catalysed acyl oxygen fission–unimolecular) :

$A_{Ac}1$ mechanism follows S_N1 pathway. In the concentrated acid medium, some special esters having high steric strain, such as esters of mesitoic acid (2,4,6- trimethylbenzoic acid) undergo this type of hydrolysis. Bimolecular attack is hindered due to steric strain.

Mesitoic acid, is stubbornly resistant to attempted esterifications under ordinary conditions, but it may be easily esterified by dissolving it in concentrated sulphuric acid and then pouring the resulting solution into cold methanol. Conversely, the methyl ester of this acid, which can be saponified only with extreme difficulty, may be hydrolysed simply by dissolving in concentrated sulphuric acid and diluting this solution with ice cold water.

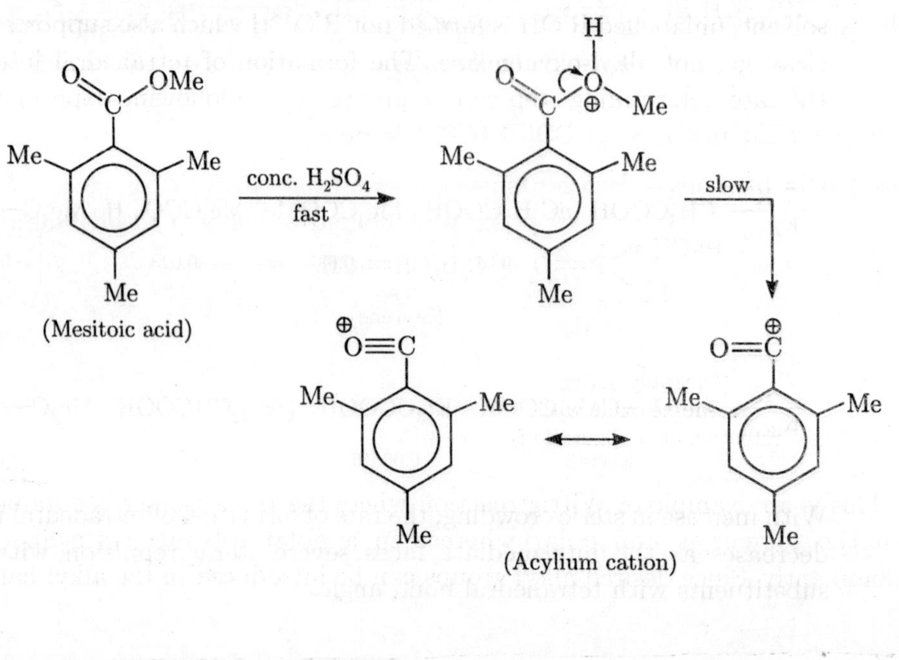

(Mesitoic acid)

(Acylium cation)

($-\overset{\oplus}{C}=O$ group is linear and lies in the plane of benzene ring and the attacking reagents may approach the carbonyl carbon perpendicular to the plane of the ring, essentially without hindrance).

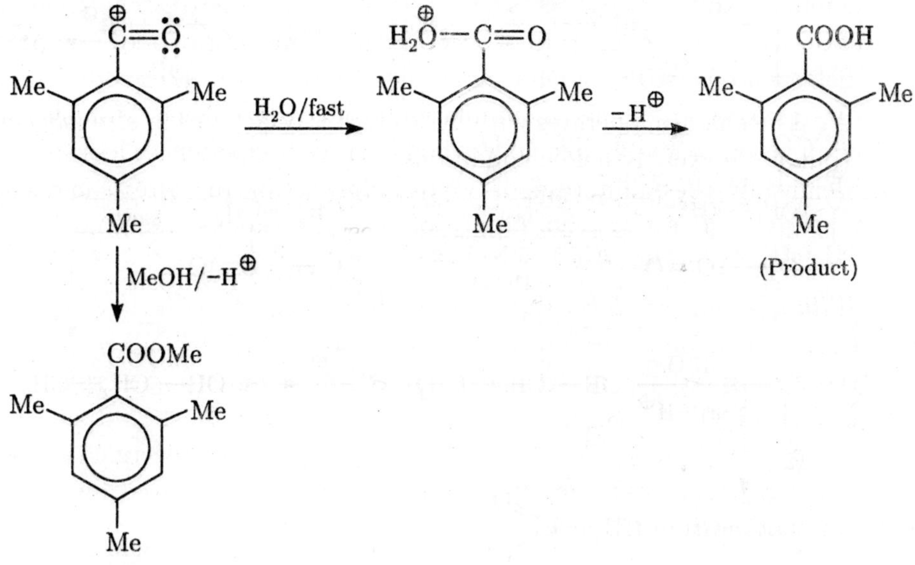

If the acyl carbocation generated gets adjacent group favourable for reaction, often ring closure occurs instead of hydrolysis.

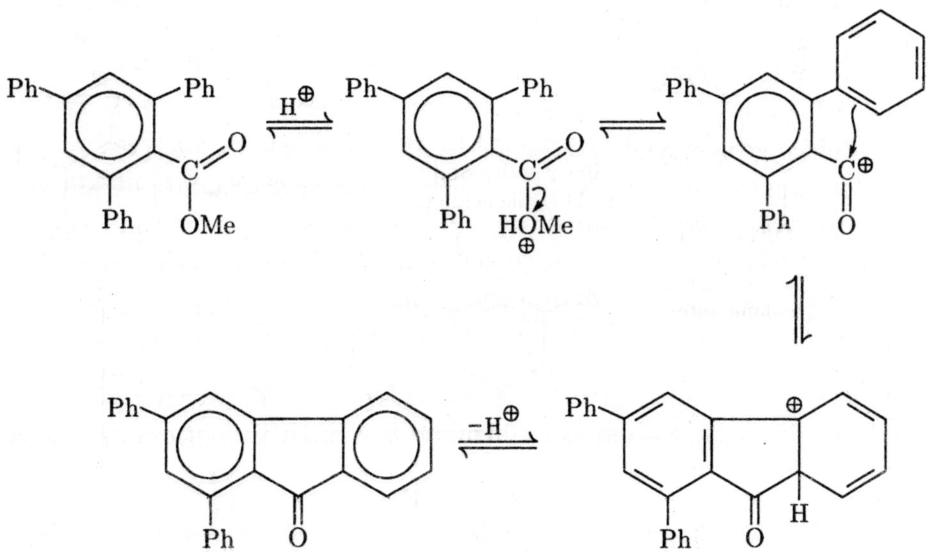

Hydrolysis of methyl benzoate and methyl *p*-toluate (p-$CH_3C_6H_4CO_2Me$) in concentrated H_2SO_4 containing small amount of water follow $A_{Ac}1$ pathway, through the formation of acylium cation.

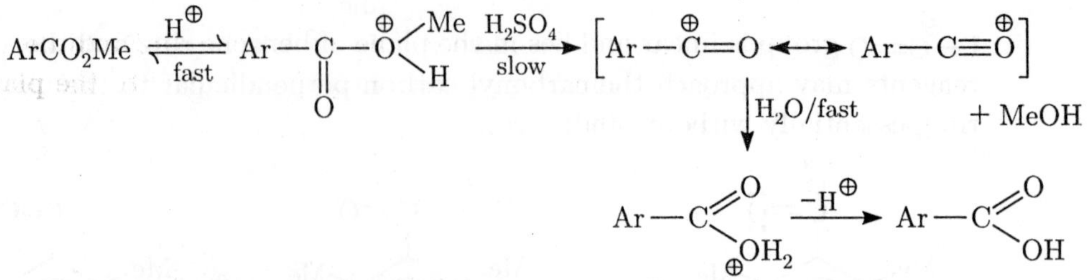

$A_{Ac}1$ mechanism operates with hydrolyses of β-lactones in *strongly acid* solutions (but *not* in weakly acidic conditions).

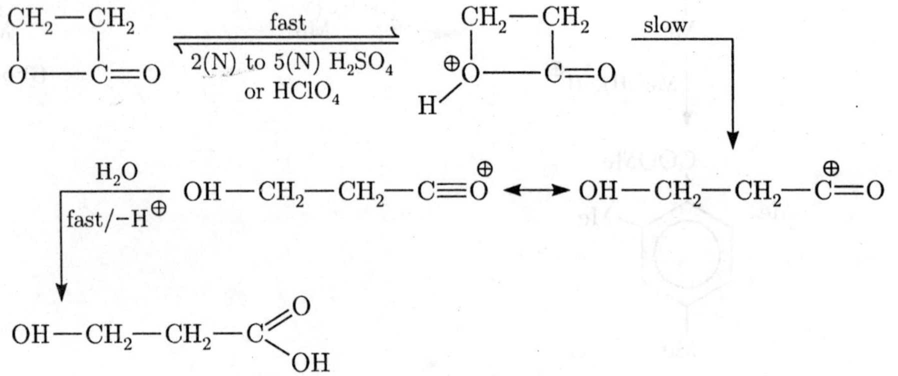

The mechanism is evident from the fact that if H_2O^{18} is used *no incorporation of* ^{18}O occurs at the *β-OH group of resulting acid.*

The following ester (structurally similar to mesitoic ester) undergoes $A_{Ac}1$ mode of hydrolysis.

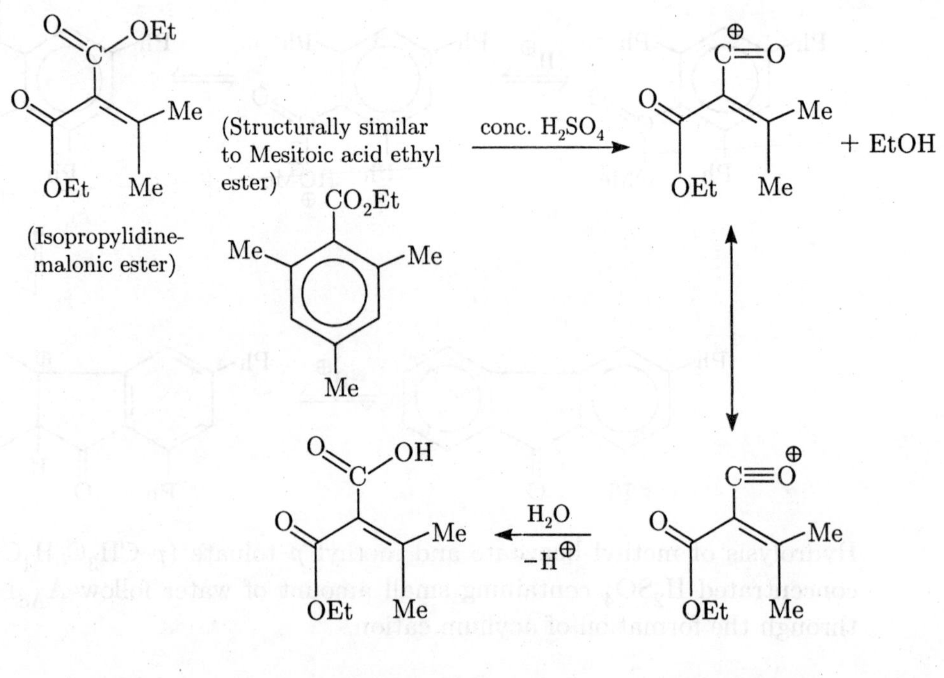

Acetates of phenols or of primary alcohols follow $A_{Ac}1$ pathway when hydrolysed under concentrated (>90%) sulphuric acid (H_2SO_4). However, under dilute sulphuric acid (H_2SO_4) conditions the mechanism followed is $A_{Ac}2$. $A_{Ac}1$ is rarely visited. When acids (or esters) are dissolved in $FSO_3H–SbF_5–SO_2$ (Olah's super acid) at 60°C, acylium cation is formed follwed by elimination of water.

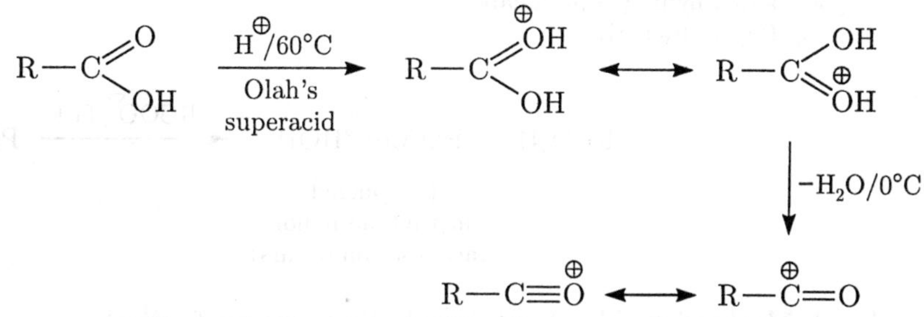

4. $B_{AL}1$ ***Mechanism*** (Base catalysed alkyl oxygen fission–unimolecular)

$B_{AL}1$ mechanism follows S_N1 pathway. When O—R′ group of the substrate esters forms a stable carbocation, *e.g.*, tertiarybutyl cation, allylic or benzylic cation, $B_{AL}1$ mechanism is followed. But even for these substrates, $B_{AL}1$ mechanism occurs only in neutral or weakly basic solution, where the rate of attack by $\overset{\ominus}{O}H$ is so slow that the normally slow unimolecular cleavage takes over. The mechanism has been established by kinetic studies, ^{18}O labelling and racemisation of R′.

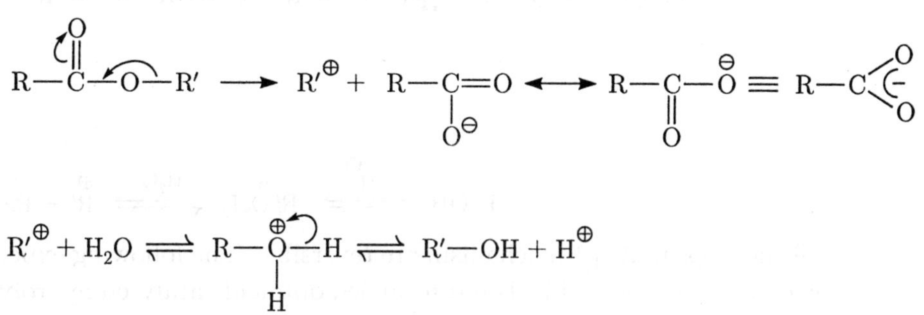

An ester containing optically active R′ group gives racemic alcohol after hydrolysis and if the reaction is carried out in presence of $H_2{}^{18}O$, $R'–{}^{18}OH$ is obtained, which favours the pathway as alkyl oxygen fission. Despite its designation, $B_{AL}1$ mechanism is actually **uncatalysed**.

Example : Hydrolysis of optically active α-phenylethyl hydrogen phthalate in *faintly alkaline* solution, the product found is racemic α-phenylethanol (phenyl-methyl methanol). Racemisation can only occur if the intermediate is an sp^2 hybridised carbocation.

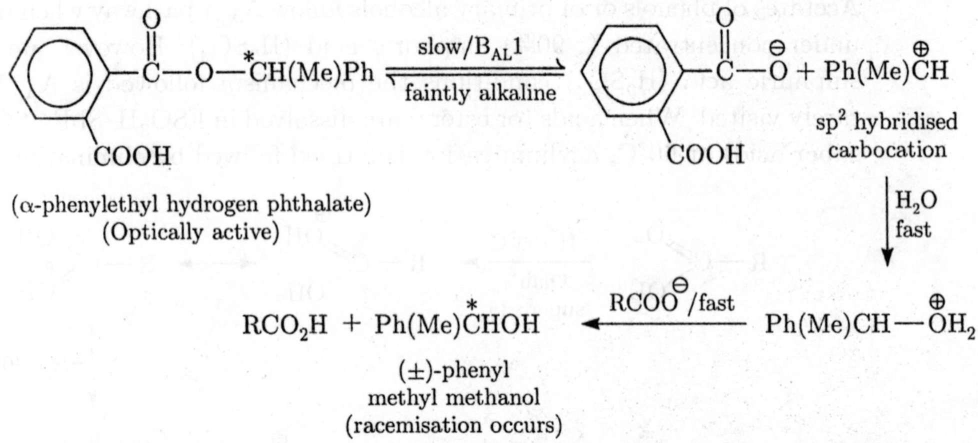

5. $A_{AL}1$ ***Mechanism*** (Acid catalysed alkyl oxygen fission) :

$A_{AL}1$ follows S_N1 pathway. Like $B_{AL}1$, the esters which undergo $A_{AL}1$ mechanism for the hydrolysis, stable carbocations are formed through alkyl-oxygen (O—R′) cleavage. Secondary benzylic acetates hydrolyse by $A_{Ac}2$ mechanism in dilute sulphuric acid (H_2SO_4), but in concentrated sulphuric acid (H_2SO_4), the mechanism changes to $A_{Al}1$. This type of hydrolysis is fairly common.

$$\text{Rate} = k[\text{ester}]$$

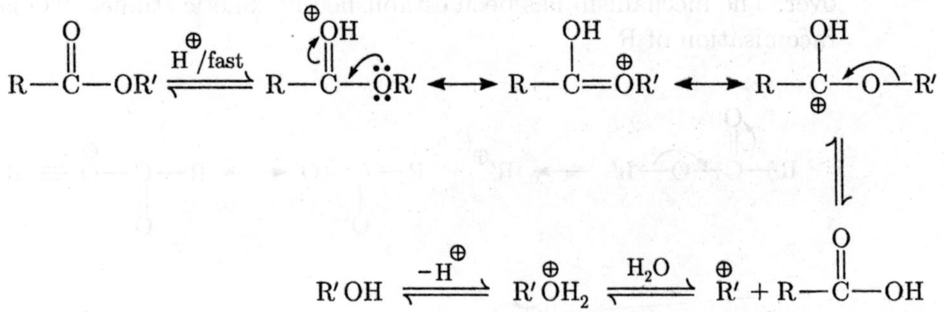

All the steps in $A_{AL}1$ mechanism are reversible. The following experiment shows evidence in support of it. Bunton carried out acid catalysed hydrolysis of *t*-butyl acetate in water enriched with ^{18}O and obtained tertiarybutanol containing ^{18}O.

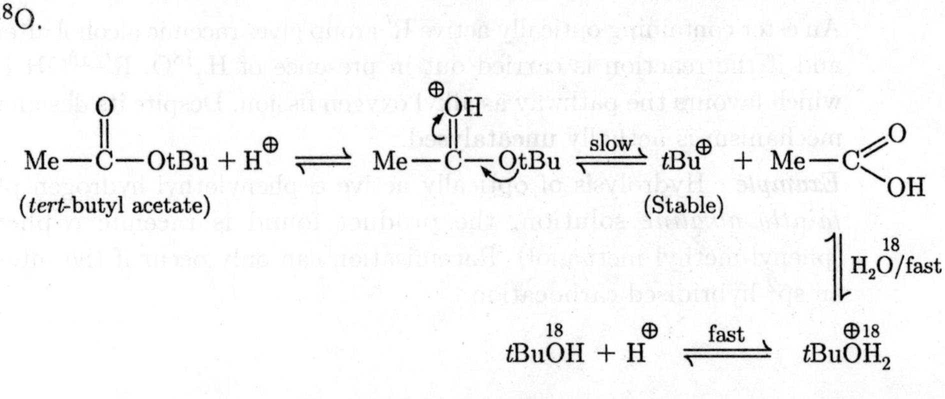

The $A_{AL}1$ mechanism is common for esters of tertiary alcohols as these form relatively stable carbocations.

6. $B_{Ac}1$ *Mechanism* (Base catalysed acyl oxygen fission unimolecular)

   This mode of hydrolysis is not observed.

7. $B_{AL}2$ *Mechanism* (Base catalysed alkyl oxygen fission-bimolecular)

   $B_{AL}2$ mechanism follows S_N2 pathway, and is very rare. $B_{AL}2$ requires $OH^{\ominus}$ ion to attack an alkyl carbon through an S_N2 pathway. $B_{AL}2$ has been seen in the hydrolysis of β-lactones under neutral conditions. Cleavage of C—O bond in the transition state opens the four-membered ring and relieves the ring strain.

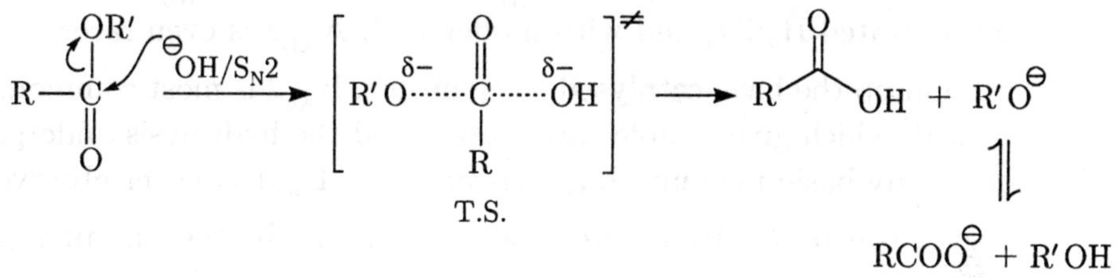

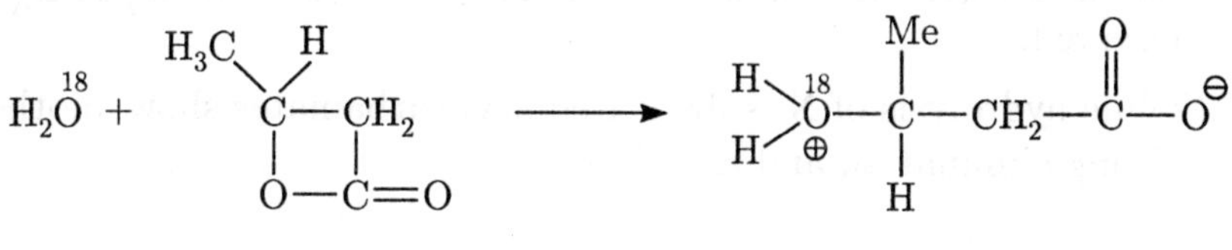

(+)-β-Bulyrolactone

Alkaline hydrolysis of methyl 2,4,6-tritertiarybutylbenzoate follows $B_{AL}2$ mechanism.

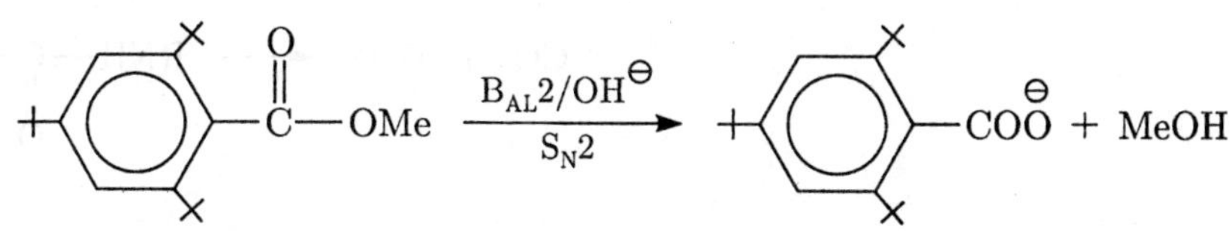

Another example is the reaction between methyl benzoate and NaOMe in MeOH (transesterification reaction). The products are dimethyl ether and sodium benzoate which can be explained by $B_{AL}2$ mechanism.

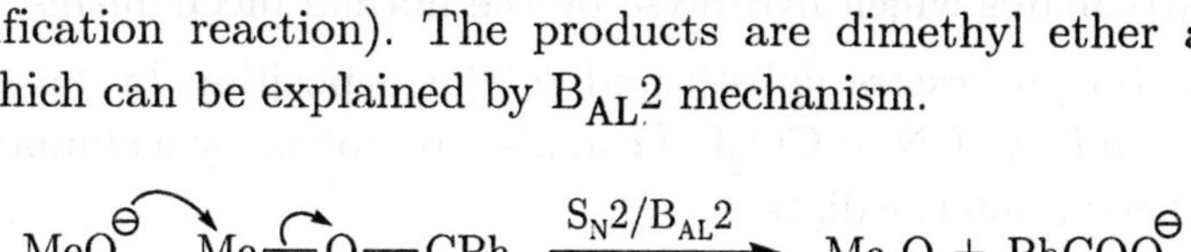

8. $A_{AL}2$ ***Mechanism*** (Acid catalysed alkyl-oxygen fission, bimolecular)

$A_{AL}2$ is very rare and requires water as a nucleophile in an S_N2 pathway.

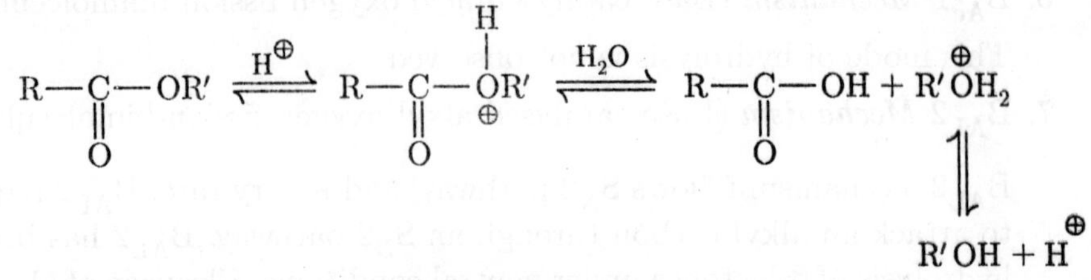

To sum up. the **acid-catalysed** mechanisms, $A_{Ac}2$ and $A_{AL}1$ are common. $A_{AL}1$ gives stable carbocation and $A_{AL}2$ is all the rest. $A_{Ac}1$ is rare, found only in concentrated H_2SO_4 and with hindered R. $A_{AL}2$ is even rarer.

To sum up the **base-catalysed** mechanisms, $B_{Ac}2$ is most common. $B_{AL}1$ occurs with R′ which gives stable carbocation and the hydrolysis undergoes in neutral or weakly basic medium. $B_{AL}2$ is very rare. $B_{Ac}1$ is never observed.

The above observations are true in solution. In the gas phase, reactions of carboxylic esters along with aromatic esters with $\overset{\ominus}{O}Me$ takes place only by $B_{AL}2$ mechanism. The reaction is actually a transsterification reaction. When $\overset{\ominus}{O}Me$ ion is solvated with a single molecule of MeOH or H_2O, $B_{Ac}2$ mechanism is observed.

Alkaline hydrolysis of N- substituted aryl carbamates show another mechanism involving elimination and addition.

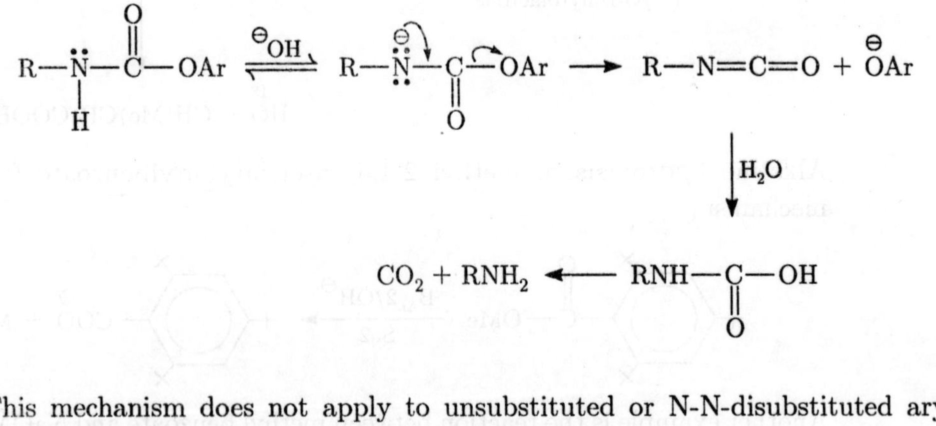

This mechanism does not apply to unsubstituted or N-N-disubstituted aryl carbamates which hydrolyse by the normal mechanisms.

Carboxylic esters substituted in the α-position by an electron- withdrawing group (*e.g.*, CN or CO_2Et) can also hydrolyse by a similar mechanism involving a ketene intermediate.

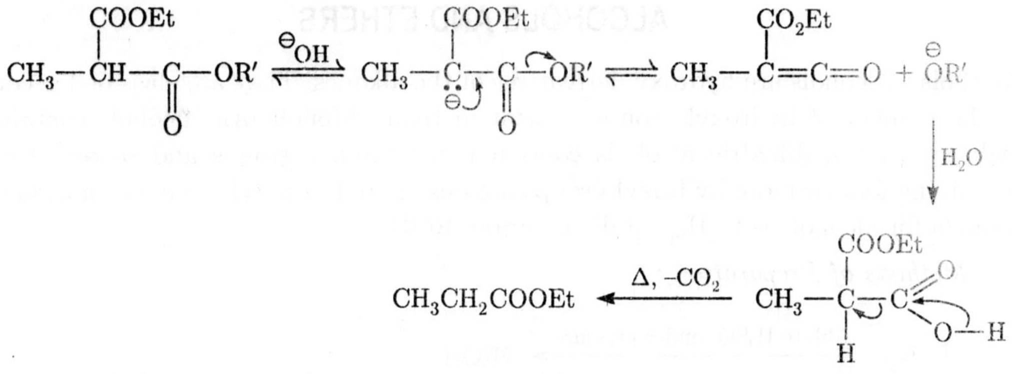

This mechanism is referred as E1cB mechanism.

β-ketoesters are hydrolysed with concommitant decarboxylation.

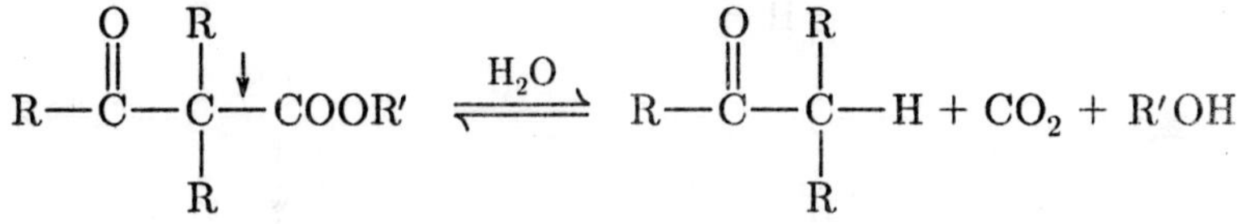

Condition is either acidic, neutral or slightly basic and the product is ketone.

ALCOHOLS AND ETHERS

Alcohols : Alcohols are hydroxy derivatives of the alkanes. They are classified according to the number of hydroxyl groups present in them. Monohydric alcohols contain one hydroxyl group, dihydric alcohols contain two hydroxyl groups and so on. Alcohols containing four or more hydroxyl groups are designated as polyhydric alcohols. General formula for alcohols is $C_nH_{2n+1}OH$ or simply ROH.

Methods of Preparation :

1. $R_2O \xrightarrow{\text{dilute } H_2SO_4 \text{ under pressure}} 2ROH$

Mechanism :

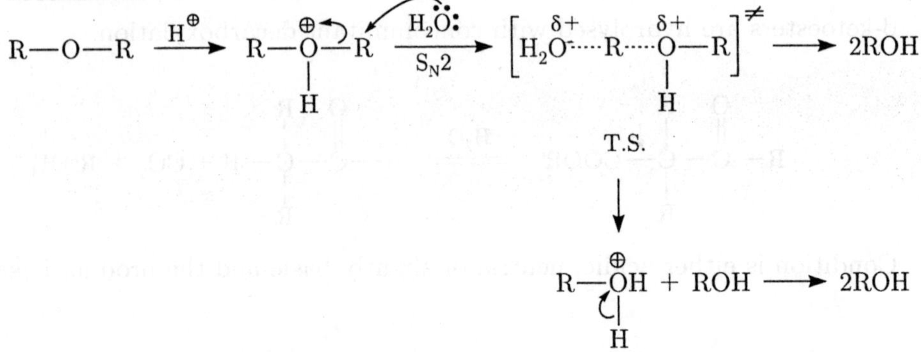

2. $\underset{\text{(Primary amine)}}{RNH_2} \xrightarrow[\text{(HNO}_2\text{)}]{\text{Aqueous NaNO}_2\text{/dil HCl/0°–5°C}} ROH + N_2\uparrow + H_2O$

Mechanism :

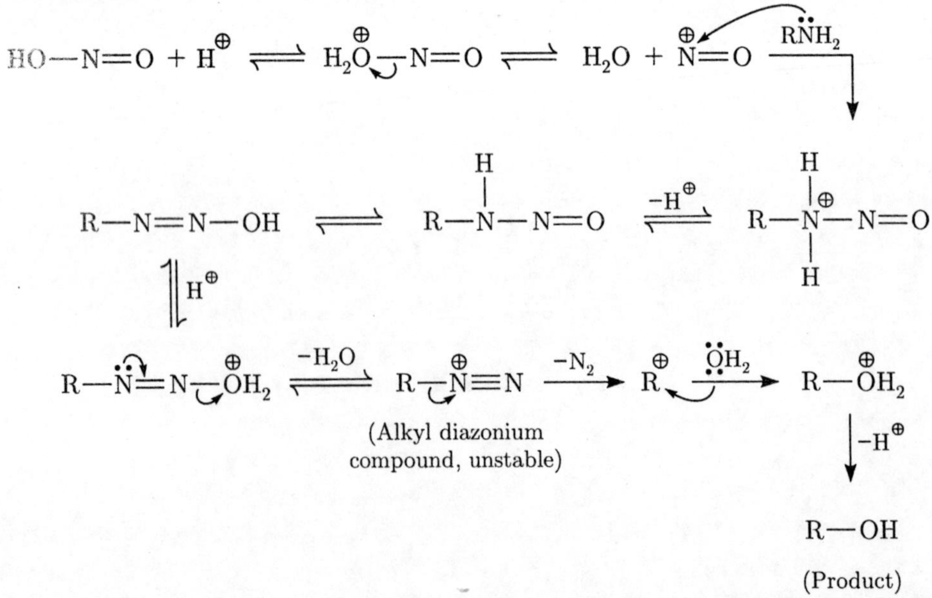

However, carbocation being the intermediate of the reaction, several side products and rearranged products are obtained.

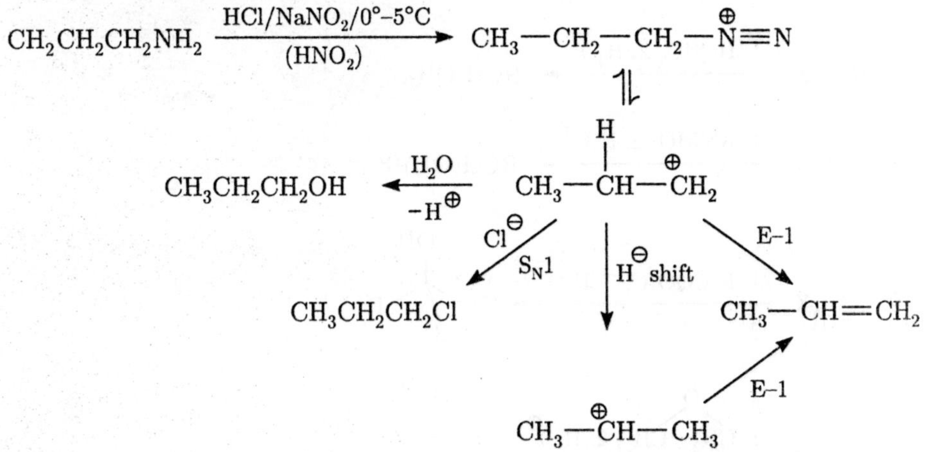

(Stable secondary-carbocation)

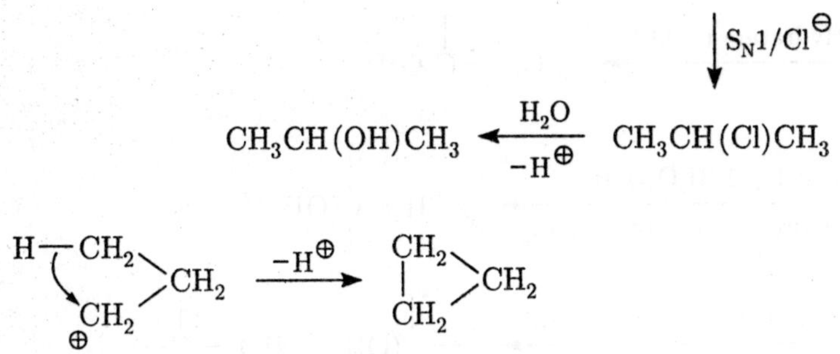

(Ring formation)

3. $RCOOR^1 \xrightarrow[\text{2. } H_3O^{\oplus}]{\text{1. hydrolysis by aqueous alkali(saponification)}} RCOOH + R^1OH$

(Carboxylic acid ester)

$\downarrow$ hydrolysis by dilute H_2SO_4

$RCOOH + R^1OH$

4. $RCHO \xrightarrow[\text{or } (Me_2CHO)_3Al\text{/isopropanol or Na/EtOH}]{LiAlH_4\text{/dry ether or } NaBH_4\text{/ether or water}} RCH_2OH$

(reduction of –CHO group to $-CH_2OH$)

5. 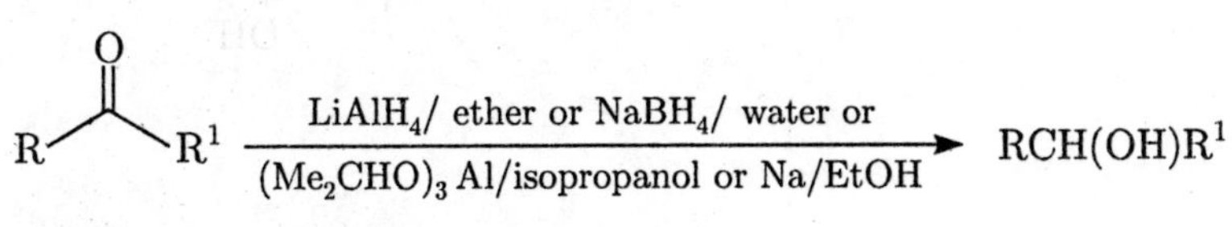

$$6.\ \ RCOOH \xrightarrow[\text{or Na/EtOH}]{1.\ LiAlH_4/Et_2O,\ 2.\ H_3O^{\oplus}} RCH_2OH + R'OH$$

$$7.\ \ RMgX \xrightarrow{1.\ HCHO,\ 2.\ H_3O^{\oplus}} RCH_2OH$$

$$8.\ \ RMgX \xrightarrow{1.\ R'CHO,\ 2.\ H_3O^{\oplus}} RCH(OH)R'$$

9. 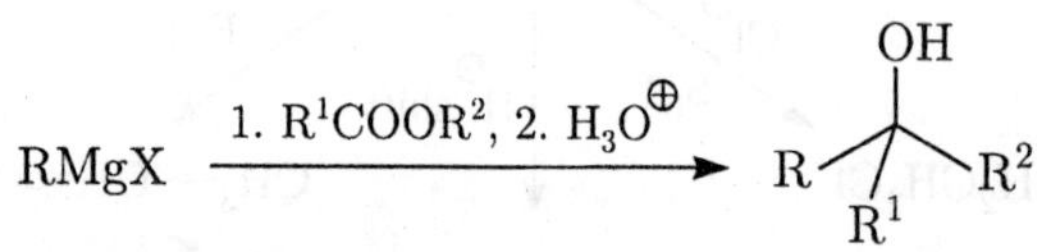

10. 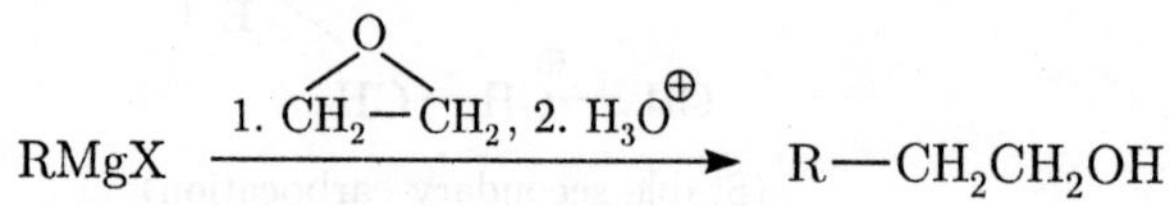

11. 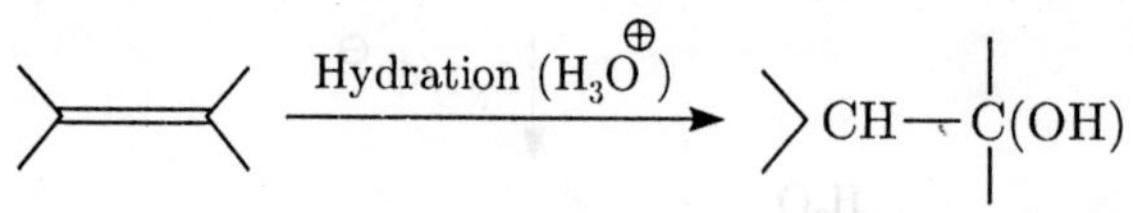

12. 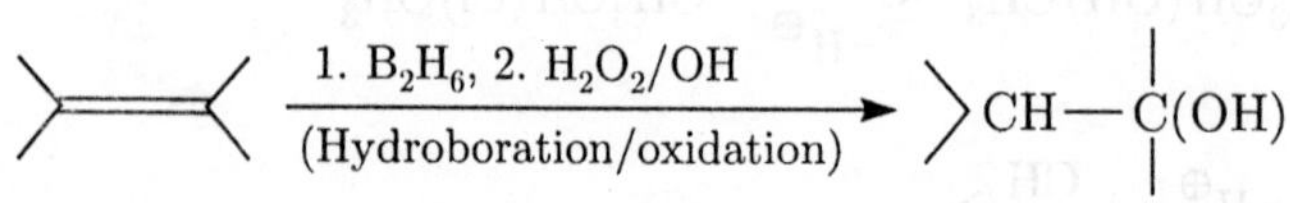

13. 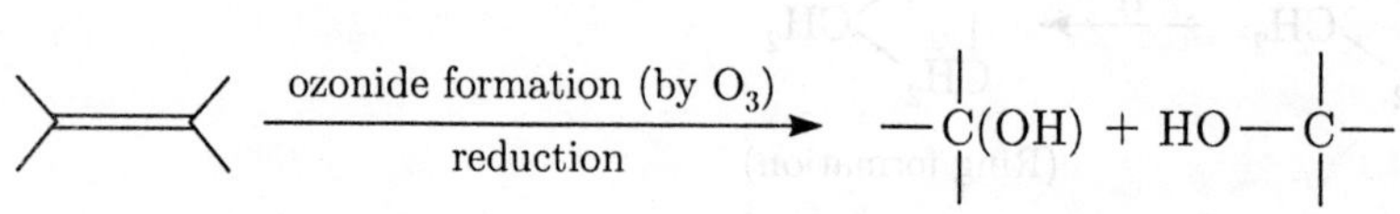

14. 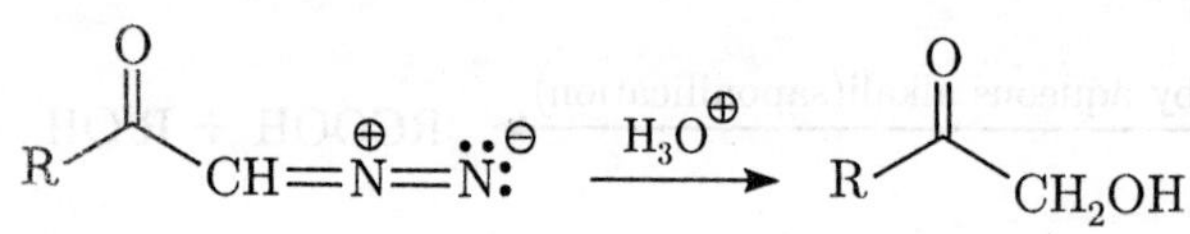

Formation of 1, 2-glycols

1. 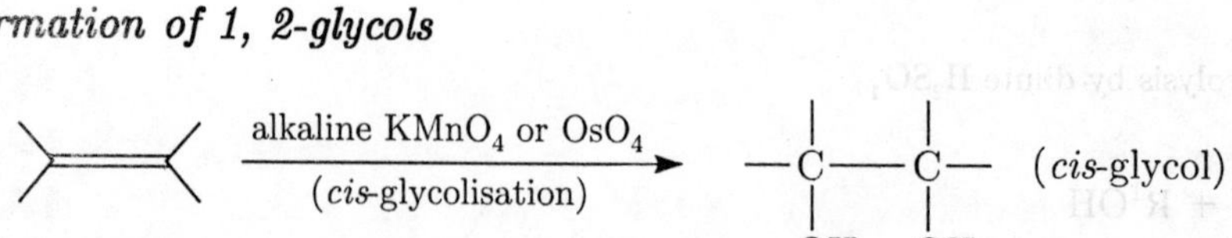

2. 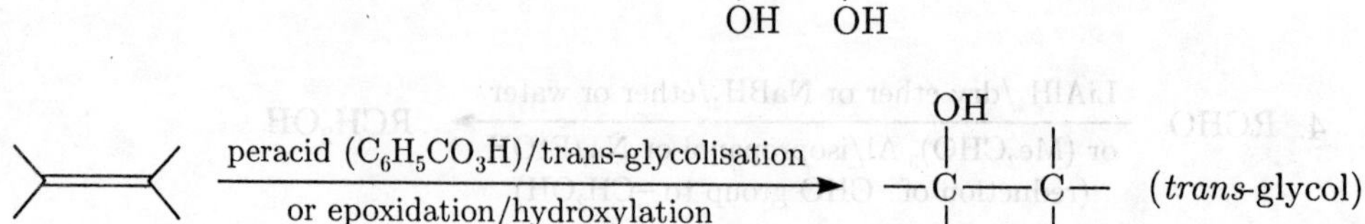

3. $CH_3-CH{=}CH_2 \xrightarrow{Cl_2/\text{polar mechanism}} CH_3CH(Cl)CH_2Cl \xrightarrow{\text{Aqueous } Na_2CO_3} CH_3CH(OH)CH_2OH$

(Propene)

4. $Me_2C{=}O \xrightarrow{1.\ Mg/\text{dry } Et_2O,\ 2.\ H_3O^{\oplus}} Me_2C(OH)-C(OH)Me_2$ (Pinacol)

(Acetone)

5. 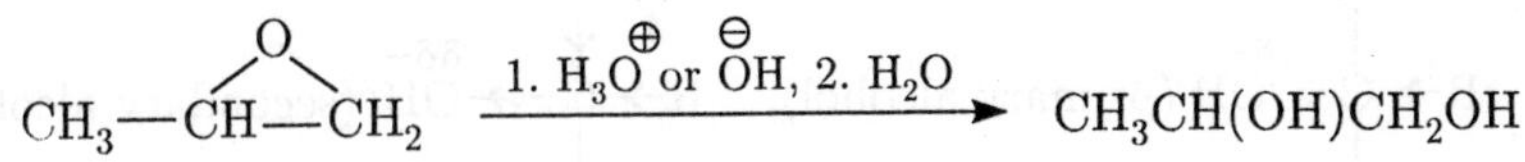

(a) Acid catalysed Mechanism :

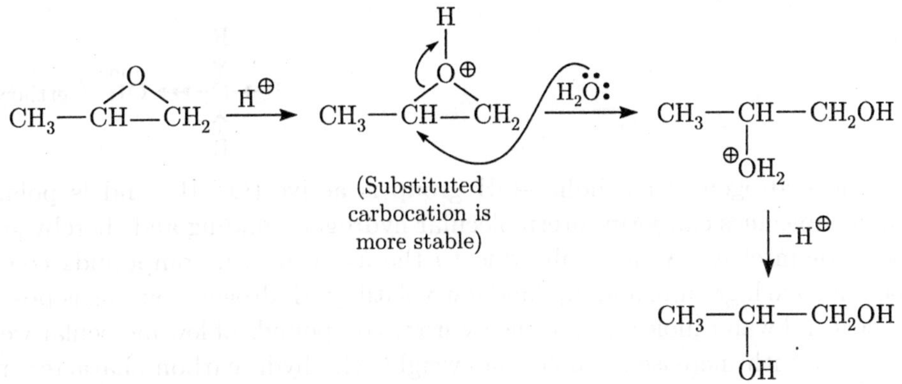

(b) Base catalysed Mechanism :

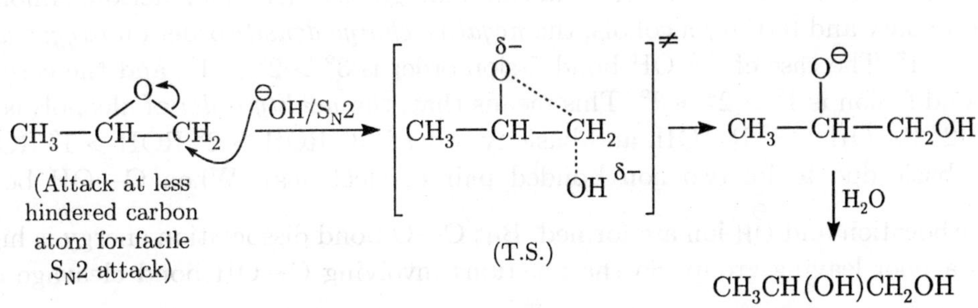

6. 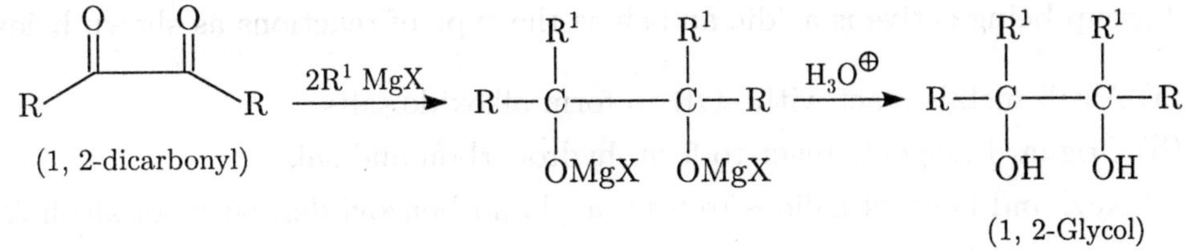

Structure, Reactivity and Physical Properties of Monohydroxy Alcohols

Alcoholic –OH group contains C—O sigma bond and O—H sigma bond and both the bonds are polar where oxygen atom is the negative pole and carbon or hydrogen is the positive pole. The carbon atom may be primary, secondary or tertiary and the alcohols are classified accordingly as primary, secondary and tertiary alcohols. The order of partial positive charge on the carbon atoms bearing the –OH group is primary > secondary > tertiary. The (+I) effect of the alkyl groups in secondary and tertiary alcohls reduces the partial positive charge on carbon.

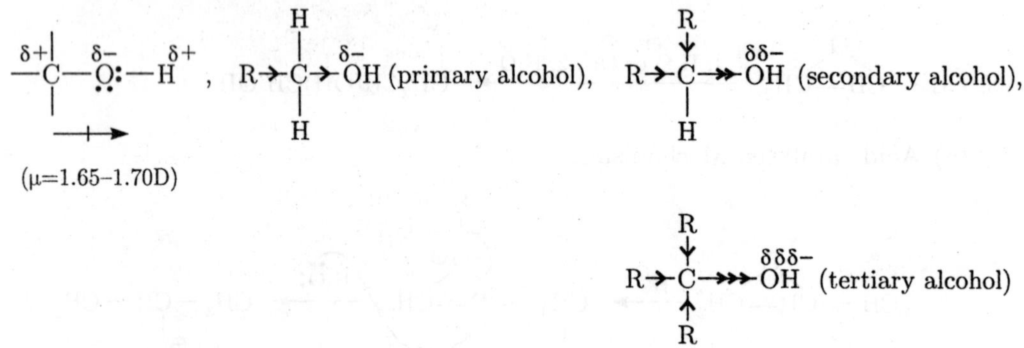

(μ=1.65–1.70D), (primary alcohol), (secondary alcohol), (tertiary alcohol)

The hydrogen of alcoholic –OH group is active (O—H bond is polar) and thus, alcohol molecules can form intermolecular hydrogen bonding and thereby get associated among themselves. As a result (due to the association), compounds containing –OH function have high m.p. and b.p. and low volatility. Hydrogen bonding is possible between alcohols and water molecules, so the hydroxy compounds of low molecular weight dissolve in water. With increase in molecular weight, the hydrocarbon character increases and *London force* (*vander Waals force*) also increases. As a result, m.p and b.p increase but solubility in water decreases. So far as the structure of C—O—H moiety is concerned, the C—OH as well as CO—H bond can undergo cleavage in a reaction. Among primary, secondary and tertiary alcohols, the *negative charge density* order on *oxygen atom* is 3° > 2° > 1°. The ease of C—OH bond fission order is 3° > 2° > 1°, and the ease of CO—H bond fission is 1° > 2° > 3°. This means that, the *acidity order* of alcohols is 1° R—OH > 2° R—OH > 3° R—OH, and basicity order is 3° ROH > 2° ROH > 1° ROH (alcohol is basic due to its two non bonded pair of electrons). When C—OH bond breaks, carbocation and $\overset{\ominus}{O}H$ ion are formed. But C—O bond dissociation energy is high and $\overset{\ominus}{O}H$ is a poor leaving group. So the reactions involving C—OH bond cleavage are usually acid-catalysed. On protonation $C—\overset{\oplus}{O}H_2$ is formed which now holds a good leaving group (H_2O) and nucleophilic substitution reactions occur readily. The hydrogen atom of O—H group being active is acidic and show the type of reactions as shown below.

(a) Alkali metals react with –OH to form alkoxide salts.

(b) Grignard reagents react to form hydrocarbon and salt.

(c) Acyl and benzoyl halides to form acyl and benzoyl derivative of alcohols.

Besides this, *β-hydrogen* of alcohols is *slightly active* because of the (–I) effect of the –OH group. For this reason, alcohols undergo *β-elimination* reactions to form *alkenes.*

Oxidation number of alcohols :

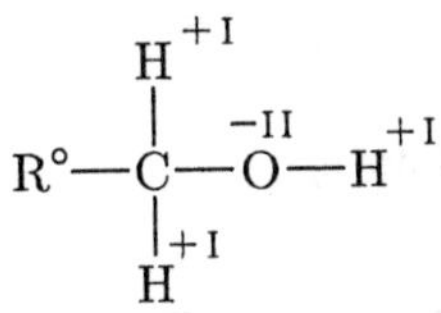

(primary alcohol)

(Oxidation number)

(O. N.) of carbon=O+I–I–I=–I

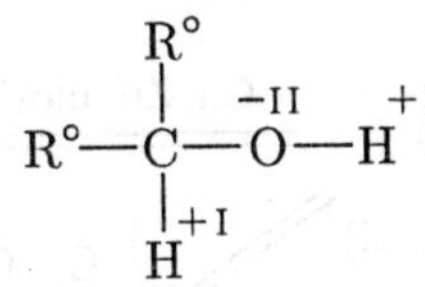

(secondary alcohol),

O. N. of carbon=+I –I+O+O=O

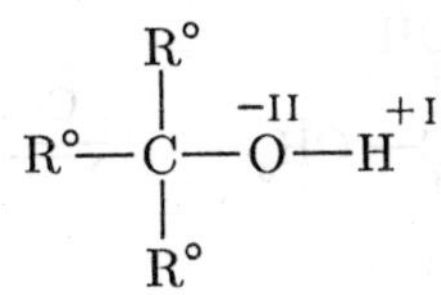

(tertiary alcohol)

O. N. of carbon=+I+O+O+O=+I

Carbon in CO_2 has maximum oxidation number (+IV) and minimum oxidation number in CH_4 (–IV). Oxidation number of carbinol carbon atom in primary, secondary and tertiary alcohols are –1, 0 and +1 respectively. Therefore alcohols may undergo *both oxidation* and *reduction reactions.*

Chemical reactions given by Alcohols

1. ***Conversion of –CH(OH) group to —CO— group by dehydrogenation*** : Catalytic removal of hydrogen from a compound is called dehydrogenation. Some metals like Cu, Fe, Pd, Ni etc. adsorb hydrogen in their metal lattices and form a solution of the gas in solid. These solutions of hydrogen in metal have strong reducing properties which indicate that the hydrogen present in the lattice is in the atomic form; these metals are capable of breaking C—H or O—H bonds. When the vapour of an alcohol is passed over copper gauze at an elevated temperature, the metal takes up two hydrogen atoms from a molecule of the alcohol by breaking the O—H bond and the other by breaking the α- C—H bond, and as a result, a *carbonyl compound* is obtained. *Primary alcohol* gives an *aldehyde, a* secondary alcohol *forms a* ketone, while a *tertiary alcohol* gives an *alkene* by dehydration since it has no α–hydrogen. In practice, instead of a pure metal, usually *zinc-copper alloy* is used. The reaction is reversible. Carbonyl compounds have lower boiling points than the parent alcohols and so can be distilled out, and the unconverted alcohols are recycled. If however, a mixture of air and the alcohol vapour is used instead of alcohol vapour alone, the oxygen of air combines with hydrogen and forms water.

(a) $$\underset{\text{(Primary alcohol)}}{R{-}CH_2OH} \xrightarrow{\text{Cu–Zn alloy, 300°–325°C}} \text{RCHO (Aldehyde)}$$

$$\underset{\text{(Primary alcohol)}}{R{-}CH_2OH} \xrightarrow{\frac{1}{2}O_2,\ \text{Cu or Ag, 600°C}} \text{RCHO (Aldehyde)} + H_2O$$

(b) $$\underset{\text{(Secondary alcohol)}}{R_2CHOH} \xrightarrow{\text{Cu–Zn alloy, 300°–325°C}} R_2CO\ \text{(Ketone)}$$

$$\underset{\text{(Secondary alcohol)}}{R_2CHOH} \xrightarrow{\frac{1}{2}O_2,\ \text{Cu or Ag, 600°C}} R_2CO\ \text{(Ketone)} + H_2O$$

(c) 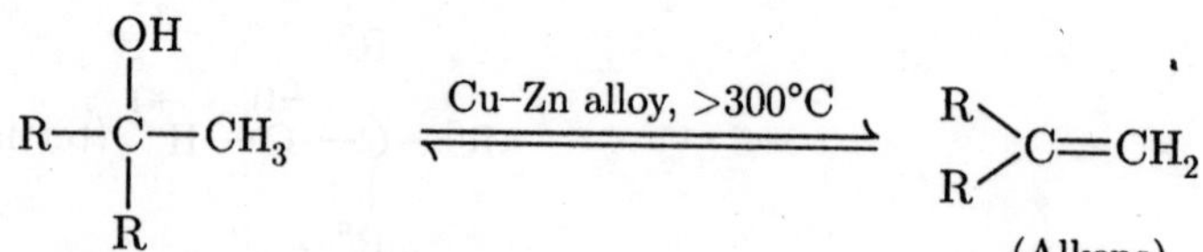

(Alkene)

(Tertiary alchol, no α–H atom)

Mechanism of dehydrogenation reaction :

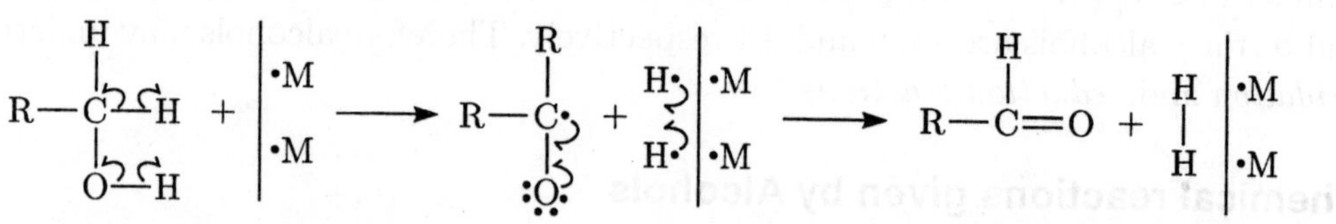

(Metal surface) (Metal surface) (Metal surface)

2. ***Oxidation of alcohols*** (***Conversion*** of ***–CHOH– group to –CO– group***) : Usually alcohols are oxidised to carbonyl compounds by $K_2Cr_2O_7$ or $Na_2Cr_2O_7$ and concentrated sulphuric acid. The carbonyl compound may undergo further oxidation to form a carboxylic acid or a mixture of acids. Primary alcohols on prolonged oxidation give carboxylic acids (*via* aldehyde) having the same number of carbon atoms as the parent alcohols. A secondary alcohol first forms a ketone which on further oxidation gives a mixture of acids each containing a fewer number of carbon atoms than the parent alcohols. On the other hand, a tertiary alcohol, being devoid of α–hydrogen gets dehydrated to the corresponding alkene, the alkene then gets oxidised to a ketone and/or an acid according to the nature of double bonded carbons. Thus, in this case, each of the ketone and the carboxylic acid contains lesser number of carbon atoms than the tertiary alcohol. The ketone so formed will undergo further oxidation to carboxylic acid or acids, each having a fewer number of carbon atoms than the parent ketone.

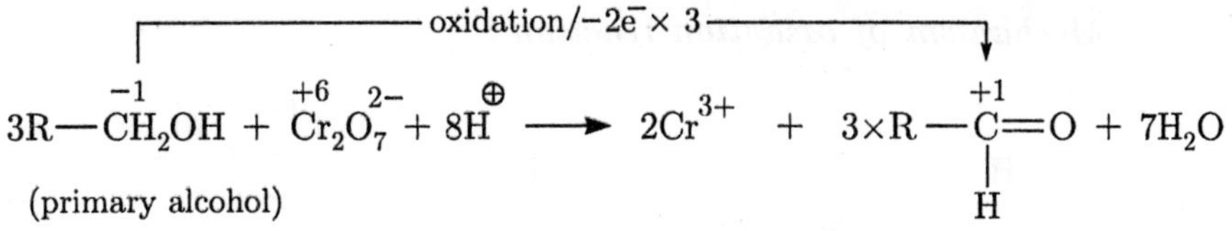

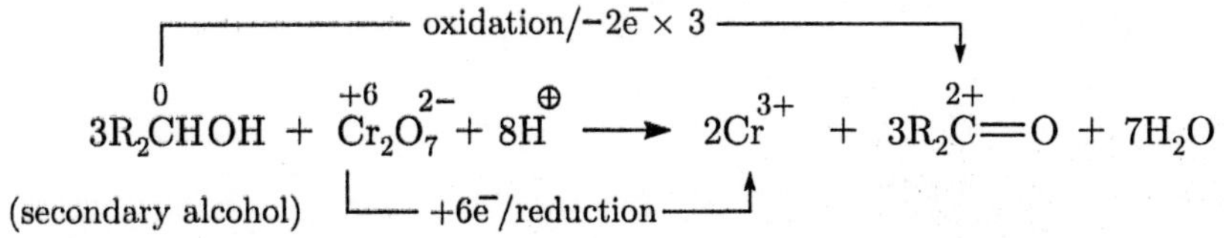

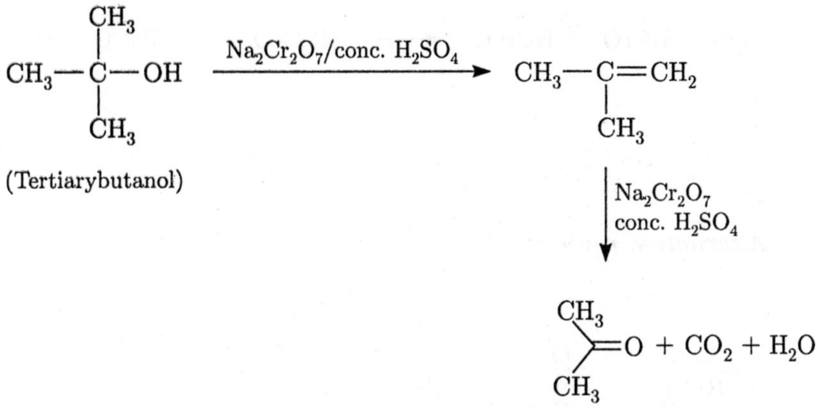

However, a *primary alcohol* may be *oxidised* to the *aldehyde* under mild conditions using *lead tetraacetate in pyridine.*

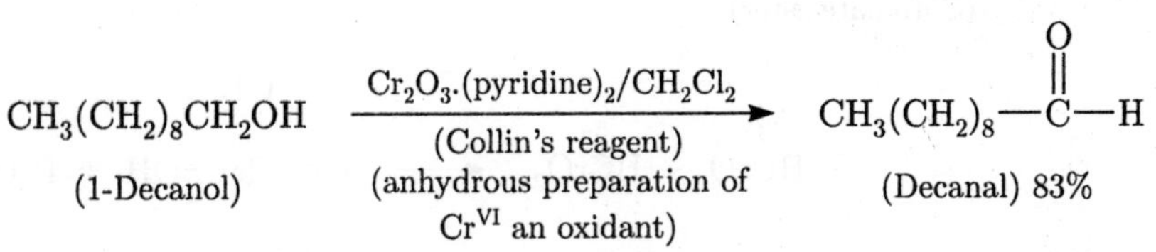

Water promotes the transformation of aldehydes into carboxylic acids because in water, aldehydes are in equilibrium with hydrates formed by addition of water across the C=O double bond.

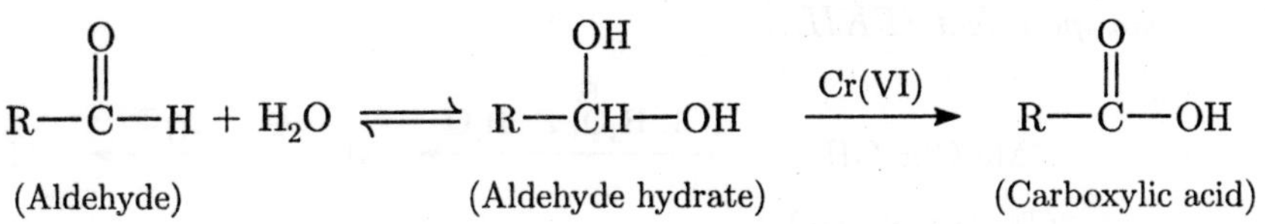

Aldehyde hydrates are really alcohols and therefore can be oxidised just like secondary alcohols. Because of the absence of water in anhydrous reagents such as the Collins reagent, a 1,1-diol does not form and the reaction stops at the aldehyde stage.

Mechanism of oxidation reaction :

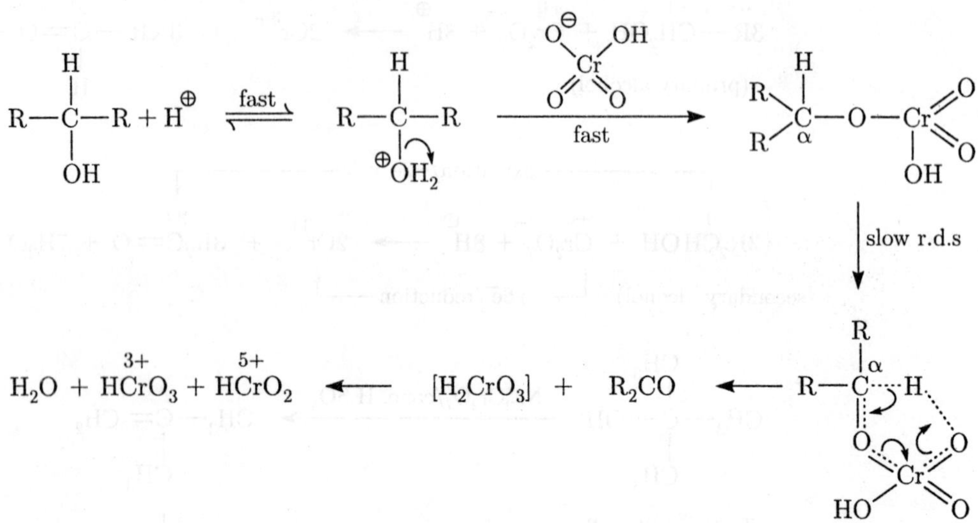

Alternative route :

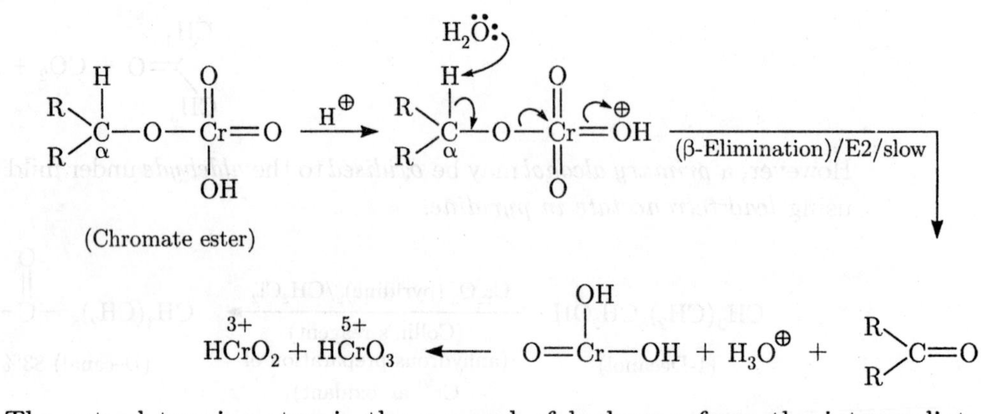

The rate determing step is the removal of hydrogen from the intermediate chromate ester. Me_2CDOH is oxidised at about $^1/_7$ th the rate of either Me_2CHOH or $(CD_3)_2CHOH$. *Thus, the rate determining step involves the fission of the C—H (α-hydrogen) bond. (K_H/K_D= 7.00), and accounts for the primary kinetic isotope effect (PKIE).*

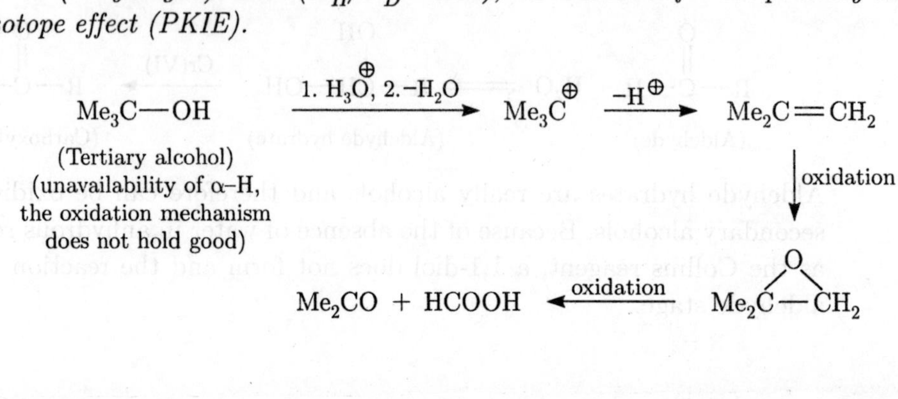

Oxidation to carboxylic acids : Primary alcohols can be oxidised to carboxylic acids using aqueous solutions of chromium (VI) such as aqueous potassium dichromate ($K_2Cr_2O_7$) in acid. Another useful reagent for oxidising primary alcohols to carboxylic acids is potassium permanganate ($KMnO_4$) *in basic solution.*

$$RCH_2OH \xrightarrow{\overset{7+}{KMnO_4}/OH^{\ominus}} R-\overset{\overset{O}{\|}}{C}-O^{\ominus} + \overset{4+}{MnO_2} \xrightarrow{H_3O^{\oplus}} RCOOH$$

Potassium permanganate is not used for the oxidation of secondary alcohols to ketones because many ketones react further with alkaline potassium permanganate ($KMnO_4$) reagent.

3. ***Dehydration of alcohols :*** Alcohols may be dehydrated to alkenes, the ease of dehydration being tertiary > secondary > primary. Dehydration may be effected by heat alone, but in the presence of a catalyst, lower temperatures may be used, *e.g.*, when passed over heated alumina (Al_2O_3) tertiary alcohols are dehydrated at about 150°C, secondary alcohols at 250°C and primary alcohols at 350°C. Also primary alcohols are dehydrated by concentrated sulphuric acid (H_2SO_4) at about 170°C, secondary and tertiary alcohols by boiling dilute H_2SO_4 (this is used to avoid polymerisation of the alkene). Isomerisation, usually occurs with dehydration by acid or alumina, but in the latter case, isomerisation is suppressed by the addition of a small amount of pyridine.

Mechanism of dehydration of primary alcohols :

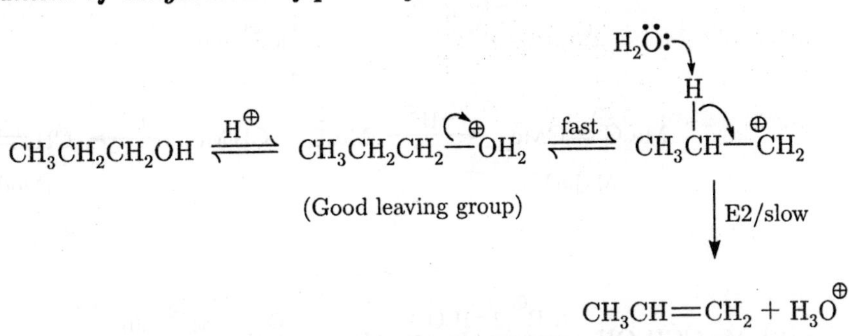

Carbocation is formed as an intermediate, so the rate and ease of dehydration $t > s > p$: this is the order of stabilities of carbocations. With secondary and tertiary alcohols, dehydration may occur in two ways.

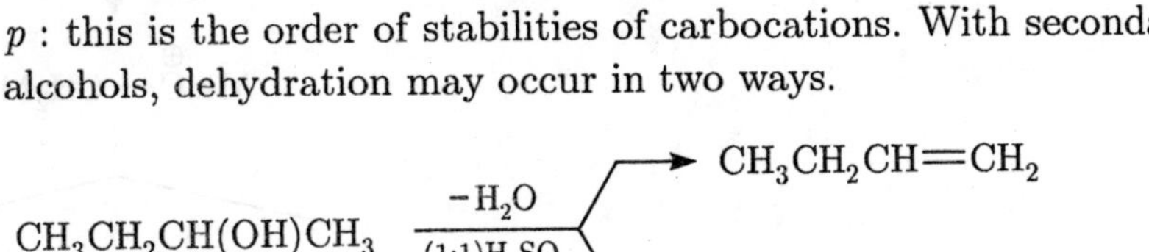

Experiments show that hydrogen attached to the adjacent carbon atom joined to the least number of hydrogen atoms is eliminated most easily. Thus, in the above reaction, the main product is but-2-ene (65–80%). This elimination therefore occurs in accordance with Saytzeff's rule for the dehydrohalogenation of alkyl halides. When thorium or lanthanide metal oxides are used as dehydrating agents, the yield of 1-alkene from secondary alcohols becomes 98%.

Rearrangement often occurs with acid-catalysed dehydration. All the three types of alcohols may behave in this way via a carbocation that may undergo methyl and/or hydride ion 1,2-shift. In the following examples, only methyl shifts are shown (all the possible hydride ion shifts lead finally to the same products resulting from some of the competiting methyl shifts.)

(a) 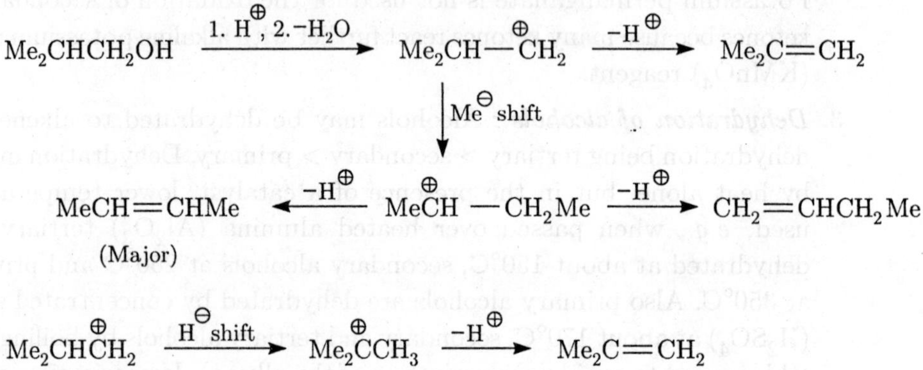

(b) 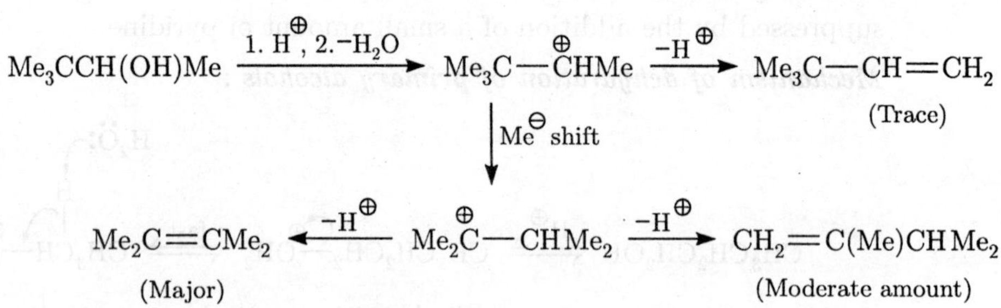

(c) 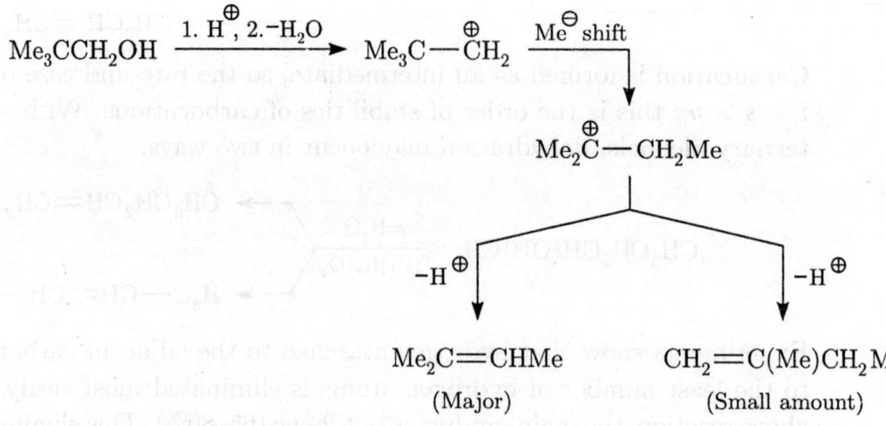

In each case, the major product is in accordance with Saytzeff's rule. The rearrangements occur extremely rapidly, infact, faster than the proton elimination. The ease of anion migration is Ph >> Me > H.

When a double bond is produced in the product accompanied by a 1,2-shift, the reaction is said to be a *retropinacol rearrangement.* This type of rearrangement when occuring in open chain compounds is also sometimes called the *Wagner Rearrangement.* Alcohols may also be converted into alkenes via their esters or xanthates, but in this case, no rearrangements occur.

$$Me_3CCH(OAc)Me \xrightarrow{\Delta} Me_3CCH{=}CH_2$$

Dehydration may be used as the first step in the conversion of a primary alcohol of suitable structure into a secondary or tertiary alcohol, or a secondary alcohol into a tertiary alcohol. Hydroiodic acid (HI) additions are in accordance with Markownikoff's rule.

(a) $MeCH_2CH_2OH \xrightarrow{Al_2O_3/350°C} MeCH{=}CH_2 \xrightarrow{1.\ HI,\ 2.\ AgOH} MeCH(OH)Me$

(b) $Me_2CHCH_2OH \xrightarrow{Al_2O_3/350°C} Me_2C{=}CH_2 \xrightarrow{1.\ HI,\ 2.\ AgOH} Me_3COH$

(c) $Me_2CHCH(OH)Me \xrightarrow{Al_2O_3/350°C} Me_2C{=}CHMe \xrightarrow{1.\ HI,\ 2.\ AgOH} Me_2C(OH)CH_2Me$

The reverse procedure, that is conversion of tertiary to secondary to primary alcohol can be carried out by hydroboronation.

$$Me_2C(OH)CH_2Me \xrightarrow{Al_2O_3/350°C/-H_2O} Me_2C{=}CHMe \xrightarrow{B_2H_6} (Me_2CH{-}CHMe\text{)}_2BH$$

$$(Me_2CH{-}CHMe\text{)}_2BH \xrightarrow{H_2O_2/OH^{\ominus}} \underset{\text{(secondary alcohol)}}{Me_2CH{-}CH(OH)Me}$$

$$(Me_2CH{-}CHMe\text{)}_2BH \xrightarrow{heat} (Me_2CH{-}CH_2{-}CH_2\text{)}_2BH \xrightarrow{H_2O_2/OH^{\ominus}} \underset{\text{(primary alcohol)}}{Me_2CH{-}CH_2CH_2OH}$$

It is also possible to step down the alcohol series by first dehydrating to the alkene which is then subjected to ozonolysis.

$$\text{(a) } RCH_2CH_2OH \xrightarrow{Al_2O_3/350°C} RCH{=}CH_2 \xrightarrow{1.\ O_3,\ 2.\ Zn/H^{\oplus}} RCHO \xrightarrow{H_2/\text{catalyst}} RCH_2OH$$

$$\text{(b) } RCH(OH)CH_3 \xrightarrow{ThO_2/300°C} RCH{=}CH_2 \xrightarrow{1.\ O_3,\ 2.\ Zn/H^{\oplus}} RCHO \xrightarrow{H_2/\text{catalyst}} RCH_2OH$$

The dehydration of alcohols is the reverse of the hydration of the alkenes. Hydration of alkenes and dehydration of alcohols are the forward and reverse of the same reaction.

Any reaction and its reverse proceed by the forward and reverse of the same mechanism. This statement is known as the "*Principle of Microscopic Reversibility*". It follows from this principle that, forward and reverse reactions must have the same intermediates and the rate limiting transition states. Thus, because protonation of the alkene is the rate determining step in alkene hydration, the reverse of this step — loss of the proton from the carbocation intermediate is rate limiting in alcohol dehydration. The principle also requires that if a catalyst accelerates a reaction in one direction, it also accelerates the reaction in the reverse direction. Thus, both hydration of alkenes to alcohols and dehydration of alcohols to alkenes are catalysed by acids. The relative rates of alcohol dehydration are in the order tertiary > secondary > primary. Application of Hammond's postulate suggests that the rate limiting transition state of a dehydration reaction closely resembles the corresponding carbocation intermediate.

Dehydration of Alcohols to form Ethers

$$\underset{\text{(Ethanol) (1°-alcohol)}}{CH_3CH_2OH} \xrightarrow{H_2SO_4/140°C} \underset{\text{(Diethyl ether)}}{CH_3CH_2{-}O{-}CH_2CH_3} + H_2O$$

Secondary and tertiary alcohols can not be used under strong acid condition because they undergo dehydration to alkenes.

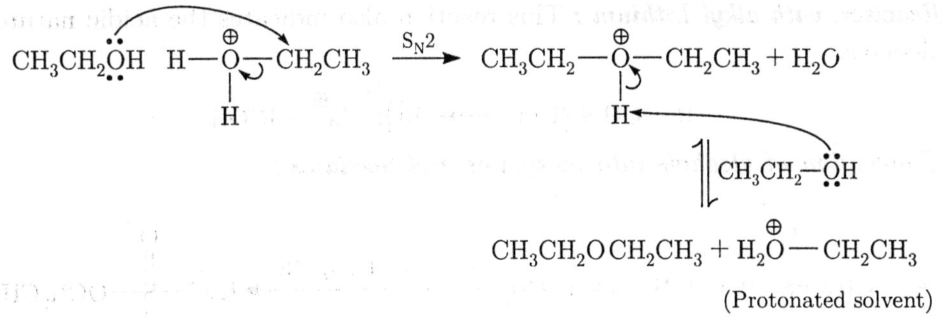

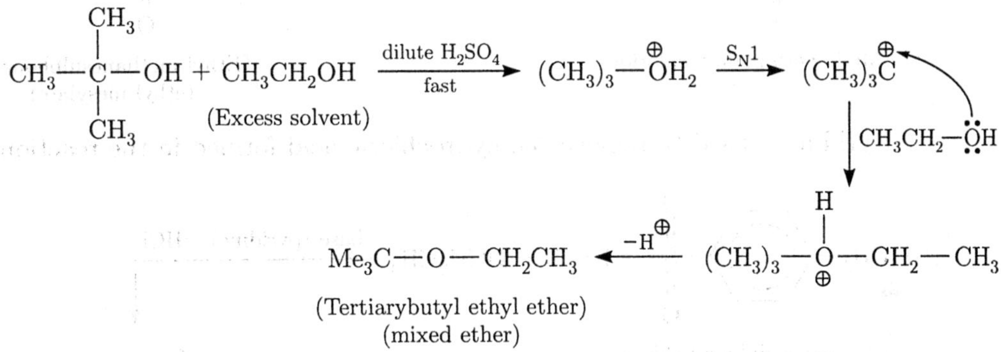

Reactions of alcohols involving O—H cleavage

1. ***Reaction with active metals*** : Sodium, calcium, aluminium etc. metals react with alcohols to form alkoxides and evolve hydrogen gas; water also reacts similarly with these metals. This reaction shows the *acid character* of the alcohols.

$$2ROH + 2Na \text{ (Electropositive metal)} \longrightarrow 2R\overset{\ominus}{O}\,\overset{\oplus}{Na} + H_2\uparrow$$

(Sodium alkoxide)

$$R\overset{\ominus}{O}\,\overset{\oplus}{Na} + H_2O \rightleftharpoons ROH + \overset{\oplus}{Na}\,\overset{\ominus}{OH}$$

Alcohols being extremely weak acids, the alkoxides hydrolyse in water to alcohols and alkalis. The reactions of an alcohol with calcium and aluminium are much slower than the reaction with sodium; the aluminium alkoxides have some synthetic use and are prepared by the action of aluminium amalgam on anhydrous alcohols. The acidity order of the three types of alcohols being primary > secondary > tertiary, a primary alcohol reacts with sodium faster than the corresponding secondary alcohol and the latter in turn reacts more readily than the corresponding tertiary alcohol.

Sodium alkoxides are used in Williamson ether synthesis and aluminium alkoxides are used in Meerwein-Pondorf-Verley reduction and Oppenaur oxidation.

Relative acidity order is as follows : $H_2O \rangle ROH \rangle R{-}C{\equiv}\overset{\ominus}{C}{:} \rangle R\ddot{\underset{..}{O}}{:}^{\ominus} \rangle {:}\overset{\ominus}{\ddot{\underset{..}{O}}}H$ in a decreasing manner.

2. ***Reaction with alkyl Lithium*** : This reaction also indicates the acidic nature of alcohols.

$$R{-}OH + R^1Li \longrightarrow R\ddot{\underset{\cdot\cdot}{O}}{:}^{\ominus}\ Li^{\oplus} + R^1OH$$

3. ***Conversion of alcohols into mesylates and tosylates*** :

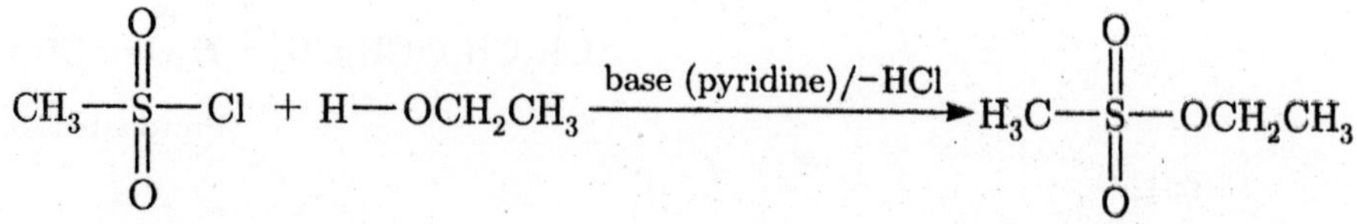

(Methanesulphonyl chloride) (Ethyl methanesulphonate) (ethyl mesylate)

Pyridine is used to remove the hydrochloric acid formed in the reaction.

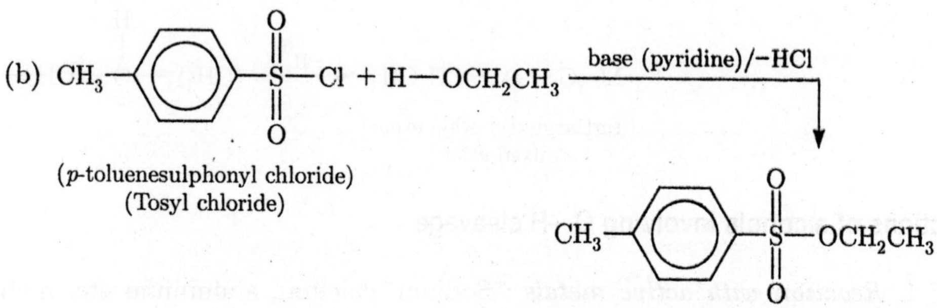

(p-toluenesulphonyl chloride) (Tosyl chloride)

(Ethyl p-toluenesulphonate) (ethyl tosylate)

These are important reactions to activate alcohols toward nucleophilic substitution and β-elimination reactions. *Sulphonate anions* are *good leaving groups* as they are *weak bases*, where arylsulphonic acids are strong acids

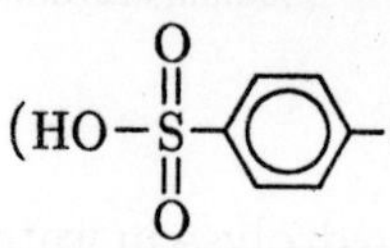 CH_3, p-toluenesulphonic acid, pH < 1).

4. ***Acylation of –OH group*** : The alcoholic –OH group can be acylated by the action of acyl halides or acid anhydrides. Alcohols form esters on acylation and is the *best method for the preparation* of *esters* in general.

$$ROH + R'COCl \xrightarrow{\text{base(pyridine)}} R'COOR + HCl$$

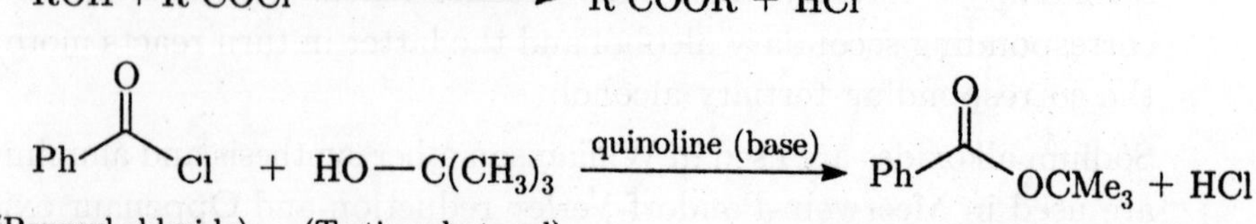

(Benzoyl chloride) (Tertiary butanol)

Pyridine and quinoline are used to remove the hydrochloric acid (HCl) formed in the reaction.

Esters of tertiary alcohols and phenols which cannot be prepared by acid-catalysed esterification, can be prepared by the following method.

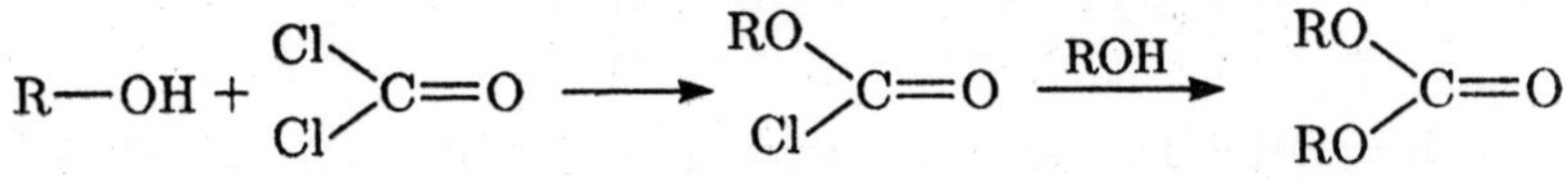

(Chloroformic ester) (Alkyl carbonate)

Benzyloxycarbonyl chloride, an important reagent for protecting the amino function of an amino acid during the synthesis of peptides is synthesized by the following reaction.

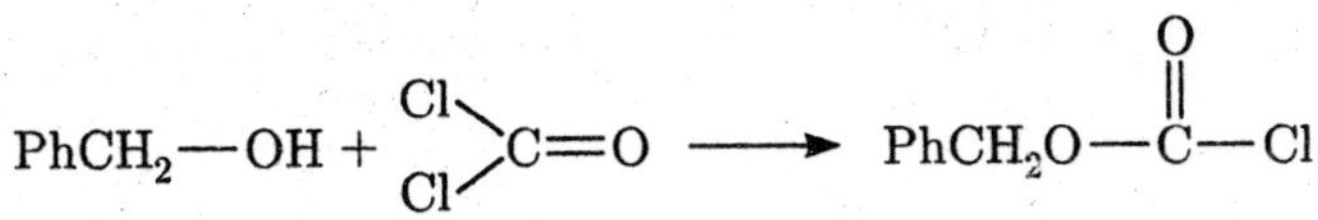

5. ***Benzoylation reaction*** :

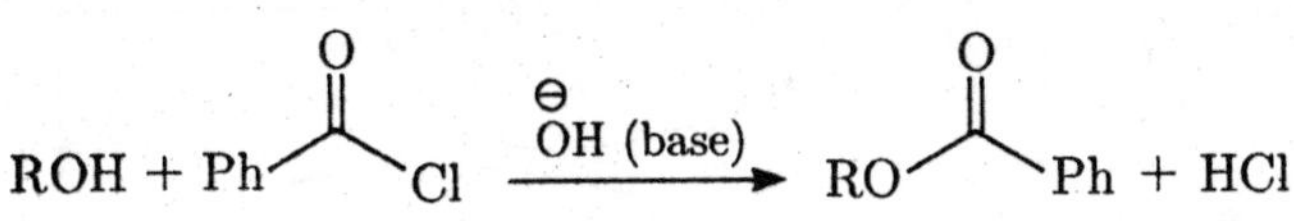

(Product)

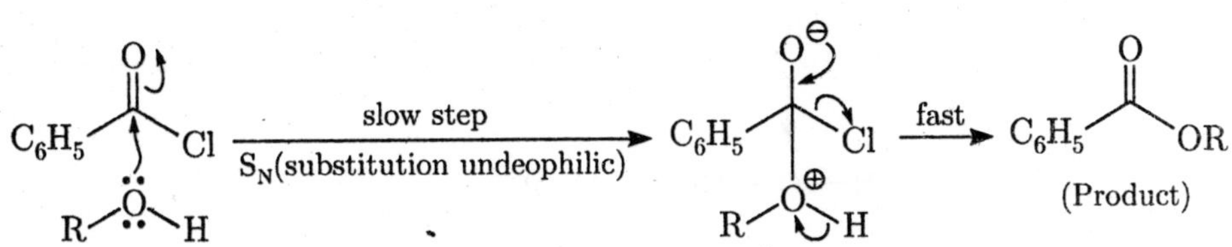

6. ***Esterification raction*** :

$$R{-}OH + CH_3COOH \xrightleftharpoons{\text{conc. } H_2SO_4/\Delta} CH_3{-}\overset{O}{\overset{\|}{C}}{-}OR + H_2O$$

7. ***Transesterification reaction*** :

$$R^1COOR^2 + ROH \xrightleftharpoons{H^{\oplus}} R^1COOR + R^2OH$$

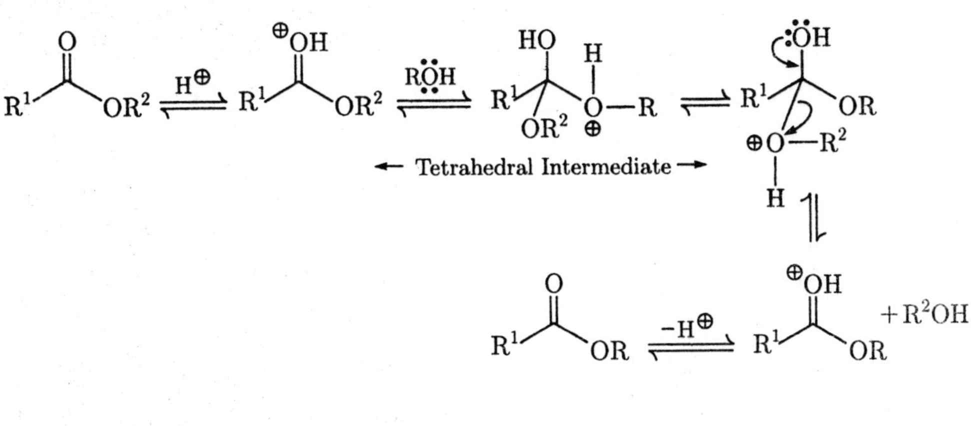

8. *D-Exchange* :

$$R{-}OH + D_2O \rightleftharpoons ROD + HOD$$

$$R{-}OH + D{-}O{-}D \rightleftharpoons R{-}\overset{\oplus}{O}(D){-}H + \overset{\ominus}{O}D \rightleftharpoons ROD + HOD$$

This reaction shows the identical polarity of O—H bond in alcohol and water.

9. ***Reaction with Diazomethane*** : In the presence of a Lewis acid, alcohols (alcoholic –OH hydrogen is only weakly acidic) react with diazomethane to form methyl ether.

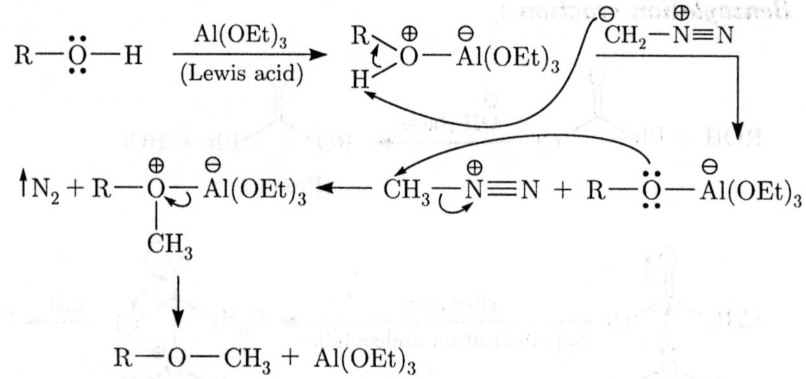

Reactions of alcohols via C—O cleavage

1. ***Reactions with epoxides*** :

(a) 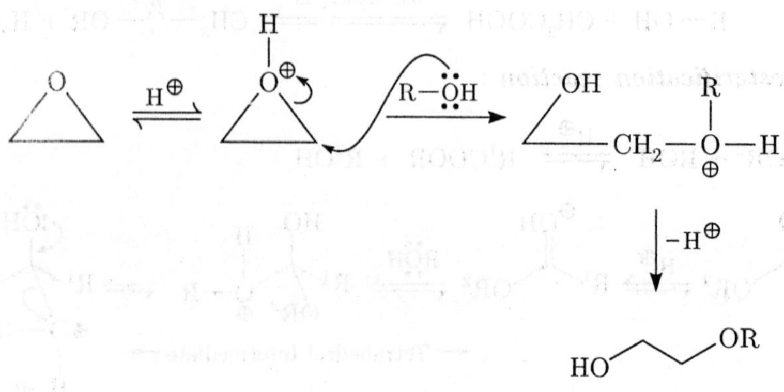

(b) 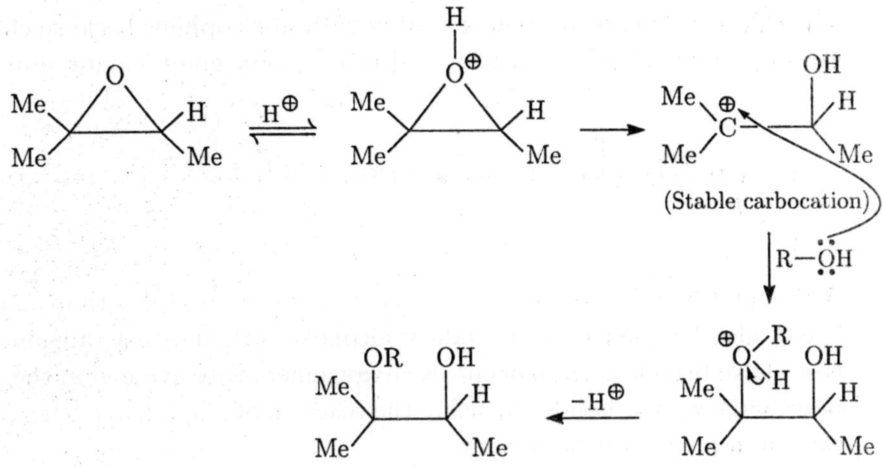

(c) 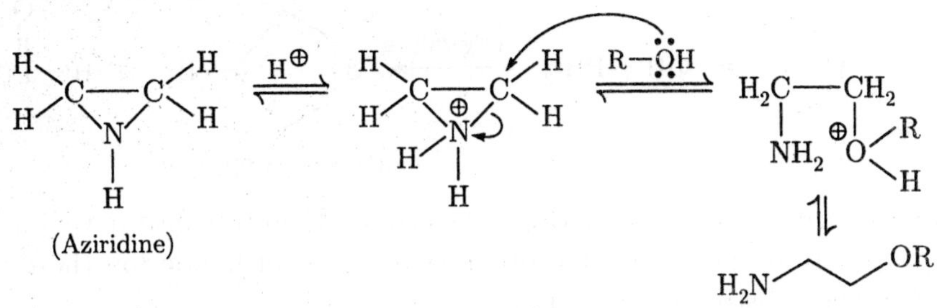

(Aziridine)

2. ***β*-Elimination reactions**

$$CH_3-CH(OH)CH_3 \xrightarrow{\overset{\oplus}{H}/350°C \text{ or } Al_2O_3/\Delta} CH_3-\underset{\overset{|}{\overset{\oplus}{O}H_2}}{CH}-CH_3 \xrightarrow{-H_2O} CH_3-\overset{\oplus}{C}H-CH_3 \xrightarrow{-H^{\oplus}} CH_3-CH=CH_2$$

3. ***Reactions of alcohols with $SOCl_2$ and PBr_3* :**

$$\underset{\text{(1–octanol)}}{CH_3(CH_2)_6CH_2OH} + SOCl_2 \xrightarrow{\text{pyridine}} \underset{\text{(1–Chlorooactane)}}{CH_3(CH_2)_6CH_2Cl} + SO_2\uparrow + HCl$$

One advantage of using thionyl chloride ($SOCl_2$) for the preparation of alkyl chlorides is that the by products of the reaction are HCl, which reacts with the base pyridine and sulphur dioxide (SO_2) (a gas). Consequently, there are no problems in the purification of the product alkyl chlorides and the reaction shifts to the product (alkyl halide) side as gaseous SO_2 escapes from the reaction mixture.

$$RCH_2OH + Cl-\overset{\overset{O}{\|}}{S}-Cl \xrightarrow{\text{pyridine}} \underset{\text{(1–Chlorosulphite ester)}}{R-CH_2O-\overset{\overset{O}{\|}}{S}-Cl} + Py.HCl$$

The chlorosulphite ester reacts readily with nucleophiles because chlorosulphite group (–OSOCl) is a weak base and thus, a very good leaving group.

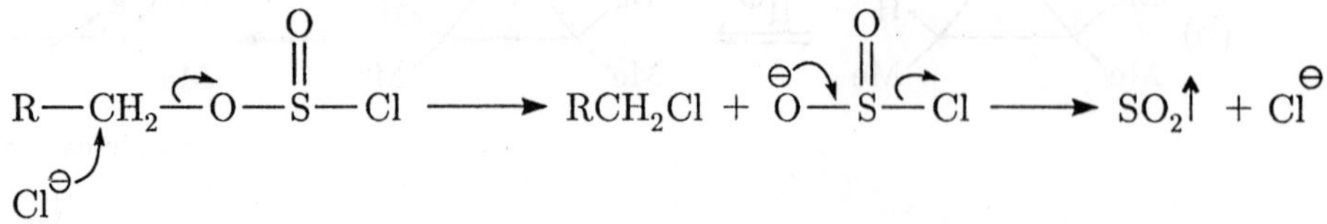

Although thionyl chloride ($SOCl_2$) method is most useful with primary alcohols, it can also be used with secondary alcohols, although rearrangements in such cases have been known to occur. Rearrangements are avoided in the preparation of secondary alkyl halides by using the reaction of a halide ion with a sulphonate ester in a polar aprotic solvent.

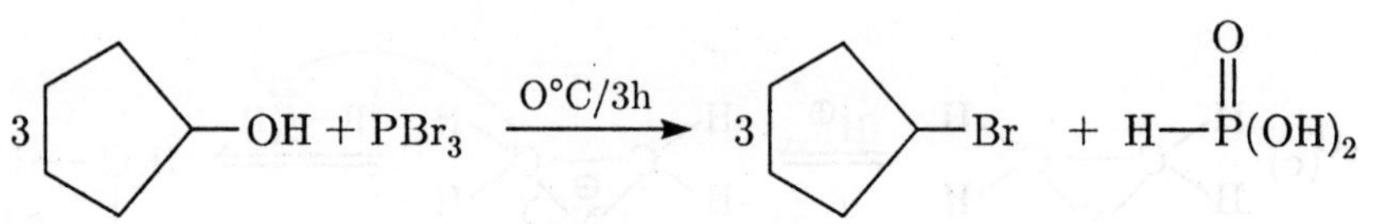

(Bromocyclopentane)

Phosphorus tribromide (PBr_3) converts –OH group into a very good leaving group and at the same time provides a source of halide ion (here it is Br^-) to effect the substitution reaction.

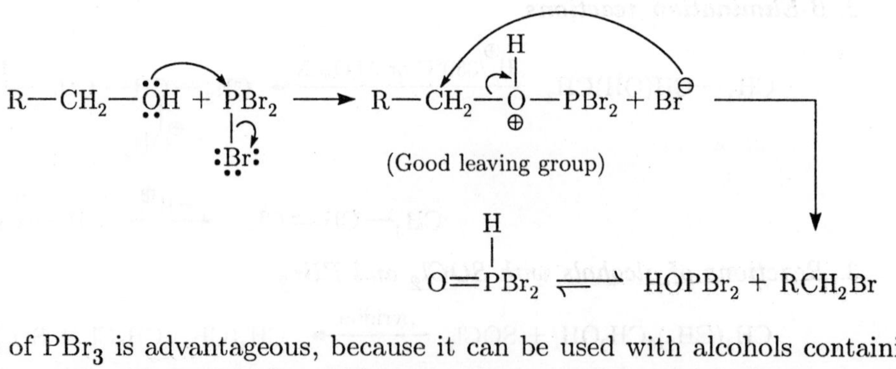

Use of PBr_3 is advantageous, because it can be used with alcohols containing acid-sensitive groups which would not survive treatment with hydrobromic acid (HBr). Also with secondary alcohols, the risk of rearrangement although not totally absent is less than that with HBr.

4. ***Reactions of alcohols with hydrogen halides :***

(a) 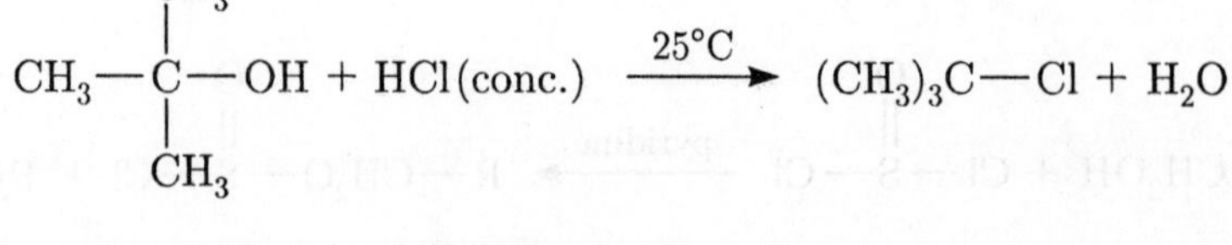

(b) $CH_3(CH_2)_3OH + HBr\,(conc.) \xrightarrow{reflux/H_2SO_4} CH_3(CH_2)_3Br$

(c) $CH_3(CH_2)_3OH + HI\,(conc.) \xrightarrow{reflux/H_2SO_4} CH_3(CH_2)_3I$

The equilibrium constant for formation of alkyl halides from alcohols is not large, so Le Chaterlier's principle is applied here. The reactant alcohols are soluble in aqueous acid (solvent) but alkyl halide not. So the separation of alkyl halides from the reaction mixture as water-insoluble layers drives the reaction to completion.

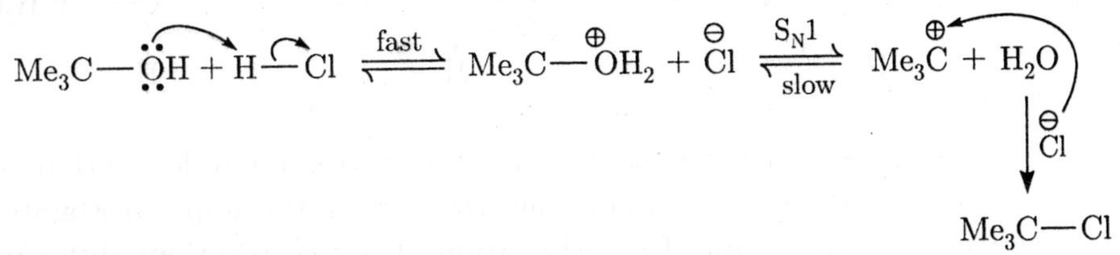

In case of primary alcohols, S_N2 reaction occurs.

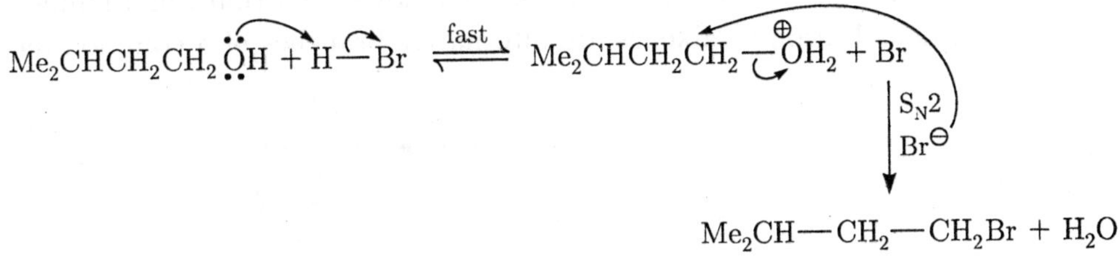

The reactions of tertiary alcohols with hydrogen halides are much faster than the reactions of primary alcohols. (room temperature for tertiary alcohols whereas reflux is needed for primary alcohols). Primary alcohols react satisfactorily with HI and HBr and very slowly with HCl.

The reaction of secondary alcohols tend to occur by S_N1 mechanism. This means that rearrangements may occur in many cases.

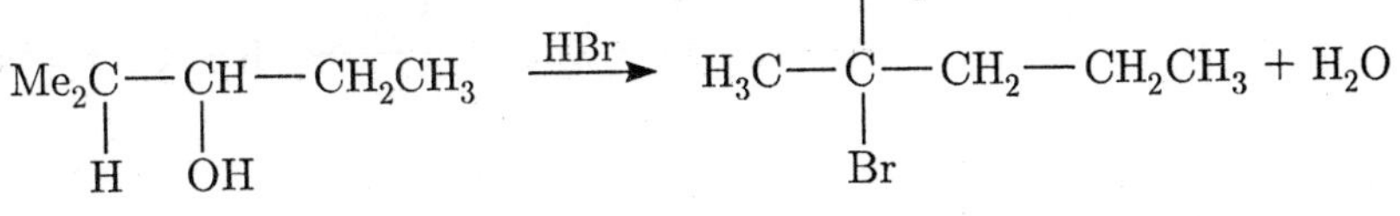

(3-methyl-3-pentanol) (2-bromo-2-methylpentane)

Dehydration of alcohols to alkenes and the reactions of alcohols with hydrogen acids (HX) have some important points in common. Both take place in very acidic solution. In both the reactions, acid converts –OH group into a good leaving group ($-\overset{\oplus}{O}H_2$). In the absence of acid, $X^{\ominus}$ would have to displace $\overset{\ominus}{O}H$ to form the alkyl halide. But this reaction does not take place because $\overset{\ominus}{O}H$ is a stronger base than any $X^{\ominus}$.

$$:\ddot{\underset{\cdot\cdot}{Br}}:^{\ominus} + CH_3-OH \not\longrightarrow Br-CH_3 + \overset{\ominus}{O}H$$ (Strong base, poor leaving group)

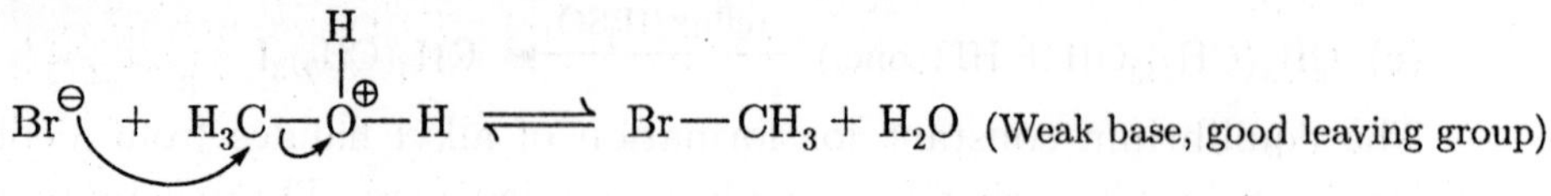

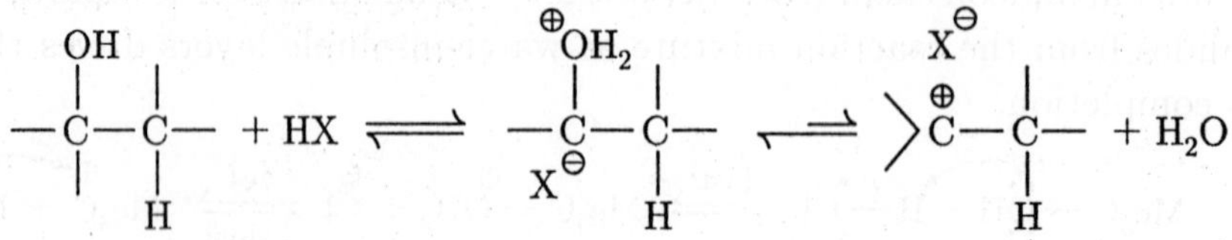

The formation of secondary and tertiary alkyl halides and dehydration of secondary and tertiary alcohols have the same initial steps, protonation of alcohol oxygen and formation of a carbocation. The two reactions differ in the fate of the carbocation. In the presence of halogen acid, HX, the halide ion is present in excess and attacks the carbocation. It follows then that alkyl halide formation and dehydration to alkenes are alternative branches of a common mechanism.

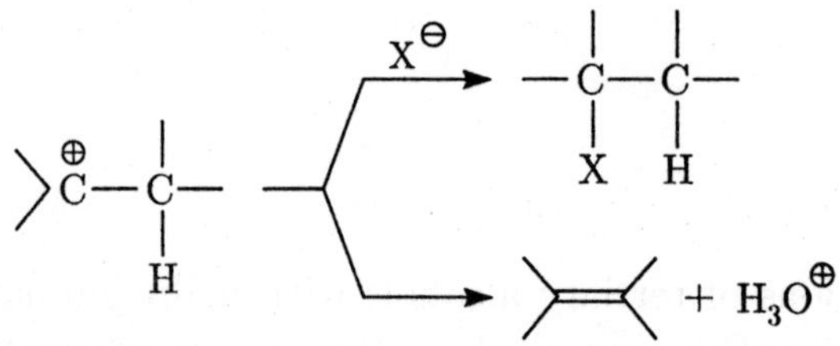

Lewis acid like $ZnCl_2$ enhances the reaction rate between primary and secondary alcohols. As $Cl^{\ominus}$ is a weaker nucleophile, does not react with primary and secondary alcohols alone.

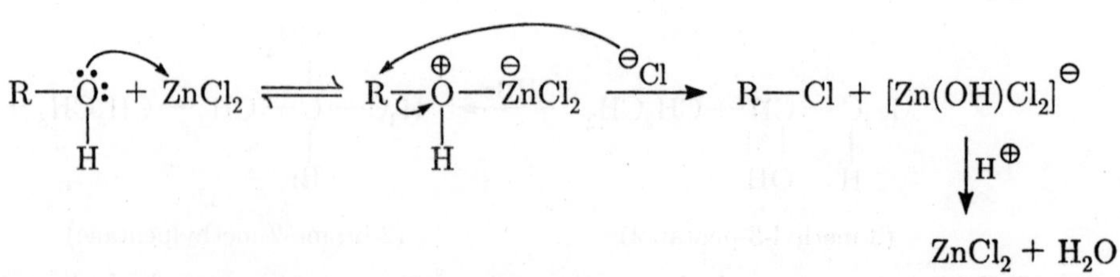

5. ***Reactivity of sulphonate and inorganic ester derivatives of alcohols*** : Sulphonate esters prepared from primary and secondary alcohols, like primary and secondary alkyl halides undergo S_N2 reactions in which a sulphonate anion serves as the leaving group. Similarly, secondary and tertiary sulphonate esters like the corresponding alkyl halides also undergo E-2 reaction with strong bases and they undergo S_N1 -E1 solvolysis reaction in polar protic solvents.

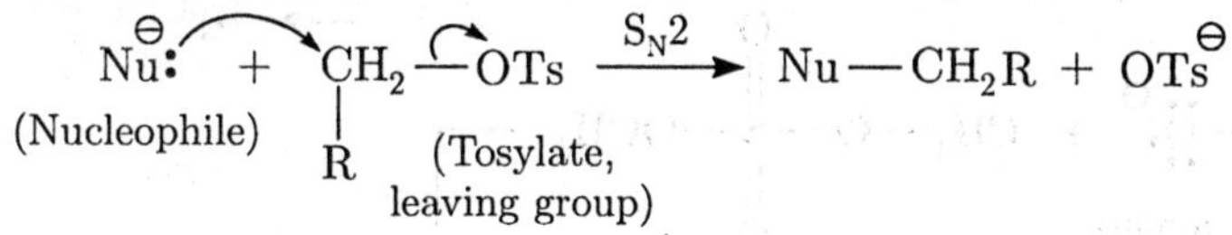

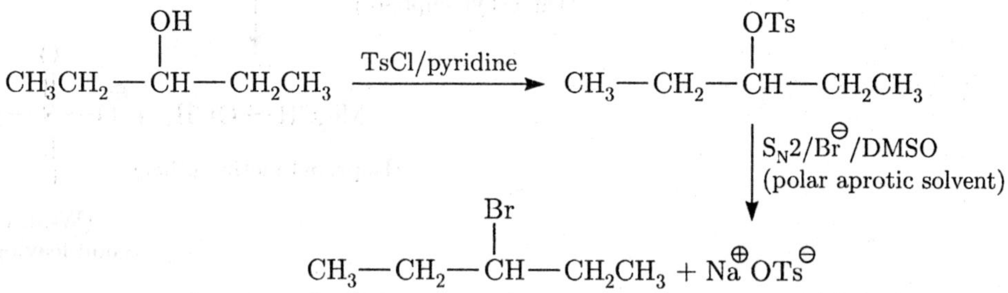

Alcohols can be converted to alkyl bromides by HBr and heat, but the secondary carbocations are prone to rearrange, so the above *method is better.* Secondary alkyl tosylates are not reactive towards S_N1 pathway. The use of polar aprotic solvent suppresses carbocation formation which would be more likely to occur in a protic solvent.

E2 Reaction :

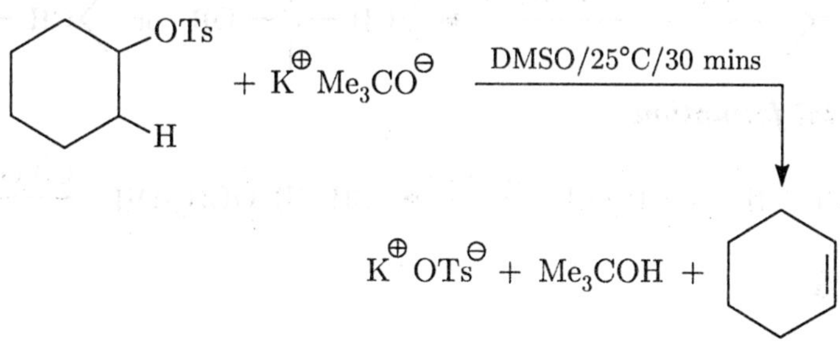

No unwanted rearrangement reactions occur.

6. ***Alkylating agent and ester derivatives of strong inorganic acids*** : Alkyl sulphonates are good alkylating agents and react rapidly with nucleophiles in S_N2 and S_N1 reactions to transfer alkyl groups.

Ester Derivatives

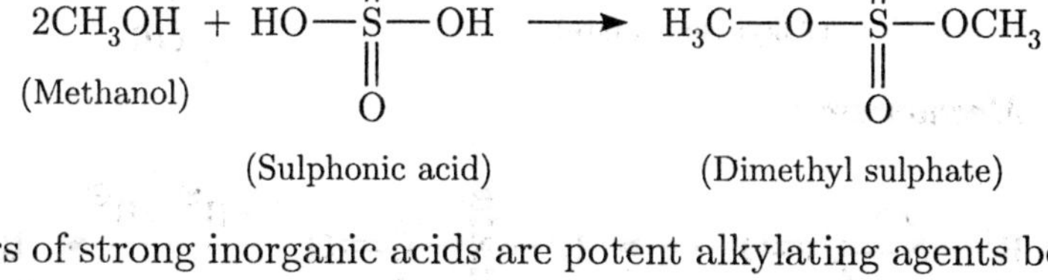

Alkyl esters of strong inorganic acids are potent alkylating agents because they contain leaving groups that are very weak bases. For example, dimethyl sulphate is a very effective methylating agent.

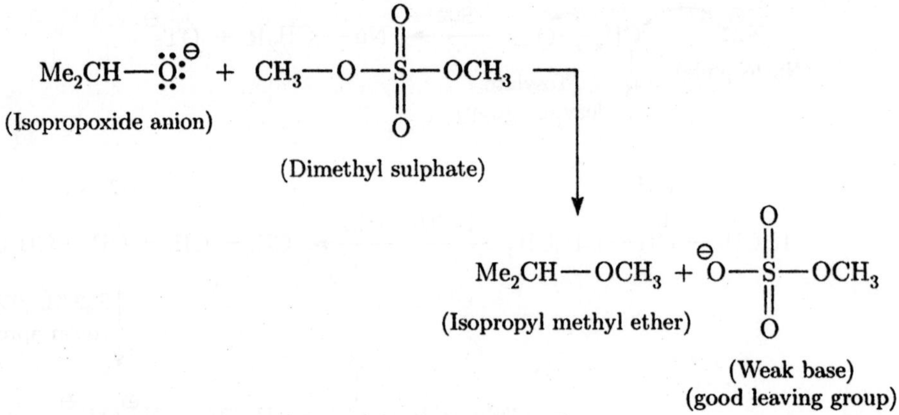

Me_2SO_4 is toxic as it reacts with nucleophilic functional groups like proteins and nucleic acids.

7. $R-OH + NH_3 \xrightarrow[\text{(under pressure)}]{Al_2O_3 \text{ or Copper chromite}} RNH_2 + H_2O$

With excess NH_3, a mixture of primary, secondary and tertiary amines are produced.

8. 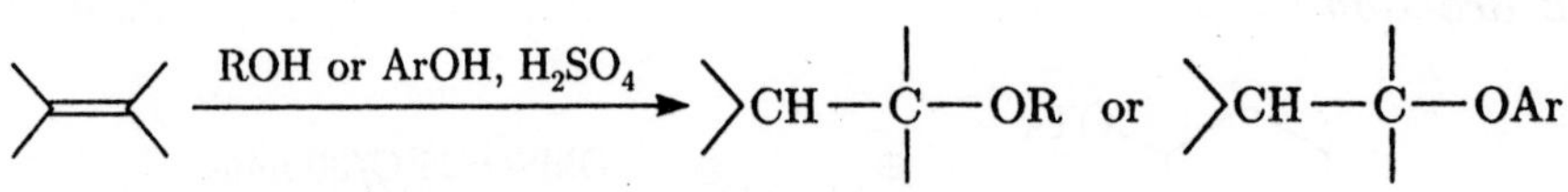

9. ***Acetal formation*** :

$$CH_3CHO + CH_3OH \xrightarrow{\text{dry HCl}} CH_3CH(OCH_3)OH \xrightarrow{CH_3OH/\text{dry HCl}} CH_3CH(OCH_3)_2$$

10. ***Reaction with isocyanates*** :

(a) 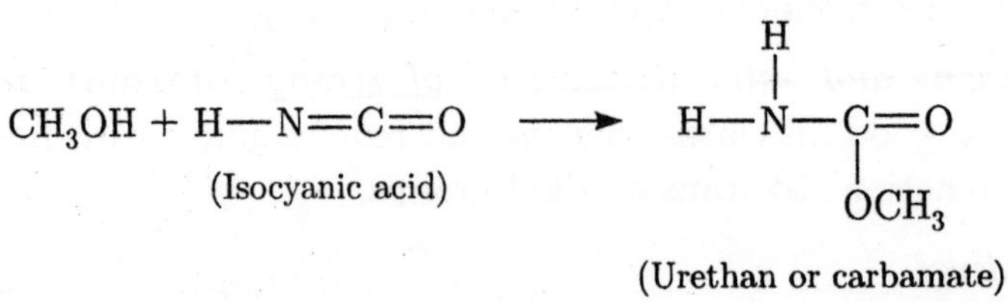

(b) 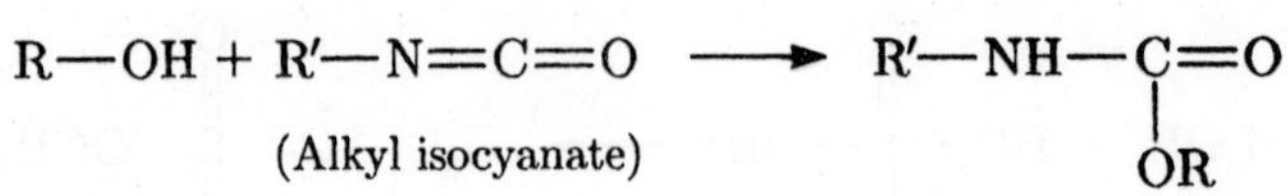

Mechanism :

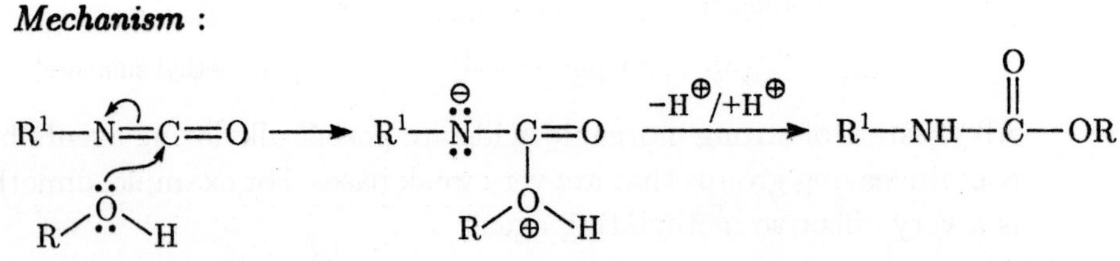

11. ***Reaction with cyanides*** : Alcohols react with cyanides (aliphatic, aromatic or heterocyclic) in the presence of dry HCl to give imino ester salts. If the alcohol is taken in excess, *ortho* esters are formed. On the other hand, when aquous HCl is used, carboxylic esters are formed.

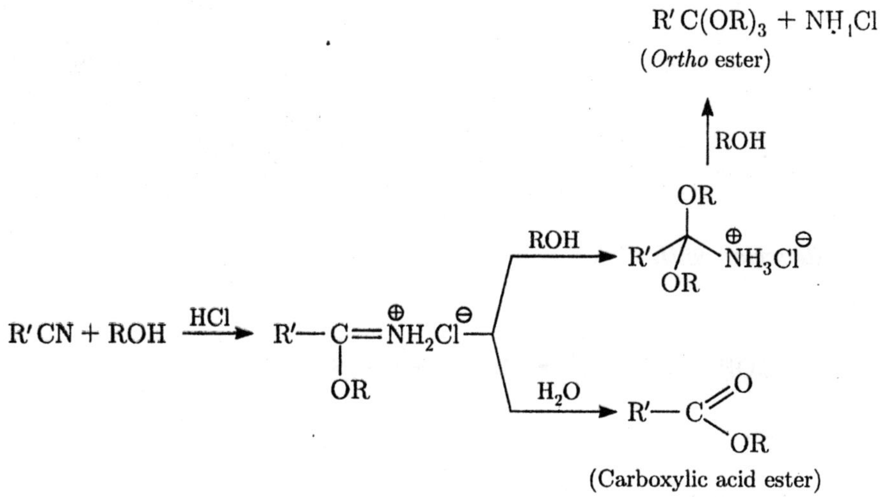

Mechanism :

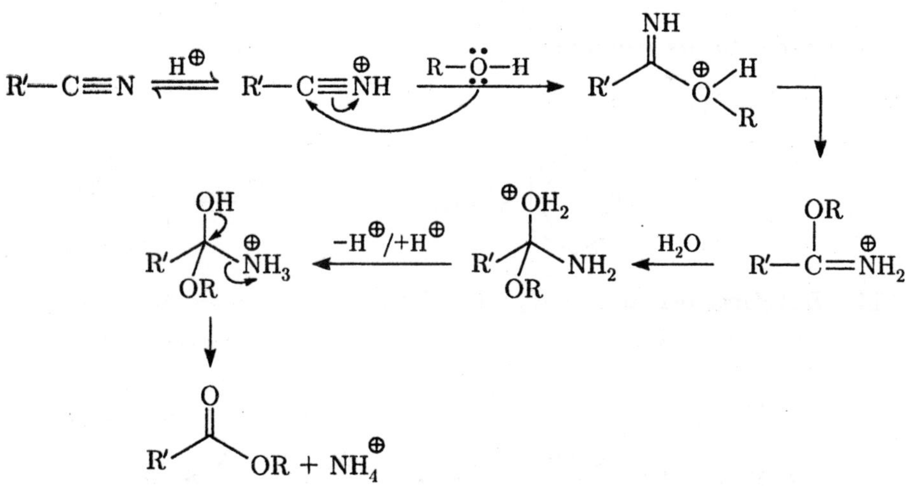

Alcohols may also be added to cyanides in the following way to form an N- substituted amide.

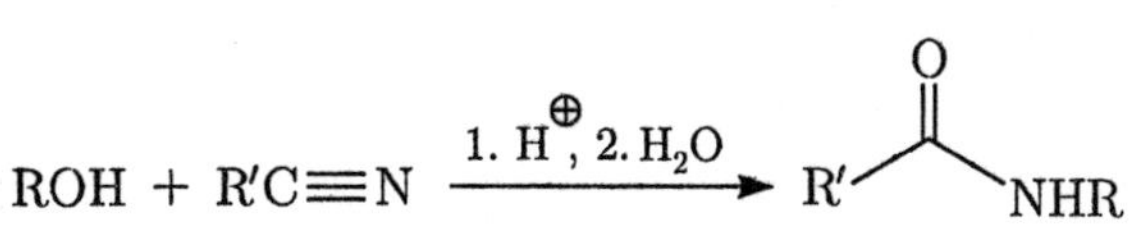

$$R{-}OH \underset{}{\overset{H^{\oplus}}{\rightleftharpoons}} R{-}\overset{\oplus}{O}H_2 \longrightarrow \overset{\oplus}{R} + H_2O$$

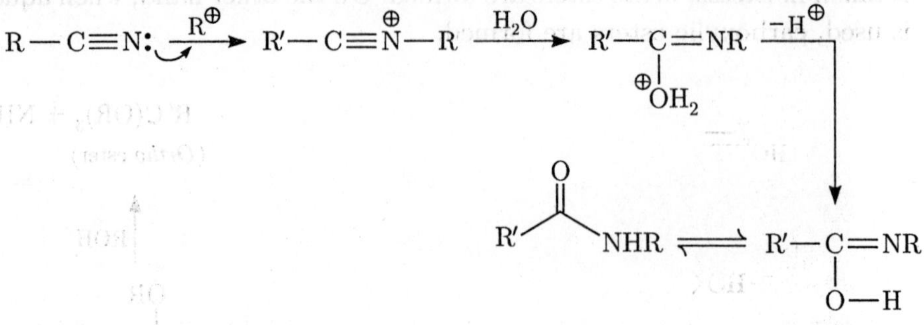

12. ***Reaction with CS_2*** :

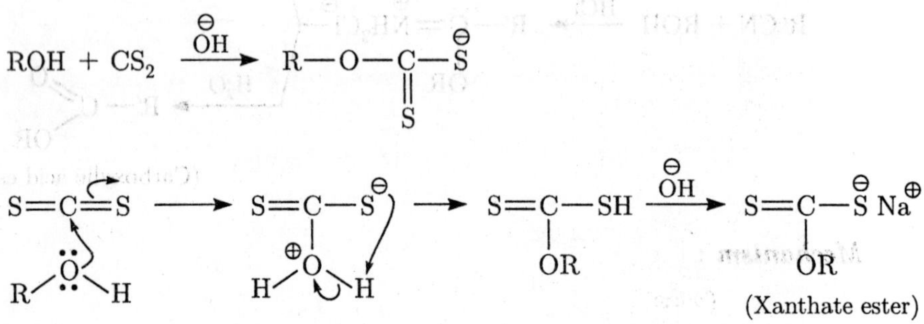

13. ***Friedel-Crafts reaction*** :

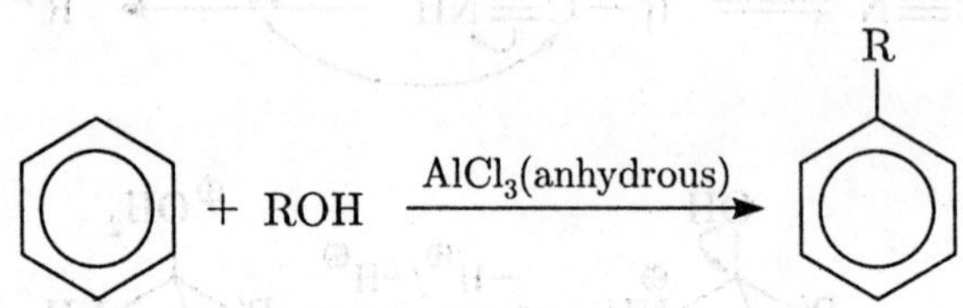

14. ***Haloform reaction*** : CH_3CH_2OH and secondary alcohols with $-CH(OH)CH_3$ group form haloform when they are treated with alkaline halogen solution.

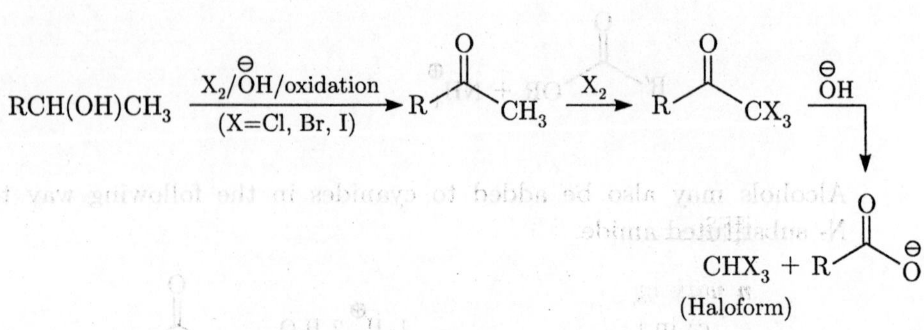

Methods of Distinguishing between the three classes of alcohols

1. ***By means of oxidation*** : The nature of oxidation products of an alcohol depends on whether the alcohol is primary, secondary or tertiary.

(a) $$CH_3CH_2OH \xrightarrow{\text{oxidation}} CH_3CHO \xrightarrow{\text{oxidation}} CH_3COOH$$

(primary alcohol)

Both aldehyde and the acid contain same number of carbon atoms as the original alcohol. A secondary alcohol on oxidation first gives a ketone with same number of carbon atoms as the original alcohol. Ketones are fairly difficult to oxidise, but prolonged action of the oxidising agents produces a mixture of acids each containing fewer carbon atoms than the original alcohol.

(b) $$CH_3CH(OH)CH_2CH_2CH_3 \xrightarrow{\text{oxidation}} CH_3-\overset{\overset{O}{\|}}{C}-CH_2-CH_2-CH_3$$

(secondary alcohol)

$$\xrightarrow{\text{oxidation}} Me_2CO + MeCOOH$$

The oxidising agents usually used for oxidising alcohols are acid/dichromate, acid or alkaline potassium permanganate ($KMnO_4$), nitric acid etc.

(c) A tertiary alcohol on oxidation gives carboxylic acids with fewer number of carbon atoms.

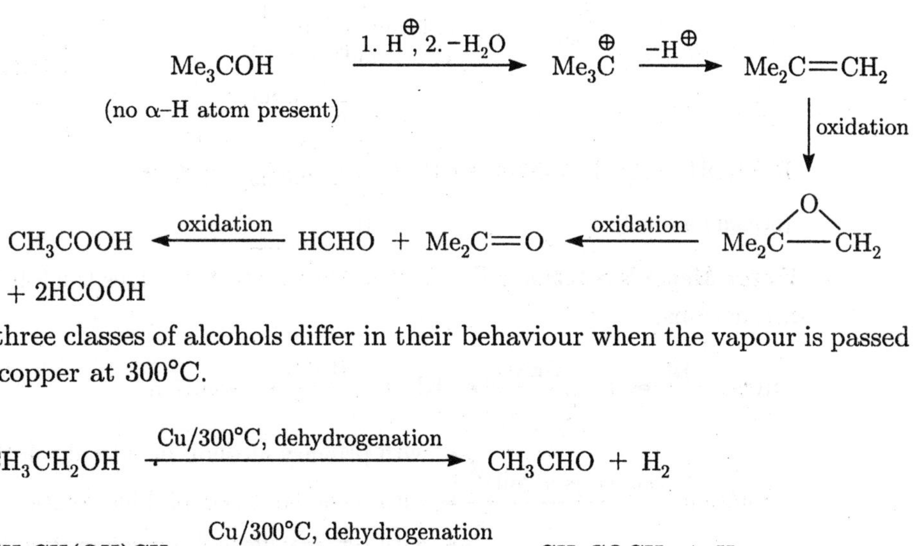

2. The three classes of alcohols differ in their behaviour when the vapour is passed over copper at 300°C.

(a) $$CH_3CH_2OH \xrightarrow{\text{Cu/300°C, dehydrogenation}} CH_3CHO + H_2$$

(b) $$CH_3CH(OH)CH_3 \xrightarrow{\text{Cu/300°C, dehydrogenation}} CH_3COCH_3 + H_2$$

(c) $$Me_2C(OH)CH_2CH_3 \xrightarrow{\text{Cu/300°C}} Me_2C{=}CHCH_3 + H_2O$$

3. ***Lucas Test***

$$CH_3CH_2OH + H_2SO_4 \xrightarrow{100°C} CH_3CH_2HSO_4 + H_2O$$

The inorganic acid (H_2SO_4) supplies the proton and the alcohol supplies the –OH group to form water. The removal of water increases the yield by stopping the hydrolysis of ester. Since R—OH supplies the –OH group by breaking C—OH bond (carbinol carbon—OH bond), the reactivity order is 3° R—OH > 2° R—OH > 1° R—OH. This reaction constitutes the *Lucas Test* which tells us whether an alcohol is primary, secondary or tertiary. The given alcohol is mixed with anhydrous zinc chloride ($ZnCl_2$) in concentrated hydrochloric acid (HCl) at room temperature. A tertiary alcohol produces cloudiness immediately, a secondary alcohol does so within five minutes but a primary alcohol does not form cloudiness at all at room temperature.

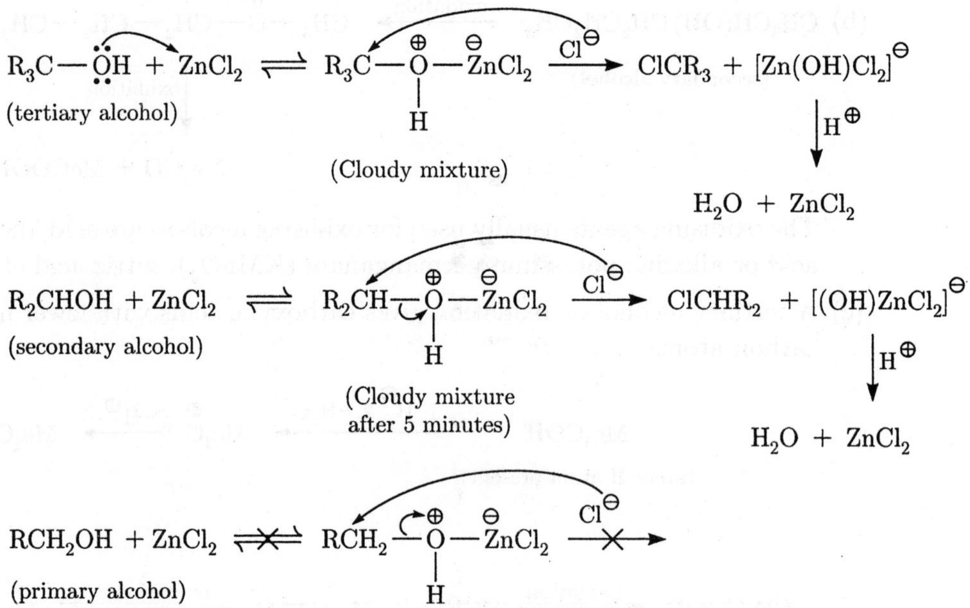

4. ***Victor Meyer's reaction*** : The Victor Meyer's test involves the following sequence of reactions.

$$ROH \xrightarrow{HI} RI \xrightarrow{AgNO_2} RNO_2 \xrightarrow{HNO_2} \text{solution}$$

Solution $\xrightarrow{\text{(aqueous alkali)}}$
- with primary alcohol, blood red solution is formed.
- with secondary alcohol, blue solution is formed.
- with tertiary alcohol, no colouration is formed.

Since, through these reactions, primary, secondary and tertiary alcohols give red, blue and colourless solutions respectively, this test is also called ***Victor Meyer's red-blue-white test.***

Mechanism of the reaction :

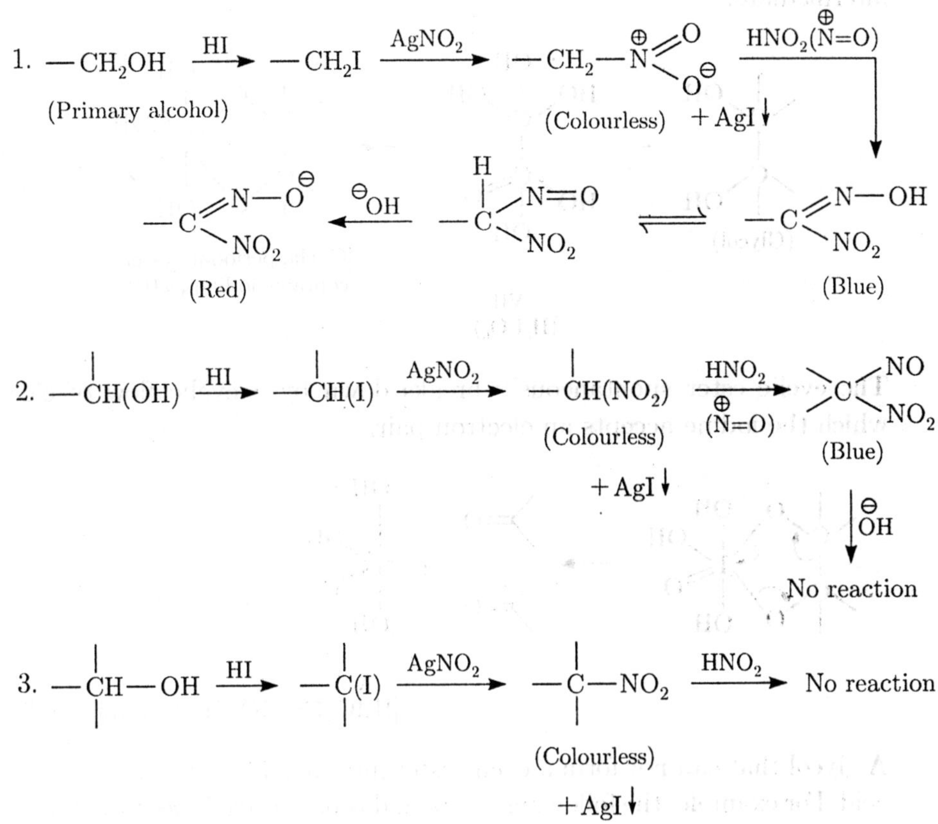

Chemical reactions of 1, 2-glycols :

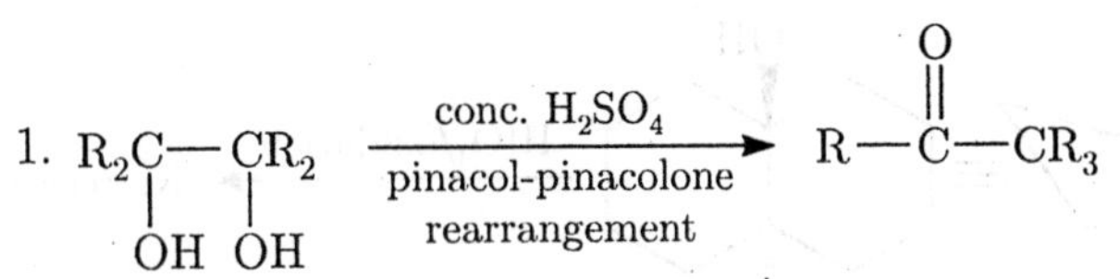

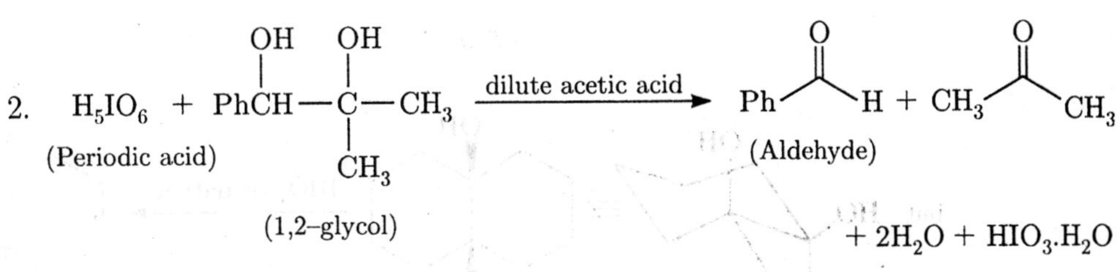

Periodic acid is the iodine analogue of perchloric acid. Periodic acid is commercially available as $HIO_4 \cdot 2H_2O$, often abbreviated as H_5IO_6. Its sodium salt, $NaIO_4$ is sometimes used. Periodic acid (HIO_4) is a fairly strong acid ($pK_a = -1.6$). Periodate cleavage reaction has been used as a test for glycols as well as for synthesis.

The cleavage of glycols with HIO_4 takes place through a cyclic periodate ester intermediate.

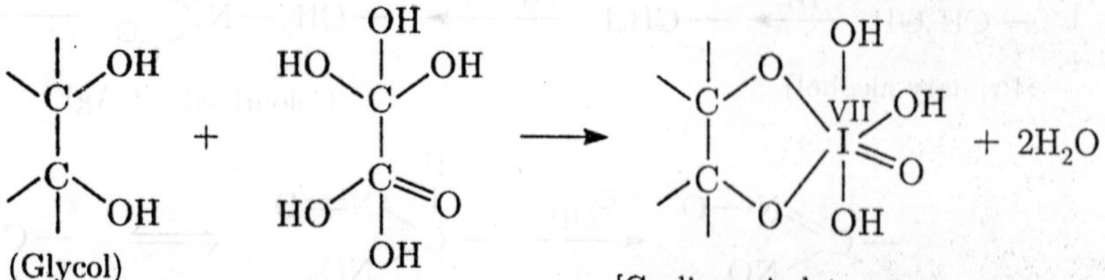

(Glycol) VII (H_5IO_6) [Cyclic periodate ester contains iodine (VII)]

The cyclic ester spontaneously breaks down by a cyclic flow of electrons in which the iodine accepts an electron pair.

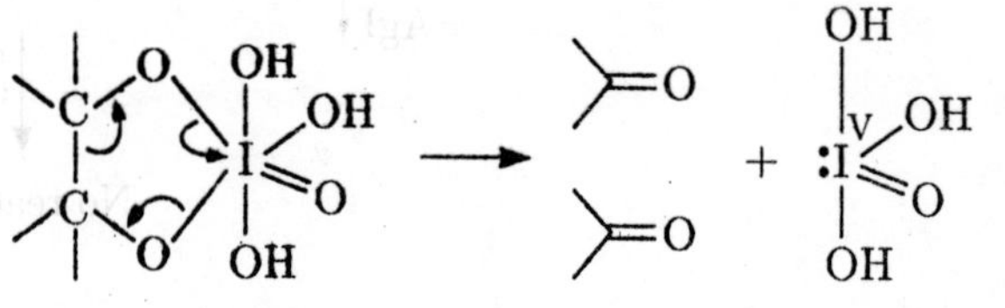

[$\overset{V}{H_3IO_4} \equiv \overset{V}{HIO_4}.H_2O$ contains iodine (V)]

A glycol that can not form a cyclic ester intermediate is not cleaved by periodic acid. For example, the following compound is not cleaved, because it is impossible for both oxygens to be part of the same cyclic periodate esters.

(a)

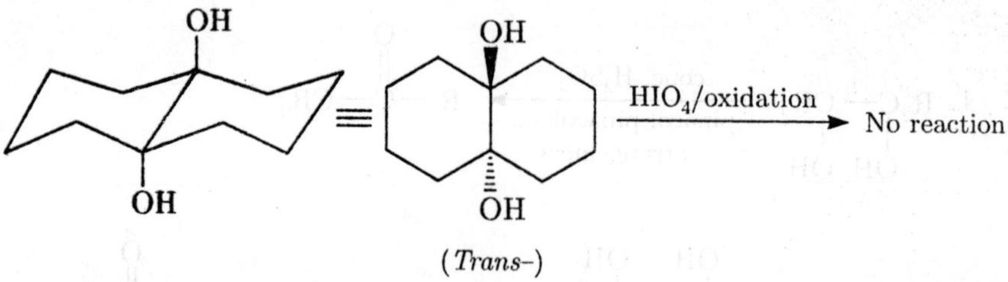

(*Trans*–)

but

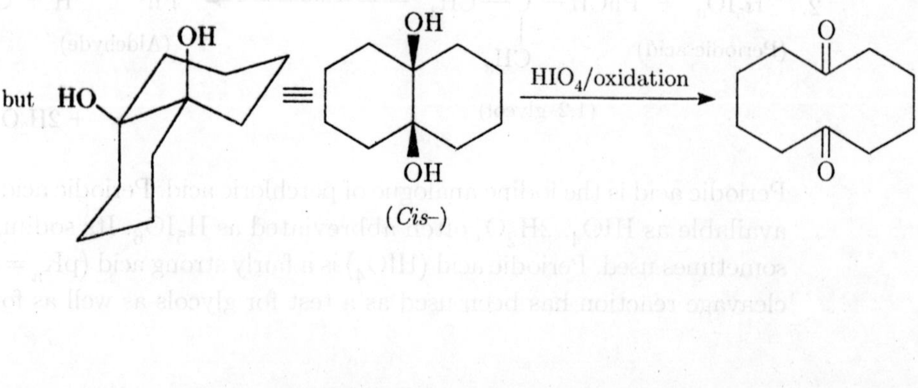

(*Cis*–)

(b) 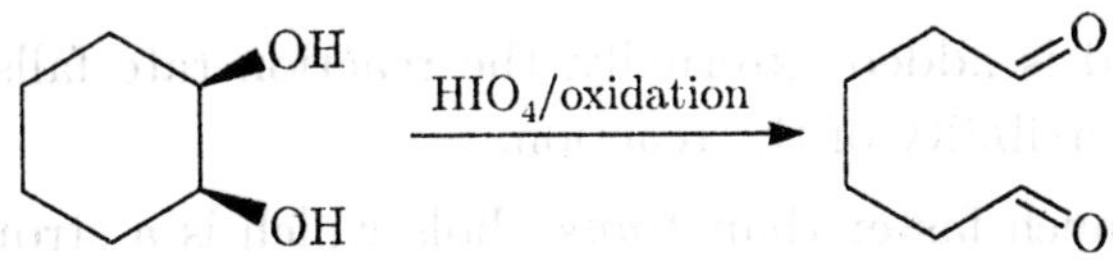

(c) 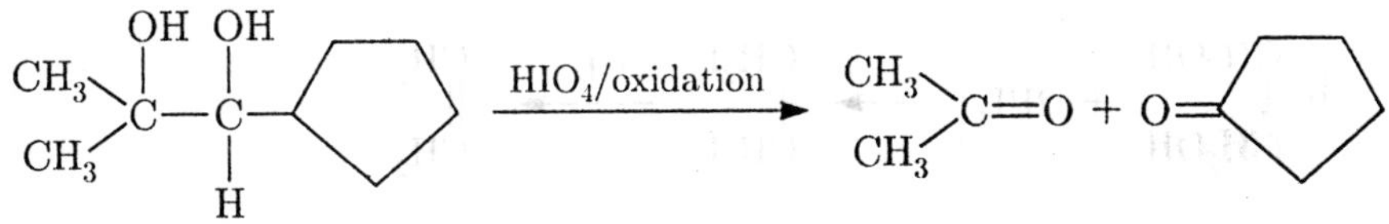

(d) 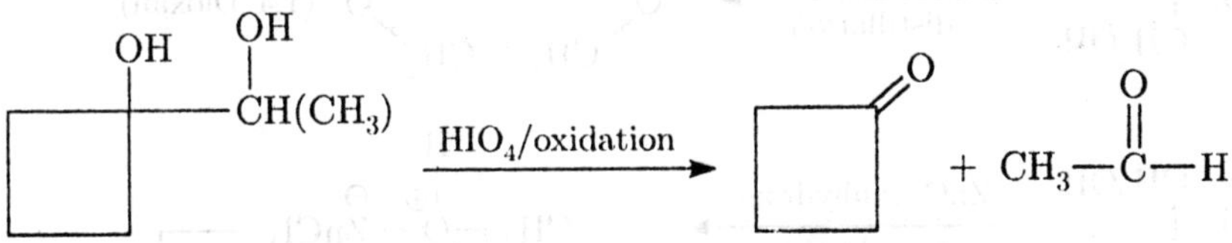

(e) 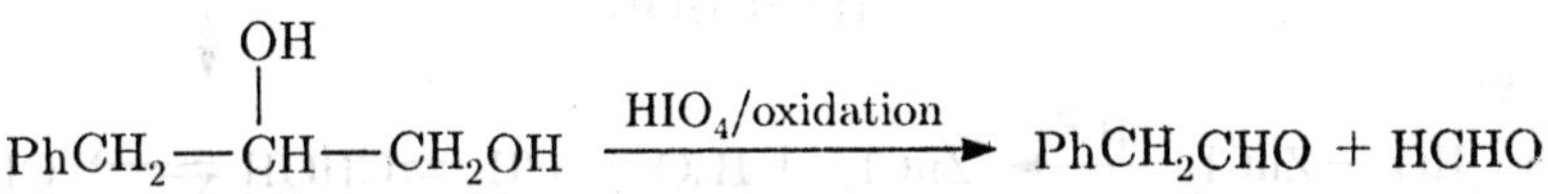

Oxidation of glycols occur because iodine is in a highly positive oxidation state and can accept an additional pair of electrons. The reduction of iodine occurs during the breakdown of a cyclic esters.

3. ***Oxidative cleavage by lead tetraacetate*** : Oxidative cleavage by lead tetraacetate shows the same mechanism *i.e.* the reaction takes place through the formation of a cyclic ester intermediate. Lead (Pb) in lead tetraacetate is in +IV oxidation state and after the oxidation of glycols, itself gets reduced to +II oxidation state.

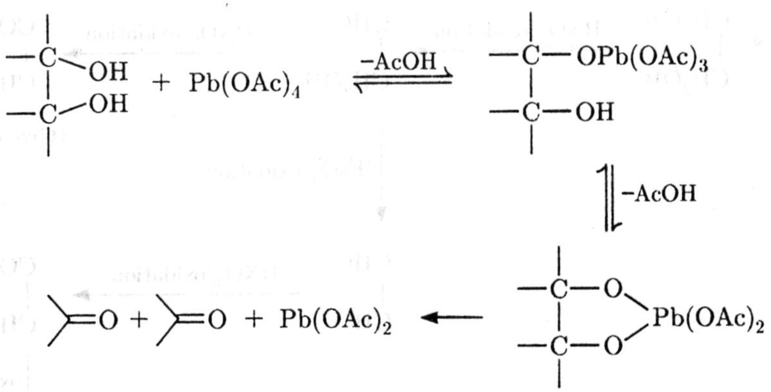

The following points are observed from the above reaction.

(a) The rate of the reaction = k[substrate] $[Pb(OAc)_4]$, which is in confirmity with the given mechanism.

(b) When acetic acid is added externally, the reaction rate falls down, which supports the reversibility of the reaction.

(c) *Cis*-diols react much faster than *trans*- diols which is a strong evidence in favour of the cyclic intermediate.

4. $$\begin{matrix} CH_2OH \\ | \\ CH_2OH \end{matrix} + 2PI_3 \longrightarrow \begin{matrix} CH_2I \\ | \\ CH_2I \end{matrix} \xrightarrow{-I_2} \begin{matrix} CH_2 \\ \| \\ CH_2 \end{matrix}$$

5. 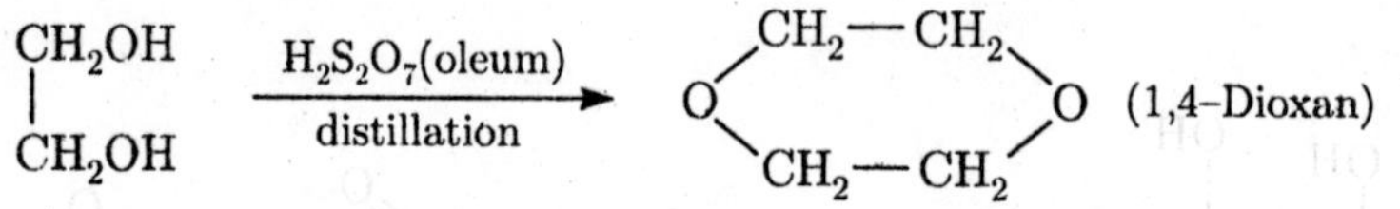

6. 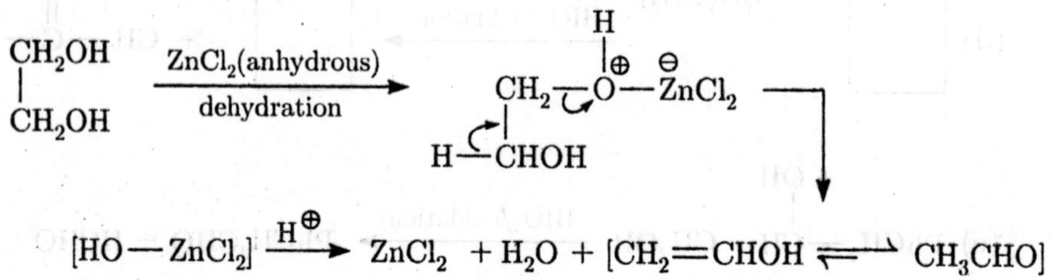

7. When 1,2-glycols are dehydrated with phosphoric acid, polymerisation occurs. For example, ethylene forms polyethlene glycol in the presence of phosphoric acid (H_3PO_4). Maximum five ethylene glycol molecules take part in the reaction.

$$2\begin{matrix} CH_2OH \\ | \\ CH_2OH \end{matrix} \xrightarrow{\text{polyphosphoric acid}} HOCH_2CH_2OCH_2CH_2OH \xrightarrow[\text{distillation}]{H_3PO_4(CH_2OH)_2} HO(CH_2)_2O(CH_2)_2O(CH_2)_2OH$$

8. 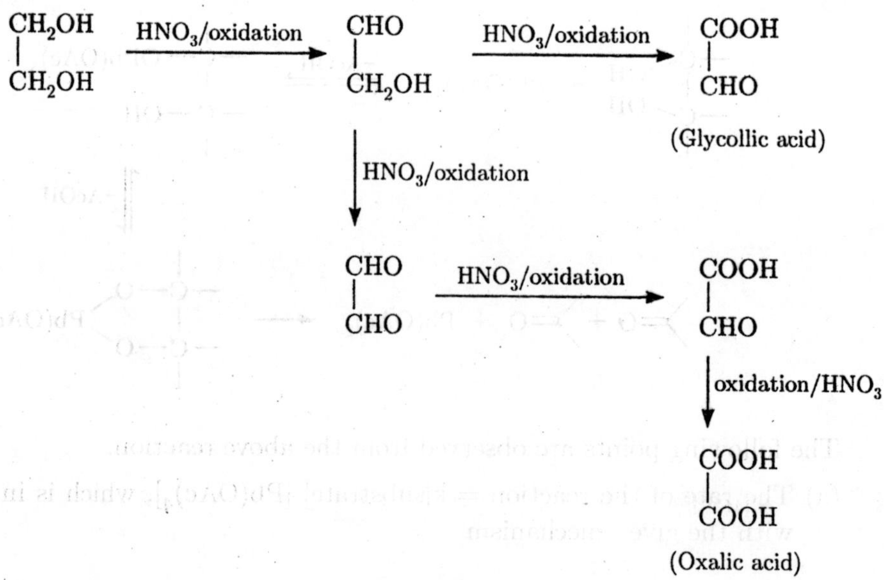

9. ***Complex formation of 1,2-glycols with boric acid*** : Boric acid is a very weak acid, but in the presence of certain organic polyhydroxy compounds such as glycerol, mannitol etc, the strength of boric acid is so much increased that it may be titrated as a fairly strong mono basic acid against sodium hydroxide solution using phenolphthalein as an indicator. The increase in strength may be due to the formation of 'chelate' complex as follows.

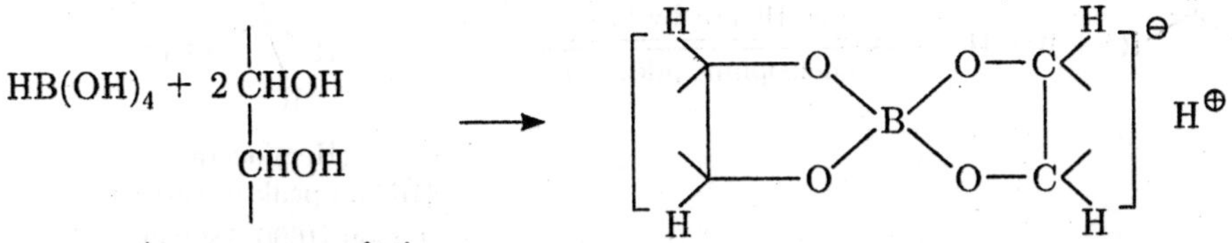

(*e.g.* aqueous solution of glycerol) (Chelate complex, higher electrical conductivity than boric acid itself, *i.e.* is a stronger acid)

The complex anion contains tetravalent boron atom (covalency of boron is maximum four) and so can not accept a proton without undergoing decomposition. The complex is believed to be a borospiranic acid in which the two rings attached to the boron atom are perpendicular to each other (hence the name spiran). This borospiranic acid is formed from α-glycols in which the two hydroxyl groups are in the *cis* configuration. Ethylene glycol apparently does not form the complex, the reason being unknown.

Catechol and salicyclic acid also form similar chelated oxyderivatives giving rise to anionic boron complex.

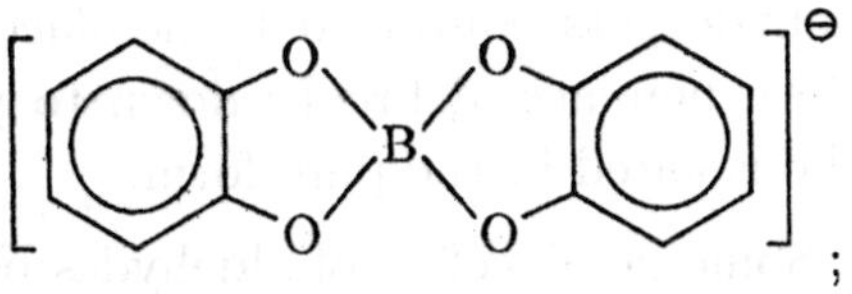

(Catechol–boric acid complex) ;

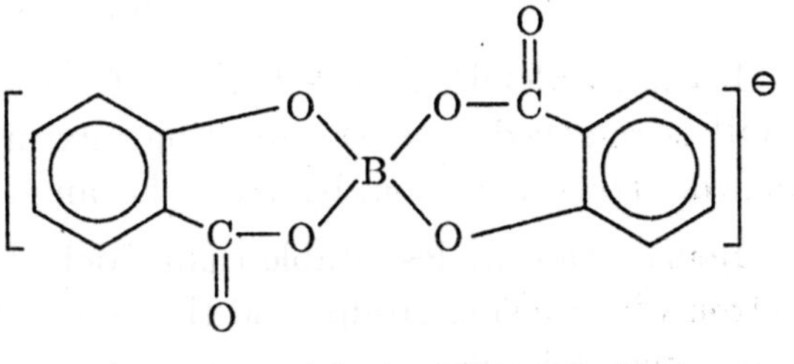

(Salicylic acid–boric acid complex)

The brucine and strychnine salts of 4-chlorocatechol and salicylic acid derivatives have been resolved into optical isomers, showing that the distribution of bond around boron is tetrahedral.

Acetals and Ketals

Alcohols add to aldehydes and ketones in the presence of specific acid catalyst to yield acetals *via* hemiacetals. Acetals are 1,1-diethers and hemiacetals are ether-alcohols, *i.e.*, half acetals.

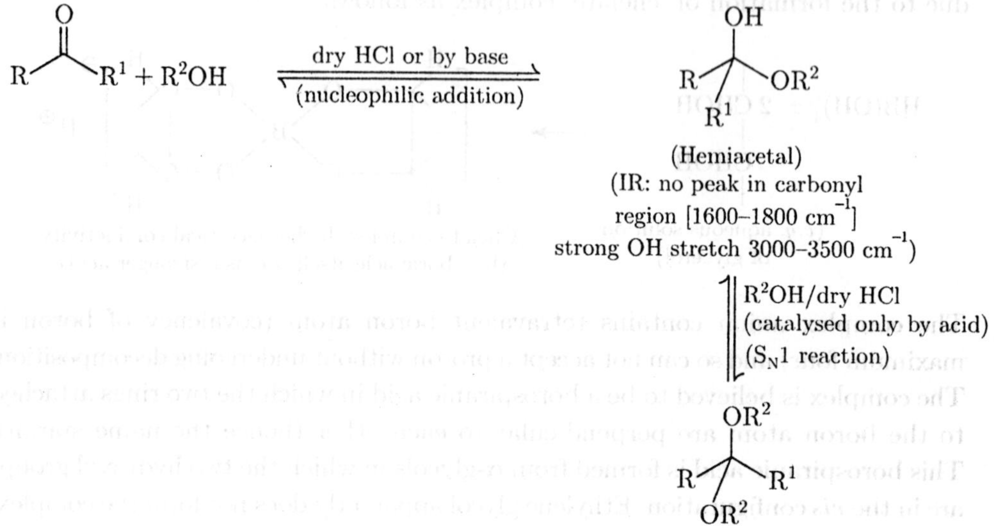

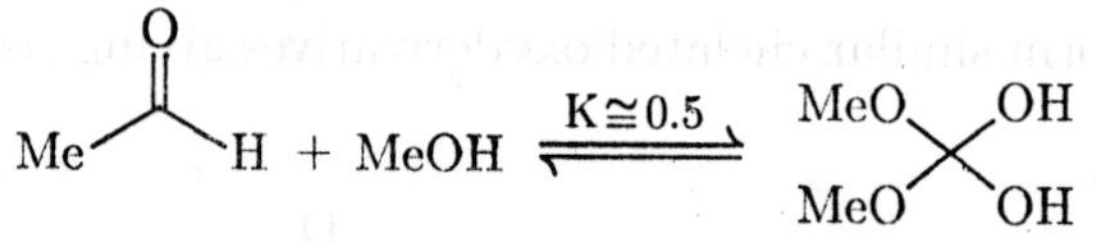

(Hemiacetal)

If excess MeOH is added most of the aldehyde gets converted to hemiacetal. If MeOH is removed from the reaction mixture, the hemiacetal breaks down to parent aldehyde. For this reason, hemiacetals can not be isolated in the pure form.

Hemiacetals are less stable than aldehydes. Some hemiacetals of aldehydes bearing electron withdrawing groups and this of cyclopropanes are stable just like the hydrates of the same molecules.

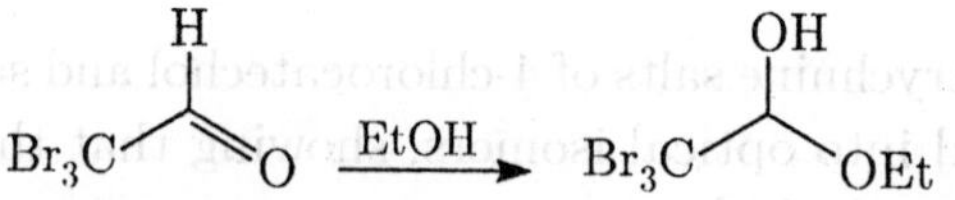

Hemiacetals that can be formed by intramolecular cyclisation of an alcohol on to an aldehyde are often stable especially if a five membered or six membered ring is formed.

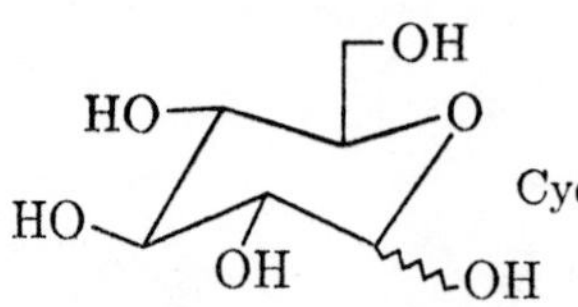

Cyclic hemiacetal (D–glycopyranose) >99%

Cyclic Hemiacetals are more stable : Part of the reason for the stability of cyclic hemiacetals concerns entropy. Formation of an acyclic hemiacetal involves a decrease in entropy (ΔS° negative) because two molecules are consumed for every one produced. This is not the case for formation of cyclic hemiacetal.

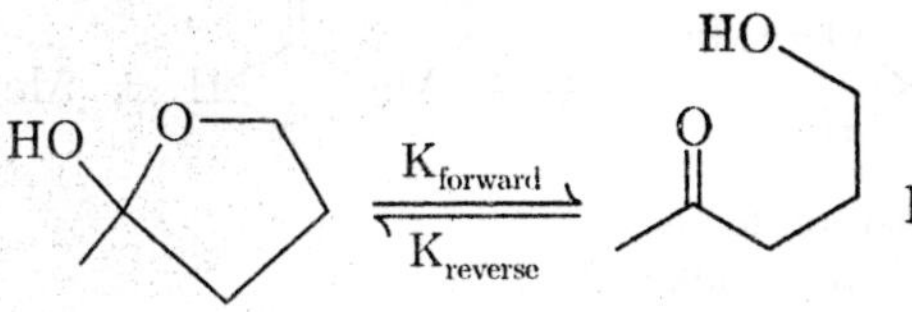

$$K = \frac{K_{forward}}{K_{reverse}} = \text{Equilibrium constant}$$

The reaction is intramolecular and fast for cyclic hemiacetals.

Acyclic hemiacetals form slowly from an aldehyde or ketone plus an alcohol, but their rate of formation is greatly increased by acid or by base.

Acid catalysed hemiacetal formation :

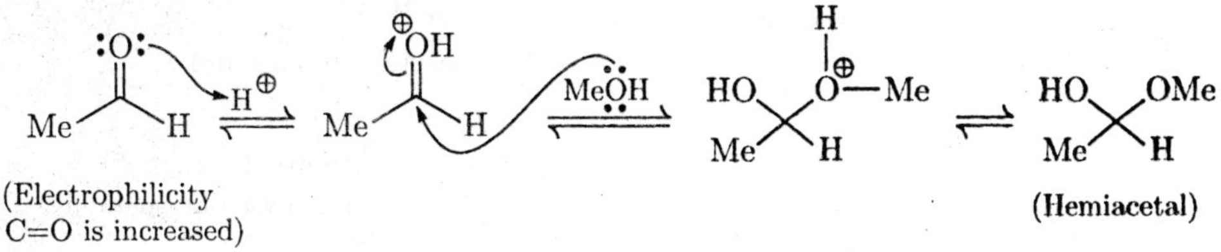

Base catalysed hemiacetal formation :

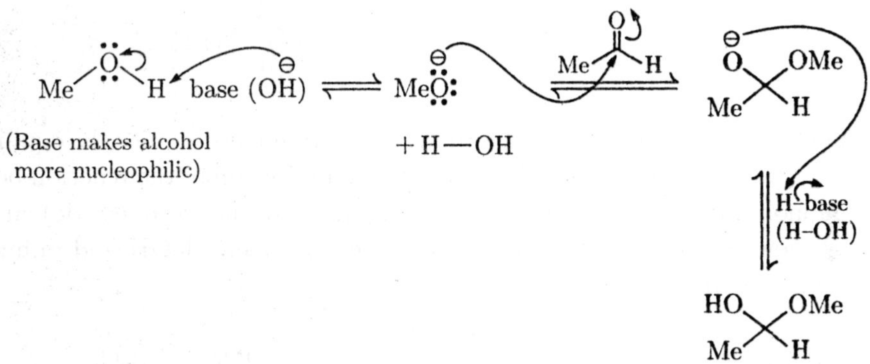

Acid or base catalyses the formation of hemiacetals, acid or base also catalyses their decomposition back to starting aldehyde or ketone and alcohol. Acid or base catalysts increase the rate of equilibration of hemiacetals with their aldehyde and alcohol components – the catalysts do not change the pattern of that equilibrium.

Acid catalysed hemiacetal decomposition :

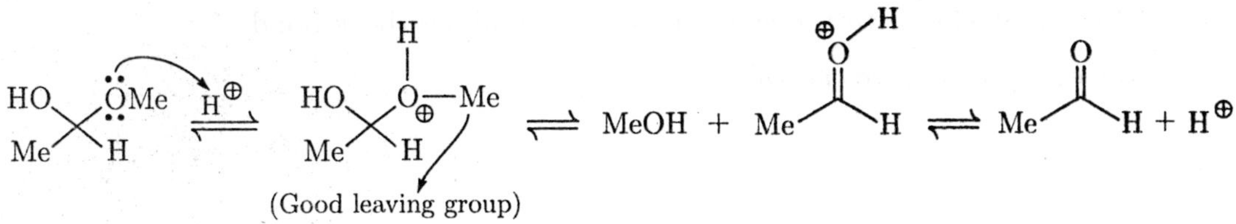

Base catalysed hemiacetal decomposition :

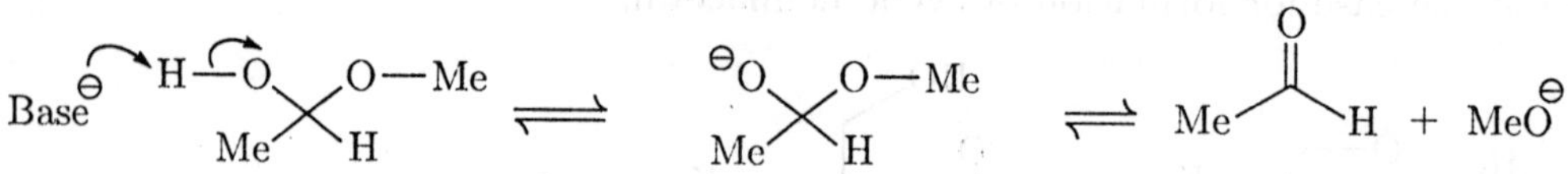

(Deprotonation forces
the alcohol to leave as alkoxide)

Acetals are formed from aldehydes or ketones plus alcohols in the presence of acid :

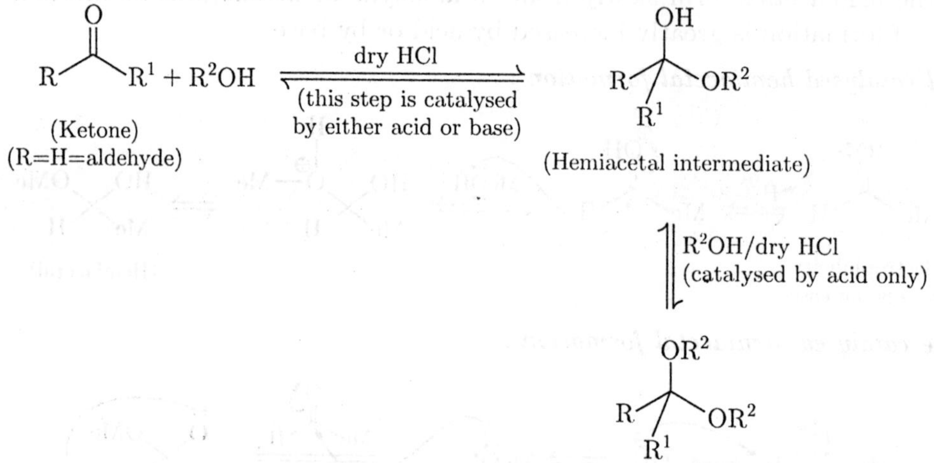

Usually aldehydes undergo the acetal formation reaction readily since the equilibrium lies to the right at room temperature. The position of equilibrium of the reaction between ketones and monohydric alcohols lies to the left (*i.e.*, to the ketone side) at room temperature. At low temperature, the ketal formation between MeOH and unhindered ketone is somewhat favourable.

$$\text{MeCOMe} + 2\text{MeOH} \xrightleftharpoons{\text{acid resin}/-27°\text{C}} \text{Me}_2\text{C(OMe)}_2 + \text{H}_2\text{O}$$

In the presence of acid (but not base) hemiacetals can undergo an elimination reaction losing the oxygen atom that once belonged to the parent aldehyde group.

The stages are –

1. Protonation of the hydroxyl group of the hemiacetals.
2. Loss of water by elimination and leads to an unstable and highly reactive oxonium ion.
3. Addition of MeOH to the oxonium ion by breaking the π-bond.
4. Loss of a proton gives acetal.

Acid catalysed acetal formation from hemiacetal :

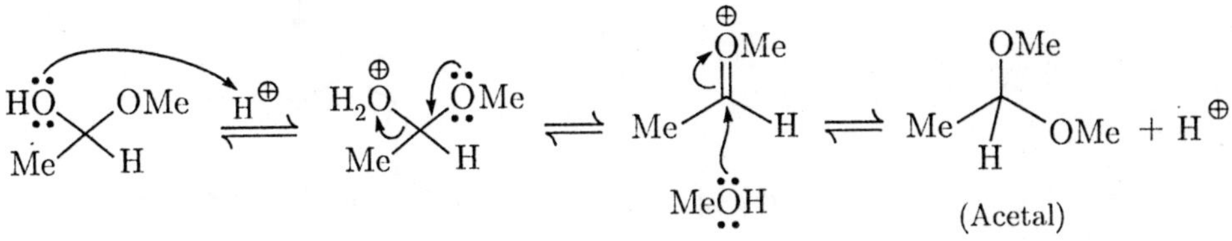

(Unstable oxonium ion)

Oxonium ions are more electrophilic just like the protonated carbonyl group and can react rapidly with a second molecule of methanol.

Acid catalysed acetal formation :

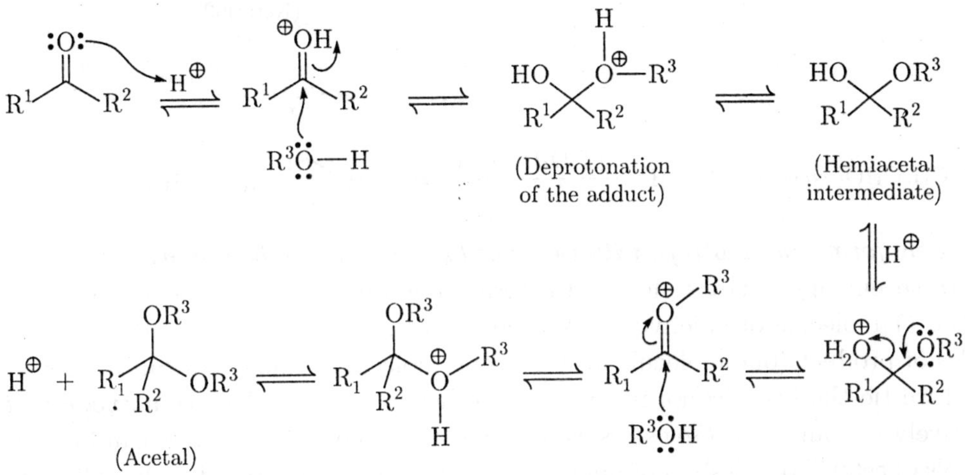

Making Acetals : Every step in the formation of an acetal is reversible. To make acetals, therefore, we must use an excess of alcohol or remove the water from the reaction mixture as it forms, by distillation.

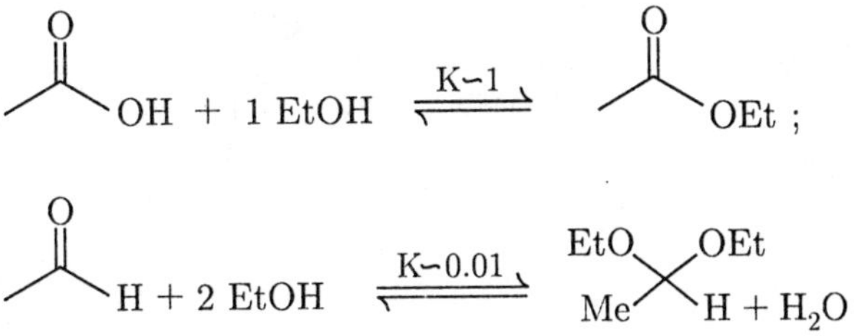

In fact, acetal formation is more difficult than ester formation and for ketones, the value is even lower. It is often very difficult to get the acetals of ketones (sometimes called ketals) to form unless they are cyclic.

(a) 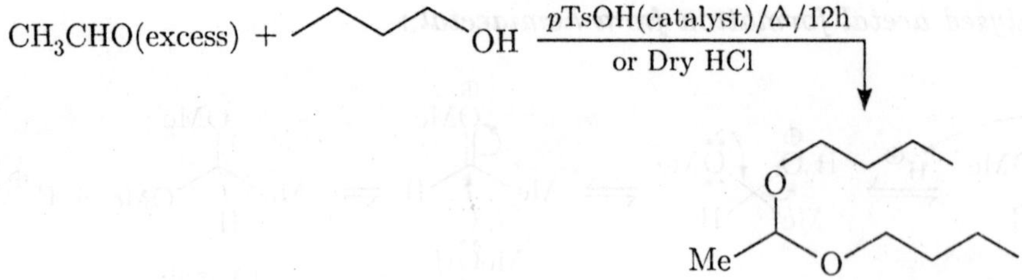

(Acetal) 50%

(b) 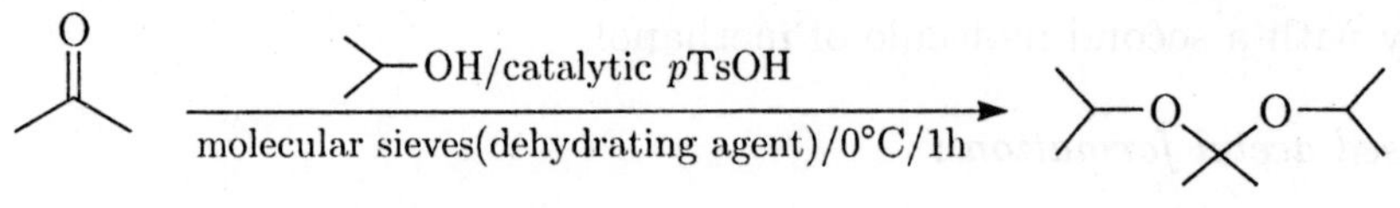

(Ketal)62%

(c) 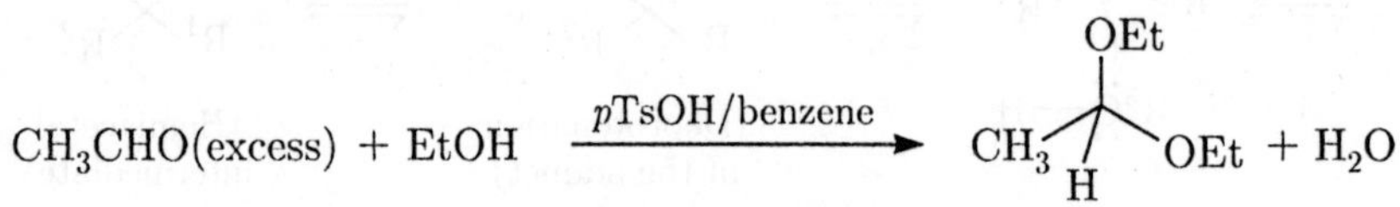

Benzene forms an azeotrope with water at 64.9°C and can be removed. There is an unfavourable entropy decrease for acetal formation when three molecules of starting compound (1 molecule of aldehyde or ketone + two molecules of alcohol) become two molecules of product (one molecule acetal + one molecule water). We can improve the matter if we tie the two alcohol molecules together in a diol and make a ***cyclic acetal.*** Alternatively we can use *ortho* esters as a source of alcohol. *Ortho* esters can be viewed as "acetals of esters" or triesters of unknown "*ortho* acid" (hydrates of carboxylic acids), for example *ortho* acetic acid [$Me_3C(OH)_3$].

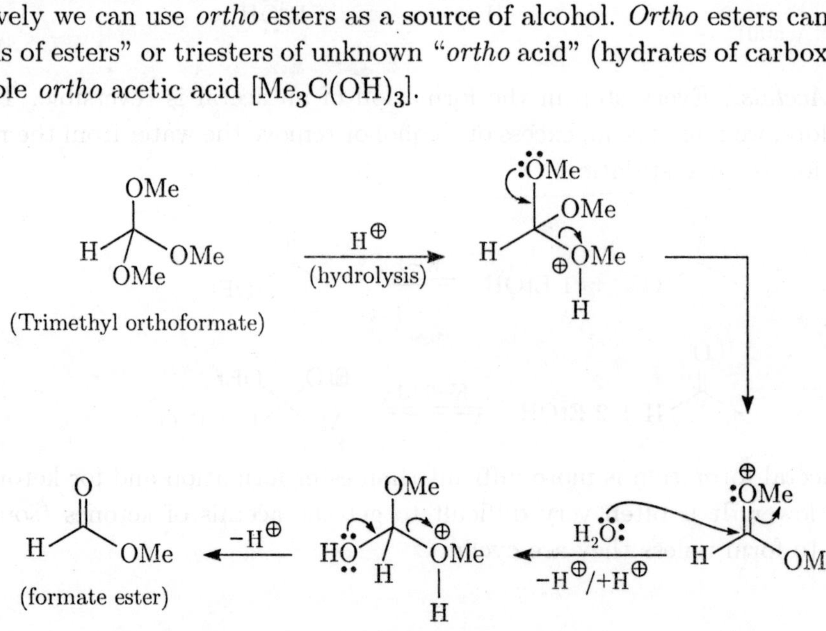

Ketones and aldehydes undergo acetal exchange with *ortho* esters. The water produced is taken out of the equilibrium by hydrolysis of the *ortho* esters.

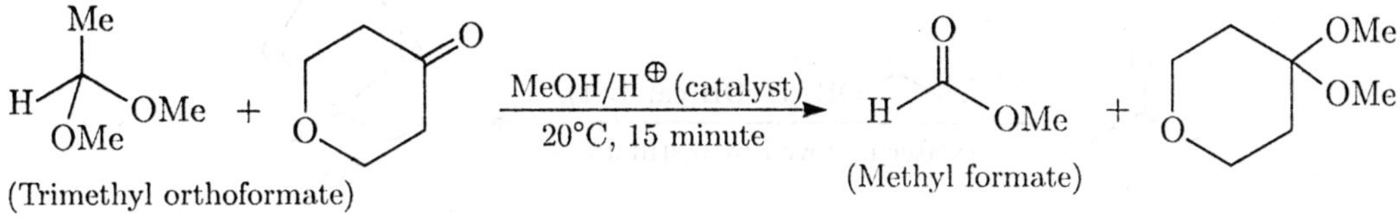

The *acetal formation* reaction is *reversible* and the hydrolysis of the acetal back to the starting carbonyl compound may easily be effected with dilute acid. The acetals do not *hydrolyse in the presence of a base.*

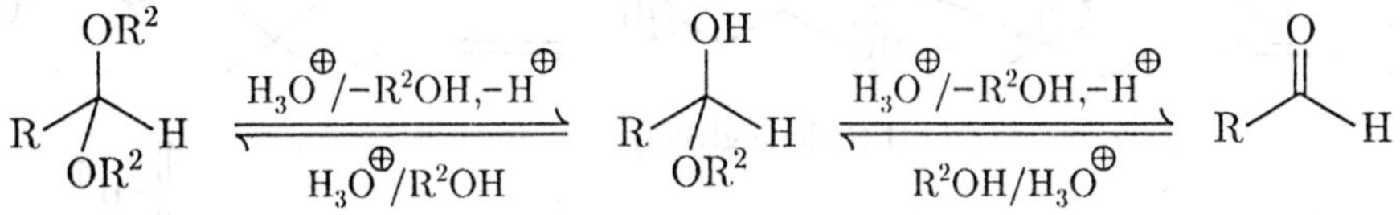

A similar reaction is the addition of thiols to carbonyl compounds in the presence of dry HCl to yield hemithioacetals and thioacetals.

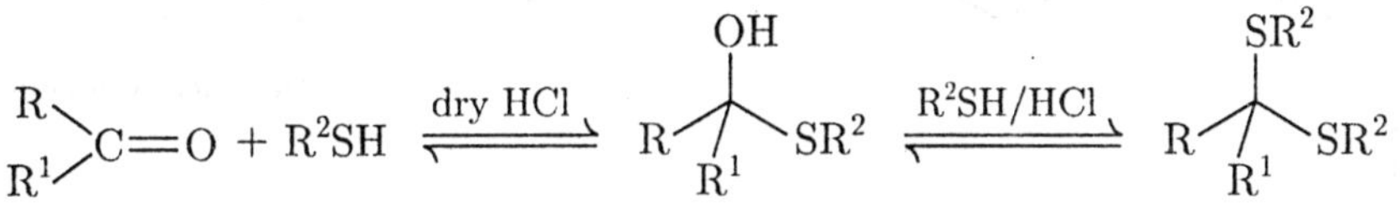

The nucleophilicity of sulphur being greater than that of oxygen, they undergo acetal formation reaction more readily than alcohols. The thioacetals are relatively stable in dilute acids and bases. However, they may be decomposed readily by $HgCl_2$ and $CdCO_3$ mixture.

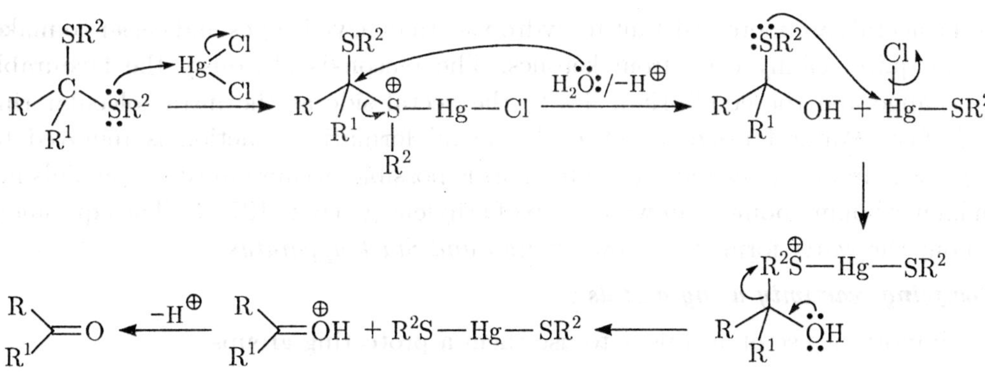

Cyclic acetals are more stable towards hydrolysis than acyclic ones : Cyclic acetals are formed by reaction of a single molecule of a diol, a compound containing two hydroxyl groups, and is favourable from the entropy point of view. Acyclic acetals are formed from two molecules of alcohols and one molecule of aldehyde or ketone (total three molecules) to give one molecule of acetal and one molecule of water (total two molecules) and thus, entropy is decreased (ΔS° negative). But with a diol, two molecules of reactants (one molecule diol + one molecule of aldehyde/ketone) forms a cyclic acetal or ketal and a molecule of water ($\Delta S°$ is zero), which is favourable from thermodynamic point of view.

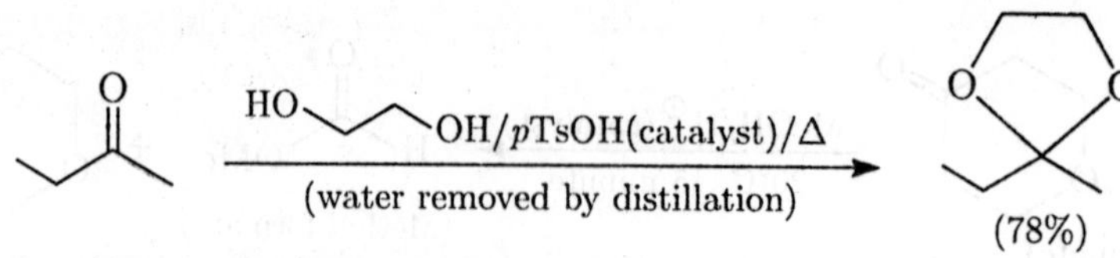

Acid–catalysed dioxolane formation :

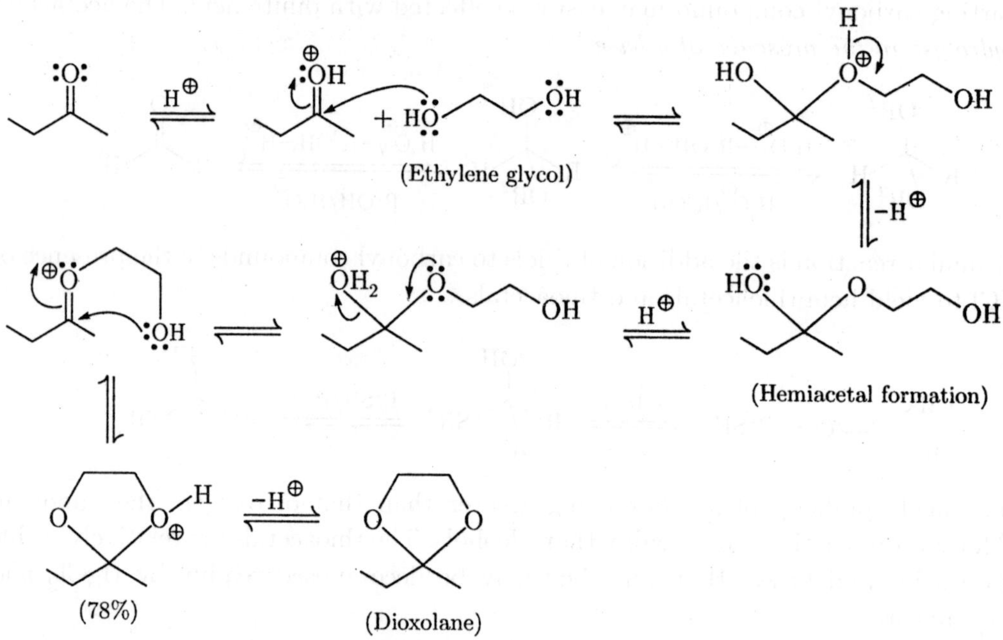

Cyclic acetals are more resistant to hydrolysis than acyclic ones and easier to make. They form quite readily even from ketones. The reason is obviously the favourable entropy change and the equilibrium lies to the acetal side as the intramolecular ring closure is fast. Water formed in the cyclic acetal formation reaction is removed by distilling out it from the reaction mixture. This is possible because most of the diols has a much higher boiling point than water (b.p of ethylene glycol is 197°C). The equipment to distil out the water formed is known "*Dean and Stark apparatus.*"

Modifying reactivity using acetals :

One important use of acetals is to use them a protecting groups.

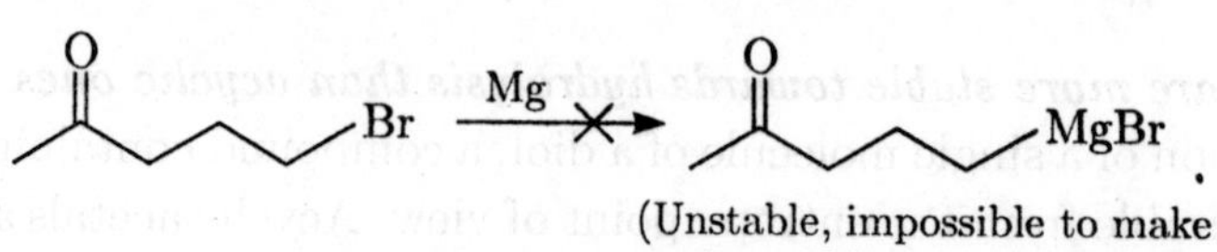

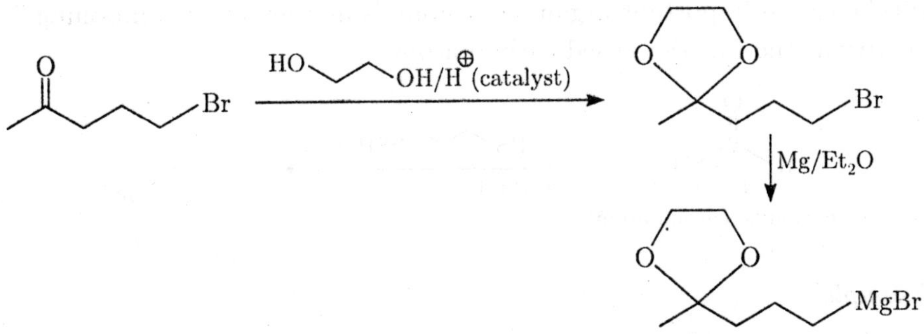

(Stable Grignard Reagent)

Acetals are stable to base, and to basic nucleophiles such as Grignard reagent and once the Grignard reagent has reacted with an electrophile, the ketone can be recovered by hydrolysing the acetal in dilute acid. The acetal is functioning here as a *protecting group* because it protects the carbonyl group from attack by the Grignard reagent.

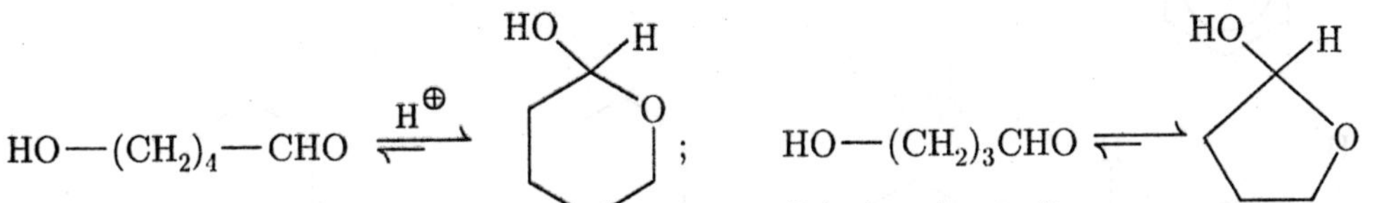

(5-hydroxypentanal) (Cyclic hemiacetal) 94% ; (4-hydroxybutanal) (Cyclic hemiacetal) 89%

Thioacetals and Cyclic Thioacetals

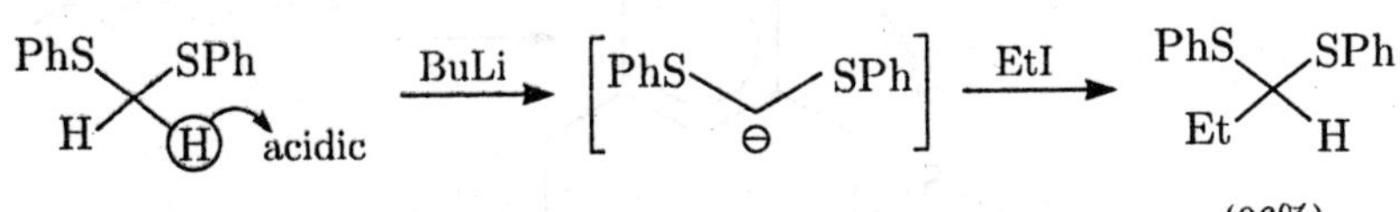

pK_a=31 (96%)

'Normal' thioacetals are prepared by treatment of a aldehyde or a ketone with a thiol and an acid catalyst, though Lewis acid such as BF_3 is preferred over protic acids.

Formation of cyclic thioacetals :

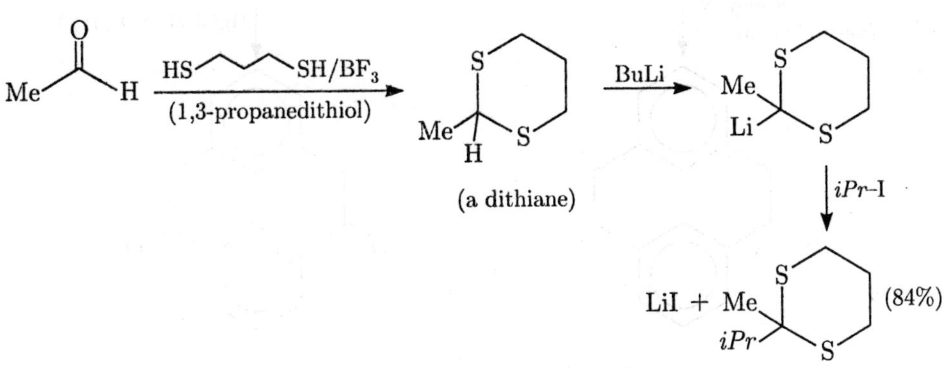

(a dithiane) (84%)

Dithianes are important organic compounds as they exert '**umpolung**,'' *i.e* inverts the polarity at the functionalised carbon atom.

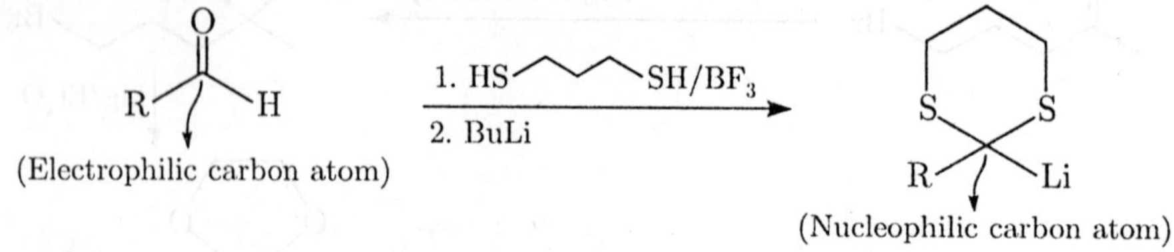

Example :

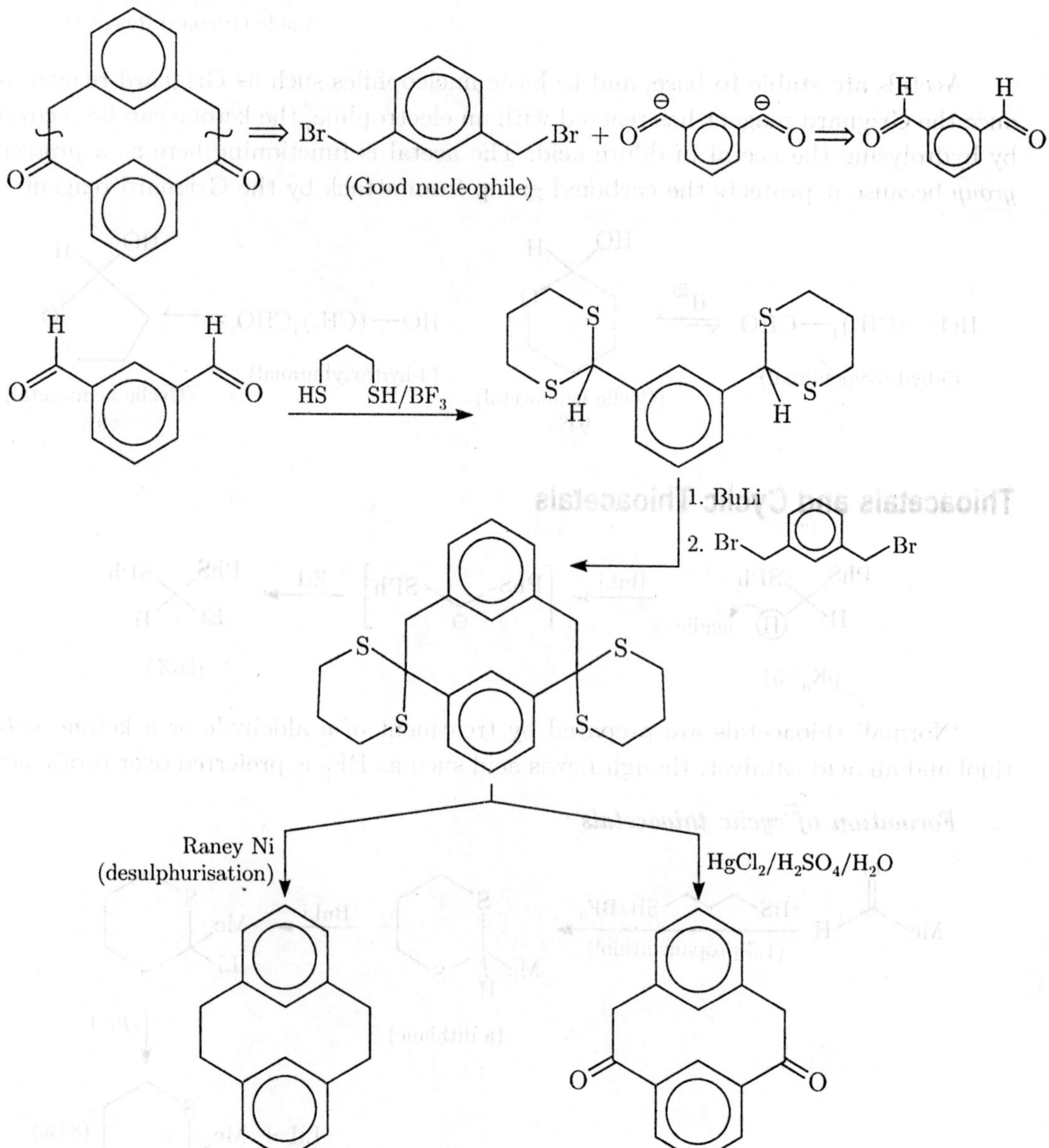

Mechanism of Hydrolysis : Dithianes are more stable than acetals and a mercury reagent has to be used to assist their hydrolysis. Hg (II) and sulphides form strong coordination complexes and Hg catalyses the reaction by acting as a sulphur selective Lewis acid.

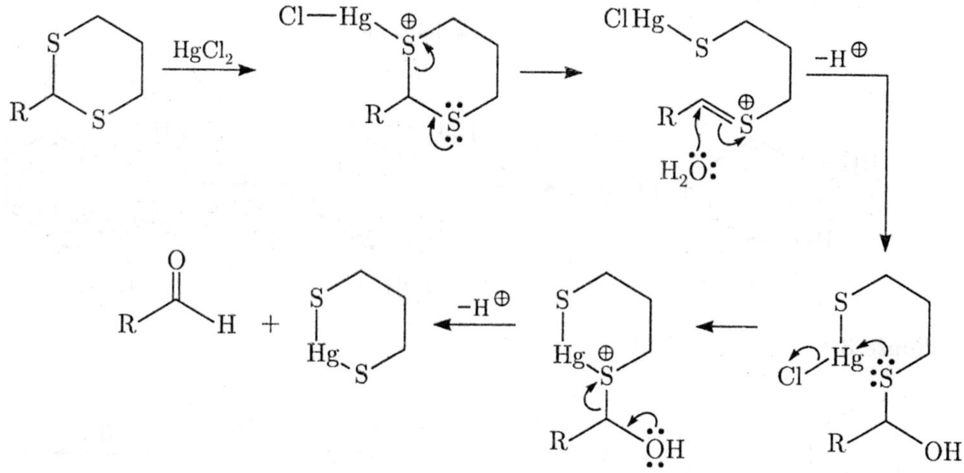

There are two reasons why the normal *acid catalysed hydrolysis of acetals usually fails* with *thioacetals.* Sulphur is less basic than oxygen, so the protonated species is lower in concentration at a given pH and the sulphur 3p lone pairs are less able to form a stable π-bond to carbon than are the oxygen 2p lone pairs 2p-3p orbital overlap is energetically forbidden.

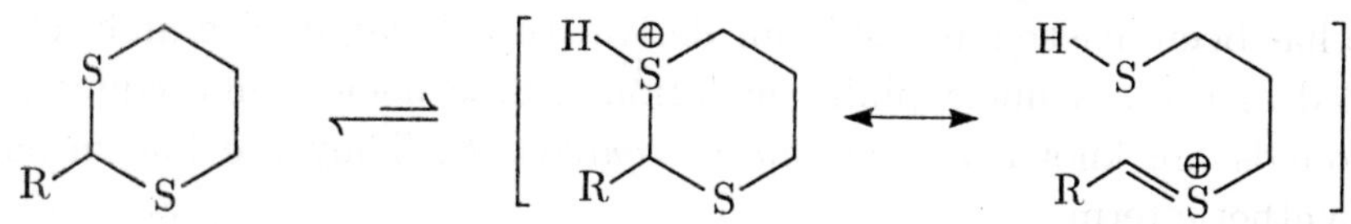

(Weakly basic lone pairs) (Low concentration) (Weak S–C π bond) (dπ–pπ)

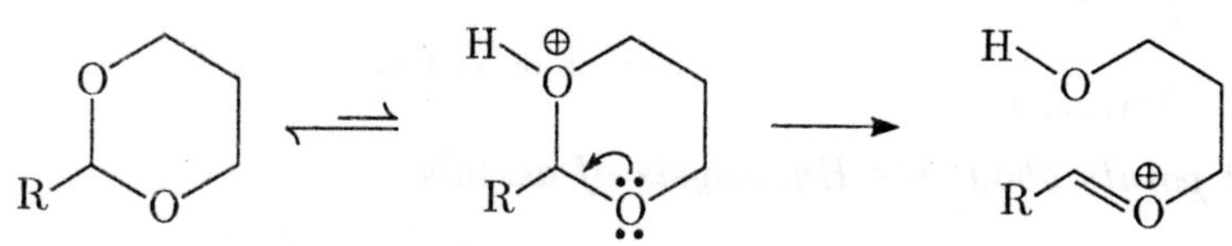

(Higher concentration) (Strong O–C π bond) (pπ–pπ bond)

Route 2 :

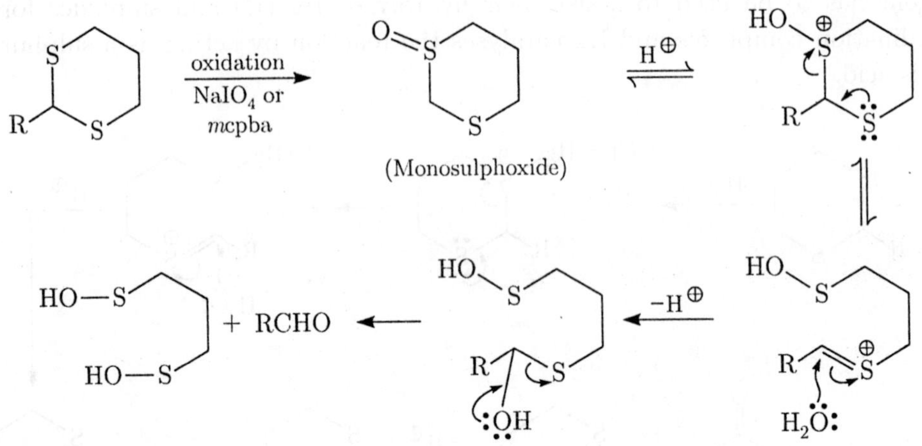

Route 3 :

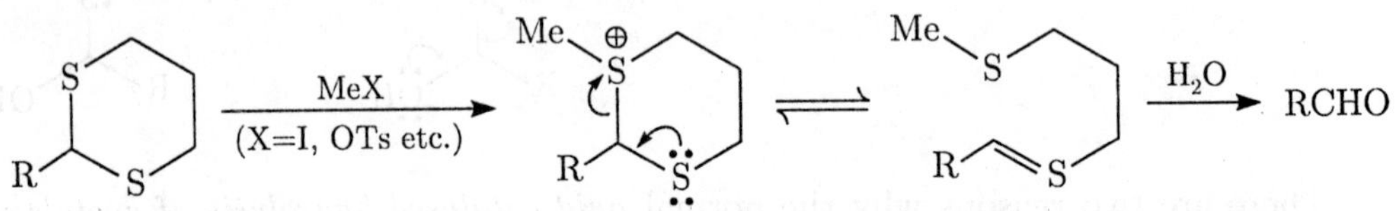

Hydrogenation of C—S bonds in thioacetals is often achieved with Raney Ni. This acetalisation followed by Raney Ni reduction is a useful way of replacing C=O group with $-CH_2-$.

Dithianes are d¹ reagents (Acyl anion equivalent) : A sequence in which a carbonyl group has been masked as a sulphur derivative, alkylated with an electrophile and then revealed again is a nucleophilic acylation. These nucleophilic equivalents of carbonyl compounds are known as *acyl anion equivalents.* They are known as d^1 reagents in retrosynthetic term.

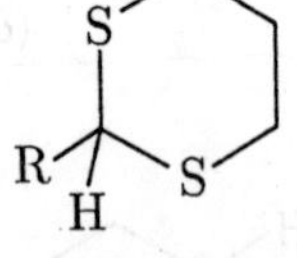

(Dithiane)

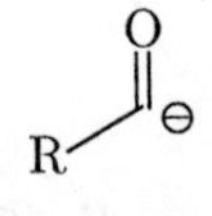

(d^1–synthon or acylanion equivalent)

Some salient points about the Hydrolysis of acetals

1. The reaction proceeds with specific acid catalyst $H_3O^{\oplus}$.
2. The reaction has been found to proceed faster with D_2O than with H_2O.
3. The R^2—O bond does not break even when R^2 is tertiarybutyl groups –confirmed by ^{18}O labelling. Therefore C—OR^2 bond breaks.
4. Acetal of an optically active alcohol does not give racemic alcohol. This indicates that $R^{2\oplus}$ is never formed.

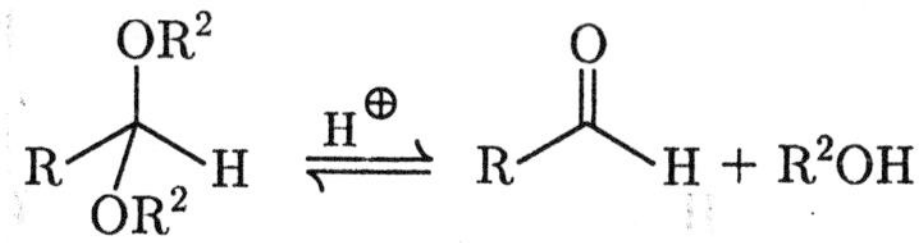

Since the hydrolysis of acetals and formation of acetals are the reverse reactions, they follow the *principle of microscopic reversibility.*

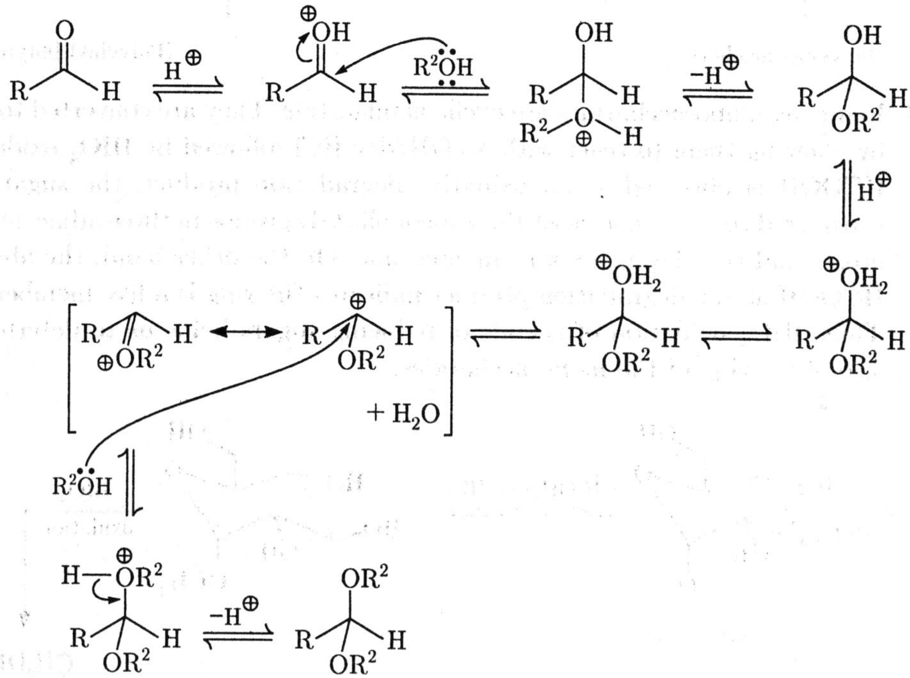

Acetals are stable towards alkali but not to acids : There is no active hydrogen in an acetal, so $^{\ominus}OH$ cannot abstract it and thus, decomposition does not take place. Again –OR group is a poor leaving group, so S_N reaction can not take place with $^{\ominus}OH$. So an acetal is stable towards alkali. $H_3O^{\oplus}$ protonates the OR group and the latter becomes $R-\overset{\oplus}{O}-H$; this is a good leaving group and thus, S_N reaction occurs with H_2O. This makes acetals unstable to acids.

Applications of acetal formation reaction :

1. ***Protecting group*** :

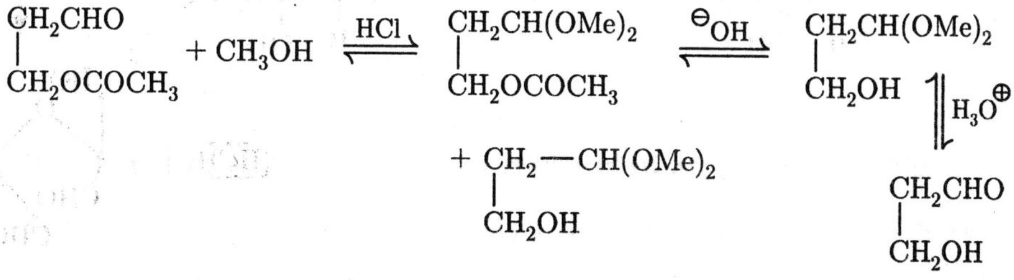

2. 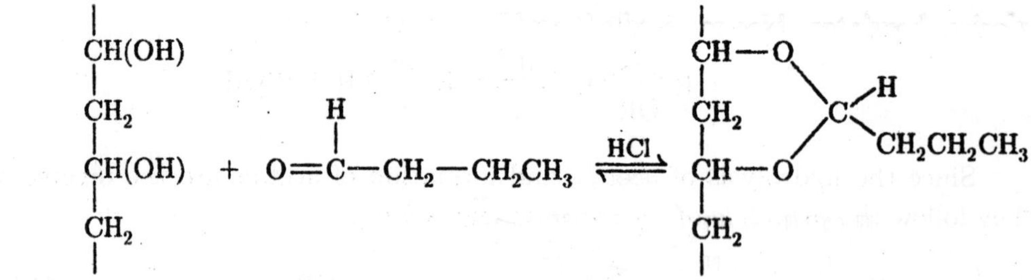

(Polyvinyl alcohol) (Polyvinyl butyral)

3. Reducing monosaccharides are cyclic hemiacetals. They are converted to acetals by allowing them to react with MeOH/dry HCl followed by HIO_4 oxidation. If HCOOH is obtained as an oxidative degradation product, the sugar ring is considered to contain at least three alcoholic OH groups in three adjacent carbon atoms and the ring is a six-membered one. On the other hand, the absence of HCOOH as the degradation product indicates the ring is a five membered one. Thus, HIO_4 oxidation of acetals of reducing sugars helps us to determine the size of the ring of the monosaccharides.

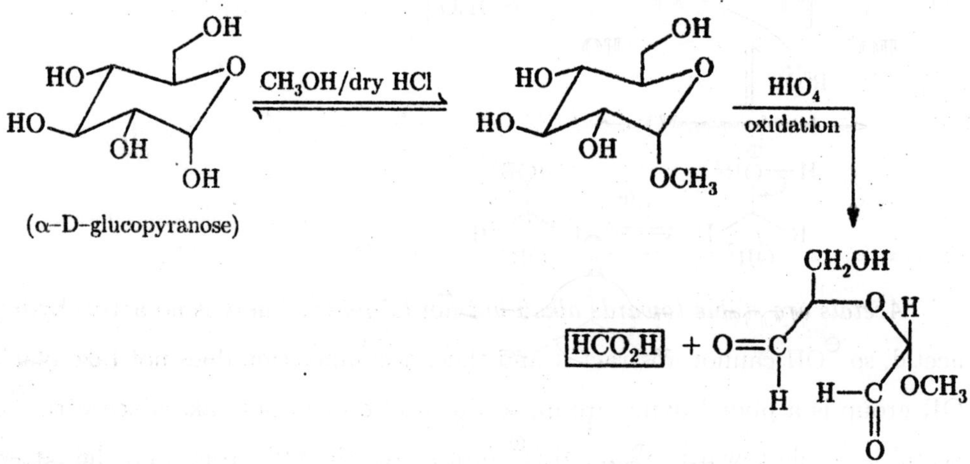

(α–D–glucopyranose)

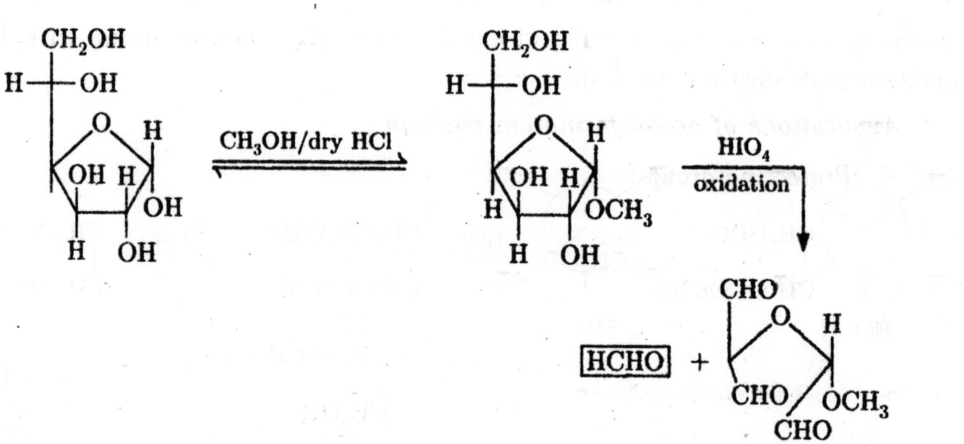

Ethers

C—O—C Linkage is known as ether linkage and compounds containing ether linkage are called *ethers.* The hydrocarbon substituents may be alkyl, aryl, cycloalkyl, allyl, benzyl etc. Depending on the nature of hydrocarbon moiety, the ethers may be classified as dialkyl ethers, alkyl aryl ethers, diaryl ethers etc. when the hydrocarbon groups of an ether are equivalent, they are called **symmetric** ethers, for example dimethyl ether ($Me-\ddot{\underset{\cdot\cdot}{O}}-Me$) or diphenyl ether ($Ph-\ddot{\underset{\cdot\cdot}{O}}-Ph$). When these hydrocarbon groups are different, they are called **mixed** ethers, like ethyl methyl ether ($Et-\ddot{\underset{\cdot\cdot}{O}}-Me$) or methyl phenyl ether ($Me-\ddot{\underset{\cdot\cdot}{O}}-Ph$) etc.

Synthesis of ethers

1. ***Williamson's ether synthesis*** : The synthesis consists of an S_N2 reaction of a sodium alkoxide with an alkyl halide, alkyl sulphonate or alkyl sulphate.

$$R-\ddot{\underset{\cdot\cdot}{O}}:^{\ominus}\;\overset{\oplus}{Na} \quad + \quad R'-L \xrightarrow{S_N2} R-\ddot{\underset{\cdot\cdot}{O}}-R' + \overset{\oplus}{Na}\;\overset{\ominus}{L}:$$

(Sodium or potassium alkoxide) (R=alkyl or aryl) — (L=Br, Cl, OSO_2R'', OSO_2OR'')

Aryl halides have partial double bond character in C—X bond, so they do not react with alkoxides or phenoxides. Primary halides are of better choice as secondary or tertiary halides may undergo E-2 elimination reaction in the presence of strong alkoxide bases. The alkoxide anion may contain secondary or tertiary group, but tertiary alkoxides react very slowly. Ar_3C-X reacts even with alcohol, a weak base, because $Ar_3\overset{\oplus}{C}$ is a very stable carbocation and the reaction here becomes S_N1.

$$R_1\ddot{\underset{\cdot\cdot}{O}}:^{\ominus} + \underset{\text{(primary halide)}}{R-X} \xrightarrow{S_N2} \underset{\text{T.S.}}{[R_1\overset{\delta-}{O}\cdots R\cdots\overset{\delta-}{X}]^{\neq}} \longrightarrow R_1OR + :\ddot{\underset{\cdot\cdot}{X}}:^{\ominus}$$

Just like typical S_N2 reactions, the transition state will be much crowded if a tertiary halide is used.

2. ***The Ullmann biaryl ether synthesis*** :

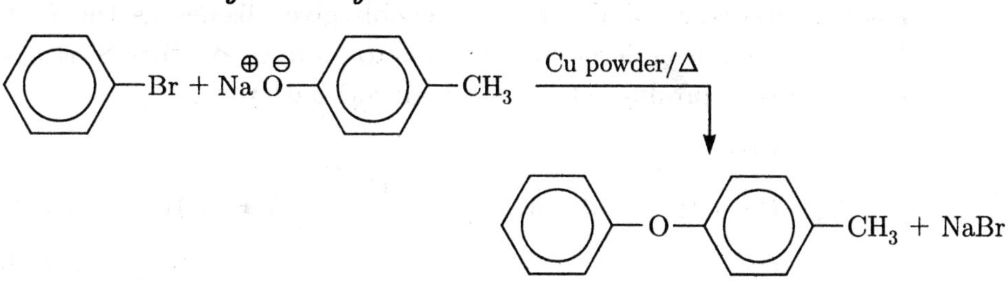

3. When an alcohol is refluxed with metallic sodium and an alkyl *p*-toluene sulphonate, a dialkyl ether is formed.

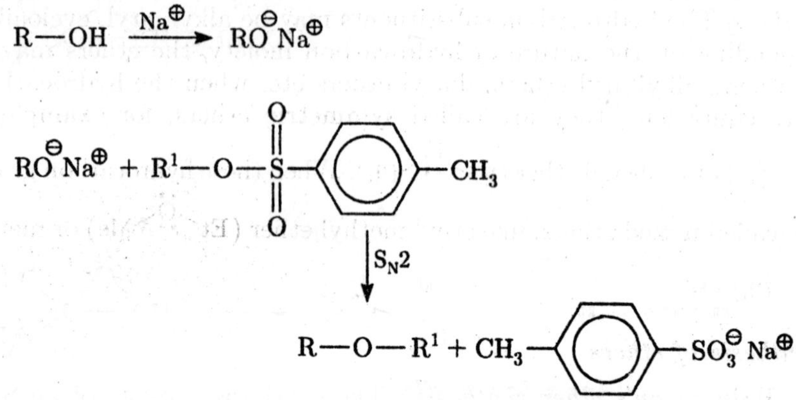

4. When alcohols are treated with CH_2N_2 (diazomethane) in the presence of a Lewis acid, $Al(OEt)_3$ or BF_3, a methyl ether is formed.

$$R{-}OH + CH_2N_2 \xrightarrow{Al(OEt)_3} R{-}OCH_3 + N_2\uparrow$$

5. Phenols react with diazomethane in the absence of any Lewis acid to form aryl methyl ether.

$$ArOH + CH_2N_2 \longrightarrow ArOCH_3 + N_2\uparrow$$

The –OH hydrogen of phenolic –OH group is sufficiently active to react with diazomethane (CH_2N_2) and no help of Lewis acid is required to activate it, where alcoholic –OH hydrogen is not that much acidic, so Lewis acid is used to activate the alcoholic –OH hydrogen to make reactive to react with diazomethane.

6. ***Dehydration of alcohols*** : When an alcohol is treated with concentrated H_2SO_4 at an elevated temperature, an ether is formed by the loss of one molecule of water from two molecules of the alcohol. The concentrated acid absorbs the water formed in the reaction and the equilibrium is shifted to the product (ether) side.

$$R{-}OH + HO{-}R \xrightarrow[\Delta]{conc.H_2SO_4} \underset{\text{(Symmetric ether)}}{R{-}O{-}R} + H_2O$$

The reactivity order of alcohol is primary alcohol>secondary alcohol>tertiary alcohol. Secondary and tertiary alcohols give alkenes as the major product. Primary alcohols undergo S_N2 reaction to produce an ether. Tertiary alcohols, if at all it works produce ethers through S_N1 pathway.

$$CH_3{-}\underset{CH_3}{\overset{CH_3}{C}}{-}OH + \underset{\text{(Solvent)}}{C_2H_5OH(excess)} \xrightarrow{\text{dilute } H_2SO_4} \underset{\text{(Tertiarybutyl ethyl ether)}}{(CH_3)_3C{-}OC_2H_5} + H_2O$$

The key to this reaction is only one of the alcohols forms stable carbocation after loss of a molecule of water and then it reacts with the other alcohol quickly to form the ether.

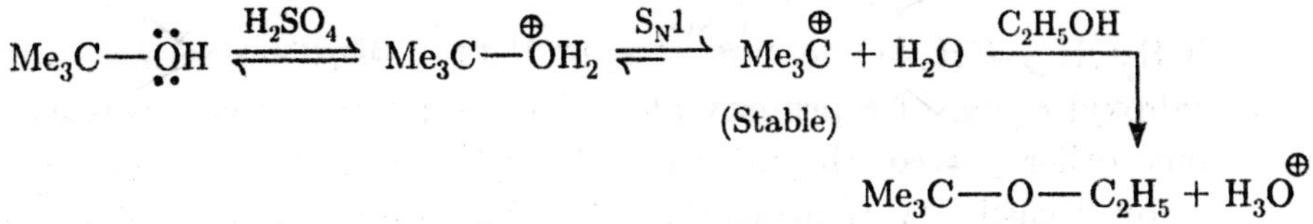

$$C_2H_5OH \overset{H^{\oplus}}{\rightleftharpoons} C_2H_5\overset{\oplus}{O}H_2 \not\longrightarrow \underset{\text{(Not Stable enough)}}{C_2H_5^{\oplus}} + H_2O$$

There is an important relationship between this reaction and alkene formation of alcohol dehydration. *Tertiary alcohols* undergo *dehydration* to *alkenes* in the presence of strong acids. *Ether formation* and *alkene formation* both involve *carbocation* intermediates. The *conditions dictate* which product is obtained. The dehydration of alcohols to *alkenes* involves relatively *high temperature (180°C)* whereas *ether formation* involves *milder temperature (140°C).*

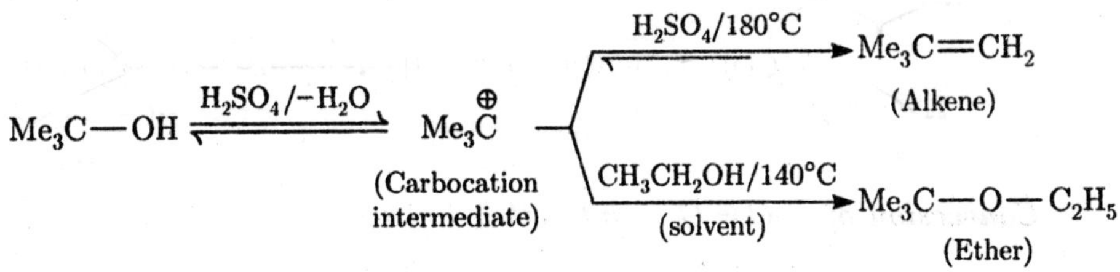

So the treatment of an alkene with a large excess of alcohol in the presence of an acid catalyst should also give an ether provided that a relatively stable carbocation intermediate is involved.

$$(H_3C)_2C{=}CH_2 + CH_3OH \xrightarrow{\text{dilute } H_2SO_4} Me_3C{-}O{-}CH_3$$

(Tertiarybutyl methyl ether) (MTBE)
(Important gasoline additive)

Mechanism of the reaction :

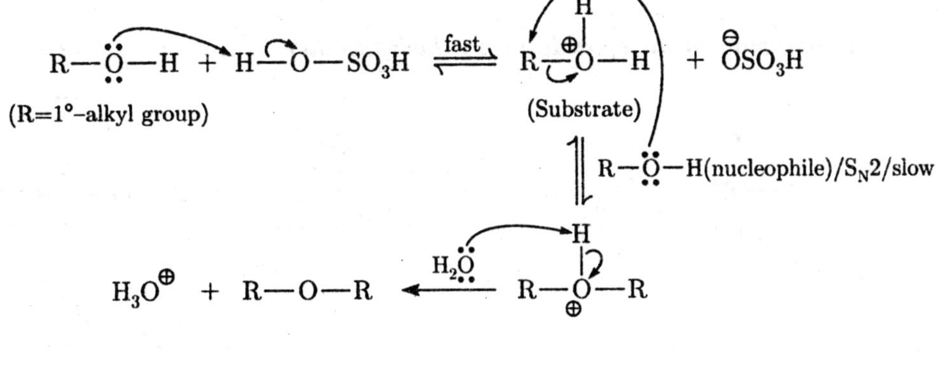

But the method is not useful for the preparatin of *unsymmetrical ethers* from primary alcohols because the reaction leads to a mixture of products.

The previous reaction, *i.e*

$RCH_2OH + CH_2{=}CMe_2 \xrightarrow{H_2SO_4} RCH_2O{-}CMe_3$ is often used to protect the hydroxyl group of a primary alcohol while another reaction is carried out on some other part of the molecule. The protecting tertiarybutyl group can be removed easily by treating the ether with dilute aqueous acid. Suppose, for example, we want to prepare 4-pentyn-1-ol from 3–bromo–1–propanol and sodium acetylide. If we allow them to react directly, the strongly basic sodium acetylide will react first with the hydroxyl group.

$$HOCH_2CH_2CH_2Br + NaC{\equiv}C{-}H \longrightarrow NaOCH_2CH_2CH_2Br + H{-}C{\equiv}C{-}H$$

However, if we protect –OH group first, the synthesis becomes feasible.

$$HOCH_2CH_2CH_2Br \xrightarrow[2.\ CH_2=CMe_2]{1.\ H_2SO_4} Me_3COCH_2CH_2CH_2Br \xrightarrow{Na-C\equiv CH} Me_3CO(CH_2)_3C{\equiv}CH$$

$$Me_3CO(CH_2)_3C{\equiv}CH \xrightarrow{H_3O^{\oplus}/H_2O} Me_3COH + HO(CH_2)_3C{\equiv}CH$$

(4-pentyn-l-ol)

7. ***Conversion of —C = C— into ether linkage*** :

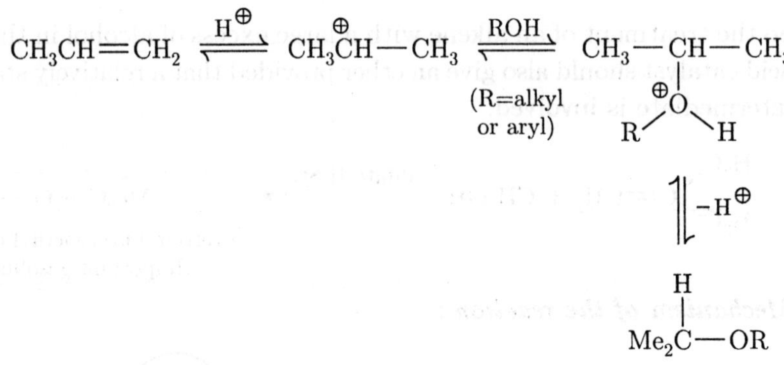

8. ***Conversion of an epoxide to a β-hydroxyether*** :

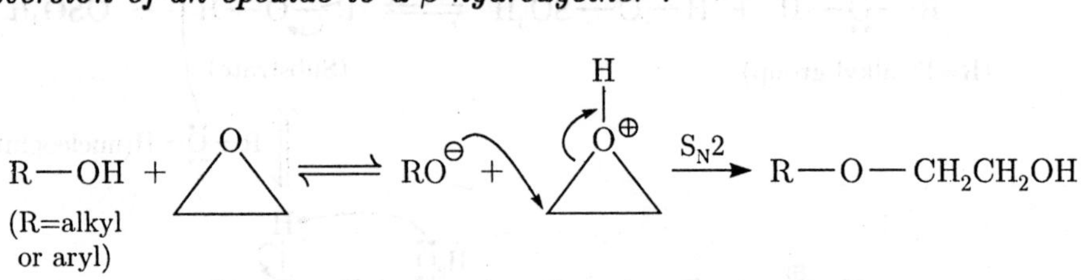

9. ***Synthesis of ethers by alkoxymercuration/demercuration*** :

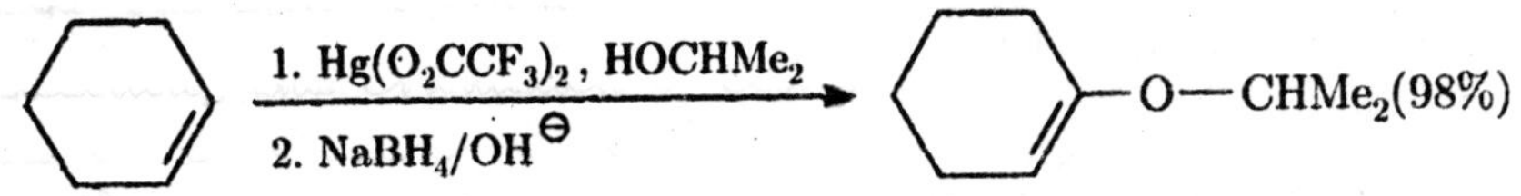

The mechanism of the reaction directly parallels hydration by mercuration/demercuration technique.

Synthesis of thioethers **(R^1–S–R^2)**

1. By heating K_2S with an alkyl halide, potassium alkyl sulphate or tosylate.

$$2\overset{\oplus}{K}S^{2-} \; R-X \longrightarrow R-\overset{\ominus}{S} + KX$$

$$R-\overset{\ominus}{S} \; R-X \longrightarrow R-S-R + X^{\ominus}$$

2. $5\,R_2O + P_2S_5 \xrightarrow{\Delta} 5\,R-S-R + P_2O_5$

(Ether) (Phosphorus pentasulphide)

3. $R^1X + R^2\overset{\ominus}{S}\overset{\oplus}{Na} \xrightarrow{\text{Williamson's synthesis}/S_N2} R^1-S-R^2 + NaX$

(Sodium mercaptide)

4. $2\,RSH \xrightarrow{\text{Alumina/ZnS, 300°C}} R_2S + H_2S$

(Thiol)

5. By the addition of thiol to an alkene in the presence of peroxides. The mechanism proceeds free radically.

$$(R_1CO_2)_2 \longrightarrow 2R_1^{\bullet} + 2CO_2$$

$$R_1^{\bullet} + R_2SH \longrightarrow R_1H + R_2S\bullet$$

$$R_3CH{=}CH_2 + R_2S\bullet \longrightarrow R_3\dot{C}HCH_2SR_2 \xrightarrow{R_2SH} R_3CH_2CH_2SR_2 + R_2S\bullet \text{ etc.}$$

6. $2\,ArH + SCl_2 \xrightarrow[\text{sulphurisation}]{2AlCl_3/\Delta} Ar\diagup^{S}\diagdown Ar + 2\overset{\oplus}{H}\overset{\ominus}{AlCl_4}$

(Sulphur dichloride)

7. $2\,RMgX(\text{excess}) + S \longrightarrow R\diagup^{S}\diagdown R + 2\overset{\oplus}{Mg}X$

8. $PhBr + \overset{\oplus}{Na}\overset{\ominus}{S}Me \longrightarrow PhSMe + NaBr$

(Aryl bromide) (aryl alkyl thioether)

9. $$2\,PhN_2^{\oplus}\,Cl^{\ominus} + K_2S \longrightarrow Ph{-}S{-}Ph + 2N_2\uparrow + 2KCl$$
(Aryl diazonium chloride)

$$PhN_2^{\oplus}\,Cl^{\ominus} + EtS^{\ominus}\,Na^{\oplus} \longrightarrow Ph{-}S{-}Et + N_2\uparrow + NaCl$$

10.

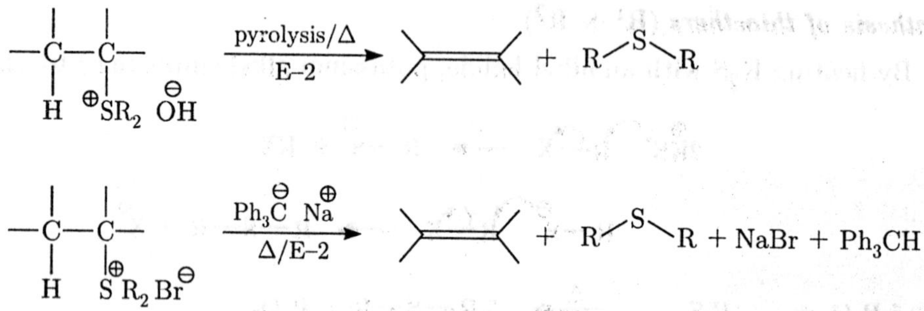

11.

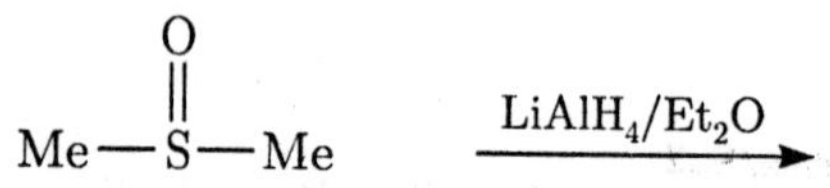

(Dimethyl sulphoxide)

Structure, reactivity and physical properties of ethers : Ether linkages have angular shape, the C—O—C bond angles are usually 110° to 118°.

The oxygen atom holds two lone pairs of electrons and due to lone pair–bond pair repulsion, the bond angle becomes like that. Moreover, due to the electronegativity of oxygen atom, C—O bond is polar. Since the shape is angular and C—O bonds are polar, the molecules contain dipole moment of the order 1.2 to 1.8 Debye.

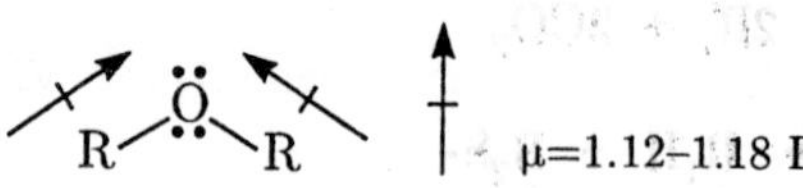

In alkyl ethers, oxygen atom is in sp^3-hybridised state, the two lone pairs belong to two sp^3 hybrid orbitals. In aryl ethers, oxygen may assume sp^2 hybridisation and hence the lone pair of electrons on the unhybrid *p*-orbital may undergo $p\pi$–$p\pi$ conjugation with the π–bonds of the aryl part.

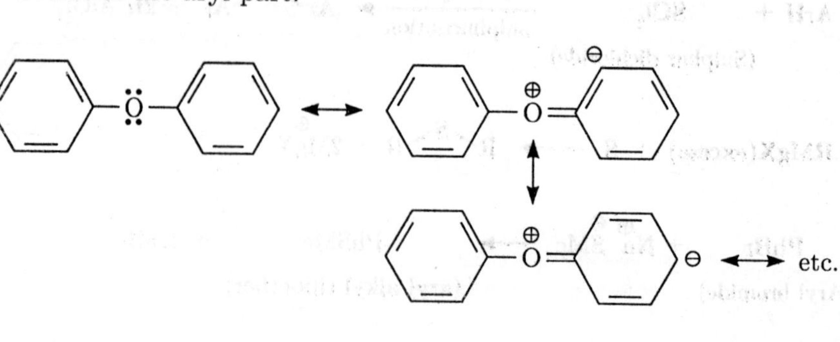

Since ethers do not have O—H bond, they can not associate amongst themselves through hydrogen bond but experience dipole dipole interaction. So ethers are low melting, low boiling and highly volatile, the m.ps and b.ps are much lower than the alcohols of comparable molecular weight. For example, dimethyl ether (b.p.–24°C), propane (–42°C) and ethanol (78°C), The m.p. and b.p. increase with increasing molecular weight. However, lower ethers are soluble in water. Ether is weakly basic and forms salts with acids. Ether can undergo reactions involving C—O bond cleavage and the cleavage requires a protonic or Lewis acid as –OR is a bad leaving group. Oxygen atom draws electrons from alkyl groups, so the α-hydrogen atoms are slightly acidic and can be substituted by electrophiles. The acidity order of α–H atom is primary > secondary > tertiary. In aryl ethers, pπ conjugation takes place; they undergo aromatic electrophilic substitution besides R—O cleavage. Ether linkage has a +R effect and so is *o/p* orienting.

***Chemical reactions given by ethers* :**

1. ***Formation of oxonium salt*** : The ethers are poorly basic (pK_a of $R-\overset{H}{\overset{|}{O^{\oplus}}}-R$ is ~35). They form salts with protonic or Lewis acid at low temperature. If the acidic hydrogen of a protonated ether is replaced by an alkyl group, the resulting compound is called an *oxonium salt.* Protonated ethers are also oxonium salts.

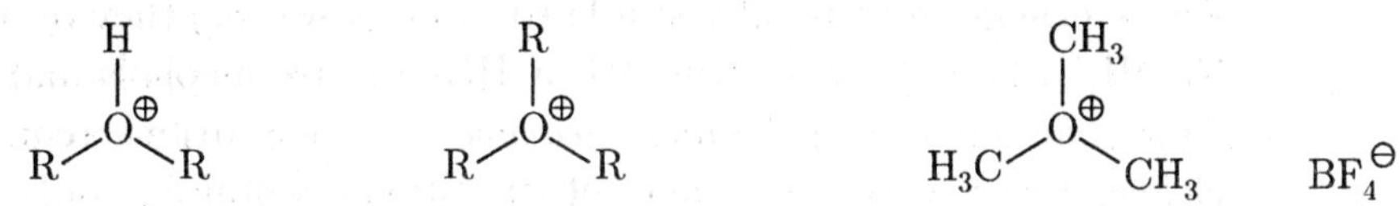

(Protonated ether) (Trialkyloxonium ion) (Trimethyloxonium fluoborate)

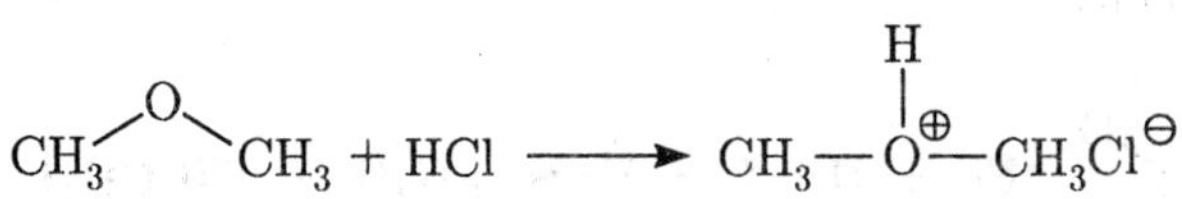

(Crystalline oxonium salt, m.p. 97°C)

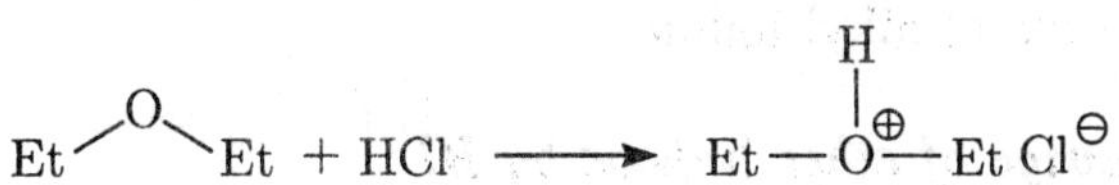

(Crystalline, m.p. 92°C)

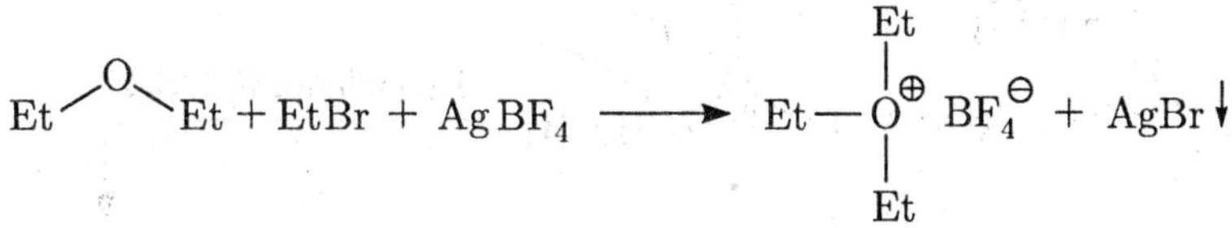

Because of salt formation, ethers are soluble in *concentrated acids (strong acids)* when the acid solution is diluted with water, ethers are thrown out of the solution. The oxonium ion gives up $H^{\oplus}$ to the water molecules as water molecules solvate proton ($H^{\oplus}$) better. Oxonium salts are amongst the most reactive alkylating agents known and they react very rapidly with most nucleophiles. For the same reason, these salts are stable when they contain counter ions which are not nucleophilic such as $BF_4^{\ominus}$ (boron has no unshared electron pair, so is not nucleophilic).

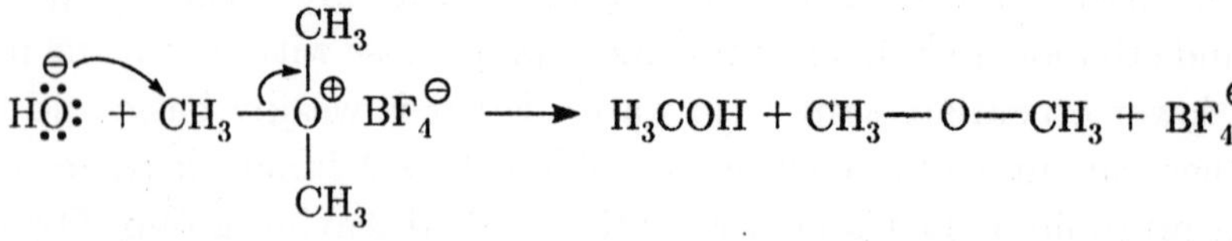

2. ***Cleavage of ethers*** :

(a) The ether linkage is relatively unreactive under a wide variety of conditions. That is why ethers are used as solvents without affecting the ether linkage. Ethers do not react with nucleophiles for the same reason as alcohols do not, an S_N2 reaction would result in a very basic leaving group. Alkoxide ions are strong bases.

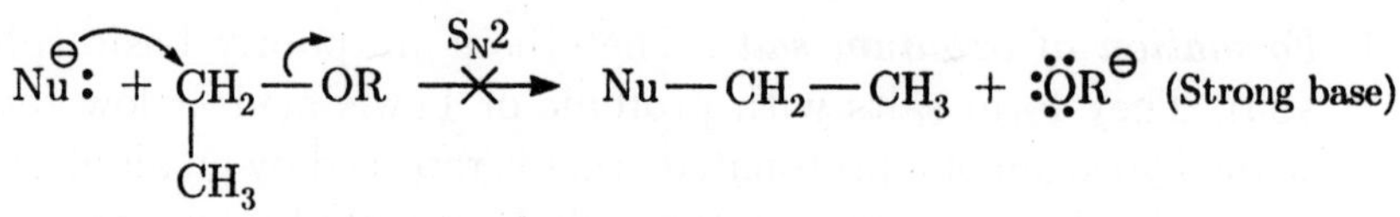

Hence ethers are generally stable towards bases, *e.g* they do not react with NaOH. Ethers do react with HI or HBr to give alcohols and alkyl halides. This reaction is called *ether cleavage.* The conditions required for ether cleavage vary with the type of ether. Ethers containing only primary alkyl groups are cleaved only under relatively harsh conditions such as concentrated HBr or HI and heat.

$$Et{-}O{-}Et + H{-}I \xrightarrow{\Delta} EtOH + CH_3CH_2I$$

The alcohol formed in the cleavage of ether can go on to react with HI to give a second molecule of alkyl halide.

Mechanism of cleavage of ether linkage by HI :

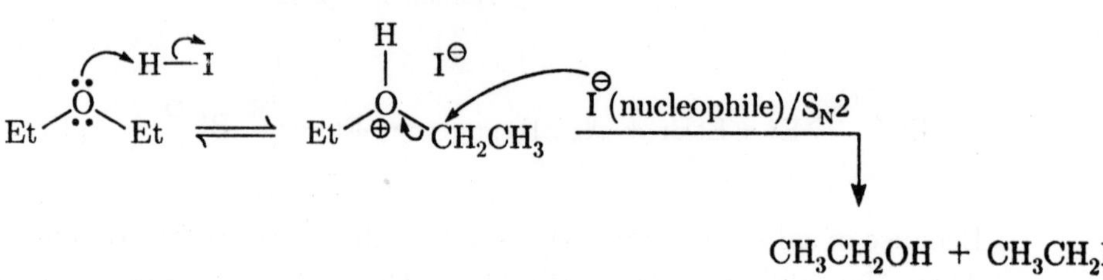

If the ether is tertiary, the cleavage occurs under milder conditions (lower temperature, dilute acid etc.

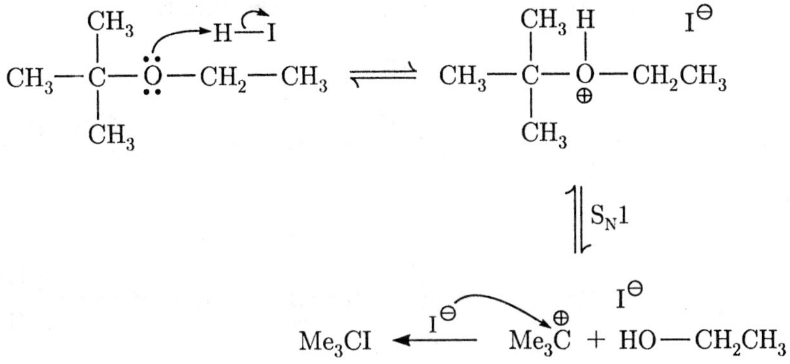

As the rate of S_N1 reaction is faster than the competing S_N2 reactions, none of the primary alkyl iodide is formed. Ethers show great similarity with alcohols regarding cleavage. In both cases, protonation converts a poor leaving group to a good one, and in case of alcohols, water (H_2O) is the leaving group and in case of ethers, alcohol is the leaving group.

$$RCH_2OH \underset{}{\overset{HI}{\rightleftharpoons}} RCH_2\overset{\oplus}{O}H_2 \xrightarrow{\overset{\ominus}{I}/S_N2} RCH_2I + H_2O$$

(primary alcohol)

$$R_3C{-}OH \overset{HBr}{\rightleftharpoons} R_3C{-}\overset{\oplus}{O}H_2 \overset{S_N1}{\rightleftharpoons} R_3\overset{\oplus}{C} + H_2O \xrightarrow{Br^{\ominus}} R_3CBr$$

(tertiary alcohol)

$$RCH_2{-}O{-}CH_2R \overset{HI}{\rightleftharpoons} R{-}CH_2{-}\overset{\oplus}{O}H{-}CH_2R \xrightarrow{\overset{\ominus}{I}/S_N2} R{-}CH_2I + RCH_2OH$$

(Diprimaryalkyl ether)

$$R_3C{-}O{-}R \overset{HBr}{\rightleftharpoons} R_3C{-}\overset{\oplus}{O}H{-}R \xrightarrow{S_N1} R_3\overset{\oplus}{C} + ROH \xrightarrow{Br^{\ominus}} R_3CBr$$

(Ether containing *t*-alkyl group)

These reaction show instability of ethers in acids.

(b) ***Reaction with dilute H_2SO_4*** :

$$R_2O + H_2O \xrightarrow{\text{dilute } H_2SO_4/\text{pressure}} 2ROH$$

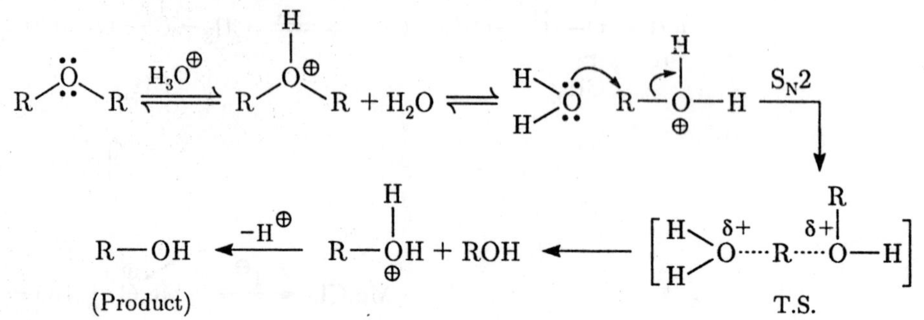

(c) ***Ethers are also cleaved by Lewis acids*** :

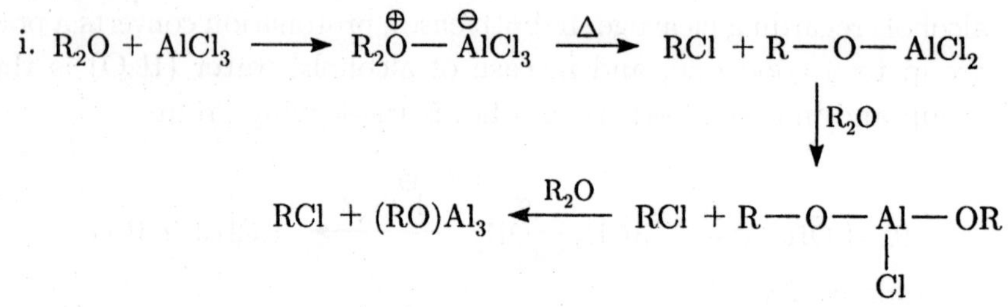

$$\text{ii. } R_2O + Ph_3PBr_2 \xrightarrow{125°C} 2RBr + Ph_3P{=}O$$

3. ***Reaction with Halogens*** : Chlorine and bromine react with ethers to form chloro– or bromo derivatives through free radical pathway. The extent of reaction depends on conditions. When diethyl ether is treated with chlorine in the dark, α,α'–dichloro derivative is obtained.

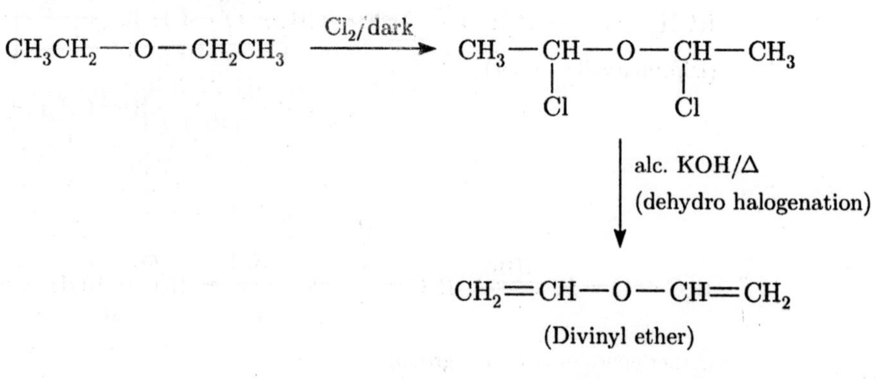

$$CH_3{-}CH_2{-}O{-}CH_2CH_3 \xrightarrow{Cl_2/\text{sunlight}} Cl_3C\,CCl_2(O)CCl_2C\,Cl_3$$

Mechanism :

$$H-CH_2-O-CH_3 + \dot{C}l \longrightarrow HCl + [\dot{C}H_2-\ddot{O}-CH_3 \longleftrightarrow CH_2=\dot{O}-CH_3]$$

(α–H free radical is stable due to resonance)

$$Cl_2 + \dot{C}H_2-O-CH_3 \longrightarrow ClCH_2OCH_3 + \dot{C}l$$

$$Cl-CH_2-O-CH_2-H + \dot{C}l \longrightarrow Cl-CH_2-O-\dot{C}H_2 + HCl$$

$$Cl-CH_2-O-\dot{C}H_2 + Cl-Cl \longrightarrow Cl-CH_2-O-CH_2Cl + \dot{C}l \text{ etc.}$$

4. ***Ester formation***

(a) In the presence of BF_3 and water ether adds to carbon monoxide (CO) to form esters.

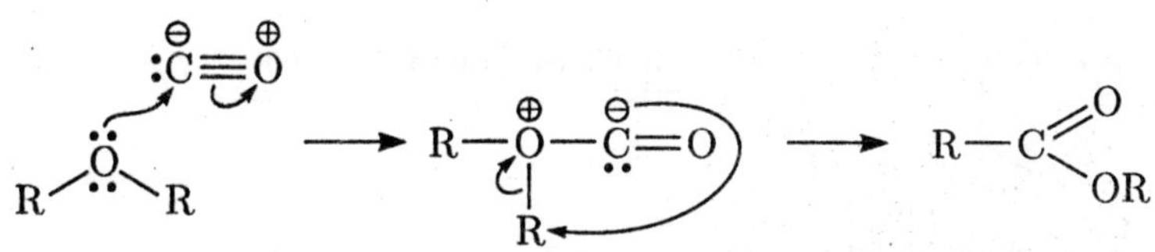

(b) When acyl halides are heated with an ether and a Lewis acid (*e.g.*, anhydrous $ZnCl_2$ or $AlCl_3$, esters and alkyl halides are formed.

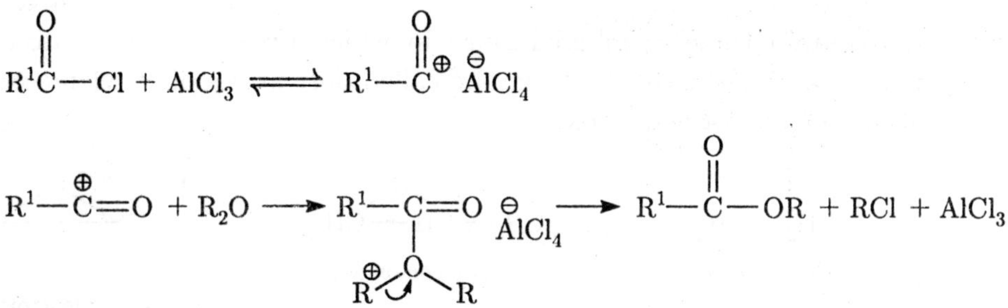

Autooxidation : When an ether is exposed to air, oxygen of the air reacts with it and forms hydroperoxide. α-Hydrogens are involved in auto oxidation.

$$Me_2CH-O-CHMe_2 + O_2 \longrightarrow Me_2CH-O-C(Me)_2-OH$$

Molecular oxygen itself is a poorly reactive radical. However, if a radical is present in any system, it reacts with O_2 molecule to form peroxy radical which then abstracts $\dot{H}$ radical to form hydroperoxide.

$$CH_3CH_2O-CH_2CH_3 \xrightarrow{h\nu} CH_3\dot{C}H-OCH_2CH_3 + \dot{H}$$

$$CH_3\dot{C}H-O-CH_2CH_3 + O_2 \longrightarrow CH_3-\underset{\substack{|\\ O-\dot{O}}}{CH}-O-CH_2-CH_3$$

$$\Big\downarrow CH_3CH_2OCH_2CH_3$$

$$CH_3-\dot{C}H-O-CH_2CH_3 \text{ etc.} \longleftarrow CH_3\underset{\substack{|\\ O-OH}}{CH}-O-CH_2CH_3$$

6. $$CH_3CH_2-OCHMe_2 \xrightarrow[\text{(oxidation)}]{K_2Cr_2O_7/\text{conc. } H_2SO_4} CH_3CHO + Me_2C{=}O + H_2O + H^{\oplus}$$

7. 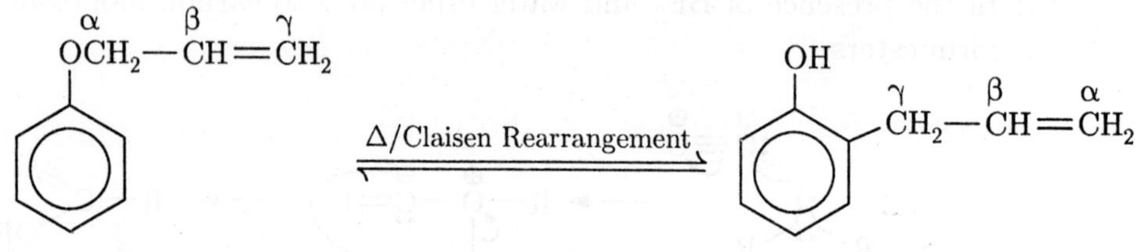

(Phenyl allyl ether) (o-allylphenol), 100%

Epoxides (Oxiranes)

Oxiranes contain three membered rings in which two are carbon atoms and one is oxygen atom and hence oxiranes may be called derivatives of ethylene oxide. They are also called epoxides or alkene oxides.

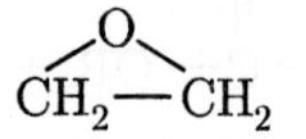

(Ethylene oxide)

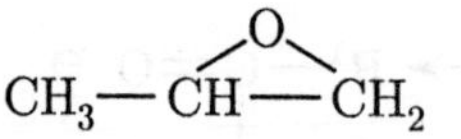

(Propylene oxide)

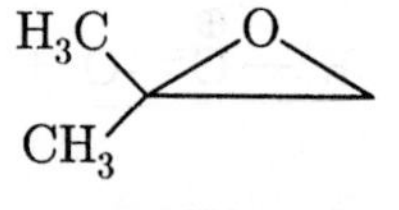

(Isobutylene oxide)

Synthesis of epoxy linkage or synthesis of epoxides :

1. 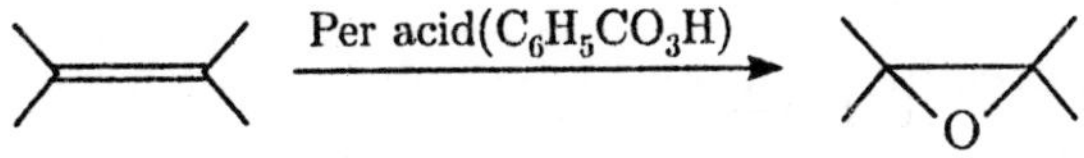

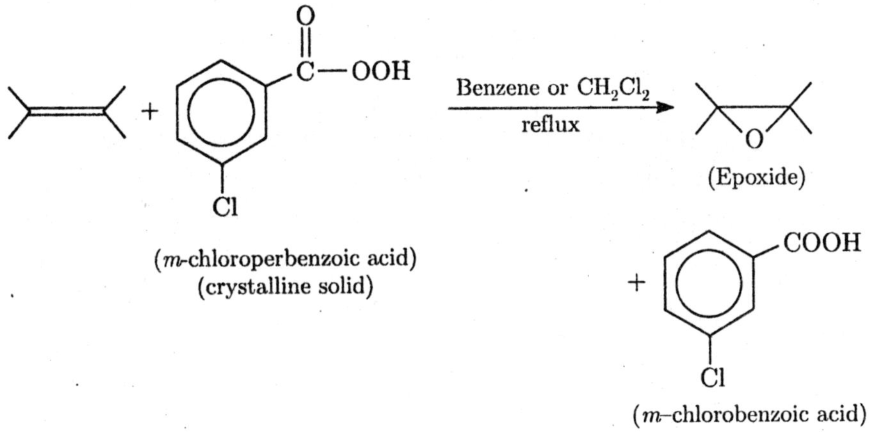

Peroxycarboxylic acids are unstable; they are prepared prior to use by mixing a carboxylic acid and hydrogen peroxide (H_2O_2).

A less hazardous peroxycarboxylic acid having the same reactivity is magnesium salt of monoperoxyphthalic acid (MMPP).

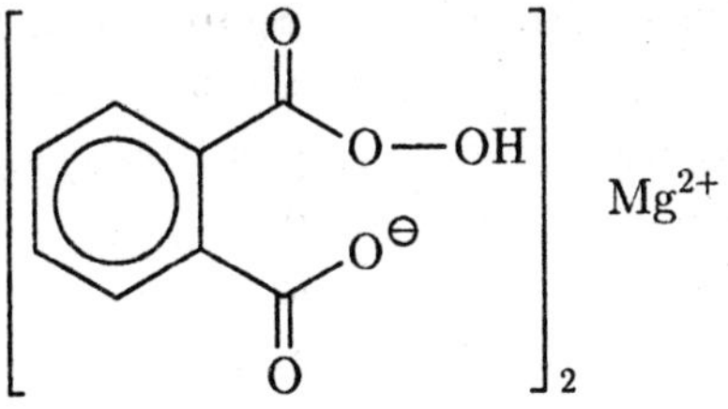

Mechanism : Epoxidation is a bimolecular concerted addition reaction as shown below.

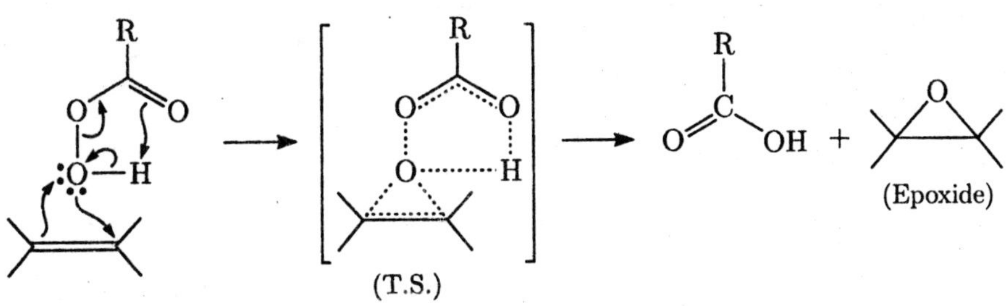

The *non-polar epoxidation* is a second order reaction, first order each with respect to the alkene and peracid respectively.

Rate = k[alkene] [peracid]

The concerted mechanism of the epoxidation reaction is supported by the following facts.

(a) The reaction takes place readily in a non-polar solvent which rules out the possibility of ionic pathway.

(b) The reaction involves the attack from one side of the double bond and thus, formation of epoxides is a stereospecific reaction.

i. 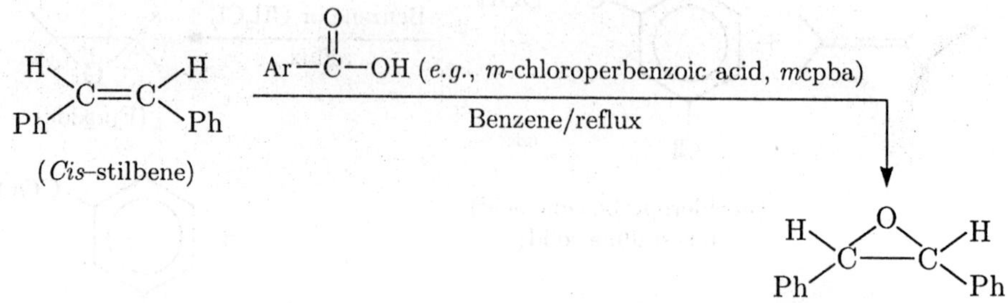

(*Cis*-stilbene)

(*Cis*-epoxide) 100%

ii. 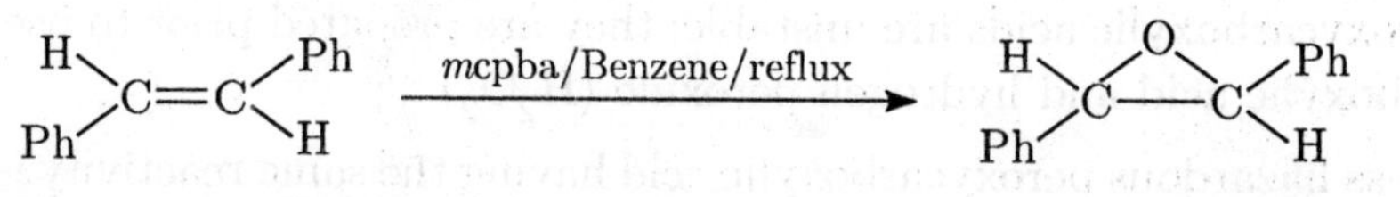

(*Trans*-stilbene) (*Trans*-epoxide) 100%

The epoxide so formed undergoes acid– or base– catalysed hydrolysis to form an anti– or *trans*– 1,2-diol. So the hydrolysis of epoxides is also a stereospecific reaction. The overall reaction may be called hydroxylation via epoxidation.

Acid catalysed hydrolysis of epoxides :

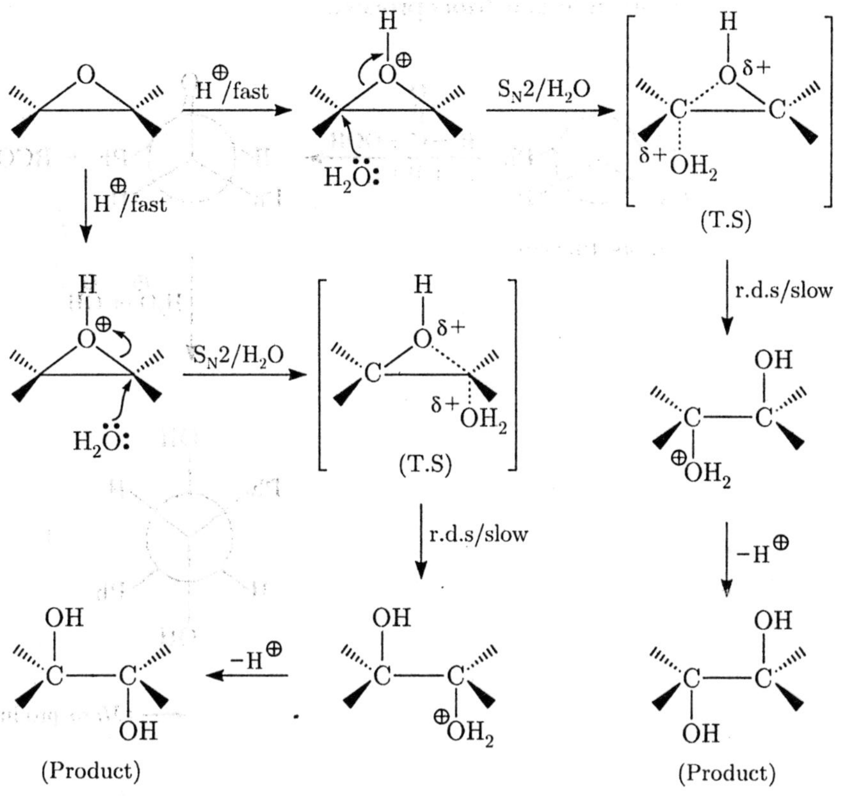

Base catalysed hydrolysis of epoxides :

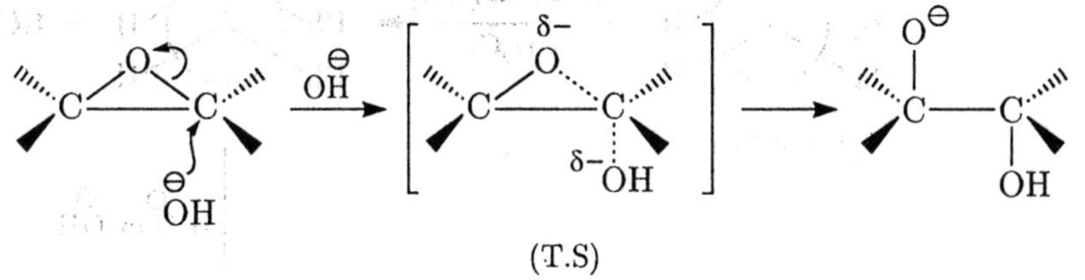

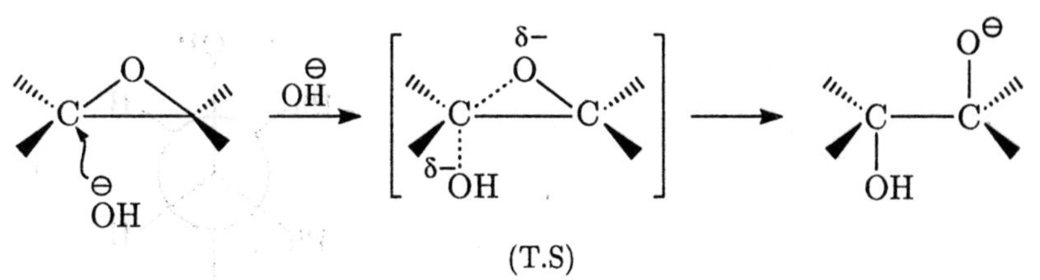

$^{\ominus}$OH attacks the less sterically hindered carbon atom more readily.

Since the nucleophilic attack by H_2O or $^{\ominus}OH$ occurs form the back side inversion of configuration occurs. Thus, the base– or acid– catalysed hydrolysis of an epoxide is a *trans* process.

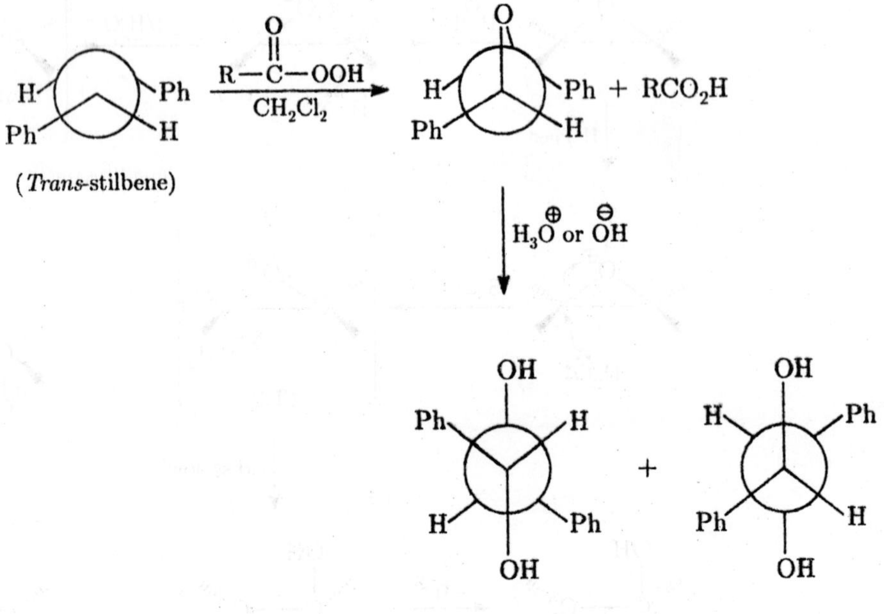

(*Trans*-stilbene)

← (*Meso*–products) →

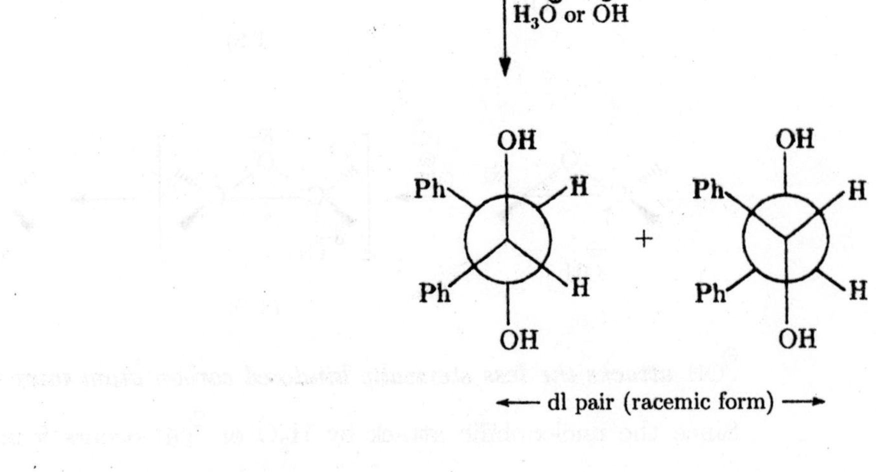

(*Cis*-stilbene)

← dl pair (racemic form) →

2. ***Formation of epoxy linkage from a-halohydrins*** : When *α-halohydrins* are treated with *bases*, α-halooxides are formed,. α-haloalkoxides then undergo *internal Williamson synthesis* to form epoxides.

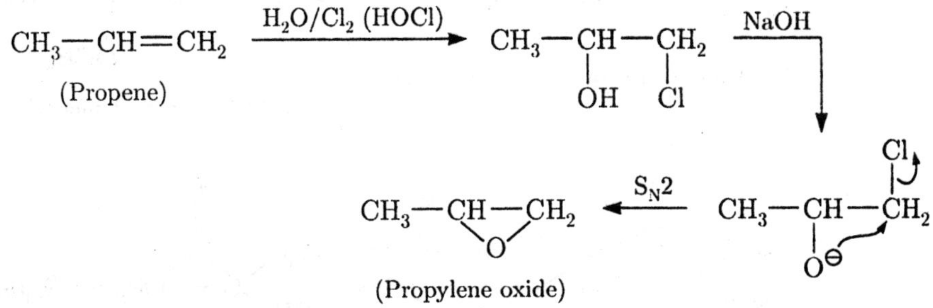

Problem 1 :

1. What is the stereochemistry of 2,3-butanediol formed when meso–2, 3-dimethyl oxirane reacts with aqueous NaOH?

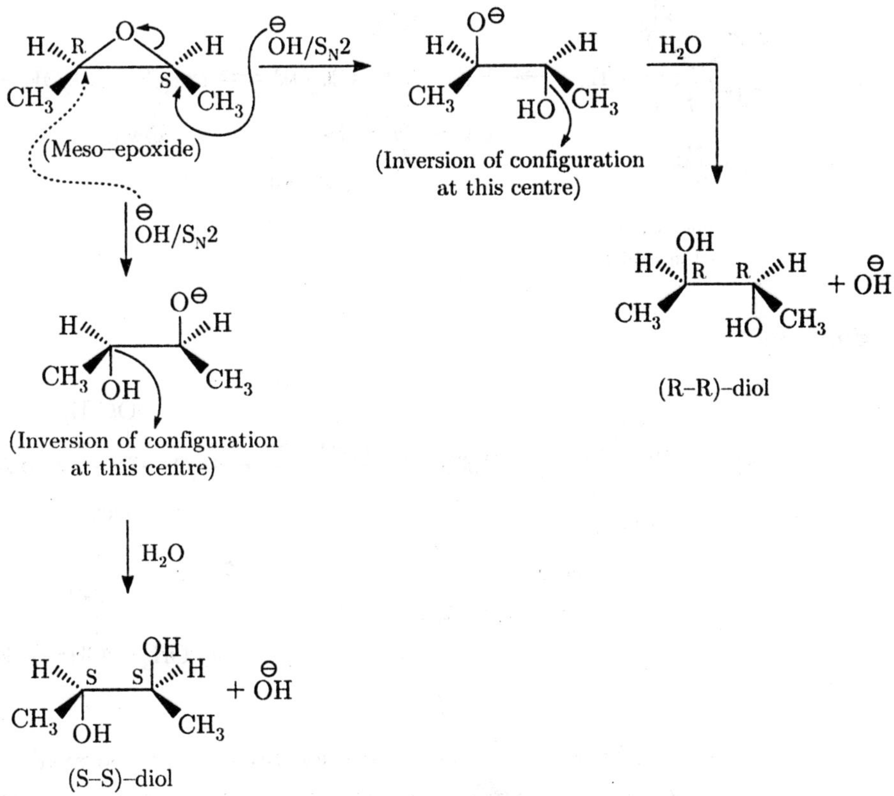

***Problem* 2 :**

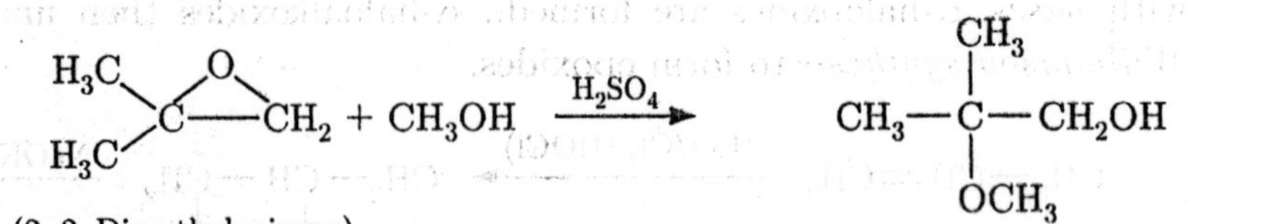

(2, 2–Dimethyloxirane) (2–Methoxy–2–methyl–1–propanol)

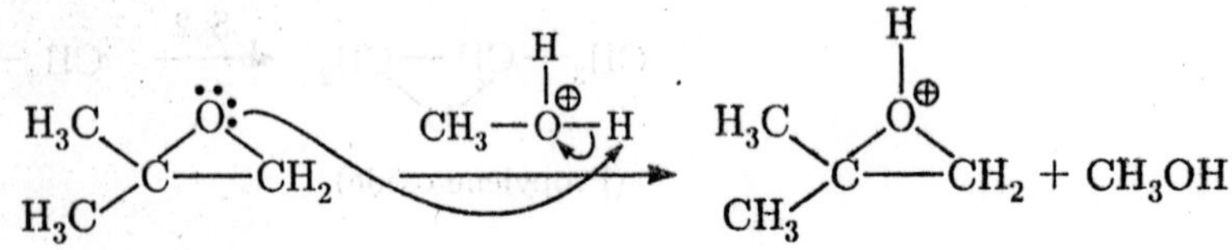

(Protonated epoxide)

Under acidic condition, the nucleophile attacks more branched carbon because the stability of carbocation follows the order 3°>2°>1°.

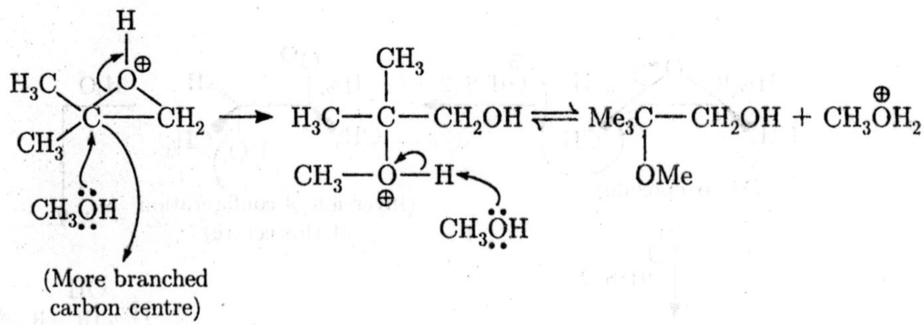

***Problem* 3 :**

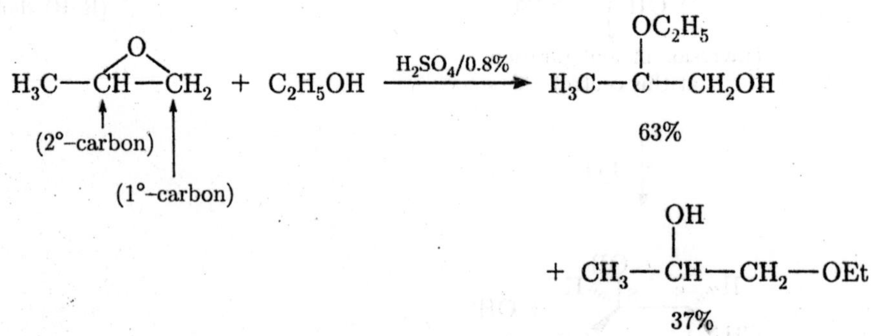

The mixture reflects the balance between opening of the weaker bond which favours attack at the more branched carbon and van der Waals repulsion with the nucleophile favours attack at the less branched carbon.

***Problem* 4 :**

(a) 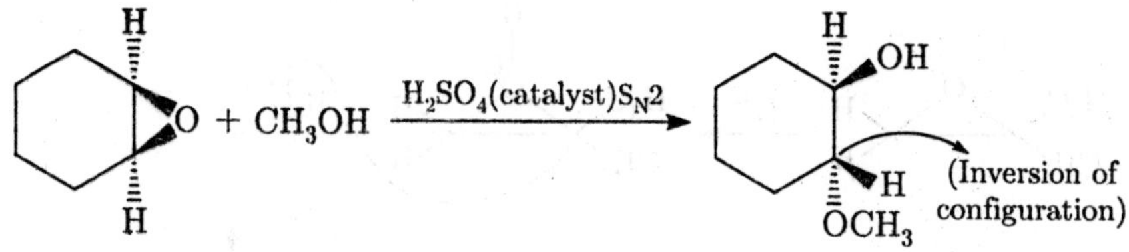

(Cyclohexene oxide)

(± *Trans*–2–methoxycyclohexanol)
(glycol)

(b) 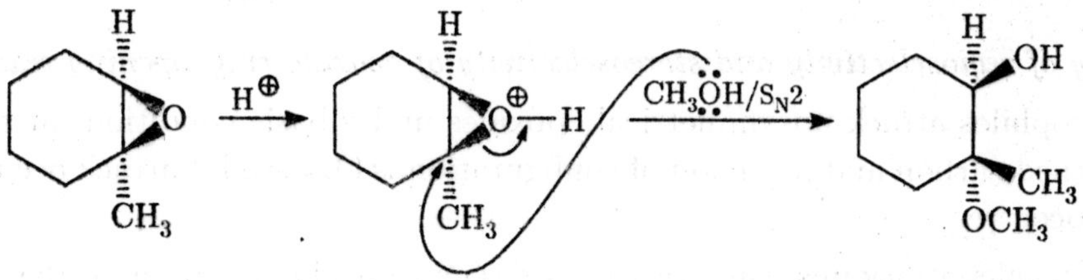

(c) 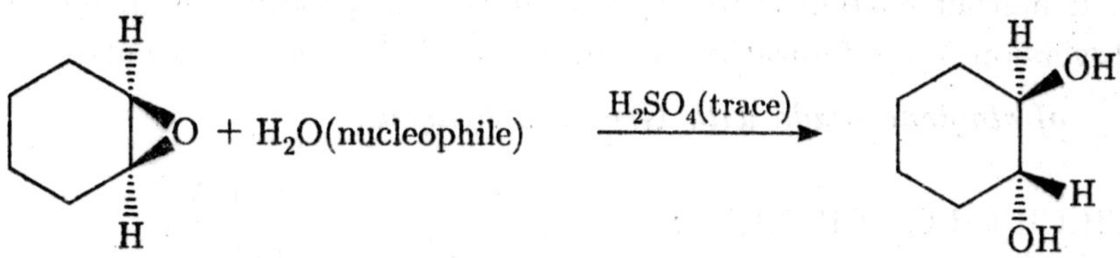

(±) *Trans*–1, 2–cyclohexanediol

Cis–1,2-cyclohexanediol can not be prepared by epoxide ring opening. Acid catalysed epoxide hydrolysis is generally a useful way to prepare glycols.

Although base-catalysed hydrolysis of epoxides also gives glycols, polymerisation sometimes occurs. So acid catalysed ring opening is preferred for the preparation of glycols.

***Problem* 5 :** 2,2–Dimethyloxirane is hydrolysed in water which is enriched with ^{18}O. Indicate how the hydrolysis product would differ under basic and acidic conditions.

(a) ***Basic condition (Attack at the less branched carbon atom)***

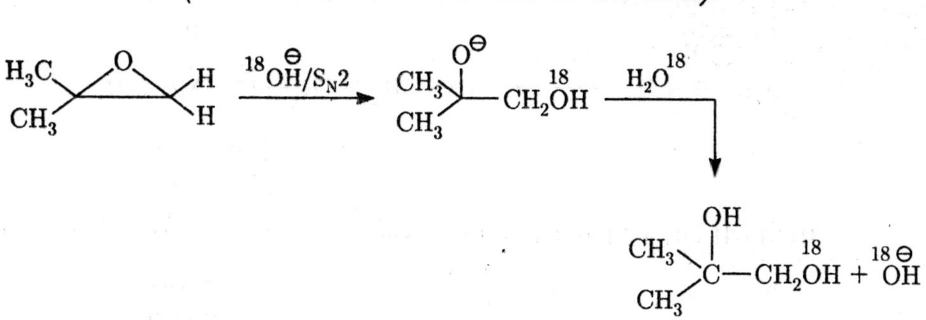

(b) ***Acidic condition (Attack at the more branched tertiary carbon, solely)***

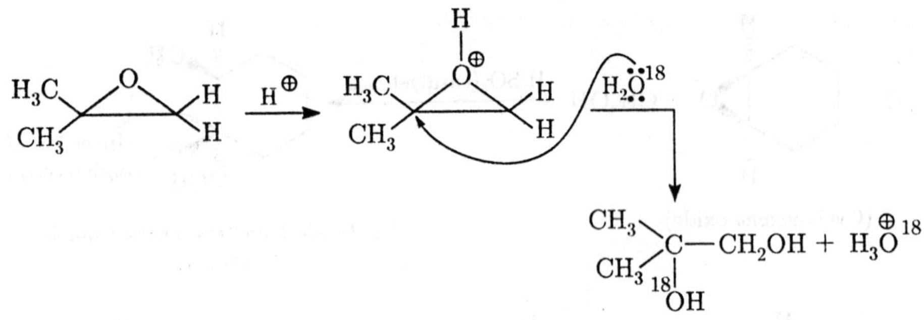

Summary of regioselectivity and stereoselectivity of epoxide ring–opening reactions :

1. Nucleophiles attack unsymmetrical epoxides under basic conditions at the less branched carbon and inversion of configuration is observed if attack occurs at a stereocentre.
2. Nucleophiles attack unsymmetrical epoxides under acidic conditions at the tertiary carbon. If neither carbon is tertiary, a mixture of products is formed in most cases. Inversion of configuration occurs if attack is at a stereocentre.

Reaction of ethylene oxide with Grignard Reagent.

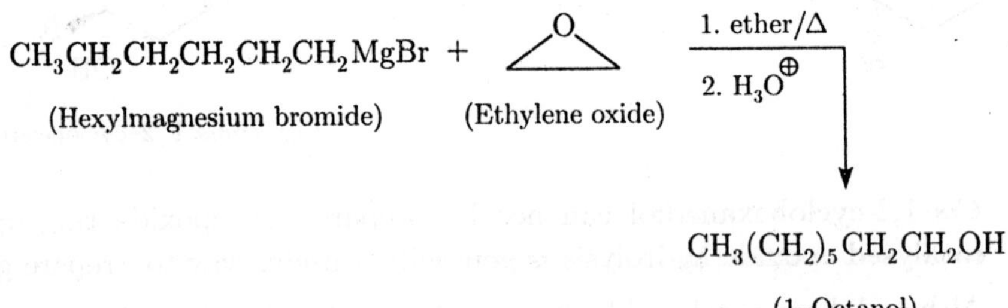

C—Mg bond of Grignard reagent has carbanion character and is therefore basic. This carbon attacks epoxide as a nucleophile and Mg of the Grignard reagent which is a Lweis acid coordinates to the epoxide oxygen, to make it a good leaving group.

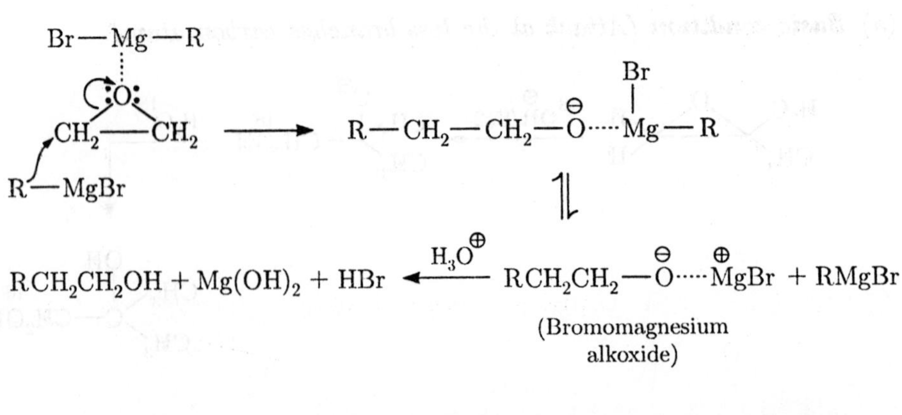

With other epoxides also, Grignard reagent react but there a mixture of products is obtained. This method provides a way for the formation of C—C bond.

Structure, Reactivity and Orientation of Oxiranes : Epoxides possess triangular ring structure. The C—O—C and O—C—C bond angles are approximately 67° and 57° respectively. The carbon and oxygen atoms both are sp^3 hybridised, therefore the expected bond angles are 109°28′. Thus, the molecules have high *I-strain (small angle or internal strain)*

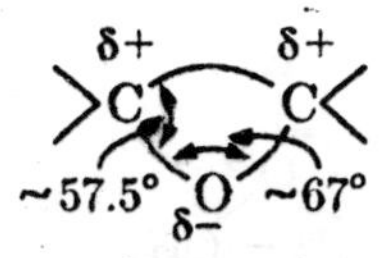

(Oxirane)

The C—C and C—O sigma bonds are formed by the overlap of sp^3 orbitals in a manner which is neither head on or nor sidewise but an intermediate between the two, commonly known as a *banana* or *bent bond.* Moreover, due to higher electronegativity of oxygen atom, the carbon atoms bear δ+ and oxygen atom bears δ− character. This polarisation along with the I– strain make oxiranes highly reactive.

Reactions of epoxy linkage :

1. (a) 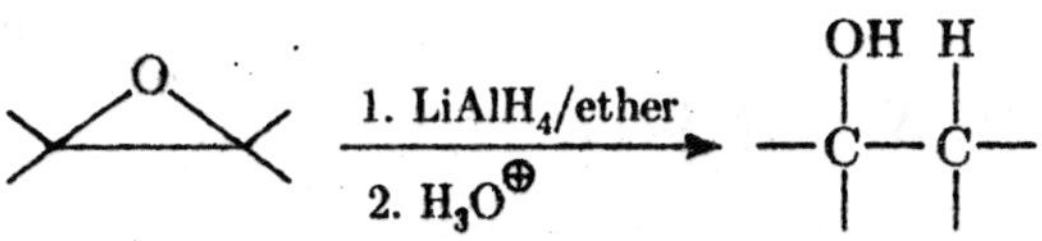

In case of an unsymmetrical epoxide, a mixture of two alcohols is obtained and the more substituted alcohol is the main product.

(b) 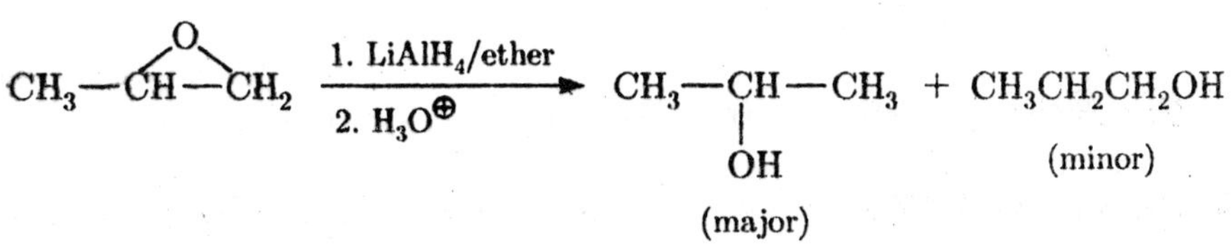

(c) 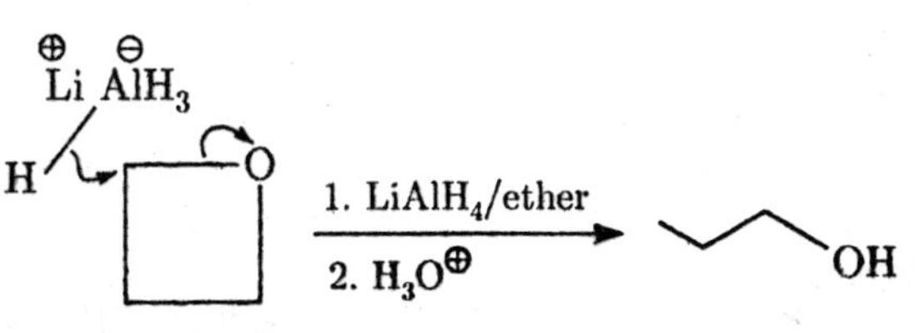

(Strained ring)

Strainless rings are however resistant, they can also be cleaved by $LiAlH_4$ in the presence of $AlCl_3$.

(d) 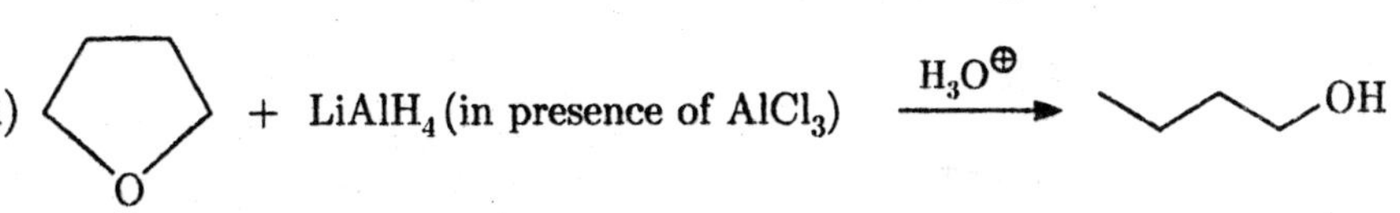

2. ***Reduction by triphenylphosphine*** :

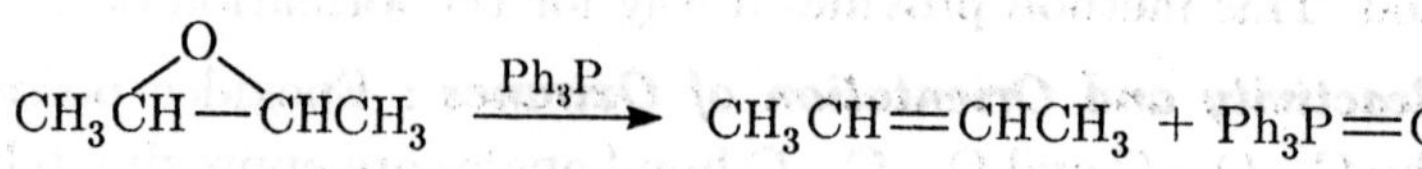

3. ***Oxidation by DMSO*** :

Epoxides are oxidised by DMSO to acyloin (α-hydroxyketones) in the presence of acids.

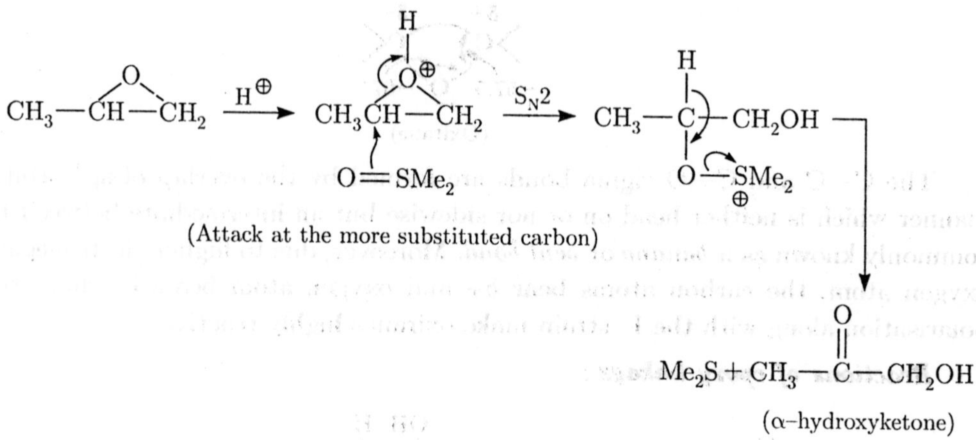

4. ***Reaction with haloacids (HX, X = Cl, Br, I)***

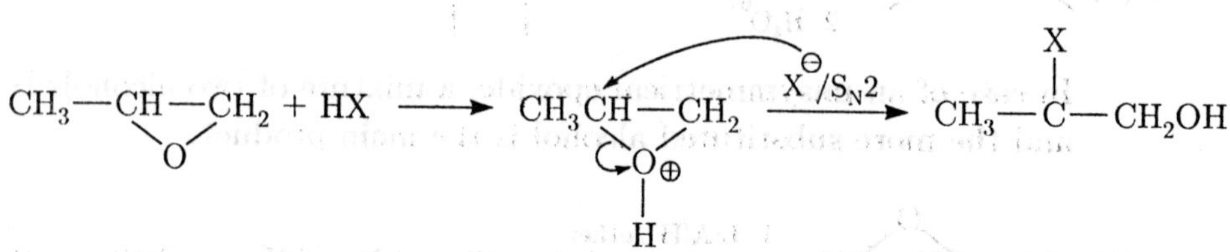

The order of reactivity : HI>HBr>HCl in a decreasing manner.

5. ***Reaction with HCN*** : In the presence of a base, HCN adds to epoxide and forms α-cyanohydrins.

$$HCN + \overset{\ominus}{O}H \rightleftharpoons \overset{\ominus}{C}N + H_2O$$

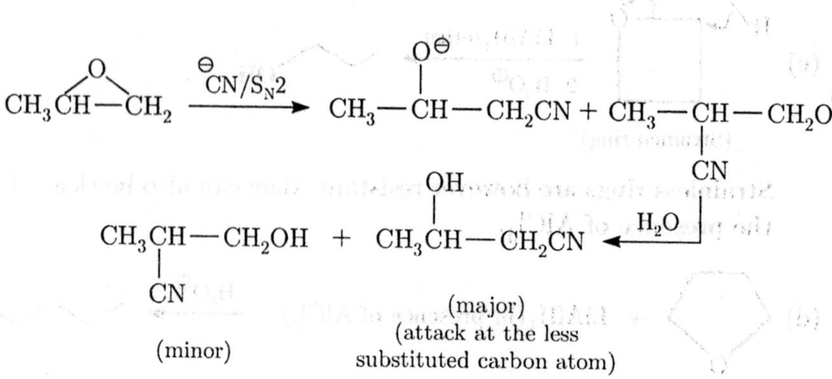

6. ***Reaction with alkoxides*** : When epoxides are treated with alkoxides, α-hydroxyalkoxides are formed.

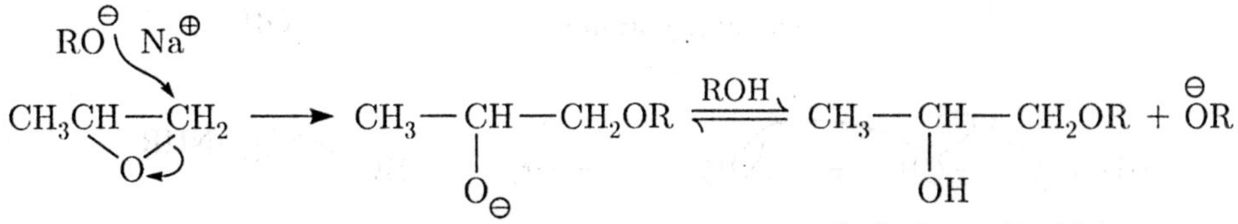

(α-hydroxyalkoxide)

7. ***Action of heat on ethylene oxide*** :

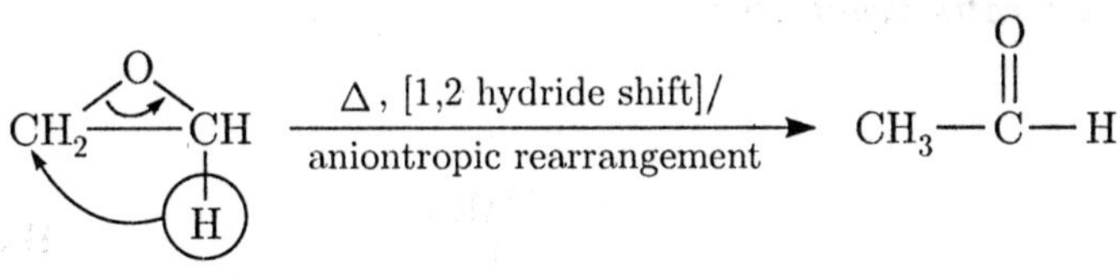

8. ***Reactions with alcohols and glycols*** :

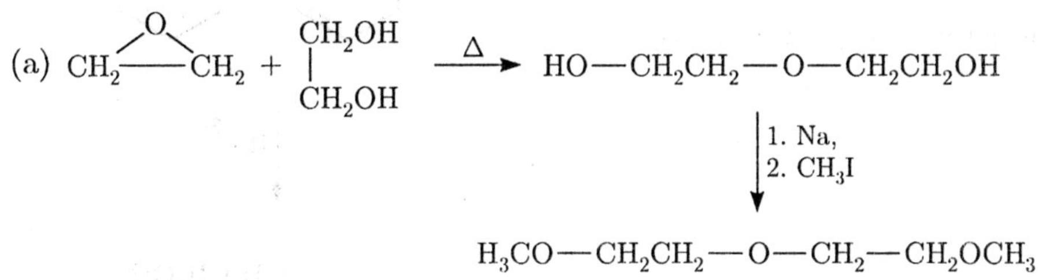

Diglyme (b.p 170°) (a solvent)

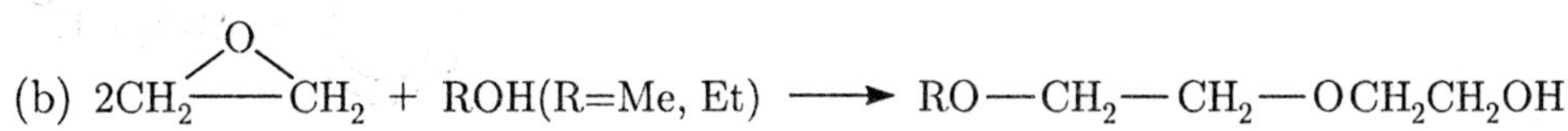

(Cellosolve, a solvent in which cellulose dissolves)

9. ***Amination of epoxy linkage*** :

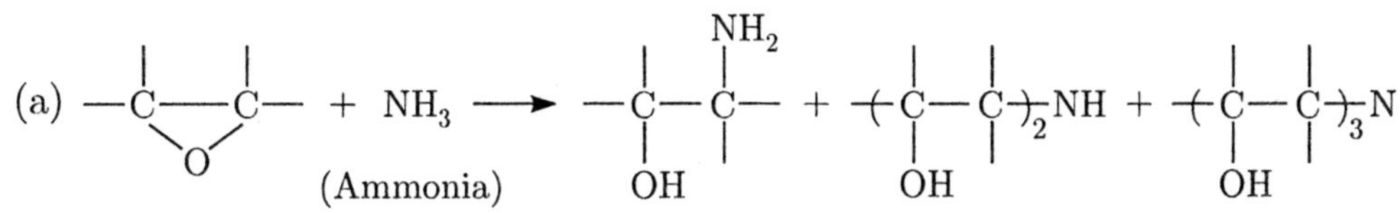

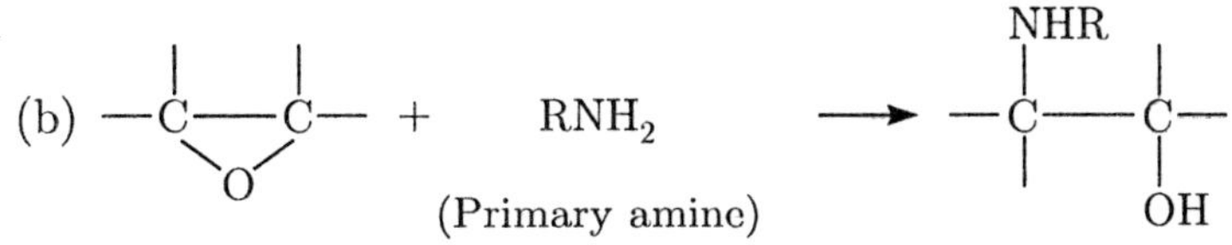

(c) 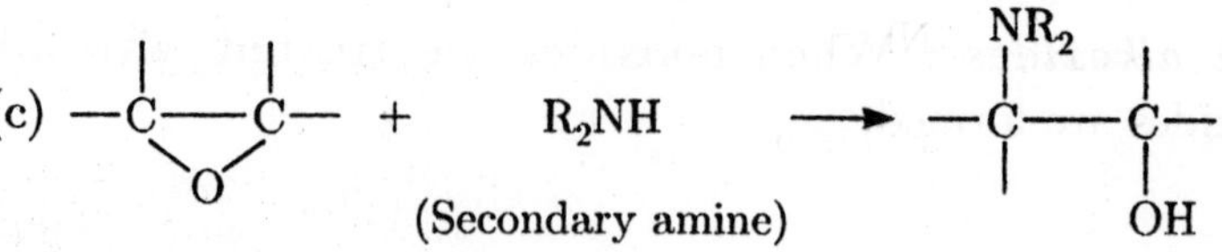

(d) 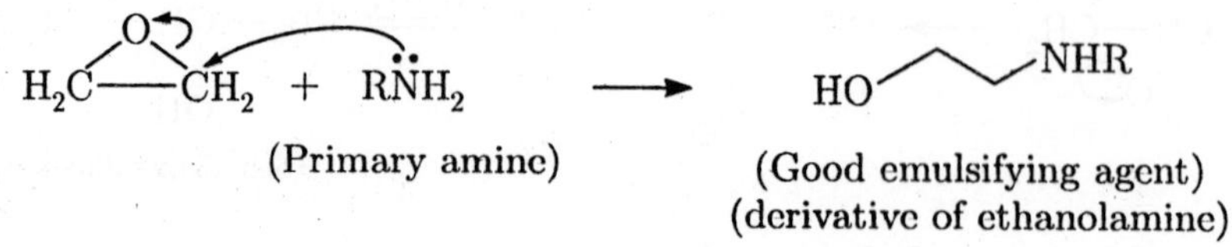

10. ***Friedel–Crafts reaction*** :

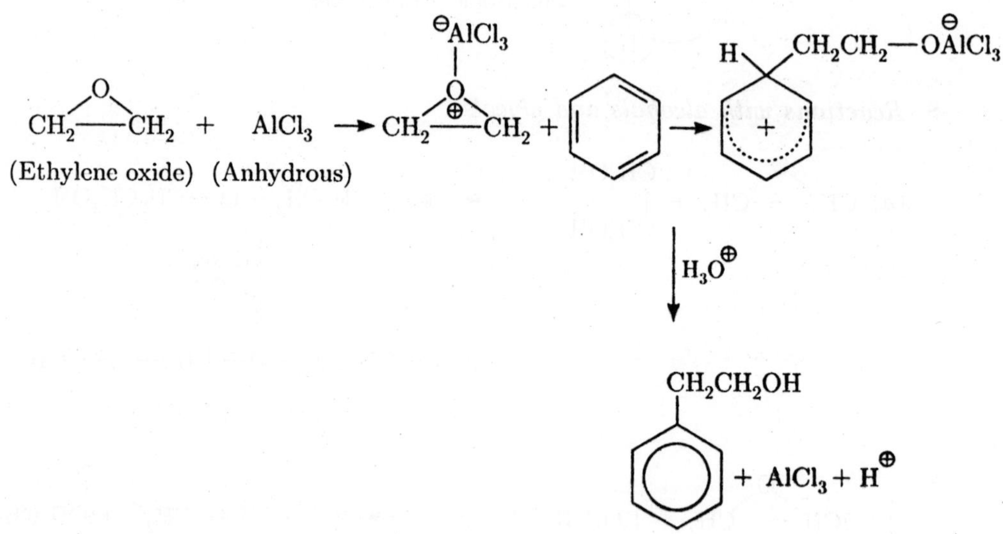

Organometallic and Organosilicon Compounds

Compounds that contain carbon-metal bonds are called organometallic compounds. The nature of carbon-metal bond varies widely, ranging from bonds that are essentially ionic to those that are primarily covalent. Whereas the structure of the organic portion of organometallic compound has some effect on the nature of the carbon-metal bond, the identity of the metal itself is of far greater importance.

Generally, carbon in organic compounds is commonly bonded to the groups which are more electronegative than carbon itself. Of course, these groups are non metallic in character when these electronegative groups accept an electron pair, carbon becomes positively charged and becomes succeptible to the attack by the *nucleophiles.*

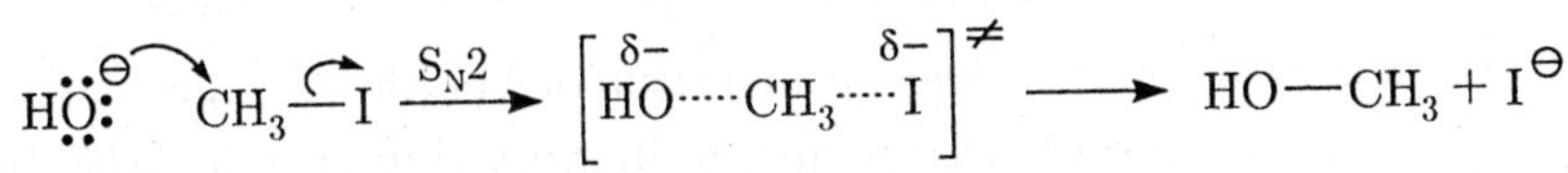

Conversely, when carbon is attached to an electropositive element, *e.g*, a metal, former becomes negatively charged, because a metal always release a pair of bonding electrons to form a cation. As a result, the *negatively charged carbon* is now succeptible to the attack by electrophiles. This is thus, an example of **umpolung** or reversal of polarity of carbon.

Organometallics are versatile reagents. Their reactivity depends on the nature of the metal atom. There is a steady decrease in the reactivity with the decrease in the electropositive character of the metal.

Metal	***K***	***Na***	***Li***	***Mg***	***Cd***
% Ionic character	51	47	43	35	15
	most reactive flamable		medium reactive Li>Mg		least reactive

Organomagnesium Compounds (Grignard Reagents)

Organomagnesium compounds are commonly known as Grignard Reagents (named after the discoverer V. Grignard, Nobel Prize, 1912). Grignard reagents have great use in organic synthesis.

1. ***Preparation of Grignard Reagents (G.R.)***

   (a) Standard method of preparation is the reaction of an organic halide in dry diethyl ether with magnesium metal (turnings, granules or powder). The reagent is not isolated but used directly in the required synthesis.

$$R—X + Mg \longrightarrow RMgX \text{ (Grignard reagent)}$$

R=alkyl, aryl, alkenyl (with special conditions)

X=Halides, reactivity order I>Br>Cl>>F in a decreasing manner.

Methyl iodide is generally used to prepare Grignard reagent as methyl chloride (CH_3Cl) and methyl bromide (CH_3Br) are gases at room temperature, and CH_3Br is again preferred over CH_3Cl. Alkyl and aryl halides react vigorously with magnesium (Mg) in dry diethyl ether. Allyl halides also form Grignard reagent in dry ether but they also react with the Grignard reagents formed. So, to keep the concentration of allyl halide minimum, addition of a dilute solution of allyl halide to a large excess of vigorously stirred suspension in dry ether is done. Vinyl chlorides are inactive in ether medium, but reactive in THF with longer time and higher temperature compared to alkyl and aryl halides.

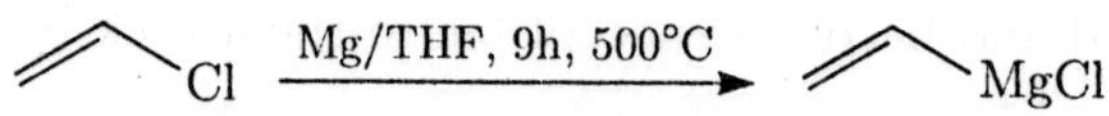

The reaction overall involves an *insertion* of Mg into the new carbon-halogen (C—X) bond. There is also a change in oxidation state of Mg, from Mg(0) to Mg(II). The reaction is therefore known as an *oxidative insertion* or *oxidative addtion.*

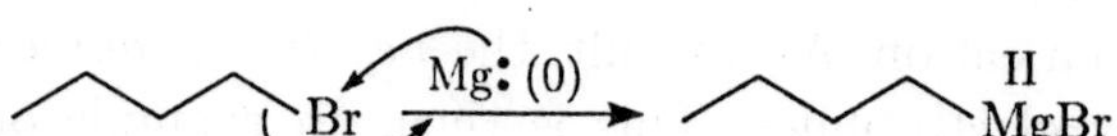

The reaction takes place not in solution but on the surface of the metal and more finely divided Mg helps to accelerate the reaction. Mg is usually covered by a thin coating of MgO and so Grignard formation requires "initiation", to allow the metal to come into contact with alkyl halide. The initiation is generally accomplished by adding a small amount of iodine (I_2) or 1,2–diiodoethane, or by using ultrasound to dislodge the oxide layer. The solvent chosen for Grignard reagent is ether, as Grignard reagents do not react with ether and they are soluble in ether. Ethers are Lewis bases which meet the Mg metal as Lewis acid and Mg (having empty 3p orbital) accepts the lone pair of electrons from oxygen atom of ether.

(b) Another method to prepare Grignard reagent by metallation procedure using a preformed Grignard reagent. The only condition is that the atom attached to magnesium in the Grignard reagent to be prepared is markedly more electronegative than that in the preformed Grignard so that equilibrium lies to the right.

$$R—H + R'MgX \text{ (preformed G. R.)} \longrightarrow RMgX \quad R'—H$$

Alkynyl Grignard reagents are normally prepared by this method.

$$R—\equiv—H + CH_3CH_2MgBr \longrightarrow R—\equiv—MgBr + C_2H_6$$

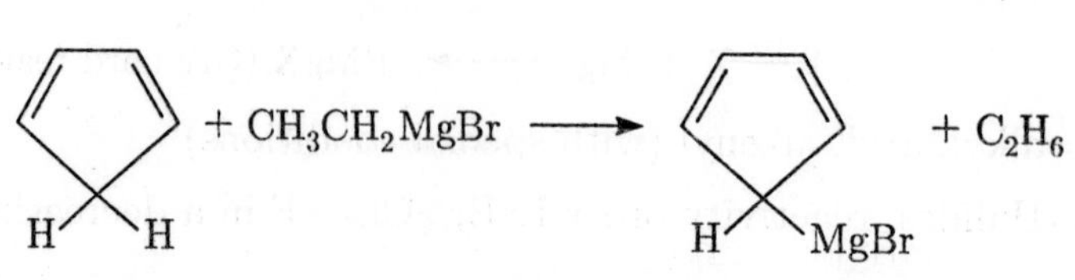

Structure of Grignard Reagent

Grignard and his coworkers attempted to isolate Grignard reagent (1901) and showed the compound contained ether (termed as "ether of crystallisation"). Although a great deal of work has been done, the structure of Grignard reagent is still not settled. According to Ashley *et al*, the structure of Grignard reagent in ether may be represented by the following equilibria.

$$\text{etc.} \rightleftharpoons \text{Dimer} \rightleftharpoons 2RMgX \rightleftharpoons R_2Mg + MgX_2 \rightleftharpoons \text{Dimer} \rightleftharpoons \text{etc.}$$

The degree of association depends on the concentration of Grignard reagent which is extensive above about 0.3 M. Each molecule of Grignard reagent coordinates with two molecules of ether in the monomer (I) and in the dimer (II), halogen atom of one unit coordinates with Mg atom of another molecule.

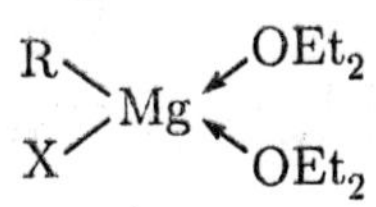

(I)

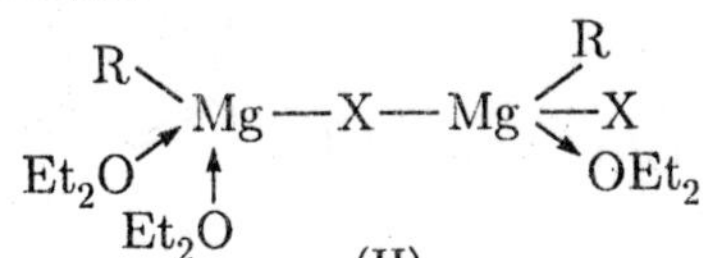

(II)

Crystalline 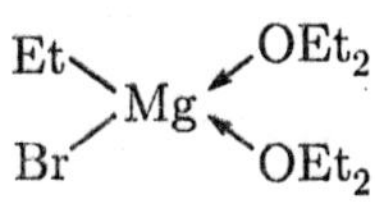 has been isolated from ether and X-ray analyses show that the four groups are arranged tetrahedrally about the magnesium atom.

Reactivity of Grignard Reagents

Grignard reagents react with all organic compounds except tertiary amines, C=C, aromatic double bonds, C≡C and ethers. So a Grignard reagent can be prepared from the compounds containing these groups only. Grignard reagent is useful in synthesising small and simple molecules and rarely used to synthesise complex molecules. *Mode of reaction of Grignard reagent is such that the magnesium atom is transferred to a more electronegative atom.*

Another type of reaction is that, *double decomposition with compounds containing an active hydrogen atom or a reactive halogen atom.* An active hydrogen atom is one, joined to oxygen, nitrogen or sulphur. When such compounds react with a Grignard reagent the alkyl group is converted into the alkane.

$$R^1H + Mg(OH)X \xleftarrow{H_2O} R^1MgX \xrightarrow{R^2OH} R^1H + Mg(OR^2)X$$

Since reactions with compounds containing an active hydrogen atom result in the quantitative yield of hydrocarbon, this type of reaction is valuable for the determination of the number of active hydrogen atoms in a compound. The procedure is known as the **Zerewitinoff Active Hydrogen Determination**. MeMgI is normally ued as the Grignard reagent and the methane which is liberated is measured by volume. One molecule of methane is equivalent to one active hydrogen atom.

$$RNH_2 + CH_3MgI \longrightarrow CH_4 + RNHMgI$$

$$R_2NH + CH_3MgI \longrightarrow CH_4 + R_2NMgI$$

Only one hydrogen atom of a primary amine reacts at room temperature. Only at an elevated temperature the active hydrogen in the magnesium derivative of the primary amine will react with a further molecule of MeMgI.

$$RNHMgI + MeMgI \longrightarrow CH_4 + RN(MgI)_2$$

It is therefore possible to estimate the number of amino and imino groups in compounds containing both. It is not possible to get a high enough temperature for the second reaction with ether; a satisfactory solvent for the complete Zerewitinoff determination is pyridine.

The enolic form of a compound, since it contains an active hydrogen atom, reacts with Grignard reagent, *e.g.*, ethyl acetoacetate and nitroethane.

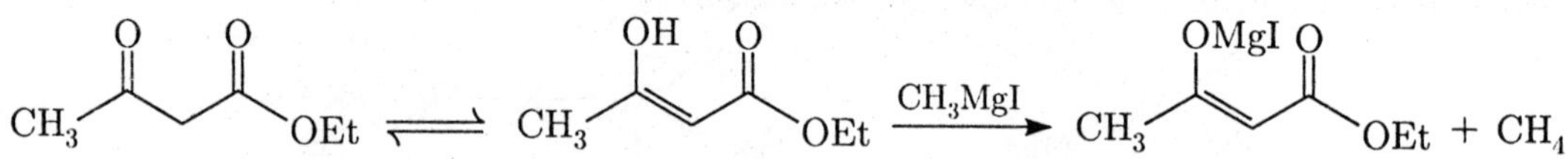

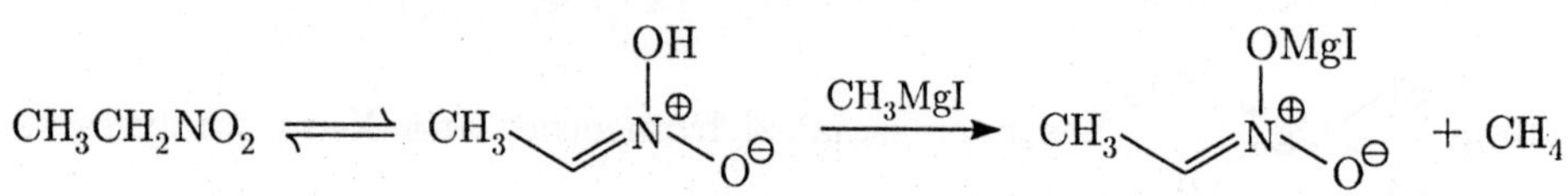

The rate of the reaction depends on the rate of keto to enol conversion. The hydrogen atom of ≡C—H group is also active with respect to G. R. since it (≡C—H) is acidic.

$$C_2H_5MgBr + H{-}C{\equiv}C{-}H \longrightarrow H{-}C{\equiv}CMgBr + C_2H_6 \xrightarrow{C_2H_5MgBr} BrMgC{\equiv}CMgBr$$

The second step of the reaction can be avoided by adding the Grignard solution to THF saturated with acetylene.

Order of Reactivity of Functional Groups : In most cases of synthesis in which a Grignard reagent is used, the other compound has only one functional group and consequently, the reaction takes place in one direction only. Occassionally it is necessary to carry out a synthesis with a compound containing two (or more) functional groups. If an excess of Grignard reagent is used then both groups react as would be expected. It has been experimentally found that the reactivity of different groups is not equal, and hence when one equivalent of Grignard reagent is added, two competitive reactions take place simultaneously, but at different rates, resulting in two products in unequal amounts. Experiments have shown that an active hydrogen reacts very much faster than any other group, a compound containing an active hydrogen and another group reacts with one equivalent of Grignard reagent as if it has only one reactive group, the active hydrogen. In general the oxo group is more reactive than the halogen of alkyl halide towards a Grignard reagent.

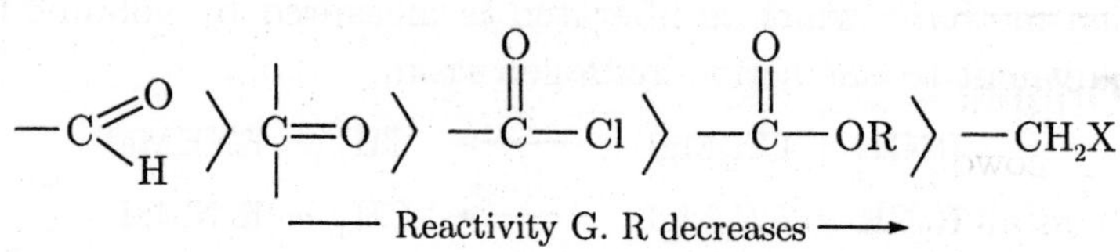

Stereoselectivity of Grignard Reactions

The reaction of a Grignard reagent with a carbonyl group can establish a stereocentre. If the *reactants are symmetric*, equal amounts of the two enantiomers are formed.

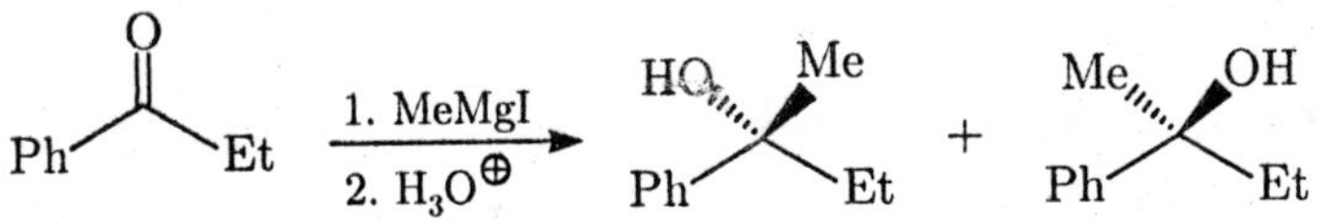

50% 50%

Since the reaction is equally likely on either face of the carbonyl group, if *one of the reactants is asymmetric*, there is as predominance of one of the two possible diastereomers. The results are in accord with Cram's rule.

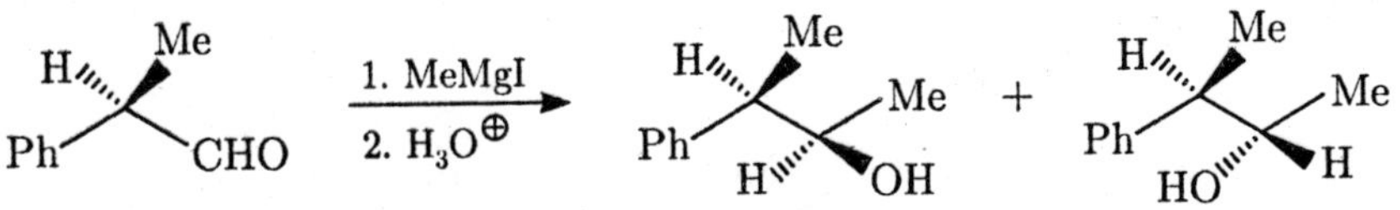

2 part 1 part

Cram's rule of Diastereoselective Synthesis

Addition of a nucleophile ($Nu^{\ominus}$:) is done to the carbonyl group of a chiral compound 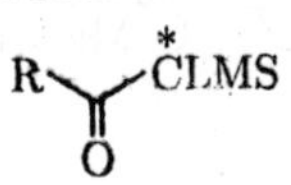 where L,M,S represent respectively the largest, medium sized and smallest of the substituents on the asymmetric carbon. The lowest energy T.S corresponds to a conformer in which in Newmann Projection, the C–L bond is perpendicular to the >=O group. The nucleophile approaches the carbonyl carbon in a plane perpendicular to that of –CO– fragment, from the side opposite to that of C–L bond and at an obtuse angle with C=O, corresponding approximately to the tetrahedral angle of Nu–C–O in the product. There may be two possibilities as follows.

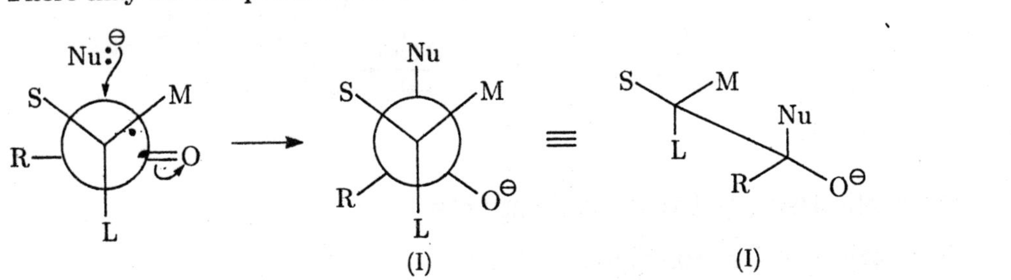

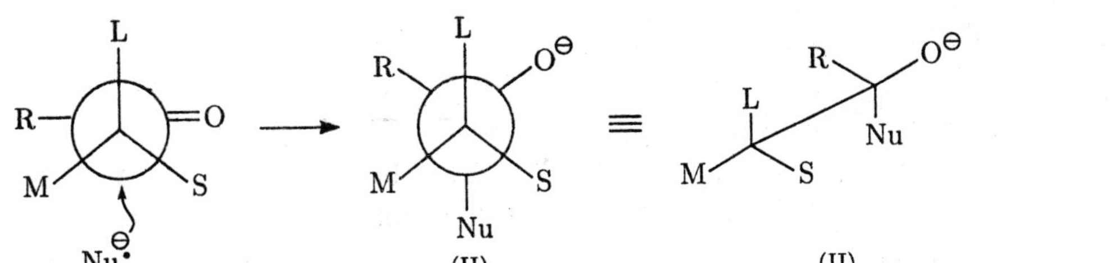

Conformation (I) is of lower energy because there is less steric interference between nucleophile (nu) and smallest group (s) than between Nu and larger group (M) in conformation II.

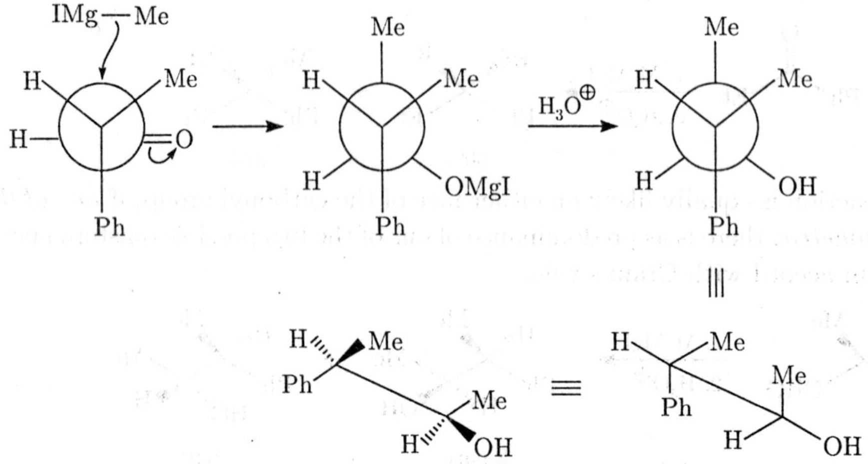

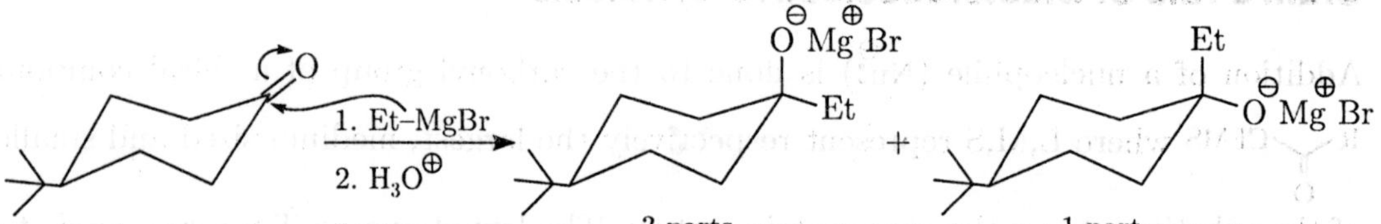

3 parts 1 part

Equatorial approach of Grignard reagent is preferred to avoid steric hindrance.

With an axial substituent at the 3-position, the stereoselectivity (approach of reagent from the equatorial side) is more pronounced.

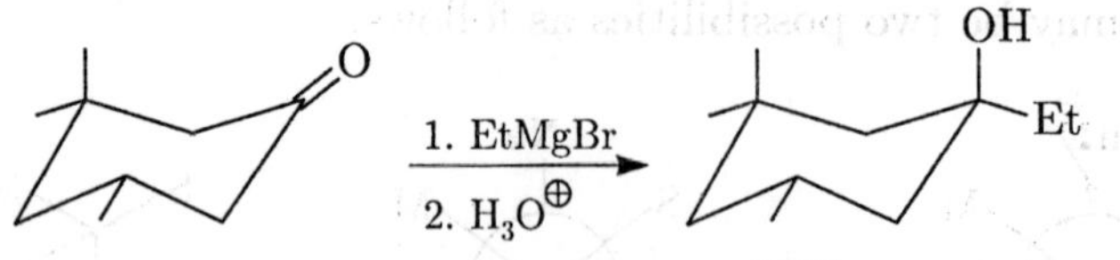

100%

Synthetic Uses of Grignard Reagents

Formation of Carbon-Carbon Bond

1. *Preparation of Hydrocarbons*

(a) RMgBr + H—OH (compound containing active H) $\xrightarrow{H^{\oplus}}$ R—H + Mg(OH)Br

G. R. (Stronger base); H—OH (Stronger acid); R—H (Weaker acid); Mg(OH)Br (Weaker base)

$$\text{(b) } RMgBr + H{-}OR \xrightarrow{H^{\oplus}} R{-}H + Mg(OH)Br$$

$$\text{(c) } XMg{-}R^1 + R^2{-}X \xrightarrow{S_N2} R^1{-}R^2 + MgX_2$$

$$\text{(d) } R{-}MgX + D_2O \longrightarrow RD + MgX(OD)$$

D is introduced in the hydrocarbon

The yield is very good if R^2 is allyl, or benzyl. This reaction also works well with α–halogenoethers. A good yield of R^1–R^2 is obtained if R^2OTs is used.

$$R^1MgI + R^2OTs \xrightarrow{S_N2} R^1{-}R^2 + MgI(OTs)$$

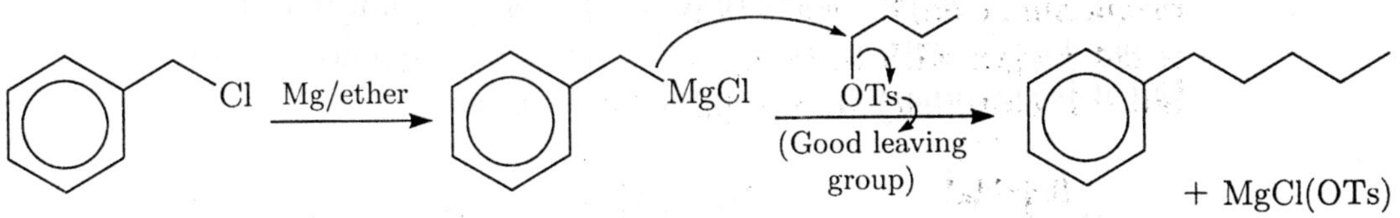

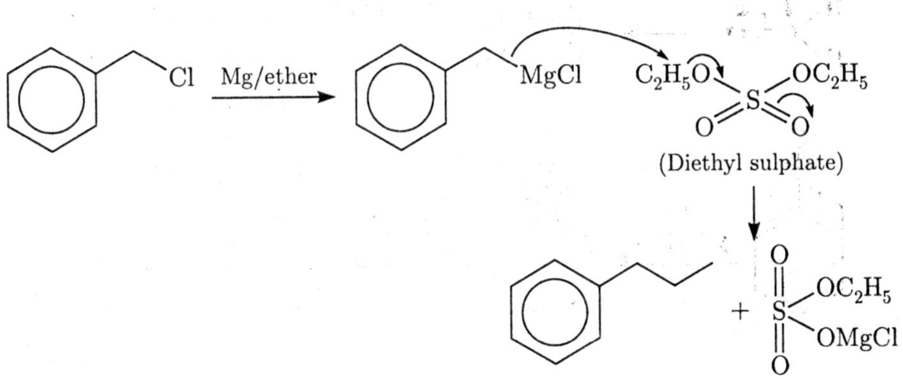

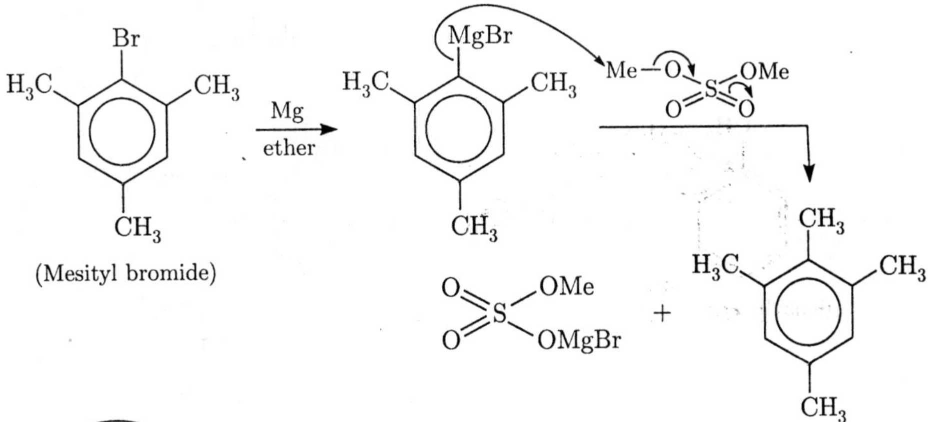

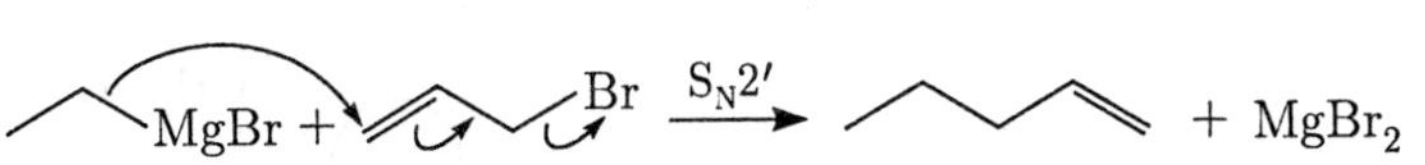

(Allyl bromide) (High yield)

2. ***Synthesis of Alcohols***

(a) *Primary Alcohols*

I. A Grignard reagent may be used to synthesise an alcohol by treating it with **dry oxygen and decomposing** the product with acid.

$$RMgX \xrightarrow{O_2} RO_2MgX \xrightarrow{RMgX} 2ROMgX \xrightarrow{H_3O^{\oplus}} 2ROH$$

This method is more useful converting aryl halides into phenols.

II. When a Grignard reagent (in ethereal solution) is treated with formaldehyd **(HCHO) gas or when** a Grignard reagent in di-n–butyl ether is refluxed with **paraformaldehyde,** a primary alcohol is obtained by decomposing the **magnesium complex** with dilute acid. The mechanism of Grignard reaction **is not known with** certainty, a complicated sequence is generally followed **but it is customary** to use simplified equations.

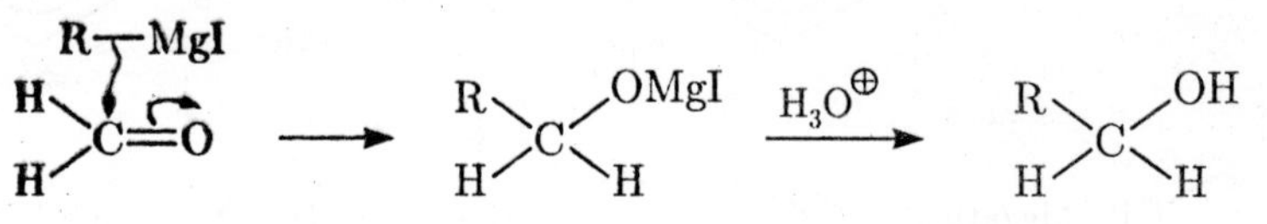

(Primary alcohol)

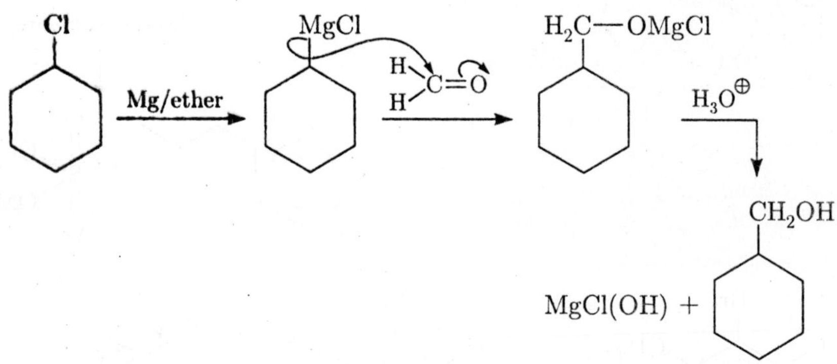

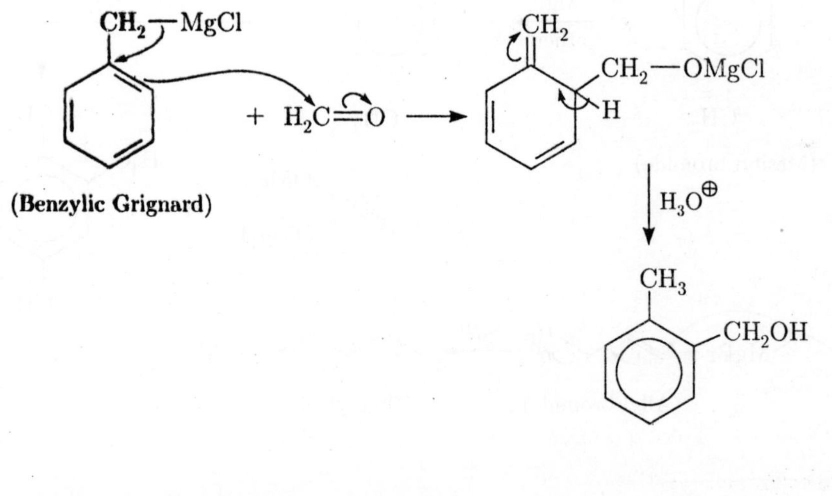

(Benzylic Grignard)

III. A primary alcohol containing *two* carbon atoms more than the Grignard alkyl group can be prepared by adding one molecule of ethylene chlorohydrin to two molecules of Grignard reagent.

$$RMgBr + ClCH_2CH_2OH \longrightarrow RH + ClCH_2CH_2OMgBr$$

$$ClCH_2CH_2OMgBr \xrightarrow{RMgBr} RCH_2CH_2OMgBr \xrightarrow{H_3O^{\oplus}} RCH_2CH_2OH$$

IV. ***Reactions of Grignard Reagents with Oxiranes (Epoxides)*** : The nucleophilic alkyl group of Grignard reagent attacks the partially positive carbon of the oxirane ring. Because it is highly strained, the ring opens, and the reaction leads to the salt of a primary alcohol. Subsequent acidification produces the alcohol.

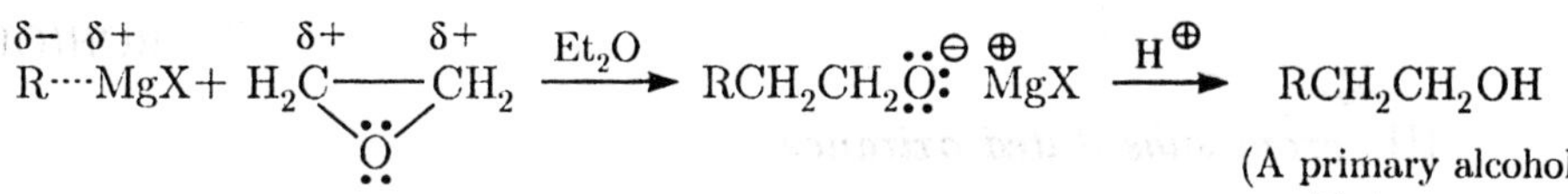

(Oxirane)

(A primary alcohol with two more carbon atoms than R)

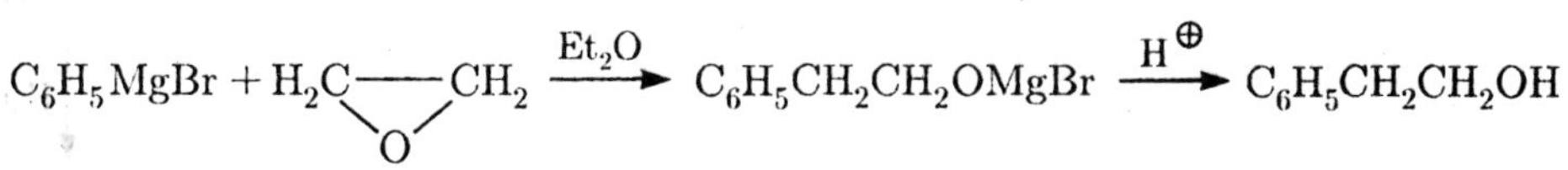

Grignard reagents react primarily at the *less substituted* ring carbon atom of substituted oxiranes. (compare with the base catalysed ring opening of oxiranes).

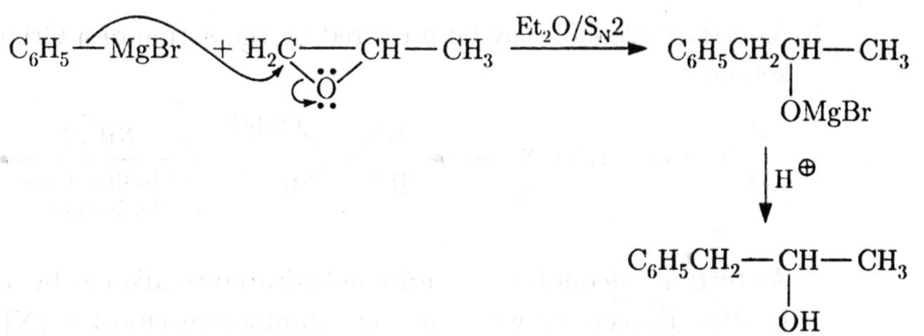

Similarly, a primary alcohol containing *three* more carbon atoms can be prepared from the Grignard reagent by using trimethylene oxide.

(b) ***Preparation of Secondary Alcohols***

I. When a Grignard reagent is treated with any aldehyde other than formaldehyde a secondary alcohol is obtained.

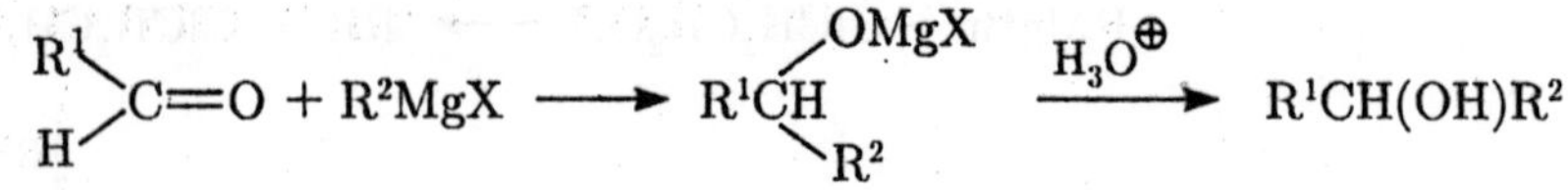

II. Secondary alcohols may also be prepared by interaction of a Grignard reagent (2 molecules) and ethyl formate (1 molecule).

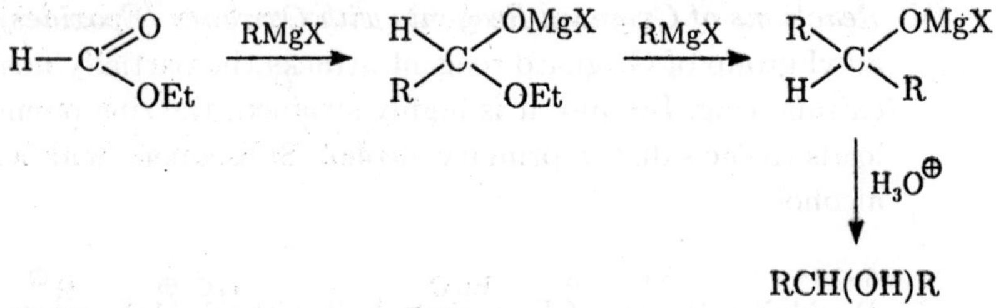

III. ***From substituted oxiranes***

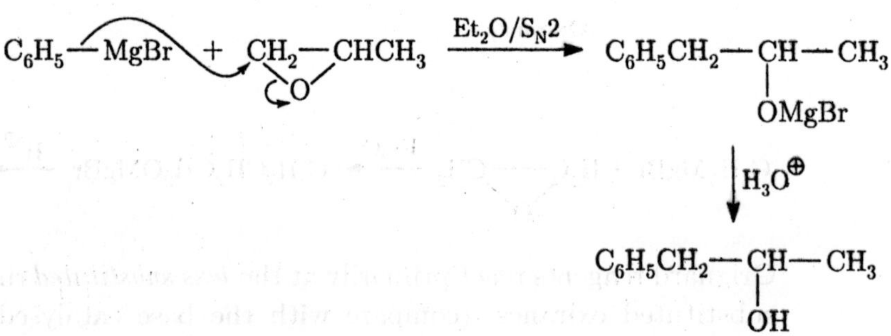

(c) ***Preparation of tertiary Alcohols***

I. A tertiary alcohol may be prepared by the action of a Grignard reagent on a ketone.

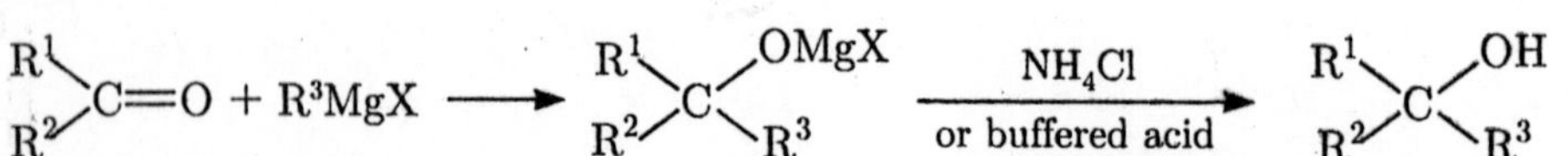

(Tertiary alcohol)

As tertiary alcohols are readily dehydrated to alkenes by acids, the complex is often broken up with aqueous ammonium chloride (NH_4Cl) or buffered acid solution.

II. Esters react with two molar equivalents of a Grignard reagent to form tertiary alcohols. When a Grignard reagent adds to the carbonyl group of an ester, the initial product is unstable and loses a magnesium alkoxide to form a ketone. Ketones are however more reactive toward Grignard reagent than esters. Therefore, as soon as a molecule of the ketone is formed in the mixture, it reacts with a second molecule of Grignard reagent After hydrolysis, the product is a tertiary alcohol with *two identical alkyl groups.*

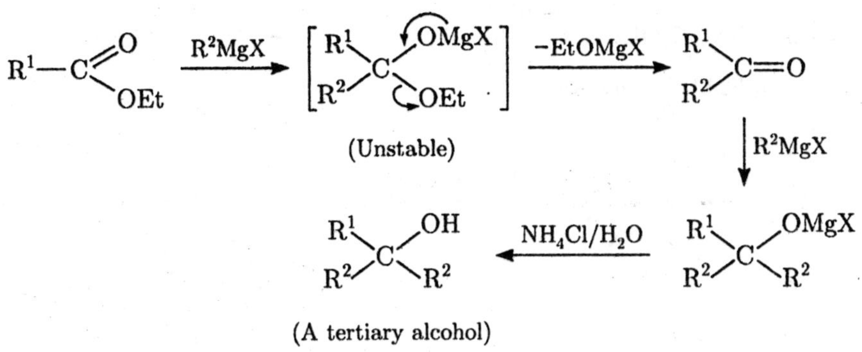

Mechanism of the Reaction :

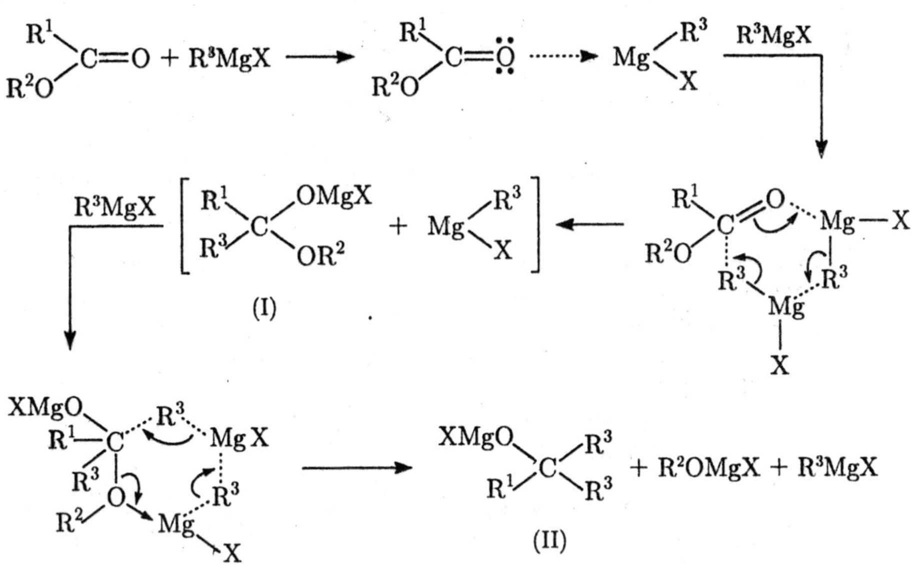

For most esters, it appears that, the step leading to (II) is much faster than that leading to(I). Thus, treatment of an ester with one equivalent of a Grignard reagent generally gives *t*–alcohol and recovery of half of the ester. If however, the Grignard reagent is added to ester (reverse addition) and the reaction is carried out at low temperatures, then reasonable yield of ketone is obtained. If the Grignard reagent or the ester is sterically hindered, *ketone and not alcohol* is the major product.

III. Tertiary alcohols containing three identical alkyl groups may be prepared by the reaction between a Grignard reagent (3 molecules) and ethyl carbonate (1 molecule).

$$3RMgX + (C_2H_5O)_2CO \longrightarrow R_3COMgX + 2Mg(OC_2H_5)X \xrightarrow{H_3O^{\oplus}} R_3COH$$

Mechanism of Reaction Between a Grignard reagent and a Carbonyl Compound (Proposed by Asby *et. al*)

$$R_2C{=}O + RMgX(OEt_2)_2 \underset{}{\overset{-OEt_2}{\rightleftharpoons}} R_2C{=}\ddot{O}: \longrightarrow MgRX(OEt_2)$$

R=Ph (G. R. Et_2O complex)

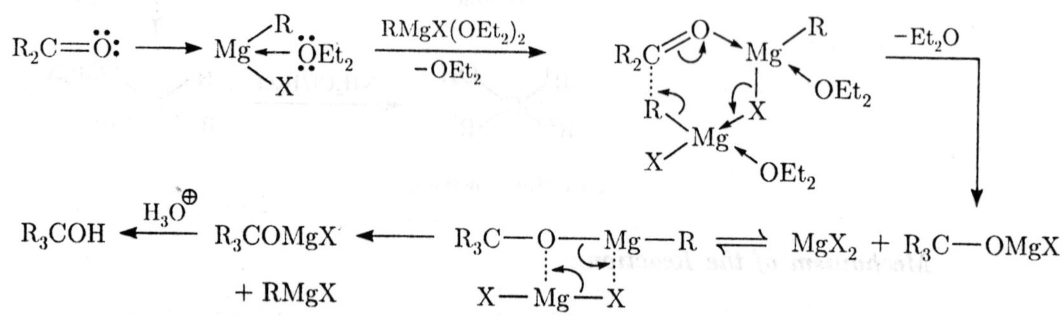

The mechanism is supported by the following facts :

1. The rate of the reaction decreases when half of Grignard reagent has been used up.
2. A mixture of alkoxy magnesium alkyl and $MgBr_2$ produces the alkoxy magnesium halide.
3. ***Synthesis of Ethers*** : Ethers may be prepared by reaction between a Grignard reagent and a monochloroether (an example of double decomposition).

$$R^1OCH_2Cl + R^2MgX \longrightarrow R^1OCH_2R^2 + MgXCl$$

$$MeOH + HCHO + HCl \longrightarrow MeOCH_2Cl + H_2O$$

$$ROH + HBr \longrightarrow RBr \xrightarrow{Mg/Et_2O} RMgBr \xrightarrow{MeOCH_2Cl} RCH_2OMe$$

$$RCH_2OMe \xrightarrow{HBr} RCH_2Br \xrightarrow{OH^{\ominus}} RCH_2OH$$

(Stepping up of both ether and alcohol series)

4. ***Synthesis of Aldehydes*** :

(a) An aldehyde may be prepared by the reaction between a Grignard reagent (1 molecule) and ethyl formate (1 molecule). If the Grignard reagent is present in excess, a secondary alcohol is formed. Hence to avoid this as much as possible, the *Grignard reagent is added to the ester.*

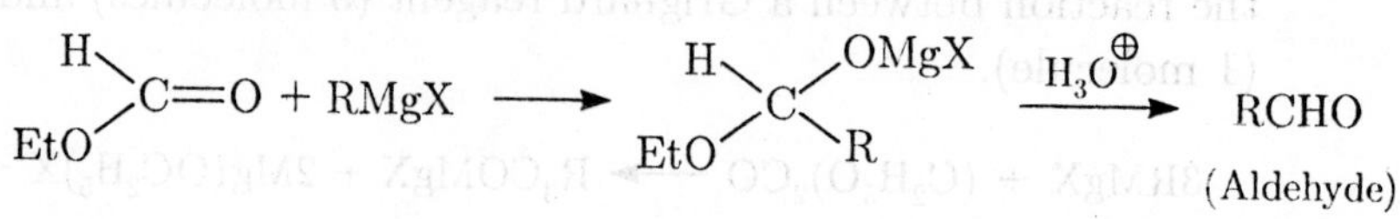

(b) A better yield of aldehyde is obtained if ethyl orthoformate is used instead of ethyl formate, since the formation of secondary alcohol is prevented by the formation of an acetal.

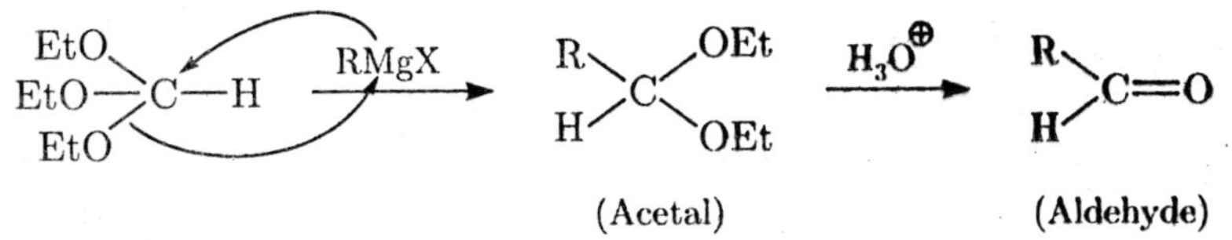

(c) Aldehydes are also prepared by the reaction between a Grignard reagent and hydrocyanic acid (HCN).

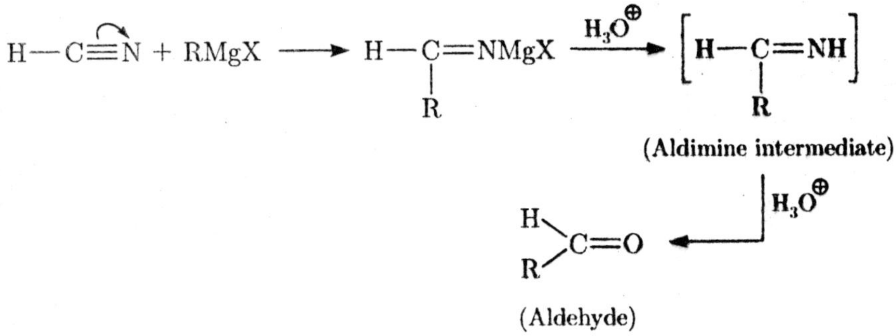

(d) 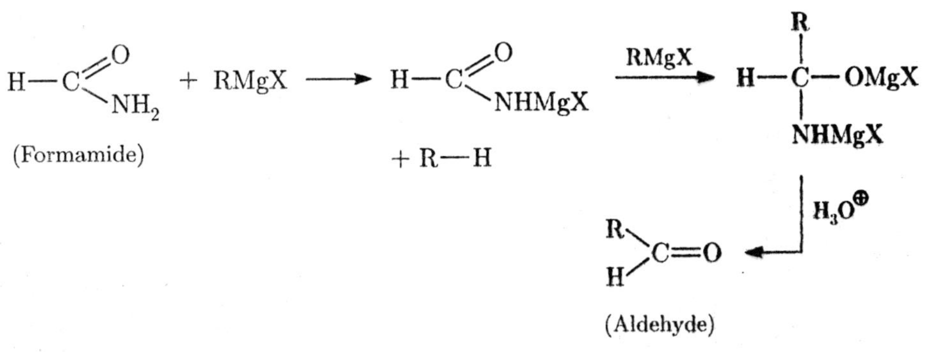

5. *Synthesis of Ketones* :

(a) Ketones may be prepared from orthoester ketals by using any ortho ester ketal other than orthoformic ester.

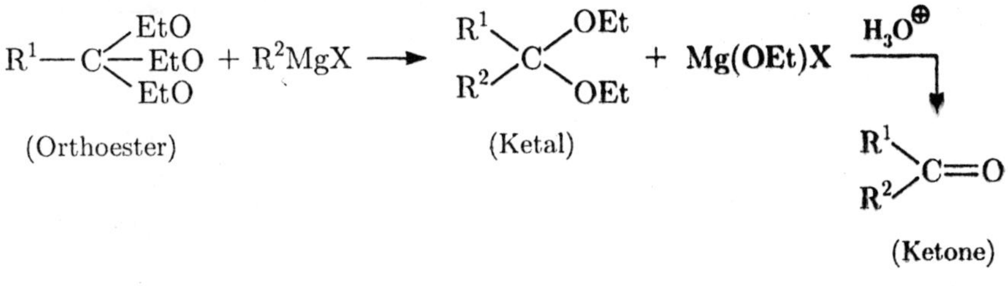

(b) 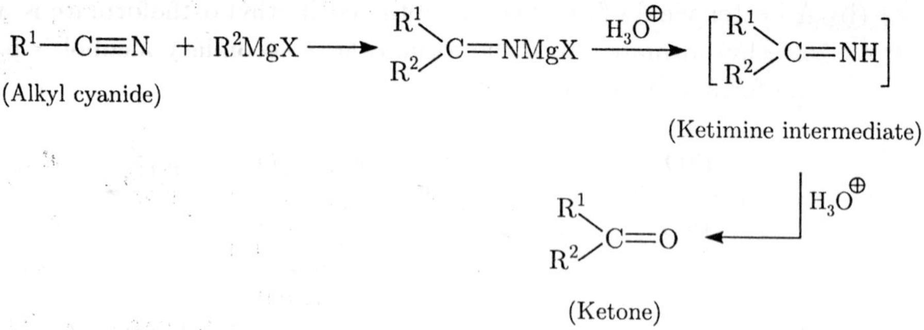

(c) Acyl chlorides (1 molecule) react rapidly with Grignard reagent (1 molecule) to form ketones.

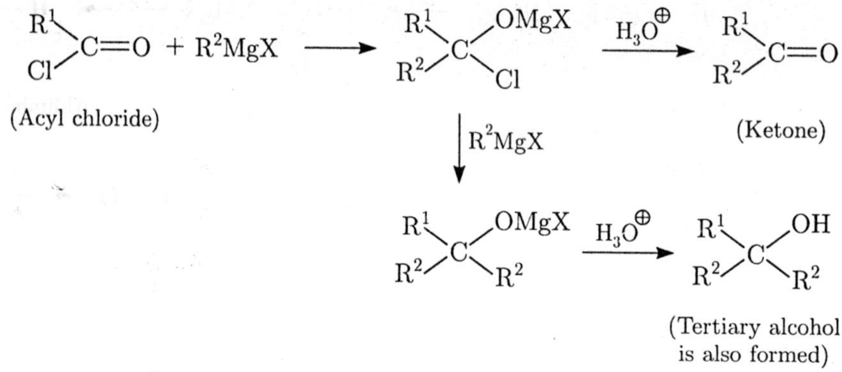

(d) $$(R^1CO)_2O + R^2MgX \xrightarrow{-70^\circ C} R^1COR^2 + R^1COOMgX$$

(Acid anhydride) (Ketone)

(e) Amides and N–substituted amides react with Grignard reagent to form ketones.

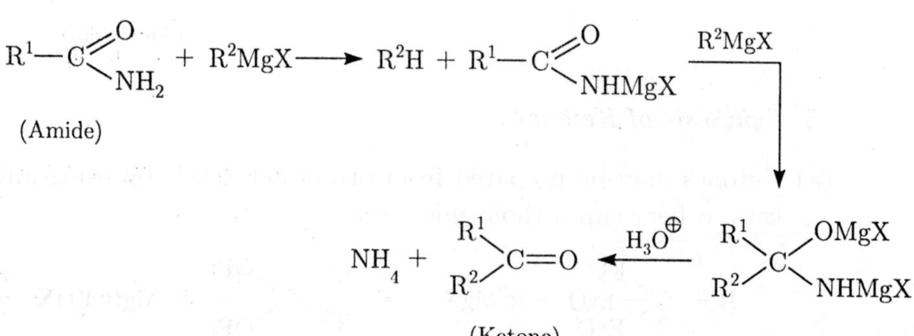

6. ***Synthesis of Acids* :**

(a) When a Grignard reagent is treated with solid carbon dioxide (CO_2) and the complex decomposed with dilute acid, a monocarboxylic acid is obtained.

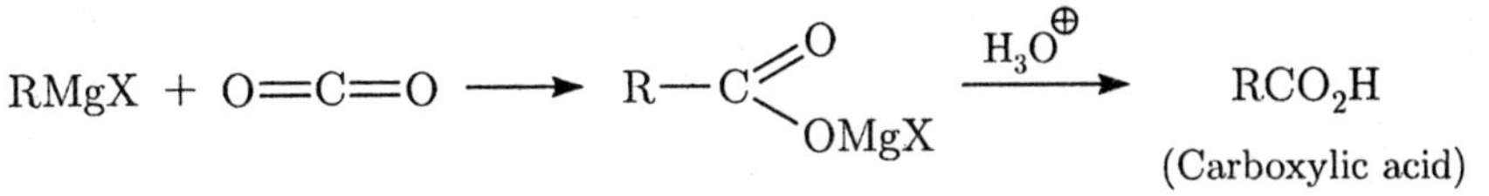

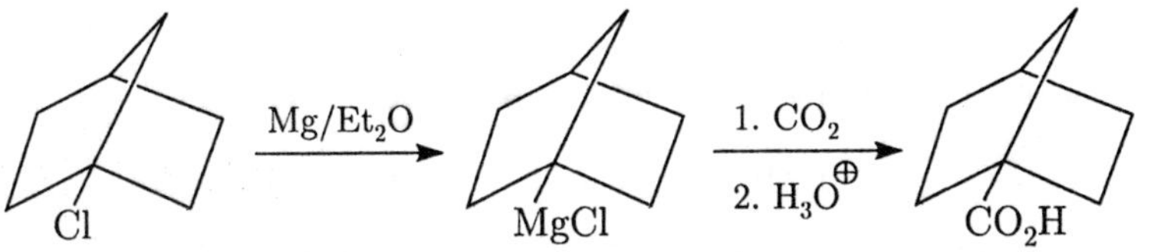

A good yield of acid may be obtained by passing carbon dioxide (CO_2) into Grignard solution cooled to 0°C. This method is particularly useful for preparing acids of the type R_3CCOOH which is othewise difficult to prepare. This method also offers a means of asceding the acid series.

(b) γ–ketoacids are prepared from cyclic anhydrides with Grignard reagents.

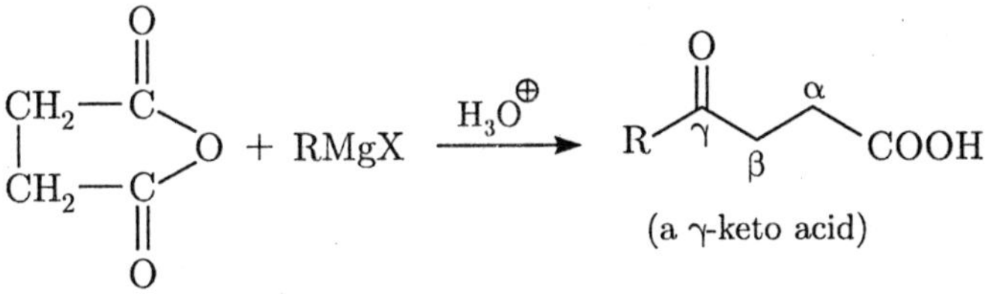

7. ***Synthesis of Esters* :**

(a) When Grignard reagent (1 molecule) reacts with ethyl chloroformate (1 molecule) an ester is formed. To avoid the reaction with the carbethoxy group, the Grignard reagent is added to the ester (reverse addition).

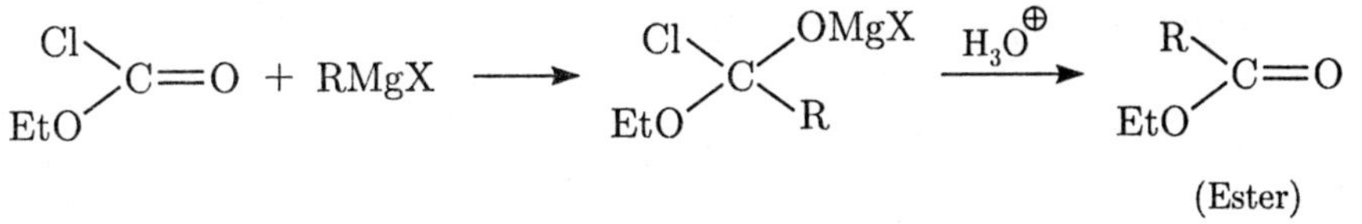

(b) Esters of tertiary alcohols are conveniently prepared as follows.

$$R^1OH + CH_3MgI \longrightarrow CH_4 + R^1OMgI \xrightarrow[2.\ H_3O^{\oplus}]{1.\ R^2COCl} R^1COOR^2$$

[R^1=t-alkyl group] (Ester)

8. *Synthesis of Alkyl Cyanides* :

(a) Cyanogen (1 molecule) reacts with a Grignard reagent (1 molecule) to form an alkyl cyanide.

$$RMgX + (CN)_2 \longrightarrow \underset{\text{(Alkyl cyanide)}}{RCN} + Mg(CN)X$$

(b) Alkyl cyanides are formed together with alkyl chloride, when a Grignard reagent (1 molecule) is added to an ethereal solution of cyanogen chloride (1 molecule). The latter should always be in excess, since the alkyl cyanide produced tends to react with the Grignard reagent.

$$RMgCl + ClCN \longrightarrow RCN + MgCl_2$$

$$RMgCl + ClCN \longrightarrow RCl + Mg(CN)Cl$$

Tertiaryalkyl cyanides are produced in good yield by this method.

9. *Synthesis of Primary Amines* :

(a) $$2RMgCl + \underset{\text{(O-methylhydroxylamine)}}{CH_3ONH_2} \xrightarrow{S_N2} RNHMgCl + RH + Mg(OCH_3)Cl$$

$$RNHMgCl \xrightarrow{H_3O^{\oplus}} \underset{\text{(Primary amine)}}{RNH_2}$$

RMgCl or RMgBr may be used but not RMgI. Tertiaryalkyl amines (Me_3CNH_2) can be prepared by this method, as it is not obtained from S_N2 reaction between *t*-alkyl halides and NH_3.

(b) $$RMgX + \underset{\text{(Chloramine)}}{ClNH_2} \longrightarrow \underset{\text{(primary amine)}}{RNH_2} + MgXCl$$

Yield is reasonable only for the tertiaryalkyl group.

10. *Synthesis of pyrrole and indole derivatives* :

(a)

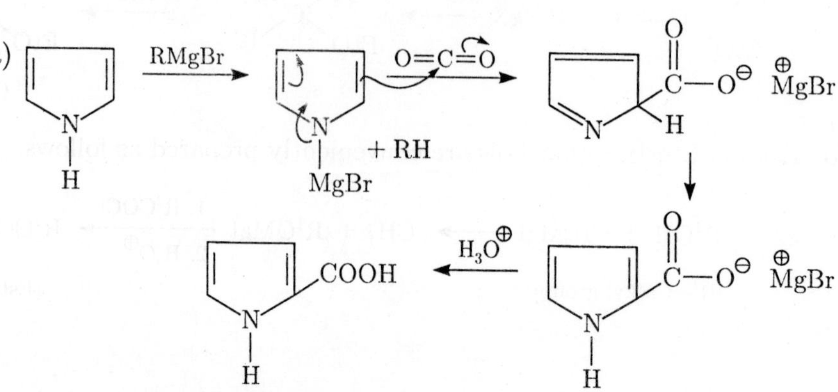

(Pyrrole-2-carboxylic acid)

(b) 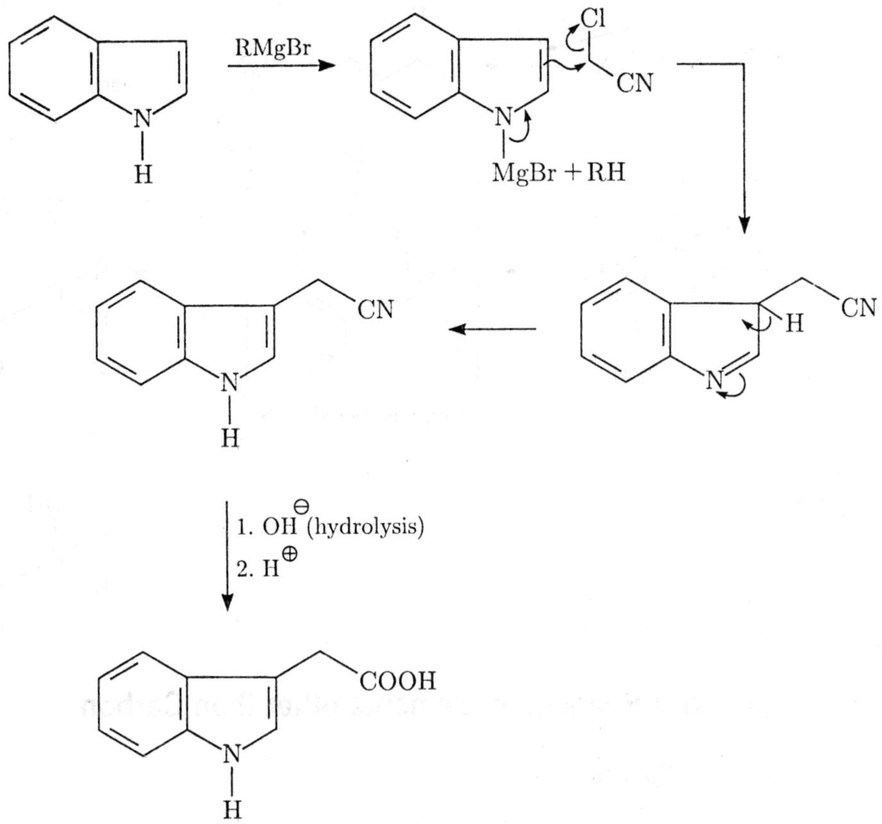

(Indole-3-acetic acid)
(Plant growth hormone, heteroauxin)

11. ***Reactions of Allyl Grignard Reagent*** : Allyl Grignard reagents exist in solutions as a mixture of isomers in rapid equilibrium.

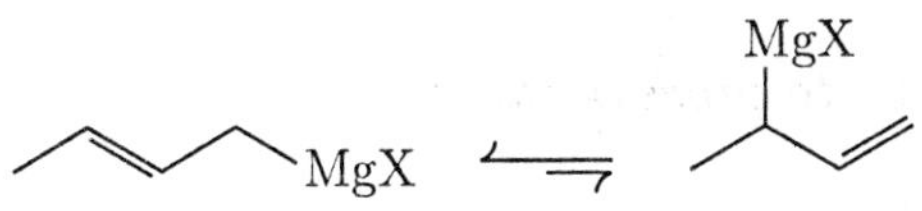

(I) (major) (II) (minor)

(I) is the major component as it contains more substituted double bond. But the product obtained on reaction is usually that corresponding to the minor isomer. Explanation is that the major isomer can result in a shift of the double bond.

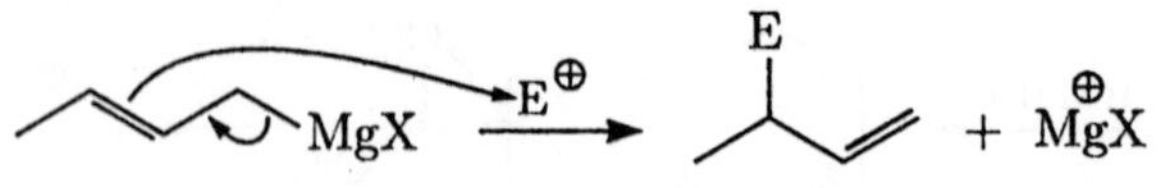

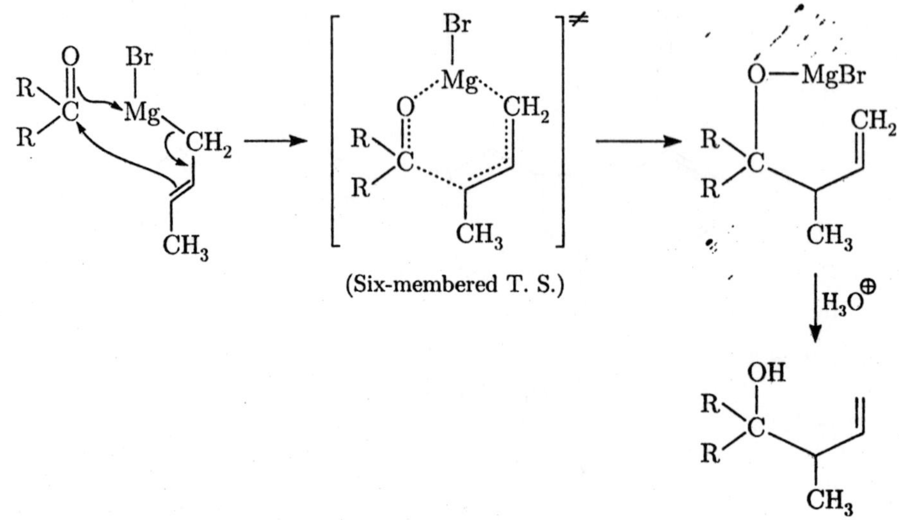

Reaction of Grignard Reagent at Elements other than Carbon

1. ***Synthesis of Hydroperoxides*** :

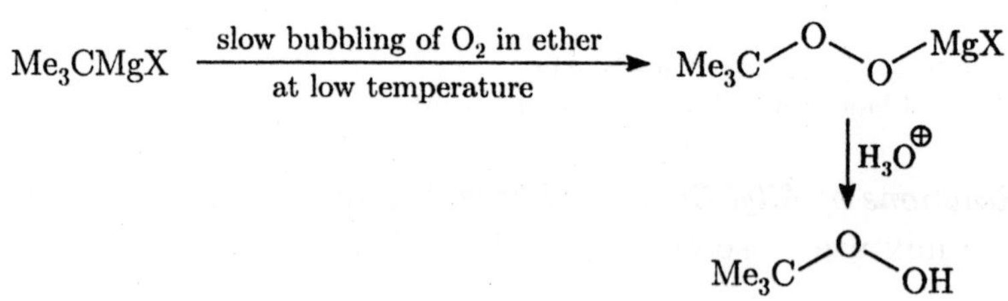

2. ***With sulphur to produce thiols*** :

$$R{-}MgX + S \longrightarrow R{-}S{-}MgX \xrightarrow{H_3O^{\oplus}} RSH$$

3. ***With SO_2 to produce sulphinic acids*** :

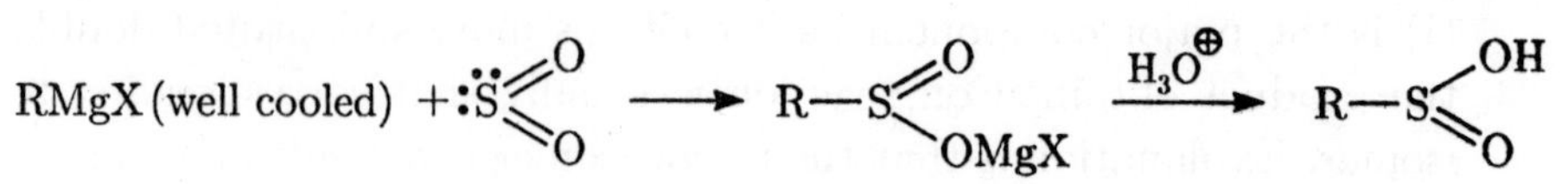

(Sulphinic acid)

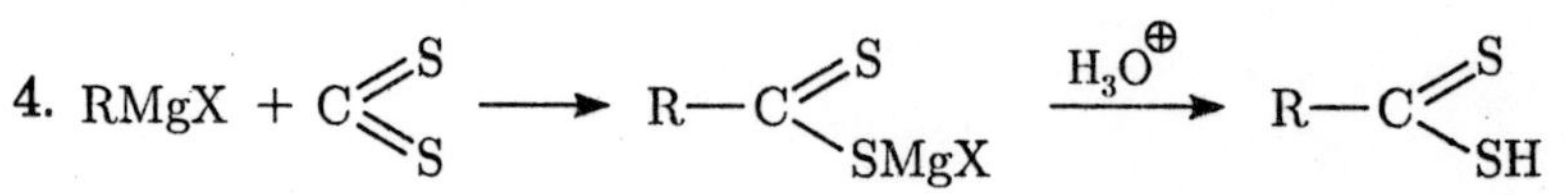

(Dithioic acid)

5. ***With I_2 to produce iodides*** :

$$MgX—R + I—I \longrightarrow R—I + MgX(I)$$

This method is useful when other methods for the preparation of iodides fail. Hindered neopentyl chloride does not form iodide with sodium iodide (NaI) but the above method fulfils the purpose of synthesising neopentyl iodide.

$$Me_3CCH_2—Cl \xrightarrow[\text{ether}]{\text{Mg}} Me_3CCH_2—MgCl \xrightarrow{I—I} \underset{\text{(Neopentyl iodide)}}{Me_3CCH_2I} + MgClI$$

Corresponding bromide (*e.g.*, neopentyl bromide) can be prepared from bromine by analogous method.

6. ***Derivatives of Phosphorus, boron and Silicon*** :

(a) $3RMgX + PCl_3 \longrightarrow R_3P + 3MgXCl$

(b) $3RMgX + BCl_3 \longrightarrow R_3B + 3MgXCl$

(c) $4RMgX + SiCl_4 \longrightarrow R_4Si + 4MgXCl$

In the last case, it is possible to isolate the intermediate silanes, $RSiCl_3$, R_2SiCl_2 and R_3SiCl, by using calculated quantities of the Grignard reagent.

7. ***Application of Acetylenic Grignard Reagent*** :

Preparation

$$Cl—CH_2—CHO \xrightarrow[\text{dry HCl}]{\text{EtOH}} \underset{\text{(Acetal)}}{Cl—CH_2—CH(OEt)_2} \xrightarrow[(\text{-HCl, -EtOH})]{NaNH_2/\text{liq. } NH_3} HC \equiv C—OEt$$

$$HC \equiv C—OEt \xrightarrow{\text{EtMgBr}} C_2H_6 + MgBrC \equiv C—OEt$$

Conversions :

(a) BrMg C≡C—OEt to α–acetylenic alcohol :

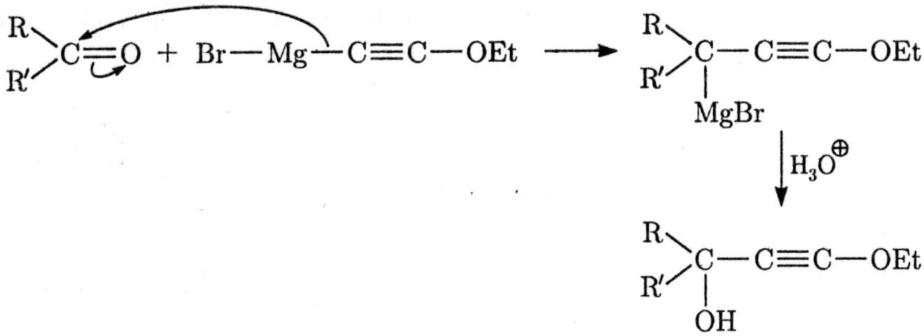

(b) BrMg–C≡C—OEt to α, β–unsaturated ester : Acid catalysed hydrolysis of α–acetylenic alcohol finally produces α, β–unsaturated ester via dehydration.

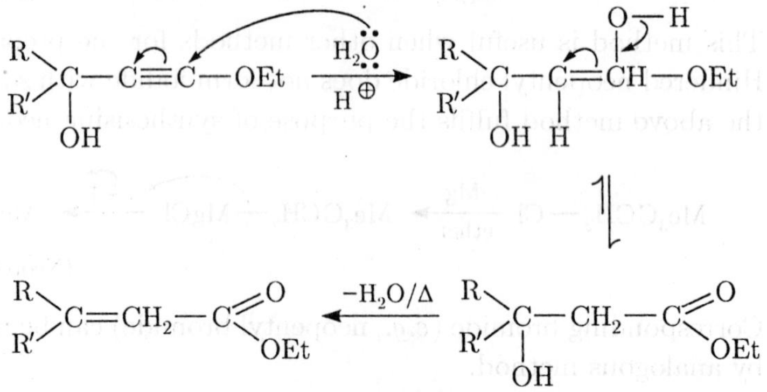

(c) BrMg–C≡C—OEt to α, β–unsaturated aldehyde : Partial catalytic hydrogenation of α–acetylenic alcohol gives a vinyl ether which is hydrolysed by mineral acids to give β–hydroxyaldehyde, dehydration of which yields α,β–unsaturated aldehyde.

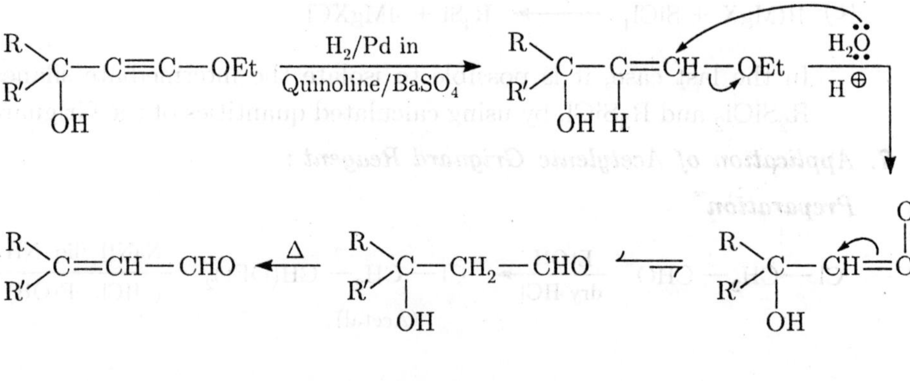

Abnormal Behaviour of Grignard Reagents

The reactions with aldehydes and ketones usually give good yields of alcohols except with ketones which contain bulky groups. For example, ditertiarybutyl ketone does not give tertiary alcohols with Grignard reagents. If the ketone contains somewhat less bulky groups, and the Grignard reagent contains a branched alkyl groups, yields are again low. Isopropyl methyl ketone reacts with MeMgI but not with tertiarybutyl magnesium chloride.

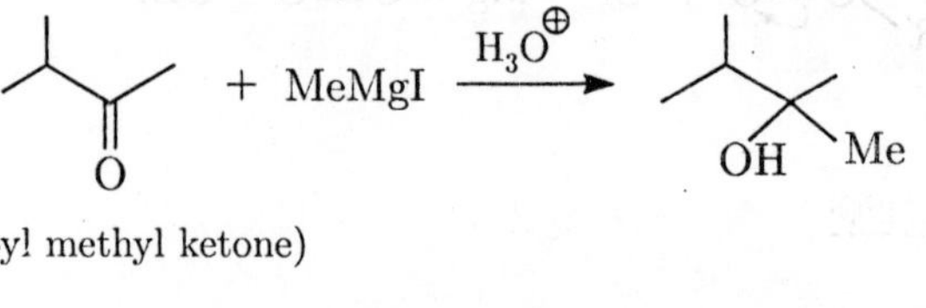

(Isopropyl methyl ketone)

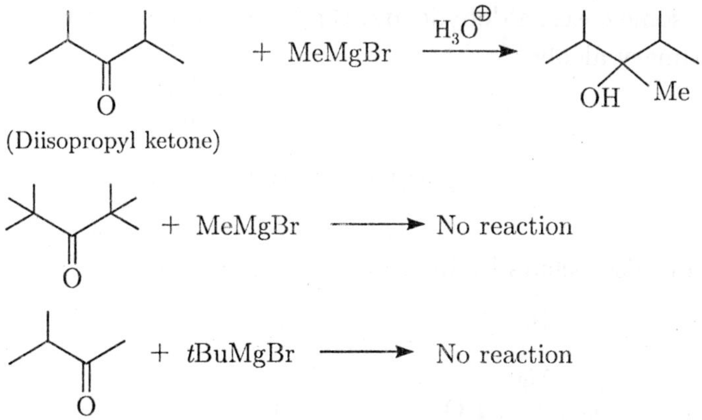

(a) In these cases one or both of two side reactions take place. If the ketone has at least one hydrogen atom on one of its two α–carbon atoms, *enolisation* can occur. The Grignard reagent acts as a base rather than as a nucleophile and abstracts an *activated hydrogen* giving the *enolate.* Treatment with acid regenerates the ketone.

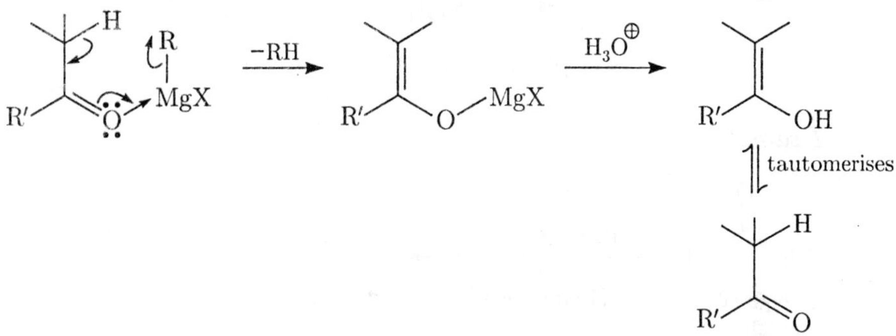

(b) If the Grignard Reagent contains at least *one hydrogen* atom on its *β-carbon atom, reduction* can occur by hydride ion transfer within a six–membered cyclic transition state (MPV reduction like).

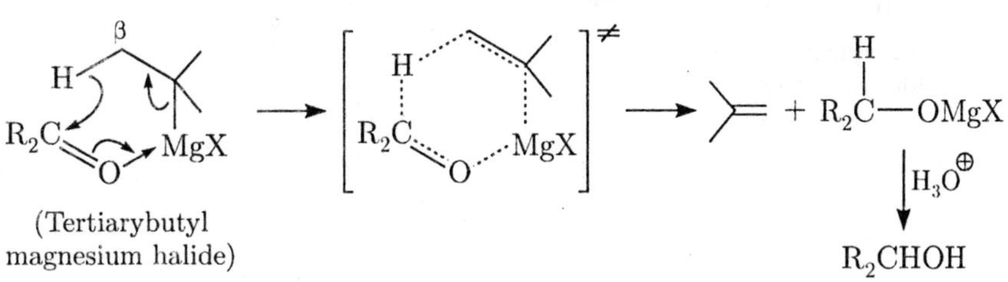

When each of these structural features (*i.e.*, the ketone containing at least one α–H which can undergo enolisation, *i.e.*, one active hydrogen is present and secondly the Grignard reagent contains a β hydrogen atom which produces secondary alcohol), enolisation and reduction are competitive. Diisopropyl ketone and tertiarybutyl magnesium bromide give 35% of enolate and 65% of the secondary alcohol.

(c) In some cases, aldehyde and the Grignard reagent interact to form ketone and a primary alcohol.

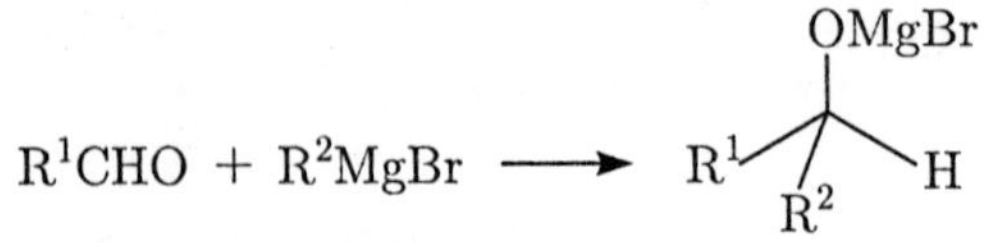

This also occurs by hydride ion transfer via a cyclic T.S.

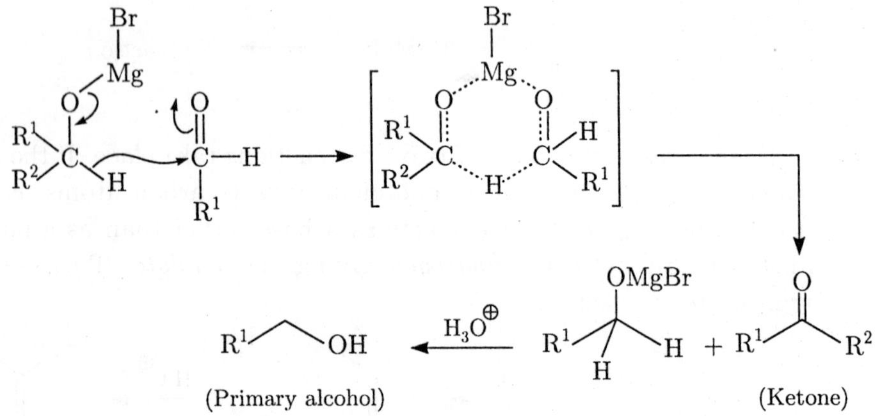

Example :

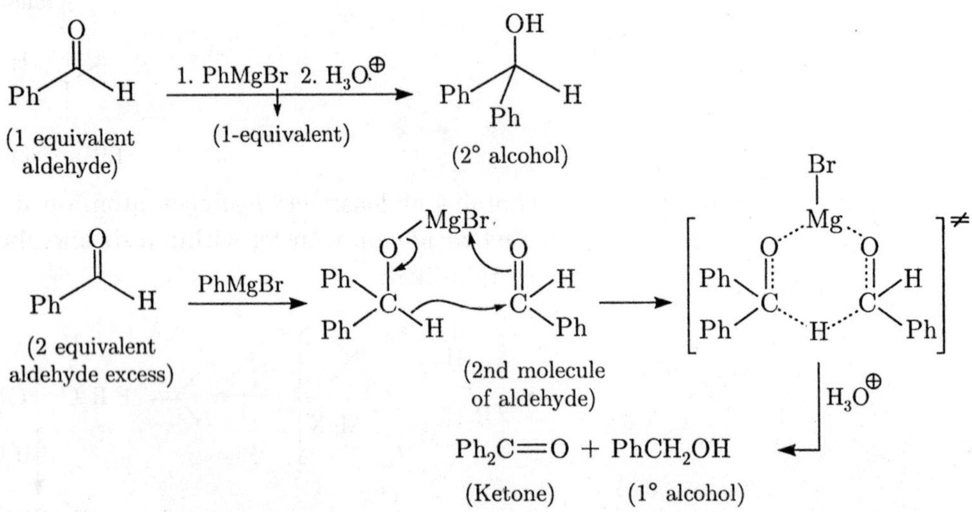

Excess aldehyde attacks the magnesium bromide complex intermediate as an electrophile and gives abnormal products, *i.e.*, a primary alcohol and a ketone. So, we find that 1 equivalent of benzaldehyde reacts with 1 equivalent of Grignard reagent to produce a secondary alcohol (normal product). But if the aldehyde and the Grignard reagent are taken in 2:1 ratio (excess aldehyde), abnormal products like a primary alcohol and a ketone are formed through a cyclic transition state.

(d) ***Reaction of Grignard reagent with α, β–unsaturated Ketone*** : α, β–Unsaturated carbonyl compounds react with a Grignard reagent in the 1,2– or 1,4–positions.

I. ***1,2–Addition***

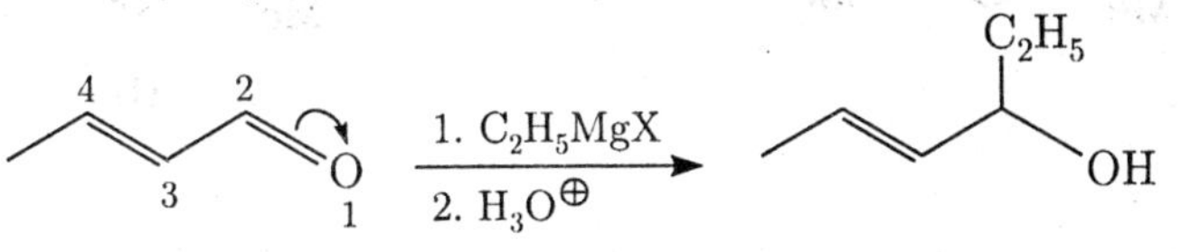

Mg used in this case is highly pure.

II. ***1,4–Addition***

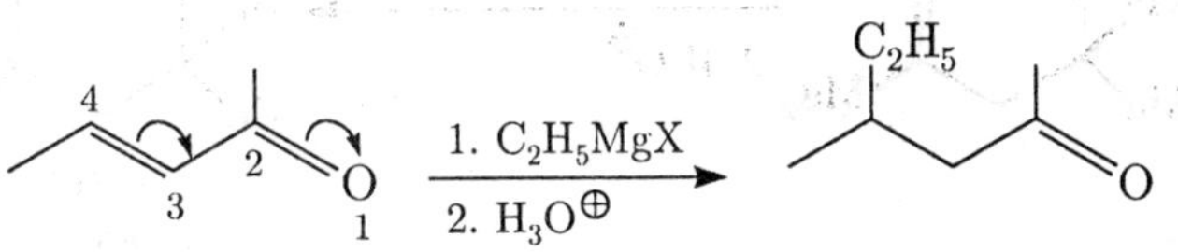

In this case, the Grignard reagent is prepared from normal comercially available magnesium.

The 1,4–addition, which passes via enolate intermediate competes increasing effectively with addition to C=O (1,2–addition) as the *sizes of the substituents at the carbonyl groups are increased.*

Mechanism of 1,4–addition (cf. Michael Reaction)

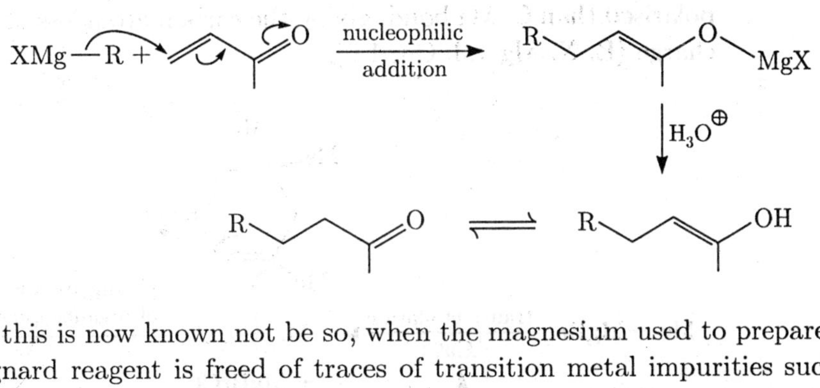

But this is now known not be so, when the magnesium used to prepare the Grignard reagent is freed of traces of transition metal impurities such as copper, only 1,2–addition occurs. Moreover, 1,4–addition is promoted compared with 1,2–addition by the addition of a catalytic quantity of Cu(I) compound such as CuBr.

Cu(I) salts have a Remarkable Effect on Organometallic Reagents : The hard Grignard reagent prefers to attack the harder C=O rather than the softer C=C electrophilic centre. But when 1% CuCl is present along with the Grignard reagent, it makes the Grignard reagent undergo conjugate addition, with only a trance of diene.

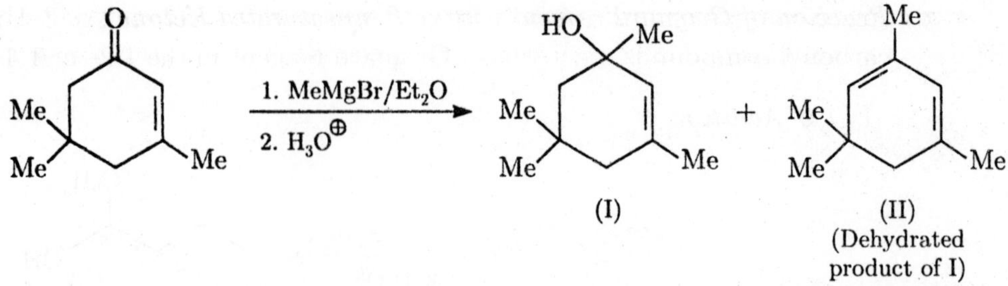

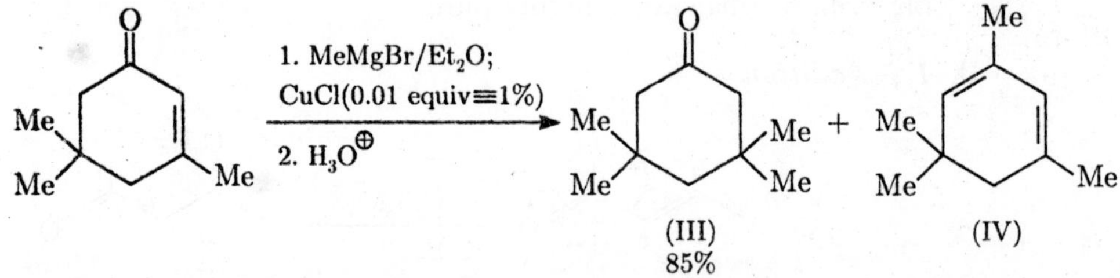

Organocopper Reagents Undergo Conjugate Addition : The copper works by transmetallating the Grignard reagent to give an organocopper reagent. Organocoppers are softer than Grignard reagent and add in a conjugate fashion to the softer C=C double bond. Once the organocopper has added, the copper salt is available to transmetallate some more Grignard and only a catalytic amount is required. Organocoppers are softer than Grignard reagent because copper is less electropositive than Mg, so C–Cu bond is less polarised than C–Mg bond, giving the carbon atom less of a partial negative charge (E. N: Mg 1.3, Cu: 1.9).

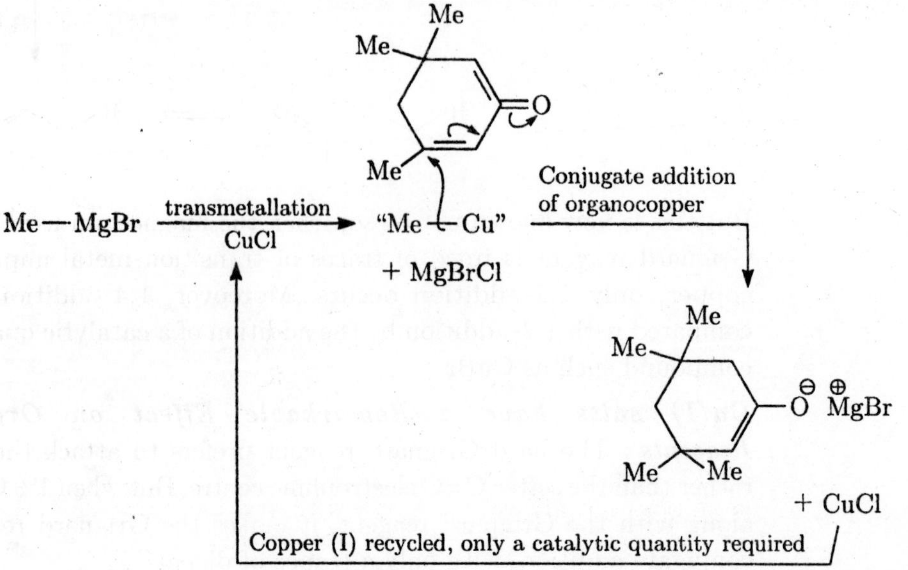

The organocopper is shown here as "Me–Cu" because its precise structure is not known. Some authors say the mechanism of 1,4–addition in the presence of CuBr is free radical.

(e) The reaction of dihalides of the type $Br(CH_2)_nBr$ with magnesium depends on the value of n. For n=1–3, no Grignard reagent is formed. For n $\gg$ 4, dimagnesium compound is obtained.

$$Br(CH_2)_5Br + 2Mg \xrightarrow{Et_2O} BrMg(CH_2)_5MgBr$$

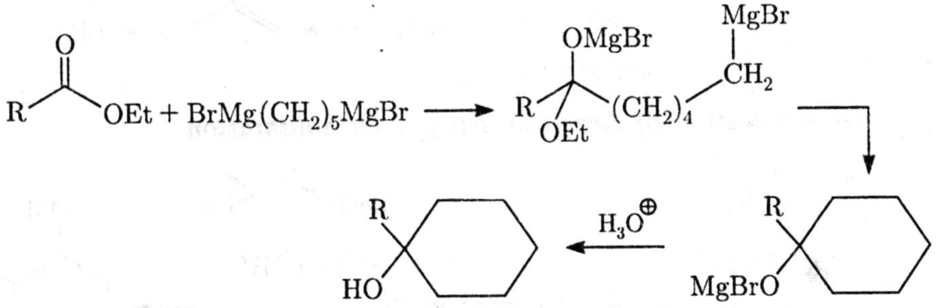

Organolithium Compounds

Organolithium compounds are more reactive than Grignard reagents but less reactive than organosodiums. The fact that they undergo same reactions of which Grignard reagents are incapable, gives them special uses in synthesis.

Methods of Preparation of Organolithium Compounds

1. Like Grignard reagents, organolithium compounds may be prepared by *oxidative insertion* reaction from Li metal and alkyl halides. Two equivalents of Li metal is needed.

$$R{-}X + 2Li \xrightarrow[-10°C]{\text{Inert atmosphere (nitrogen or argon)}} RLi + LiX$$

Because of the reactivity of organolithiums with oxygen, the reaction is carried out in an atmosphere of nitrogen or argon. Organolithium compounds are more reactive than Grignard reagent towards alkyl halides, and it is advantageous to cool the reaction mixture to about –10°C to minimise the extent of Wurtz coupling reaction.

$$RLi + RX \longrightarrow R{-}R + LiX$$

Li metal does not always react well with aryl and vinyl halides.

2. ***Halogen–Metal Exchange*** : Aryl and vinyl lithium compounds can be conveniently prepared by metal–halogen exchange reaction using *e.g.*, preformed butyllithium.

$$R{-}Br + BuLi \longrightarrow RLi + BuBr$$

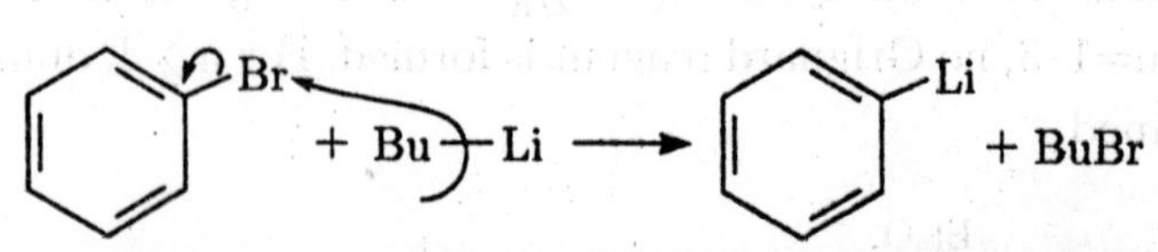

$Bu:^{\ominus}$, pK_a=50(more basic)

$Ph:^{\ominus}$, pK_a=43(Less basic)

So the reaction proceeds in the forward direction.

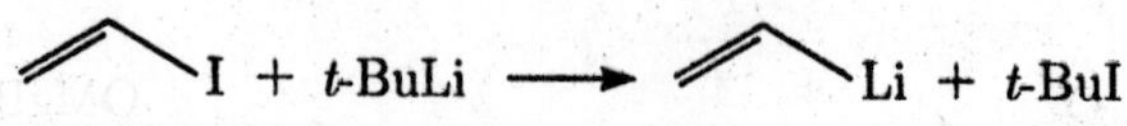

(Vinyl iodide)

3. ***Deprotonation of Aromatic Rings*** : ***Ortholithiation*** :

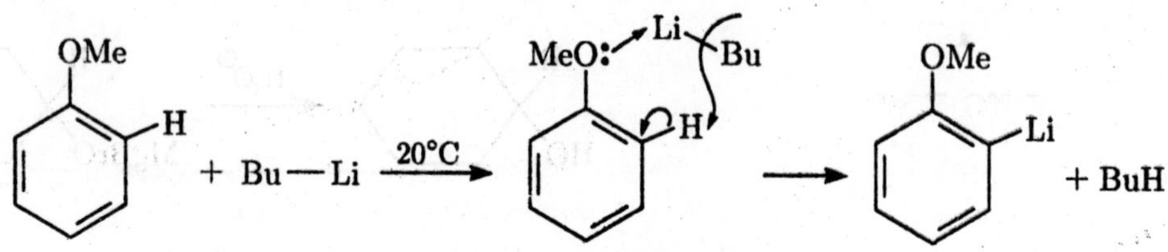

(Complexation between oxygen and Lewis acid Li)

BuLi deprotonates sp^2 hybrid carbon, as protons attached to sp^2 carbons are more acidic than those attached to sp^3 carbon.

4. ***Metallation Reaction*** : The metallation reaction is suitable for the preparation of lithium derivatives of comparatively acidic hydrocarbons.

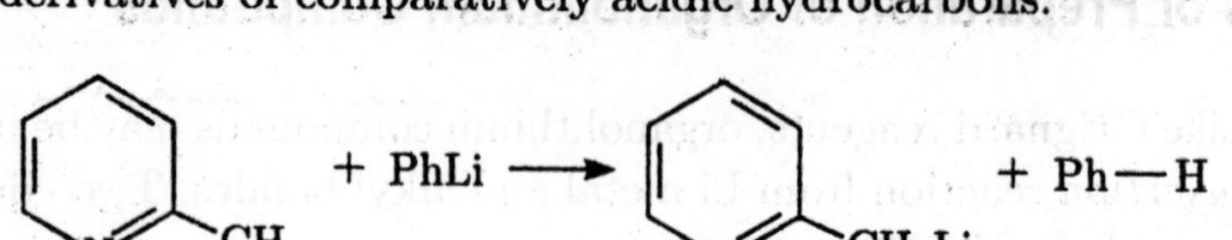

(α–picoline)

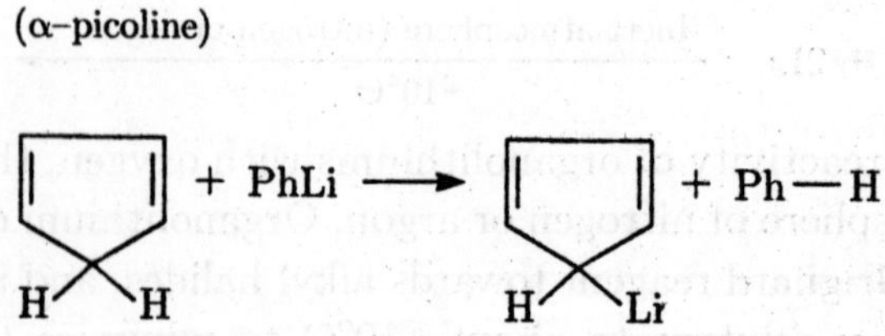

5. ***Deprotonation of Alkynes*** :

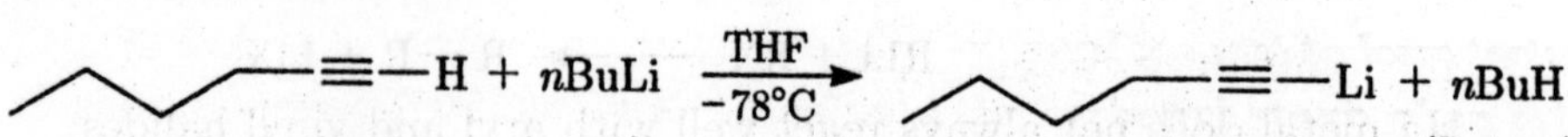

(1–hexyne) (pK_a=26) (1–hexyne) (pK_a=50) (Butane)

Structure of Organolithium

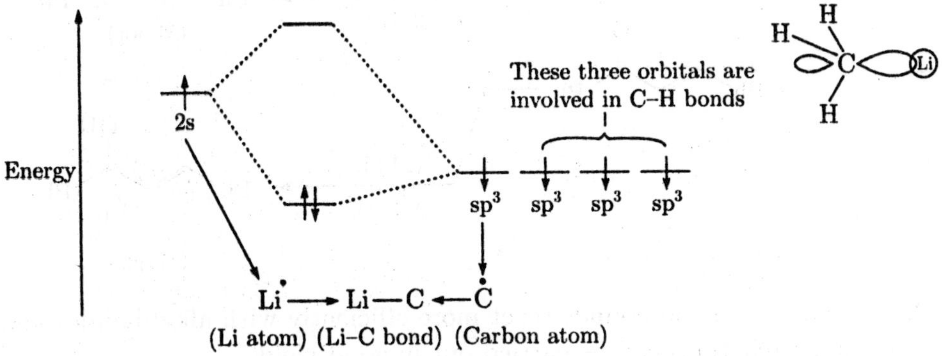

Fig. 2.5 :

Orbital Diagram for the C–Li Bond of MeLi : The more electronegative an atom is, the lower in energy its atomic orbitals. The filled C–Li σ orbital that arises is closer in energy to the carbon's sp^3 orbital than to the lithium's 2s orbital. So we can say that carbon's sp^3 orbital makes a greater contribution to the C–Li σ bond. Reactions involving the filled s orbital will therefore take place at C rather than Li. Because carbon's sp^3 orbital makes a greater contribution to the C–Li σ bond, the s bond resembles a *filled C–sp³ orbital.* In other words, it *resembles a lone pair of electrons* on carbon.

$$\underset{\text{(Organolithium)}}{R{-}Li} \longrightarrow \underset{\text{(Carbanion)}}{\overset{\ominus}{R:}} + \underset{\text{(Metal cation)}}{Li^{\oplus}}$$

Reactions of Organolithium

Most of the reactions of organolithium run parallel with Grignard reagent, but only those are emphasised which Grignard reagents fail to undergo.

1. Lithium compounds are less readily prevented by steric hindrance from reacting at carbonyl groups. Isopropylmagnesium bromide does not add to diisopropyl ketone, but brings about enolisation and reduction, isopropyllithium adds successfully.

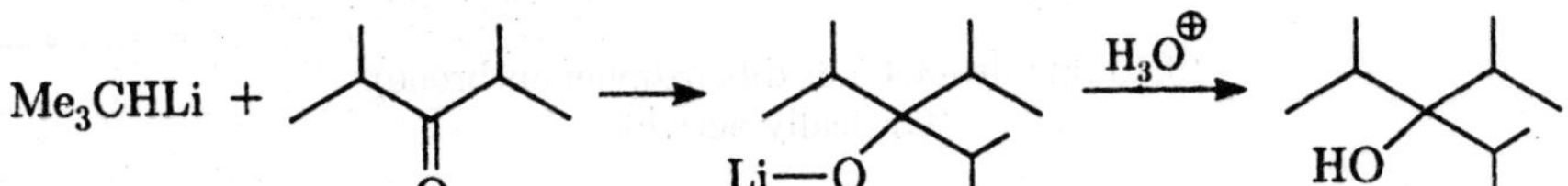

2. Whereas Grignard reagents often react with α,β-unsaturated ketones predominantly by 1,4–addition, lithium compounds react predominantly by 1,2-addition.

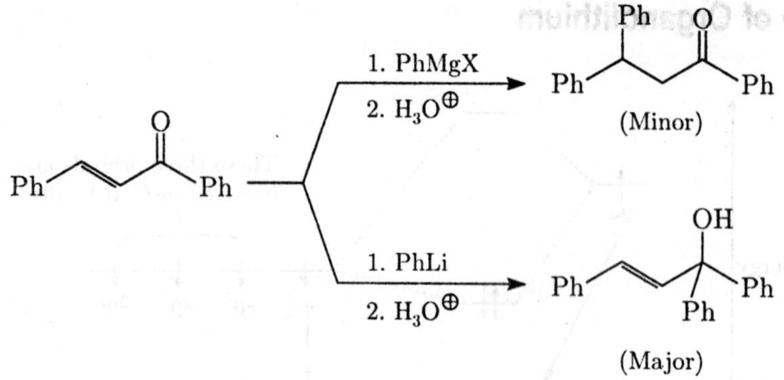

3. Organolithium compounds react more efficiently with alkyl halides and Wurtz coupling reactions can be carried out in good yield.

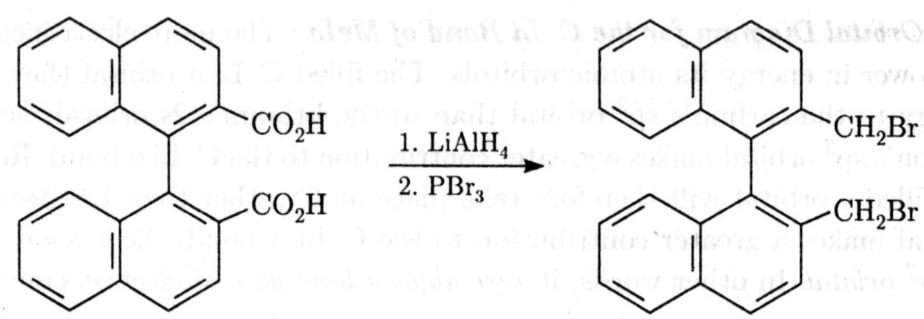

(1,1′-binaphthyl –2,2′-dicarboxylic acid)
(Optically active)

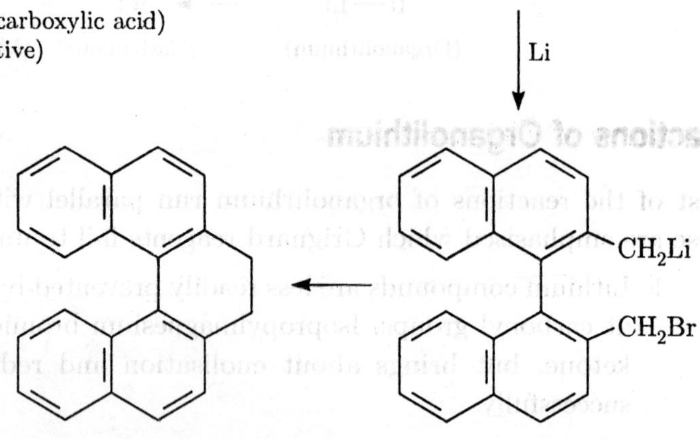

(9,10-dihydro-3,4,5,6 -dibenzophenanthrene)
(Optically active)

The product is optically active. Repulsion between the perihydrogen atoms forces the lower left-hand Benzenoid ring to lie somewhat above or below the upper left-hand ring, giving the two enantiomers. The molecule thus, has a spiral shape.

4. Carbon dioxide (CO_2), which reacts with, Grignard reagent to give carboxylic acids, react with organolithium compounds to give *ketones.*

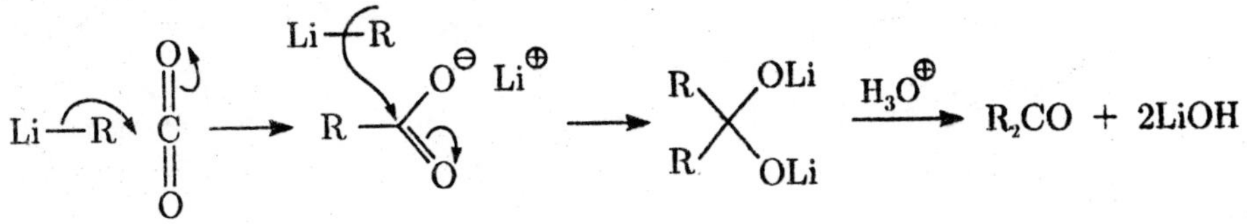

The lithium compounds being more strongly nucleophilic than Grignard reagent are able to react with the intermediate resonance stabilised carboxylate anion.

5. Carboxylic acids may be converted into ketones.

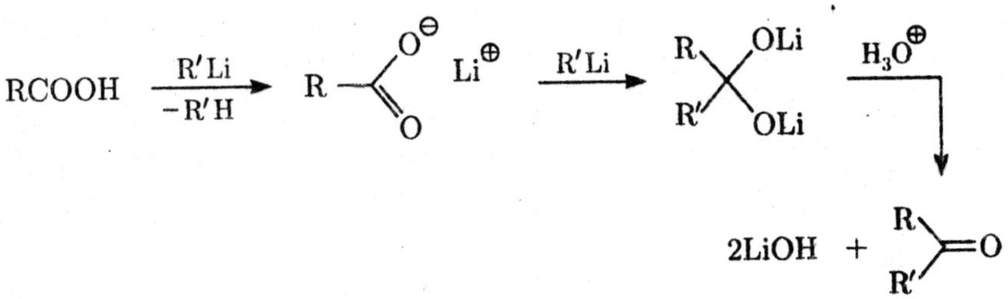

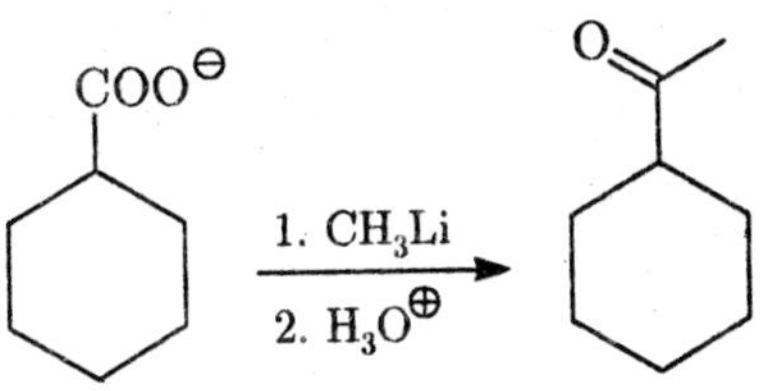

6. Organolithium compounds unlike Grignard reagent, react with C=C bonds. Primary alkyllithiums and simple alkenes such as ethylene react only at high pressures (100–500 atom) and give mixtures of compounds of different chain length.

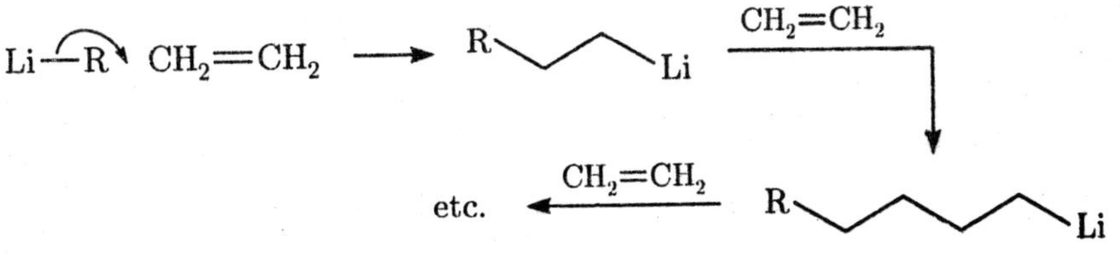

But secondary and tertiary alkyllithiums react efficiently with ethylene at low temperatures to give monomeric products.

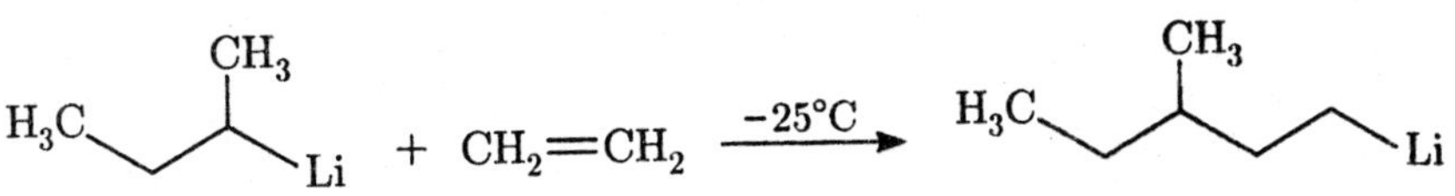

Conjugated alkenes react with primary alkyllithiums under mild conditions to give monomeric products.

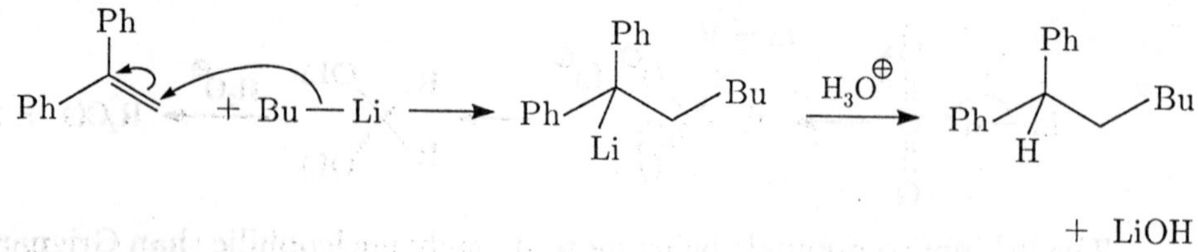

7. Unlike Grignard reagents, lithium compounds are sufficiently nucleophilic to react at the nuclear carbon atoms of aromatic systems which are activated to nucleophiles.

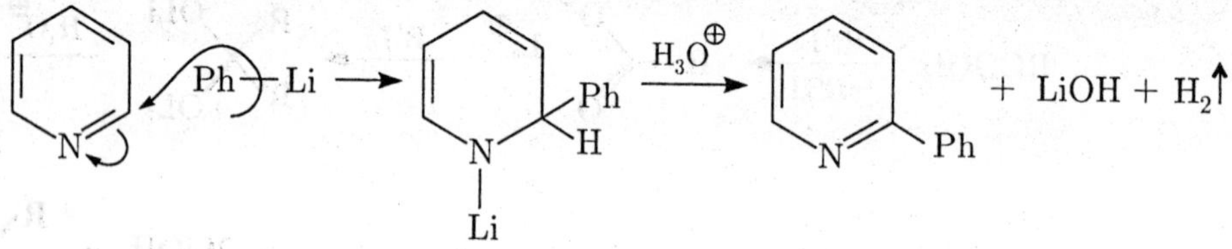

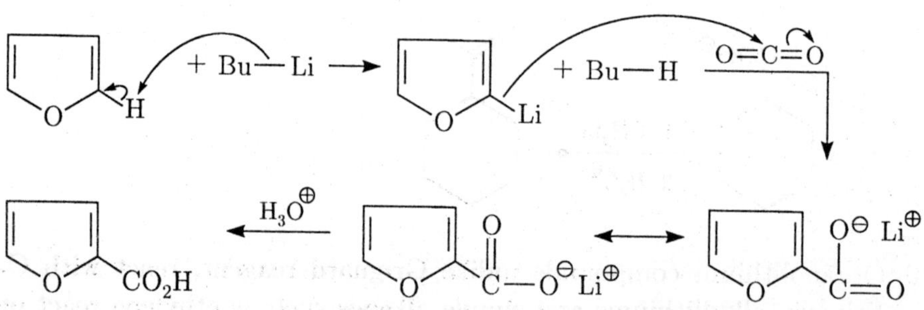

8. Unlike Grignard reagent, butyllithium (organolithium) attacks ether via metallation reaction.

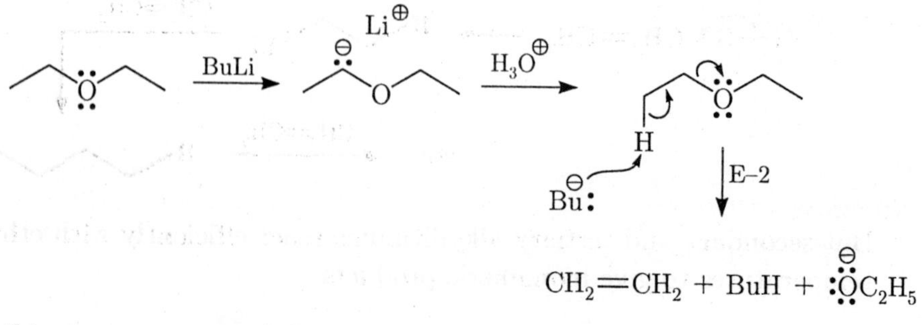

For this reasons, organolithiums are *not stored* in ether but used immediately after preparation. Organolithiums are much more stable in hydrocarbon solvents.

Organocopper Compounds

Preparation of Organocopper Compounds : Two types of copper (I) compounds are of value in synthesis, organocopper compounds, RCu and lithium organocuprates, R_2CuLi, where R is alkyl (1°, 2° or 3°), alkenyl or aryl. The compounds of the type R_2CuLi (lithium organocuprates) are also known as **Gilman cuprates.**

$$RLi + CuI \xrightarrow{Et_2O/\text{Inert atmosphere } (N_2)} RCu + LiI$$

$$2RLi + CuI \xrightarrow{Et_2O/\text{Inert atmosphere } (N_2)} \underset{\text{(Gilman cuprate)}}{R_2CuLi} + LiI$$

Acetylene reacts with organocopper compound or an organocuprate with *100% syn stereoselectivity.*

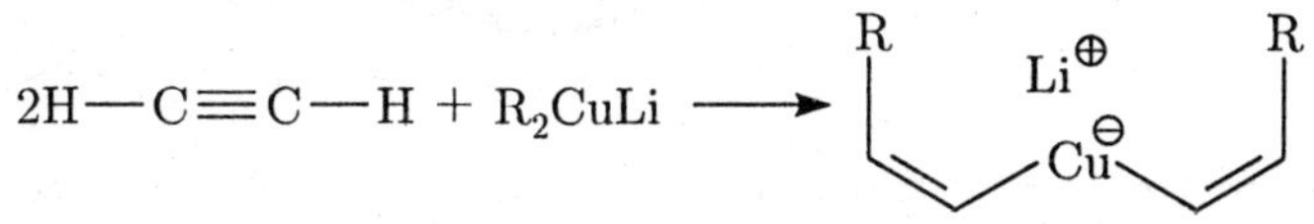

Mechanism :

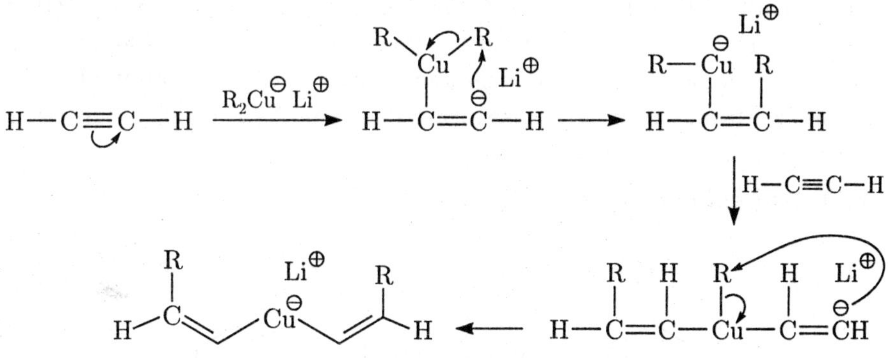

Alkynes of the type RC≡CH reacts with complex of RCu and $MgBr_2$ (but not with R_2CuLi) with both regioselectivity (copper atom attached to less substituted carbon atom) and *syn* stereoselectivity.

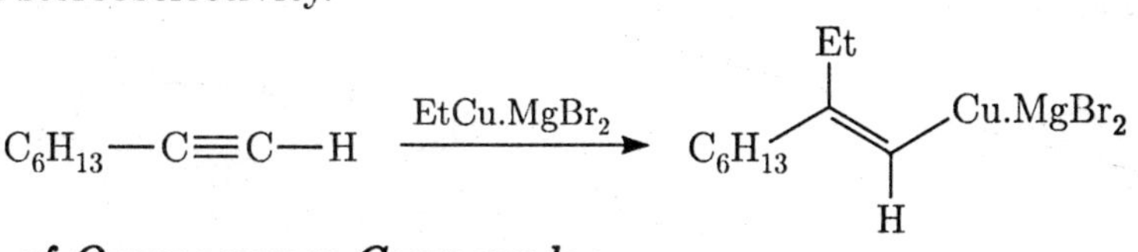

Reactions of Organocopper Compounds :

1. ***With α, β-Unsaturated carbonyl compounds*** : The reaction takes place in 1,4-or conjugate manner.

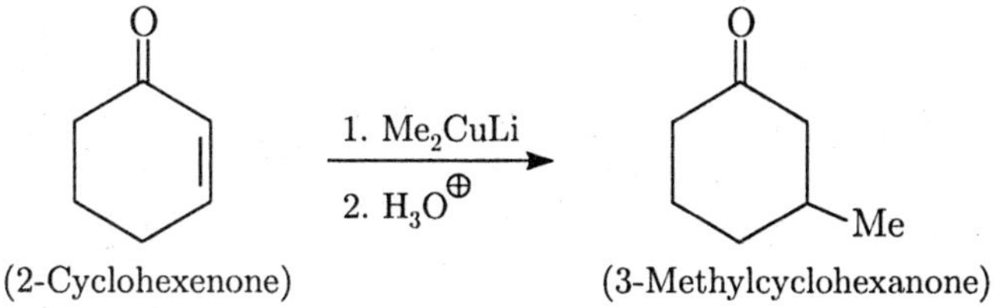

(2-Cyclohexenone) (3-Methylcyclohexanone)

But the mechanism of the reaction is totally different from that shown by Grignard reagents. Organolithiums give only 1,2-adduct.

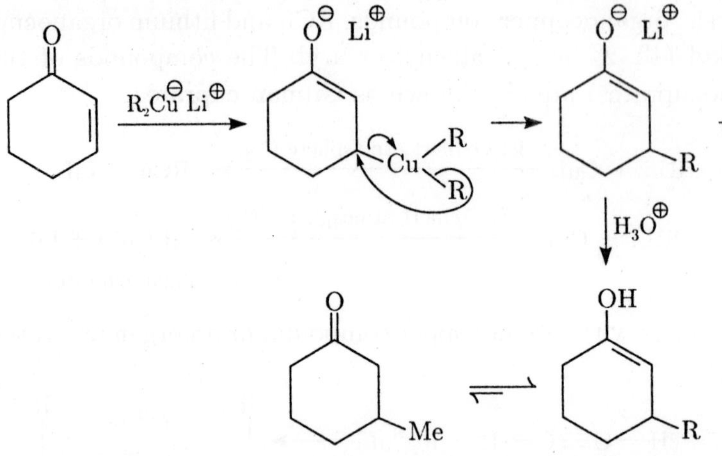

Organocuprates react more rapidly and usually give better yields than organocopper. One of the R groups in R_2CuLi is wasted as R—H which becomes indispensible if R is difficult to synthesise or expensive to be obtained. So mixed organocuprate is employed. One of the R groups is *1-pentynyl* which may be used as a member of mixed organocuprates. Generally alkynyl group is not transferred from Cu to α, β–unsaturated system. As a result, 1-pentyne is wasted as a byproduct.

2. ***With Acid halides to form ketones*** :

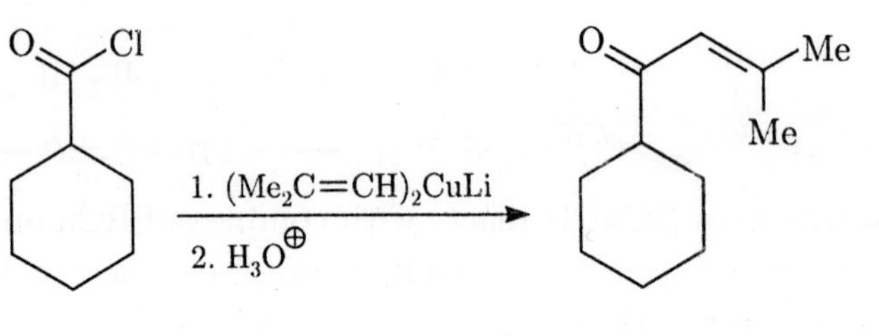

Mechanism :

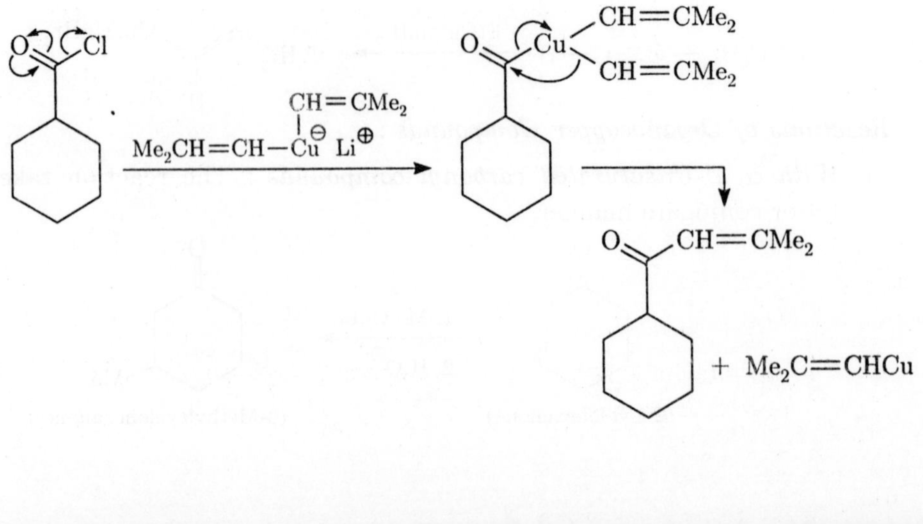

3. ***With Epoxides to form Alcohols*** : S_N2 mode with inversion of configuration and the *less substituted carbon* atom of epoxide is attached.

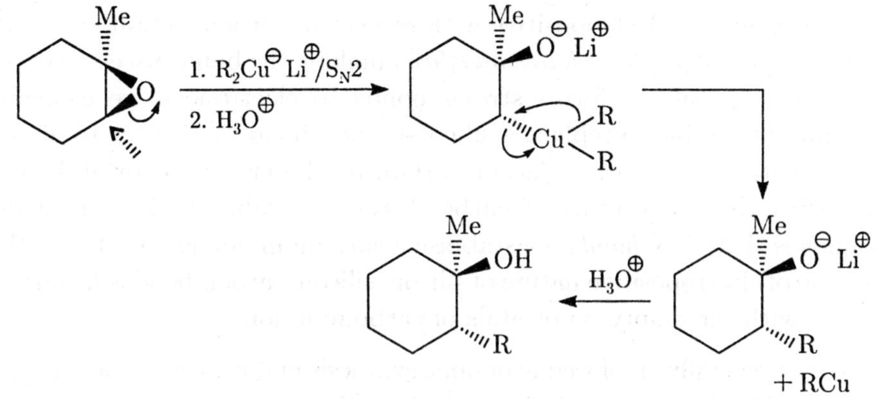

4. ***With Halides*** : Organocuprates react with alkyl (1° or 2°) alkynyl and aryl bromides and iodides but not chlorides.

(a)

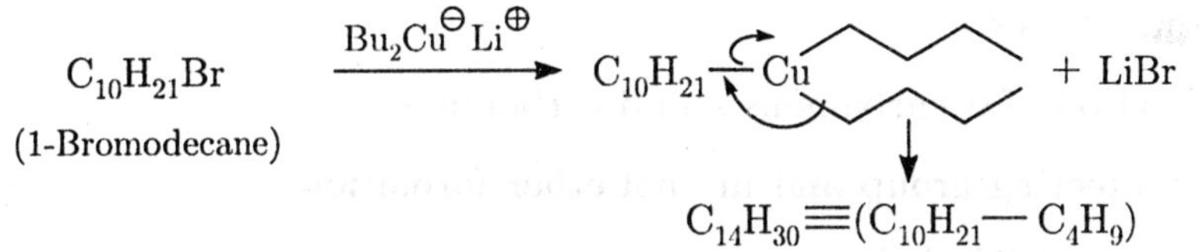

(b)

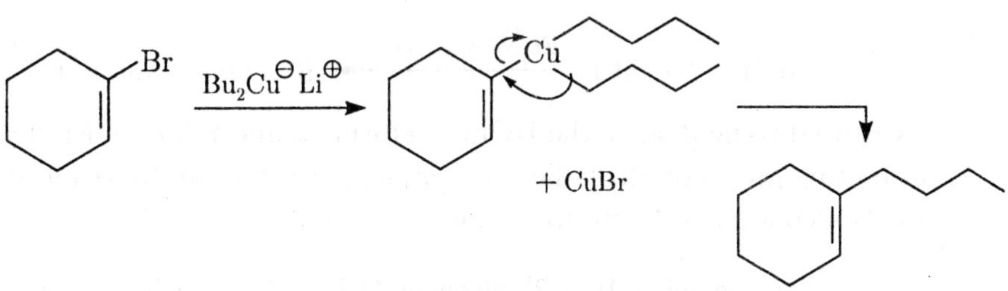

(c)

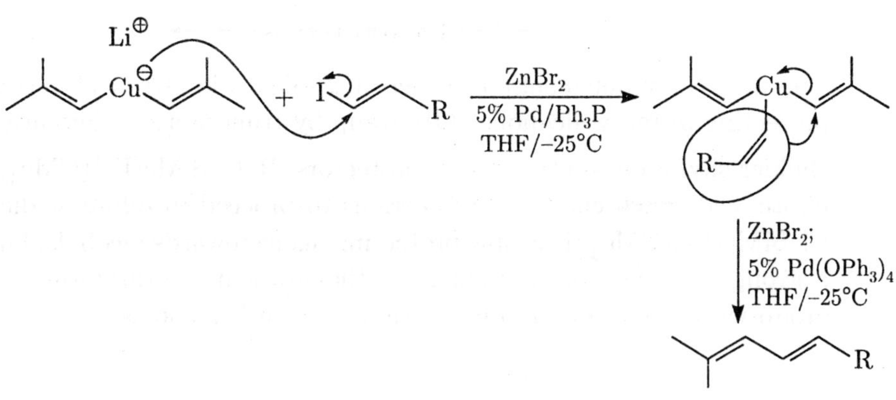

(E)–Isomer (99.5%)

Mechanism shown in (c) is unclear. Reaction pathway does not suggest a pure S_N2 process.

Organosilicon Compounds

Silicon is an inorganic element whose derivatives are of value in organic synthesis apart from boron. Silicon is electropositive with respect to carbon so that silicon-carbon bond is polarised with the *positive charge on silicon* making the bond susceptible to nucleophilic attack at silicon. Silicon forms strong bonds to electronegative elements and it is energetically profitable to replace a silicon-carbon bond to Si–O or to Si–F. Silicon can stabilise negative charge on adjacent carbon as the empty 3d orbitals of silicon may interact with the 2p orbitals of carbon. Another valuable feature of organosilicon compounds is that C–Si *bond* may stabilise a carbonium ion adjacent to carbon (*i.e*, β to Si), because of electropositive nature of silicon, silicon–carbon bond is favourably polarised to interact with the empty 2p orbitals of carbonium ion.

Silicon is generally employed in organic synthesis in the form of a trialkylsilyl functional group (often Me_3Si) and in this form, it plays *three* main roles.

1. As a protecting group and in reactive intermediate such as silyl enol ethers.
2. To form alkenes.
3. Stabilisation of α-carbanions and β-carbonium ions.

1. As a protecting group and in enol ether formation :

(a) ***Protection of Alcohols***

$$ROH + Me_3SiCl \xrightarrow{Et_3\ddot{N}\text{(weak base)}} R—O—SiMe_3 + Et_3\overset{\oplus}{N}H\overset{\ominus}{Cl}$$

Et_3N is used to neutralise the HCl thus formed, and trimethylsilyl group acts as a protecting group of alcoholic functionality. Protection by trimethylsilyl group towards alcoholic –OH groups follows the trend :

$$1°\text{–alcoholic OH} > 2°\text{–alcoholic OH} > 3°\text{–alcoholic OH group}$$

$$\xrightarrow{\text{Reactivity Decreases}}$$

One may carry out reactions either at 2°-alcoholic OH or 3°–alcoholic OH by protecting primary alcoholic –OH group by trimethylsilyl derivative.

Bulkier silyl groups are stronger protectors. R–O–SiMe(Et)(CMe_3) is stable in dilute acid which enables the reactions to proceed in dilute acidic conditions. Cl–SiMe(Et)(CMe_3) is a slow protecting agent towards alcohols, but imidazole, a stronger nucleophile (particularly in the protonated form) forms a good leaving group with the former and now reactive towards alcohols.

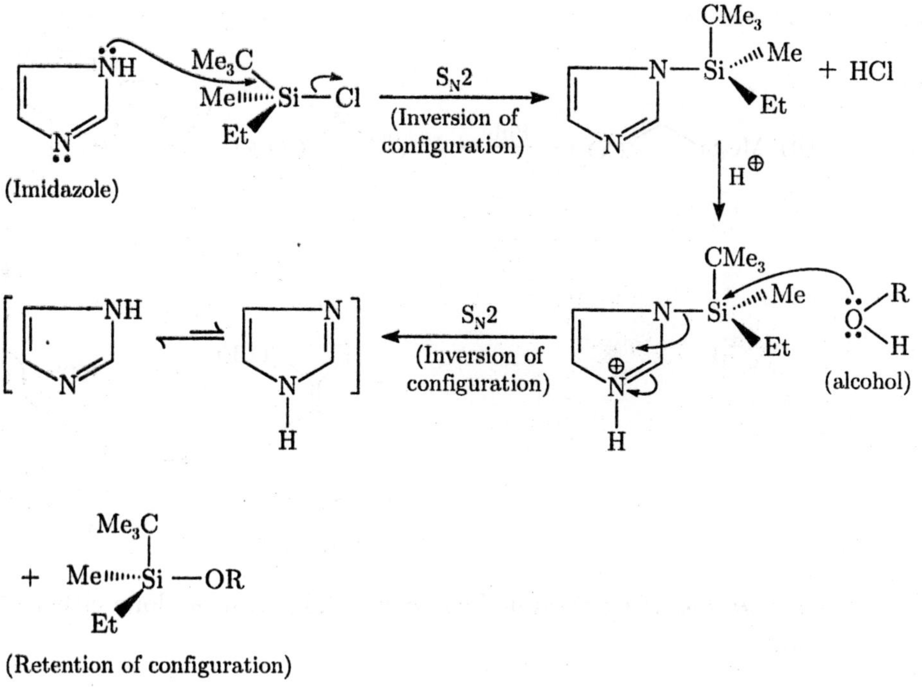

2. Synthesis of Alkenes :

(a) This reaction closely resembles Wittig reaction for the synthesis of alkenes.

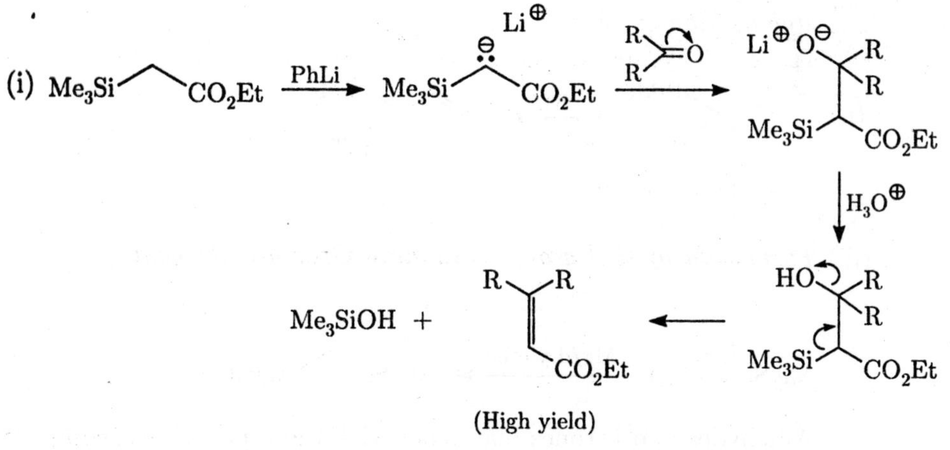

(ii) 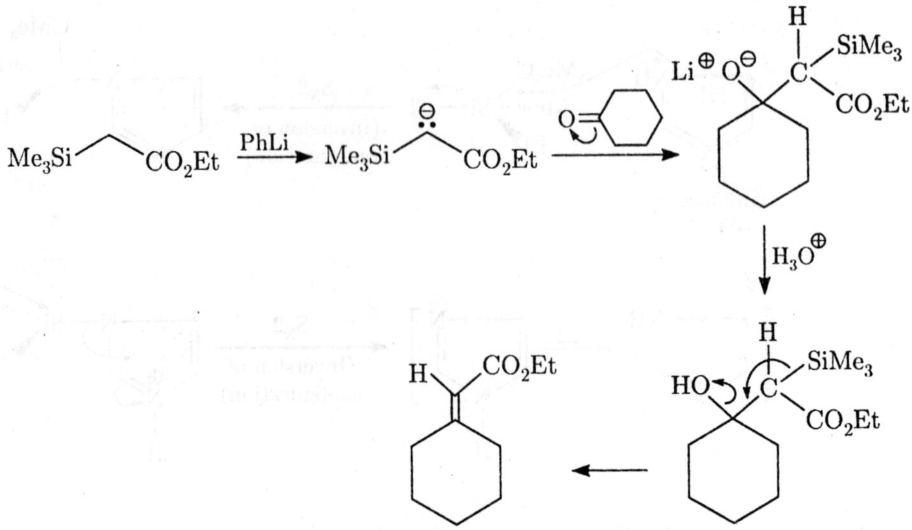

(Product)

(b) ***Formation of Carbanion Equivalent*** : This can be done either of the following ways.

(i) 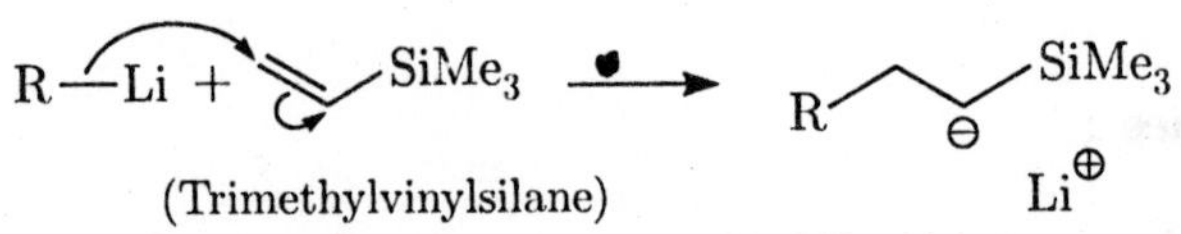

(Trimethylvinylsilane)

The regioselectivity (addition of R) of the reaction is due to *α-carbanion stabilisation* by Si.

(ii) 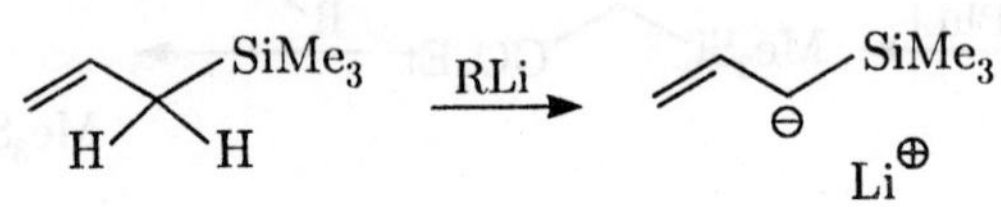

(Trimethylallylsilane)

(iii) ***Formation of silyl group containing Grignard Reagent*** :

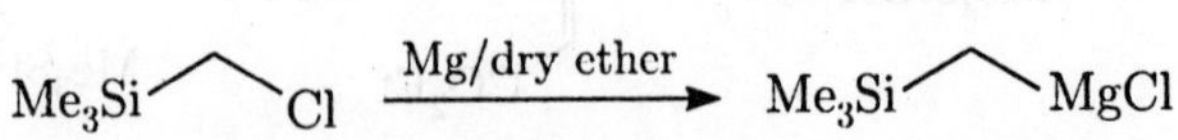

Aldehydes and ketones may react with the types of silyl compounds shown above and depending on the base employed (usually NaH or KH in Et_2O) or acid ($BF_3.Et_2O$), *syn (with base)* or *anti (with acid) elimination* is favoured.

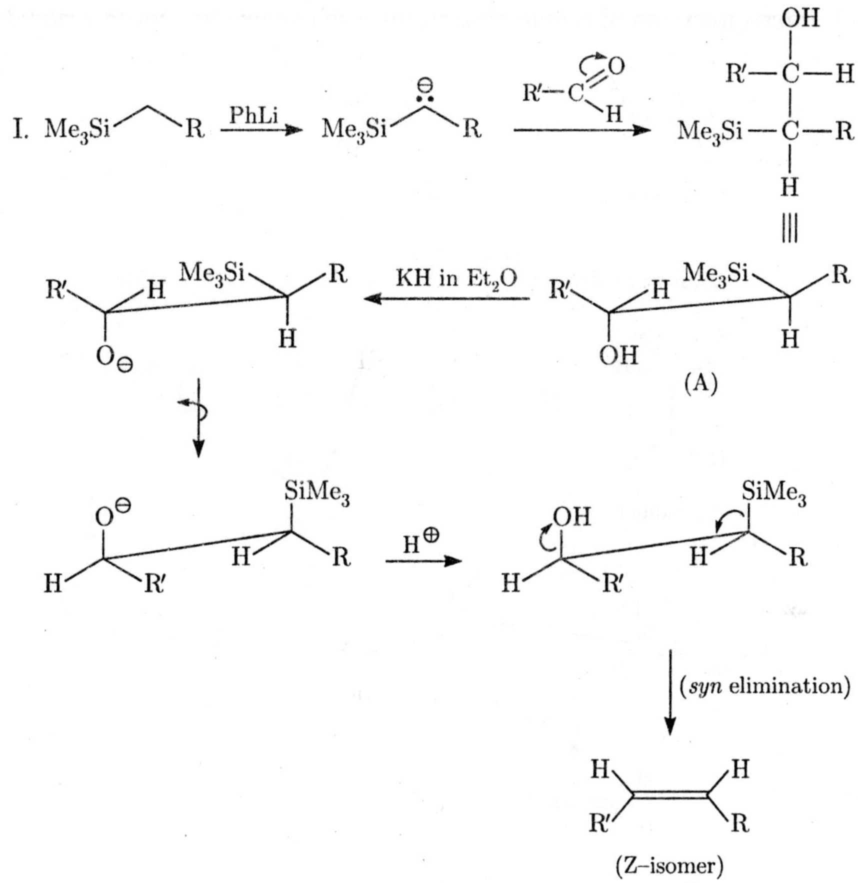

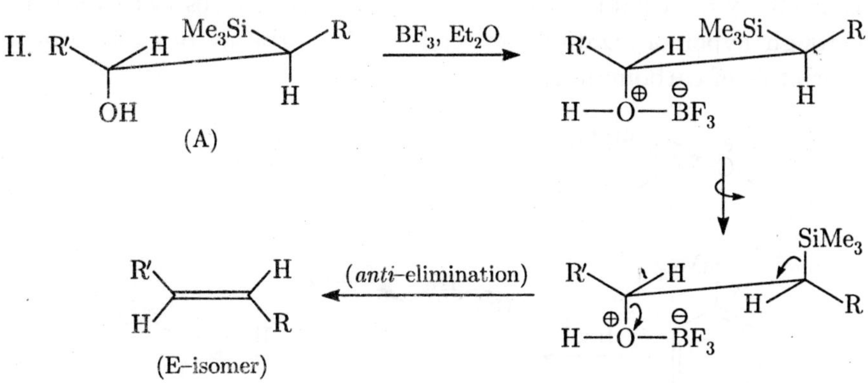

(iv) ***Interconversion** of **geometrical isomers of alkenes by trimethylsilyl derivatives.***

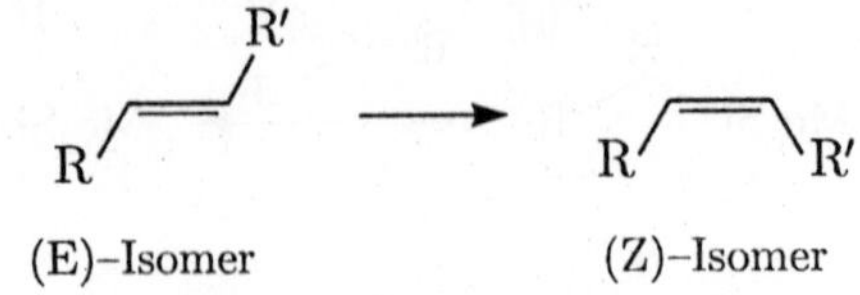

$$Me_3Si{-}SiMe_3 \xrightarrow{NaOMe} SiMe_3^{\ominus}\,Na^{\oplus} + Me_3Si^{\oplus}\,\overset{\ominus}{O}Me$$

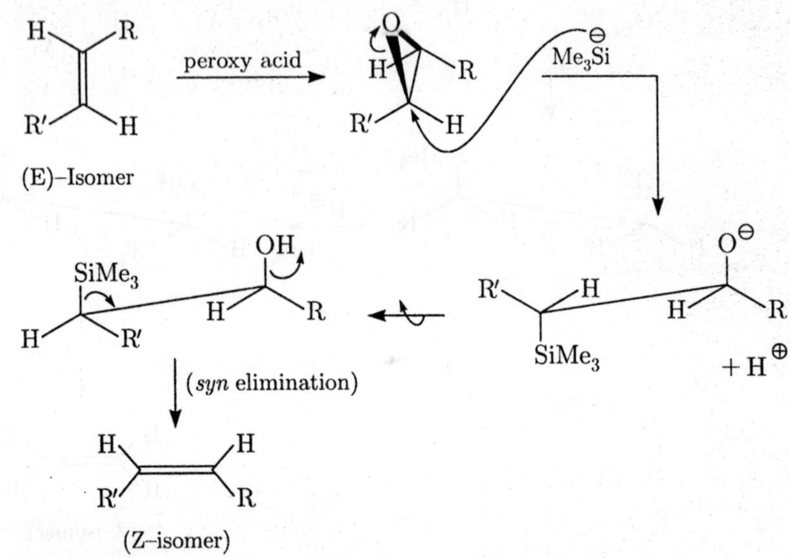

3. Directive Influence of $-SiR_3$ in Electrophilic Reactions :

A trialkylsilyl group stabilises a *β-carbonium ion.* Carbon-silicon bond is positively polarised towards silicon and negative charge resides on carbon α to silicon. Expectedly α-carbanion and β-carbonium ion (with respect to Si) are stabilised through hyperconjugation between filled p orbitals of carbanion and empty p orbitals of carbonium ion.

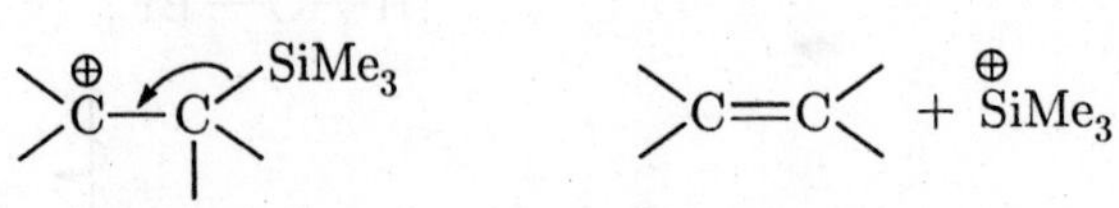

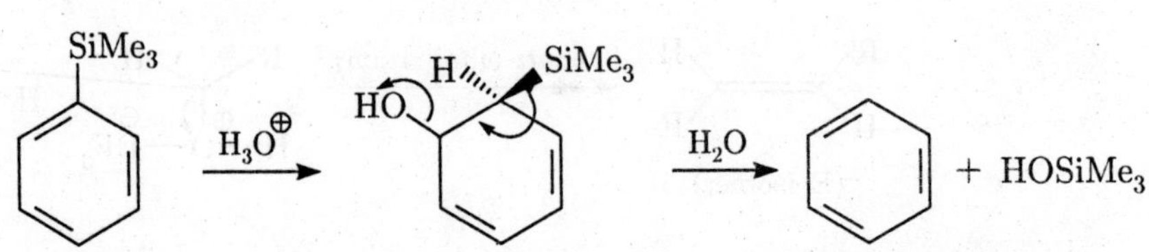

This reaction proceeds **10^3 times** faster that proton (H^+) displaced from benzene.

(a) ***Ipso-substitution in arylsilanes*** :

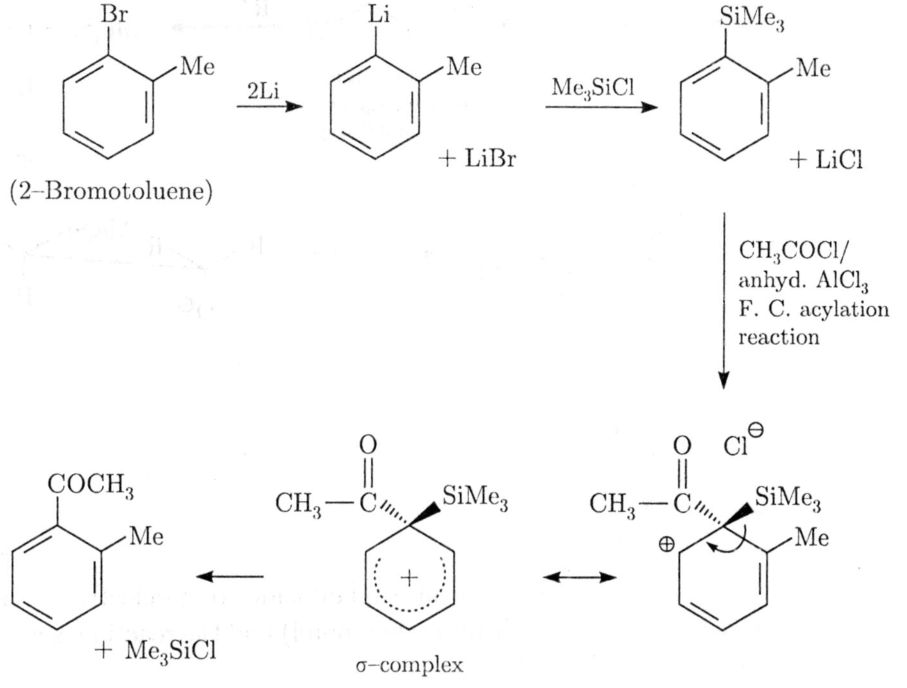

A carbonium ion, β with respect to silicon is stabilised.

(b)

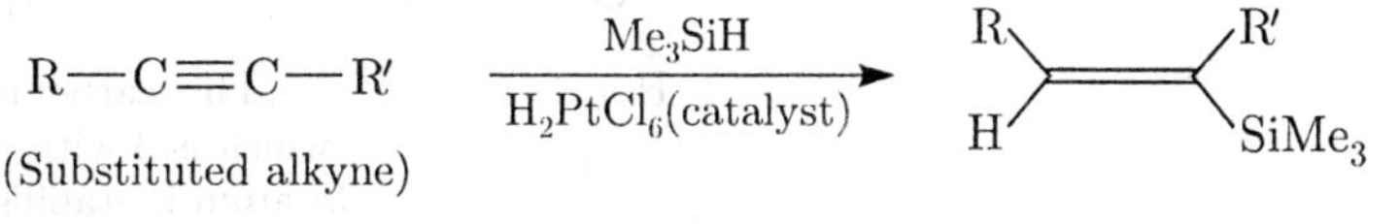

(c)

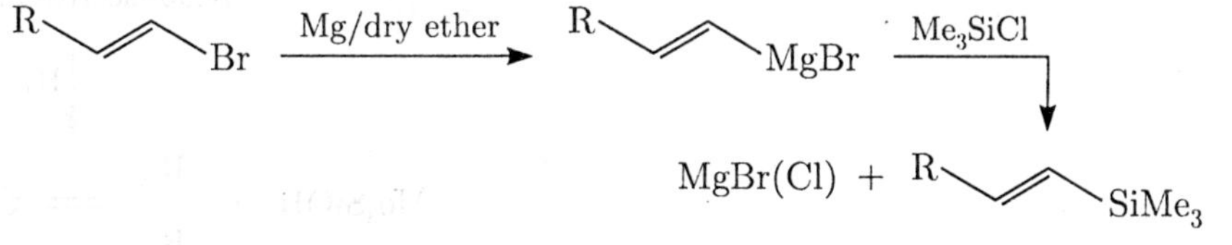

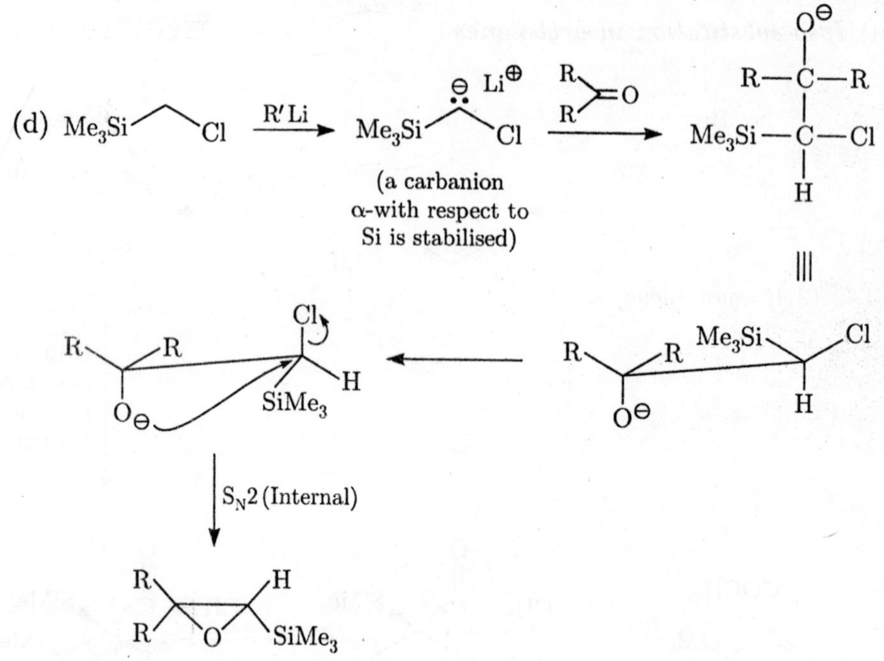

Ketones may be formed from silyl epoxides regioselectively (stabilisation of β-carbonium ion by silicon-carbon bond) and the reaction is an acid catalysed one.

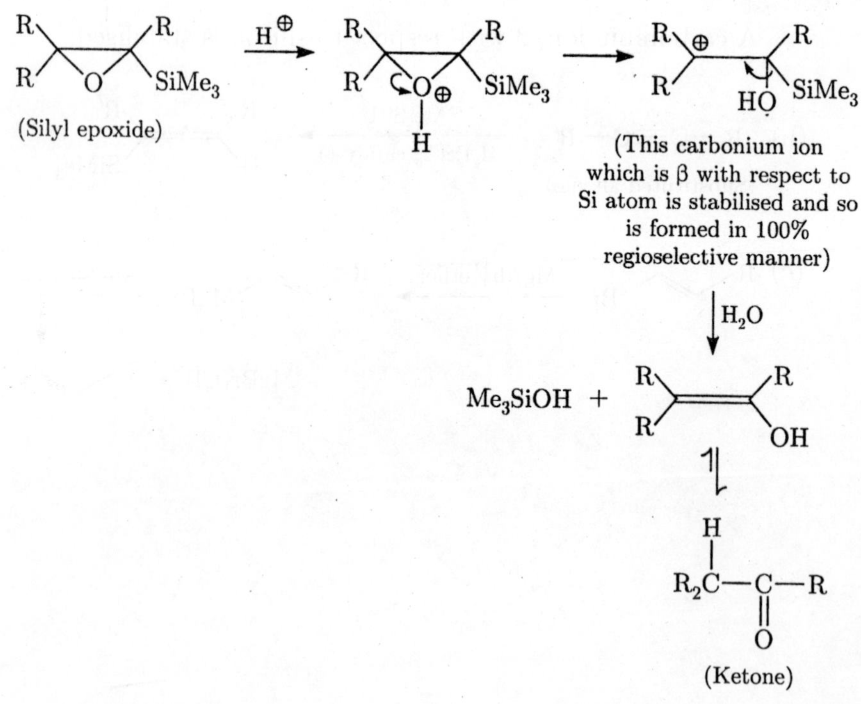

(e) 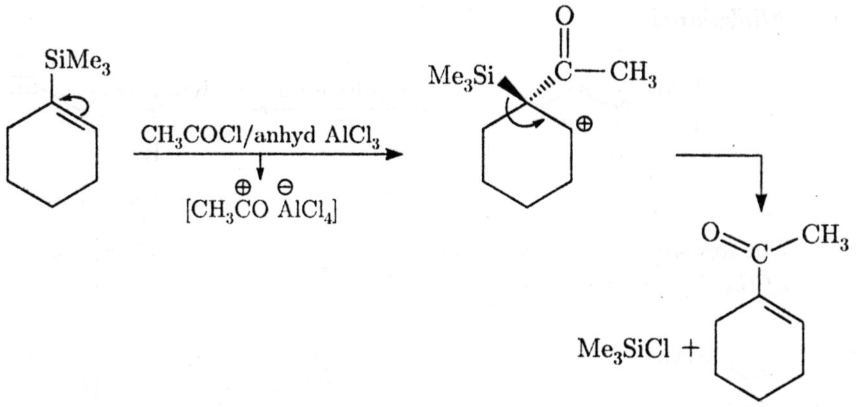

(f) 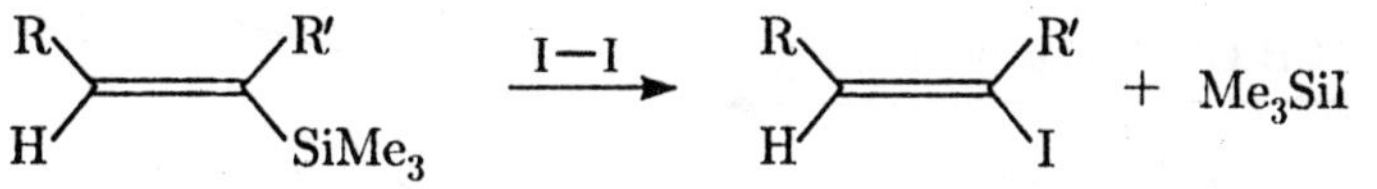

The carbocation formed with an electrophile ($E^{\oplus}$) undergoes rotation about new C—C bond which results in the stabilising interaction between unoccupied 2p orbital and C—Si bonding orbital.

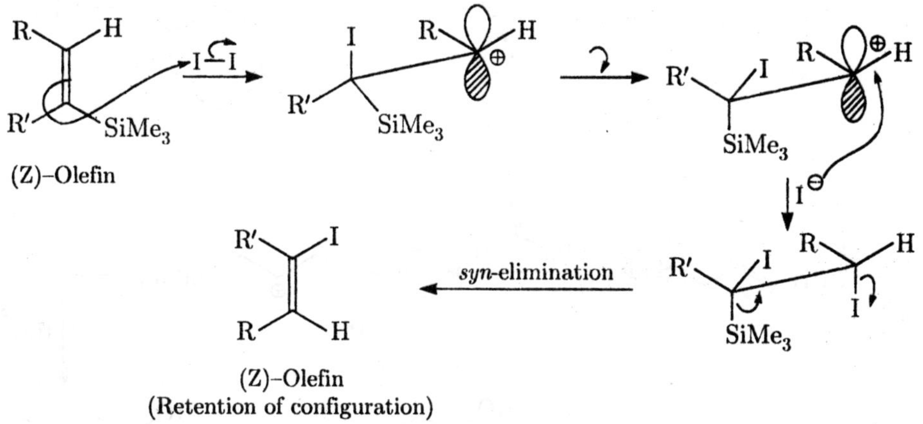

Sometimes *inversion of configuration* is also observed.

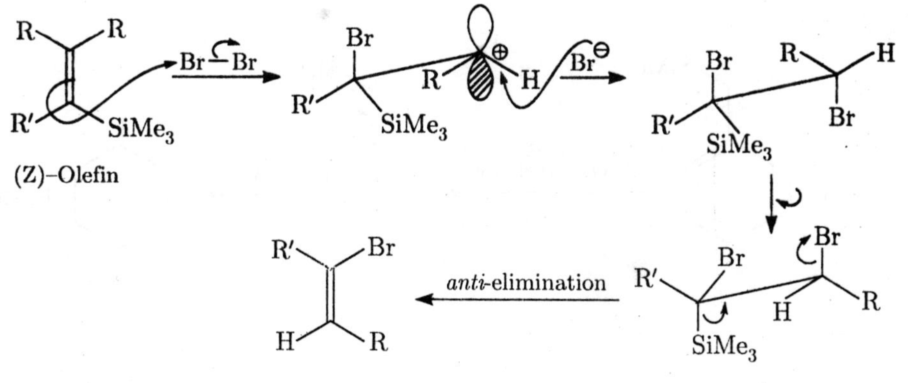

(g) ***Allylsilanes***

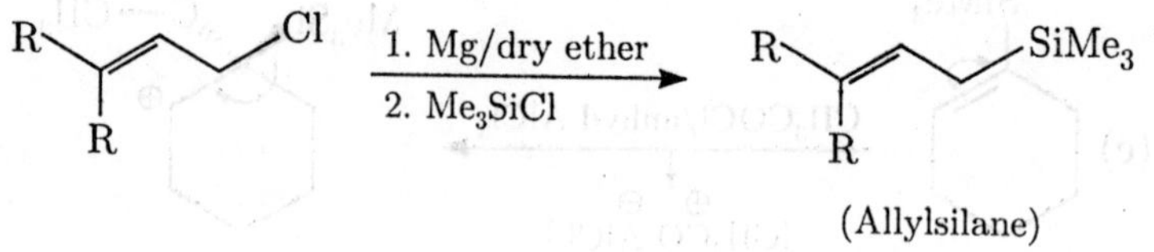

The driving force of the following reactions using allylsilanes is the *stabilisation of the β-carbonium ion by C—Si bond.*

(i)

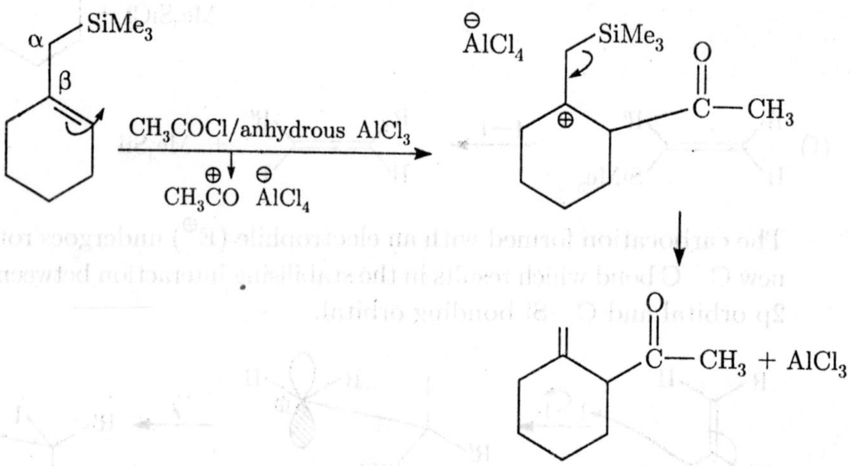

(ii)

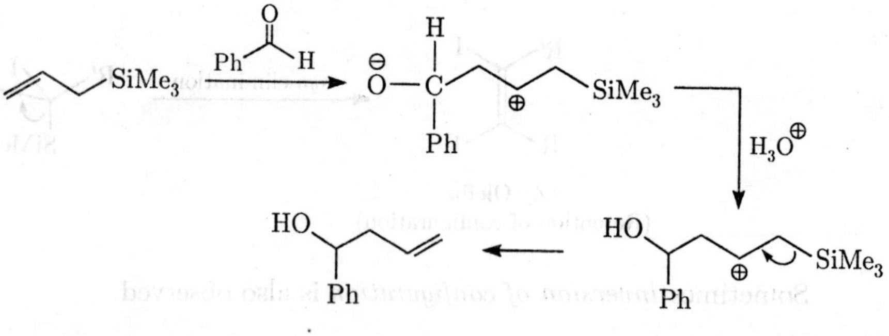

(iii)

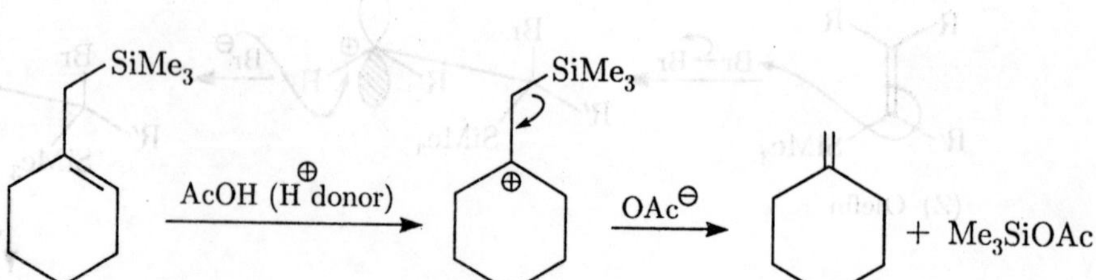

Uses of Some Organometallics

A. Butyllithium

Preparation of Butyllithium : $BuCl + 2Li \xrightarrow[-10°C]{N_2/hexane} Buli + LiCl$. Low temperature condition is necessary to avoid Wurtz coupling as a side reaction ($BuLi + BuCl \rightarrow Bu\text{-}Bu + LiCl$)

Uses :

1. Butyllithium is used to prepare other organolithium compounds where a metal-exchange reaction takes place.

$$\underset{(R=\text{vinyl or aryl})}{R—O} + BuLi \longrightarrow \underset{(R=\text{vinyl or aryl})}{RLi} + BuBr$$

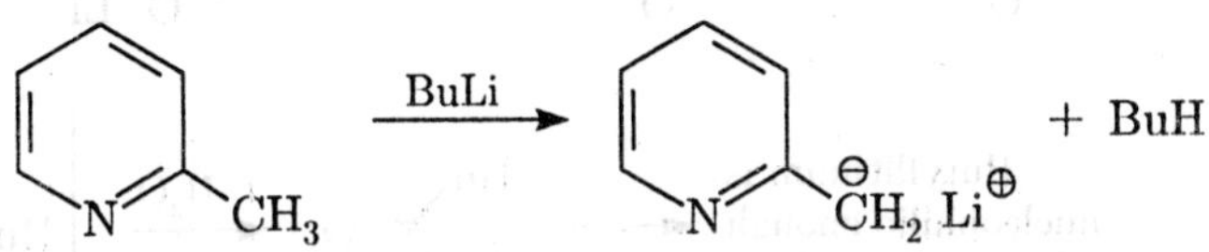

2. Unlike Grignard reagent, butyllithium attacks ethers *via* metallation reaction.

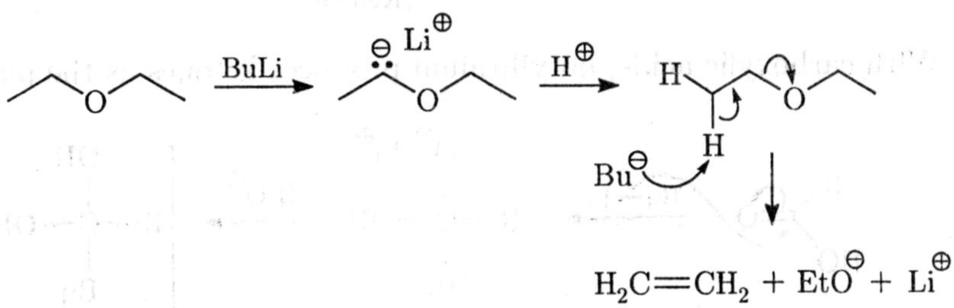

3. Butyllithium is less prevented by steric hindrance from reacting at the carbonyl functionality where Grignard reagents are incapable.

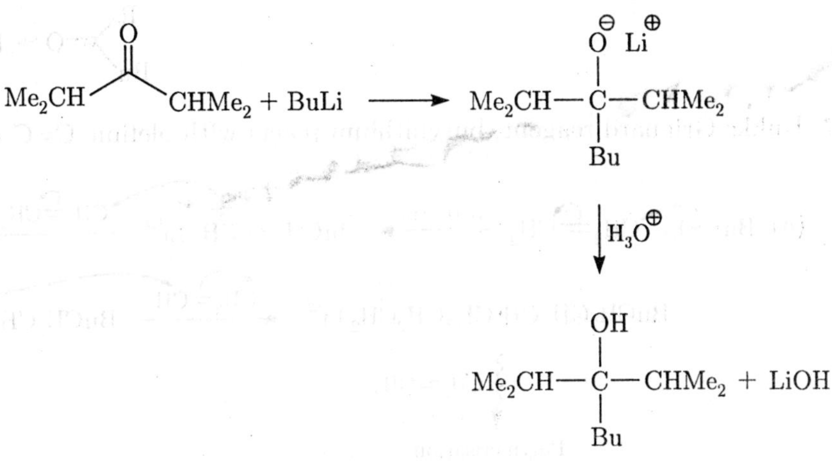

4. Butyllithium reacts with α, β-unsaturated ketones to give *1,2-adduct* where Grignard reagents predominantly produce *1,4-adduct.*

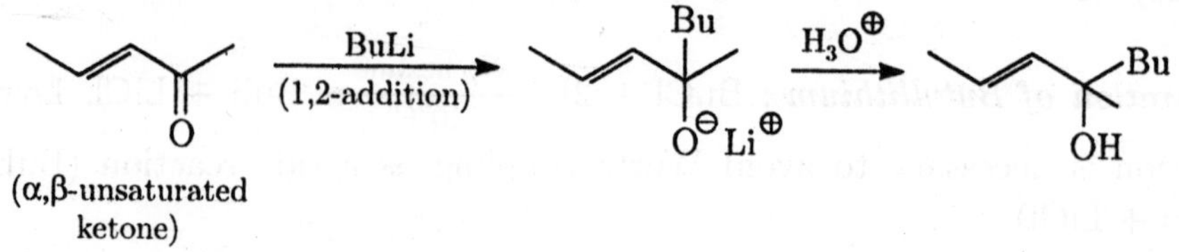

5. Unlike Grignard reagents, butyllithium reacts with CO_2 to form *ketones* where the former produces a carboxylic acid.

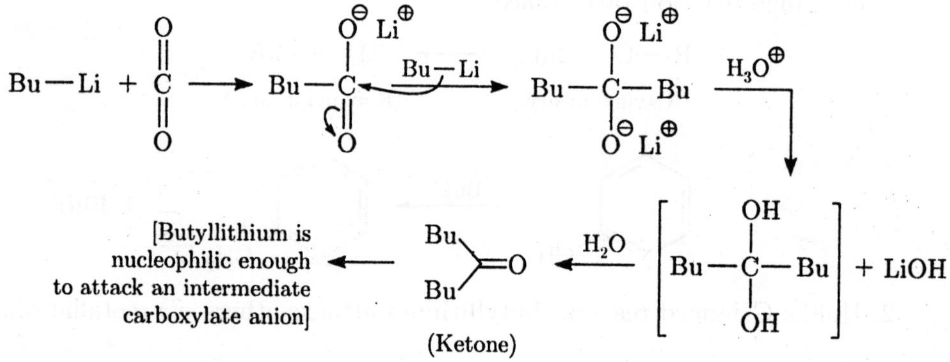

6. With carboxylic acids, butyllithium produces ketones as the major products.

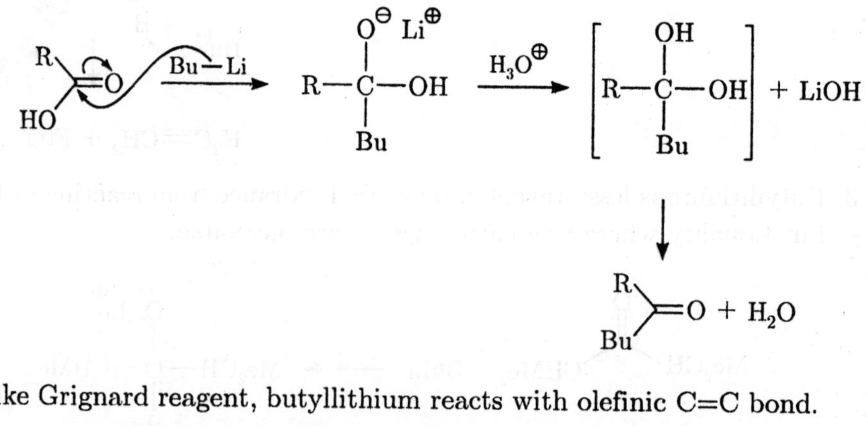

7. Unlike Grignard reagent, butyllithium reacts with olefinic C=C bond.

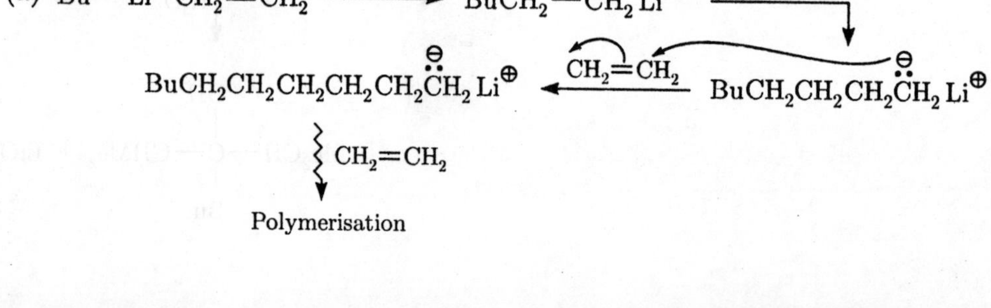

(b) 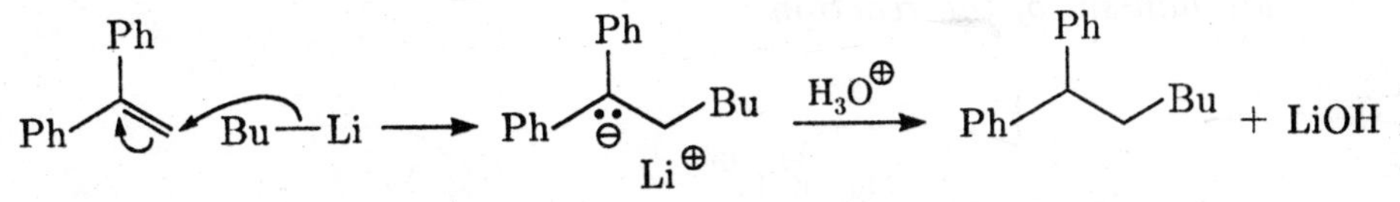

Steric bulk of the alkene permits only monomeric product.

8. BuLi is sufficiently nucleophilic to attack at the nuclear carbon of an aromatic system which is activated to be reacted by a nucleophile.

(a) 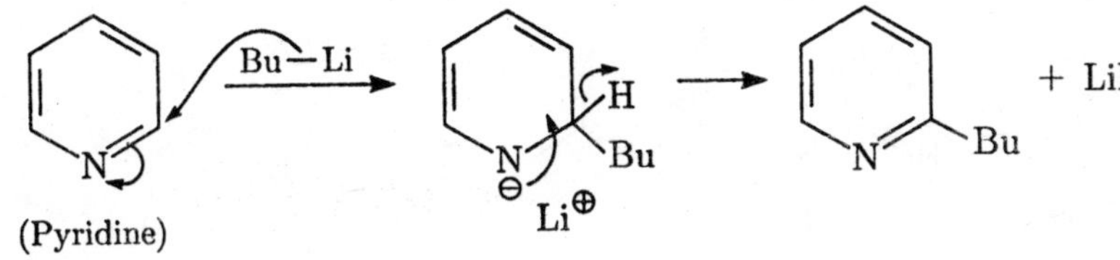

(Pyridine)

(b) 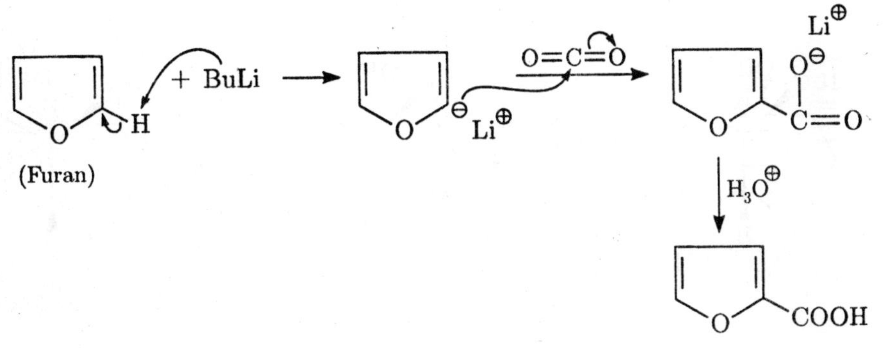

(Furan)

(Furan-2-carboxylic acid)

B. Lithium Dimethylcuprate (Gilman Cuprate)

Lithium dialkylcuprate is more stable and reactive than other organocopper (I) reagents like $RCu.MgBr_2$. It is prepared *in situ* and *not isolated*, most convenimently by the reaction of two equivalents of an organolithium compound with cuprous iodide in ether.

$$CH_3Li + CuI \xrightarrow{Et_2O} \underset{+\ LiI}{CH_3Cu} \xrightarrow{CH_3Li} (CH_3)_2CuLi$$

In ethereal solution, Me_2CuLi exists as a dimer like $[LiCuMe_2]_2$

Uses of Lithium Dimethylcuprate :

1. Acetylene reacts with Me_2CuLi with 100% syn stereoselectivity.

$$2H{-}C{\equiv}C{-}H + Me_2CuLi \longrightarrow$$ 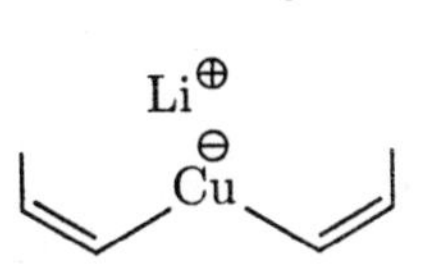

Mechanism of the reaction :

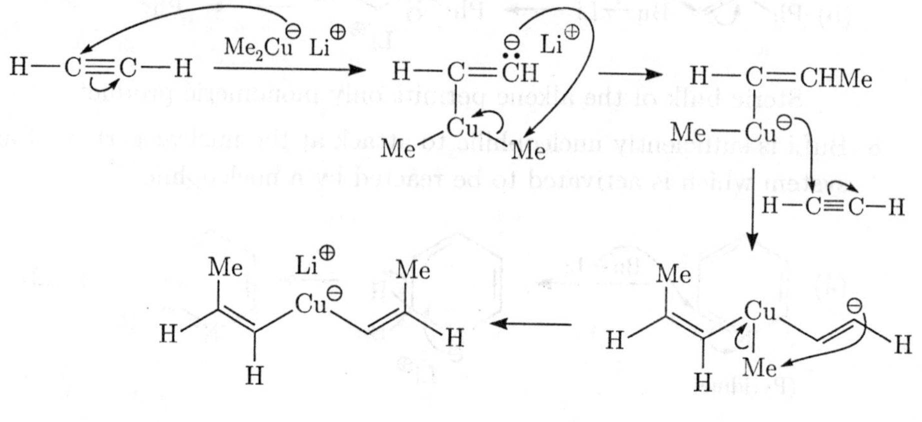

2.

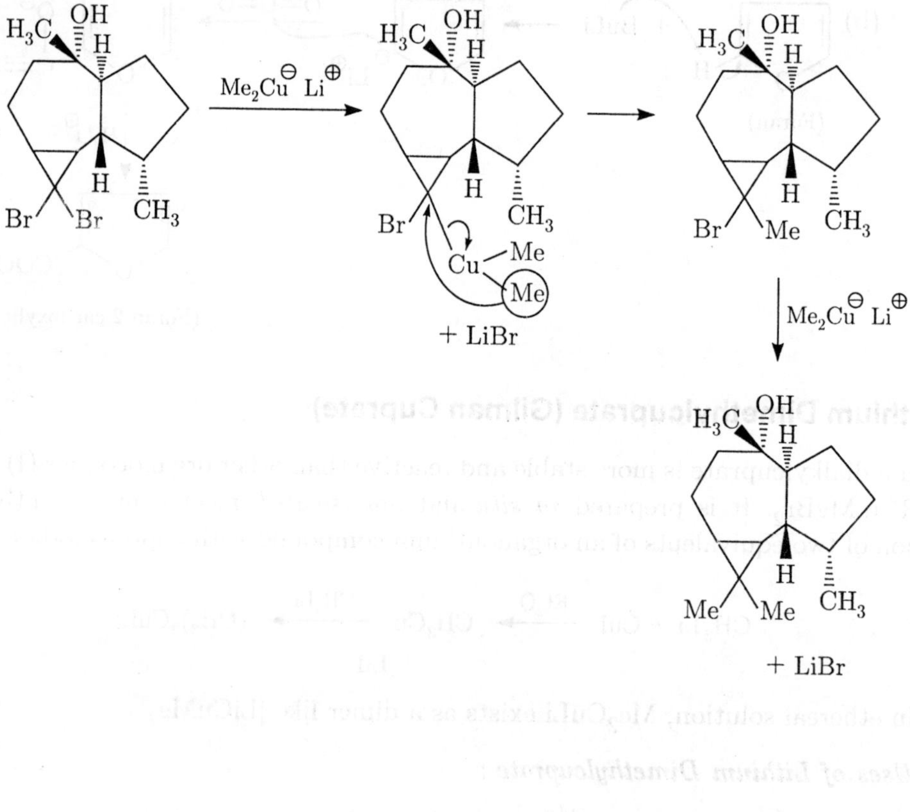

3. With α, β-unsaturated carbonyl compounds, Me_2CuLi reacts in *1,4-manner.*

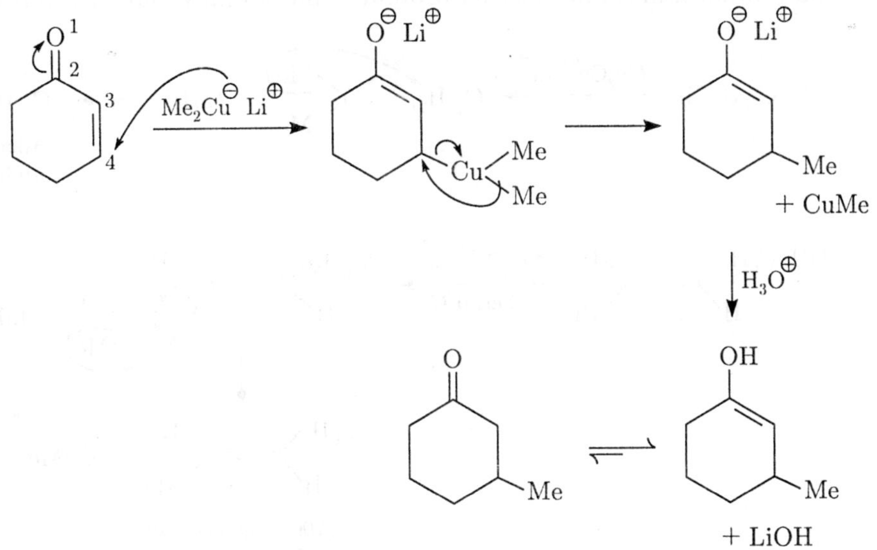

The reaction is rapid and of higher yield than any other organocopper reagents.

4. Formation of *ketones* is possible when dimethyllithium cuprate reacts with acid chlorides.

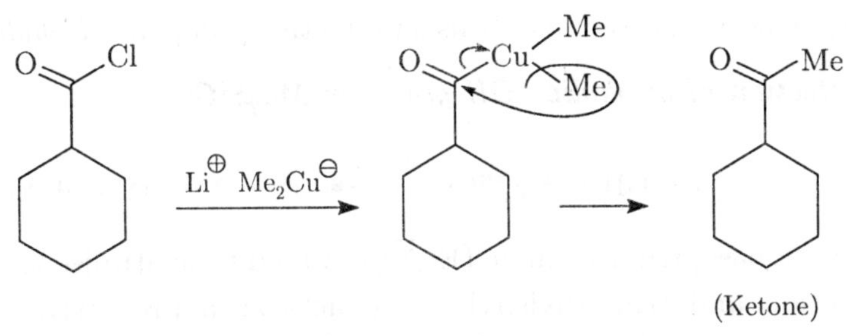

5. Lithium dimethylcuprate reacts with epoxides to form alcohols.

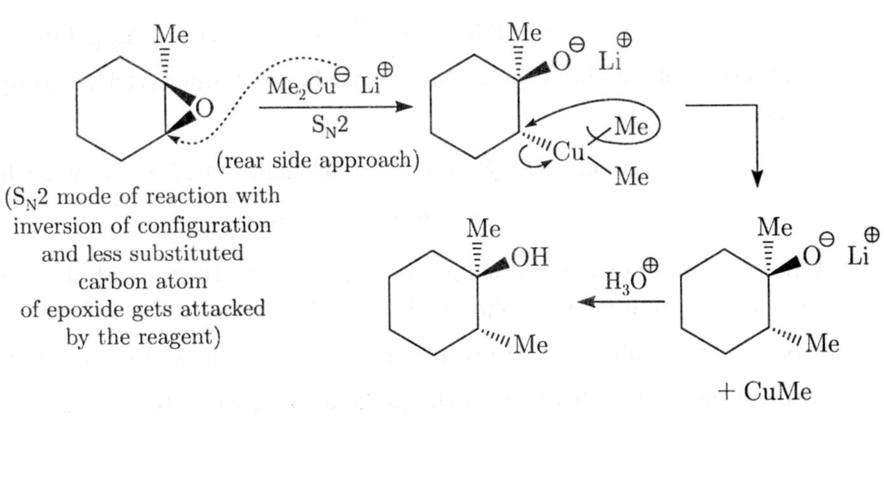

6. Lithium dimethylcuprate reacts with primary and secondary alkyl bromides and iodides; aryl and alkynyl bromides and iodides, but *not chlorides.*

(a) 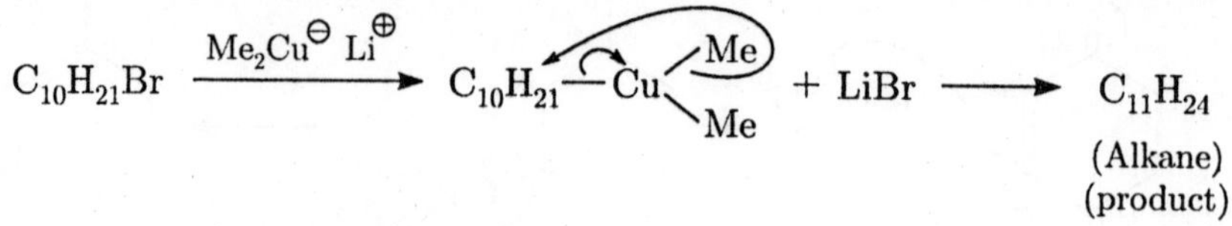

(b) 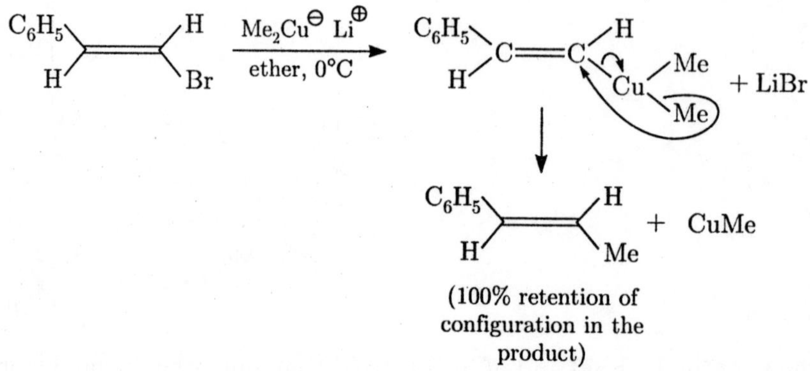

C. Trimethylsilyl Chloride (TMS–Cl)

Trimethylsilyl chloride is used mainly as a protecting group for *alcoholic–OH* functionality.

1. ***Protection of alcoholic –OH group by Me_3SiCl***

$$R—OH + Me_3SiCl \xrightarrow{Et_3N} R—O—SiMe_3 + Et_3\overset{\oplus}{N}H\ \overset{\ominus}{Cl}$$

A weak base, triethylamine ($Et_3\ddot{N}$) is added to neutralise the HCl formed in the reaction and trimethylsilyl group acts as a protective block for alcoholic functionality. Trimethylsilyl group is deprotected by adding dilute acid (dil HCl for example).

$$R—O—SiMe_3 \xrightarrow{\text{dil HCl}} R—OH + Me_3SiOH$$

Protection of alcoholic –OH functionality by trimethylsilyl group follows the trend :

Primary alcoholic –OH ≫ Secondary alcoholic –OH > Tertiary alcoholic –OH

—— Reactivity decreases ⟶

One may carry out reactions at secondary or tertiary alcoholic –OH groups by protecting primary alcoholic –OH group by trimethylsilyl chloride.

Apart from alcoholic –OH group, amino and terminal alkyne functionalities are also protected by Me_3SiCl, in the presence of a weak base ($Et_3\ddot{N}$ or pyridine), or from a metallic derivative of alkynes. Protected alkynes are used to prepare polyalkynes and the silyl group can be easily deprotected by employing methanol or aqueous sodium hydroxide. *Large trimethylsilyl group musks* the *neighbouring triple bond* and so selective hydrogenation of any other triple bond present in the molecule possible.

$$BrMgC{\equiv}C{-}C{\equiv}C{-}H \xrightarrow{Me_3SiCl} Me_3SiC{\equiv}C{-}C{\equiv}C{-}H$$

$$\downarrow \text{hydrogenation}$$

$$\underset{\text{(Product)}}{H{-}C{\equiv}C{-}CH_2CH_3} \xleftarrow[\text{by MeOH}]{\text{Deprotection}} Me_3SiC{\equiv}C{-}CH_2CH_3$$

2. ***Regiospecific formation of α–substituted carbonyl compounds***

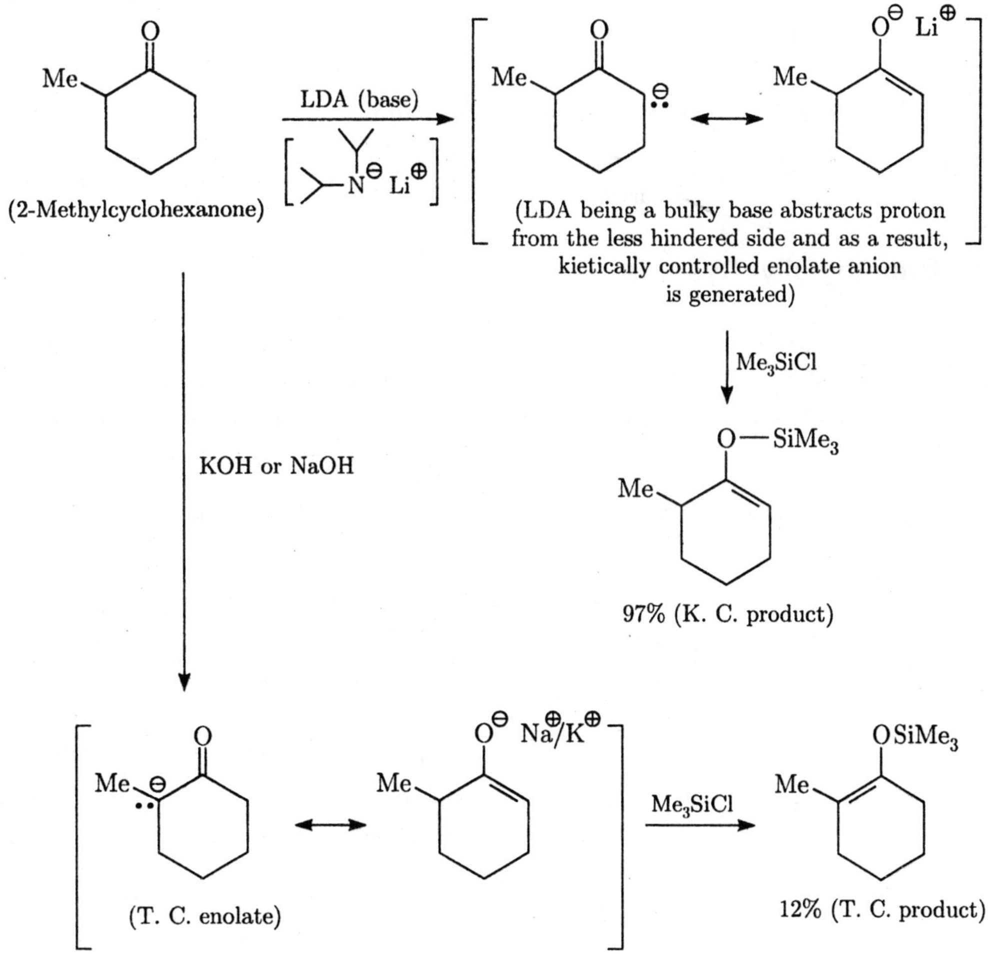

3. Arylsilanes show *ipso* substitution reactions.

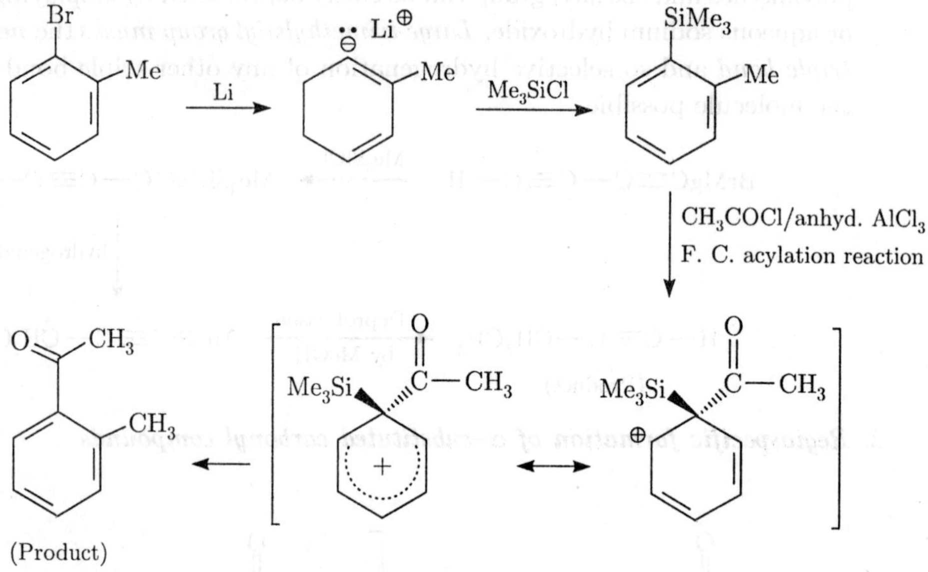

4. Trimethylsilyl chloride forms alkenylsilanes.

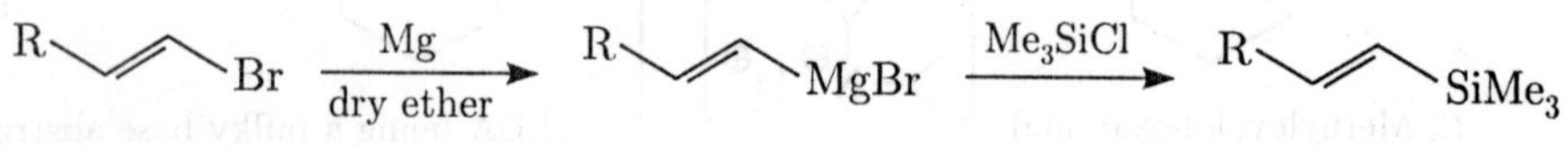

D. Trimethylsilyl Cyanide

1. Trimethylsilyl cyanide is a useful silicon reagent which reacts readily with aldehydes and ketones in the presence of catalytic amounts of Lewis acids or cyanide ion to give the trimethylsilyl ethers of the corresponding cyanohydrins.

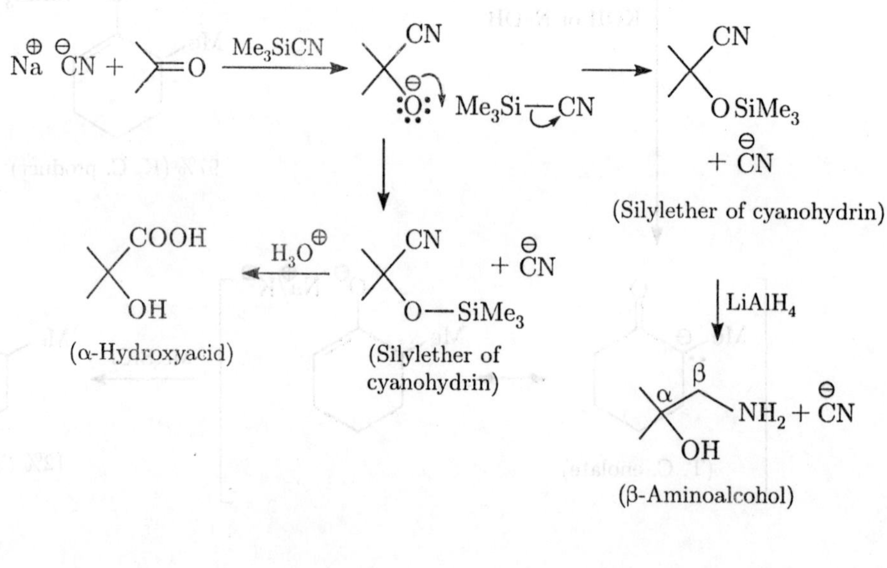

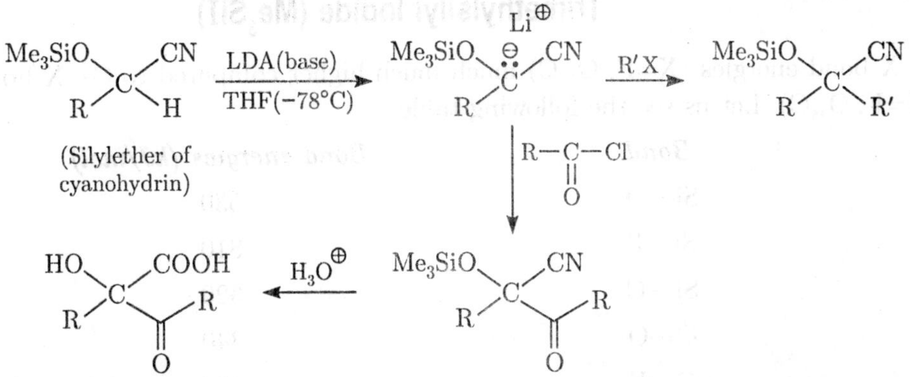

Even normally unreactive ketones react readily with Me_3SiCN due to the formation of strong Si–O bond. *Base-catalysed* addition of hydrogen cyanide to carbonyl compounds gives poor yield but Me_3SiCN affords a good yield. Tetralone, which does not form cyanohydrin but gives trimethylsilyl derivative in excellent yield. The silylated cyanohydrins can be hydrolysed to α–hydroxyacids and on reduction with $LiAlH_4$ they afford corresponding β–aminoalcohols in excellent yield. The derivatives from aromatic aldehydes are excellent acyl anion equivalents.

2. 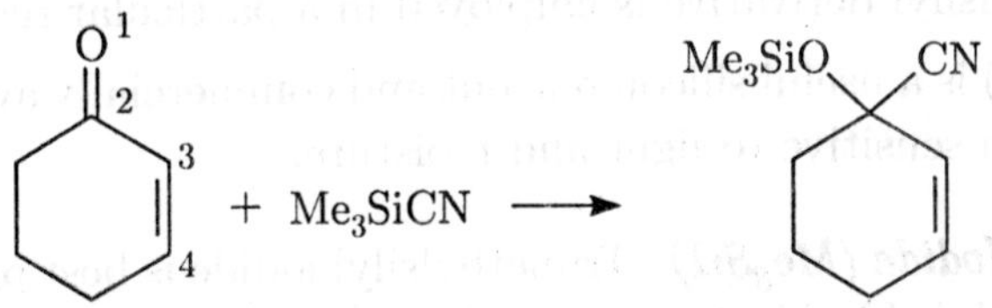

Only **1,2-adduct is formed with no 1,4-addition compound**. Generally, base catalysed addition of HCN to α,β–unsaturated carbonyl compounds give 1,4-adduct.

3. In the reaction with quinones, selective protection of one of the carbonyl groups can be achieved and subsequent transformations, lead to quinols in excellent yield.

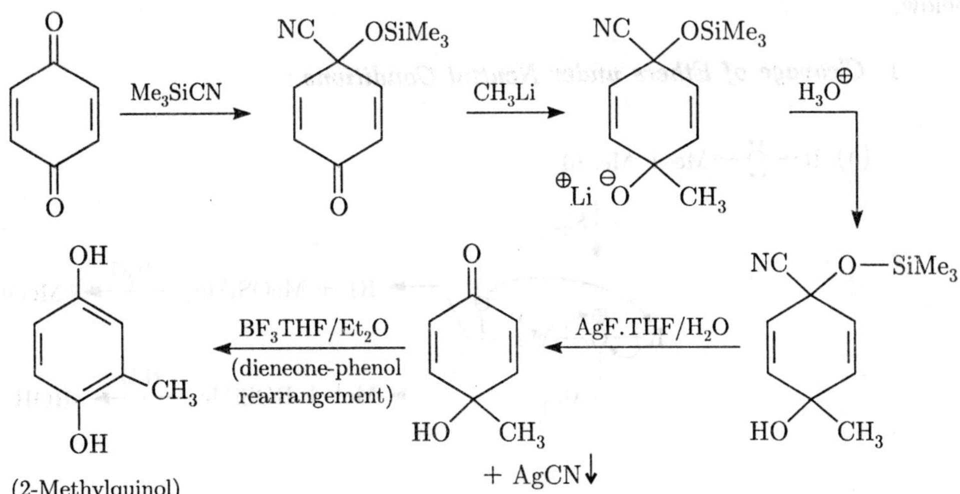

(2-Methylquinol)

Trimethylsilyl Iodide (Me_3SiI)

Si–X bond energies (X=F, O, C) much much higher compared to C—X bond energies (X=F, O, C). Let us see the following table.

Bond	*Bond energies (kJ/mol)*
Si—O	530
Si—F	810
Si—C	320
C—O	340
C—F	450
C—C	335

So the bond strengths of Si—O, Si—F and Si—C bonds are quite high those compared with C—O, C—F and C—C bond strengths. Trialkylsilyl groups are important in organosilicon chemistry (most common derivative is trimethylsilyl one, Me_3Si). Me_3Si group is sterically *less* crowded compared to Me_3C group (tertiarybutyl group) as C—Si, bond length is longer than the C—C bond length. As a result, steric congestion is experienced less when trimethylsilyl derivative is employed in a particular reaction.

Trimethylsilyl iodide (Me_3SiI) is a useful silicon reagent and commercially available. But it is expensive and very much sensitive to light and moisture.

Preparation of trimethylsilyl Iodide (Me_3SiI) : Trimethylsilyl iodide is best prepared *in situ* from reaction of trimethylsilyl chloride and sodium iodide in acetonitrile solution.

$$Me_3SiCl + NaI \xrightarrow{CH_3CN(\text{solvent})} \underset{\text{(Trimethylsilyl iodide)}}{Me_3SiI} + NaCl$$

Silicon atom having vacant 3d orbitals mostly acts as an *electrophile* as shown below.

1. ***Cleavage of Ethers under Neutral Conditions*** :

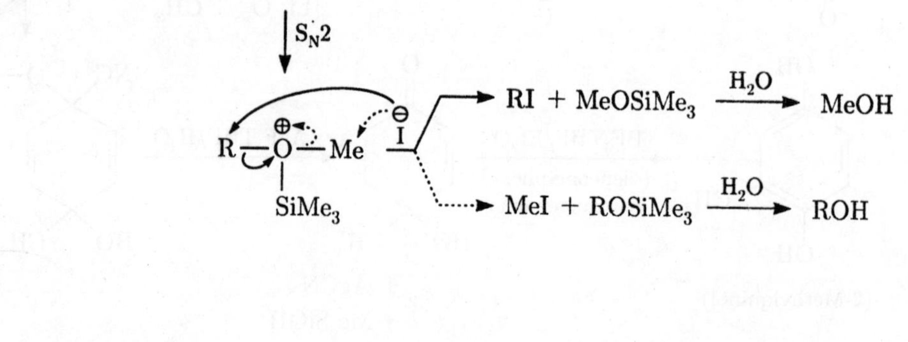

So ethers are cleaved into *alcohols.*

(b) 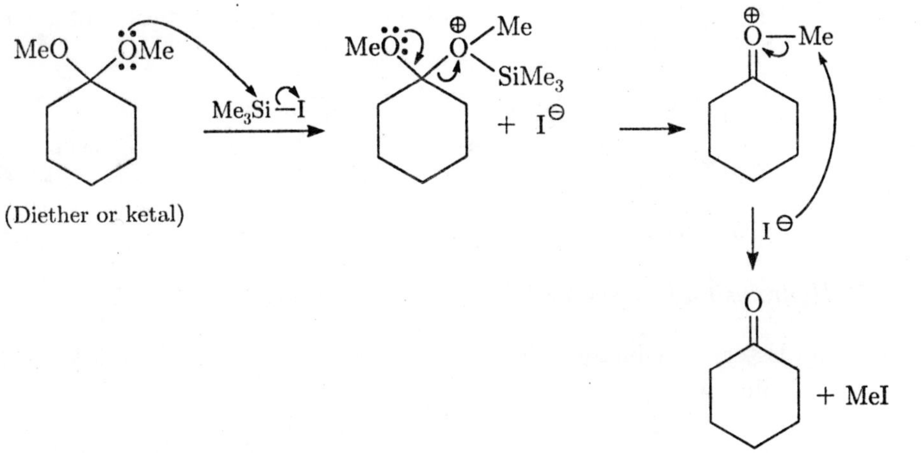

So, acetals and ketals are cleaved to corresponding aldehydes and ketones.

(c) 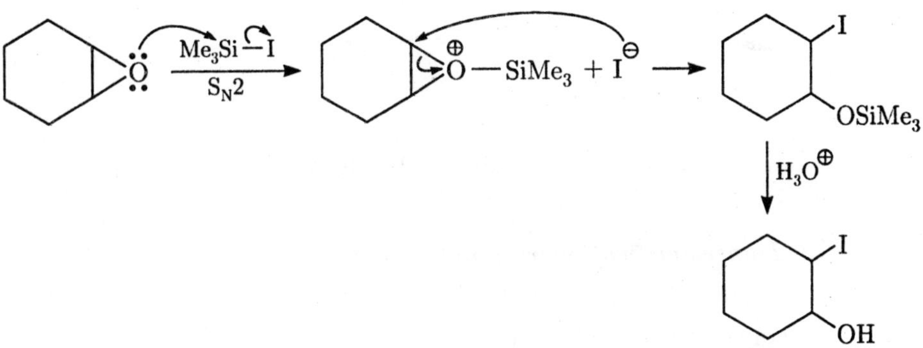

(d) 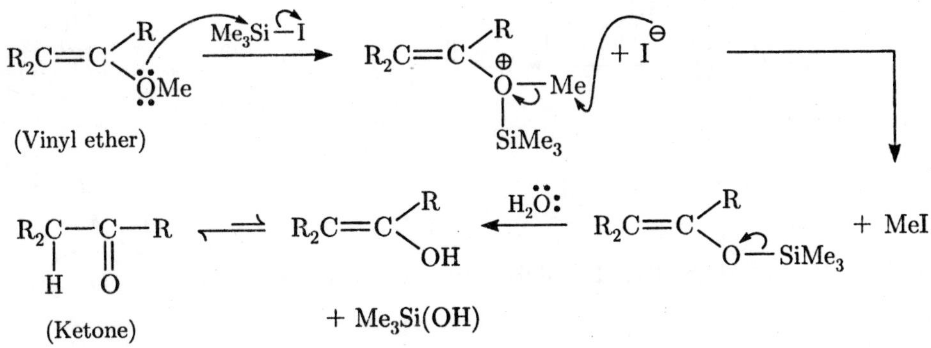

2. ***Alcohols to halides through S_N2 reactions***

(a) 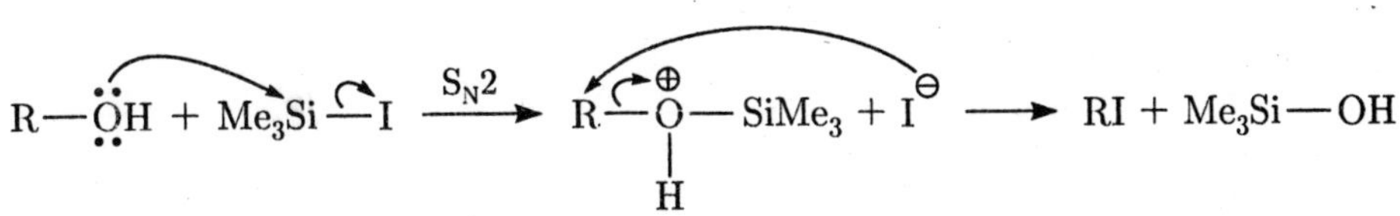

If the R group is asymmetric, then the resulting halide (iodide) is formed with inversion of configuration, *e.g,* (R)-2-butanol can be converted to (S)-2-butyl iodide.

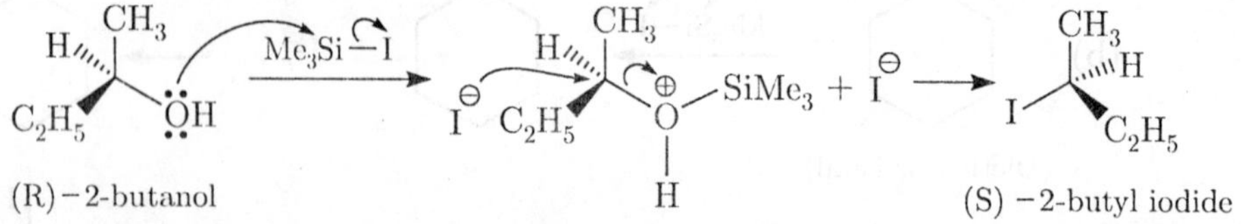

3. ***Hydrolysis of esters under neutral conditions***

(a) Esters may be hydrolysed under neutral conditions using Me_3SiI, in aqueous solution.

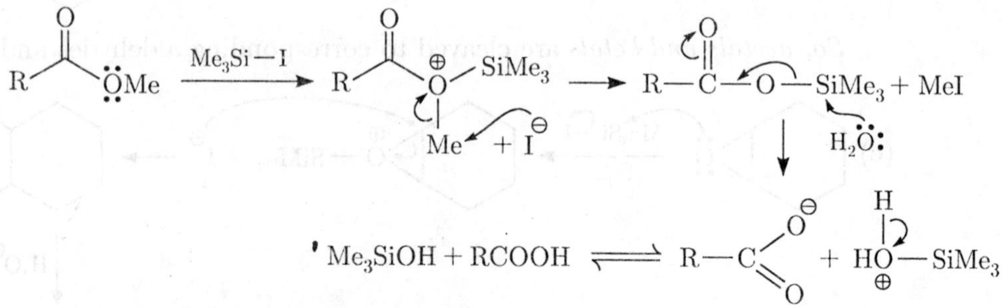

(b) ***Transesterification reaction*** : Interconversion of esters can be done using Me_3SiI or Me_3SiCl in alcohols under neutral conditions. For example, conversion of RCO_2Me to RCO_2Et in neutral medium.

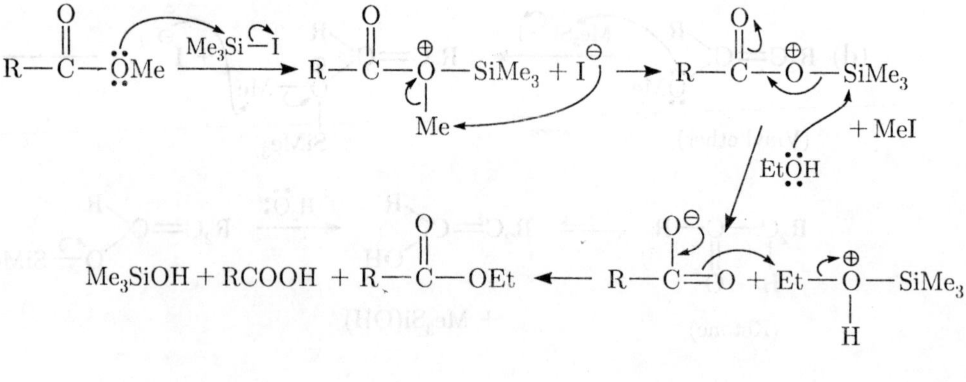

4. ***In lieu of Enamine Reaction***

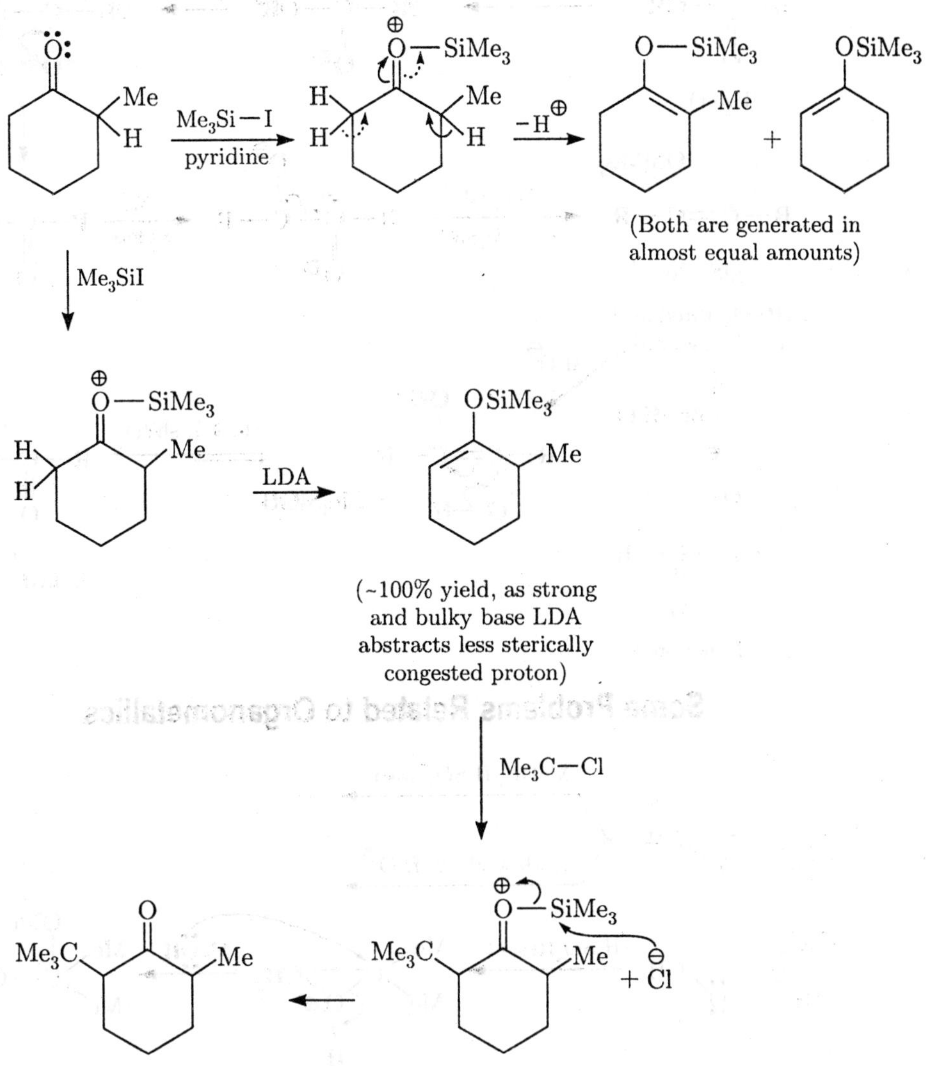

(2-methyl-6-*t*-butylcyclohexanone)

5. ***Acyloin Condensation*** : Use of Me_3SiI or Me_3SiCl stabilises the dianion formed as bissilyl enol ether which can be isolated and can be subsequently hydrolysed to the corresponding acyloin. Use of silyl halides particularly inhibit Dieckmann condensation reaction which always competes with acyloin condensation. As a result, the yield of acyloin product increases, in particular where generation of four- or five-membered ring (cyclic) acyloins occur.

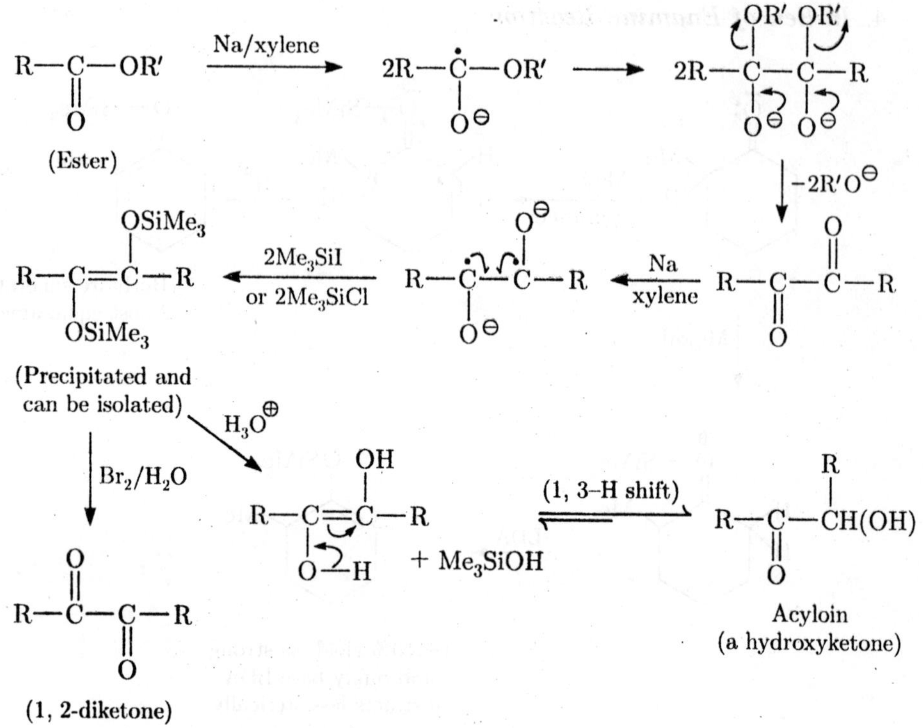

Some Problems Related to Organometallics

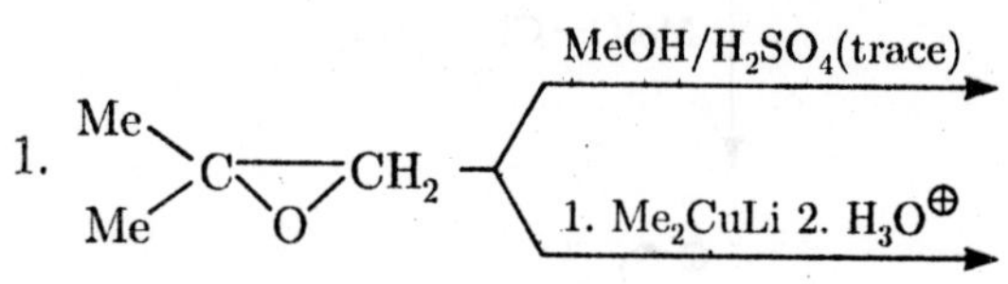

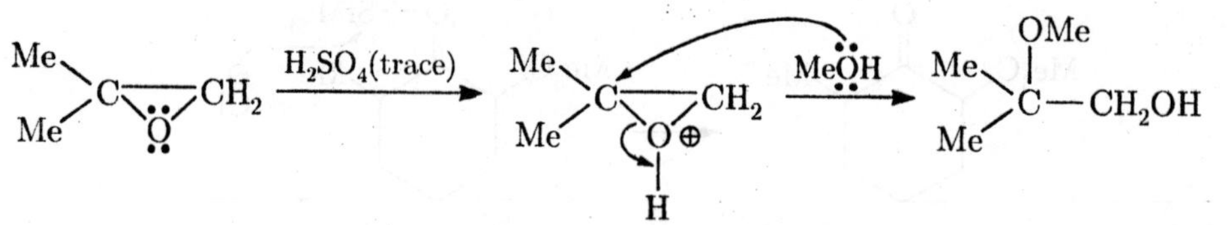

It is an example of acid catalysed ring opening of epoxides where the most substituted carbocation is formed due to its greater stability. Here bond breaking exceeds bond making. So MeOH attacks more hindered carbon.

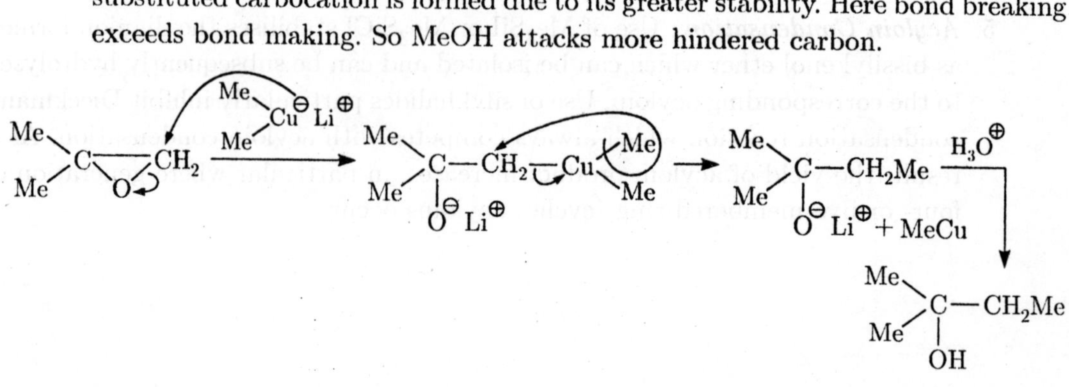

Here, bond making exceeds bond breaking. So, Me_2CuLi attacks on that carbon where partial negative charge gets stabilised, *i.e.*, on the less hindered carbon atom.

2. 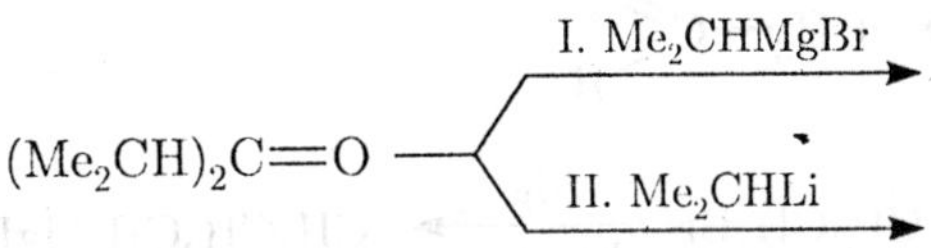

I. 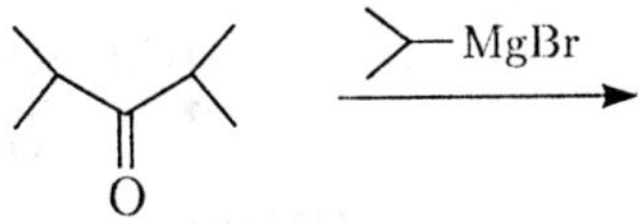

Due to bulk of isopropyl group, Grignard reagent cannot react with carbonyl group.

Two side reactions may take place.

(a) 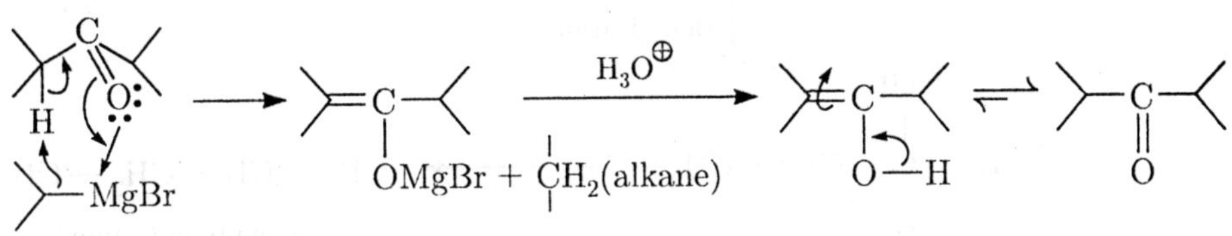

Here Grignard reagent acts as a base rather than a nucleophile.

(b) Hydride ion transfer from β-carbon of Grignard reagent occurs to reduce the carbonyl group.

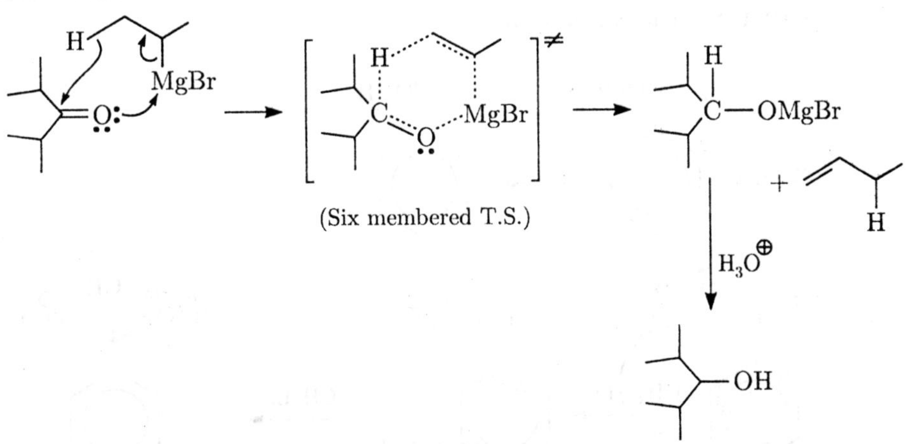

With organolithium, steric factor is of little importance, and organolithium attacks the carbonyl carbon to get the corresponding tertiary alcohol.

II. 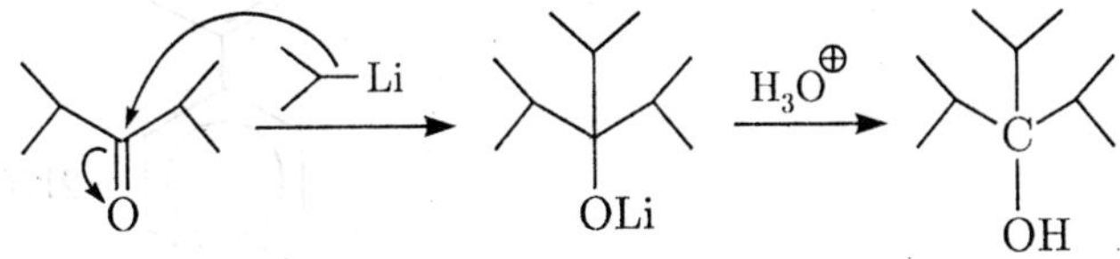

3. Outline the best possible route for the preparation of 2-pentene starting with ethanol and 1-propanol *via* Grignard reagent.

$$CH_3CH_2OH \xrightarrow{K_2Cr_2O_7/H_2SO_4} CH_3-CHO$$

$$\underset{\text{(1-propanol)}}{CH_3CH_2CH_2OH} \xrightarrow{PBr_5} CH_3CH_2CH_2Br \xrightarrow[\text{dry ether}]{Mg} CH_3CH_2CH_2MgBr$$

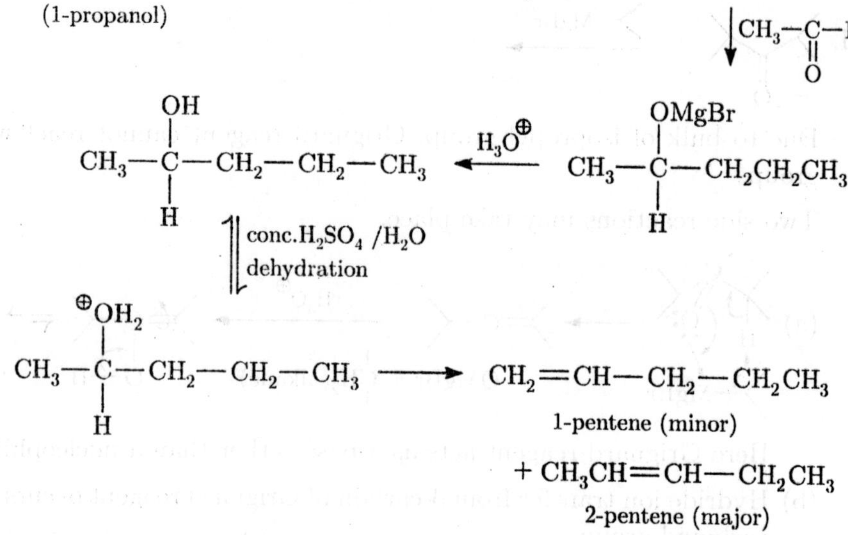

2-pentene is the major product as it is stabilised by more hyperconjugative structures than 1-pentene.

4. Convert 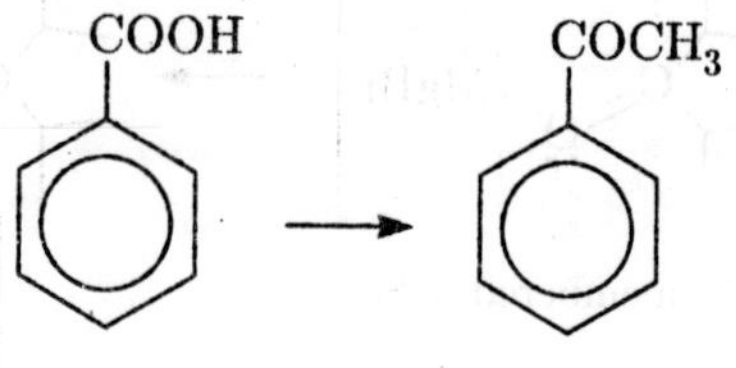

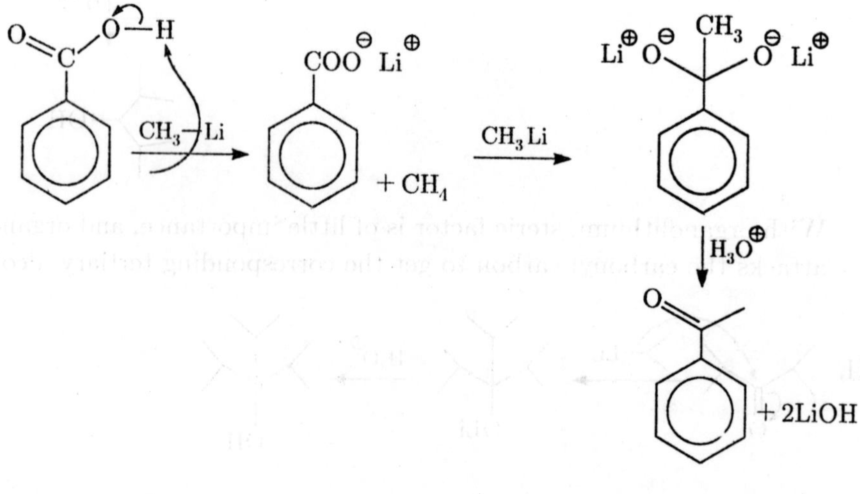

5. Using alkyl halides having not more than four carbons, synthesise 2,2,3-trimethyl -butane *via* an organocopper compound.

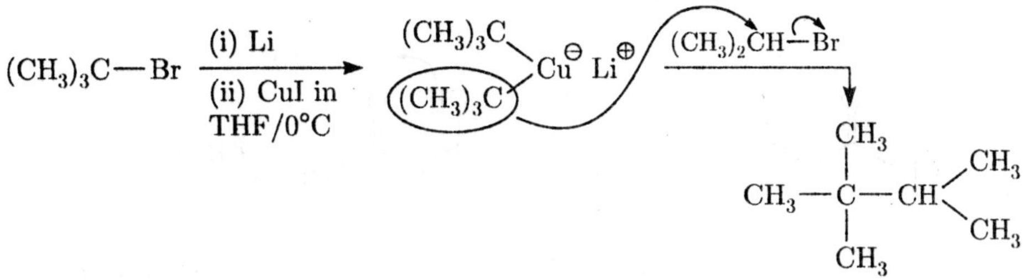

(2,2,3-trimethylbutane)

6. What happens when 1 equivalent of MeCH=CHCOMe in Et_2O is separately treated with one equivalent of the following reagents?

   a. EtMgBr in ether
   b. Et_2CuLi in ether
   c. EtLi in ether

(a) 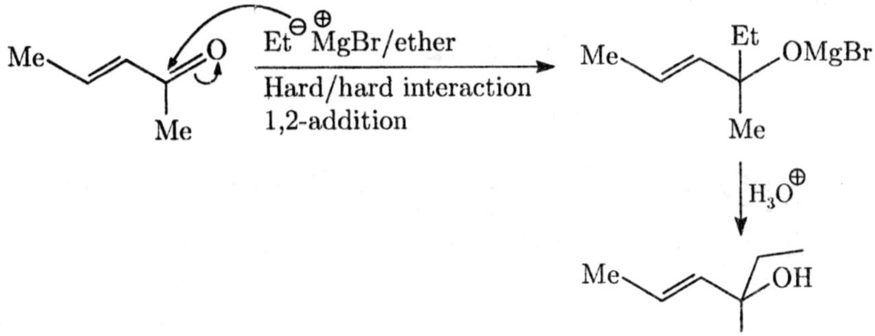

(b) 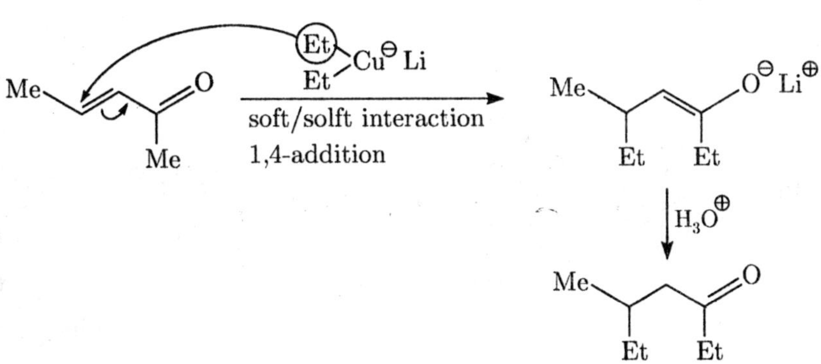

(c) In ether, Et–Li reacts with the solvent ether not with Me_2CH=CHCOMe.

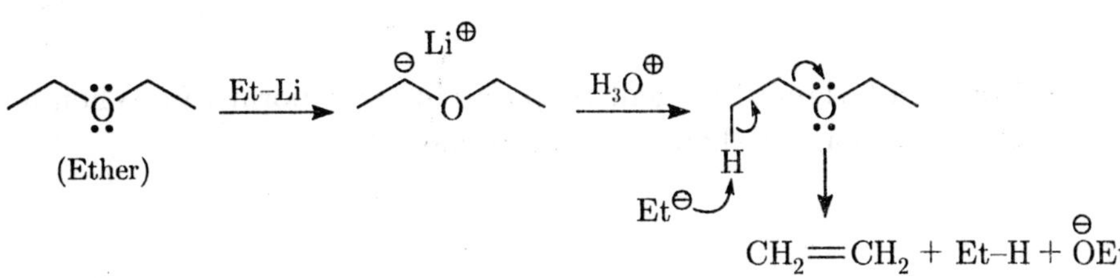

7. 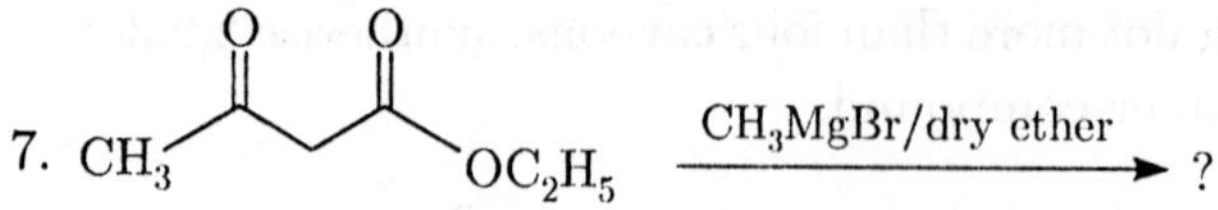

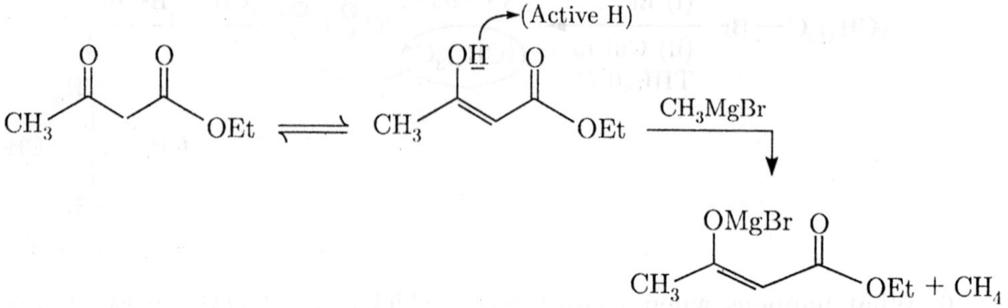

8. Indicate the products and mention the predominant one. Give mechanism.

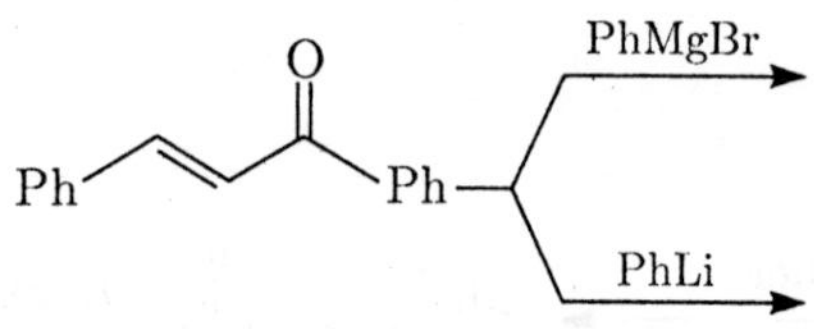

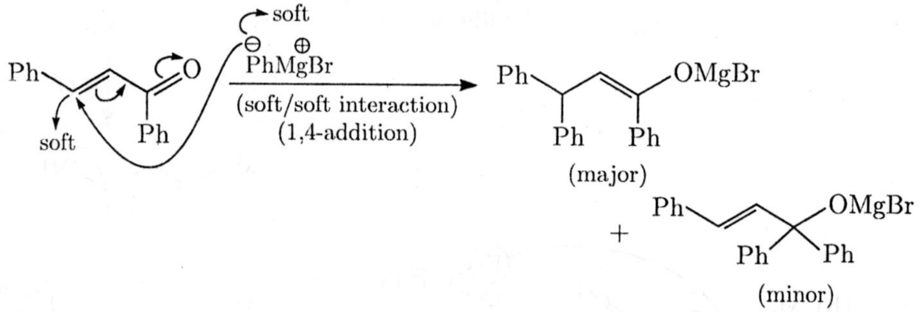

(major)

(minor)

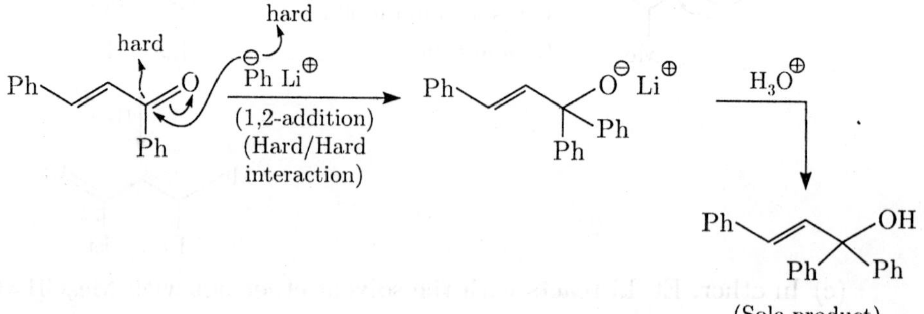

(Sole product)

9. How is a Grignard reagent prepared in the laboratory? When and how does a Grignard reagent show reducing property?

Laboratory method of preparation of Grignard reagent :

$$\underset{\text{(Alkyl halide)}}{R{-}X} + Mg \text{ (turnings or ribbon)} \xrightarrow[\text{like THF or } Et_2O \text{, reflux}]{\text{anhydrous ether}} \underset{\text{(G. R.)}}{RMgX}$$

X=Cl, Br, I
Reactivity order of halides : I>Br>Cl

When a Grignard reagent contains at least one β-hydrogen atom, then reduction may occur by hydride ion transfer *via* a six-membered cyclic transition state.

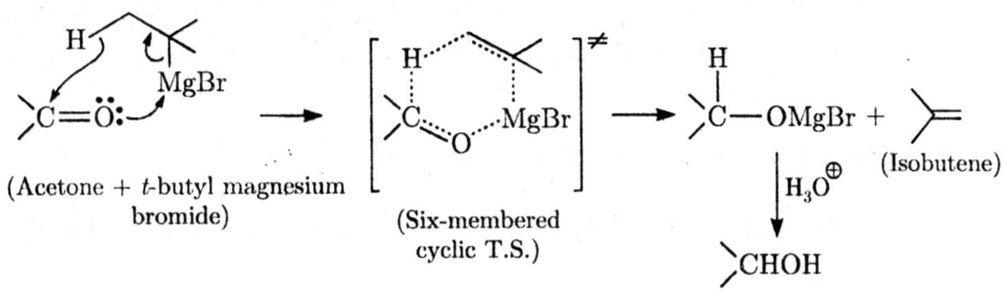

10. Comment on the following reaction sequence.

$$HOCH_2CH_2COCH_2CH_2CO_2Et \xrightarrow[\text{1 eqv}]{RMgX} \xrightarrow[\text{1 eqv}]{RMgX} \xrightarrow[\text{2 eqv}]{RMgX}$$

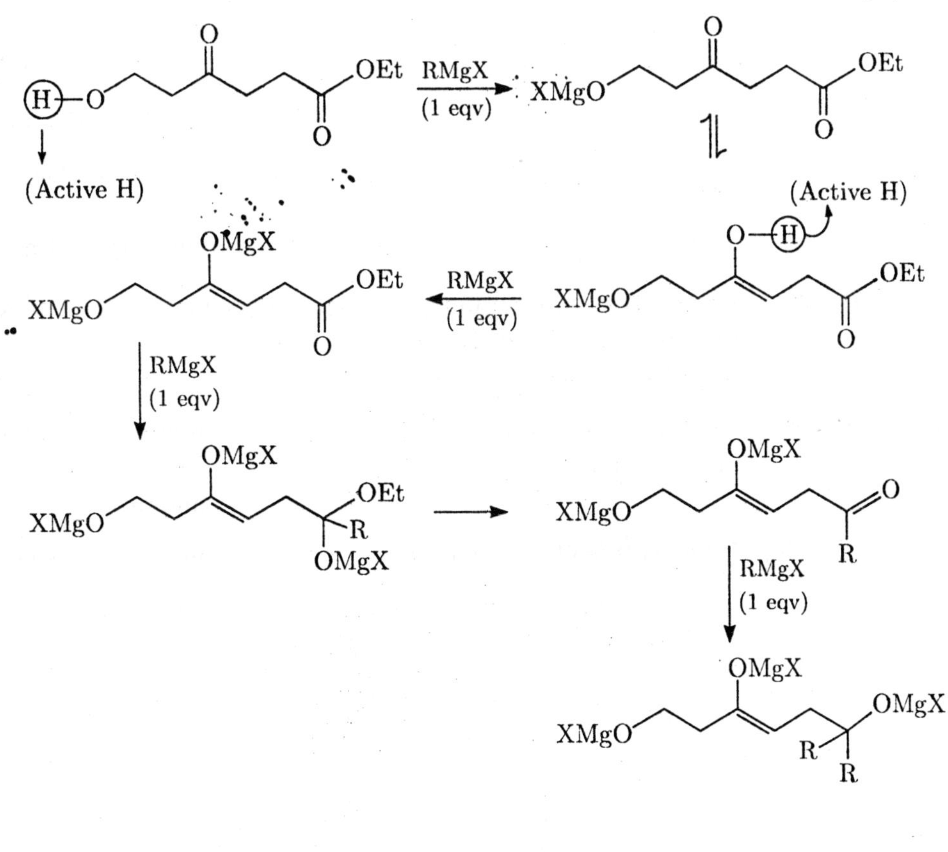

11. Indicate the products formed.

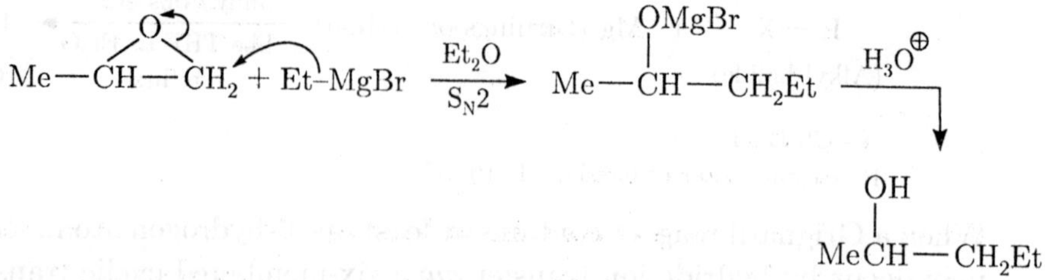

Grignard reagent attacks the carbon which is less hindered. Bond making step exceeds bond breaking step so $Et^{\ominus}$ attacks that carbon which can stabilise the partial negative charge.

12. $R^1CH{=}CHCOR^2 + R^3MgX \longrightarrow$

How would the ratio of products change in this reaction if R_2=Et, *i*Pr, and *t*Bu?

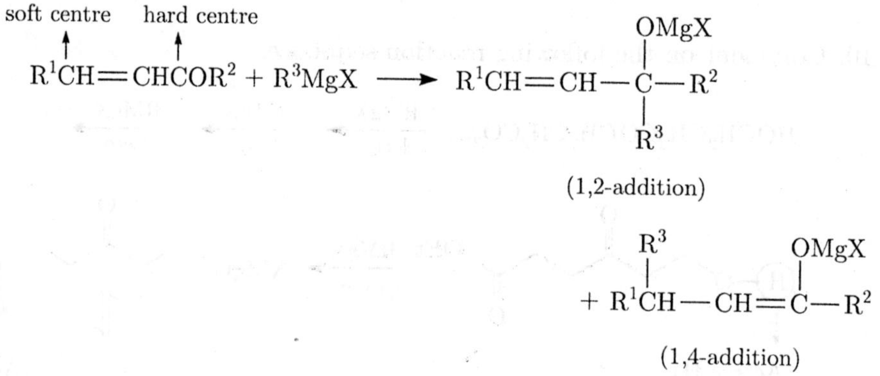

		(1,2-addition)	1,4-addition)
Et=R_2	(Hard/Hard interaction predominates due to small size of Et, by which it becomes electron dense)	major	minor
*i*Pr=R_2	(Soft/soft interaction predominates as *i*Pr group is larger in size)	minor (little amount)	major
t-Bu=R_2	(Only soft/soft interaction as *t*-butyl group is bulky enough)	nil	sole product

13. 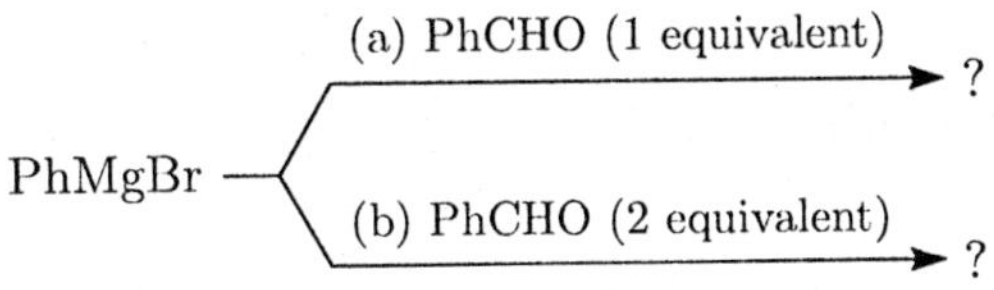

Ans. :

(a) 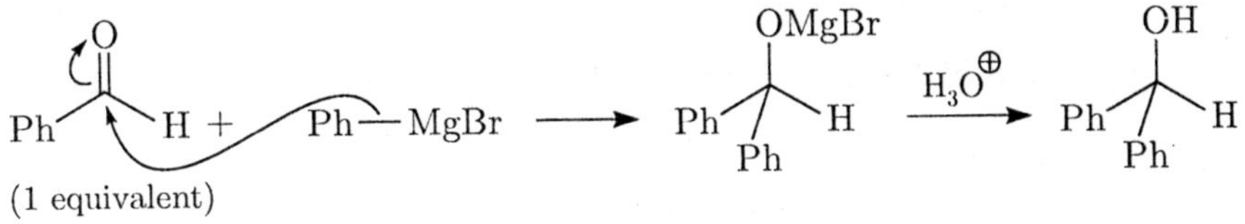

(b) 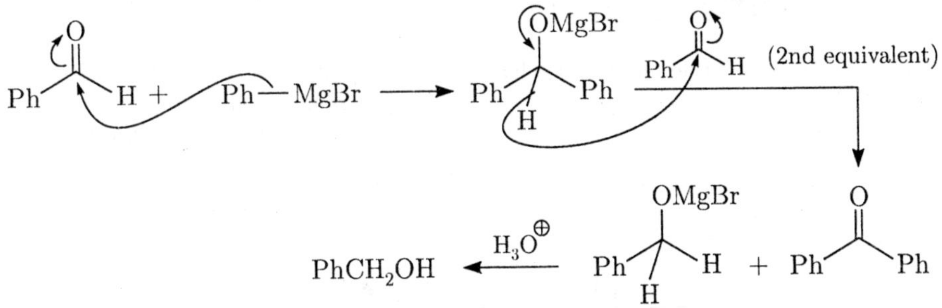

14. What product would you expect from the reaction of diethyl carbonate $(EtO)_2C{=}O$ with excess of MeMgI. Give mechanism.

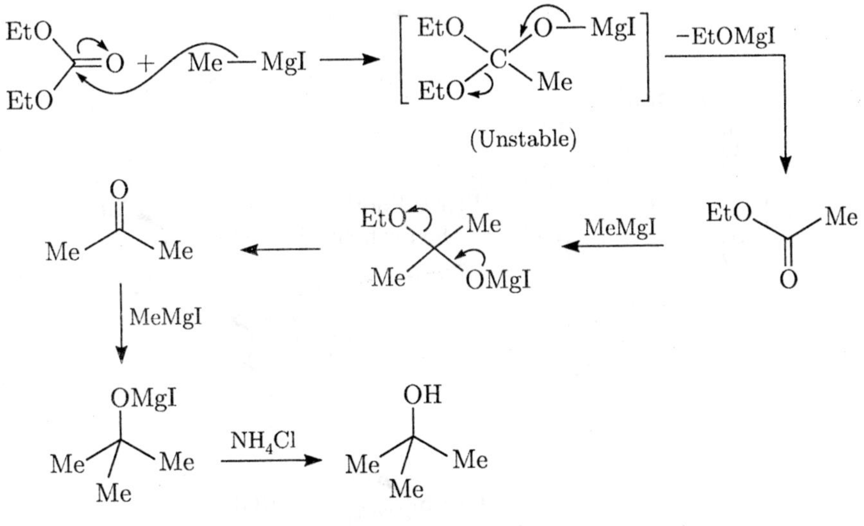

(NH_4Cl is used instead of H_3O to avoid elimination which may lead to the formation of an alkene)

15. 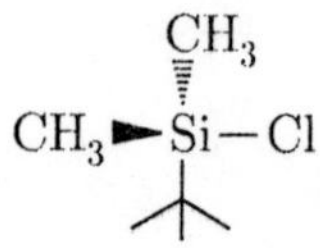 (tertiarybulyldimethylsilyl chloride) is a stronger protecting agent than Me_3SiCl and is quite stable in dilute acid medium. But in the presence of base, like NaOMe, the molecule breaks down. Show the fate of the reagent in the presence of (a) KF/18-crown-6, (b) Na^+OMe^- and (c) $nBu_4N^{\oplus}F^{\ominus}$.

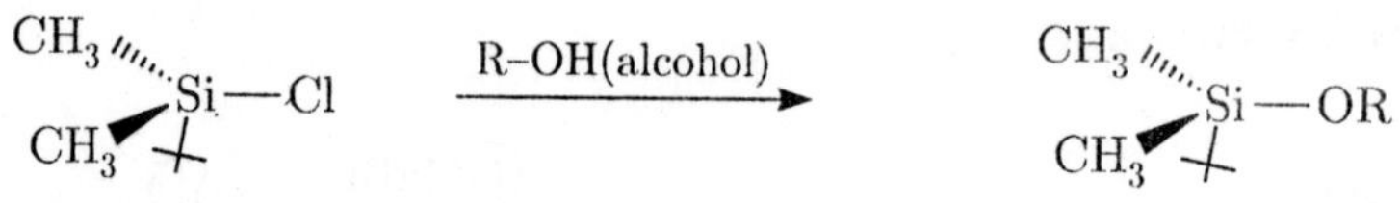

(Tertiarybutyldimethylsilyl chloride)

(Alcohol protected by tertiarybutyl-dimethylsilyl group and the molecule is quite stable in dilute acid)

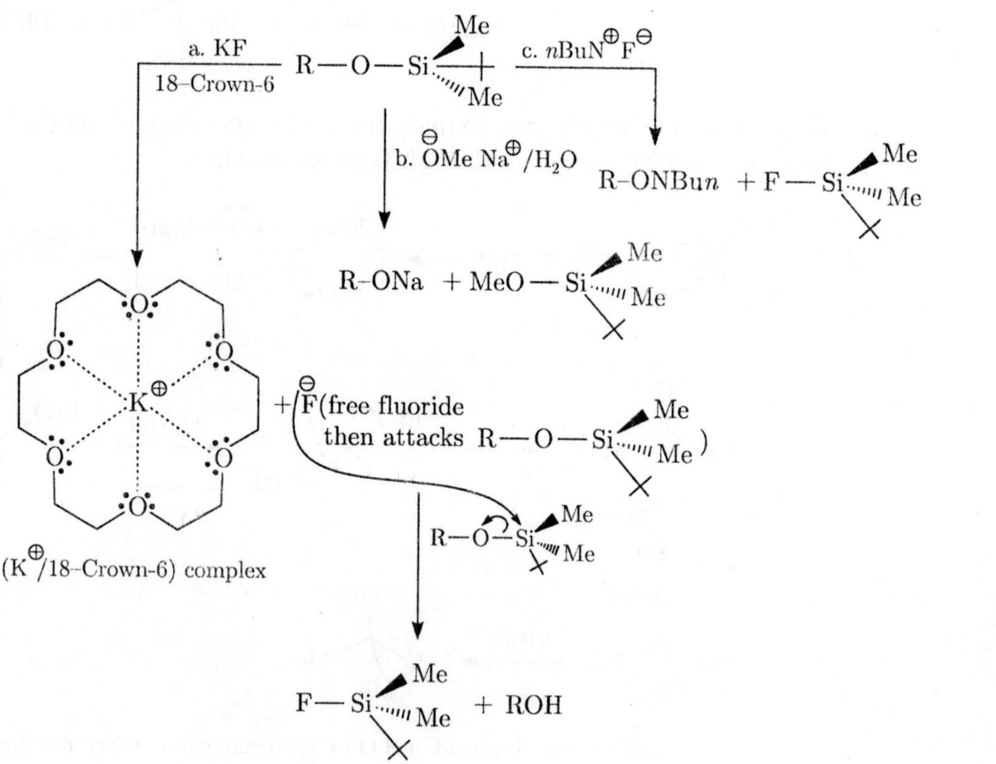

16. Why Zn metal is used instead of magnesium in Reformatsky reaction?

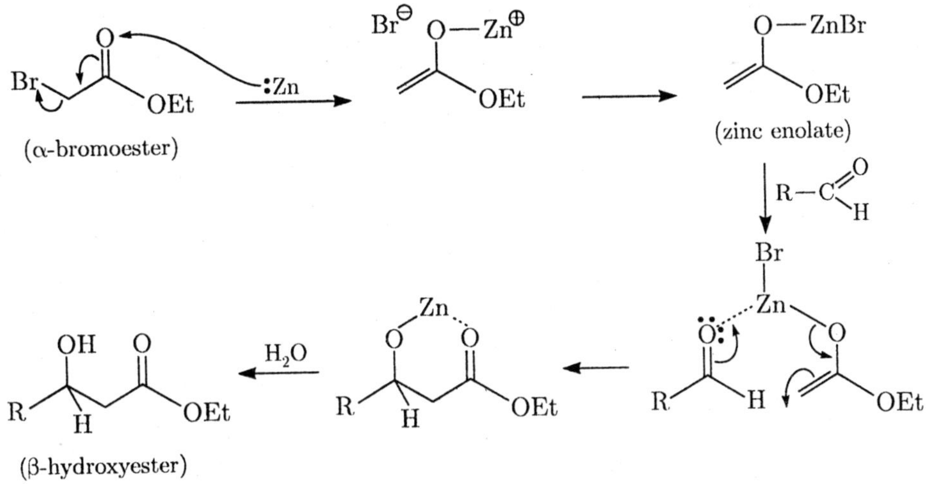

Elimination does not occur with Reformatsky reaction as no base is present in the reaction dium.

Zinc (Zn) in *much less electropositive* than magnesium (Mg) metal. Zn is used instead of Mg in Reformatsky reaction, due to its much more electropositivity (more reactivity of Mg is thus, expected) not only attacks the carbonyl group of the carbonyl compound but also attacks the ester functionality in both substrate (α–haloester) and product (β–hydroxyester). On the other hand Zn attacks only the carbonyl carbon of carbonyl compounds and ester carbonyl functionality remains undisturbed. So with Mg, we won't be able to get our desired product-β–hydroxy ester in Reformatsky reaction; which is only achieved if we use *Zn metal,* which is much less electropositive and hence much less reactive than Mg metal.

17. What happens when $Et-CH=CH-\underset{\underset{O}{\|}}{C}-Et$ is treated with two equivalents of Grignard reagent?

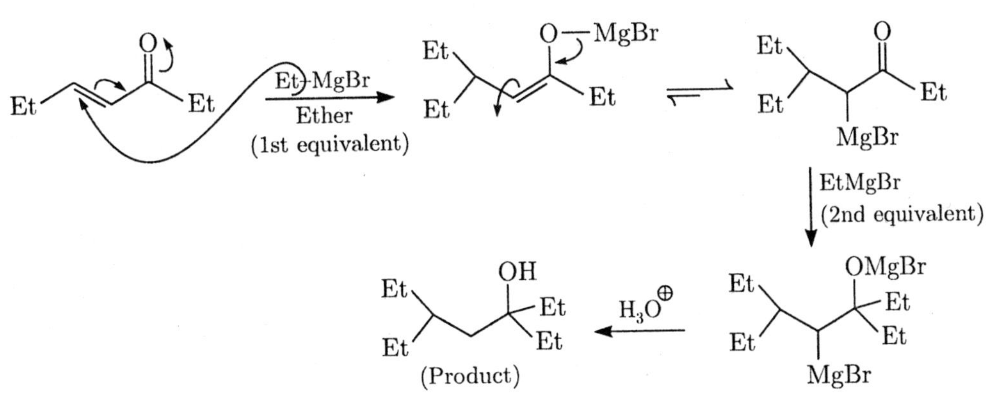

3 Aromatic Electrophilic and Nucleophilic Substitution Reactions

An electrophilic substitution reaction may be represented as —

$$R—L + E^{\oplus} \longrightarrow R—E + L^{\oplus}$$

Here the leaving electrophile or better electrofuge is $L^{\oplus}$ gets displaced by $E^{\oplus}$ the incoming electrophile. This $E^{\oplus}$ may be $\overset{\oplus}{N}O_2$, $\overset{\oplus}{N}O$, $Br^{\oplus}$, $Cl^{\oplus}$, $I^{\oplus}$, $R^{\oplus}$, $R\overset{\oplus}{C}O$, *i.e.*, positively charged species or electron deficient uncharged species like SO_3, BF_3 etc.

The weakest Lewis acids are the best electrophiles since they can exist best without a pair of electrons, which are required to fill the valence shell. However proton is the usual electrofuge in aromatic electrophilic substitution reactions, although metal ions, SO_3H, $X^{\oplus}$ etc. also act as leaving groups.

Aromatic hydrocarbons are known as arenes. The most characteristic reactions of benzenoid arenes are that they react with electrophilic reagents, but with a different pathway than those of aliphatic electrophilic substitutions.

An aromatic ring has negative charge cloud below and above its plane. Electrophiles, being either positively charged or electron deficient species, are very much prone to attack this negative charge cloud of delocalised π-electrons. So its expected that, electrophilic reactions will occur on aromatic rings much readily. But an aromatic molecule on the other hand wants to preserve its aromatic character and stability and so is reluctant to utilise it is π-electrons. For this reason, electrophiles react with aromatic compounds in a *slow manner.* The most important type of electrophilic substitution found in aromatic compounds is ArS_E2 (aromatic substitution electrophilic bimolecular).

Aromatic electrophilic substitution reaction (ArS_E2 reaction) is supposed to proceed through the following steps :

Step **1 :** Formation of π complex (pi-complex)

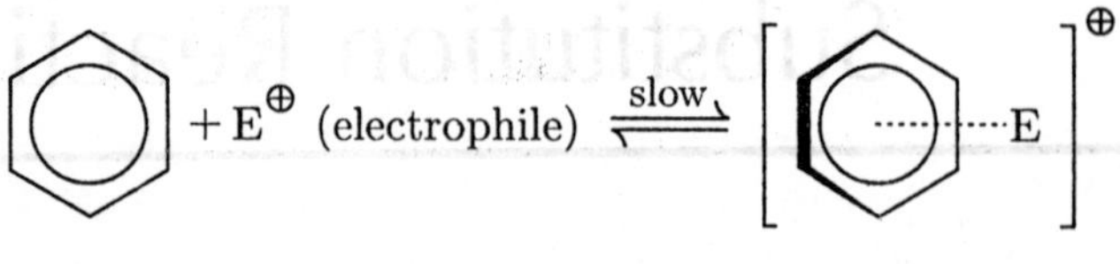

π–complex

Step **2 :** Conversion of a π complex into a σ-complex (sigma complex).

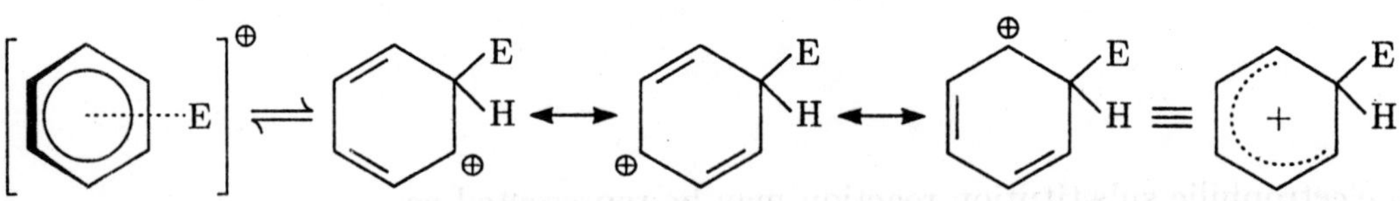

σ–complex

Step **3 :** Conversion of the σ-complex to a new π-complex.

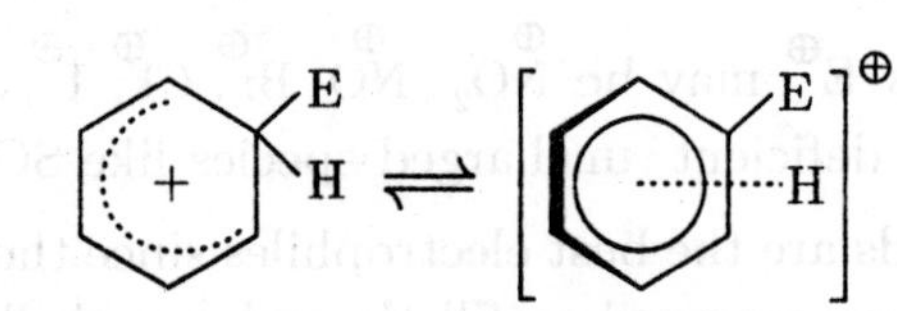

Step **4 :** Decomposition of π complex to products.

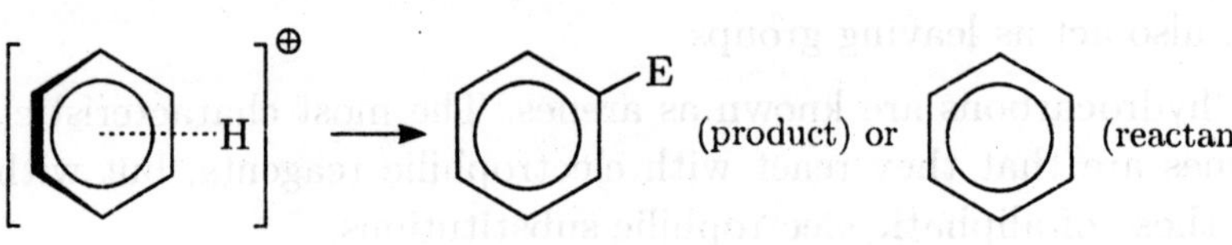

The σ-complex contains the electrofuge (here H) and electrophile both attached to an sp^3 carbon atom, and there is a possibility that both may be eliminated at the aromatisation step. Which group, *i.e.*, either E or H will be eliminated depends on the following factors:

(a) The polarisability of the bond attached to the electrofuge, and

(b) The stability of electrofuge.

Generally H atom attached to an sp^3 carbon atom of a σ-complex is acidic as the σ-complex being positively charged is electron attracting. As a result, C—H bond polarisability becomes more than the polarisability of C—E bond. Moreover the stability of $H^{\oplus}$ is in general more than that of $E^{\oplus}$. As a result, $H^{\oplus}$ is eliminated quickly as soon as the σ-complex is formed.

Two situations may arise :

Case 1 : Chlorination, bromination or nitration reactions where

$$E^{\oplus}=Cl^{\oplus}, Br^{\oplus}, NO_2^{\oplus}, \text{etc.}$$

$Cl^{\oplus}$, $Br^{\oplus}$, $NO_2^{\oplus}$, etc. are poor electrofuges, so $H^{\oplus}$ is eliminated fast as an electrofuge. As a result, chlorination, bromination and nitration reactions are *irreversible* in nature.

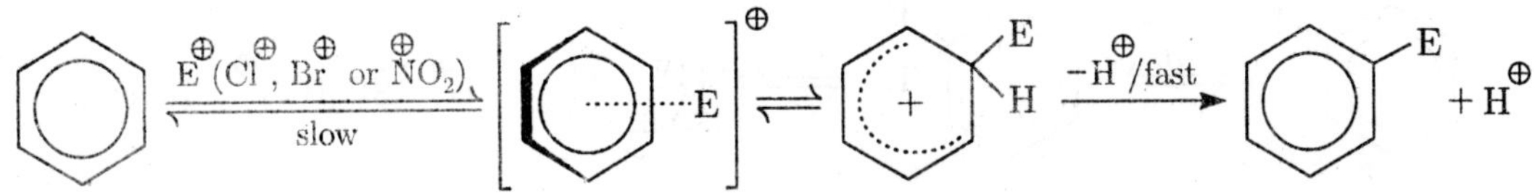

$\Delta G^{\neq}$ (activation energy) is too high for the reverse process due to poor electrofugacity of $NO_2^{\oplus}$, $Br^{\oplus}$, or $Cl^{\oplus}$ and thus, the reactions become *irreversible* in nature. The aromatisation step, *i.e.*, where $H^{\oplus}$ is eliminated is a fast step, so we donot observe any PKIE (primary kinetic isotope effect) for these type of reactions.

Energy profile diagram of an irreversible ArS$_E$2 reaction :

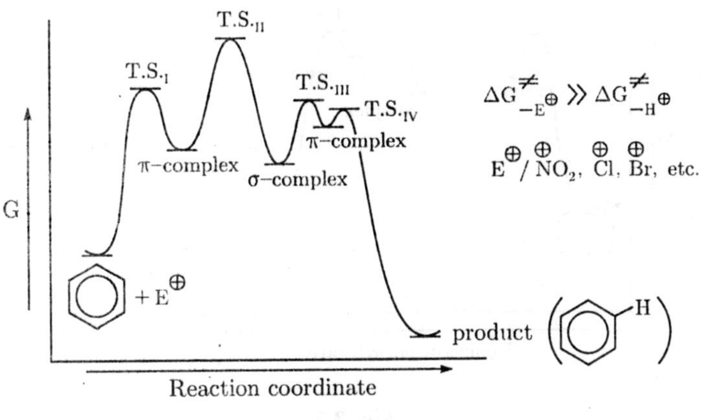

Fig. 3.1 :

Case 2 : There are some electrophiles which take part in ArS$_E$2 reactions may eliminate as $E^{\oplus}$ because these electrofuges are stable and C—E bond has high polarisability. As a result, $\Delta G^{\neq}_{-E^{\oplus}}$ becomes less than $\Delta G^{\neq}_{-H^{\oplus}}$. Ultimately there is a competition between the two processes, *i.e.*, elimination of $H^{\oplus}$ and elimination of $E^{\oplus}$ both take place and the reaction becomes *reversible* is nature. This type of ArS$_E$2 reactions includes alkylation, sulphonation, iodination etc. of aromatic systems, where the active electrophiles are $R^{\oplus}$, $^{\oplus}SO_3H$, $I^{\oplus}$ etc. These electrofuges are quite stable and the bond polarisability of C—E bond is quite high, even higher than C—H bond. As a result $\Delta G^{\neq}_{-H^{\oplus}}$ becomes somehow higher than the $\Delta G^{\neq}_{-E^{\oplus}}$. Expectedly C—H bond breaking step becomes slow and it becomes the rate determining step. In other words, alkylation, sulphonation and iodination in aromatic systems show primary kinetic isotope effect (PKIE). For example the rate of sulphonation of hexadeuterobenzene is less than that of benzene ($K_H/K_D>1$) but the rate of chlorination or nitration of benzene and hexadeuterobenzene shows the same rate. In the former case C—H bond breaking step is slow and reversible whereas in the latter it is a fast step. Naturally sulphonation reaction shows a prominent PKIE, whereas no PKIE is observed for nitration or chlorination reactions.

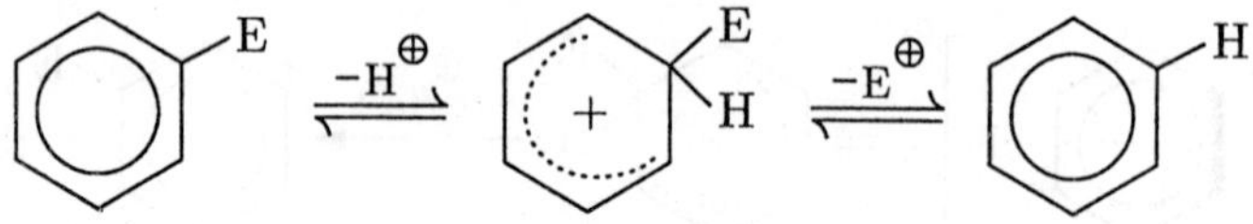

$\overset{\oplus}{E} = \overset{\oplus}{S}O_3H, \overset{\oplus}{I}, \overset{\oplus}{R}$ etc.

[Iodination of benzene is an exothermic reaction; so direct iodination of benzene is not possible. If the benzene nucleus is activated, *i.e.*, contains –OH, –NH_2 etc. groups with +R effect, then iodination can be done with poor electrophiles.]

The energy profile diagram of a reversible ArS_E2 reaction :

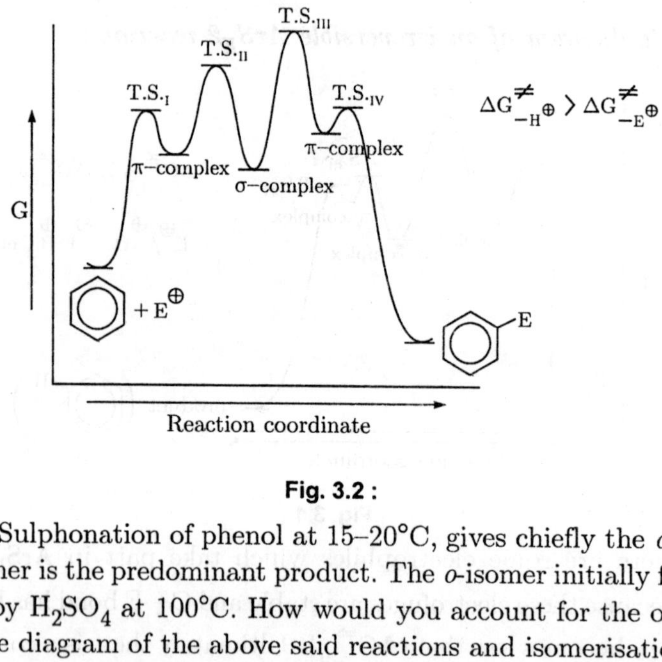

Fig. 3.2 :

Problem 1 : Sulphonation of phenol at 15–20°C, gives chiefly the *o*-isomer, while at 100°C, the *p*-isomer is the predominant product. The *o*-isomer initially formed isomerises to the *p*-isomer by H_2SO_4 at 100°C. How would you account for the observation? Give the energy profile diagram of the above said reactions and isomerisation.

Ans. : Here the active electrophile is $\overset{\oplus}{S}O_3H$ which can also behave as an electrofuge. As a result, the elimination of proton ($H^{\oplus}$) and elimination of $\overset{\oplus}{S}O_3H$ ($E^{\oplus}$) from the intermediate carbocation (σ-complex) competes and the reaction becomes *reversible.* Again *o*-phenolsulphonic acid isomerises to *p*-phenolsulphonic acid at 100°C.

$$H_2S_2O_7 \equiv HO—SO_2—O—SO_2OH \rightleftharpoons \overset{\oplus}{HOSO_2} + \overset{\ominus}{HSO_4}$$

Active electrophile

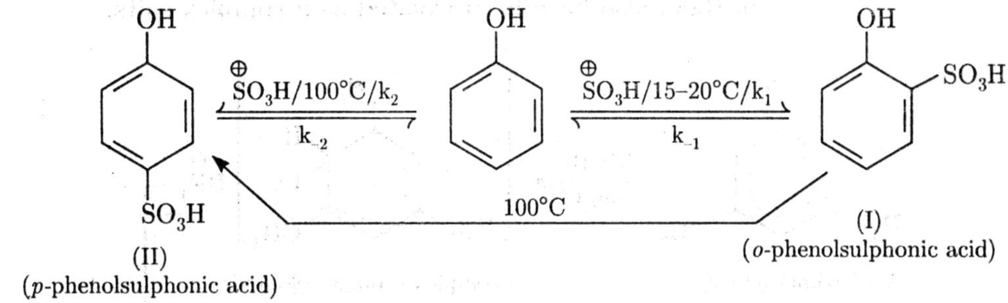

(I) is kinetically controlled product and (II) is thermodynamically controlled product. The instability of product (I) may be due to the steric repulsion present between bulky –OH and –SO_3H groups at the *ortho* positions.

(I) is K. C. product, so $k_1 > k_2$ and therefore $\Delta G^{\neq}_1 < \Delta G^{\neq}_2$. Also since (II) is the T. C. product, $\Delta H_2 > \Delta H_1$. It therefore follows that the rate of reverse (desulphonation reaction) reaction; (I) → phenol is much greater than that of another reverse reaction, *i.e.*, (II) → phenol. It follows that, $\Delta G_{-2} >> \Delta G_{-1}$ and $k_{-1} >> k_{-2}$.

At low themperature, the equilibrium between I and II is reached very slowly. Hence, if the reaction is stopped long before the equilibrium is reached, (I)>(II), since $k_1 > k_2$. If one waited long enough for equilibrium to be reached, then (II)>(I). This is due to the fact that since $k_{-1} >> k_{-2}$, (I) reforms phenol much faster than (II) and hence (II) accumulates at the expense of (I). Because rising the temperature speeds up a reaction, equilibrium is reached far more quickly at higher temperature, the production of (II) (*p*-phenolsulphonic acid) which is also the thermodynamically controlled product is facilitated.

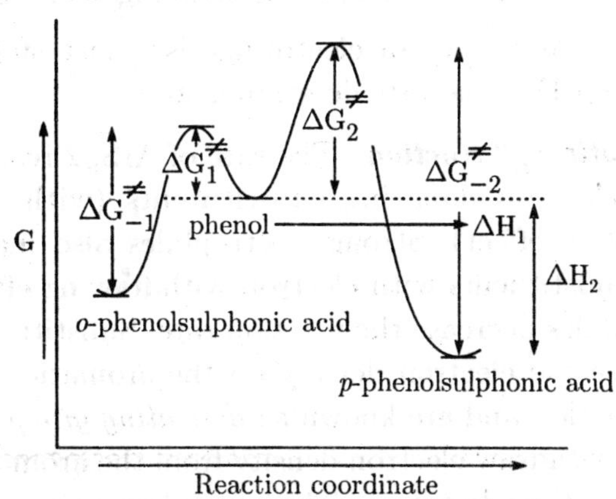

Fig. 3.3 :

Evidences in favour of ArS$_E$2 mechanism

(a) ***Detection and isolation of σ-complexes*** : A large number of σ-complexes as intermediates in ArS$_E$2 reactions have been detected by NMR spectroscopic studies. Some of them also have been isolated as σ-complex salts.

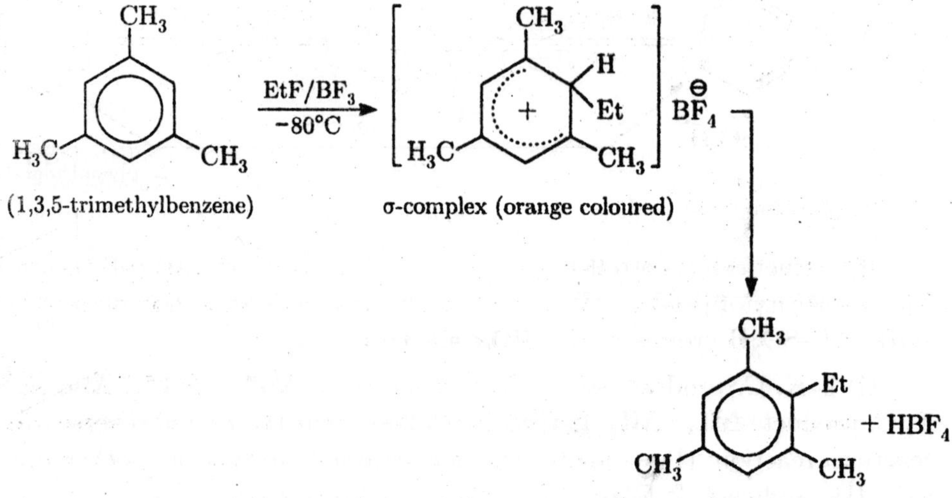

The σ-comlex formed by the action of HCl on benzene in the presence of $AlCl_3$ is red oil which conducts electricity.

(b) ***Primary kinetic isotope effect (PKIE)*** : Displacement of a H (or D) atom of C_6H_6 (or C_6D_6) by a nitronium ion ($\overset{\oplus}{N}O_2$ ion) is an ArS$_E$2 reaction which is irreversible in nature. It has been found that, the rate of formation of $C_6H_5NO_2$ from C_6H_6 is almost equal to the rate of formation of $C_6D_6NO_2$ from C_6D_6 under the same reaction conditions. It implies that the rate of breaking of C—H bond is equivalent to the rate of breaking of C—D bond. This proves that the elimination of $H^{\oplus}$ as an electrofuge is a fast step and the formation of σ-complex (step 1) is the rate determing step.

Rate of aromatic S$_E$2 reaction : The rate of ArS$_E$2 reaction is enhanced by the presence of electron donating substitutents (with +I and +R effect and hyperconjugative effect). Strong electrophiles also increase the rate. On the other hand, substituents with electron withdrawing effect (–I, –R effects) and weak electrophiles decrease the reaction rate. Substitutents with +I and or +R effects increase the electron density on the aromatic ring, thereby facililating the ArS$_E$2 reaction and are known as *activating groups.* The substituents with –I/–R effects withdraw electron density from the aromatic ring and thereby the rate of the reaction decreases. These substituents are known as *deactivating groups.*

Effect of substituents on the rate of ArS_E2 reaction (standard of comparison is H atom) :

Nature of group	*Decreasing order of rate*	*Electrical effect*
(a) Activating	(i) $:\ddot{\underset{\cdot\cdot}{O}}:^{\ominus} > \ddot{N}R_2 > -\ddot{N}R_2 > -\ddot{\underset{\cdot\cdot}{O}}H >$	$+R > +I$
	$:\ddot{O}R > \ddot{N}HCOR > -\ddot{\underset{\cdot\cdot}{O}}COR$	
	(ii) Ar	Conjugative effect
	(iii) R	+I and hyperconjugative effects
(b) Deactivating	(i) $-\ddot{\underset{\cdot\cdot}{X}}:$	$-I > +R$
	(ii) $-CX_3$	$-I$
	(iii) $-CHO > -CO_2H > -COCH_3 > -CN > -SO_3H > NO_2$	$-I$ and $-R$ effects
	(iv) $\overset{\oplus}{S}R_2$, $\overset{\oplus}{N}R_3$	$-I$ effect

The rate of ArS_E2 reaction depends on the stability of transition state. If the free energy of activation for the formation of the transition state is lower, greater will be the stability. In ArS_E2 reaction the transition state is σ-complex like as the formation of σ-complex is endothermic (Hammond's postulate). Therefore, the stability of the transition state may be determined by considering the factors which stabilise or destabilise the σ-complex (an intermediate). Since the σ-complex bears positive charge, it is assumed that, the transition state leading to the formation of σ-complex is partially positively charged and so the substituents containing +I, +R and hyperconjugative effects will bring stability to the transition state by making $\Delta G^{\neq}$ low, and thereby the rate of the reaction increases. On the other hand, electron withdrawing or deactivating substituents decrease the rate of reaction by destabilising the transition state which is reflected by more $\Delta G^{\neq}$ needed to reach it. So we see the following order of nitration which is justified.

Toluene > benzene > nitrobenzene

—— rate of nitration decreases ⟶

In case of toluene, the electron density on the aromatic ring is increased by hyperconjugative effect and shows maximum rate regarding nitration. $-NO_2$ group in nitrobenzene deactivates the benzene ring by withdrawing electron density from the aromatic nucleus and so the rate of nitration becomes minimum. Benzene being neither activated nor deactivated falls in between.

Since (I) effects are reasonably strong upto two carbon atoms (C_2) and virtually becomes zero after four carbon atoms (C_4), a +I effect activates *ortho* positions more than the *para* position and a –I effect deactivates *ortho* positions more than the *para* position. Therefore, an aromatic compound with +I substituent will undergo electrophilic substitution more readily if only this electronic effect (I effect) is taken into consideration, at the *ortho*-position. Similarly with substituents having –I effect deactivates the *ortho*-positions strongly, and so the substitution occurs mainly at *ortho*-position. For this reason, toluene is nitrated mainly at *ortho*-position (CH_3 group contains +I, +R effects) and chlorobenzene is nitrated chiefly at the *para*-position (Cl has –I effect). But this explanation is over simplified, as with increase in the bulk of substituents and attacking electrophiles the percentage formation of *ortho* product decreases, whatever may be the electronic effects, *i.e.*, +I or –I or +R or –R. The reason is steric in nature, known as *ortho* effect.

Orientation of the attacking electrophile : By orientation of the attacking electrophile in an aromatic electrophilic substitution is meant by assigning its position in the aromatic ring in which the attacking electrophile attaches itself. When benzene undergoes electrophilic substitution, only one monosubstituted derivative of benzene is obtained, since all the six hydrogen atoms of benzene are equivalent. The electrophile joins a substituted benzene ring at positions where electron density is relatively high.

Orientation in monsubstituted benzenes : When a monosubstituted benzene molecule undergoes an electrophilic substitution reaction, the incoming electrophile ($E^{\oplus}$) may have three orientations *viz. ortho*, *meta* and *para* with respect to the substituent already present in the ring.

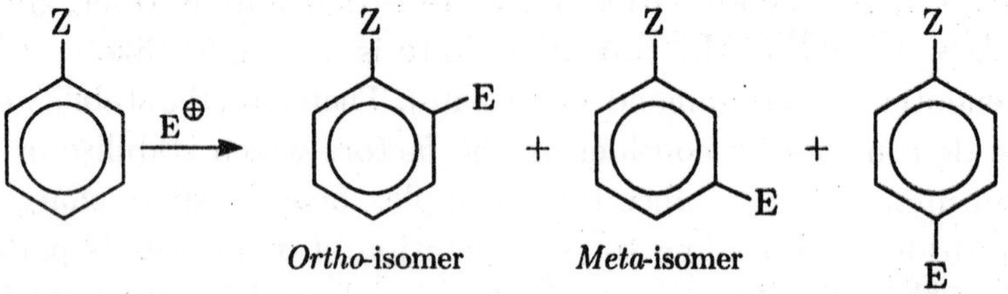

Ortho-isomer *Meta*-isomer *Para*-isomer

There are some groups which direct the incoming electrophile to take *o*- and *p*- positions and the substituents are called activating or *o*-/*p*-directing groups. Deactivating substituents (excluding halogens) direct the incoming electrophile to acquire *m*-position and are known as *m*-directing groups.

	Groups	*Electronic effect*	*Directing nature*
a.	$:\ddot{O}:^{\ominus}$	+R	*o*/*p*
	$-\ddot{N}R_2$, $\ddot{N}H_2$, $\ddot{O}H$, $\ddot{N}HCOR$	–I, +R	*o*/*p*
	$-\ddot{O}R$, $\ddot{S}R$, $\ddot{O}COR$, $:\ddot{F}:$, $\ddot{S}R$	–I, +R	*o*/*p*
b.	$-Me$, $-CH_2Me$, $-CHMe_2$	+I, hyperconjugative	*o*/*p*
	$-CMe_3$	+I	*o*/*p*
	$-CH{=}CH_2$	+I	*o*/*p*

Groups	*Electronic effect*	*Directing nature*
c. $\overset{\oplus}{N}H_3$, $\overset{\oplus}{N}R_3$, $\overset{\oplus}{S}R_2$, $\overset{\oplus}{P}R_3$	–I	*m*
CF_3, CCl_3		
d. NO_2, CN, SO_3H, COOH, SO_3R, COOR	–I, –R	*m*
$-B(OH)_2$, –CHO, –COR		

The *o/p* or *m*-directing nature of different groups may be explained by–

(a) Explanation on the basis of the stability of σ-complexes, and

(b) Explanation on the basis of charge distribution in the substrate.

1. ***Stability of the σ-complex and orientation effect*** : The greater is the stability of the σ-complex, the lower is the energy of activation of transition state and higher is the rate of reaction.

(i) *Ortho-para* directing groups have one electronegative element possessing at least a pair of non-bonded electrons in p-atomic orbital which undergoes pπ-pπ conjugation involving the aromatic ring but the electronegative element should not have any π-bond.

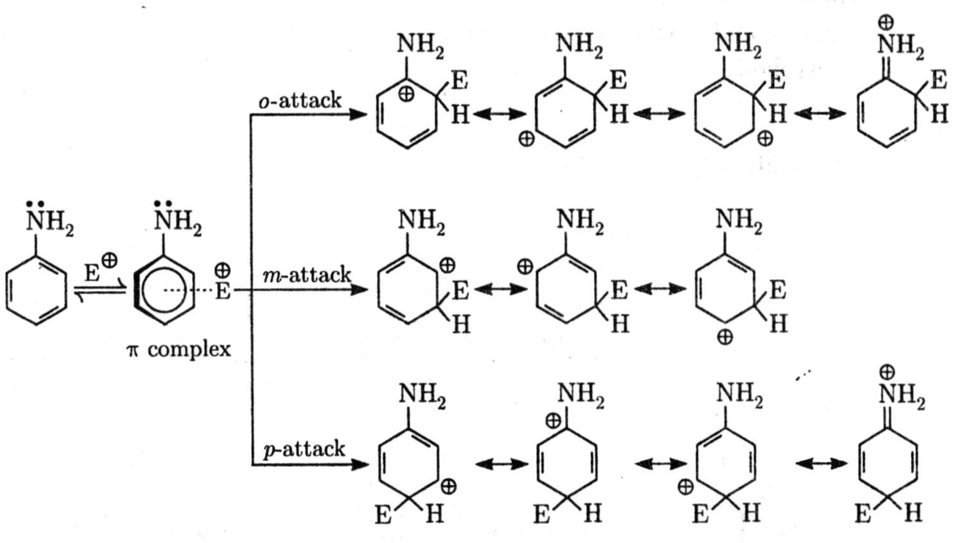

For *ortho* and *para* attack, higher number of resonating structures (four) are there compared to attack at the *meta* position (three resonating structures) for the sigma complex. So $\overset{\oplus}{E}$ will preferably attack *ortho* and *para* positions.

(ii) ***ortho-para directing nature due to hyperconjugation***

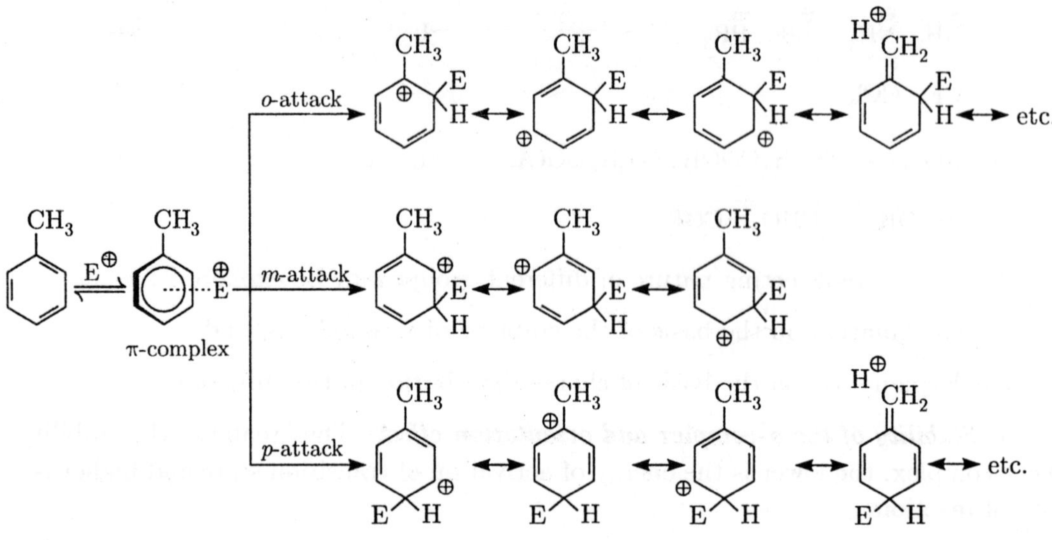

Here, *ortho* and *para* attack provide extra stable hyperconjugated resonating forms of σ-complex which are absent with *m*-attack, making *ortho*- and *para*-disubstituted product in major amount.

(iii) ***Ortho-para directing nature due to +R/–I effect of substituents*** : Nitration of chlorobenzene in the presence of concentrated HNO_3 and concentrated H_2SO_4 (mixed acid). Nitration reaction is an irreversible reaction and so is kinetically controlled.

$$HNO_3 + 2H_2SO_4 \rightleftharpoons \overset{\oplus}{N}O_2 + H_3\overset{\oplus}{O} + 2H\overset{\ominus}{S}O_4$$

(Active electrophile)

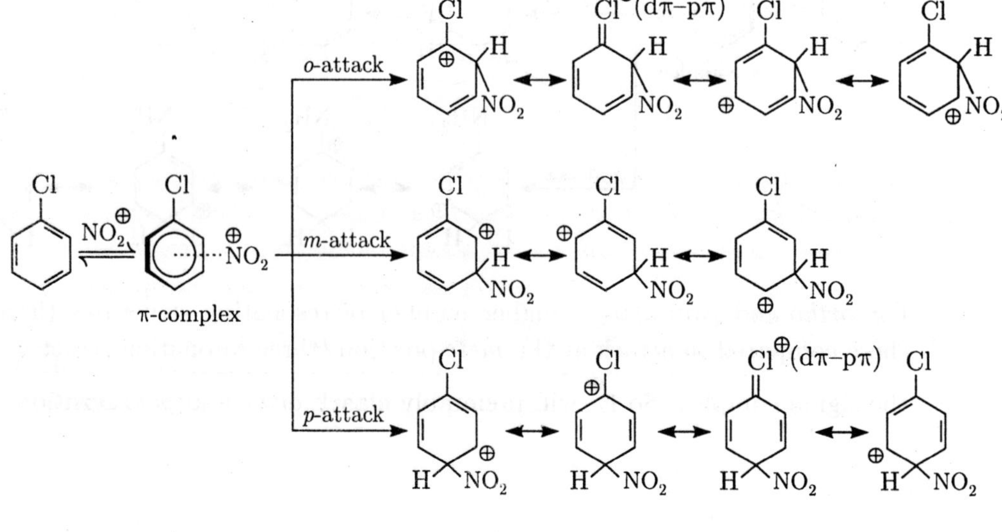

The stability of σ-complex due to *p*-attack is maximum as it contains more canonical structures (four), where one of the forms has extended delocalisation of positive charge. Regarding the difference in stability of the σ-complexes between *p*- and *o*- attack (both of them have four resonating structures), the former is more stable and requires less $\Delta G^{\neq}$ to be formed. The σ-complex formed by the *o*-attack experiences (1) steric interaction between the *ortho* groups, and (2) Less polarisability of the double bond due to –I effect of Cl atom. So the order of $\Delta G^{\neq}$ for the formation of three σ-complexes is as follows.

$$\Delta G^{\neq}_{para} < \Delta G^{\neq}_{ortho} < \Delta G^{\neq}_{meta}$$

The percentage of disubstituted products experimentally found is as follows.

para (~74%), *ortho* (~25%) and *meta* (~1%)

When Cl and other halogens like Br and I (exception is F) are present in the aromatic nucleus are known as groups which are *deactivating* (due to their –I effect) but *o/p*-directing.

Energy profile diagram for the nitration of chlorobenzene :

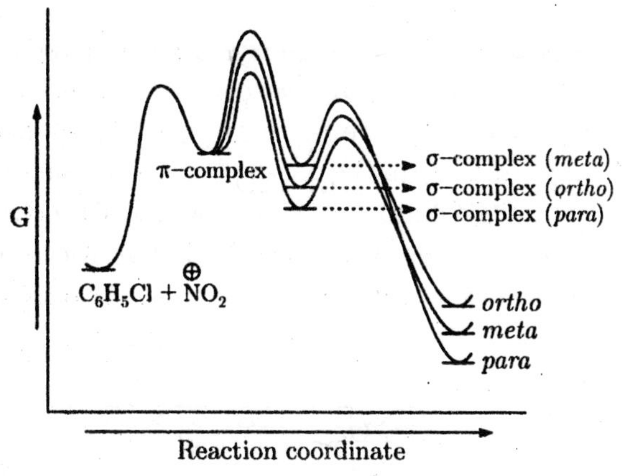

Fig. 3.4 :

(iv) ***Meta directing nature due to –R/–I containing substituents***

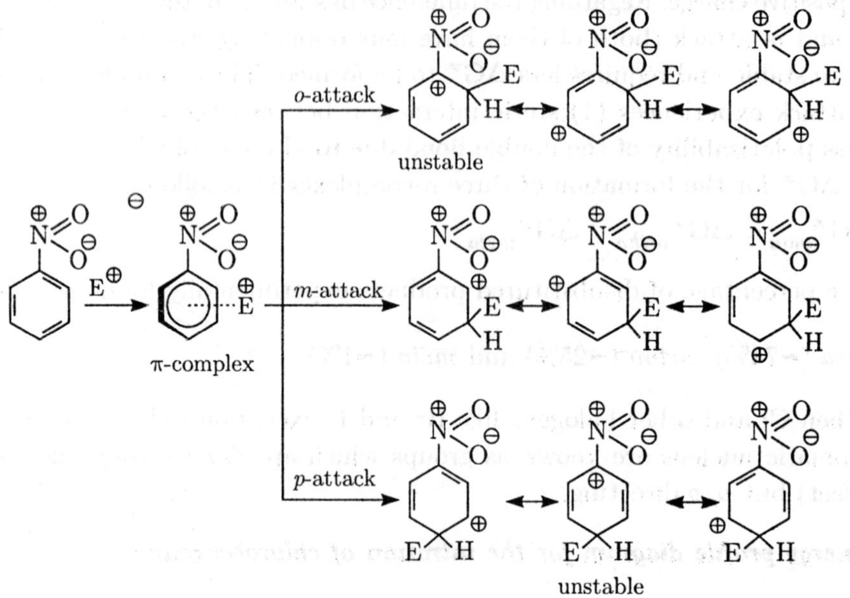

So we see that the stability of σ-complex due to *m*-attack is more compared to the σ-complexes formed by *ortho* and *para* attack. In the former case, there is no such unstable cannonical structure where two positive charges reside on adjacent atoms. So $\Delta G^{\neq}$ required to form the σ-complex is minimum for the *m*-substitution and *m*-isomer becomes the major product. If we consider the canonical structures of the substrate (nitrobenzene), we will find that the *m*-position is relatively electron dense and so electrophilic substitution is favoured at this position.

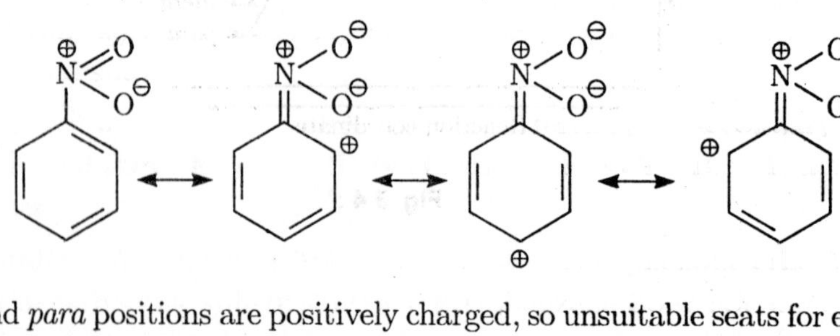

Ortho and *para* positions are positively charged, so unsuitable seats for electrophilic substitution but the *m*-position, which is electrically neutral, comparatively more electron dense with respect to *o*- and *p*-positions. This makes the *m*-substitution more preferable for nitrobenzene. $-NO_2$ group may be replaced by groups with –R effect like $-B(OR)_2$, $\overset{\oplus}{P}R_3$, $\overset{\oplus}{S}R_2$, –CHO, –COR, –COOH, $-CO_2R$, –CN, $-SO_3H$, $-SO_2Cl$ etc.

***Problem* 1** : The spectrum of chlorination of ^{14}C–labelled benzene is as follows.

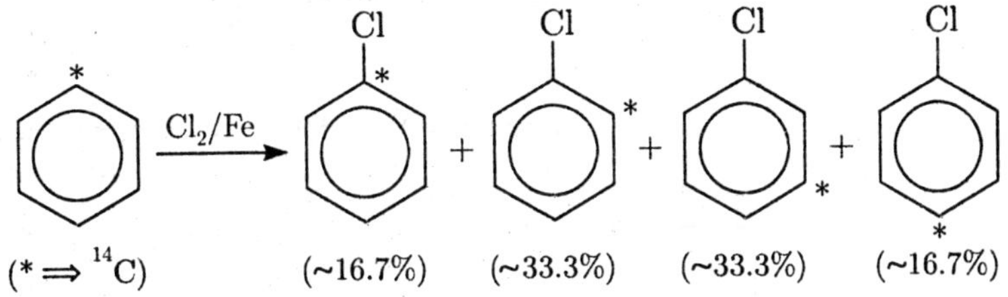

Explain the nature of scattering of labelled carbon

Ans. : As all the six carbon atoms of a benzene molecule are equivalent, monochlorination occurs with equal probability at all the six carbon atoms. Two equivalent *ortho* positions, two equivalent *meta* positions, one *para* position and one labelled carbon atom are there where chlorination is done with equivalent probability. Thus, the spectrum of chlorination of benzene is justified.

***Problem* 2** : Reaction of methyl chloride (CH_3Cl) with toluene in the presence of $AlCl_3$ as a Lewis acid catalyst. Predict the major product with reason.

Ans. : In presence of $AlCl_3$ (a Lewis acid catalyst), the reaction between CH_3Cl and toluene is of *reversible nature*, and the three isomeric products are *o*-xylene, *m*-xylene and *p*-xylene, $H^{\oplus}$ may react again with these xylenes. The σ-complex which leads to the formation of *m*-xylene is the most stable one as the positive charge is stabilised by +I effect of two adjacent methyl groups and hyperconjugative effects. On the other hand, σ-complexes leading to *o*- and *p*- xylenes are stabilised by only one methyl group. At room temperature, alkylation of aromatic nucleus is a thermodynamically controlled reaction and so *meta*-xylene forms the corresponding σ-complex most rapidly in the equilibrium.

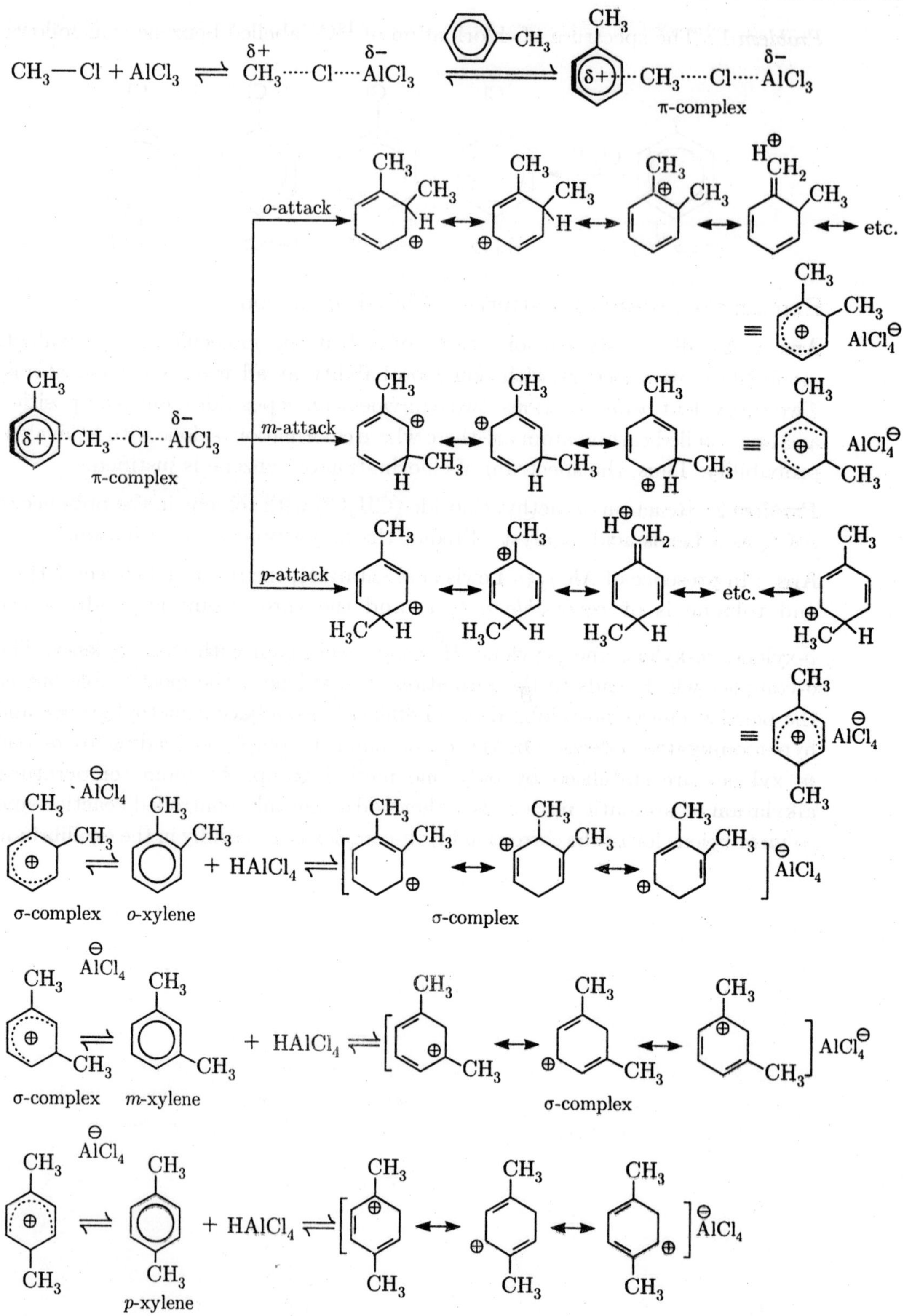
π-complex
o-attack
m-attack
p-attack
etc.
σ-complex
o-xylene
m-xylene
p-xylene

After the completion of the reaction, we get *m*- xylene as a chief product in the equilibrium upon addition of water.

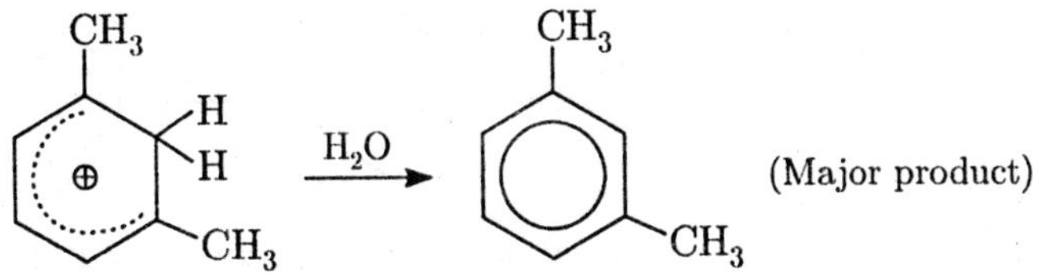

As alkylation reaction is reversible, three *situations* may arise.

(a) One isomer may get converted to another by [1, 2]-shift.

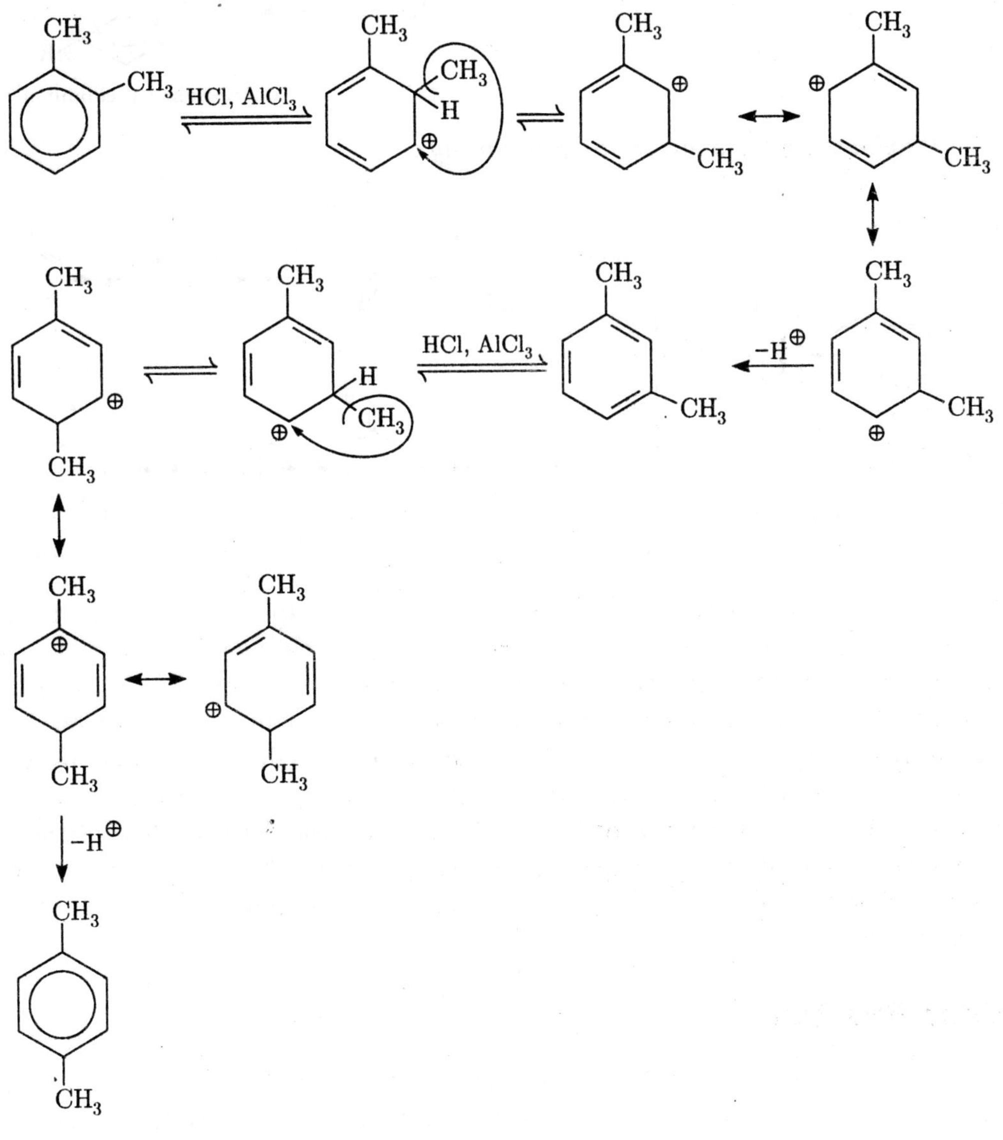

(b) Dealkylation reaction may occur to produce lower homologue.

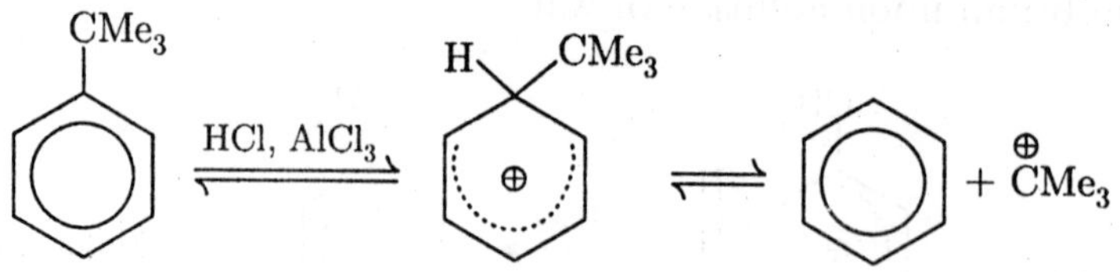

(c) The carbocation produced upon dealkylation reaction can react further to produce a higher homologue.

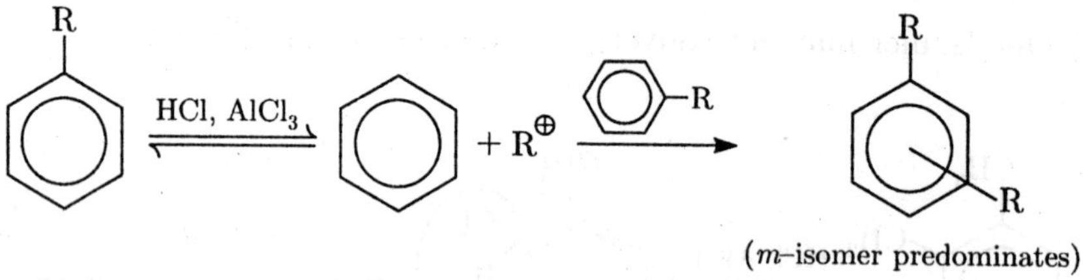

Vinyl and aryl groups are o-/p-orienting :

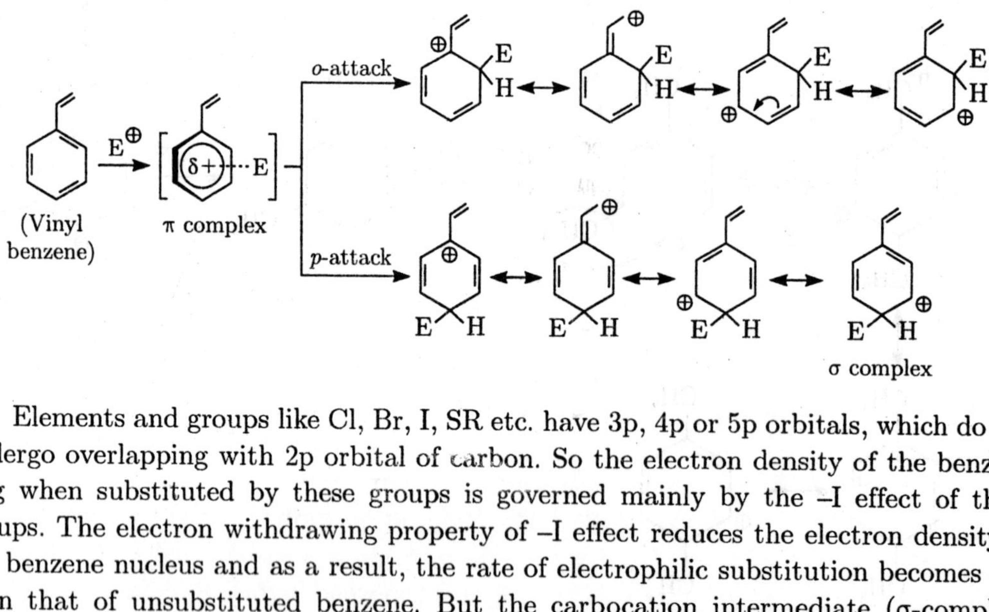

Elements and groups like Cl, Br, I, SR etc. have 3p, 4p or 5p orbitals, which do not undergo overlapping with 2p orbital of carbon. So the electron density of the benzene ring when substituted by these groups is governed mainly by the –I effect of these groups. The electron withdrawing property of –I effect reduces the electron density of the benzene nucleus and as a result, the rate of electrophilic substitution becomes less than that of unsubstituted benzene. But the carbocation intermediate (σ-complex) polarises the 3p or 4p orbitals of Cl, Br, SR etc. and the delocalisation of the positive charge occurs by sidewise overlap. So although Cl, Br, SR, I etc. reduce the reactivity of benzene ring towards electrophilic substitution when present as substituents, they are all *o-/p*-orienting.

Ortho–Para Ratio

When a benzene ring contains a substituent which is *o-/p*-directing, the ratio of *o*-product to *p*-product in an ArS_E2 reaction depends on the following factors :

(a) ***Statistical factor*** : Regarding the probability of collision between aromatic substrate and electrophile at the *ortho-* and *para* positions is 2:1. When both the aromatic substrate and the electrophile are reactive, the rate of product formation depends on the probability of collision between the two and so the production of *ortho* isomer becomes higher. At a higher temperature, the energy levels of both substrate and electrophile get increased and energy difference between the transition state and substrate or electrophile decreases. As a result, the statistical factor becomes important and the rate of formation of *o*-product increases.

(b) ***Relative charge density*** : The relative charge densities at the *o-* and *p-* positions are controlled by the electronic factors of the substituents already present in the ring and the difference between the bond polarisabilities at the two positions. If the electron density increases, then the polarisability increases (as σ-complex is positively charged) and the rate of the reaction also increases. On the other hand, with poor electron charge density, the polarisability of the bond decreases ($\Delta G^{\neq}$ becomes higher) and the rate of the reaction decreases. For example, the rate of production of *o-* and *p-* nitrohalobenzene depends on the relative electron density at the *o-* and *p-* positions of halobenzene. Halogens have –I effect, so the electron density at the *o-* position becomes less dense compared to that in the *p-* position. Depending on the type of halogen atom (*i.e.*, with increasing –I effect), the electron density at the *o-* position decreases and the percentage of production of *p-* product increases.

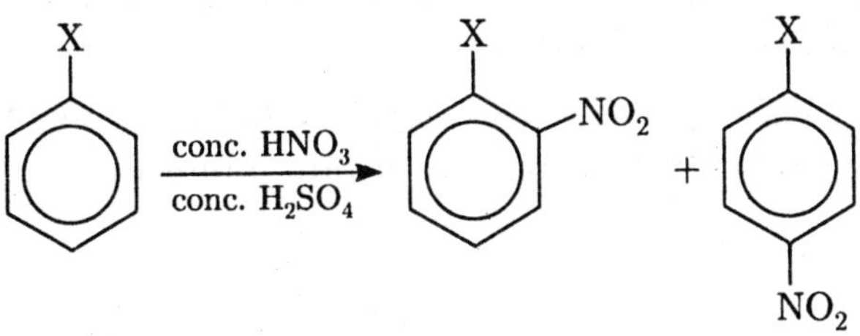

X	*o*	*p*
F	16%	84%
Cl	25%	75%
Br	30%	70%
I	35%	65%

(c) ***Steric interaction*** : The percentage of production of *o-* product may decrease due to steric repulsion between the substituent and attacking electrophile at the *o-* position (*ortho* effect).

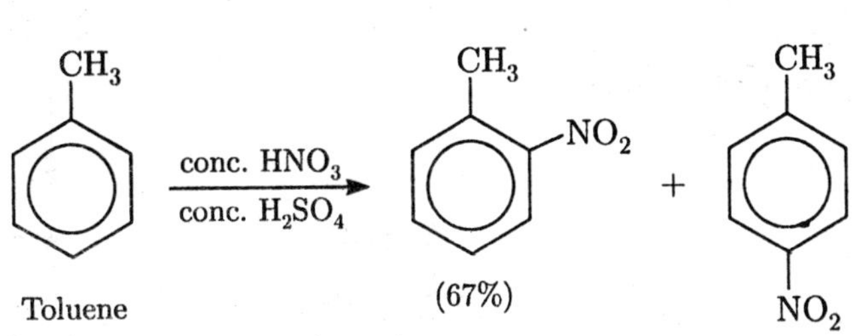

Toluene (67%) (33%)

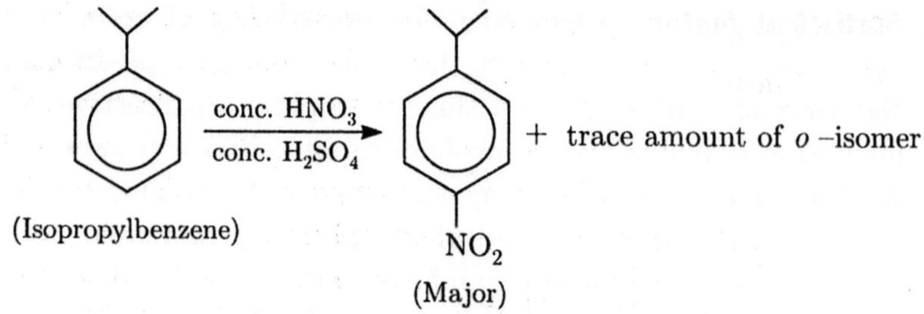

(d) ***Electrostatic factor*** : The incoming electrophile and the substituent already present may face electrostatic force of attraction before the bond breaks. As a result, the rate of formation of *ortho* prouct increases.

When sodium phenoxide reacts with carbon dioxide (CO_2), mainly sodium salicylate is produced. CO_2 gets absorbed by the electric field of $Na^{\oplus}$ ion and the *ortho* product predominates through the formation of a six-membered chelate.

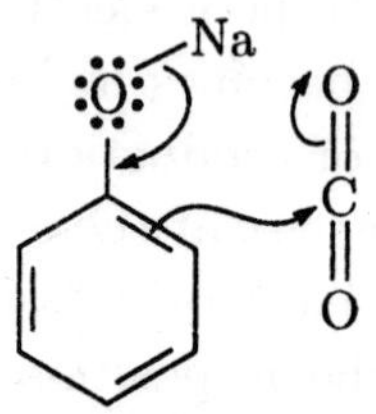

But potassium phenoxide in a similar reaction produces *p*- product as the major one. The size of $K^{\oplus}$ being large, the effect of electric field becomes poor and as a result, CO_2 can not get absorbed.

If the group attached to the benzene nucleus has nucleophilic character, then nitration with nitric anhydride or acyl nitrate produces *o*- nitrobenzene as the major product.

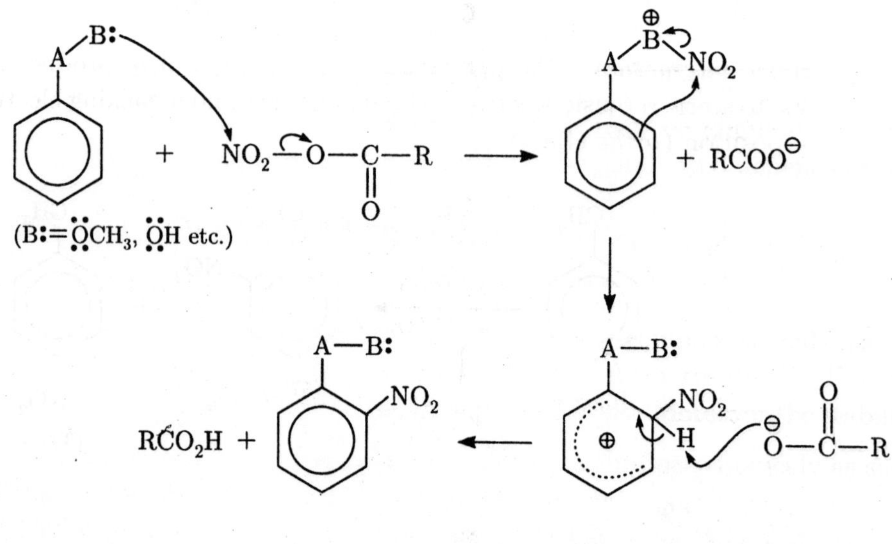

This is the reason why

(i) When $C_6H_5CH_2\ddot{\underset{..}{O}}CH_3$ is nitrated with mixed acid (conc. HNO_3+ conc. H_2SO_4), *p*-nitro derivative is formed as the major product but with (Ac_2O + conc. HNO_3) as nitrating agent, *o*-isomer becomes the major product.

(ii) Acetanilide reacts with HNO_3 and Ac_2O to produce mainly *ortho*- nitroacetanilide but produces *p*-nitroacetanilide with mixed acid (conc. HNO_3 + conc. H_2SO_4). Again if the latter nitration (with mixed acid) is carried out at room temperature, *p*-isomer still remains the major product but the percentage of *o*-product increases.

(e) ***Stability of the intermediate*** : If the intermediate in an ArS_E2 reaction gets stability on chelation through hydrogen bonding, then *ortho* product will predominate. Sodium phenoxide reacts with CO_2 to produce sodium salicylate as the major product, where the intermediate gets stabilisation through chelation.

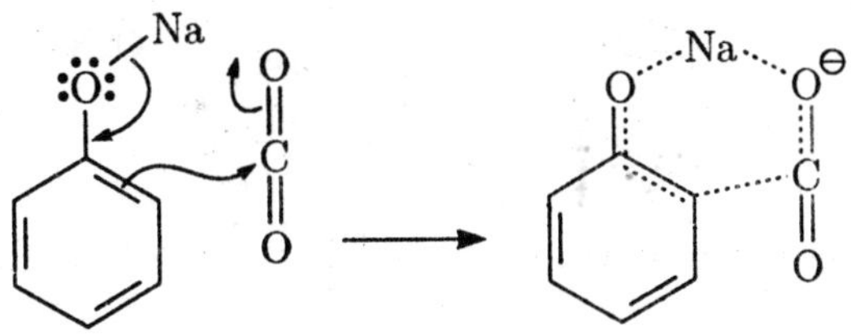

(Intermediate chelate)

The intermediate formed from potassium phenoxide cannot have an intermediate chelate. The size of $K^{\oplus}$ being larger than $Na^{\oplus}$, it can not substitute itself in a small cagelike intermediate as shown above. For this reason, potassium phenoxide reacts with CO_2 to form potassium parahydroxybenzoate as the major product.

Polysubstitution in Aromatic Compounds

(a) If two substituents are present in the benzene ring, then further substitution will be controlled by the more electron donating group. For example in *p*- chlorophenol, OH group is more electron donating than Cl although both of them are *o*/*p*- orienting. So, when *p*- chlorophenol is nitrated with mixed acid, 4-chloro-2-nitrophenol will be the major product.

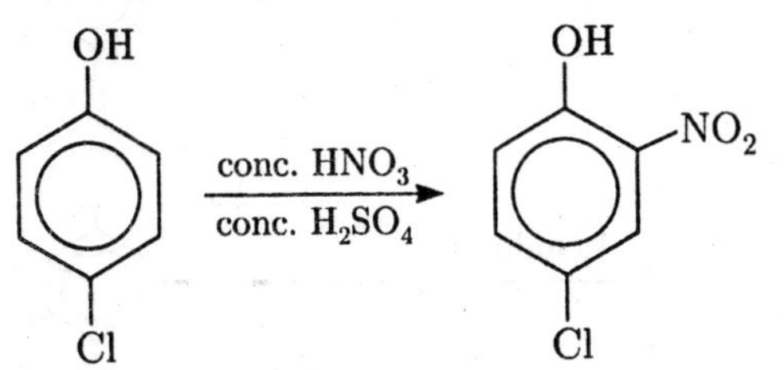

(b) If the benzene nucleus contains two electron withdrawing substituents then the positions *o*- and *p*- to the more electron withdrawing group will have low electron density and so the rate of electrophilic substitution will be less. In these cases, further substitution occurs at the *m*- position to the more electron withdrawing substituent.

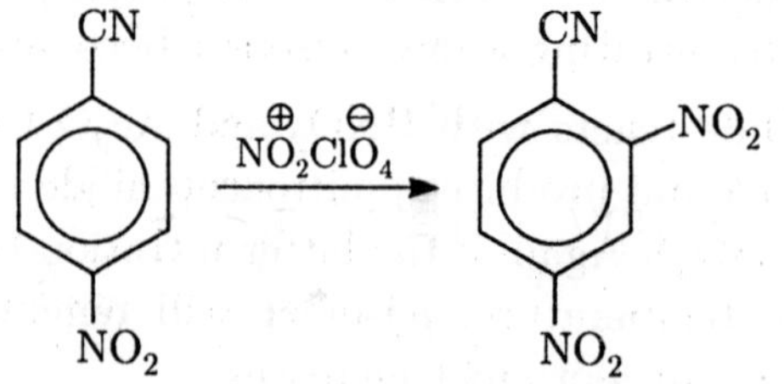

(c) If the benzene ring contains one electron donating and another electron withdrawing substituent, then further substitution will be controlled by electron donating group.

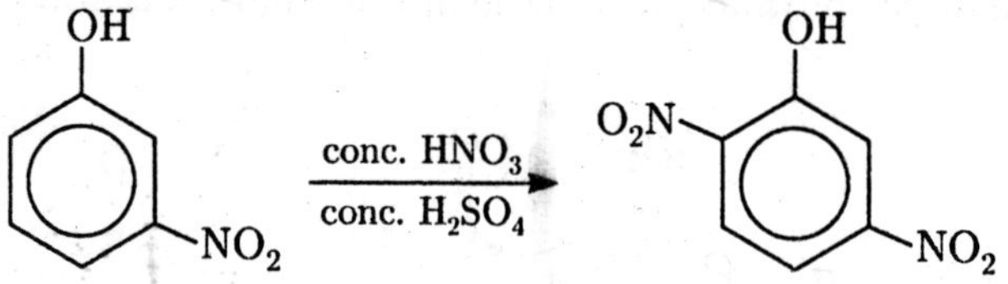

(d) Apart from electronic factors, steric factors also play important roles.

(i)

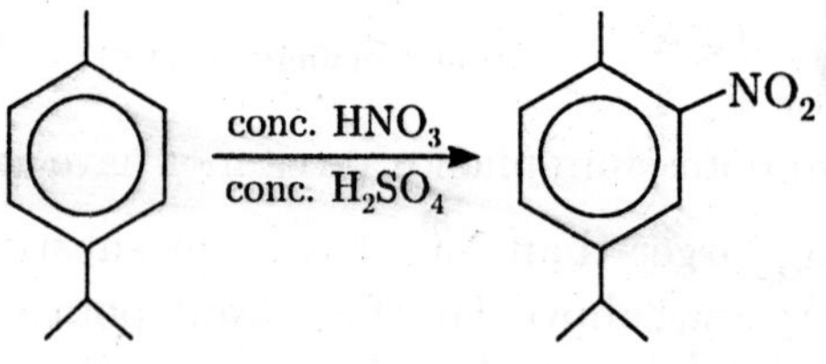

(ii)

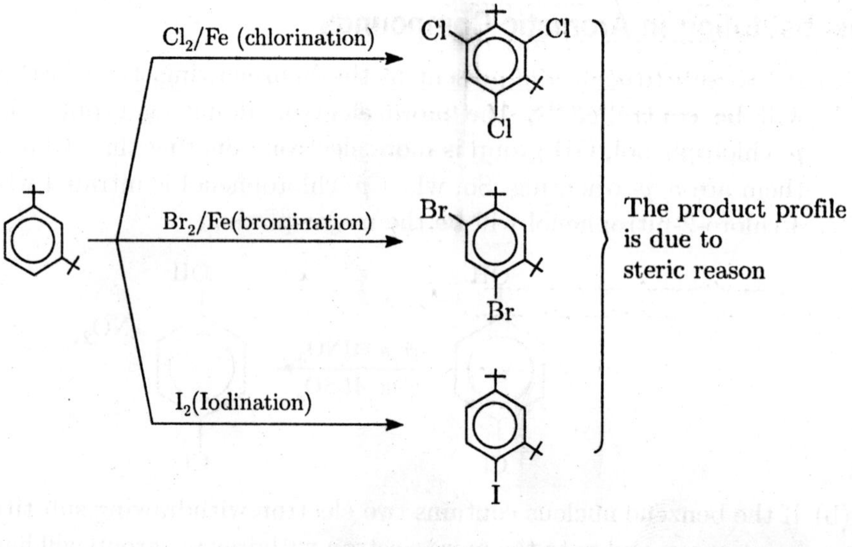

(e) If the substrate contains more than one aromatic rings, then the position of electrophilic substitution will be determined either by chemical reactivity or relative electron density of a particular benzene ring.

4-nitrobiphenyl on nitration produces dinitrobiphenyl where second $-NO_2$ group joins the benzene ring which does not contain electron withdrawing NO_2 group. Nitrophenyl group is *o*/*p*- orientating, so the major product becomes 4,4′–dinitrobiphenyl.

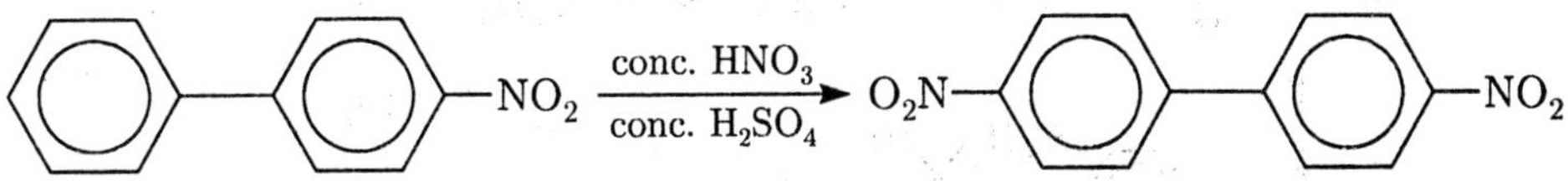

(4–4′–dinitrobiphenyl)

Radical Addition to the Aromatic π-Bonds

(a) If the attacking radical is reactive, the addition of radical occurs in a stepwise manner.

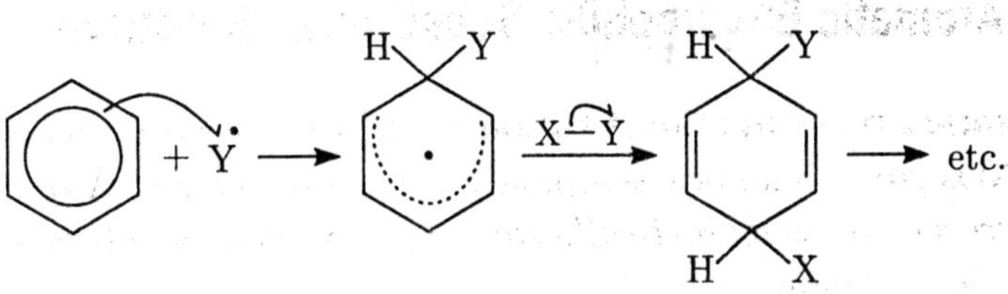

Example :

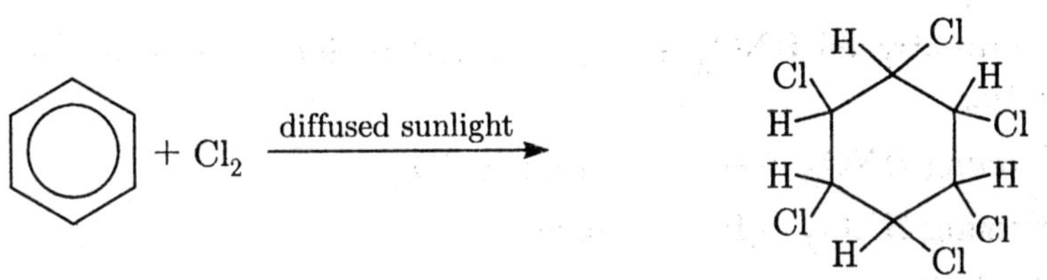

(1,2,3,4,5,6 – hexachlorocyclohexane)

(b) 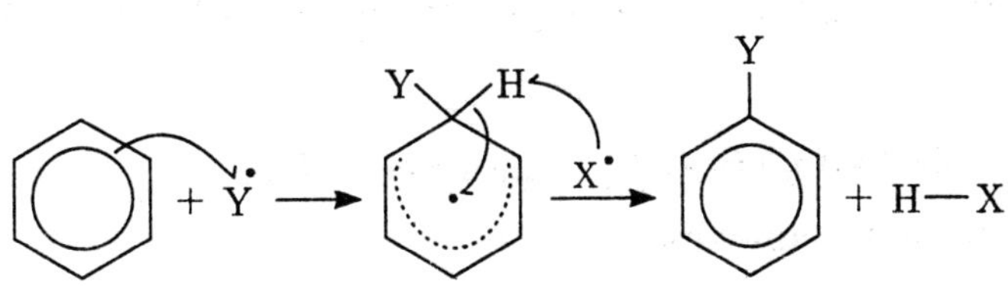

Example :

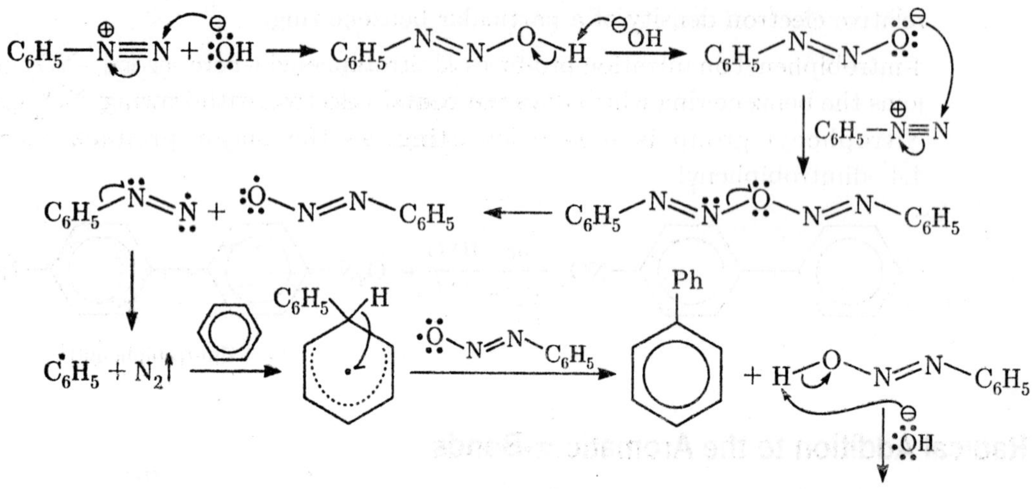

etc. (chain reaction)

Individual Aromatic Electrophilic Substitution Reactions

1. ***Nitration reaction*** : Substitution of a hydrogen atom in an aromatic nucleus by a $-NO_2$ group is known as aromatic nitration reaction. Aromatic nitration reaction is *irreversible and kinetically controlled.* Several *nitrating agents* for the reaction are gieven below.

   (a) concentrated HNO_3 + glacial acetic acid

   (b) Dilute nitric acid

   (c) (concentrated HNO_3 + concentrated H_2SO_4) is mixed acid (M. A.) in 1:1 ratio.

   (d) Fuming HNO_3 + concentrated H_2SO_4

   (e) Fuming HNO_3 + fuming H_2SO_4

   (f) Acyl nitrate (*e.g.*, acetyl nitrate or benzoyl nitrate) in organic solvents

   (g) Nitronium salts like $\overset{\oplus}{N}O_2\overset{\ominus}{BF_4}$ (nitronium fluoborate) or nitronium perchlorate $(\overset{\oplus}{NO_2}\,\overset{\ominus}{ClO_4})$

   (h) Nitrogen pentoxide (N_2O_5) in CCl_4 in presence of P_2O_5

   (i) Fuming HNO_3 in acetic anhydride

   Among the nitrating agents, **mixed acid** (concentrated HNO_3 + concentrated H_2SO_4) is the most **common nitrating agent**, while the others are used depending on varying substrates.

A wide range of aromatic substrates undergo nitration reaction, *e.g.*,

(a) aromatic hydrocarbons like benzene, toluene, naphthalene etc.

(b) Halobenzenes, phenols, phenolic ethers, amines, amides.

(c) Nitrobenzene, aromatic carboxylic and sulphonic acids.

(d) Heterocyclic compounds like furan, pyridine, thiophene, quinoline etc.

The nitrating agents and conditions vary from substrate to substrate. Benzene nucleus containing activating group requires mild nitrating agents and conditions, while aromatic compounds containing deactivating groups demand strong nitrating agents and vigorous conditions.

Some examples of aromatic nitration reaction

1.

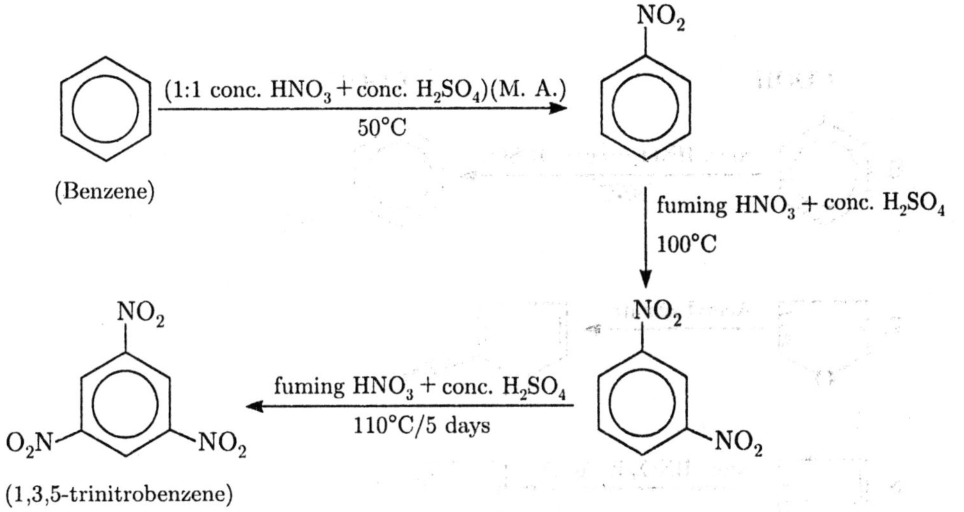

2.

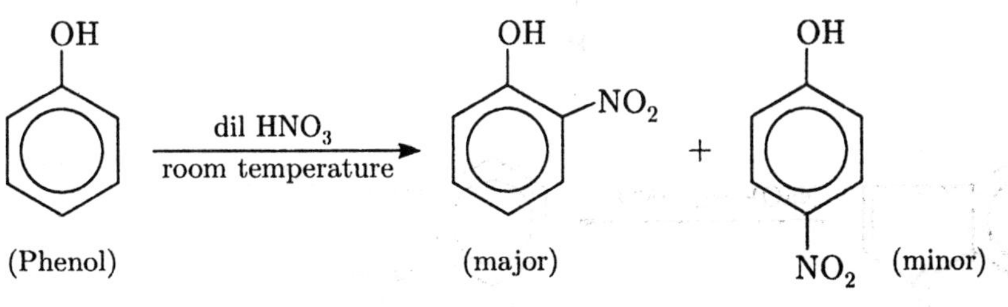

3.

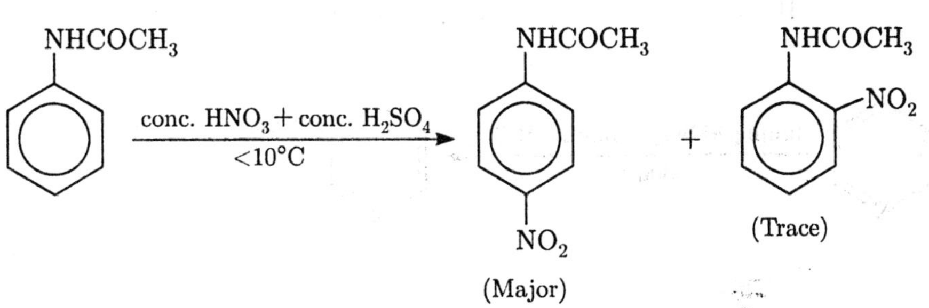

4. 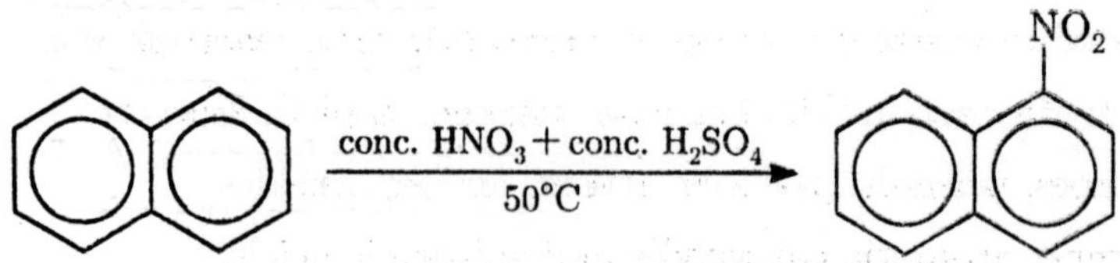
NO$_2$
conc. HNO$_3$ + conc. H$_2$SO$_4$
50°C

5. 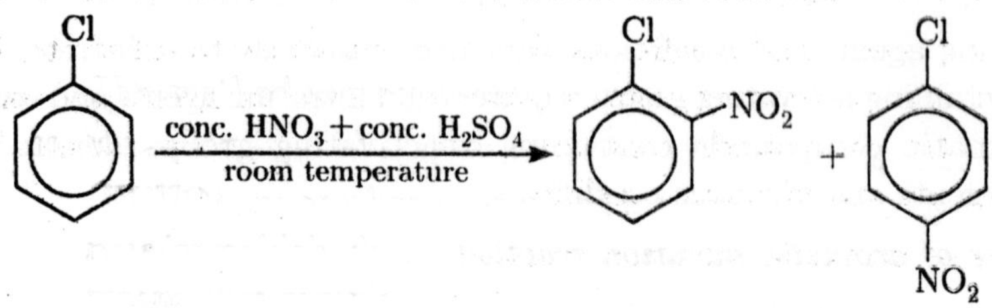
Cl
conc. HNO$_3$ + conc. H$_2$SO$_4$
room temperature
Cl
NO$_2$
+
Cl
NO$_2$

6. 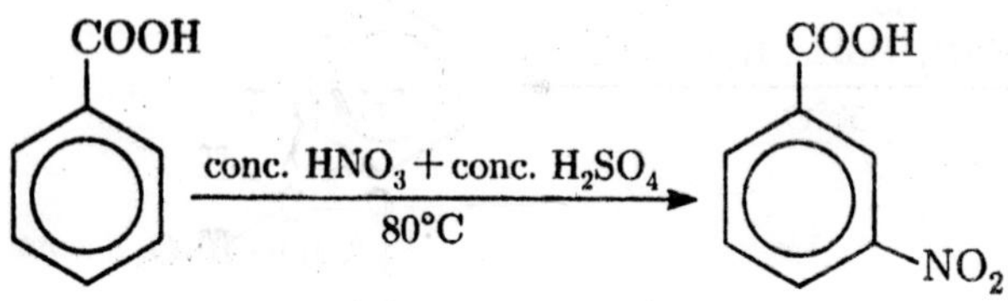
COOH
conc. HNO$_3$ + conc. H$_2$SO$_4$
80°C
COOH
NO$_2$

7. 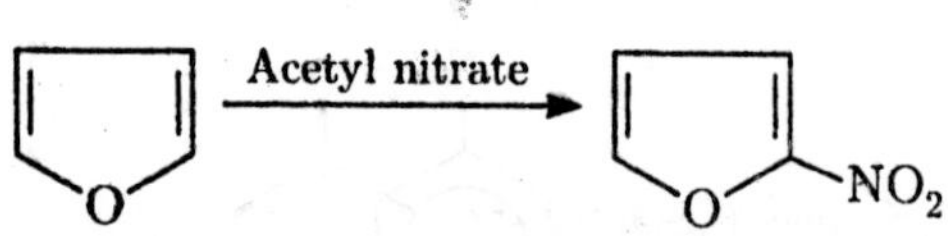
O
Acetyl nitrate
O
NO$_2$

8. 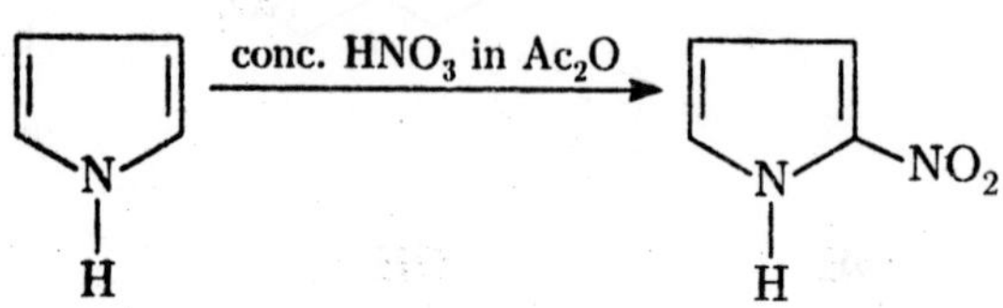
N
H
conc. HNO$_3$ in Ac$_2$O
N
H
NO$_2$

9. 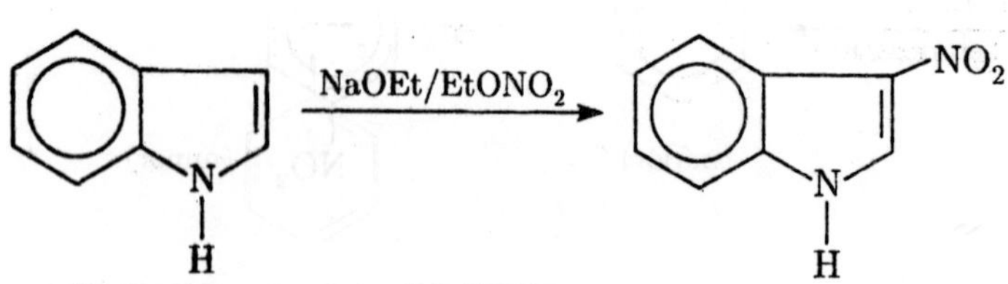
N
H
NaOEt/EtONO$_2$
NO$_2$
N
H

10. 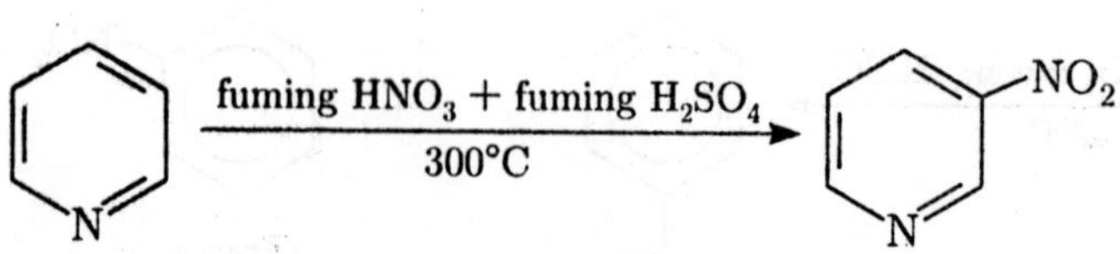
N
fuming HNO$_3$ + fuming H$_2$SO$_4$
300°C
NO$_2$
N

11. 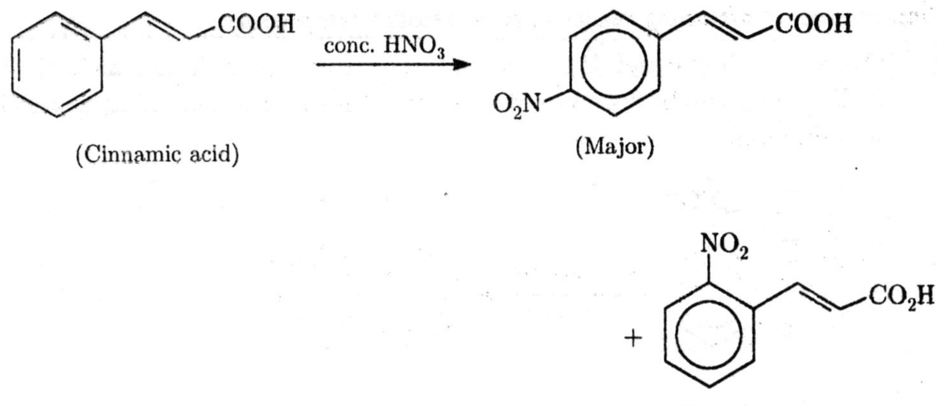

Cinnamic acid on nitration gives *o*- and *p*- nitrocinnamic acids (major is *p*-isomer), although $-CO_2H$ group is *meta* directing.

Mechanism of nitration of cinnamic acid : In order to explain the formation of *o*- and *p*-nitrocinnamic acid, we have to consider the stability of various carbonium ions.

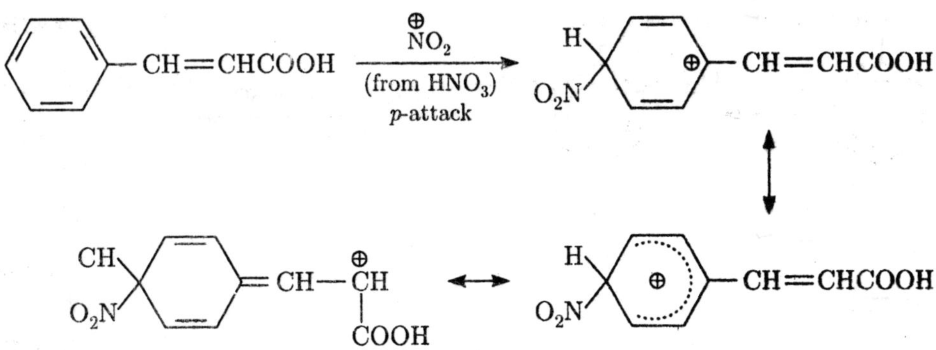

Only in the *o*- and *p*- carbonium ions, the spreading of positive charge to the side chain possible, not in *m*-caronium ion. As a result, *o*- and *p*- carbonium ions are more stable.

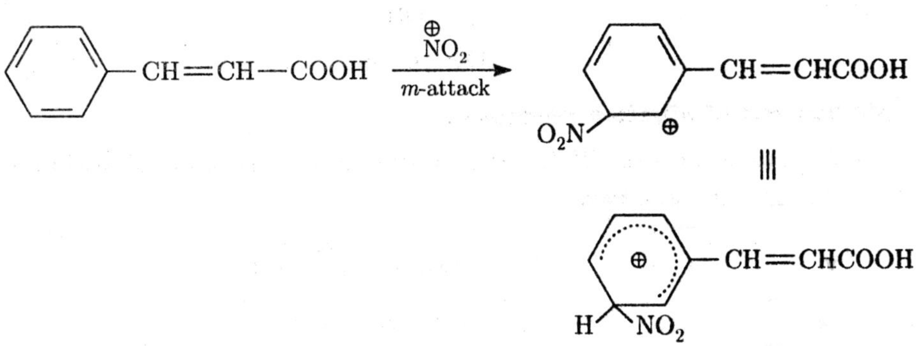

(This σ-complex is not formed)

Importance of nitration reaction in aromatic compounds :

(a) There is no simple and direct method of introducing $-NH_2$ group in the benzene nucleus. This can be done first by nitration (introduction of $-NO_2$ group) followed by reduction.

(i) 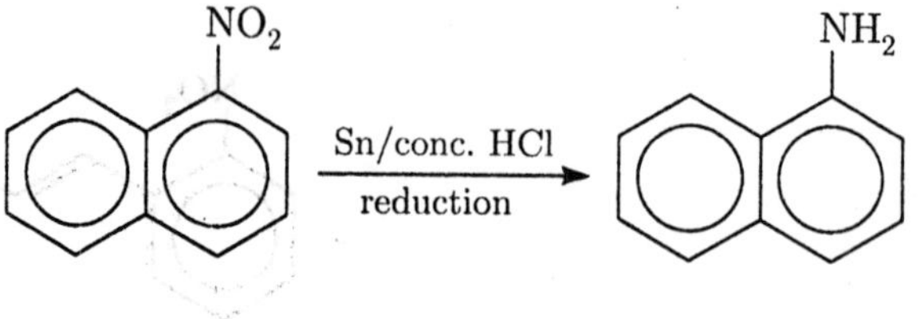

(ii) 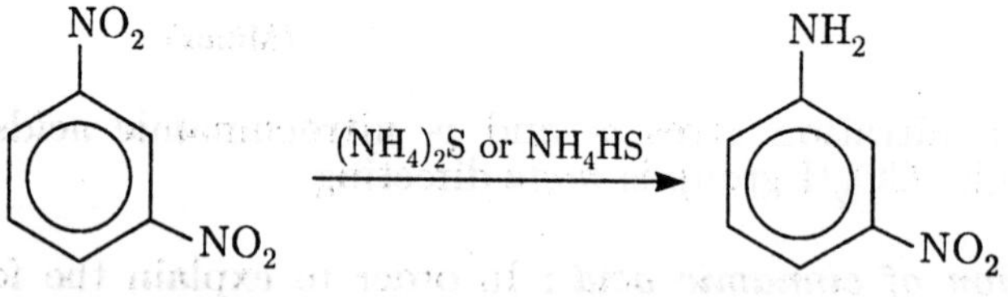

(iii) Preparation of phloroglucinol

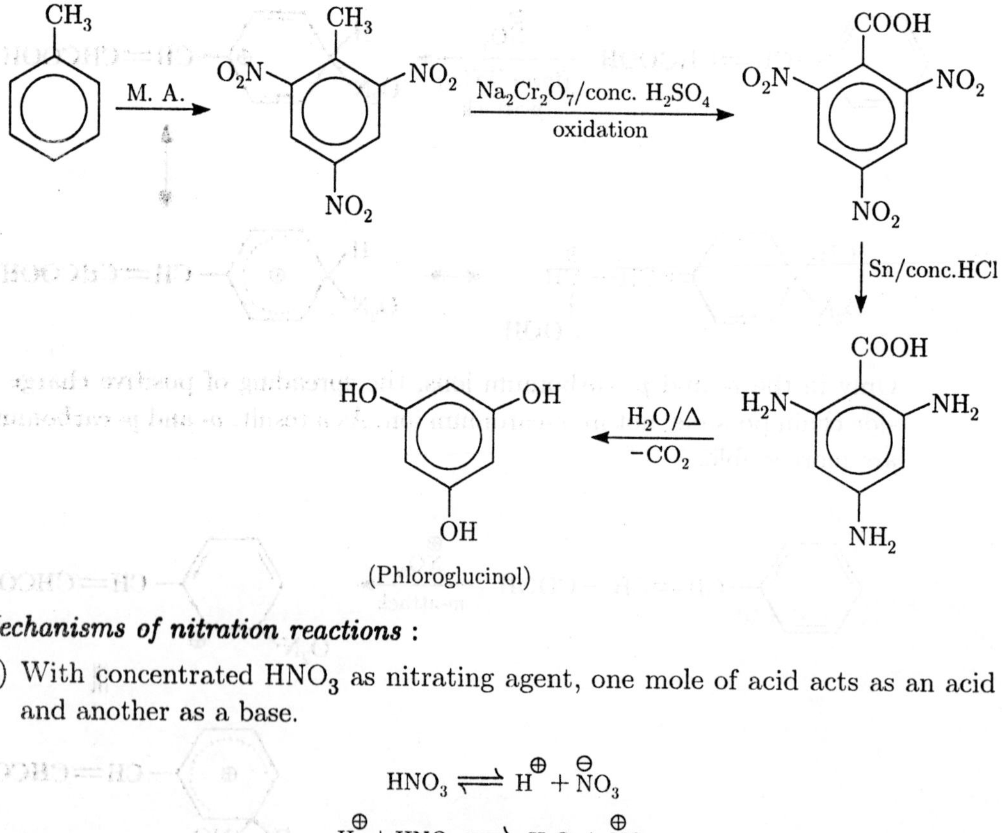

Mechanisms of nitration reactions :

(a) With concentrated HNO_3 as nitrating agent, one mole of acid acts as an acid and another as a base.

$$HNO_3 \rightleftharpoons \overset{\oplus}{H} + \overset{\ominus}{NO_3}$$

$$\overset{\oplus}{H} + HNO_3 \rightleftharpoons H_2O + \overset{\oplus}{NO_2}$$

$$2HNO_3 \rightleftharpoons \overset{\ominus}{NO_3} + H_2O + \overset{\oplus}{NO_2}$$

Although the equilibrium shifts to the left, enough nitronium ions are always there ($\overset{\oplus}{N}O_2$ ion) to ensure nitration reaction.

(b) With mixed acid (concentrated HNO_3 + concentrated H_2SO_4), an acid base reaction is found. Here H_2SO_4 acts as an acid and HNO_3 acts as a base. The ionisation in both the cases is essentially complete.

$$H_2SO_4 \rightleftharpoons \overset{\oplus}{H} + HSO_4^{\ominus}$$

$$HNO_3 + \overset{\oplus}{H} \rightleftharpoons H_2O + \overset{\oplus}{N}O_2$$

$$H_2O + H_2SO_4 \rightleftharpoons H_3O^{\oplus} + HSO_4^{\ominus}$$

$$HNO_3 + 2H_2SO_4 \rightleftharpoons H_3O^{\oplus} + \overset{\oplus}{N}O_2 + 2H_2SO_4^{\ominus}$$

(c) With dinitrogen pentoxide as nitrating agent, the electrophile ($\overset{\oplus}{N}O_2$) is generated through spontaneous dissociation.

$$N_2O_5 \rightleftharpoons \overset{\oplus}{N}O_2\,\overset{\ominus}{N}O_3 \rightleftharpoons \overset{\oplus}{N}O_2 + \overset{\ominus}{N}O_3$$

(d) Nitronium fluo-or hydrofluoborate or nitronium perchlorate dissociates to produce $\overset{\oplus}{N}O_2$ ion, the active electrophile.

$$\overset{\oplus}{NO_2}\,HBF_4^{\ominus} \rightleftharpoons \overset{\oplus}{N}O_2 + H\overset{\ominus}{B}F_4$$

$$\overset{\oplus}{NO_2}\,\overset{\ominus}{ClO_4} \rightleftharpoons \overset{\oplus}{N}O_2 + \overset{\ominus}{Cl}O_4$$

(e) Nitration with acyl nitrate (*e.g.*, acetyl nitrate $-HNO_3/Ac_2O$), the mechanism of nitration is uncertain due to uncertainty of nature of nitrating species.

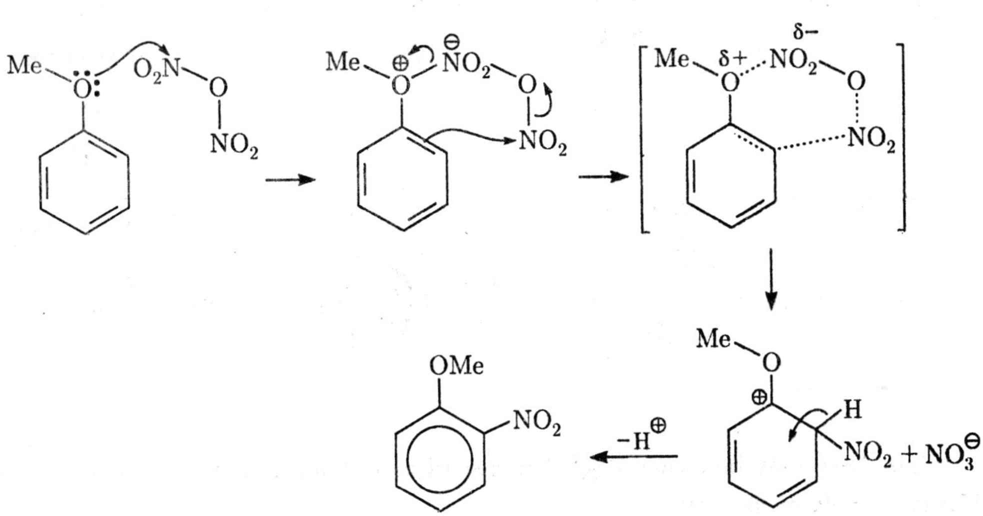

The followings have been proposed like CH_3COONO_2, $CH_3CO\overset{\overset{H}{|}\oplus}{O}—NO_2$, N_2O_5, $NO^{\oplus}$ etc. An interesting feature of this reagent is the unusually high percentage of *o*-isomer that is obtained when the side chain contains a heteroatom. Anisole with mixed acid forms 31% *o*-nitroanisole but with HNO_3/Ac_2O 71% *o*-nitroanisole is formed. One explanation is the involvement of dinitrogen pentoxide as an active electrophile which reacts *via* a six centre rearrangement.

(f) When the reagent is dilute HNO_3, nitrosonium ion ($NO^{\oplus}$) is formed, which is the active electrophile.

$$HNO_3 \rightleftharpoons \overset{\oplus}{H} + \overset{\ominus}{NO_3}$$

HNO_3 + organic compound → HNO_2 + oxidised organic compound.

$$HO—N{=}O + H^{\oplus} \rightleftharpoons \underset{\text{(Nitrosonium ion)}}{\overset{\oplus}{NO}} + H_2O$$

(g) With more dilute HNO_3, probably nitracidium cation is involved in nitration reaction, Nitracidium cation is less active than nitronium cation.

$$2HNO_3 \rightleftharpoons \underset{\text{(Nitracidium cation)}}{H_2NO_3^{\oplus}} + NO_3^{\ominus}$$

Mechanistic pathway :

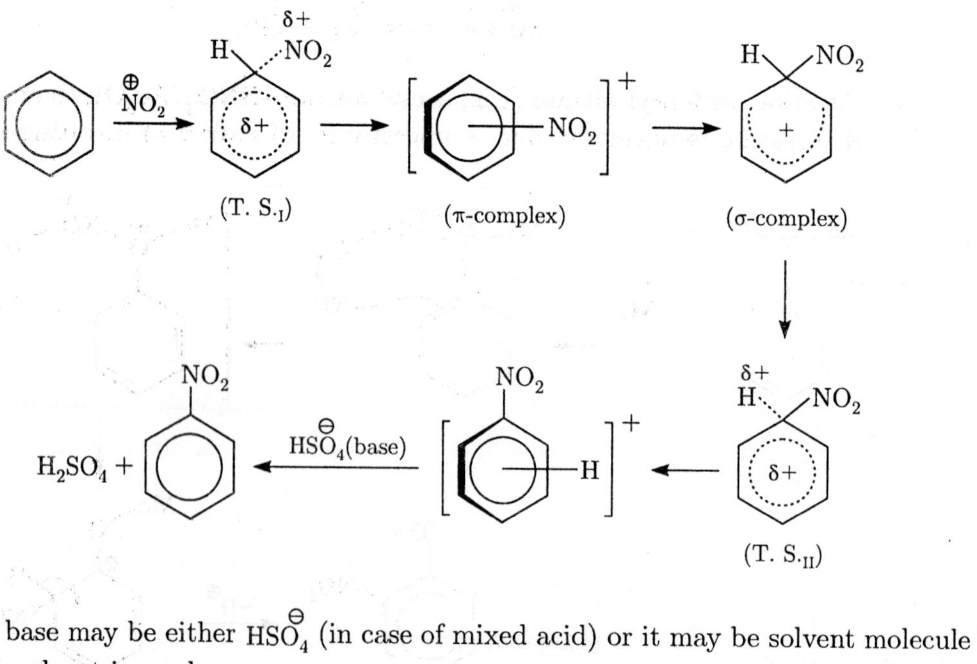

The base may be either $\overset{\ominus}{HSO_4}$ (in case of mixed acid) or it may be solvent molecule if organic solvent is used.

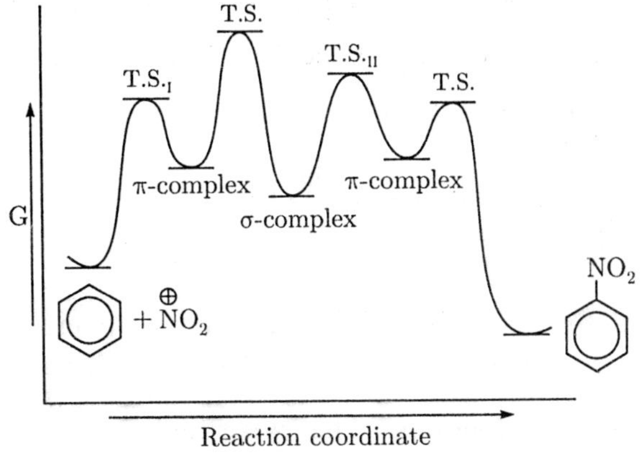

Fig. 3.5 :

The order of nitration reaction in aromatic compounds may follow zero order, first order or fractional order depending on the nature of the substrate.

(a) The zero order or pseudo zero order reacn is followed by substrates which are more reactive than benzene itself. Here, the reversible formation of $NO_2^{\oplus}$ ion is *slower* than the electrophilic attack step. As a result, the formation of nitronium ion becomes rate limiting. Electrophilic attack by $NO_2^{\oplus}$ becomes insignificant and the reaction follows a zero order reaction. Toluene and xylene show zero order regarding their nitration reactions.

(b) First order reaction is followed by the substrates which are less reactive than benzene. In this case, formation of nitronium ion is fast and electrophilic attack by $NO_2^{\oplus}$ ion is slow. So the electrophilic attack step is rate limiting and a first order kinetics is observed with respect to substrate.

Rate=k[substrate]

Nitration of ethyl benzoate, nitrobenzene.etc. follow first order kinetics.

(c) Fractional order kinetics (between 0 and 1) is followed by substrates of intermediate activity. Nitration of chlorobenzene follows fractional order kinetics.

Supports in favour of $NO_2^{\oplus}$ ion as an attacking electrophile :

(a) When concentrated HNO_3 is added to a cold solution of H_2SO_4, the freezing point of H_2SO_4 gets lowered by four fold. Four ions are detected in the mixed acid solution.

$$HNO_3 + 2H_2SO_4 \longrightarrow 2HSO_4^{\ominus} + \overset{\oplus}{N}O_2 + H_3\overset{\oplus}{O}$$

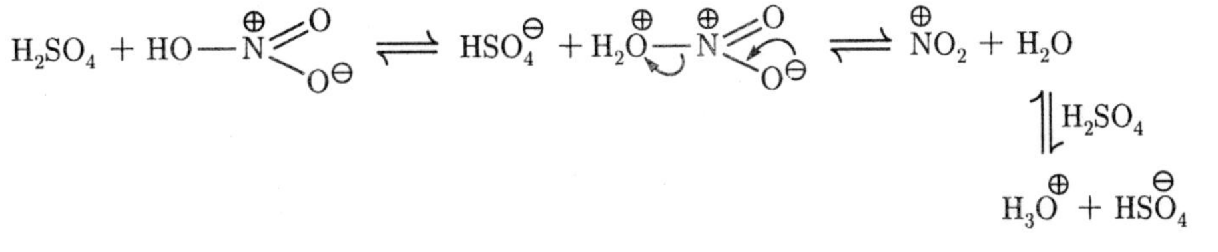

(b) Nitric acid shows a characteristic peak in the Raman spectrum. In mixed acid the peak disappears and two new peaks corresponding to $NO_2^{\oplus}$ ion (1400 cm^{-1}) and $HSO_4^{\ominus}$ ion (1050 cm^{-1}) appear.

(c) X-ray crystallographic studies of $\overset{\oplus}{N}O_2BF_4^{\ominus}$ (nitonium fluoborate) show that it contains $NO_2^{\oplus}$ ion.

(d) The intermediate σ-complex of the reaction between trifluoromethylbenzene and nitronium fluoborate has been isolated. The product is *m*-nitrotrifluoromethylbenzene. This experiment supports the evidence for $\overset{\oplus}{N}O_2$ ion as an active electrophile and also the formation of σ-complex as an intermediate.

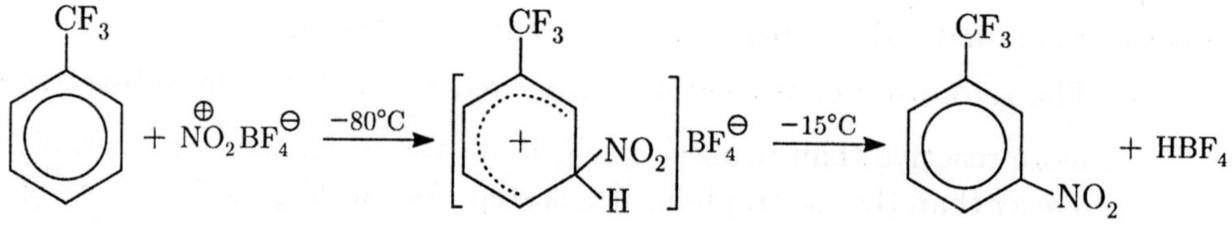

Nitration reaction does not show PKIE, *i.e.*, the rate of nitration of C_6H_6 and C_6D_6 are the same. This shows that C—H bond breaking is not rate limiting but attack of electrophile is the rate determining step.

Some Examples :

1. ***Nitration of phenol in dilute HNO$_3$*** : Dilute nitric acid always contains some nitrous acid (HNO_2) which forms $NO^{\oplus}$ (nitrosonium ion) in presence of strong acid H_2SO_4 as follows :

$$H_2SO_4 \rightleftharpoons \overset{\oplus}{H} + HSO_4^{\ominus}$$

$$HNO_2 \rightleftharpoons HO—N{=}O \text{ (a little amount)}$$

$$\overset{\oplus}{H} + HO—N{=}O \rightleftharpoons H_2\overset{\oplus}{O}—N{=}O \rightleftharpoons H_2O + \overset{\oplus}{N}{=}O \text{ (nitrosonium ion)}$$

$$H_2O + H_2SO_4 \rightleftharpoons \overset{\oplus}{H_3O} + \overset{\ominus}{HSO_4}$$

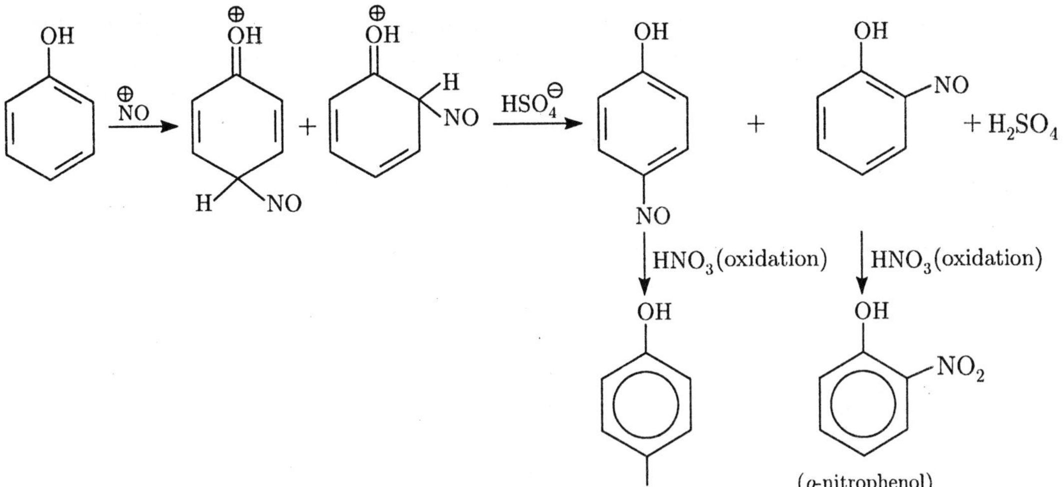

(p-nitrophenol) (minor)

(o-nitrophenol) (major)

2. ***Preparation of aromatic nitrocompounds from arenediazonium salts***

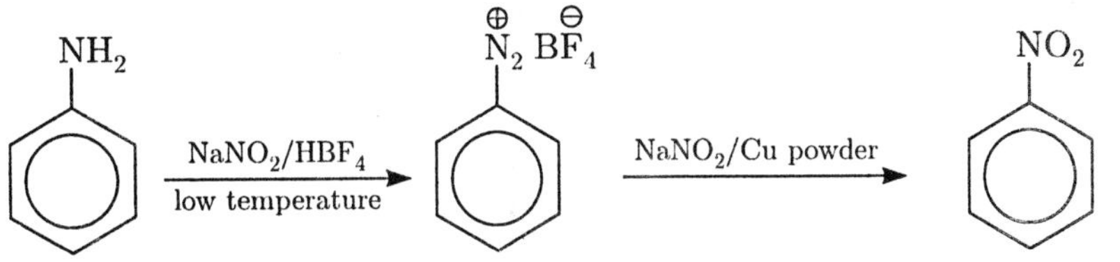

(Aniline) (Nitrobenzene)

3. ***Aromatic sulphonation reaction*** : The process of introducing a $-SO_3H$ group into an aromatic nucleus by the action of concentrated H_2SO_4 or fuming H_2SO_4 [oleum ($H_2S_2O_7$ – sulphur trioxide in H_2SO_4)] or SO_3 in organic solvent (nitromethane, pyridine etc.) or chlorosulphonic acid in carbon tetrachloride (CCl_4) is known as *aromatic sulphonation reaction.*

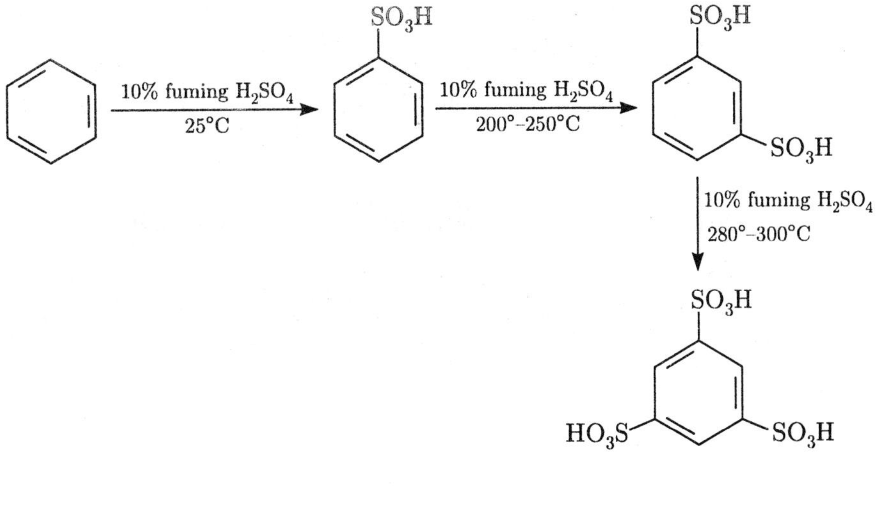

Alkylbenzenes, aromatic amines, phenols, phenolic ethers, thiophene, furan, pyridine, naphthalene etc. undergo the aromatic sulphonation reaction.

(i) 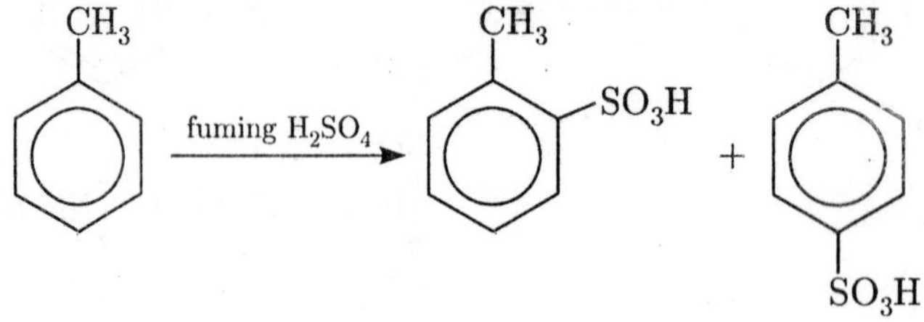

(ii) 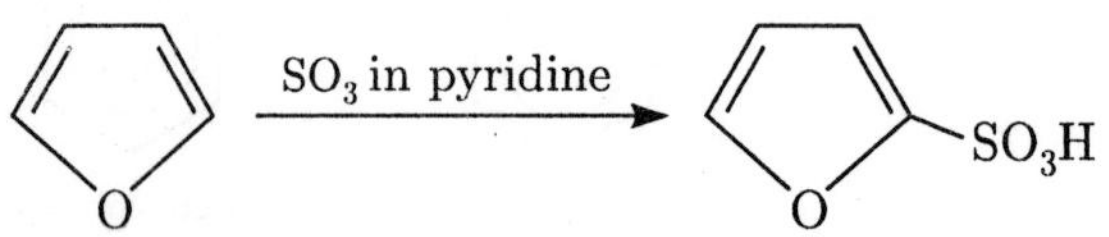

(iii) a. 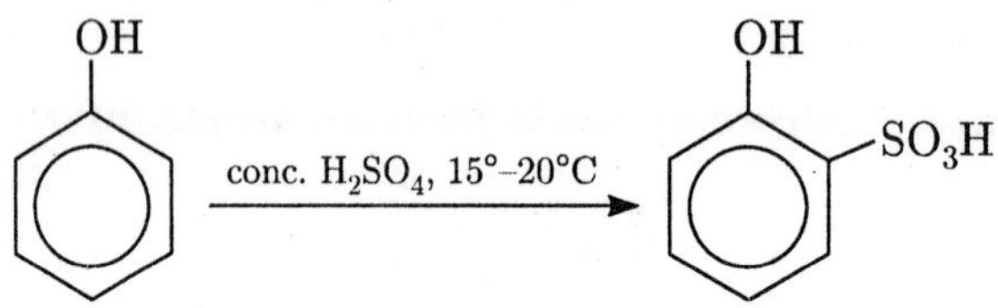

b. 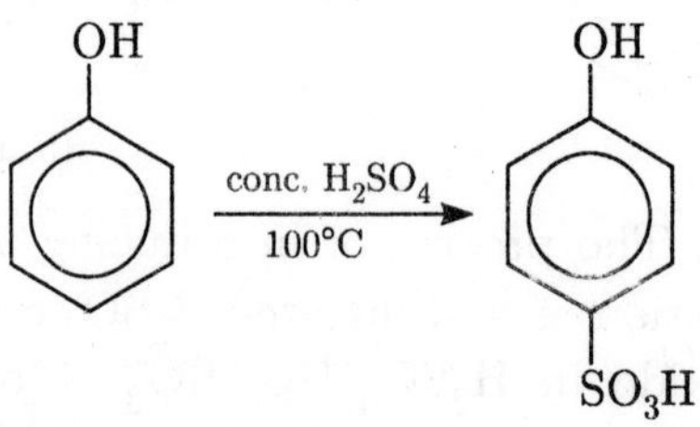

(iv) 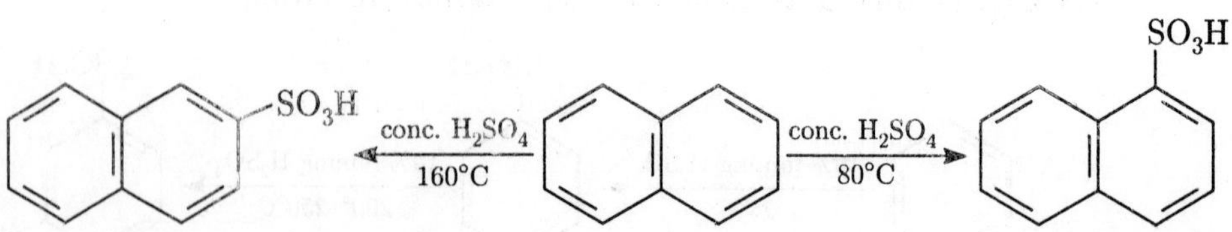

(v) 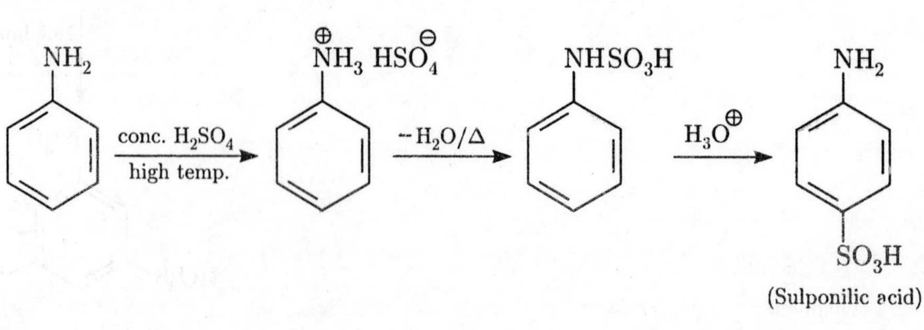

(Sulponilic acid)

The orientation depends on the nature of substituent already present in the ring. Usually at a lower temperature, the kinetically controlled product is obtained, while at an elevated temperature, the thermodynamically controlled product is formed. Since SO_3H is a bulky group, there is a steric interaction present in the *ortho* compound and so becomes less stable compared to the *para* product.

Aromatic sulphonation reaction is a reversible reaction at a high temperature. At low temperature the reaction proceeds to form the kinetically controlled product (*o*-isomer), and as the activation energy needed for desulphonation reaction is quite high at that temperature, the reaction seems to operate irreversibly. At higher temperature, this energy barrier is overcome and both sulphonation and desuphanation occurs to make the process reversible. Reversibility of aromatic sulphonation reaction has got some synthetic values. Several aromatic sulphonic acids and 2-substituted naphthalene are prepared by the help of sulphonation/desulphonation reactions. Desulphonation is usually done by heating the sulphonic acid derivative with dilute hydrochloric acid at a high temperature.

Some examples of utility of sulphonation reaction :

1. ***Synthesis of o-bromotoluene***

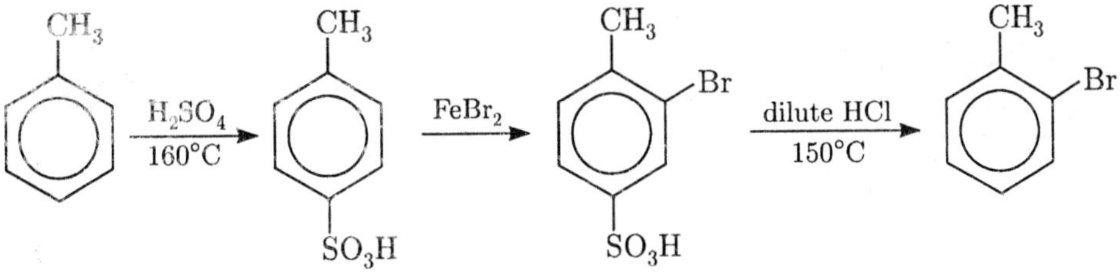

2. ***Synthesis of o-bromophenol***

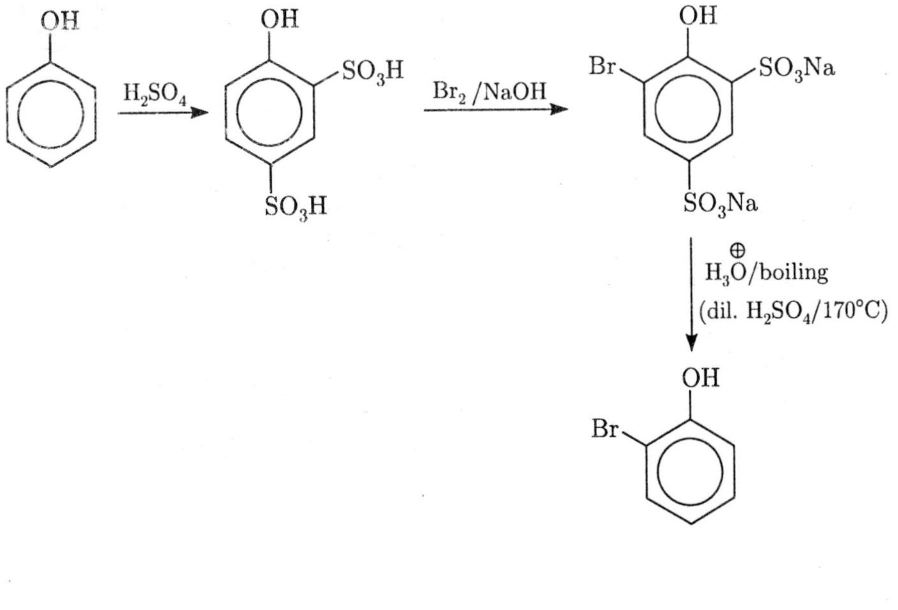

3. ***Synthesis of* o*-bromoaniline***

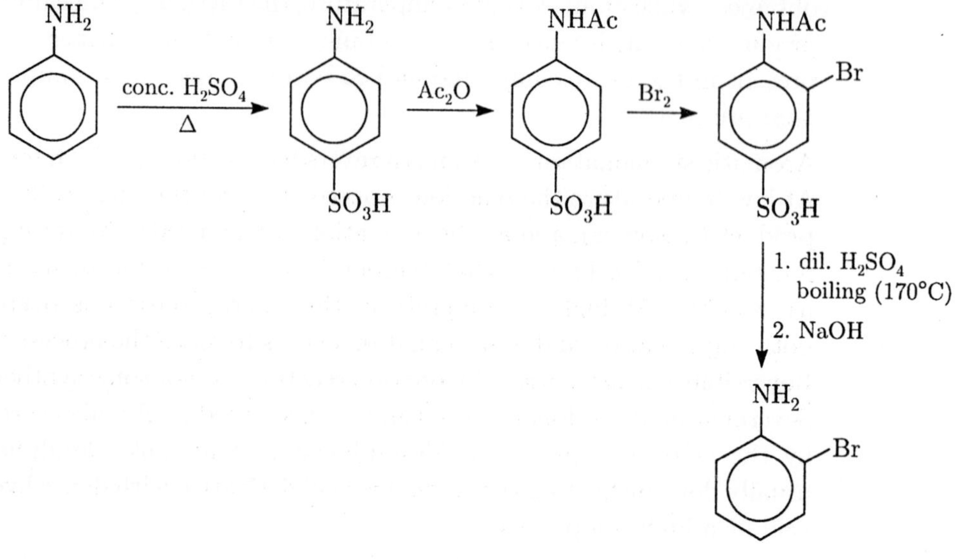

4. ***Synthesis of β-naphthol and other β-substituted naphthalenes***

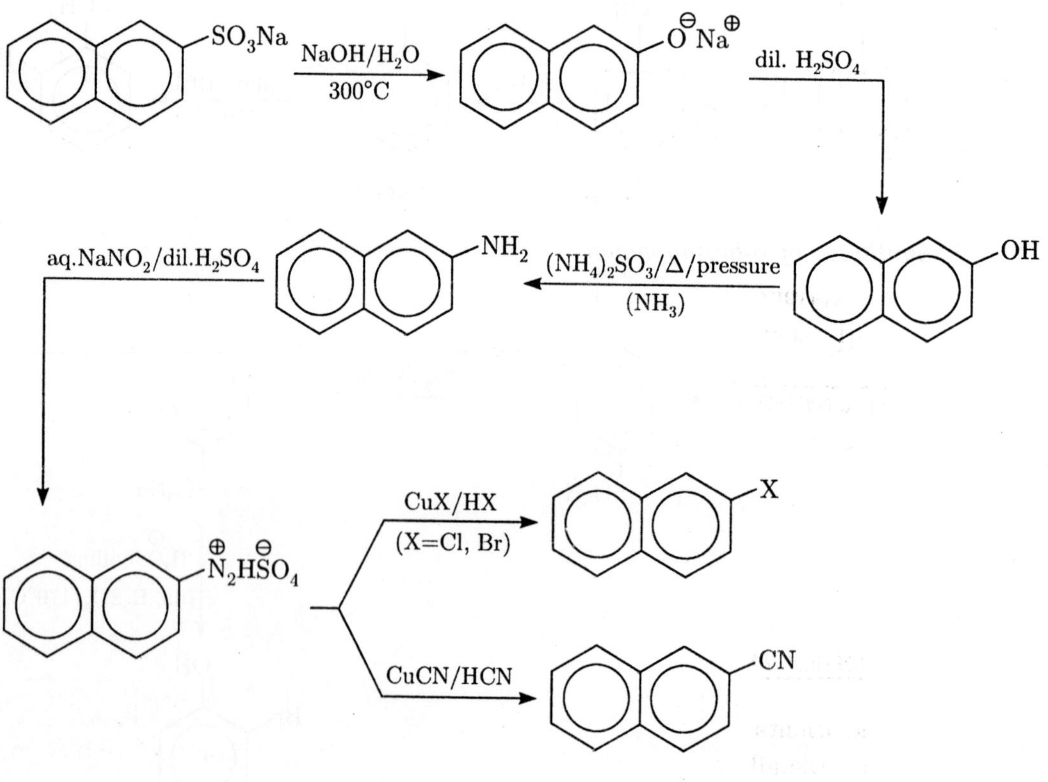

5. ***Synthesis of* o-*nitrotoluene***

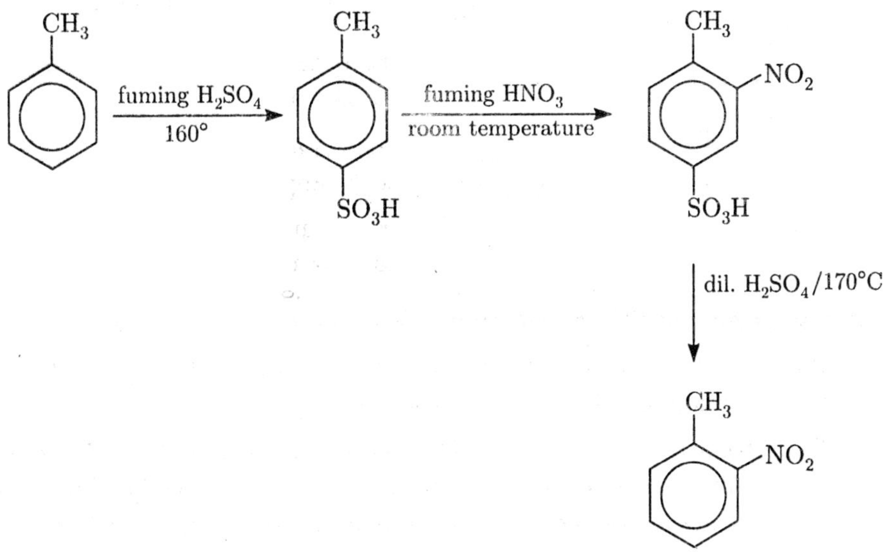

Mechanism of sulphonation reaction : When the sulphonating reagent is concentrated H_2SO_4 or fuming H_2SO_4 or SO_3 in organic solvent, the electrophile is SO_3.

$$2H_2SO_4 \rightleftharpoons SO_3 + H\overset{\ominus}{S}O_4 + H_3O^{\oplus}$$

$$H_2S_2O_7 \text{ (oleum)} \rightleftharpoons H_2SO_4 + SO_3$$

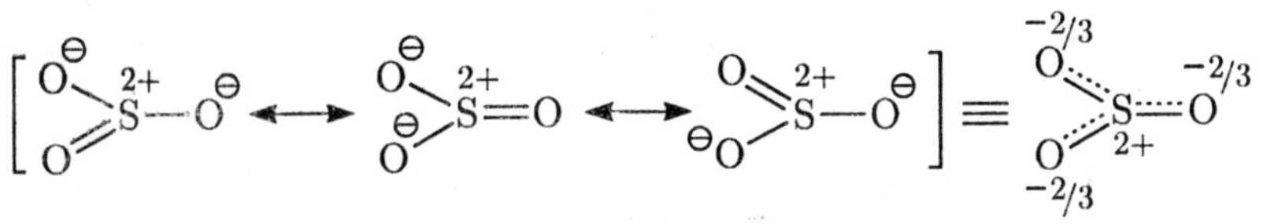

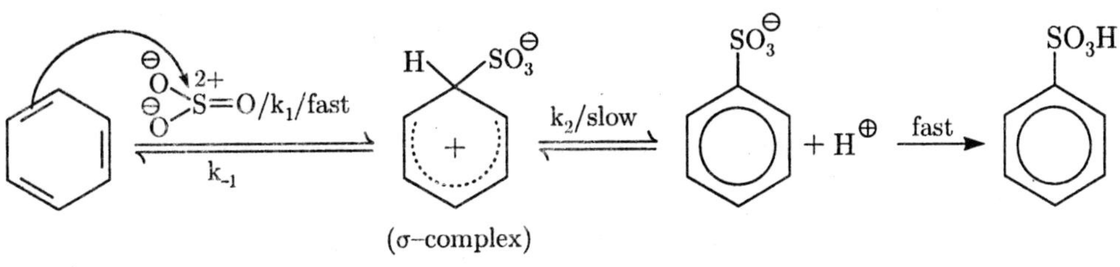

(σ–complex)

Here deprotonation step is rate determining step, not the formation of σ-complex which is observed in irreversible ArS_E2 reactions. This is proved by primary kinetic isotope effect.

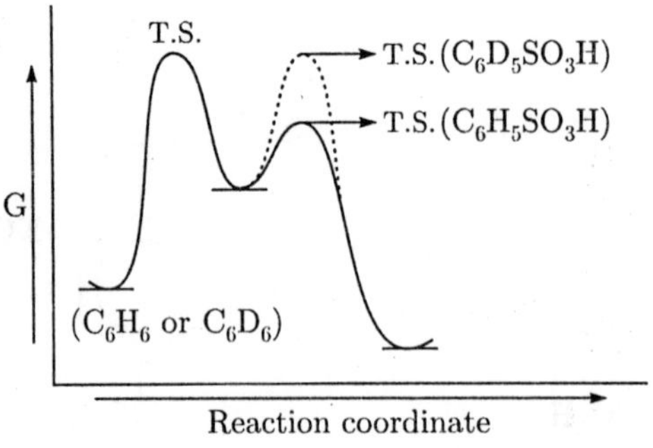

Energy profile of aromatic sulphonation reaction in C_6H_6 and C_6D_6

Fig. 3.6 :

Evidences for the SO_3 as attacking electrophile :

1. Rate of sulphonation is higher with SO_3 compared to H_2SO_4. The reaction rate is proportional to the concentration of SO_3.
2. Deprotonation step shows PKIE. This indicates that C—H bond breaking is involved in rate determining step, *i.e.*, $k_{-1} > k_2$, and the heights of two transition states being almost equal, and the reaction becomes reversible.

Synthetic applications of aromatic sulphonation reaction :

(a)

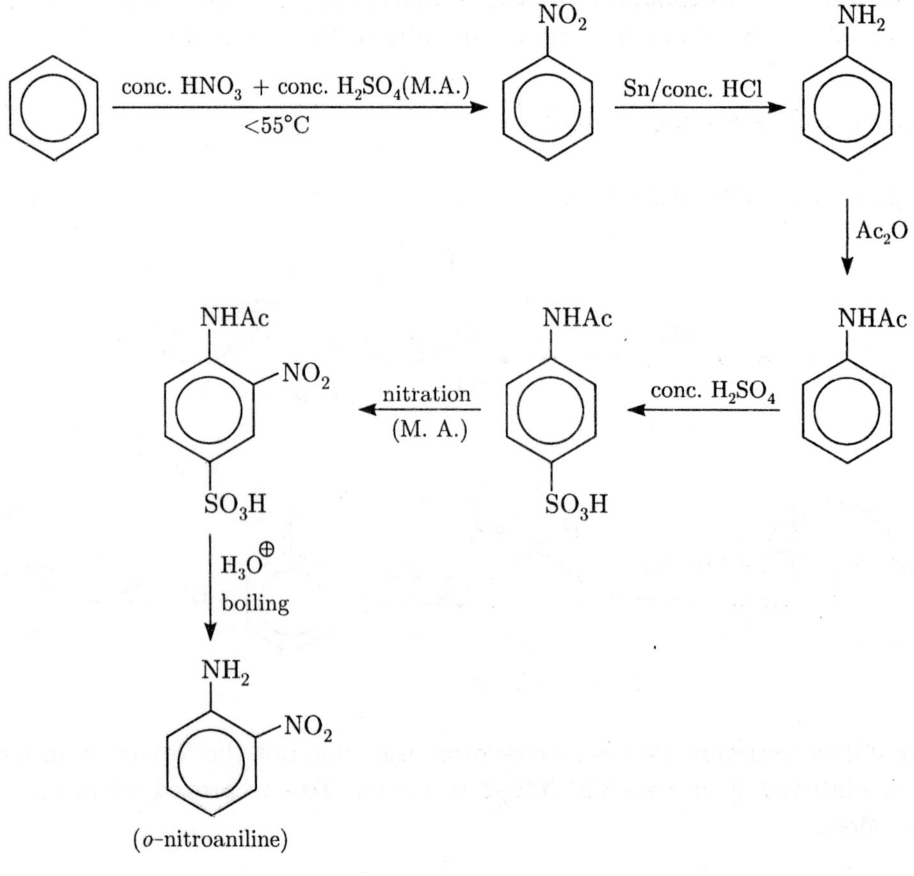

(*o*-nitroaniline)

(b)

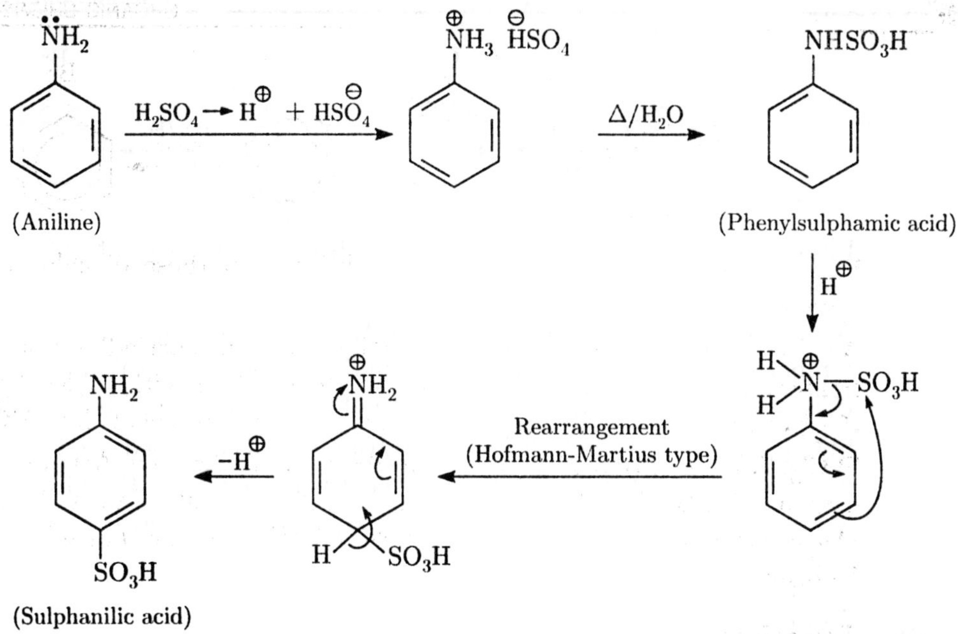

Desulphonation and its Mechanism : Unlike most substitutions, sulphonation is reversible. Thus SO_3H group can be eliminated easily by heating the sulphonic acid with dilute H_2SO_4 at 170°C, because at elevated temperature, rate constant for backward reaction becomes slightly higher than that of forward reaction, as the eliminating SO_3 is a gas and leaves the system so that the equilibrium is driven towards desulphonation at a comparatively faster rate.

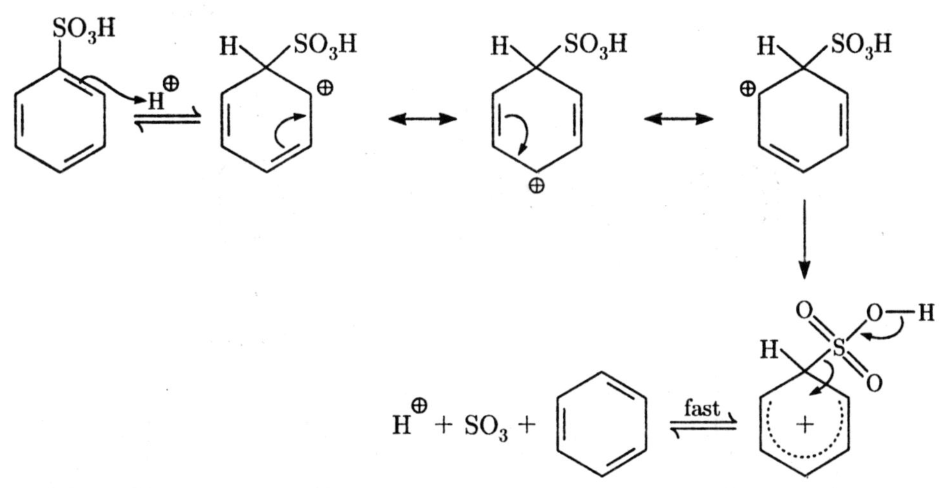

3. ***Aromatic halogenation reaction*** : Replacement or substitution of a hydrogen atom from an aromatic nucleus by a halogen atom is called aromatic halogenation reaction.

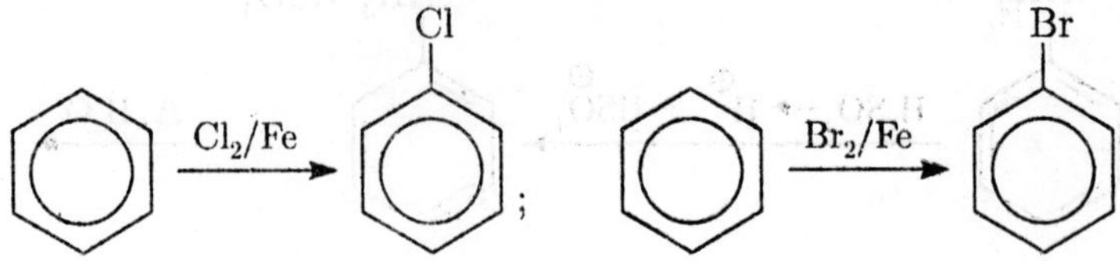

Fluorination and iodination processes differ from those of chlorination and bromination.

Aromatic chlorination and bromination may be carried out at ordinary temperature by allowing the compound to reaction with molecular chlorine (Cl_2) or bromine (Br_2) in the presence of Fe or a Lewis acids like $AlCl_3$, $AlBr_3$ $SbCl_5$, $SbBr_5$ etc. $HOCl/Cl^{\ominus}$ or $HOBr/Br^{\ominus}$ may also be used. Activated aromatic compounds like phenols, amines etc. react with molecular Br_2 or Cl_2 even in the absence of Lewis acid. Interhalogens like ICl, IBr etc. and I_2 itself can act as a halogen carrier.

Examples :

(i) 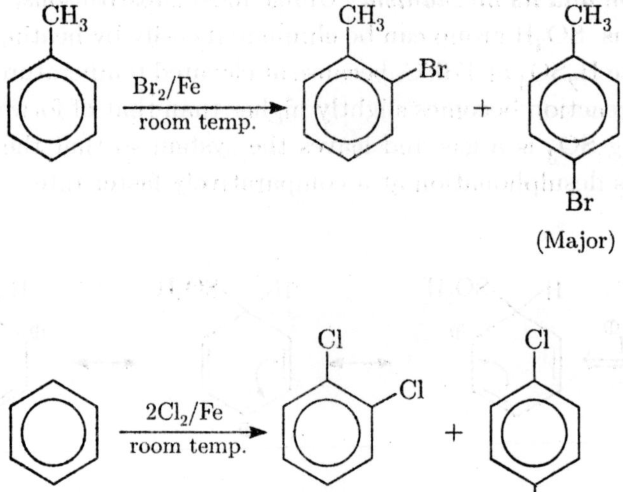

(ii) 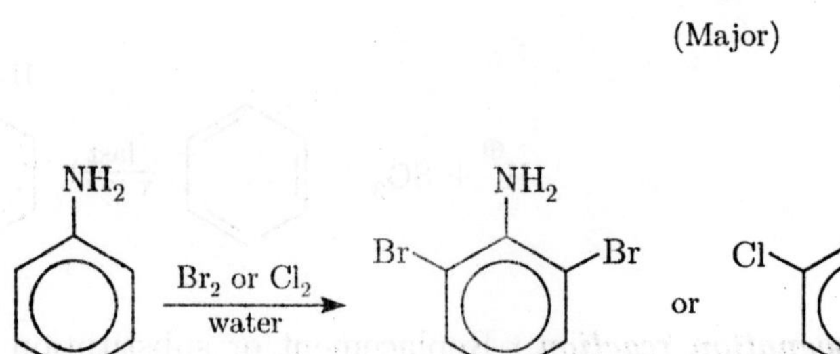

(iii) 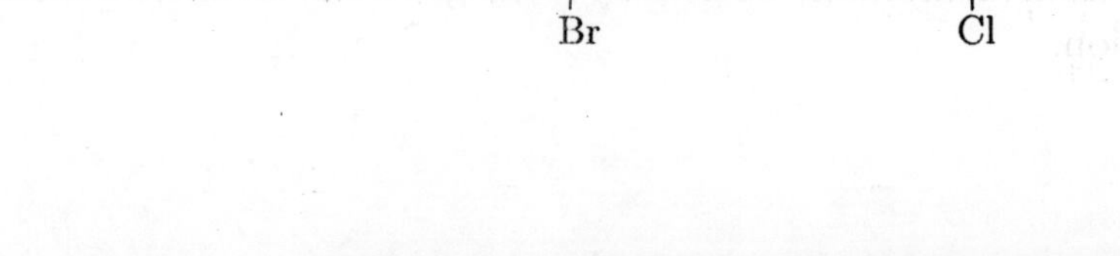

(iv) 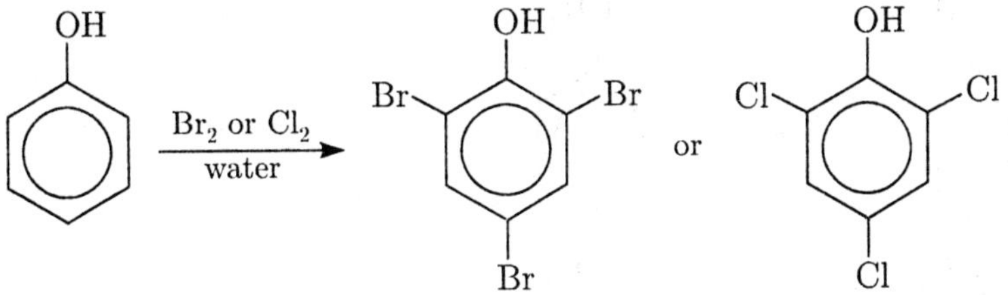

(v) 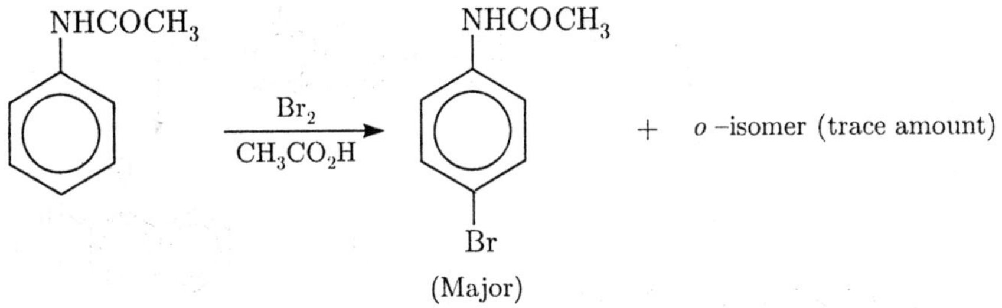

(vi) 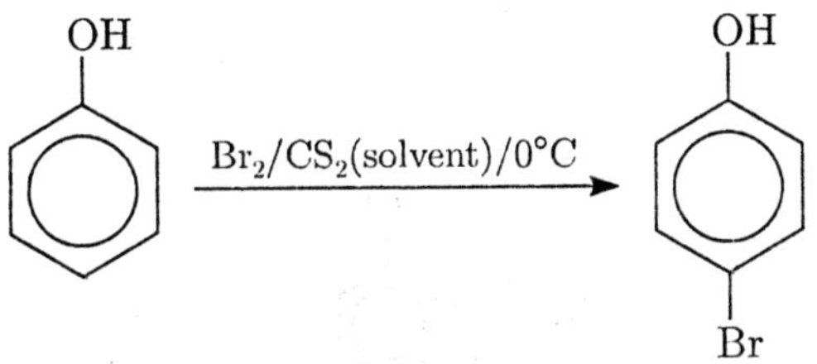

(vii) 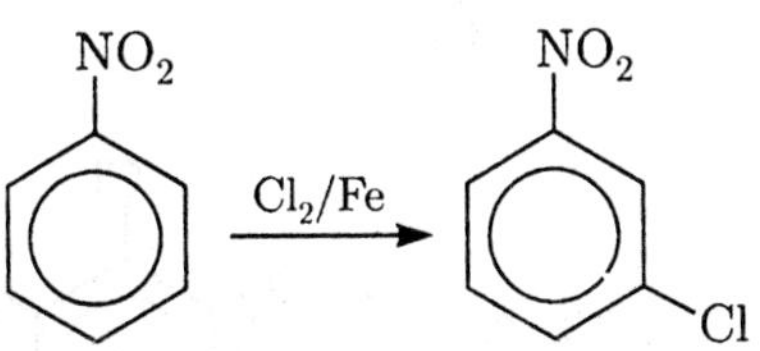

(viii) 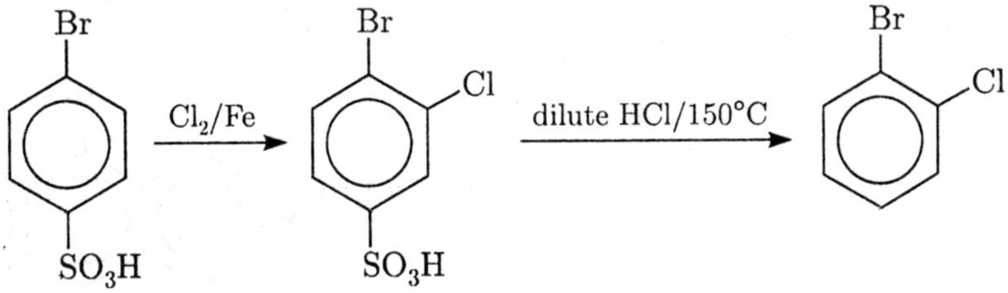

(ix) 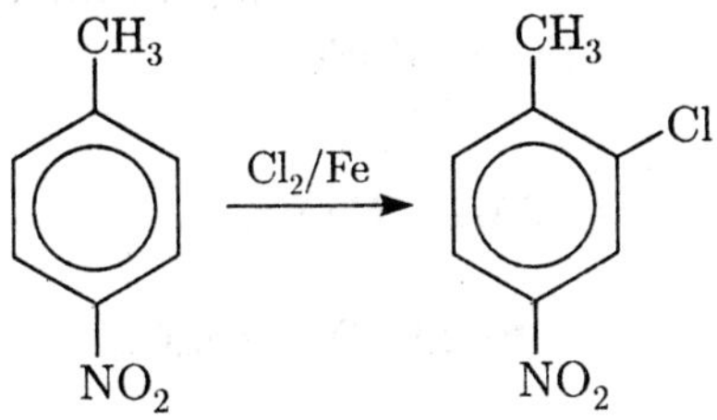

(x)

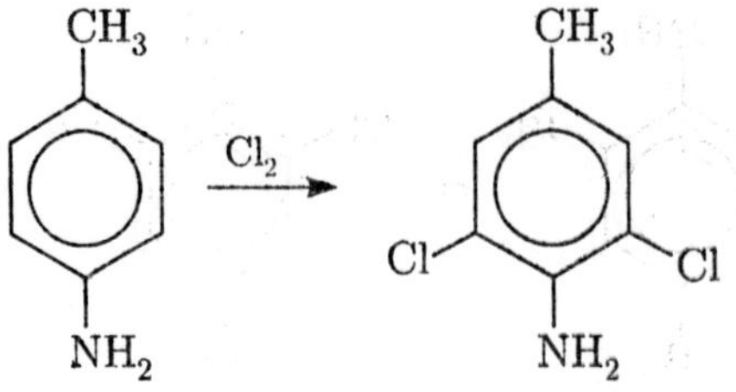

(xi)

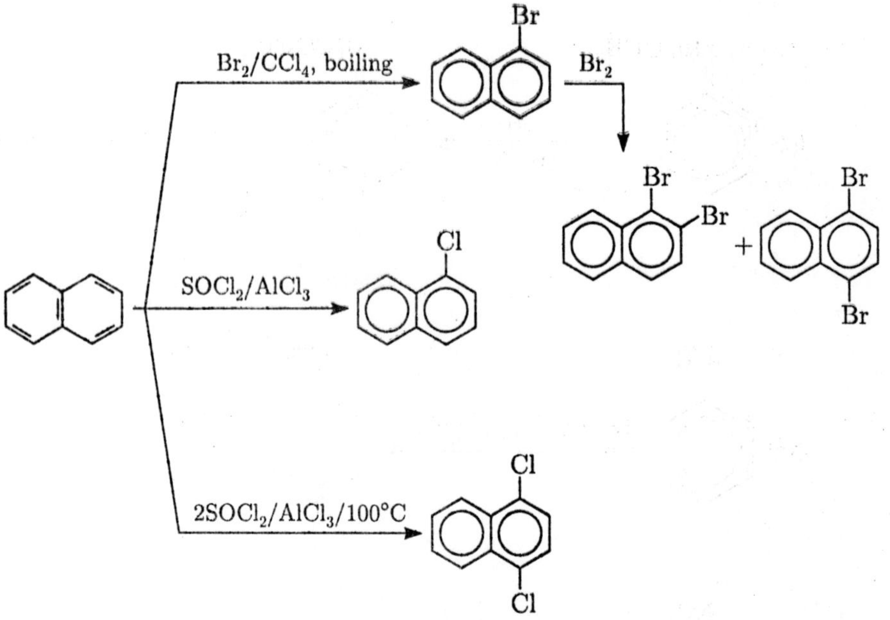

(xii)

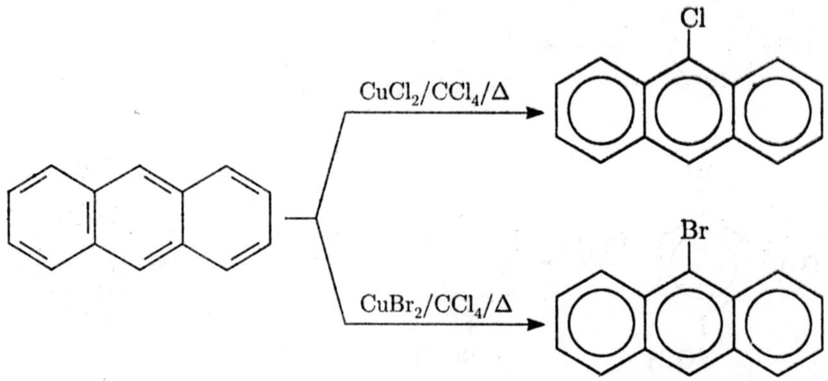

Chloroarenes are easily converted to iodoarenes and aryl cyanides by the action of Cu_2I_2 and CuCN respectively in DMF or DMSO.

$$2ArCl + Cu_2I_2 \xrightarrow{DMF} 2ArI + Cu_2Cl_2$$

$$2ArCl + 2CuCN \xrightarrow{DMSO} 2ArCN + Cu_2Cl_2$$

DDT (dichlorodiphenyltrichloroethane), an insecticide is prepared from chlorobenzene.

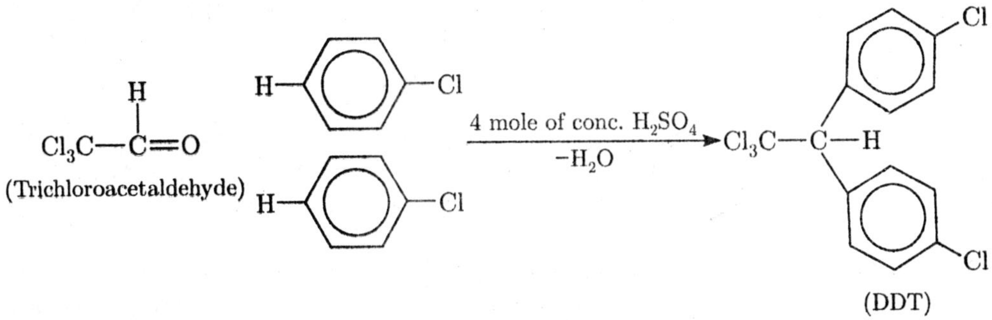

Mechanisms of aromatic halogenation reaction :

(a) *Halogenation with halogen and iron as halogen carrier* :

$$2Fe + 3X_2 \longrightarrow 2FeX_3$$

$$:\ddot{X}-\ddot{X}: + FeX_3 \rightleftharpoons \overset{\oplus}{X}-\overset{\ominus}{X}-FeX_3 + :\ddot{X}^{\oplus} + Fe\overset{\ominus}{X_4} \quad (X=Cl, Br)$$

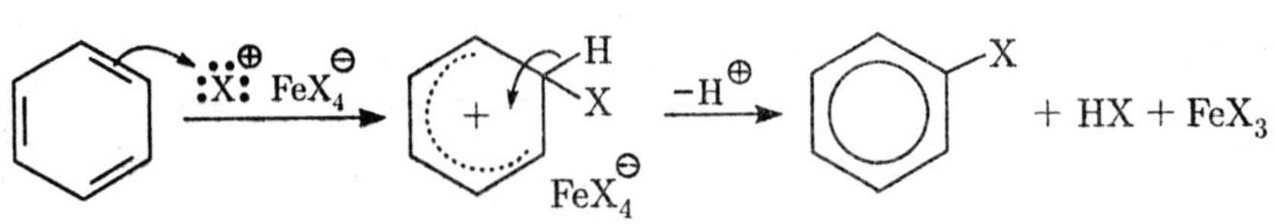

Alternative mechanism : Molecular halogen forms a π-complex with the aromatic compound, the Leiws acid then pulls in X^- part of the complex and thus, a σ-complex is formed.

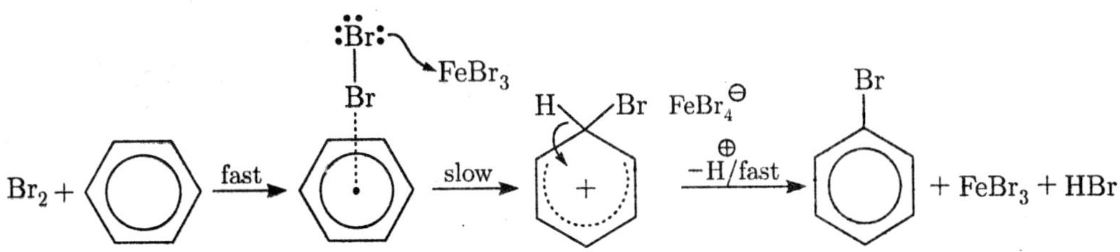

Rate=k [substrate] [halogen] [Lewis acid]

No PKIE is observed, so C—H bond breaking step is a fast step.

(b) *Halogenation with hypohalous acid and halide ion* :

$$H-OX \rightleftharpoons \overset{\oplus}{H} + \overset{\ominus}{O}X$$

$$2\overset{\oplus}{H} + \overset{\ominus}{O}X + \overset{\ominus}{X} \longrightarrow H_2O + X_2$$

The molecular halogen then forms π-complex with the π-electron cloud of the substrate which leads to a σ-complex and a haloarene is produced.

(c) *Halogenation with hypohalous acid and a strong acid* :

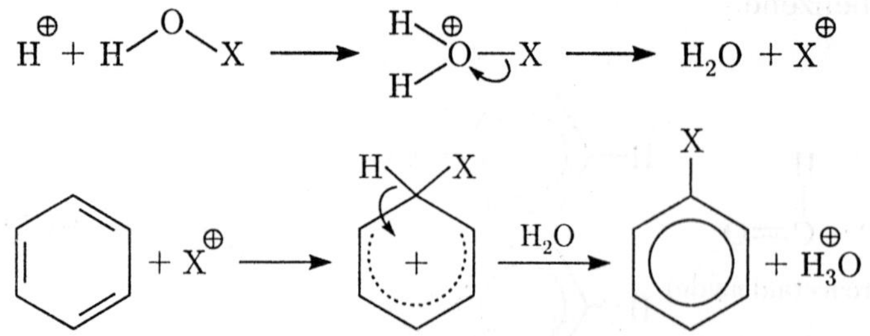

With activated aromatic molecules like phenols, amines etc. the reaction is zero order with respect to substrate; with relatively unreactive substrates like nitrophenols, the halogenation reaction is first order with respect to substrate.

Examples :

(a) *Bromination of phenol in water or CCl_4*

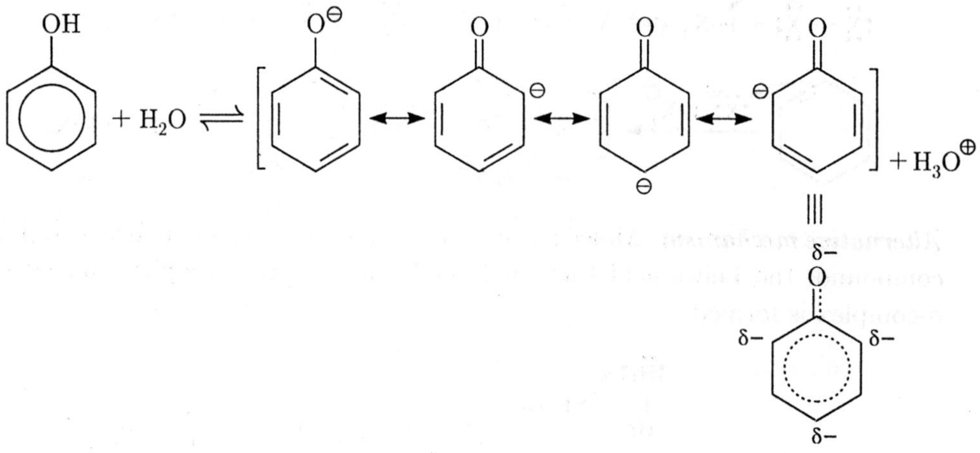

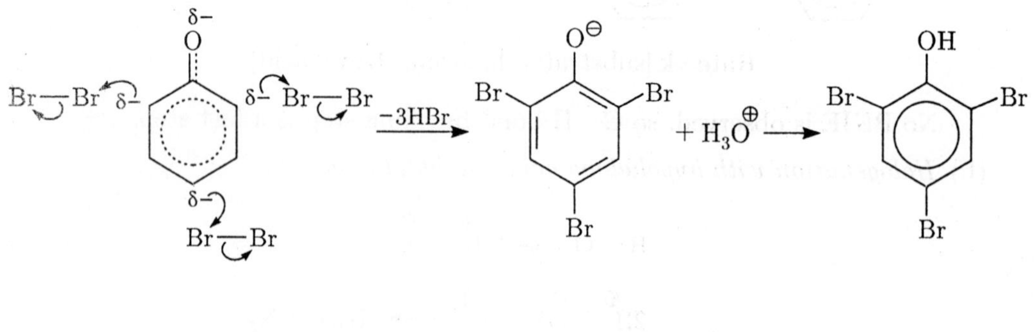

When excess bromine is used the following reaction takes place.

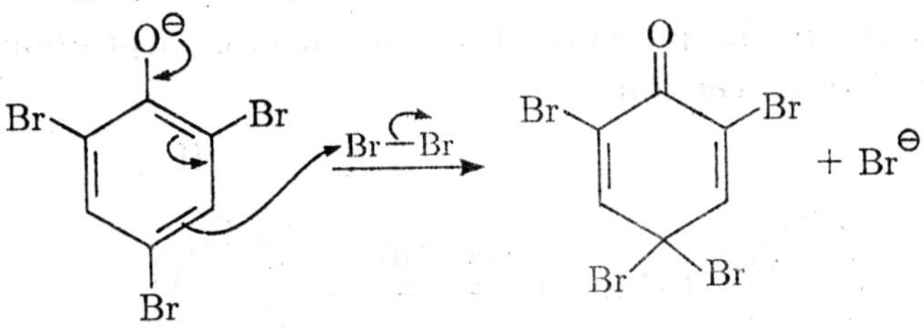

(b) In carbon disulphide (CS_2) medium, phenol forms *p*-bromophenol (major) with a little amount of *o*-bromophenol.

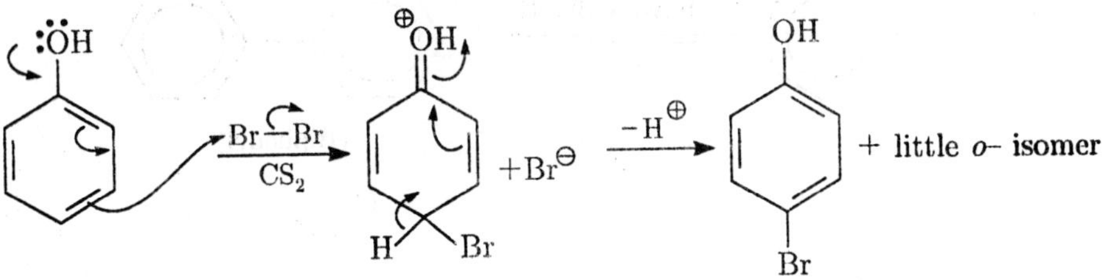

Iodination reaction : Iodination reaction unlike chlorination and bromination is reversible in nature. ICl may be used as iodionating agent. $I^{\ominus}$ in the presence of oxidising agents like HNO_3, HIO_3, H_2O_2, etc. which oxidise $I^{\ominus}$ to I_2 are also used as iodinating agents. Activated aromatic compounds like phenols, amines etc. react with iodine in water where $I^{\oplus}$ is the attacking electrophile. *Para* product is the major product in the reaction.

Fluorination reaction : The F—F bond energy is only 154.4 kJ/mol.$^{-1}$ when fluorine is allowed to react with benzene, free radical addition takes place and polyfluorocyclohexane is formed. The best method to prepare fluorobenzene is as follows.

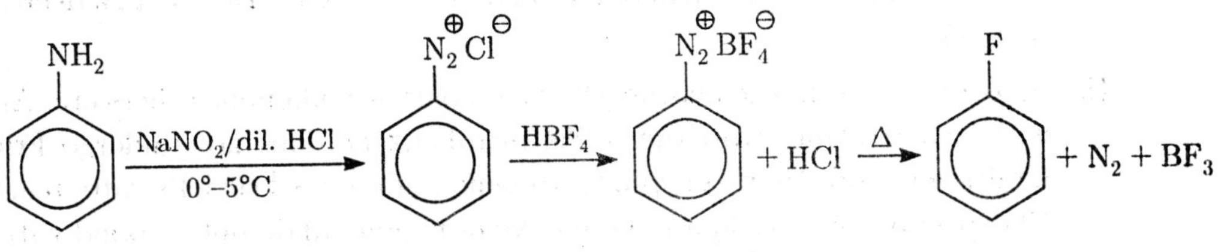

The Friedel-Crafts reaction : Introduction of an alkyl or an aryl or acyl group into an aromatic nucleus in the presence of a Lewis acid or a protonic acid as catalyst is known as Friedel-Crafts reaction.

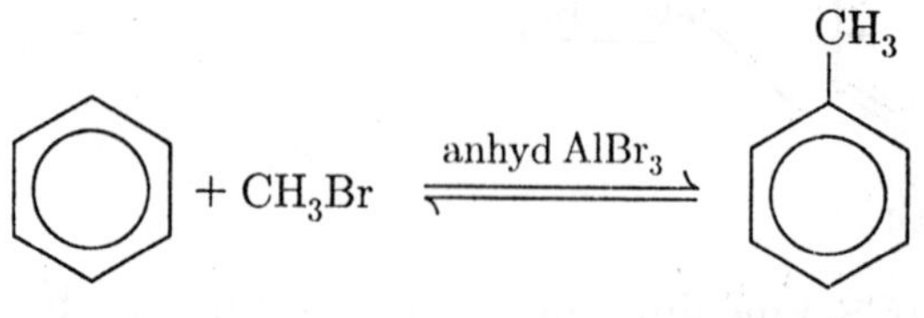

(Toluene)

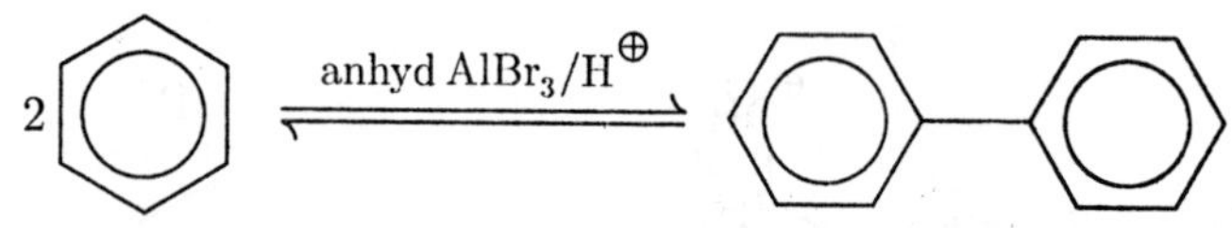

(Biphenyl)

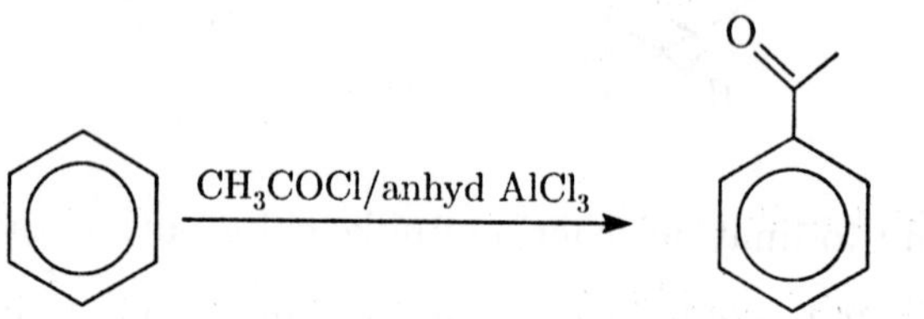

(Acetophenone)

Fridel-crafts reaction can be of two types –

(a) Friedel–Crafts alkylation reaction, and

(b) Friedel–Crafts acylation reaction.

(a) Friedel–Crafts alkylation reaction

(i) *Alkylating agents* : Alkyl halides, alkenes, alcohols, mercaptan, inorganic esters and sulphides.

The order of reactivity : allyl, benzyl > tertiary > secondary > primary halides and the order of reactivity of halides : $F^- > Cl^- > Br^- > I^-$ in a decreasing manner.

(ii) *Substrates* : Aromatic hydrocarbons, haloarenes, phenolic ethers etc. Arenes with deactivating substituent like nitrobenzene does not undergo Friedel-Crafts reaction. However, *p*-nitrotoluene undergoes Friedel-Crafts reaction. Phenols give poor yield and heterocycles in general do not respond with two exceptions like furan and thiophene.

(iii) *Acid catalysts* : $AlCl_3$, $SbCl_5$, BF_3, HF, H_2SO_4, H_3PO_4, $FeCl_3$, $SnCl_4$, $ZnCl_2$, are generally used with alkyl halides and alkenes.

HF, BF_3, H_2SO_4 etc. are used when alcohols are used as alkylating agents.

The reactivity of catalysts in alkylations follows the order,

$AlCl_3 > SbCl_5 > FeCl_3 > SnCl_4 > ZnCl_2$ in a decreasing manner.

(iv) *Solvents* : Carbon disulphide and nitrobenzene. When the substrate itself is a liquid is may act as a solvent when taken in excess dichloromethane and *n*-hexane also act as solvents.

Examples (Applications of Friedel-Crafts reaction)

(a) 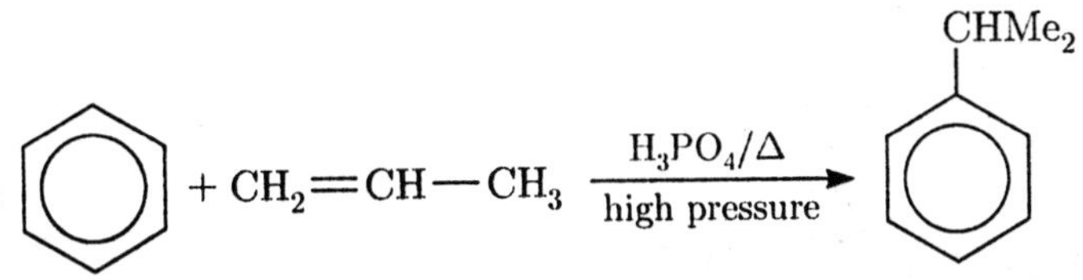

(Cumene)

(b) 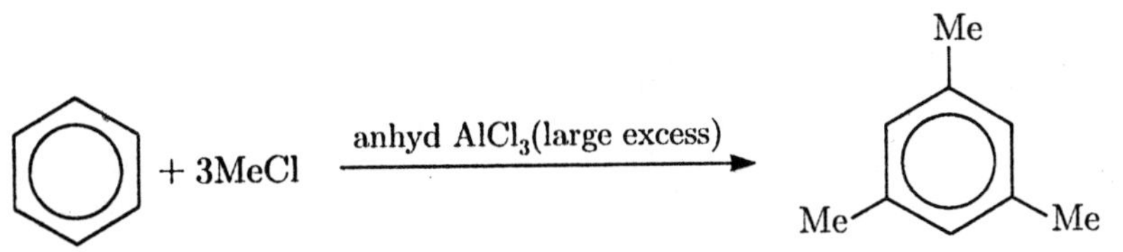

(Mesitylene)

(c) 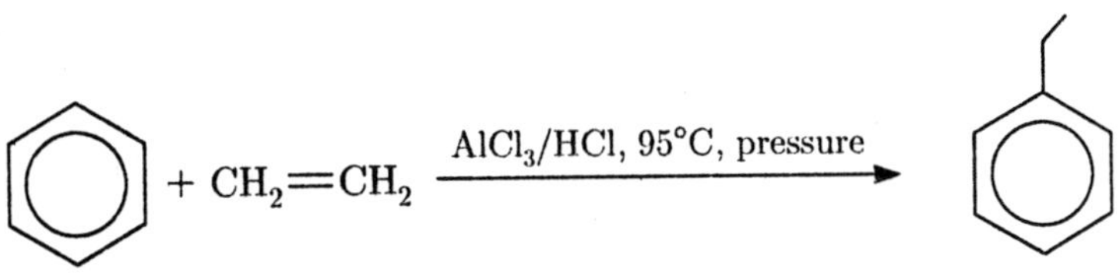

(Ethylbenzene)

(d) 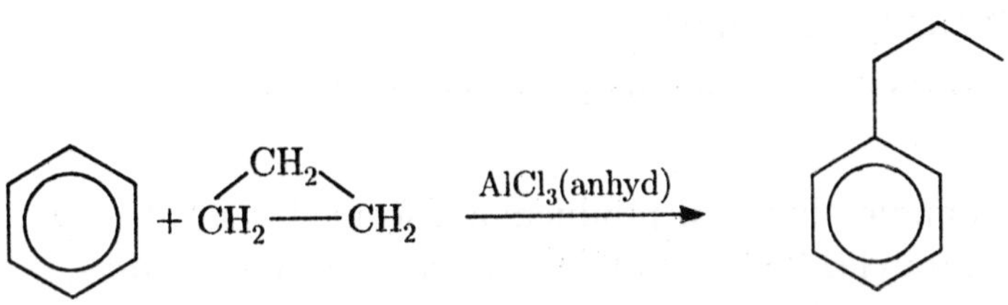

(*n*-propylbenzene)

(e) (i) 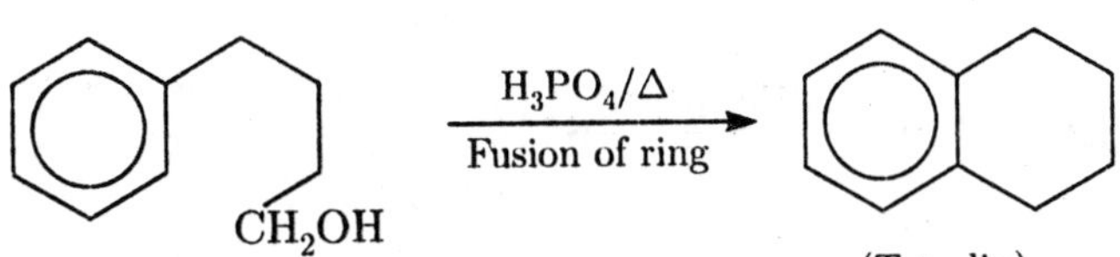

(Tetralin)

(ii) 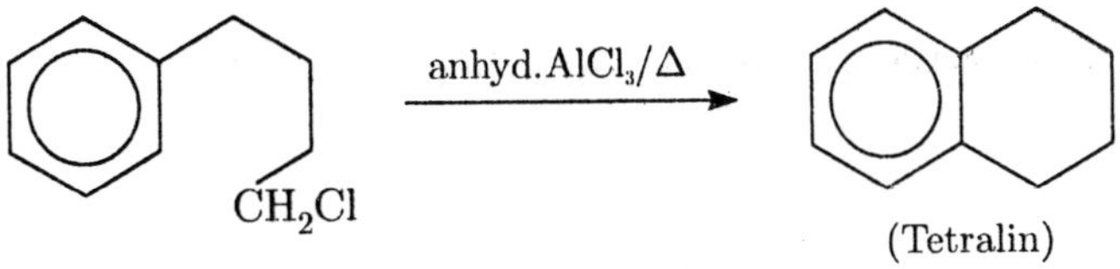

(Tetralin)

(iii) 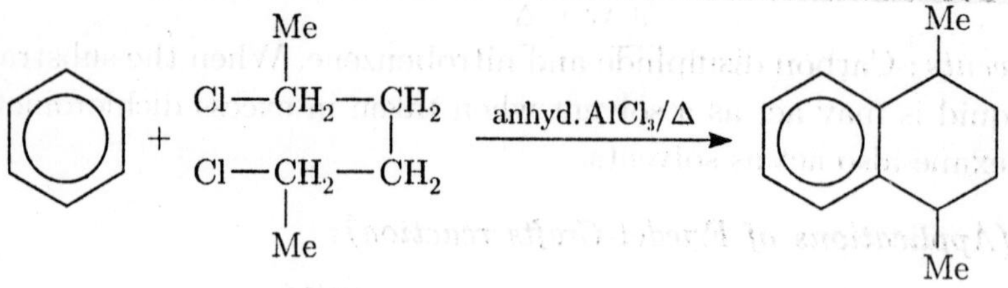

f. 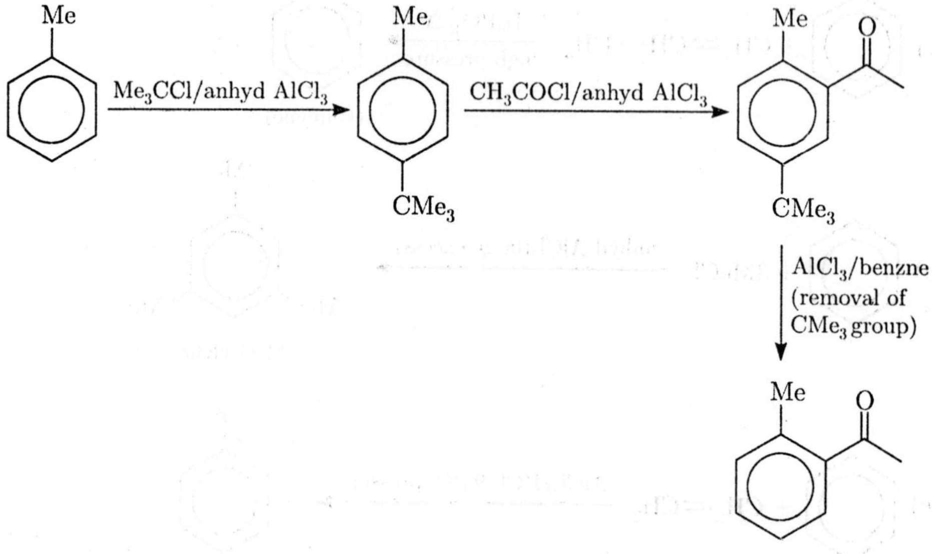

Reaction f. shows the reversible nature of Friedel-Crafts reaction

Limitations of Friedel–Crafts reaction :

1. Activated aromatic hydrocarbons undergo polyalkylation reaction instead of monoalkylation.
2. In many cases, isomeric alkylated products are formed instead of the desired product. When *n*-propyl chloride is used to prepare *n*-propylbenzene, isopropylbenzene is obtained as the major product.

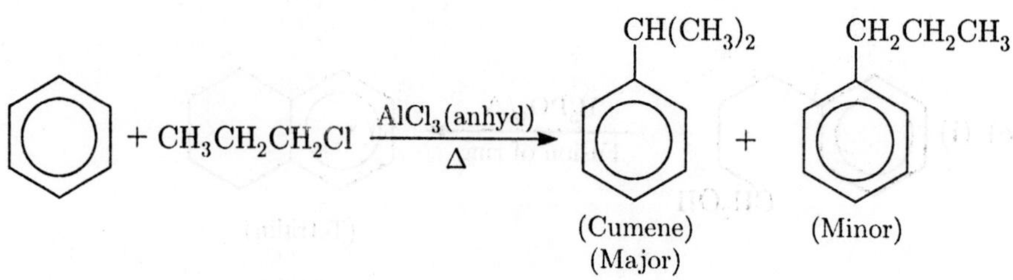

[$\overset{\oplus}{C}HMe_2$ is a more stable secondary carbocation than the primary carbocation $CH_3CH_2\overset{\oplus}{C}H_2$]

3. If the alkylating agent is highly reactive, it attacks the substrate less selectively and a mixture of products are formed.

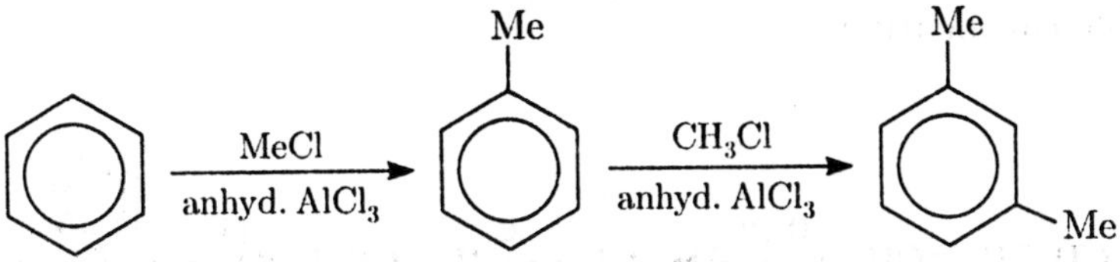

4. When a deactivating substituent is present in the aromatic ring, the reaction does not occur. Nitrobenzene fails to respond Friedel-Crafts reaction.

Mechanism of Friedel–Crafts reaction :

(a) *Alkyl halides as alkylating agents :*

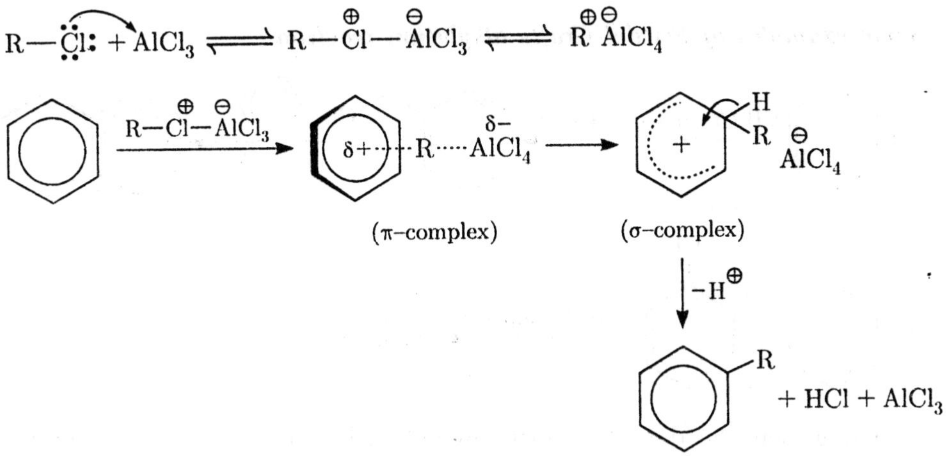

(b) *Alcohols as alkylating agents*

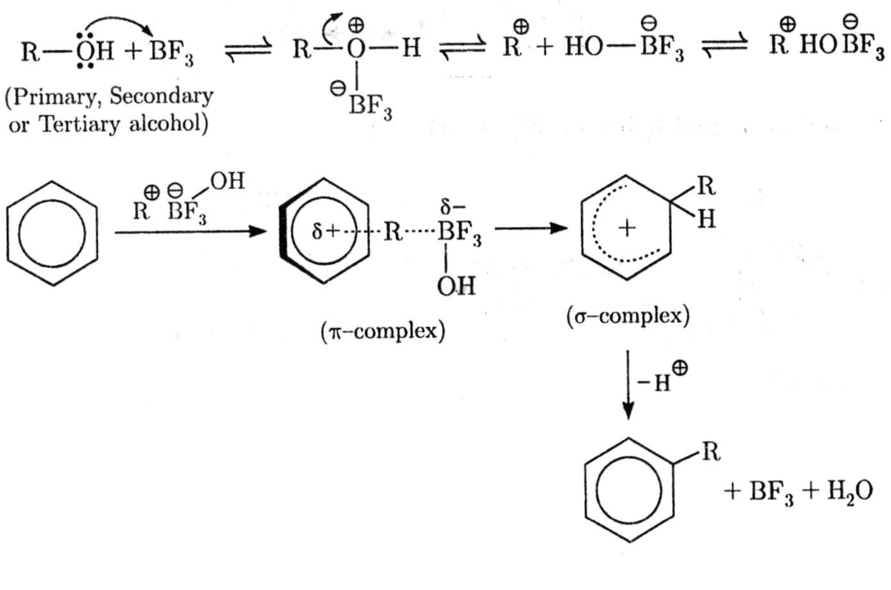

(c) *Alkenes as alkylating agents :* Alkenes undergo Fridel–Crafts alkylation in presence of in organic acids like 85% H_3PO_4. The initial step involves the formation of a stable carbocation.

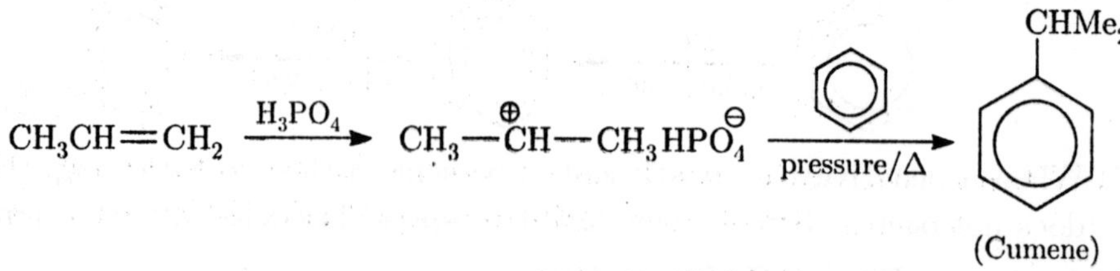

Friedel-Crafts alkylation reaction is kinetically controlled at a low temperature but is thermodynamically controlled at higher temperature.

Some examples of Friedel-Crafts alkylation reaction :

(a) 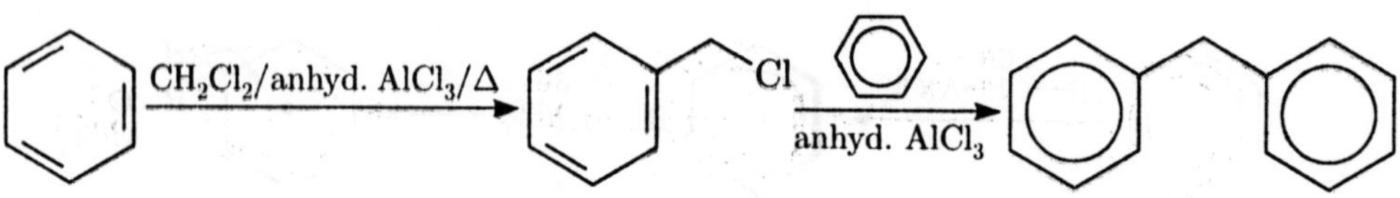

(b) 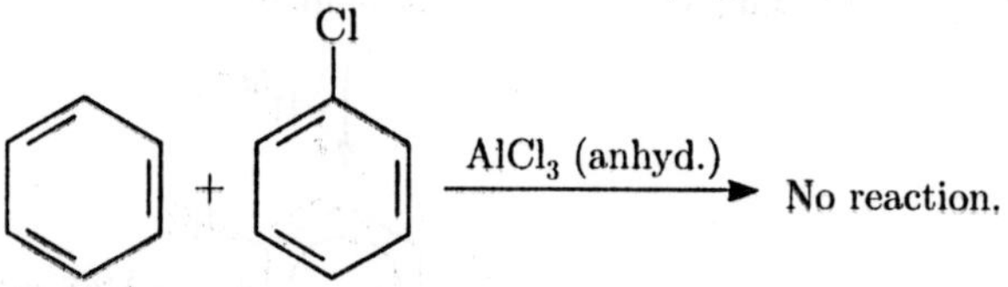

Chlorobenzene does not form phenyl cation, because C—Cl bond attains a double bond character through resonance as follows.

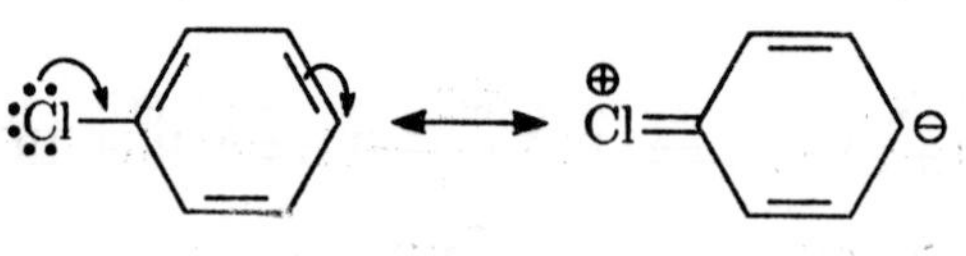

and also vinyl halides ($CH_2 = CH—Cl$).

(c) 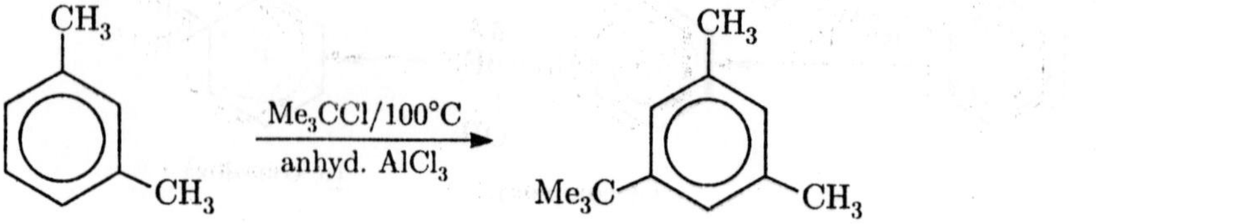

(*m*-xylene)

At high temperature, thermodynamically controlled product *i.e.*, *m*-product will be formed. The tertiarybutyl group takes up the *m*-position with respect to two CH_3 groups in order to avoid steric strain though CH_3 group is *o*/*p* directing.

(d)

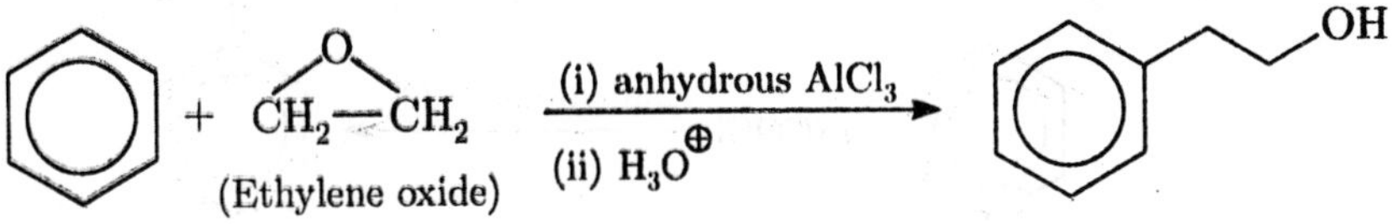

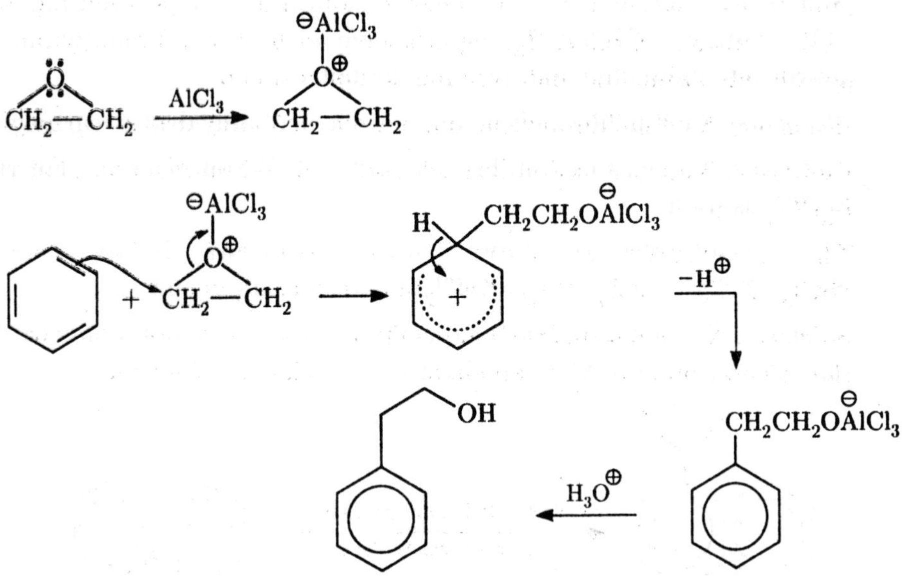

(e)

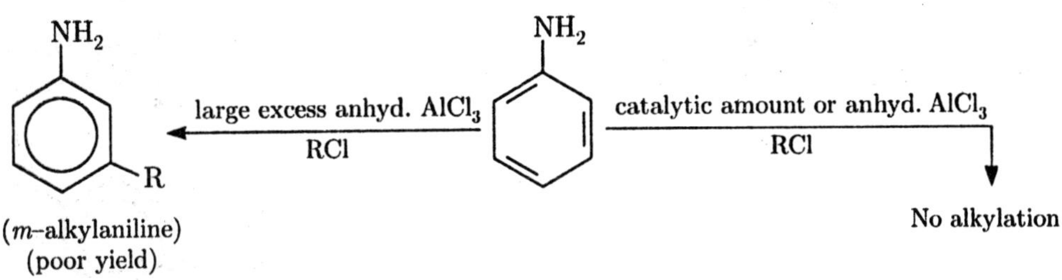

Aniline is a base as the $-\ddot{N}H_2$ contains a lone pair of electrons. So a Lewis acid/Lewis base complex is formed, between aniline and $AlCl_3$ where the latter is a Lewis acid. When $AlCl_3$ is used in catalytic amount, no $AlCl_3$ is left to activate the alkyl halide for Friedel-Crafts reaction.

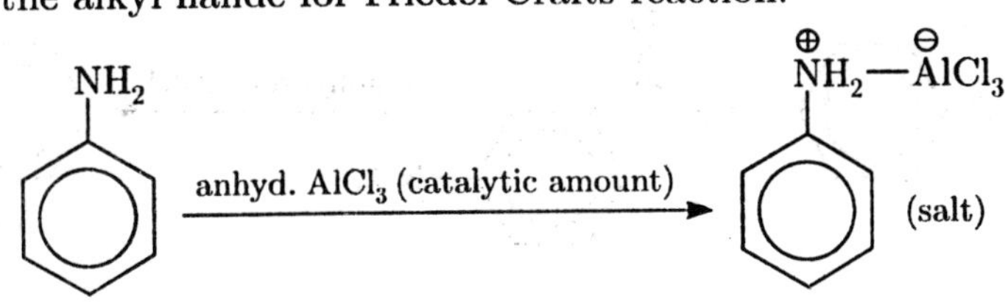

When an excess of $AlCl_3$ is used, *m*-alkylaniline is formed in poor yield as $>\overset{\oplus}{N}H_2$ group is *m*-directing.

Friedel–Crafts acylation reaction :

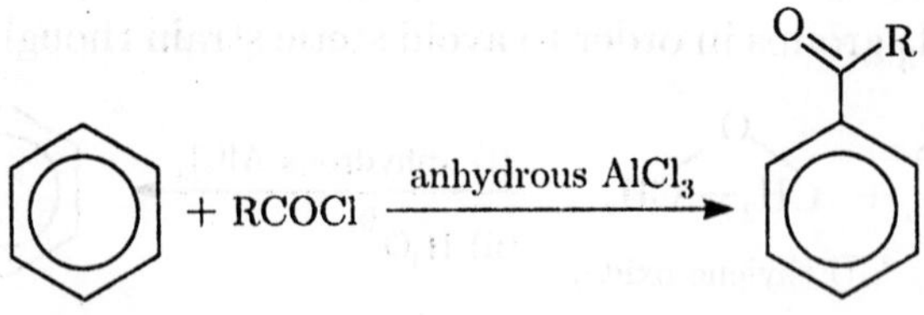

Substrates : Derivatives of benzene containing *o*/*p*-directing groups like –OH, –OR, X, –$NHCOCH_3$, naphthalene, anthracene, furan, pyran, thiophene, pyrrole etc. Quinoline and pyridine do not respond.

Reagents : Acyl halides, cyclic and acyclic acid anhydrides, carboxylic acids.

Catalysts : Same as used in Friedel-Crafts alkylation reaction. For ring closure, H_3PO_4 is used.

The reactivity of Lewis acid catalysts follow the order : $SbCl_5 > FeCl_3 > AlCl_3 > BF_3 > ZnCl_2$ in a decreasing manner.

Solvents : Nitrobenzene, carbon disulphide and tetrachloroethylene. Sometimes the orientation of acyl group changes with change of solvent.

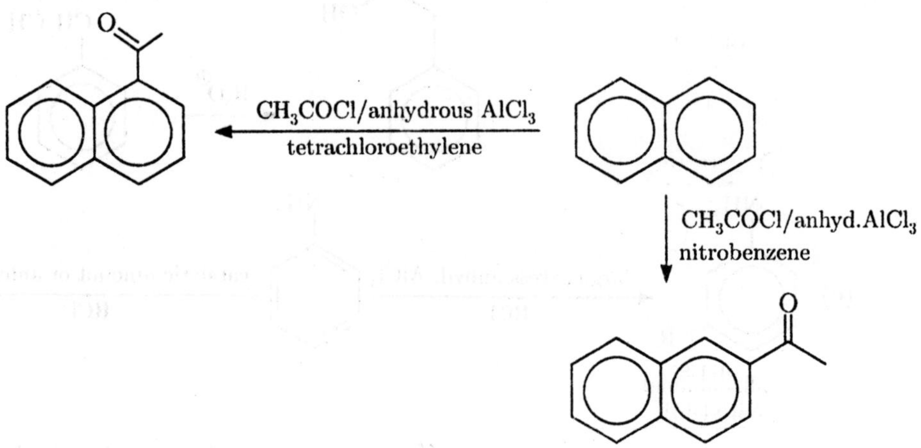

Utilities of Friedel-Crafts acylation reaction :

1. Friedel-Crafts acylation reaction is used to prepared aromatic ketones.

(a) 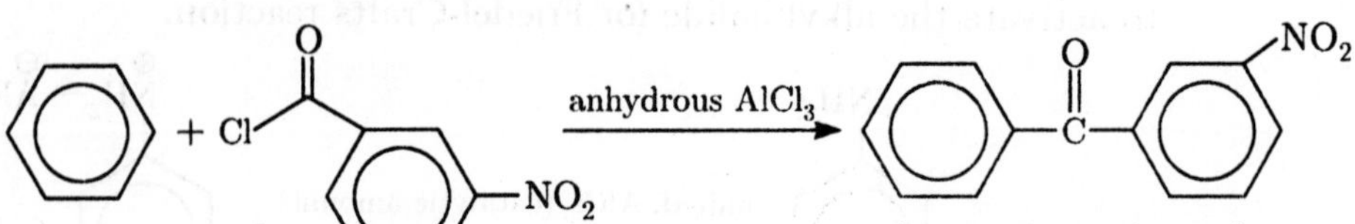

(*m*–nitrobenzophenone)

(b) 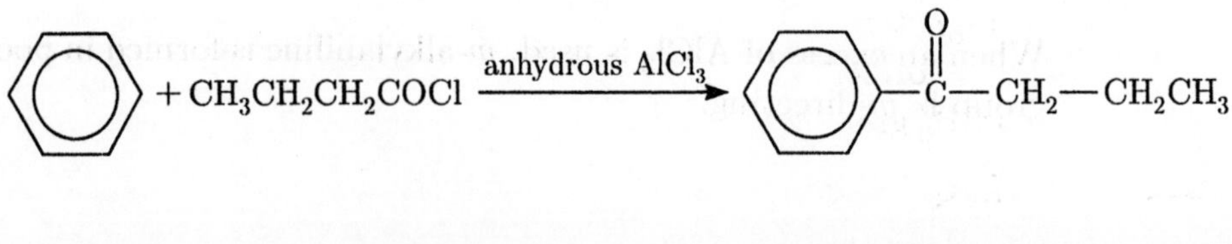

(c) 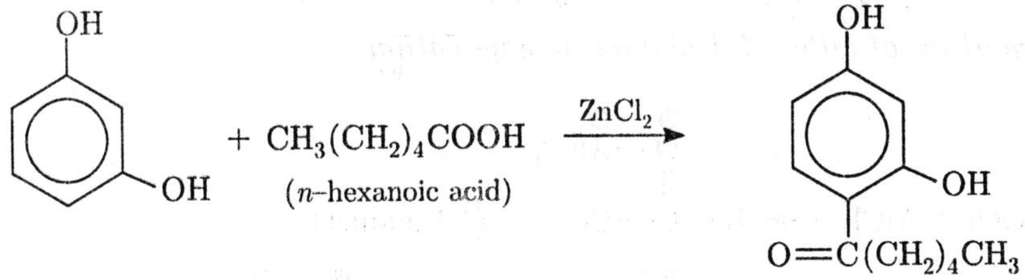

2. Friedel-Crafts acylation reaction is a good method for synthesising polynuclear hydrocarbons like naphthalene, anthracene and phenanthrene.
3. Friedel-Crafts alkylation reaction on fused ring systems give rise to polyalkylated products. But one Friedel-Crafts acylation reaction followed by reduction of carbonyl group, desired mono alkylation is possible.

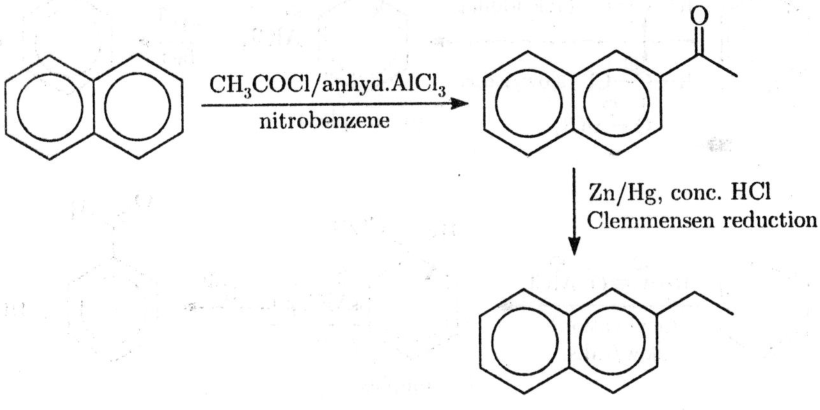

4. Acylation of heterocycles :

(a) 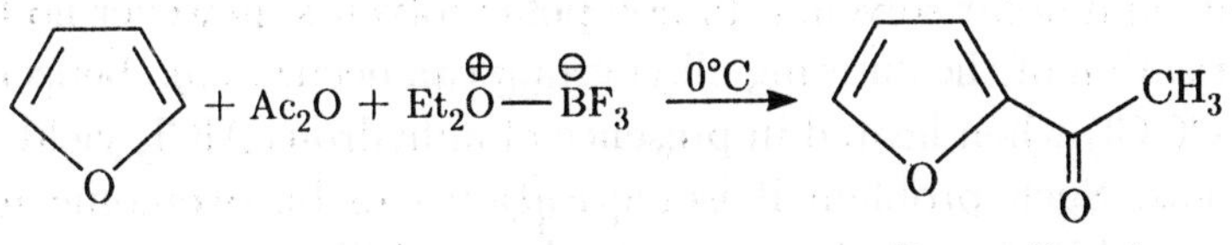

(2-acetylfuran)

(b) 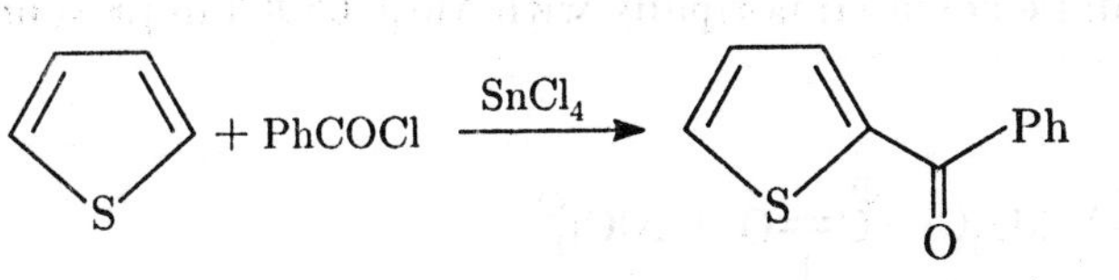

(2-benzothiophene)

5. 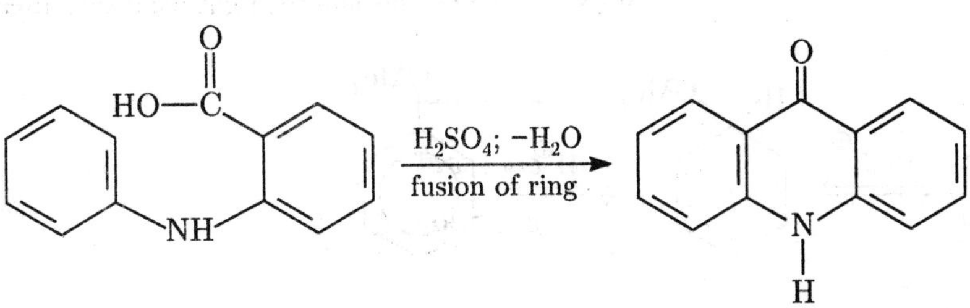

Mechanism of Friedel–Crafts acylation reaction :

Formation of either 1:1 adduct or acyl cation.

$$\mathrm{RCOCl + AlCl_3 \longrightarrow R{-}C(={\overset{\oplus}{O}}{-}\overset{\ominus}{A}lCl_3){-}Cl} \quad \text{(1:1 adduct)}$$

$$\mathrm{RCOCl + AlCl_3 \longrightarrow R{-}\overset{\oplus}{C}{=}O \longleftrightarrow R{-}C{\equiv}\overset{\oplus}{O} + \overset{\ominus}{A}lCl_4}$$
(acyl cation)

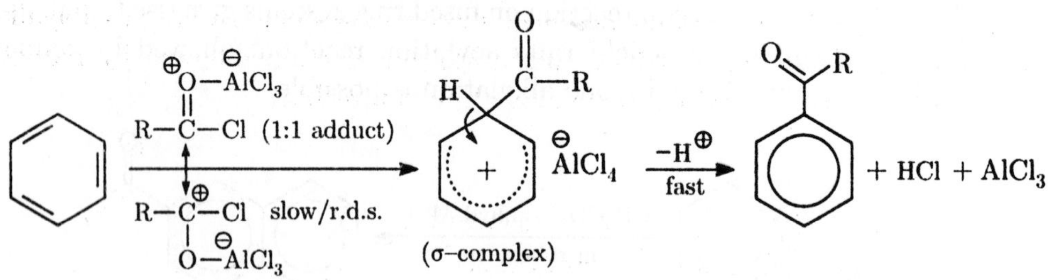

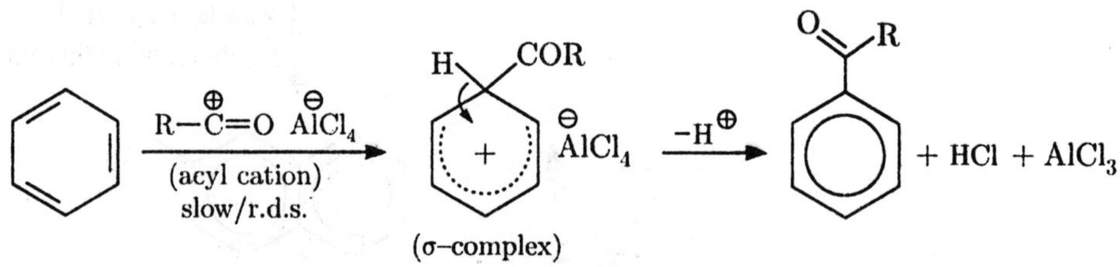

The presence of free acyl cation has been detected by IR spectroscopy in the cases of liquid reagents and polar solvents. In non polar solvents, however no free acyl cation is found. Isomerisation of the entering alkyl group can occur : *e.g.*, benzene and pivoloyl chloride (Me_3CCOCl) when heated in presence of anhydrous $AlCl_3$ yield *t*-butylbenzene liberating CO gas. Such problem if isomerisation can be overcome if the aromatic compound taken is highly reactive towards electrophilic substitution *e.g.*, anisole or N,N–dimethylaniline can be acylated normally with Me_3CCOCl in presence of anhydrous $AlCl_3$.

$$\mathrm{Me_3CCOCl \xrightleftharpoons{AlCl_3} Me_3C{-}\overset{\oplus}{C}{=}O + AlCl_4^{\ominus}}$$
$$\downarrow$$
$$\mathrm{Me_3C^{\oplus} + CO\uparrow}$$ [Leaves as a gas, hence the equilibrium favours the right hand side direction]

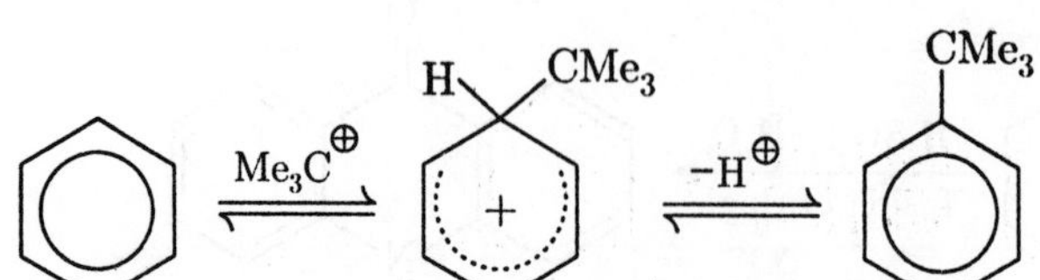

$$Me_3C{-}COCl \xrightleftharpoons{AlCl_3} Me_3C{-}\overset{\oplus}{C}{=}O + AlCl_4^{\ominus}$$

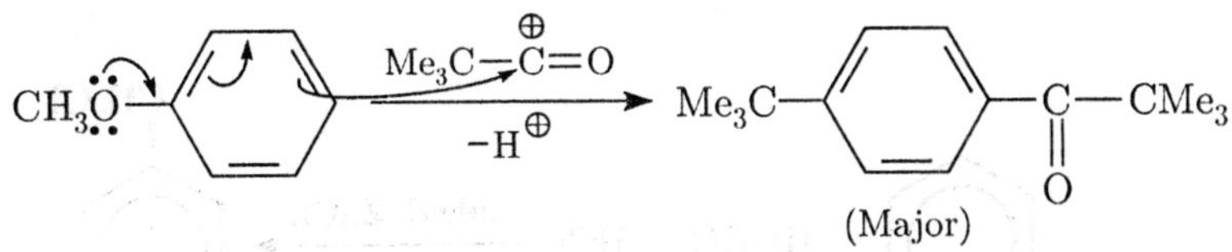

Here the reactivity of anisole towards C–acylation overrules elimination of CO.

***Extension of Friedel–Crafts acylation reaction* :**

1. ***Houben–Hoesch Reaction***

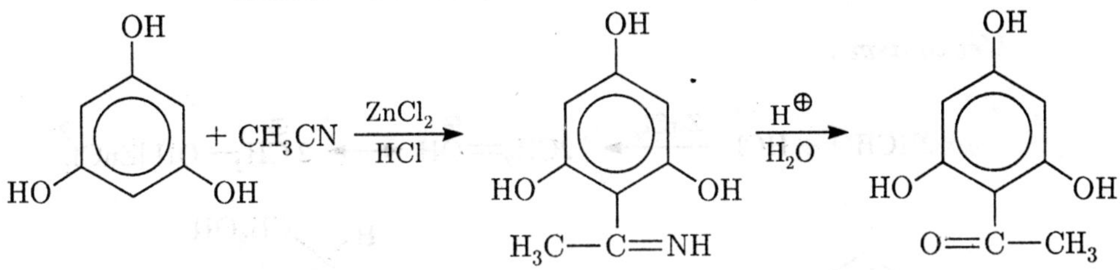

***Mechanism* :**

$$R{-}C{\equiv}N + HCl \rightleftharpoons R{-}C{\equiv}\overset{\oplus}{N}HCl^{\ominus} \longleftrightarrow R{-}\overset{\oplus}{C}{=}NHCl^{\ominus}$$

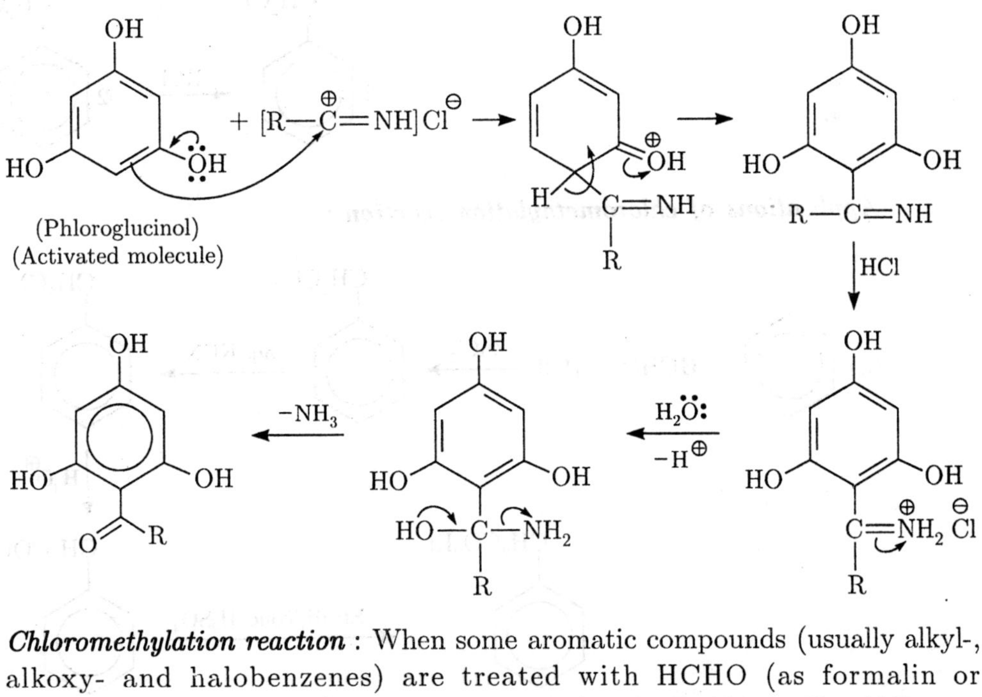

2. ***Chloromethylation reaction* :** When some aromatic compounds (usually alkyl-, alkoxy- and halobenzenes) are treated with HCHO (as formalin or paraformaldehyde) in the presence of catalysts like $ZnCl_2$, $SnCl_4$, $AlCl_3$ etc.

(Lewis acid), one hydrogen (H) atom of the aromatic nucleus gets replaced by chloromethyl (CH_2Cl group) and the reaction is known as chloromethylation reaction.

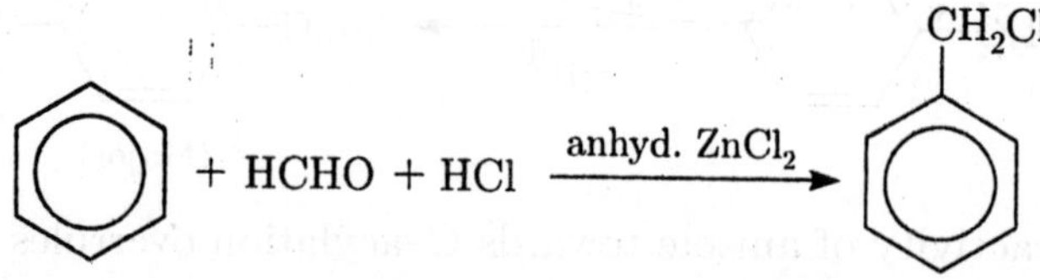

Formaldehyde (HCHO) may be replaced by other aldehydes and HCl by HBr or HI.

Amines and phenols are very reactive and form polymers. The presence of deactivating group retards or even stops the reaction.

Mechanism :

$$2HCHO + HCl \xrightarrow{ZnCl_2} [\,2CH_2{=}\overset{\oplus}{O}H \longleftrightarrow 2\,\overset{\oplus}{C}H_2{-}OH\,]ZnCl_4^{2-}$$

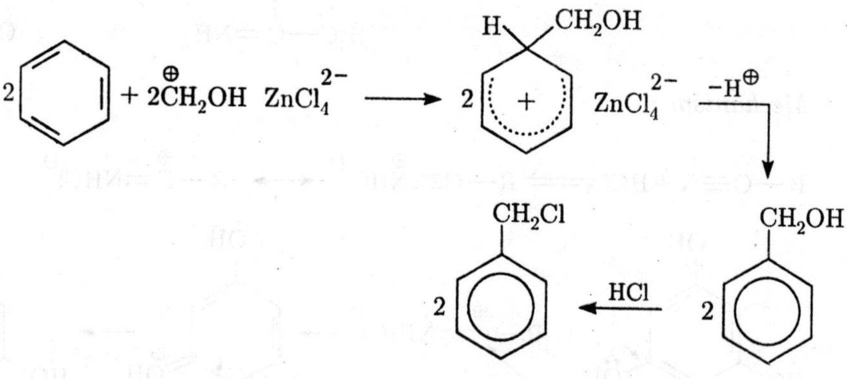

Applications of chloromethylation reaction :

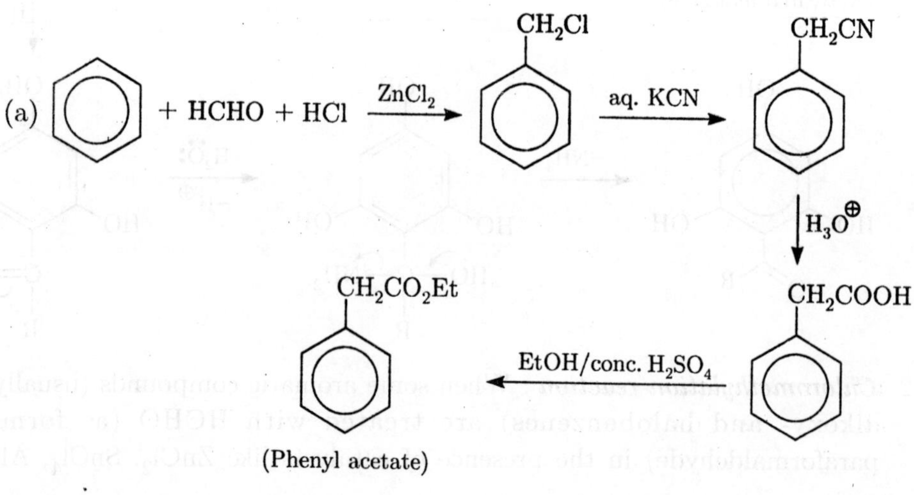

(Phenyl acetate)

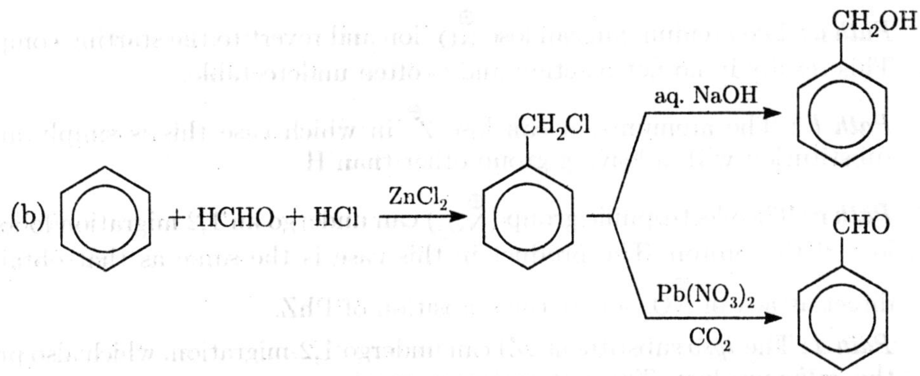

Ipso Substitution

Electrophilic attack can also occur at a position already occupied by a substitutent and this type of substitution is known as *ipso substitution* ("*ipso*" – a Latin word, means "the same"). *Ipso* substitutions are not very common, but they are industrially useful.

Electrophilic ipso substitution : There are at least five possible products for electrophilic ipso substitution shown below.

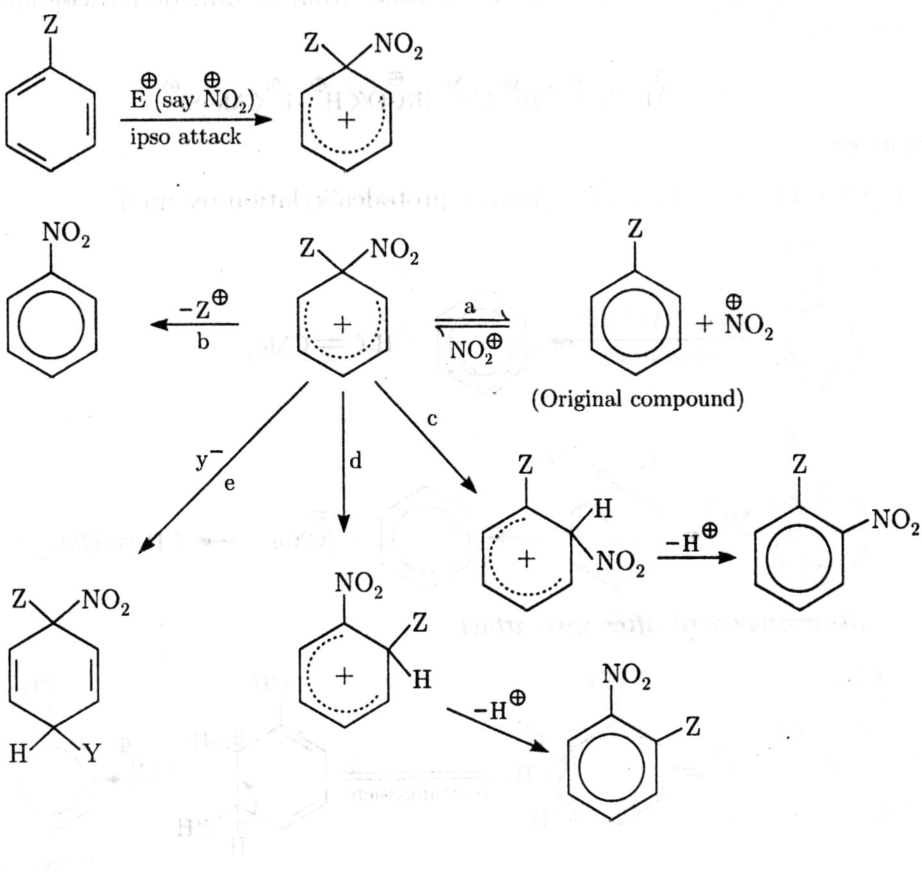

Path a : The arenium ion can lose $\overset{\oplus}{NO_2}$ ion and revert to the starting compounds. This results in no net reaction and is often undetectable.

Path b : The arenium ion can lose $Z^{\oplus}$ in which case this is simply aromatic substitution with a leaving group other than H.

Path c : The electrophilic group ($\overset{\oplus}{NO_2}$) can undergo an 1,2 migration followed by loss of the proton. The product in this case is the same as that obtained by direct attack of $\overset{\oplus}{NO_2}$ ion at the *o*-position of PhZ.

Path d : The *ipso* substituent (Z) can undergo 1,2-migration, which also produces the *ortho* product. This pathway is very minor.

Path e : Attack of a nucleophile on σ-complex gives rise to cyclohexadiene derivatives (1,4–addition to the aromatic ring).

Effect of leaving group in ipso substitution :

1. For leaving groups that depart without assistance (S_N1 process with respect to the leaving group)

$$\overset{\oplus}{NO_2} < iso\text{-}\overset{\oplus}{Pr} \sim \overset{\oplus}{SO_3} < t\overset{\oplus}{Bu} \sim Ar\overset{\oplus}{N_2} < Ar\overset{\oplus}{C}HOH < \overset{\oplus}{NO} < \overset{\oplus}{CO_2}$$

2. Leaving groups that depart with assistance from an outside nucleophile. (S_N2 process).

$$\overset{\oplus}{Me} < Cl^{\oplus} < Br^{\oplus} < D^{\oplus} \sim R\overset{\oplus}{C}O < H^{\oplus} \sim I^{\oplus} < Me_3Si^{\oplus}$$

Examples :

1. Reverse Friedel–Crafts alkylation or protodealkylation reaction.

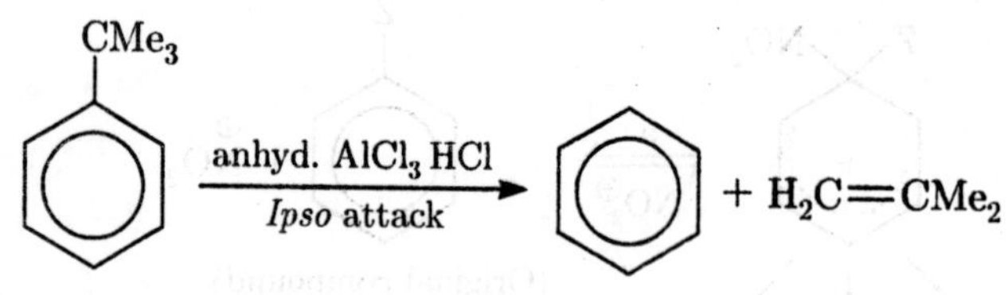

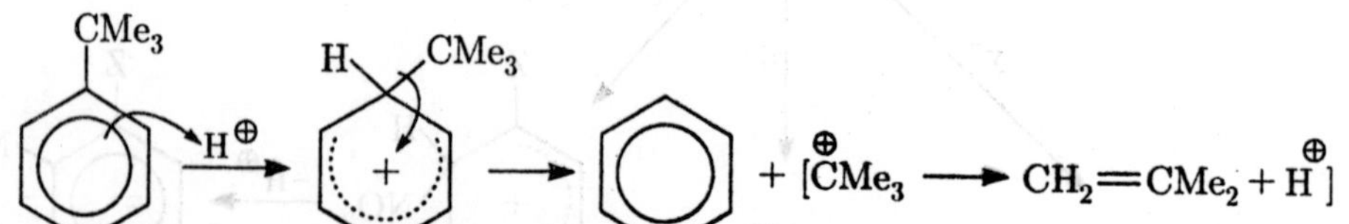

2. (a) ***Rearrangement after ipso attack***

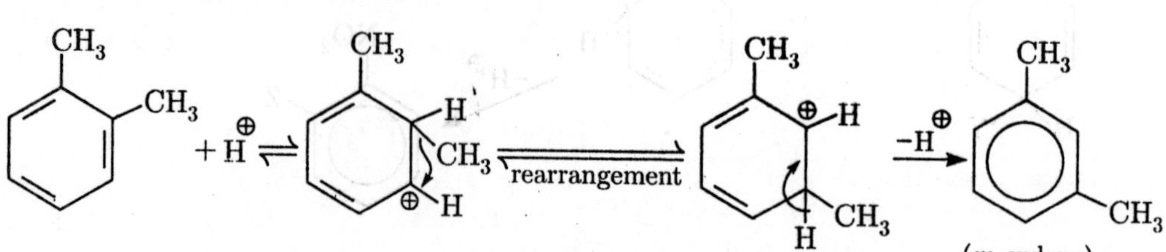

(*m*–xylene)

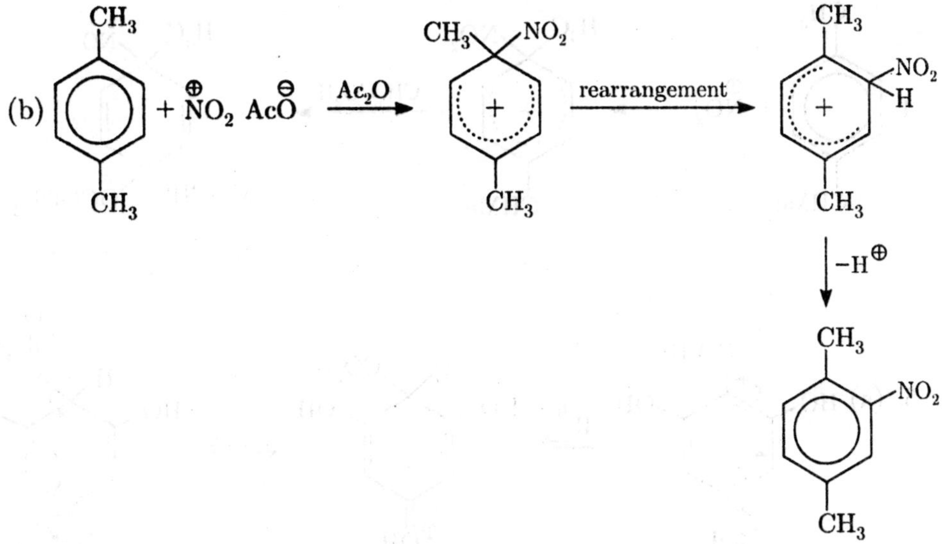

3. ***Nucleophilic aromatic ipso substitution***

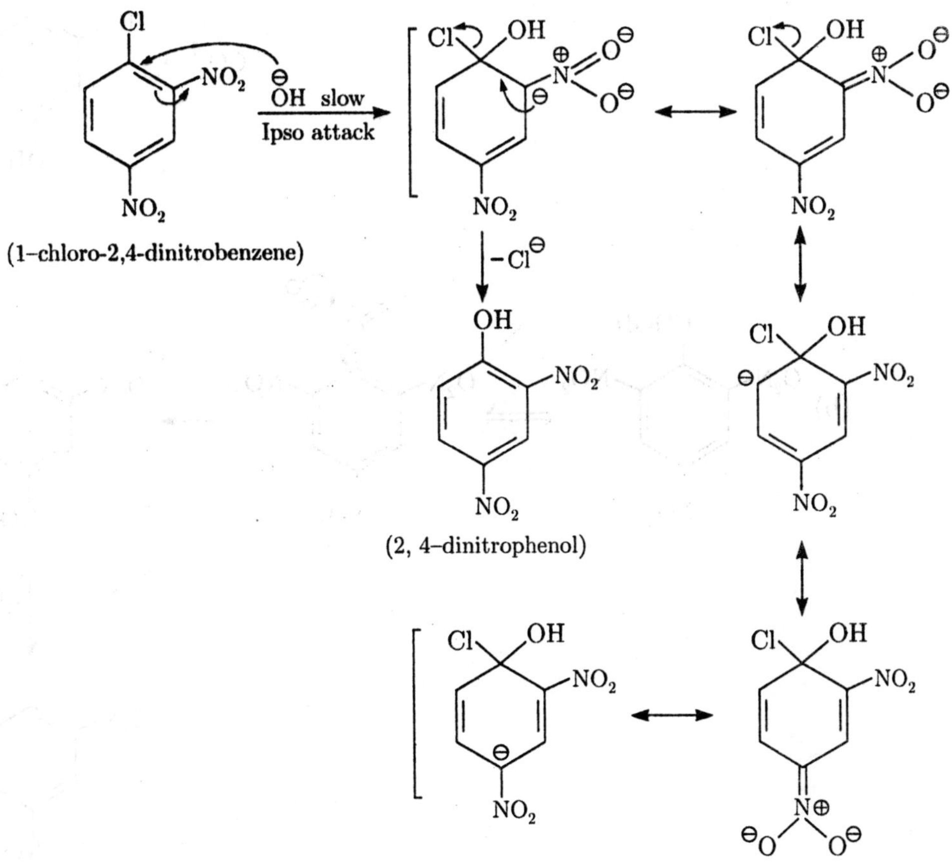

4. 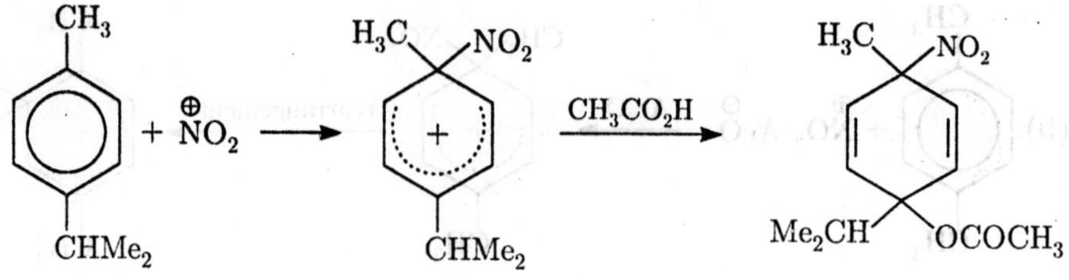

5. (a) 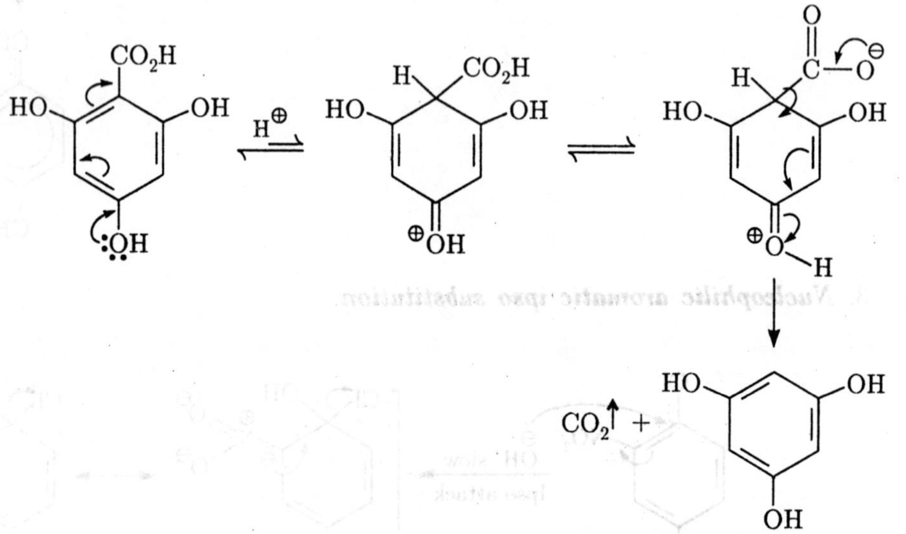

(b) 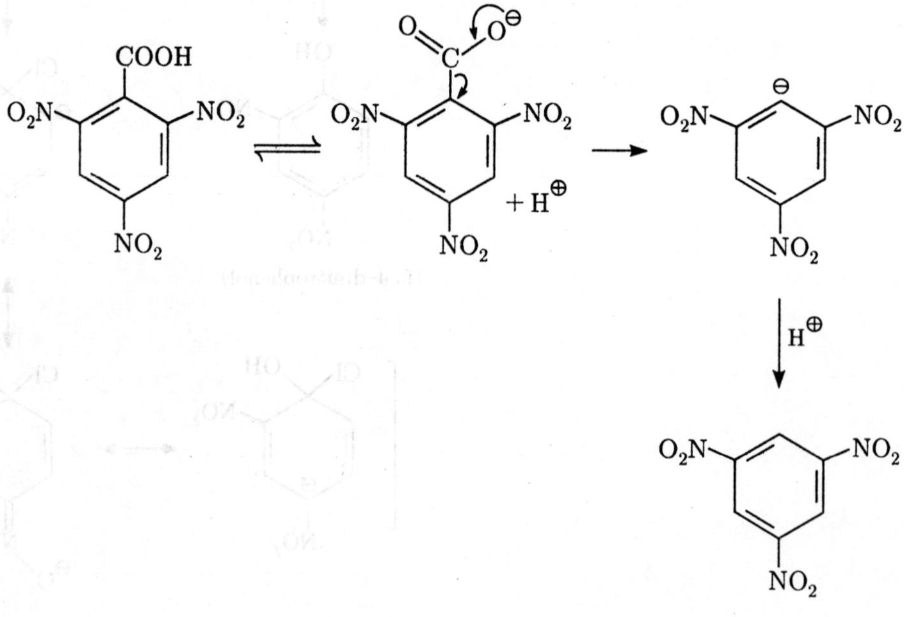

6. (a) 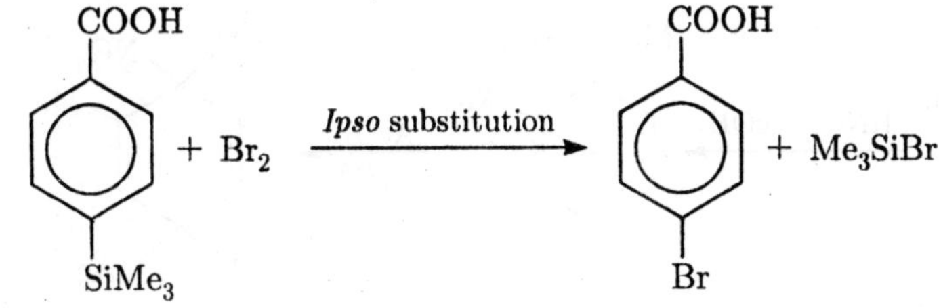

(Arylsilane)

(b) 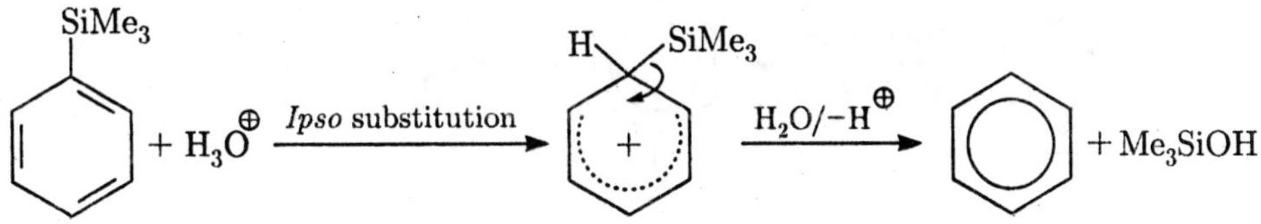

(c) 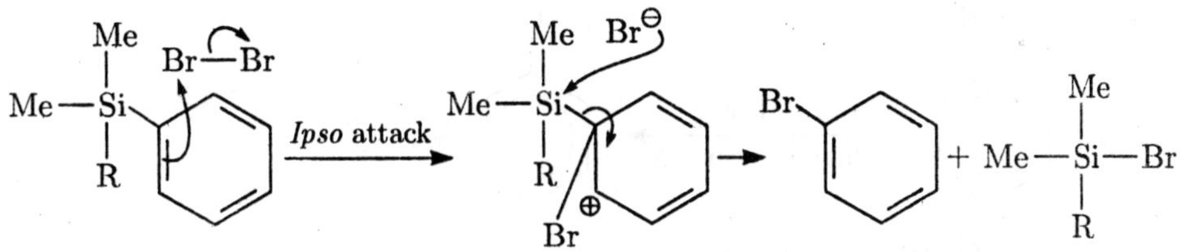

(d) 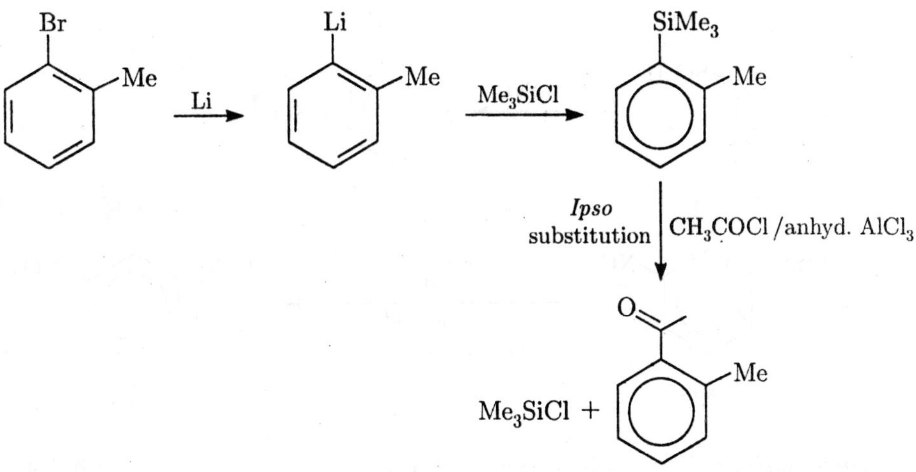

7. 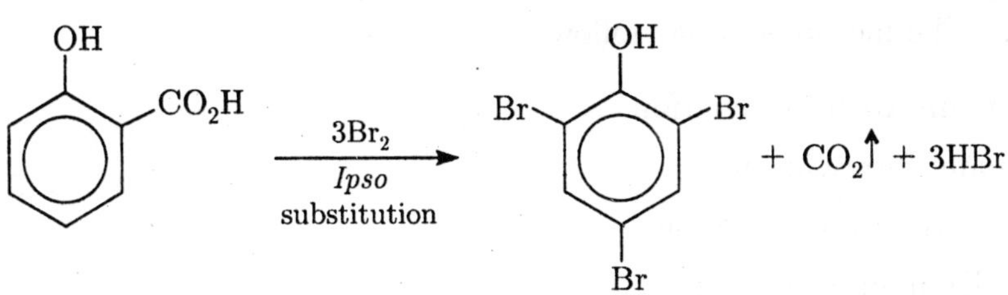

8. 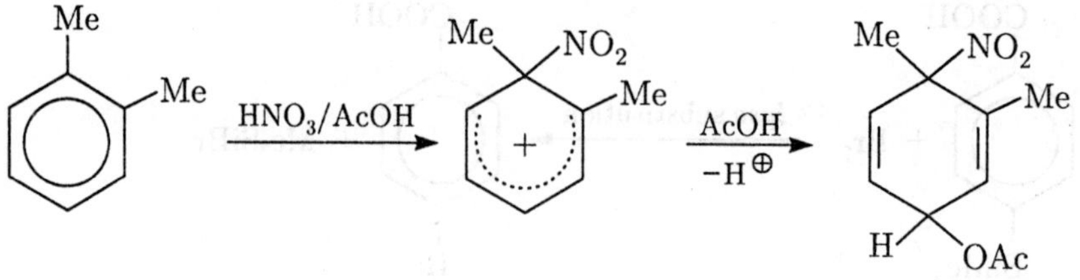

(*cis* and *trans*) 50%

9. 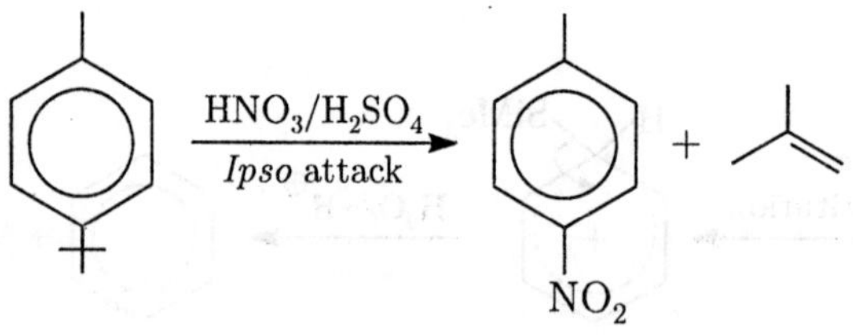

10. 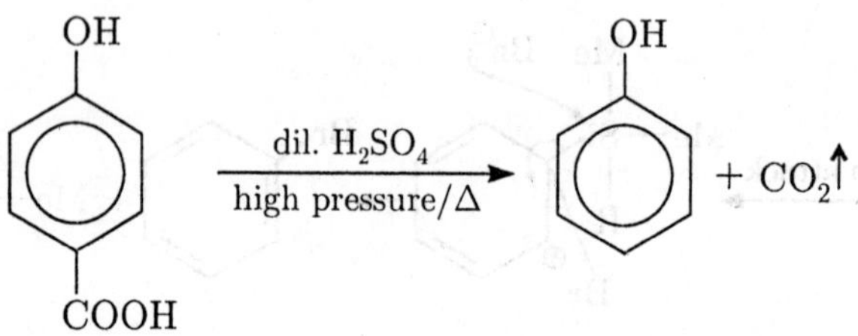

11. 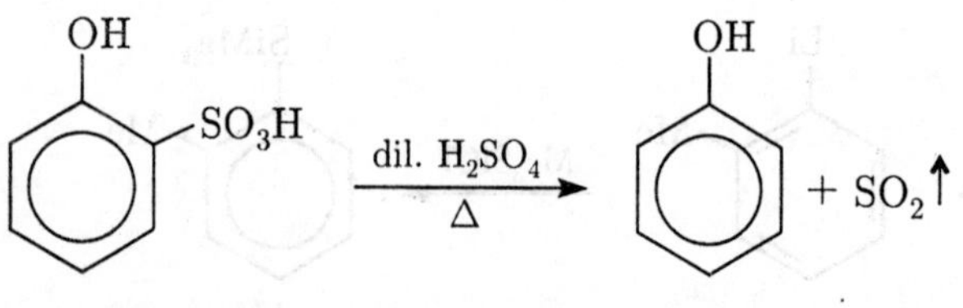

12. 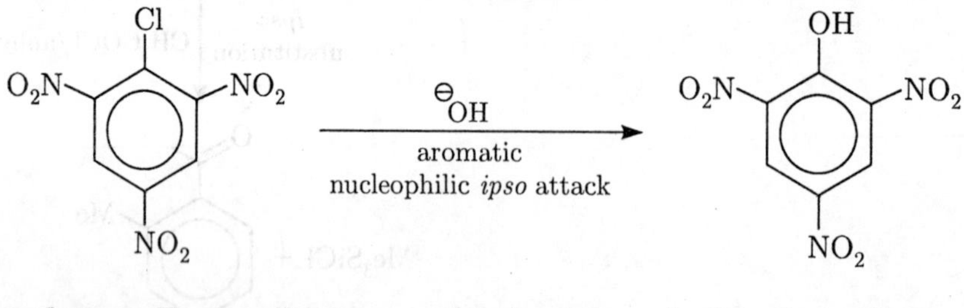

Formylation : Four well known methods of formylation are available. The method which is to be applied, very much depends upon the reactivity of the aromatic compound to be formylated. The methods are as follows.

1. Gattermann–Koch formylation
2. Gattermann formylation
3. Vilsmeyer–Haack formylation
4. Reimer–Tiemann formylation

1. ***Gattermann–Koch formylation*** : The formyl group (–CHO) may be introduced into aromatic nucleus by treatment of the aromatic compound with CO and concentrated HCl in presence of a Lewis acid like anhydrous $AlCl_3$. The reaction is carried out either under pressure or in presence of $Cu^{\oplus}$ ion (generally Cu_2Cl_2).

$$Ar—H + CO \xrightarrow[Cu_2Cl_2]{HCl + \text{anhydrous } AlCl_3} ArCHO$$

Mechanism : Originally it was thought that the reaction occurs through the formation of formyl chloride (HCOCl) from the reaction between CO and HCl followed by a Friedel–Crafts acylation catalysed by a Lewis acid. But now it is proved that the active electrophile here is the formyl cation which is formed without the mediation of formyl chloride, as follows.

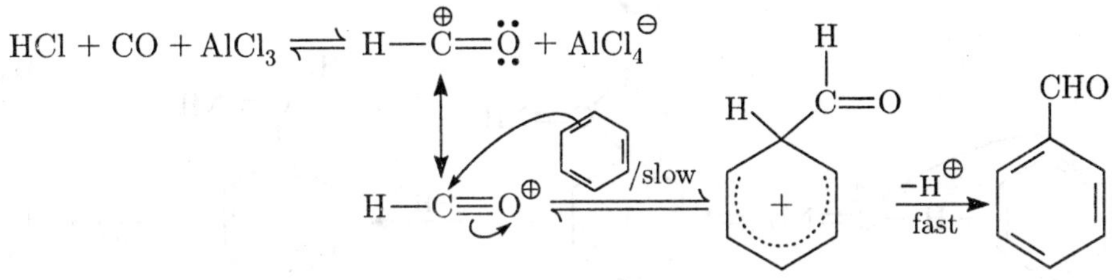

The role of Cu_2Cl_2 may be to aid the reaction between CO and HCl *via* a complex which it forms with CO.

Application and Scope : Gattermann–Koch formylation can not be applied to compounds of lower reactivity than halogenobenzenes. Nitrobenzene is inert and it can be used as a solvent for this reaction. It is also unsuccessful with phenols and phenolic ethers because the Lewis acid used for this reaction form complexes with the phenolic oxygen. Another drawback of this reaction is that polyalkylated benzenes undergo rearrangement during formylation by this process. *e.g*, *p*-xylene gives 2,4-dimethylbenzaldehyde with Gattermann–Koch formylation.

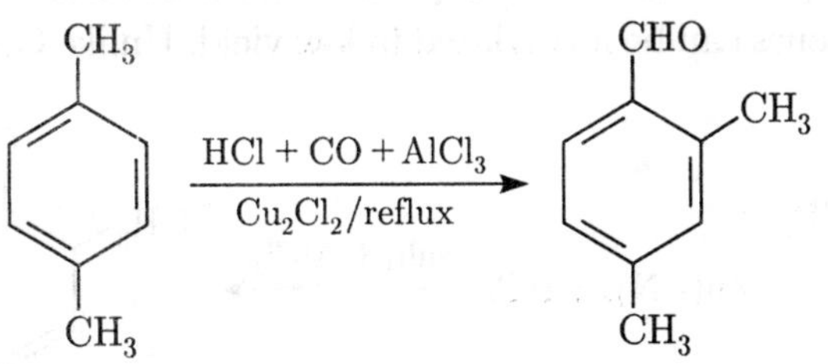

Gattermann Reaction : This method of formylation is a modification of Gattermann–Koch method of formylation. In this method the aromatic compound is treated with HCN and HCl in presence of a Lewis acid catalyst like anhydrous $AlCl_3$. Initially, an imminium hydrochloride is formed which is converted to the aldehyde by treatment with dilute mineral acid like dilute hydrochloric acid. It is convenient to use $Zn(CN)_2$ instead of direct use of HCN and here, HCN is generated *in situ* from the reaction between $Zn(CN)_2$ and HCl.

$$\text{Ar—H} + \text{HCN} + \text{HCl} \xrightarrow{\text{anhydrous AlCl}_3} \text{Ar—CH}_2\text{=}\overset{\oplus}{\text{N}}\text{H}_2\text{Cl}^{\ominus} \xrightarrow{\text{HCl/H}_2\text{O}} \text{Ar—CHO} + \text{NH}_4\text{Cl}$$

Mechanism : In Gattermann reaction, under the influence of a strong acid (HCl), the nitrogen of HCN becomes protonated to generate an ionic species $\text{H—}\overset{\oplus}{\text{C}}\text{=NH}$ analogous to the formyl, cation, $\text{H—}\overset{\oplus}{\text{C}}\text{=O}$.

$$\text{H—C}\equiv\ddot{\text{N}} + \text{H}^{\oplus} \rightleftharpoons \text{H—C}\equiv\overset{\oplus}{\text{N}}\text{H} \longleftrightarrow \text{H—}\overset{\oplus}{\text{C}}\text{=NH}$$

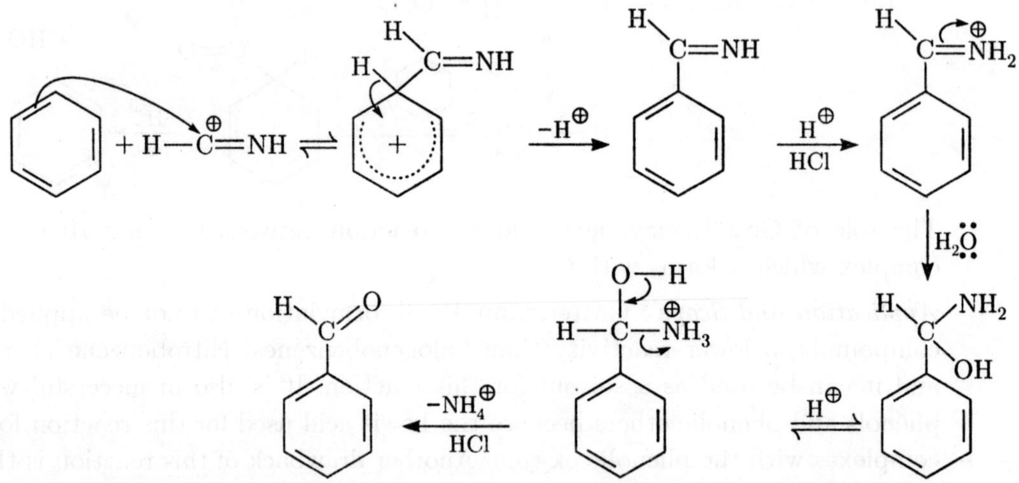

Application and Scope : This reaction is unsuccessful with compounds like nitrobenzene or cyanobenzene. Compounds with moderate reactivity such as benzene and halogenobenzenes can be formylated in low yield. Unlike Gattermann–Koch formylation,

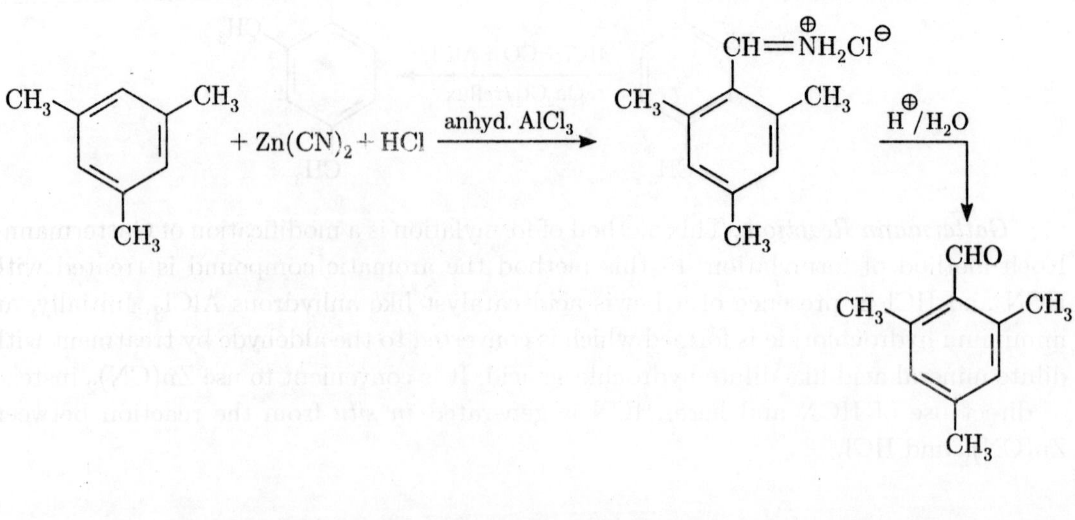

Gattermann reaction is successful with phenols and phenolic ethers, *e.g*, anisole can be made to undergo Gattermann reaction in quantitative yield in presence of anhydrous $AlCl_3$. To avoid the use of HCN it is better to use $Zn(CN)_2$ which form HCN *in situ* by reaction with HCl. This reaction can be successfully used to prepare sterically hindered aldehydes, *e.g.*, mesitaldehyde can be prepared from mesitylene by treatment of $Zn(CN)_2$ and anhydrous $AlCl_3$ in presence of concentrated HCl in carbon tetrachloride solvent.

Vilsmeyer–Haack Formylation

In this reaction, the aromatic compound is made to react with a secondary amine and formic acid in presence of phosphorus oxychloride. The intermediate, N,N–dimethylimminium chloride, when decomposed with HCl, forms the aldehyde.

$$\text{Ar—H} + R_2NH \xrightarrow[HCOOH]{POCl_3} \text{Ar—CH}{=}\overset{\oplus}{N}R_2Cl^{\ominus} \xrightarrow[H_2O]{H^{\oplus}} \text{Ar—CHO} + R_2\overset{\oplus}{N}H_2Cl^{\ominus}$$

Mechanism : In Vilsmeyer method, formic acid first reacts with the secondary amine under the influence of heat to give N–formylamine which in its turn generates the formylating electrophilic species with $POCl_3$.

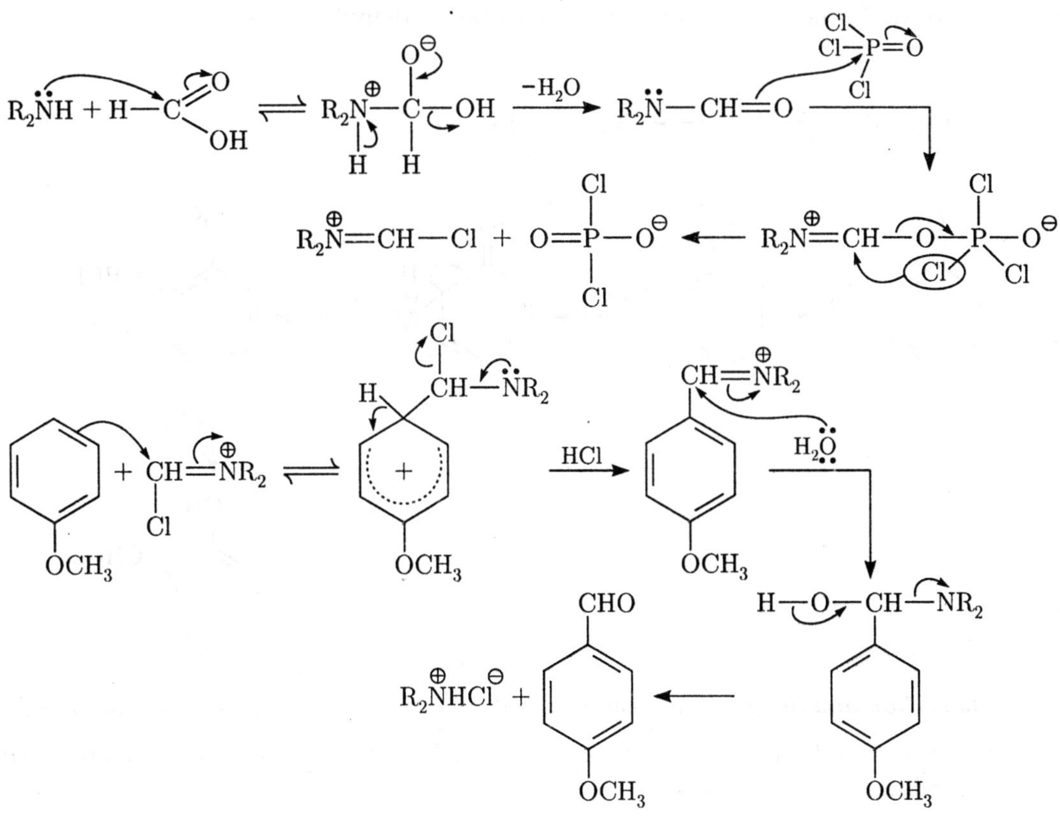

Application and Scope : Only most reactive aromatic compounds like anisole or N,N–dimethylaniline can be formylated under this process, but benzene is inert, *e.g.*, N,N–dimethylaniline gives *p*-N,N–dimethylaminobenzaldehyde by Vilsmeyer–Haack reaction.

Riemer–Tiemann Reaction

This is a method of formylation of phenols in general. When phenol is treated with chloroform ($CHCl_3$) in strong alkaline solution, salicylaldehyde is obtained as a major product, together with some *p*-hydroxybenzaldehyde.

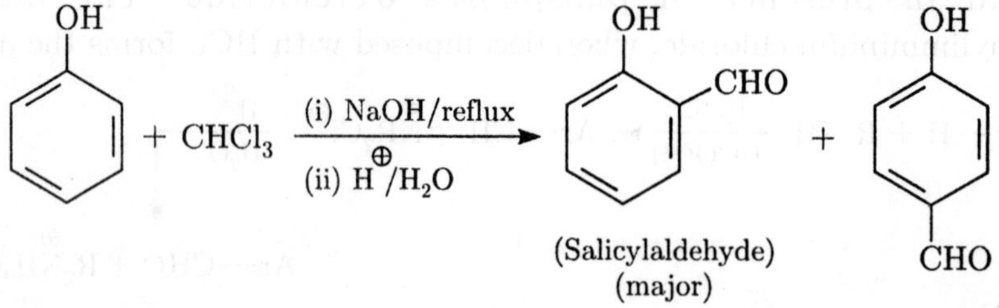

Mechanism : The reaction is believed to occur *via* the formation of dichlorocarbene from the reaction between $CHCl_3$ and NaOH. The carbene (electron deficient), acts as an electrophile though weak, to the strongly activated nucleophile, phenoxide ion. The benzal chloride formed, on acidification, gives benzaldehyde.

$$OH^{\ominus} + H—CCl_3 \longrightarrow :CCl_2 + H_2O + Cl^{\ominus}$$

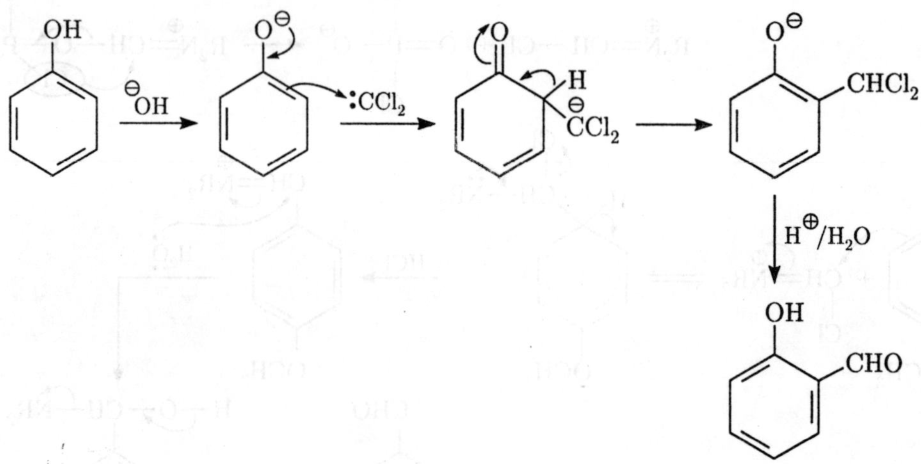

Application and Scope : This reaction gives mainly *o*-aldehyde because the phenolic oxygen forms a stable six membered complex with $Na^{\oplus}$ and carbonyl oxygen of the CHO group as follows.

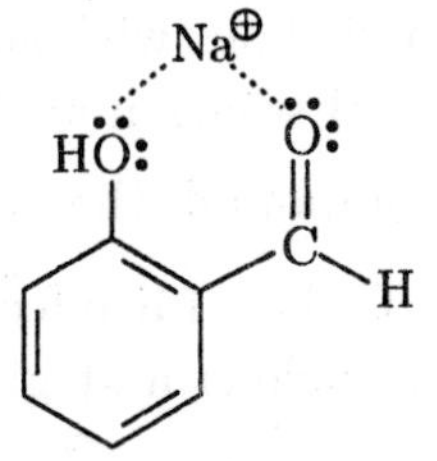

Only very activated nuclei can be formylated by this process because the carbene species is a very weak electrophile. Phenols with blocked *o*-position gives cyclohexadienone derivative in which the two chlorine atoms being in neophntyl type environment, are resistant to alkaline hydrolysis and remain intact.

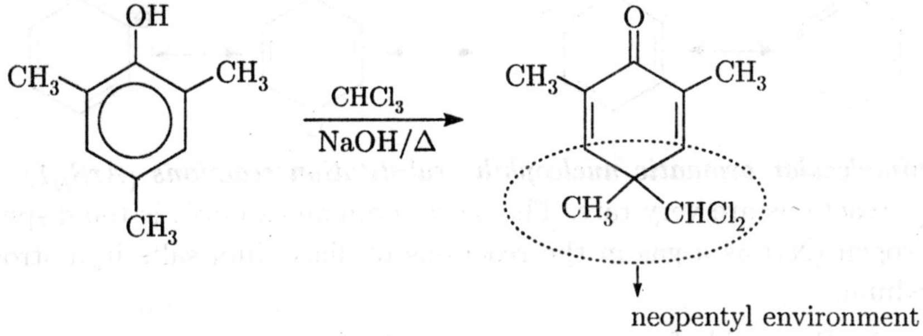

When KOH is used instead of NaOH, the major product obtained is *p*-hydroxybenzaldehyde. This is due to the fact that, larger size of $K^{\oplus}$ prevents the formation of intramolecular chelate and thus, most of the electrophilic attack takes place at the sterically more free *para*-position at which the activation energy of the transition state is also lower due to more delocalization in the transition state.

Aromatic Nucleophilic Substitution

Aromatic systems have π-electron cloud above and below the aromatic nucleus due to the delocalisation of π-electrons. When any nucleophile approaches the nucleus of an aromatic system, an electronic repulsion may occur. So any nucleophilic attack on the aromatic system is very difficult. Substituted aromatic compounds having strongly electron withdrawing substituents like F, $-NO_2$, Cl, –OH, etc. or aromatic nucleus containing heteroatom (O, N, S etc.) undergo nucleophilic substitution with less difficulty as these groups withdraw electrons towards themselves making the nucleus electron deficient. In other words, the aromatic nucleus must be *deactivated* in order to follow an aromatic nucleophilic substitution reaction.

Three types of aromatic nucleophilic substitution reactions are found to occur in practice.

1. Unimolecular reaction *via* a carbocation intermediate (ArS_N1).
2. Bimolecular reaction *via* an intermediate complex anion (ArS_N2).
3. Elimination-addition type *via* an aryne intermediate (*cine* substitution).

Hydrolysis of ethyl chloride is carried out with aqueous Na_2CO_3 solution but that of chlorobzenzene requires aqueous NaOH solution at 360°C at 320 atmospheric pressure.

Chlorobenzene is an aromatic compound, the delocalised π-electron cloud of which repels a nucleophile ($\overset{\ominus}{O}H$) ion here. Cl has +R effect and can form dπ–pπ overlapping with carbon atom of the aromatic nucleus and gives rise to a partial double bond character. So a drastic condition is needed for $\overset{\ominus}{O}H$ anion to act as a nucleophile for chlorobenzene. This situation does not occur with ethyl chloride and so it gets hydrolysed readily.

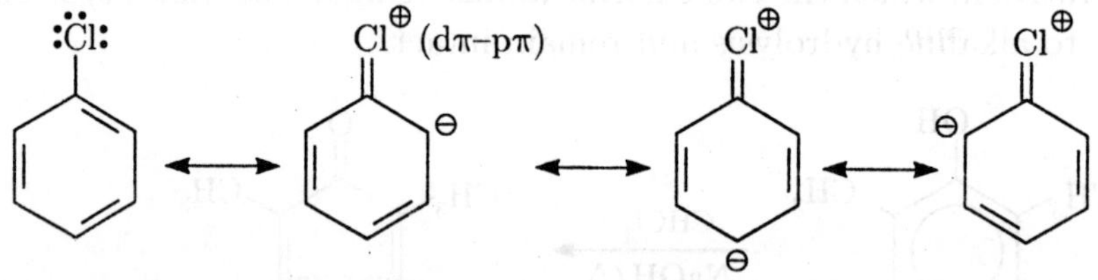

1. ***Unimolecular aromatic nucleophilic substitution reactions ($Ar S_N 1$)*** : Aromatic S_N1 reactions are very rare. The most common example is the displacement of nitrogen (N_2) as a gas in the reactions of diazonium salts in a strongly polar medium.

Step 1 : Reversible formation of aryl cation.

$$Ar{-}\overset{\oplus}{N}{\equiv}N \underset{}{\overset{\text{slow; r.d.s.}}{\rightleftharpoons}} Ar^{\oplus} + N_2\uparrow$$

The reversible formation of aryl cation is proved by using $Ar{-}\overset{15\oplus}{N}{\equiv}N$. The decomposition product is found to contain not only $Ar{-}\overset{15\oplus}{N}{\equiv}N$ but also $Ar{-}\overset{\oplus}{N}{\equiv}N^{15}$. This is possible only if $Ar^{\oplus}$ and N≡N recombines. The aryl cation formed is very unstable, since the positive charge can not get delocalised (positive charge remains in a vacant sp^2 orbital which is perpendicular to the π-electron cloud, and so delocalisation becomes impossible.)

Step 2 : Nucleophilic attack on the cationic carbon

$$Ar^{\oplus} + Nu{:}^{\ominus} \xrightarrow{\text{fast}} Ar{-}Nu$$

Rate of the reaction = $k[Ar{-}\overset{\oplus}{N}{\equiv}N]$ (First order kinetics). Addition of different nucleophile only changes the products into various kinds but the

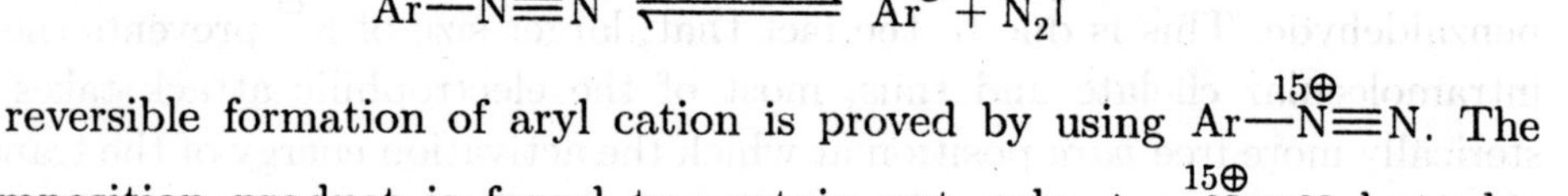

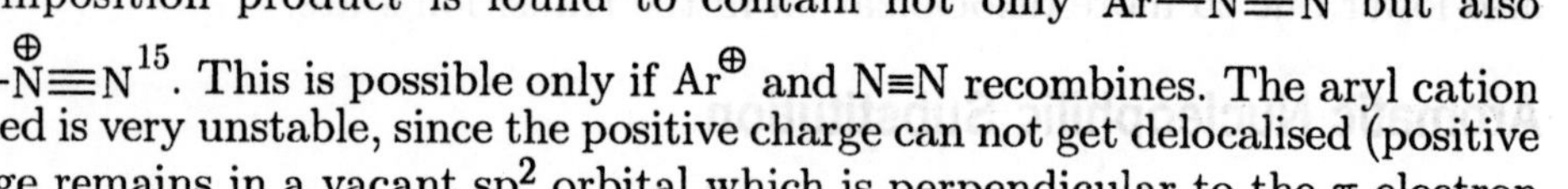

rate of the reaction remains unimolecular. Aryl cation, although it is very unstable is generated here as nitrogen(N_2) is eliminated which is incidentally the most effective leaving group.

2. ***Bimolecular aromatic nucleophilic substitution reaction (ArS_N2)*** : This is the most common type aromatic substitution reaction. $R\overset{\ominus}{O}$, $O\overset{\ominus}{H}$, $\overset{\ominus}{N}H_2$ etc. are common nucleophiles and F, Cl, Br, I, SO_3^{2-}, $R_2\overset{\ominus}{N}$, $\overset{\ominus}{H}$, etc. are the important leaving groups.

Mechanism of bimolecular aromatic nucleophilic substitution reactions :

Step **1** : The aromatic ring contains electron withdrawing group(s), so that the π-electron density of the aromatic nucleus decreases and the incoming nucleophile can attack. An intermediate carbanion known as *Meisenheimer salt* is formed which is resonance stabilised. This step is slow and hence is rate determining.

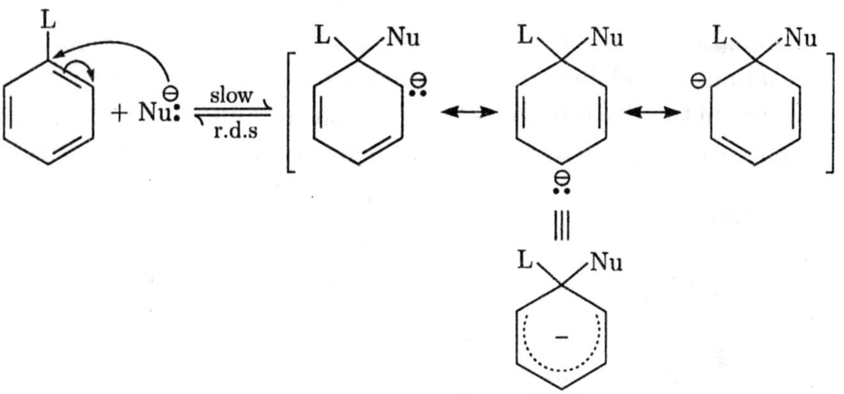

(Meisenheimer complex)

Step **2** : Loss of leaving group from the intermediate anion to yield the product.

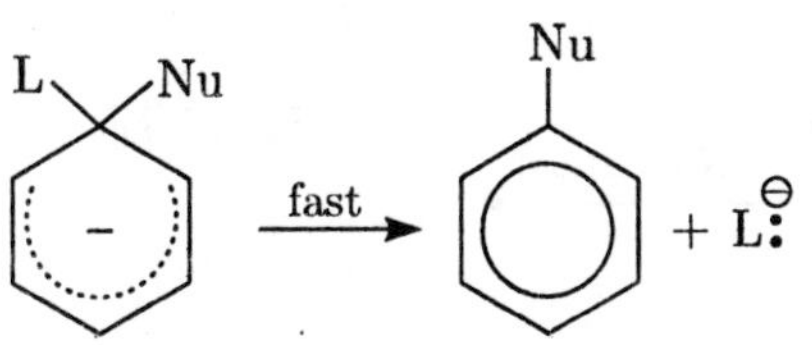

Step 1 is slow and rate determining. As this step involves both substrate and nucleophile the reaction rate becomes bimolecular.

Energy profile for ArS_N2 reaction :

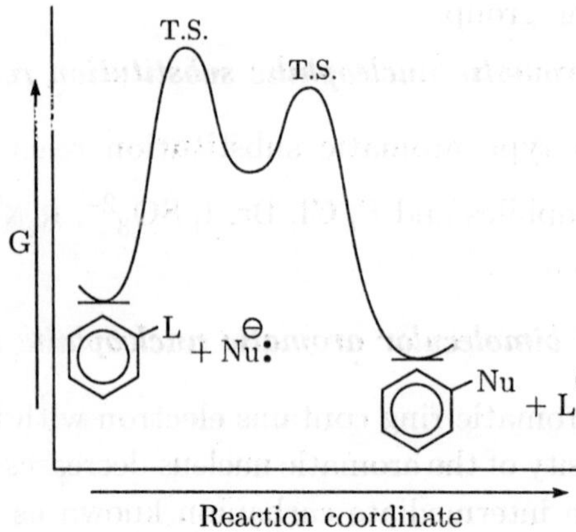

Fig. 3.7 :

Aromatic S_N2 reactions differs from aliphatic S_N2 reactions. In aromatic S_N2 reactions, bond breaking and making are do not occur in a single step but rather in two discrete steps. Moreover in the aliphatic S_N2 reactions, nucleophile approaches from back side which is not a factor in aromatic S_N2 reactions.

Examples :

1. 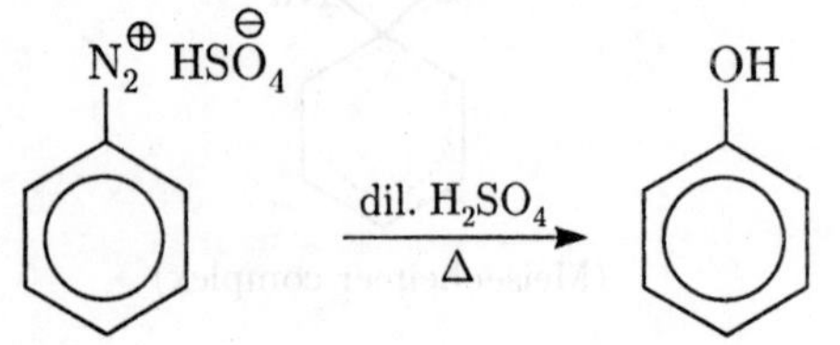

2. 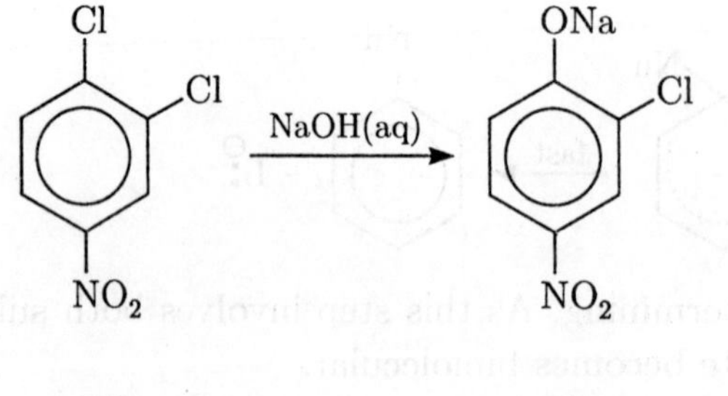

3. 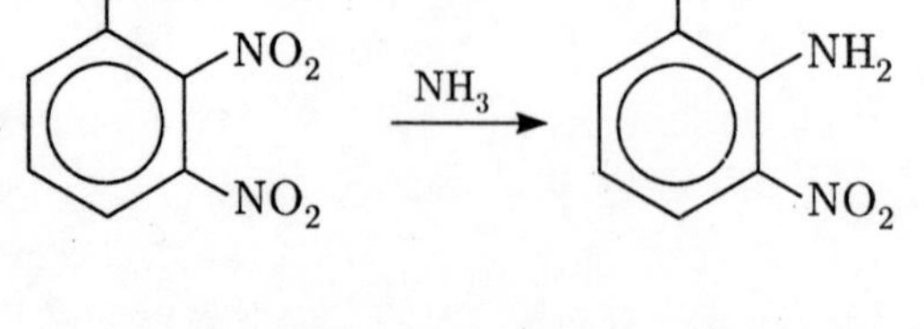

4. 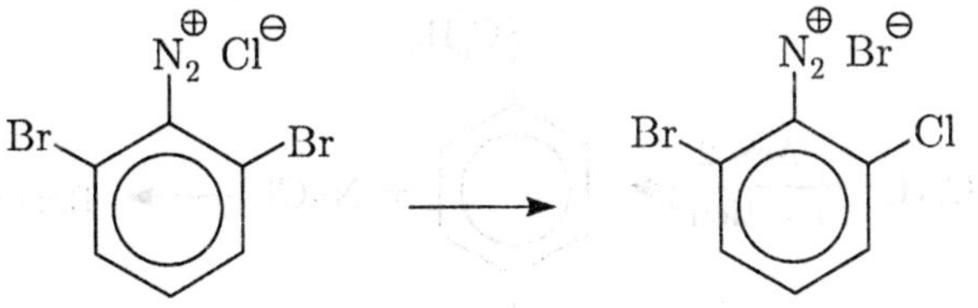

Evidences in favour of ArS$_N$2 reaction :

1. The rate equation of an ArS$_N$2 reaction is as follows.

$$\text{Rate} = k[\text{substrate}]\,[\text{nucleophile}]$$

So with increase in concentration of substrate or nucleophile or both the rate of the reaction increases.

2. Isolation and detection of the intermediate carbanion (Meisenheimer complex) [1902].

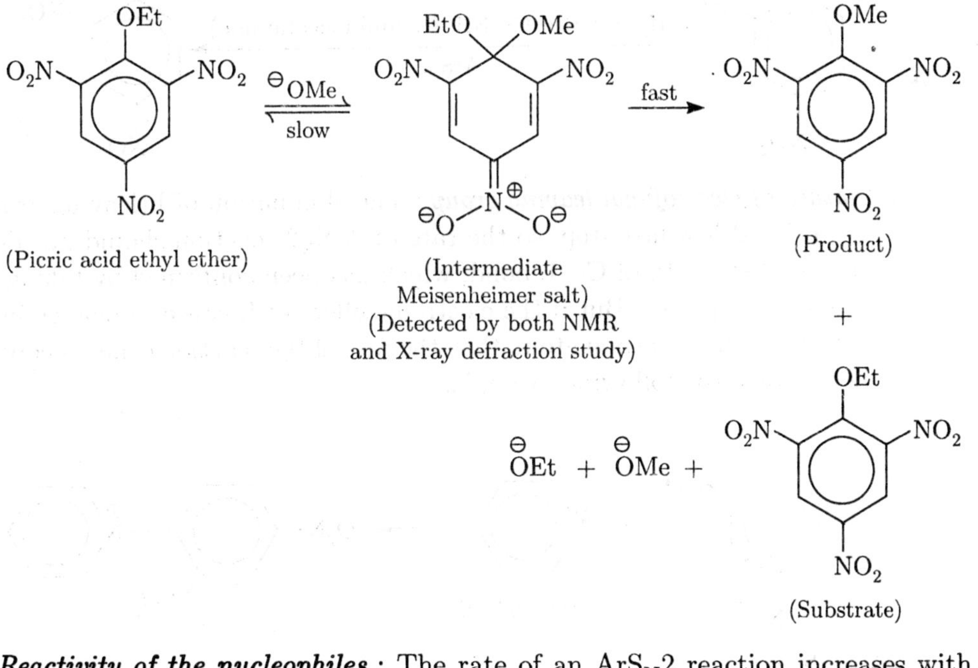

3. ***Reactivity of the nucleophiles*** : The rate of an ArS$_N$2 reaction increases with increase in reactivity of nucleophiles.

Example :

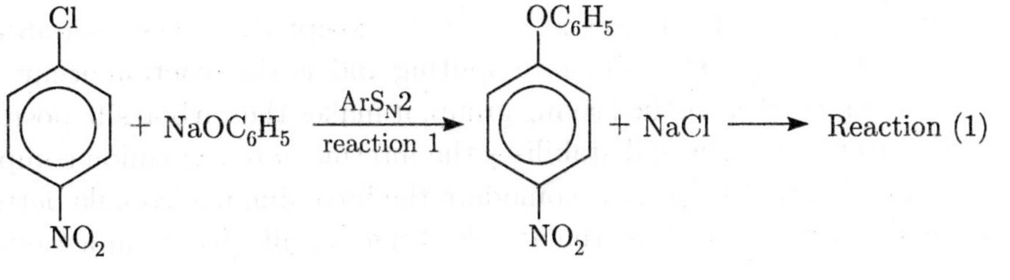

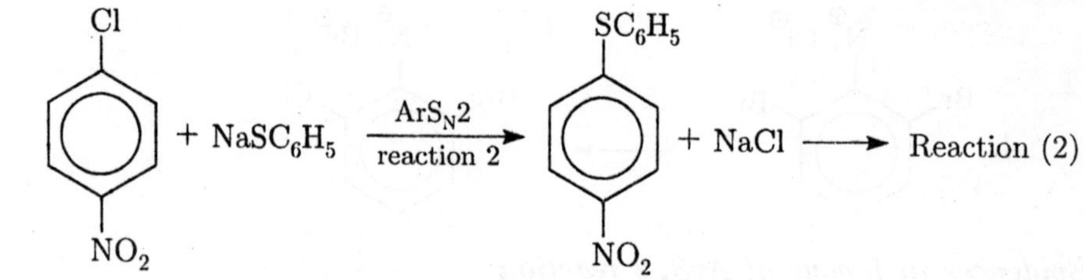

As the reactivity of $NaSC_6H_5$ as a nucleophile is higher than that of $NaOC_6H_5$, the rate of reaction (2) is higher than that of reaction 1. If the nucleophile is an ambident type, then the more nucleophilic entre mainly participates in the reaction.

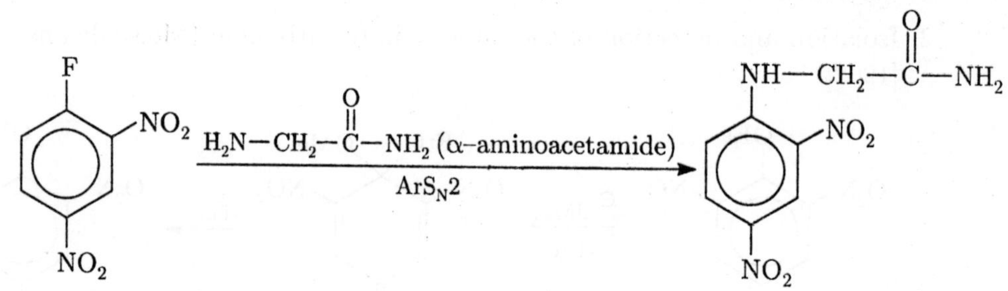

4. ***Nature of electrofugal leaving group*** : The elimination of L(leaving group) from C—L bond is a fast step, so the rate of ArS_N2 reaction should not depend on the bond strength of C—L bond, which has been confirmed by taking different leaving groups (L). But if the electronic effect of L causes a change in electron density at the α-carbon atom, then the rate of the reaction changes considerably. Let us take the following example.

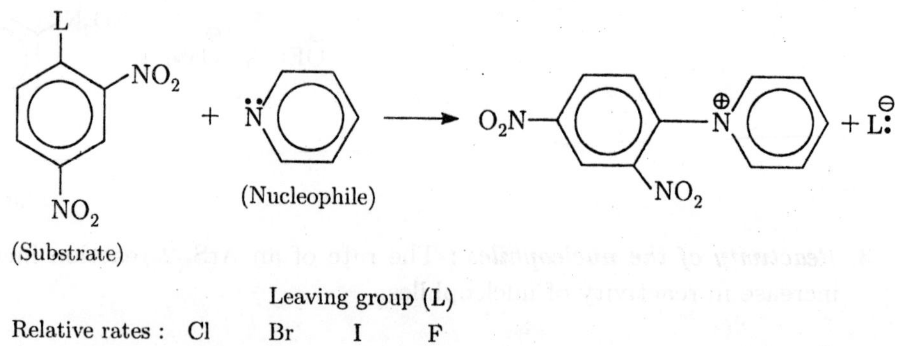

	Leaving group (L)			
Relative rates :	Cl	Br	I	F
	4.3	4.3	1.0	3,300

The negligible differences in the rates (except F) proves undoubtedly that the bond breaking step is not rate limiting and so the reaction occurs in two steps. When F is taken as the leaving group, it makes the carbon site positively charged due to its –I effect and stabilises the intermediate carbanion complex and least size of F–atom helps to accomodate the incoming nucleophile better in the rate determining step Thus, the attack of nucleophile occurs in a facile manner.

Example 2 :

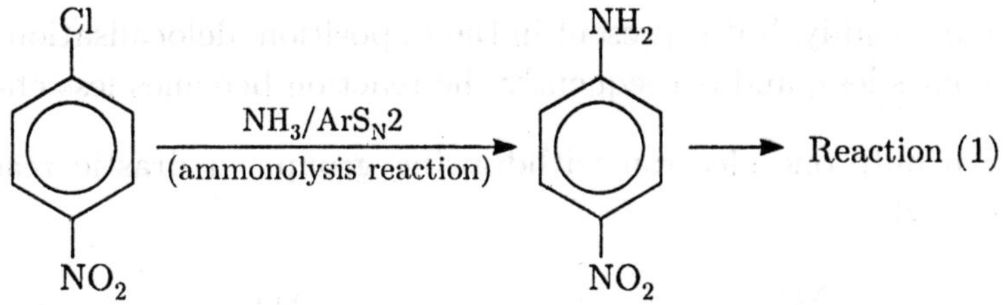

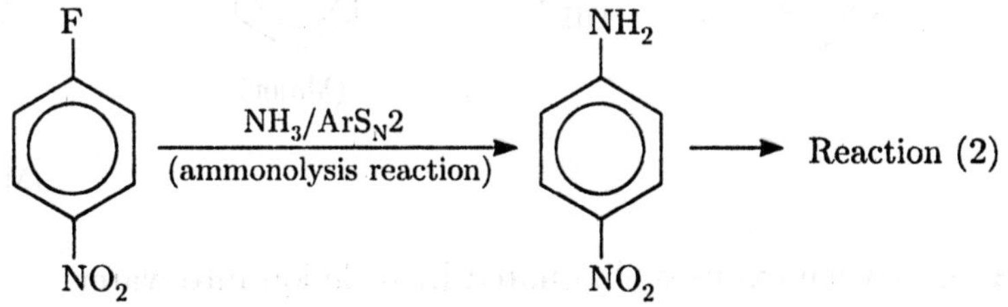

The rate of ammonolysis of reaction (2) is more than that of reaction(1). This is due to stronger –I effect of F by which the intermediate carbanion gets stabilised through effective delocalisation.

5. ***The effect of substrate*** : Arene derivatives should contain at least one electron withdrawing substituent in order to undergo ArS_N2 reaction.

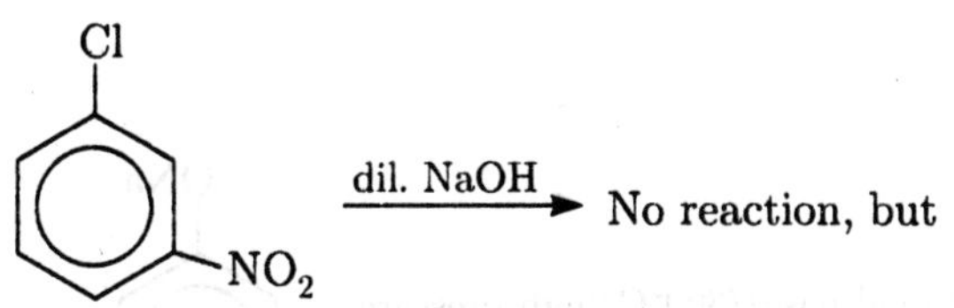

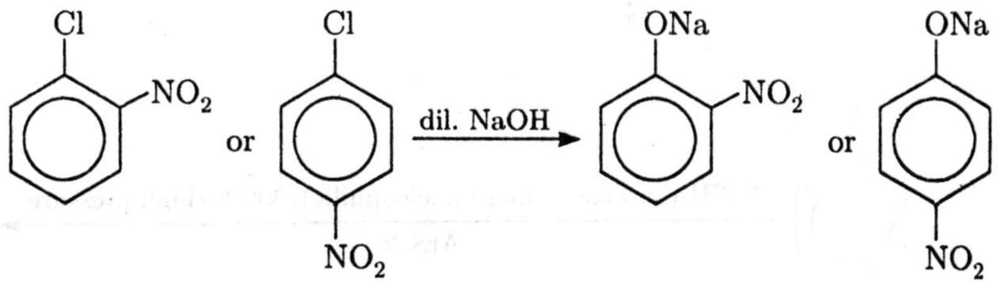

increasing number of electron withdrawing substituent(s), the rate of ArS_N2 reaction increases, as the $\Delta G^{\neq}$ of the reaction decreases, because of the greater stabilisation of intermediate carbanion. The extent of delocalisation of negative charge depends on the position of electron withdrawing group. If the latter is present at the *o*- and *p*-positions with respect to the leaving group, the negative charge of intermediate carbanion gets delocalised substantially and the reaction occurs readily. If it is present in the *m*-position, delocalisation of negative charge becomes less, and consequently the reaction becomes less effective.

With only one electron withdrawing group, a drastic reaction condition is required.

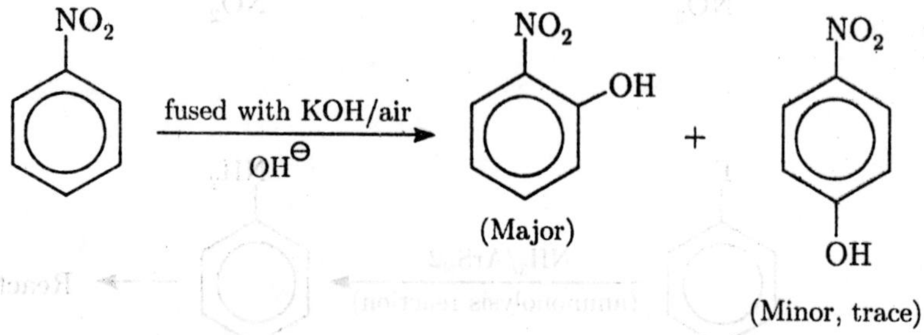

Aerial oxygen oxidises eliminated hydride ion into water.

If the aromatic nucleus does not contain any electron withdrawing group, nucleophiles with *high electron density* and a high temperature and high pressure (as organic compounds are mostly volatile) are to be used for ArS_N2 reaction. Again nucleophiles with high electron density implies to greater basicity and with increase in basicity of nucleophiles another parallel reaction namely addition elimination reaction occurs alongwith ArS_N2 reaction.

Example 1 :

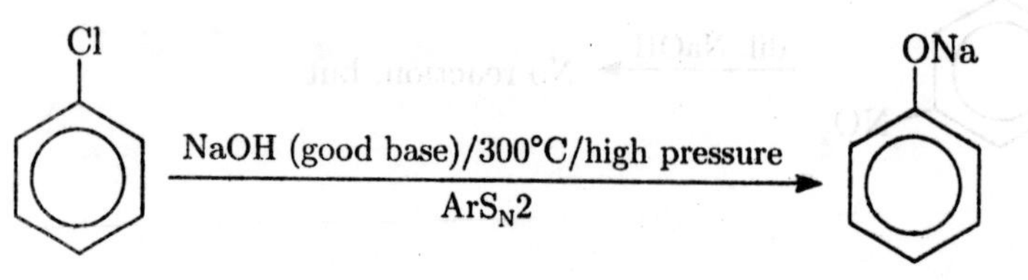

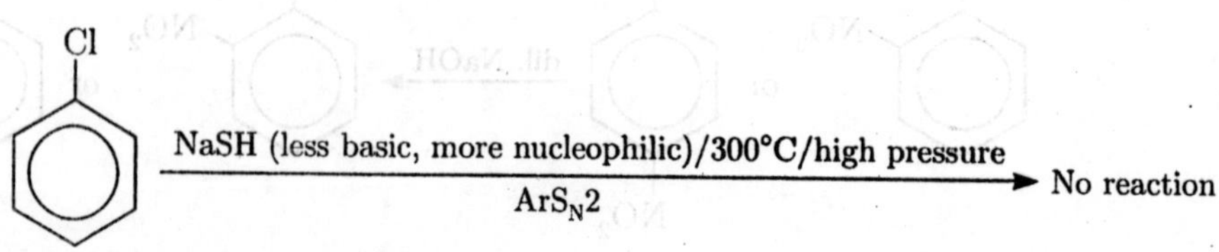

Example 2 : The rate of ammonolysis reaction of 2,4,6-tirnitrochlorobenzene is more than that of *p*-chloronitrobenzene.

The rate of ArS_N2 reaction is justifiably more in case of 2,4,6-trinitrochlorobenzene as the aromatic nucleus is more activated towards ArS_N2 reaction due to the presence of three strongly electronwithdrawing $-NO_2$ groups, whereas in *p*-chloronitrobenzene, there is only one $-NO_2$ group present in the nucleus.

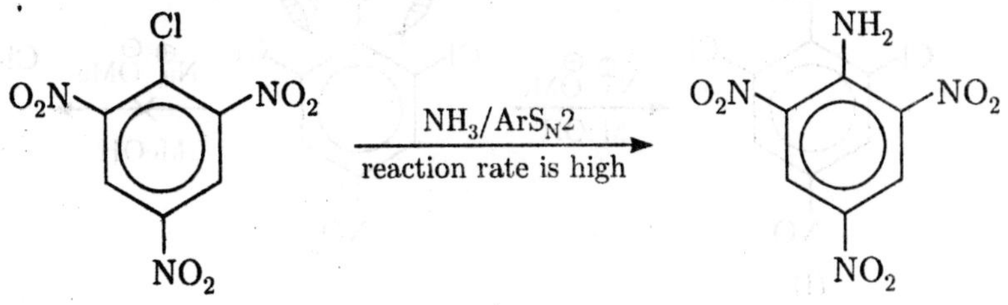

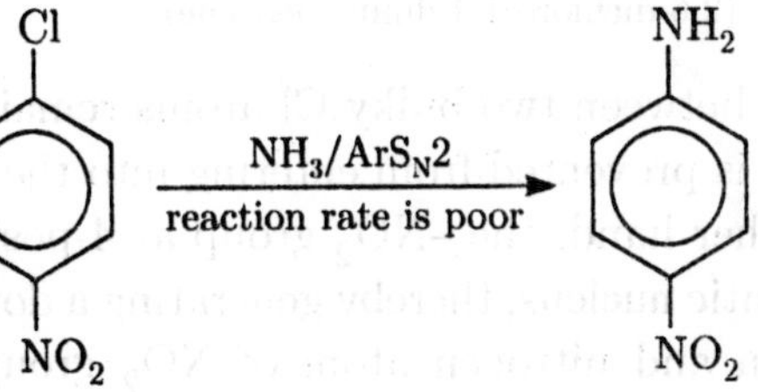

***Example* 3 :**

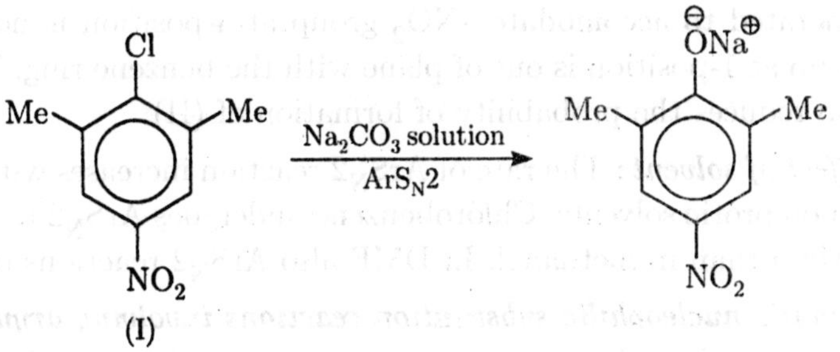

(I)

but

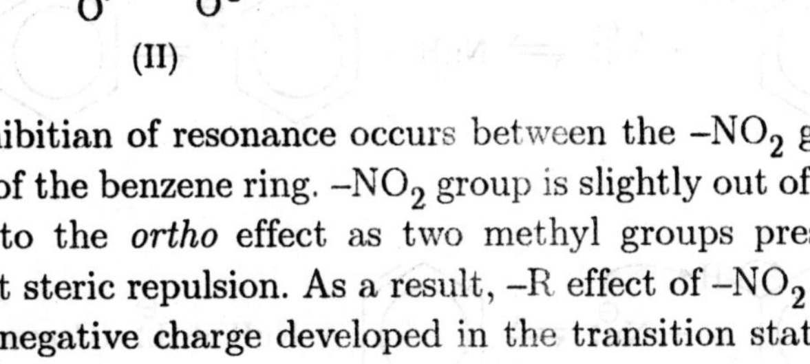

(II)

In (II), steric inhibitian of resonance occurs between the $-NO_2$ group and the π-electron cloud of the benzene ring. $-NO_2$ group is slightly out of the plane the benzene of due to the *ortho* effect as two methyl groups present *ortho* to $-NO_2$ group exert steric repulsion. As a result, –R effect of $-NO_2$ group cannot operate and the negative charge developed in the transition state can not get delocalised. The net effect is that the ArS_N2 reaction does not occur here.

***Example* 4 :**

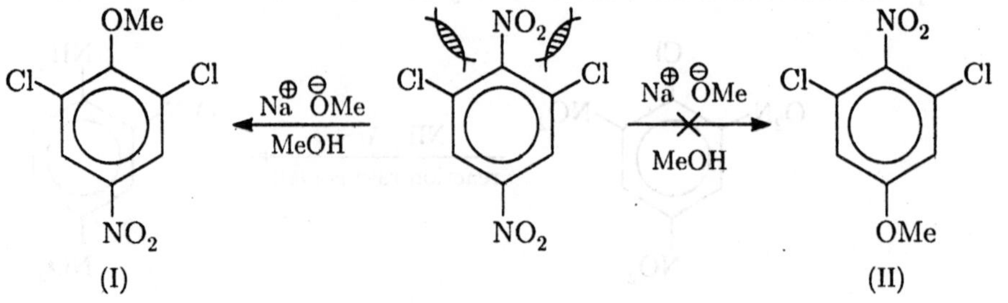

(2,6-dichloro-1,4-dinitrobenzene)

The nitro group flanked between two bulky Cl atoms remains out of plane due to *ortho* effect and thus, is prevented from entering into the resonance with the benzene ring. On the other hand, the $-NO_2$ group at 4-position can enter into resonance with the aromatic nucleus, thereby generating a double bond character between the ring carbon and nitrogen atom of NO_2 group. As a result, the approach of incoming nucleophile $\overset{\ominus}{O}Me$ is prevented and $\overset{\ominus}{O}Me$ can not replace the $-NO_2$ group at 4-position and product (II) is not formed. The carbanion generated to accomodate $-NO_2$ group at 4-position is not stabilised as $-NO_2$ group at 1-position is out of plane with the benzene ring. This electronic factor also reduces the probability of formation of (II).

6. ***Effect of solvent*** : The rate of ArS_N2 reaction increases with increase in polarity of non protic solvents. Chlorobenzene undergoes ArS_N2 reaction more readily in DMSO than in methanol. In DMF also ArS_N2 reactions occur readily.

3. ***Aromatic nucleophilic substitution reactions involving arynes as intermediates*** : If the aromatic nucleus does not contain any strong electron-withdrawing group, then nucleophiles should contain high electron density to polarise the aromatic π-electron cloud in order to facilitate ArS_N2 reactions. But the basicity of the nucleophiles increases as the electron density of the nucleophiles increases and another mechanism becomes operative along with ArS_N2 reactions known as *cine substitution* or *addition-elimination metchanism.*

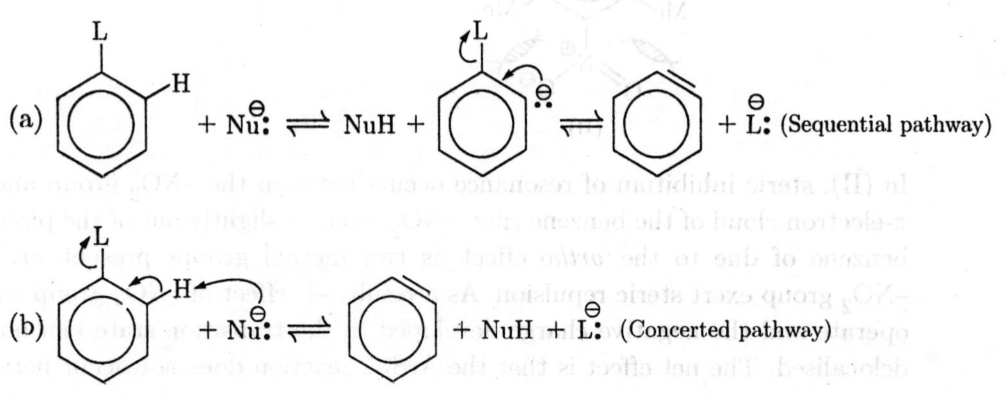

If L has strong –I effect and the bond energy of C—L bond is quite high, then the elimination reaction follows the sequential pathway. The intermediate carbanion is stabilised by –I effect of L and the elimination reaction proceeds *via* E1cB type pathway. For example, $NaNH_2$ (a strong base) reacts with fluorobenzene in liquid ammonia and elimination occurs through a sequential pathway, following the formation of a carbanion. This carbanion gets stabilised by strong –I effect of F atom. But if the leaving group (L) has not much strong –I effect and C—L bond strength is comparatively less, the elimination reaction follows a concerted pathway where E2 type reaction mechanism is followed. For example, bromo- and iodobenzene follows elimination through concerted pathway with $NaNH_2$ in liquid ammonia.

The intermediate formed upon this type of elimination reaction is known as *aryne*. If the aromatic nucleus does not contain any substituent other than hydrogen, it is called *benzyne*.

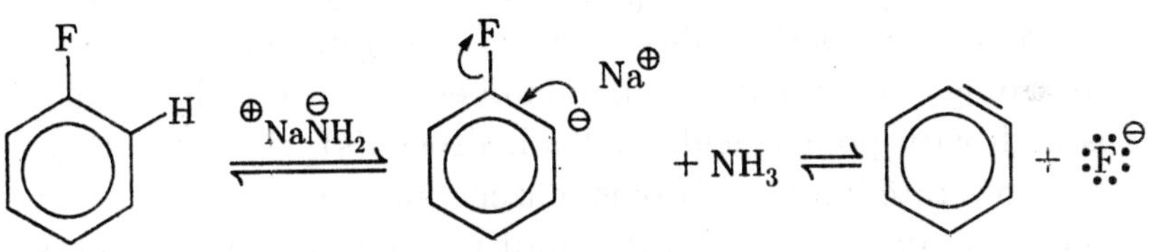

(Benzyne)

Apart from aryl halides, their alkyl and alkoxy derivatives with at least one *ortho* hydrogen, are also substrates for this type reactions and can form an aryne. Arynes are not very stable and can act as an intermediate. Substitution by nucleophiles occurs followed by elimination and the reactions are commonly known as *elimination addition reactions* or *cine substitution.*

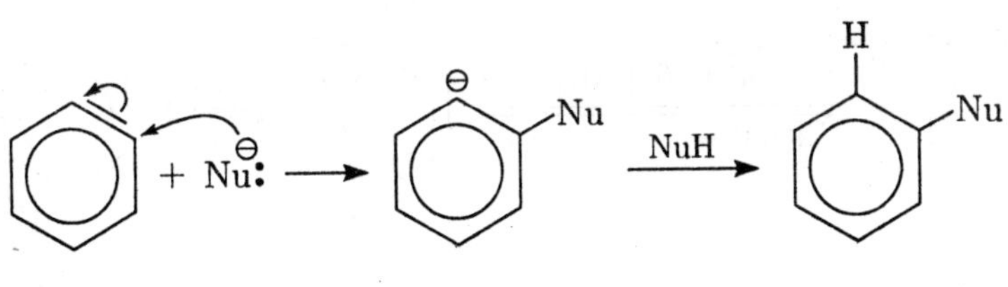

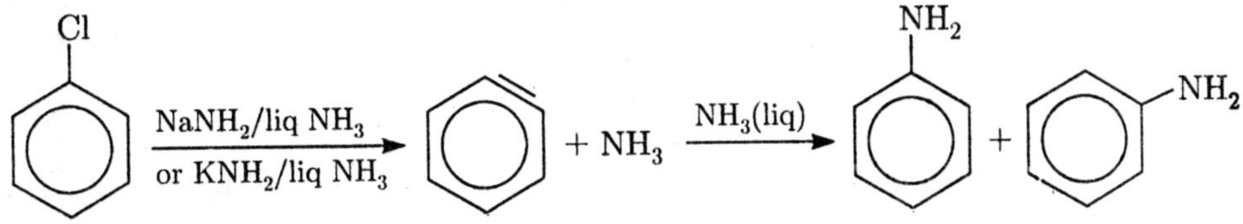

(Chlorobenzene) (Aniline)

Instead of KNH_2 or $NaNH_2$, alkyl or aryllithium can be used as bases to form aryne intermediate.

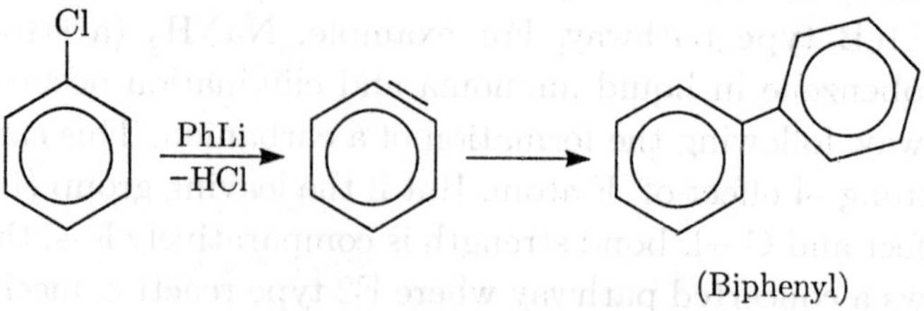

Mechanism of cine substitution reactions : Generally the formation of aryne intermediate is rate limiting. But if the leaving group (L) has strong –I effect so that C—L bond has poor polarisability, then C—L bond breaking step may become rate limiting during benzyne formation. The rate of *cine* substitution reaction for C_6H_5F and C_6H_5Cl with KNH_2/liquid NH_3 follows the order $C_6H_5F << C_6H_5Cl$. With C_6H_5F, the *ortho* hydrogens are quite acidic and C—F bond has low polarisability. So C—F bond breaking step becomes rate limiting regarding *cine* substitution in fluorobenzene. But if the C—L bond polarisability is high with poorly acidic *ortho* hydrogen(s), then (C—H bond breaking step becomes rate limiting. Bromobenzene undergoes *cine* substitution where C—H bond breaking step is rate limiting. The order of *cine* substitution with halobenzenes and $NaNH_2$ or KNH_2 in liquid NH_3 follows the order :

$$C_6H_5F \ll C_6H_5Cl < C_6H_5I < C_6H_5Br$$

Rate increases ⟶

(a) Mechanism of *cine* substitution through sequential pathway.

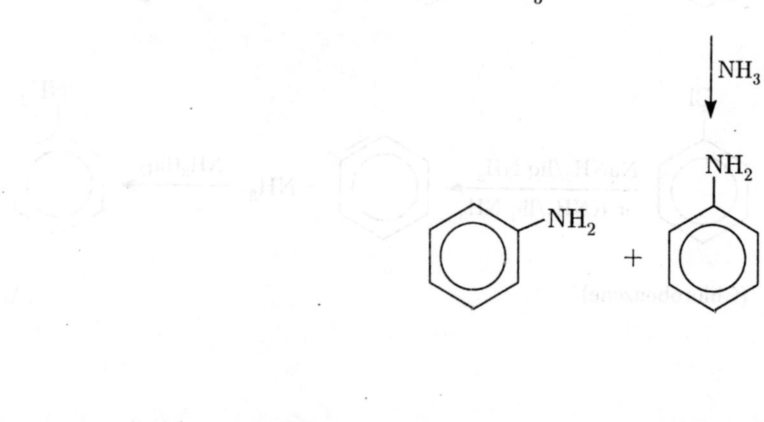

(b) Mechanism of *cine* substitution through concerted pathway :

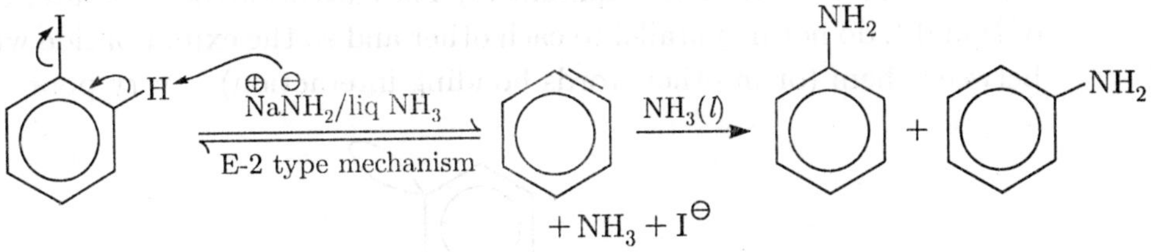

The reactions follow *cine* substitution can be proved by radio-isotope labelling experiment.

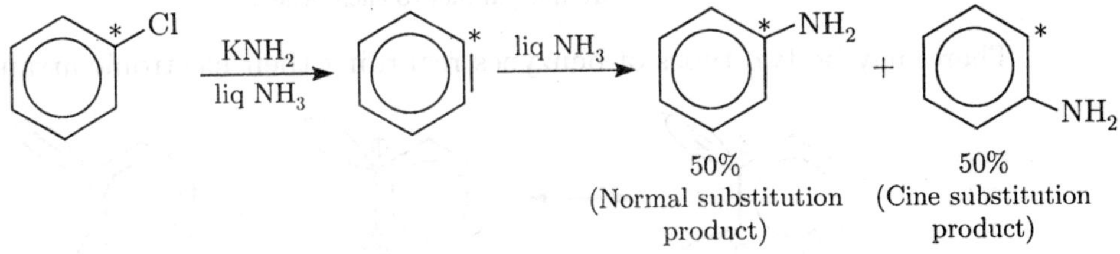

Since the aryne intermediate possesses two identical triple bonded carbon atoms the nucleophilic attack by the base may occur at either carbon atom of aryne which leads to the formation of 50% normal substitution product and 50% cine substitution product.

When benzyne is formed from a substituted halobenzene, at least one *ortho hydrogen* should be there with respect to the nucleofuge. Again if there are *two ortho* hydrogens available with respect to the nucleofuge, the *more acidic* hydrogen will be eliminated to form the aryne. The aryne may again form two carbanions upon nucleophilic attack and the more stable carbanion will be formed in major amount. The stability of carbanion is solely determined by the *inductive effect* (+I or –I effect) of the substitutent present in the benzene ring. The resonance effect (+R or –R) has no effect regarding the stability of the carbanion formed. The orbital containing unshared pair of electrons lie *perpendicular* to the p orbital of the benzene nucleus and hence can not take part in resonance.

The C—H bond breaking step is rate limiting in case of chlorobenzene (also true for bromobenzene), so far as *cine* substitution is concerned can be proved by the following experiment. Chlorobenzene reacts 10^6 times faster with $NaNH_2$/liquid NH_3 compared to *ortho* deuterochlorobenzene and also a strong PKIE is found. This unequivocally proves that C—H bond breaking step is the rate limiting step as otherwise PKIE would not have been observed.

Structure of aryne (benzyne) : Benzyne is a highly reactive intermediate. The extra bond in benzyne is a result of the overlap of sp^2 orbitals on adjacent carbons of the ring. The aromatic framework of six π electrons is arranged perpendicular to the two reactive and poorly overlapping additional hybrid orbitals which make up the distorted triple bond. Normal requirement for alkyne is to adopt a linear rather than a bent structure. Due to the cyclic structure, benzyne can not meet that requirement. The axes of two orbitals after elimination of H and L do not lie parallel to each other and so the extent of side wise overlap between them (or in other words bonding interaction) is very poor.

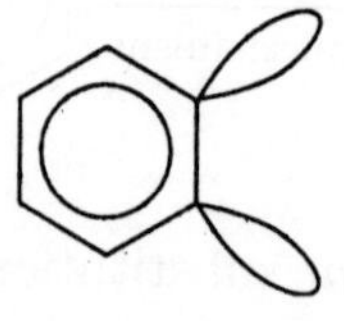

(The axes of two sp^2 orbitals are not parallel to each other)

There may be two types of benzynes regarding their electronic arrangement.

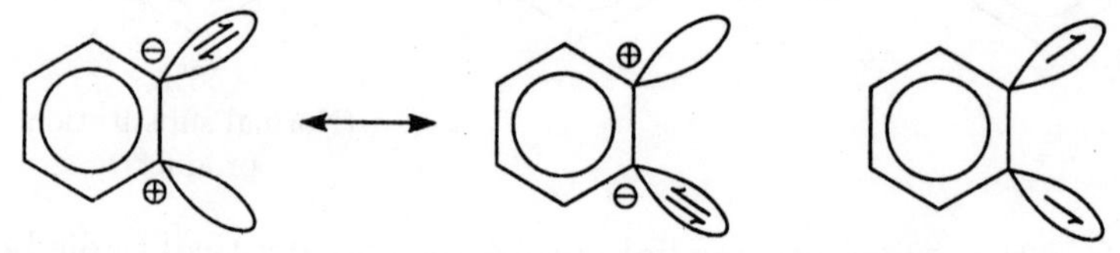

(Singlet benzyne) (Triplet benzyne)

Benzynes are highly reactive and so could not be isolated as such. However there are trapping experiments by which the formation of benzynes could be detected.

(a) 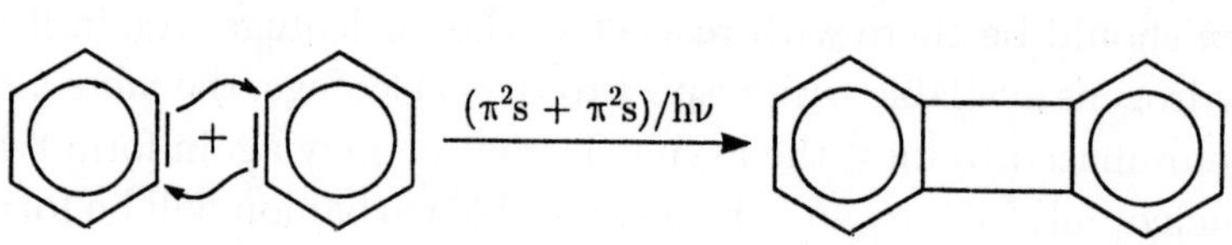

(b) 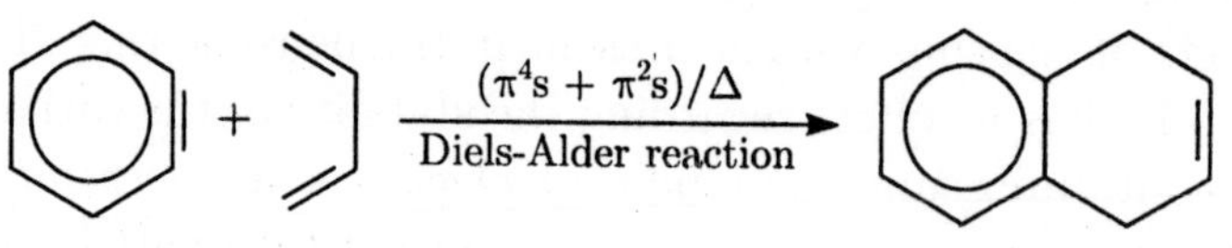

(c) 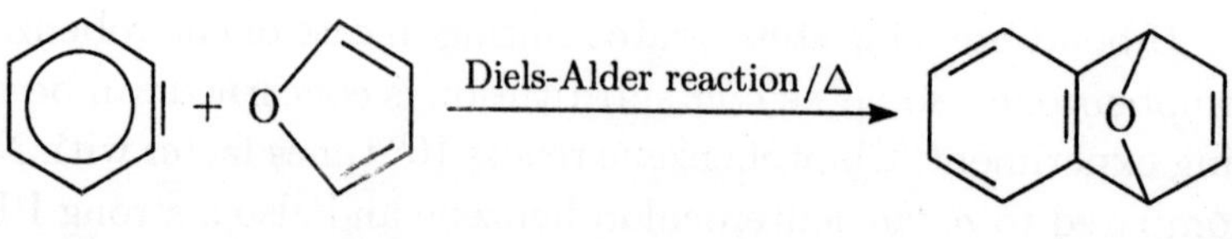

Different ways for the formation of benzynes :

1. 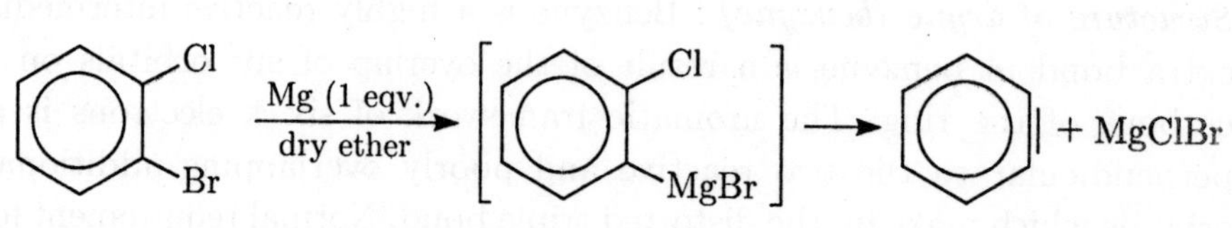

2. 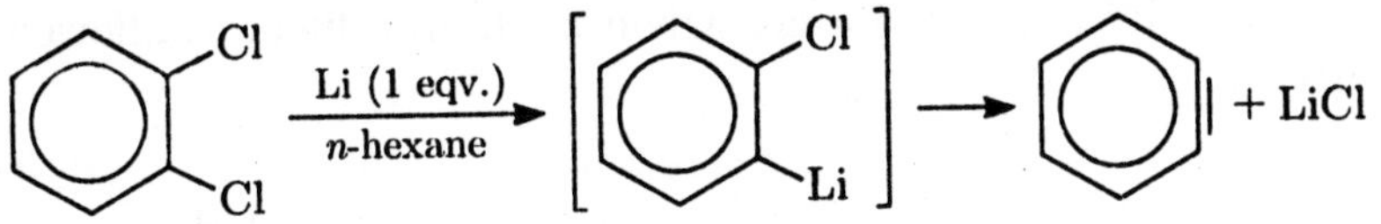

3. 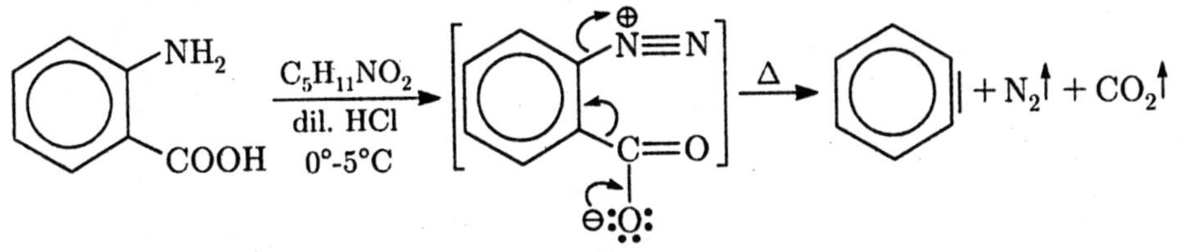

4. 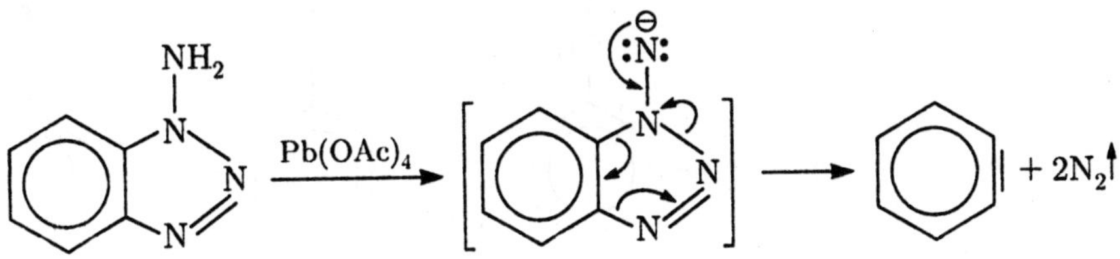

5. *Meta*-anisidine is formed when *o*-chloroanisole reacts with $NaNH_2$ in liquid NH_3.

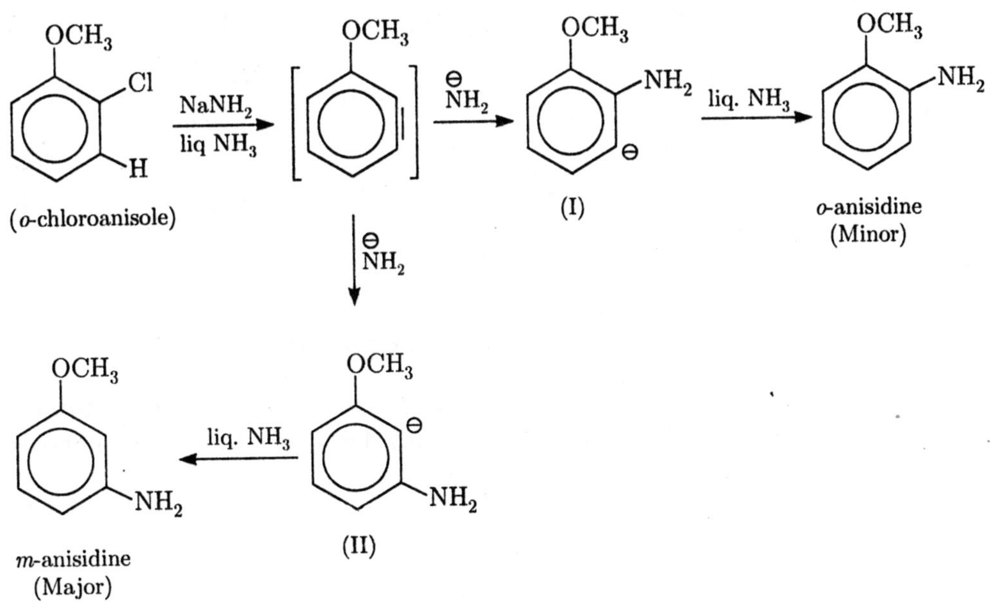

Carbanion (II) is more stable than (I) as –I effect of $-OCH_3$ group is more pronounced in case of (II) which stabilises the carbanion. As a result, *m*-anisidine is formed in major amount.

6. Three isomeric toluidines are formed when *m*-chlorotoluene is allowed to react with $NaNH_2$ in liquid ammonia.

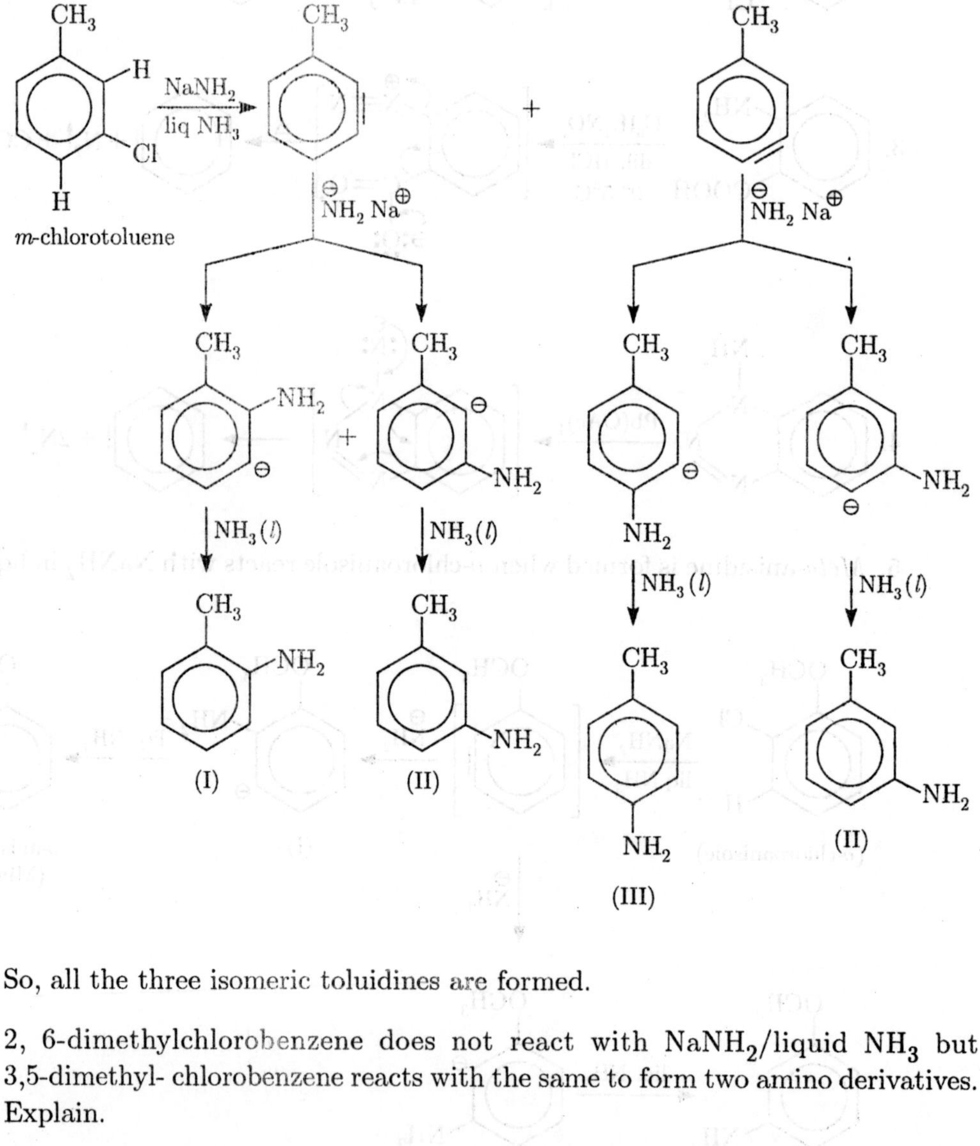

So, all the three isomeric toluidines are formed.

7. 2, 6-dimethylchlorobenzene does not react with $NaNH_2$/liquid NH_3 but 3,5-dimethyl- chlorobenzene reacts with the same to form two amino derivatives. Explain.

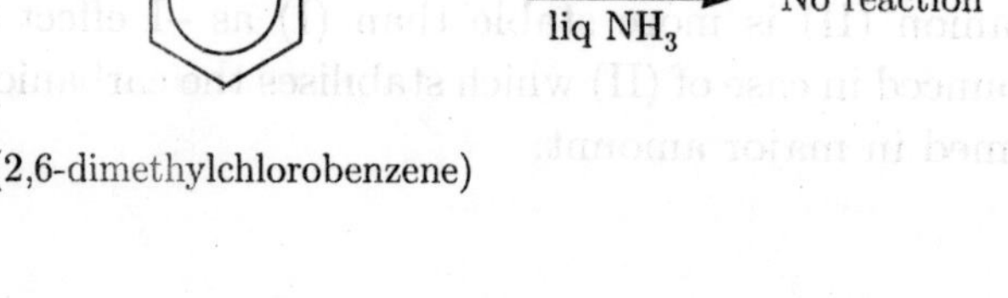

(2,6-dimethylchlorobenzene)

There is no *o*-hydrogen available to the nucleofuge (Cl) to be abstracted by the base ($NaNH_2$) and aryne intermediate is not formed to undergo a *cine* substitution.

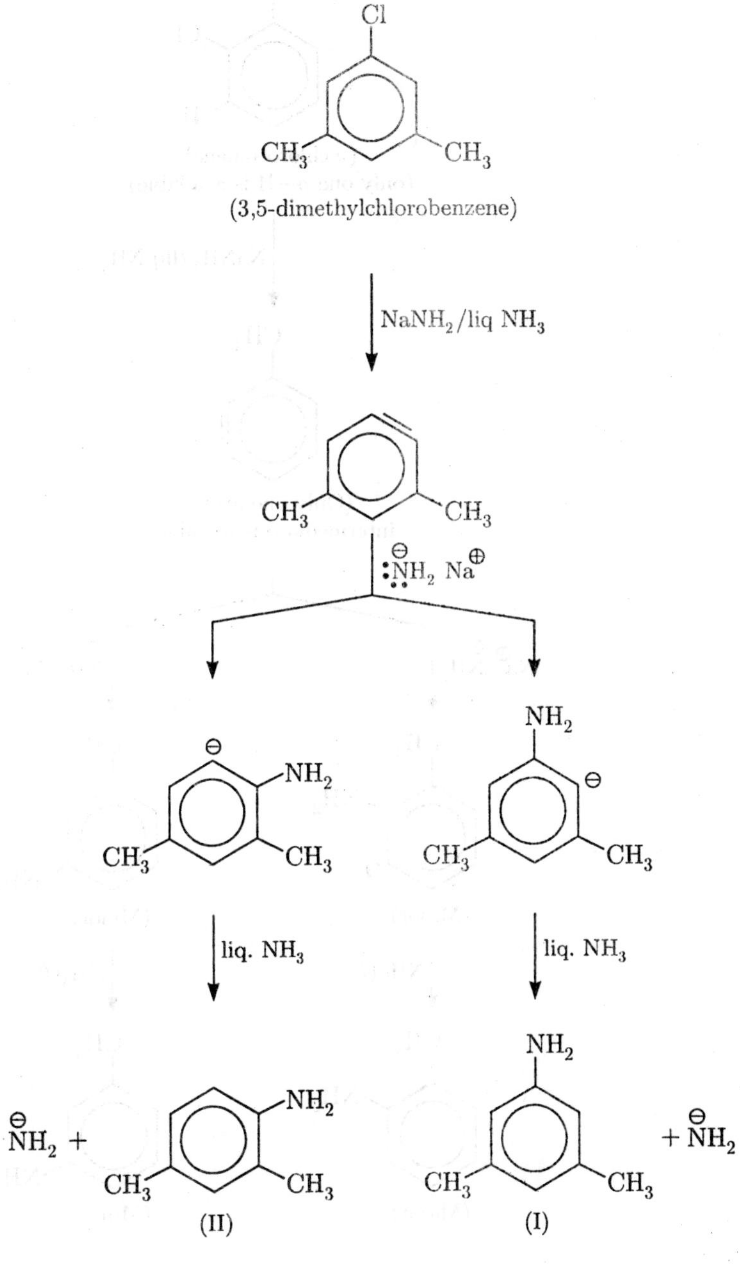

Two amine derivatives namely (I) and (II) are formed from 3,5-dimethylchlorobenzene.

8. When *o*-chlorotoluene is treated with $NaNH_2$/liquid NH_3 the products are 45% *o*-toluidine and 55% *m*-toluidine. Explain.

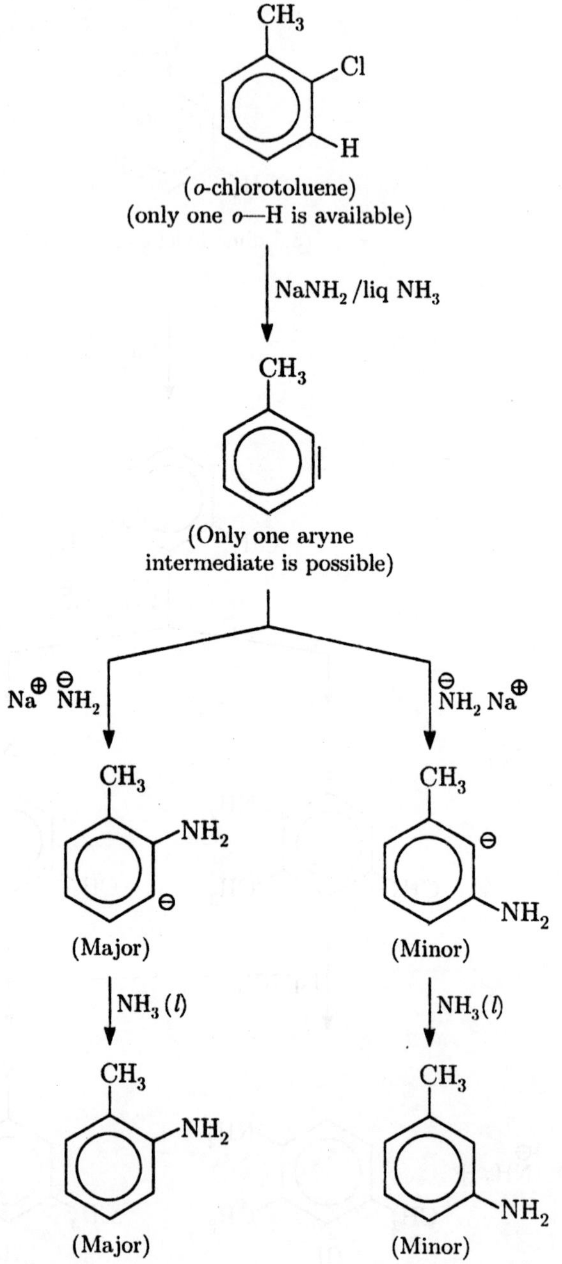

(+I) effect of CH_3 group destabilises the carbanion which leads to *m*-toluidine and as a result *m*-toluidine is formed in 45% yield. On the other hand, the carbanion which produces *o*-toluidine is comparatively stable and so *o*-toluidine is formed in 55% yield.

9. 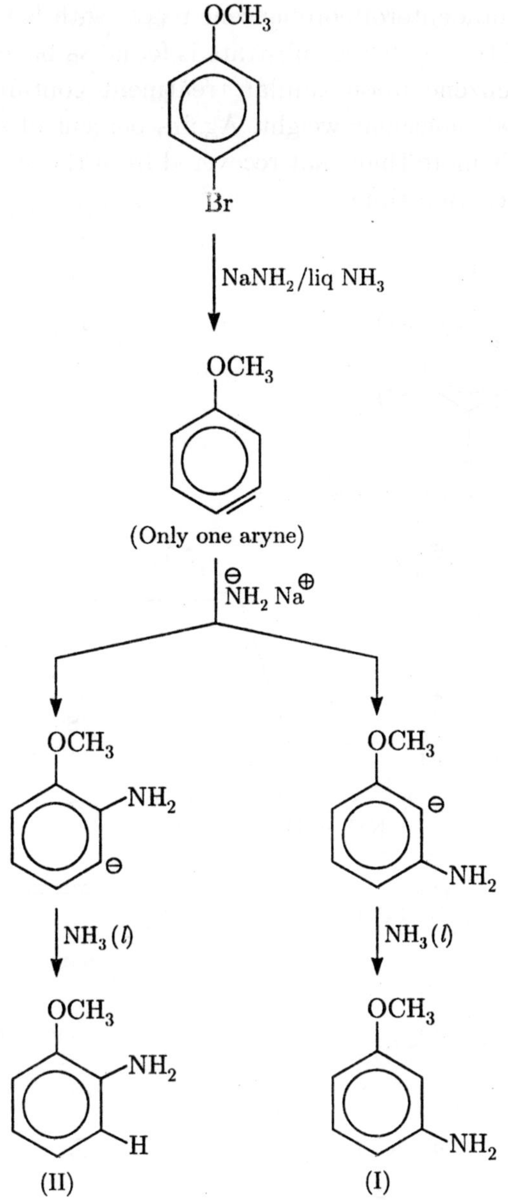

meta toluidine (I) is formed as the major product as the corresponding carbanion gets stabilisation by –I effect of $-OCH_3$ group.

10. 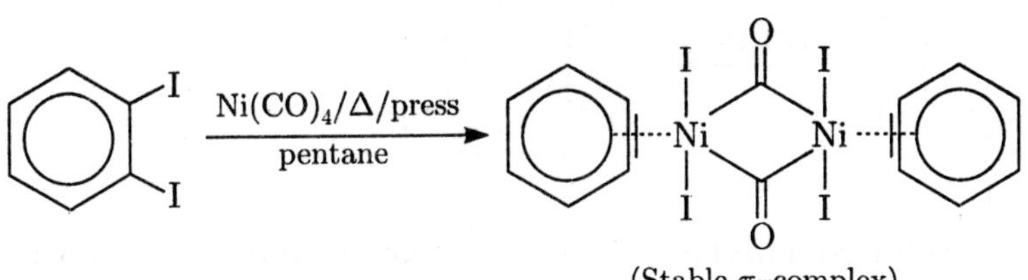

11. When pentadeuterofluorobenzene reacts with KNH_2/liquid NH_3, the molecular weight of the recovered substrate is found to have decreased. But pentadeutero-bromobenzene upon similar treatment contains unreacted substrate with unchanged molecular weight. Again, percent of substrate recovered from first reaction is more than that recovered from the second reaction during the same span of reaction time.

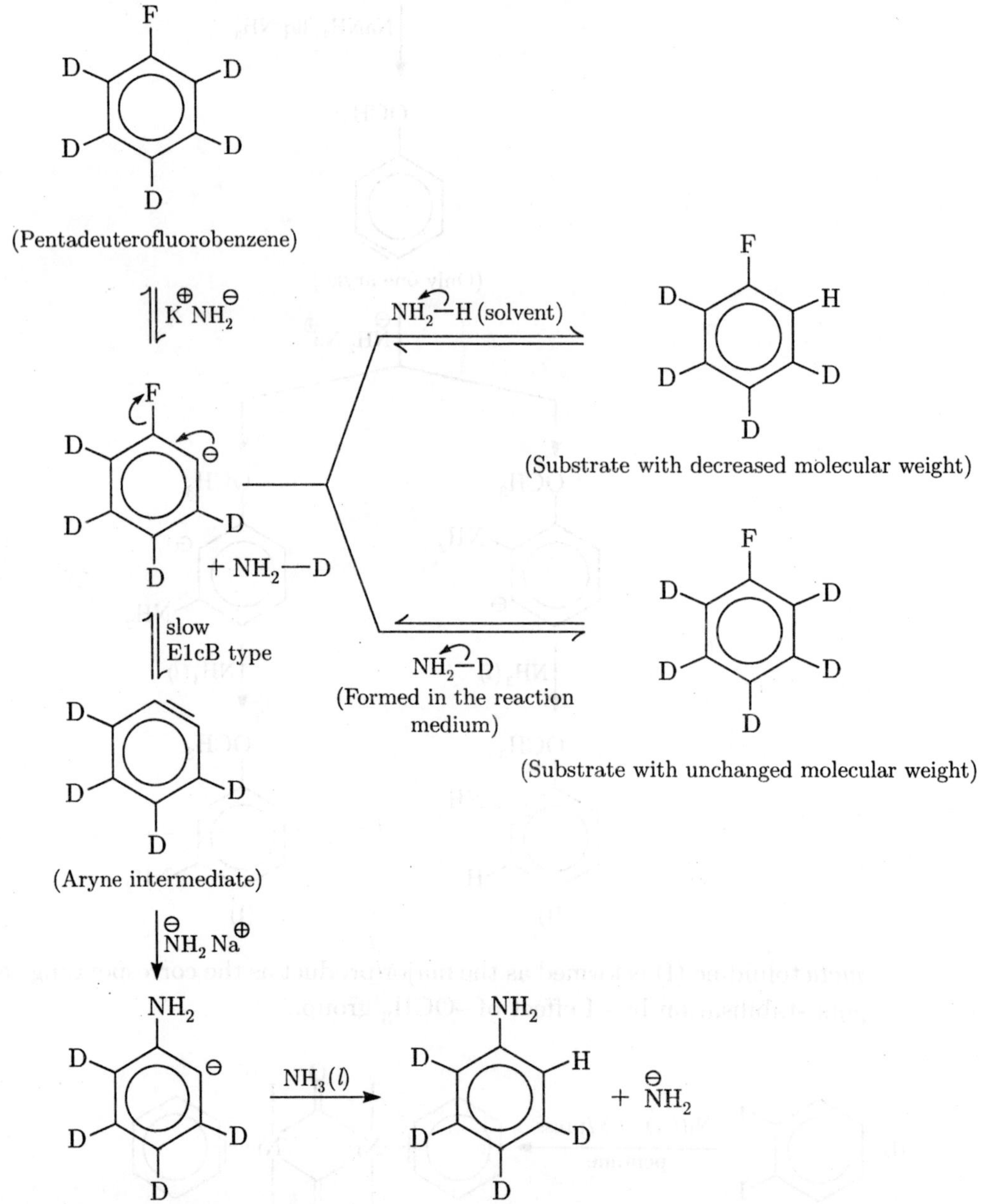

In pentadeuterofluorobenzene C—F bond breaking step is rate-limiting and the reaction mechanism is of E1cB type. The intermediate carbanion gets stabilised by –I effect of F. Due to the sequential nature of the reaction, the aryne formation becomes reversible and we get tetradeuterofluorobenzene as a substrate (lower molecular weight than pentadeuterofluorobenzene) along with the normal substrate (pentadeuterofluorobenzene) when recovered from the reaction mixture.

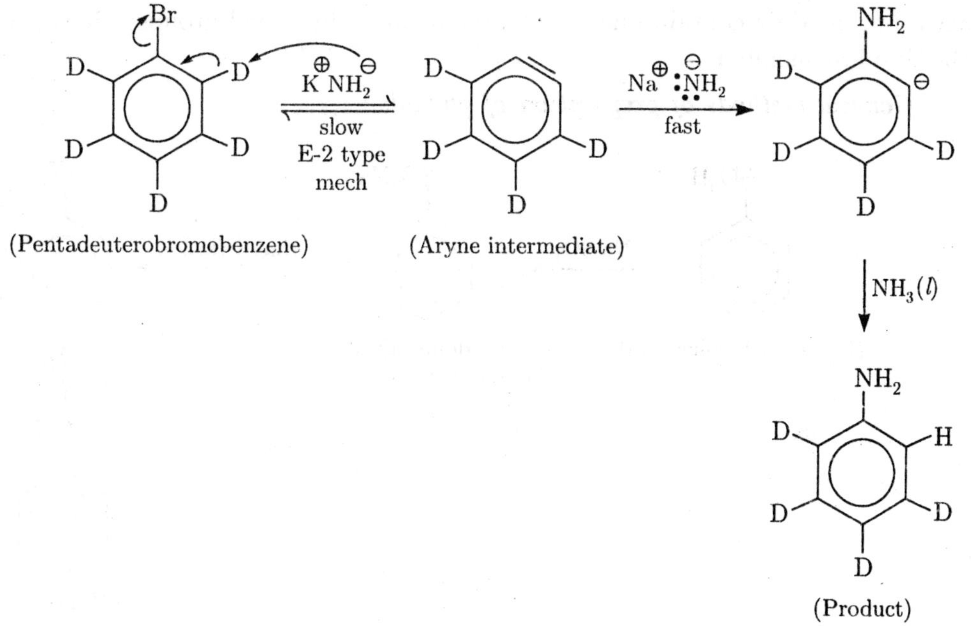

Br atom is far less electronegative than F atom, so if any carbanion be formed can not get stabilised. So here, the mechanism followed is similar to E2 type and the nature of mechanistic pathway is concerted. [From the mechanism of the reaction (as shown above) it is evident that no substrate with lower molecular weight (*i.e.*, in which one hydrogen is incorporated) is possible.]

In case of pentadeuterobromobenzene, the amount of substrate recovered is less. Arynes are reactive, so the aryne formed from pentadeuterated bromobenzene instantaneously forms the product due to the irreversible nature of the reaction. With pentadeuterofluorobenzene, the reaction is of reversible type where the carbanion reverts back to the substrate in the solvent. For this reason, the amount of recovered substrate is more with pentadeuteroflurorobenzene compared to that of pendeuterobromobenzene. In other words, the yield of product is more with pentadeuterobromobenzene.

PHENOLS

Phenols are compounds of general formula ArOH where Ar stands for phenyl, substituted phenyl, naphthyl etc. Phenols differ from the alcohols in having the –OH group attached directly to an aromatic ring. Phenols are classified as mono–, di–, tri– or polyhydric according as they contain one, two, three or more hydroxyl groups; phenol itself being the simplest member.

General methods of preparation of phenols :

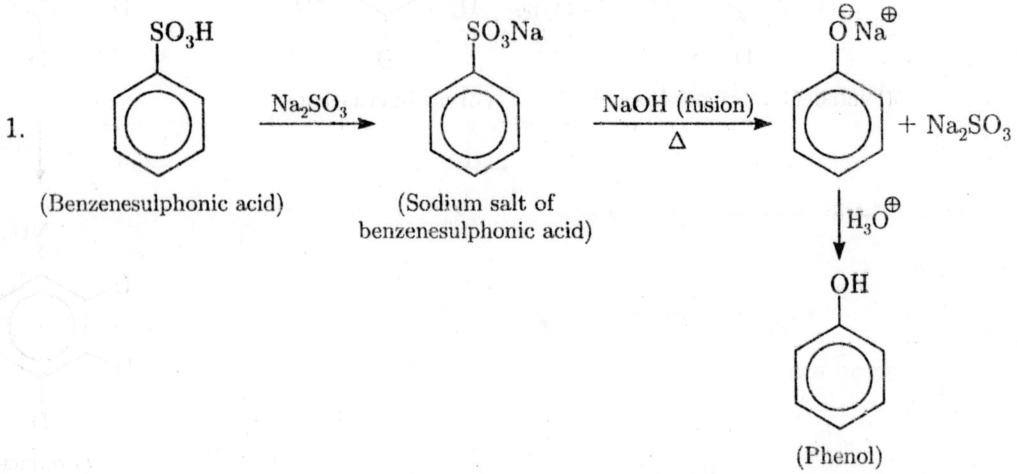

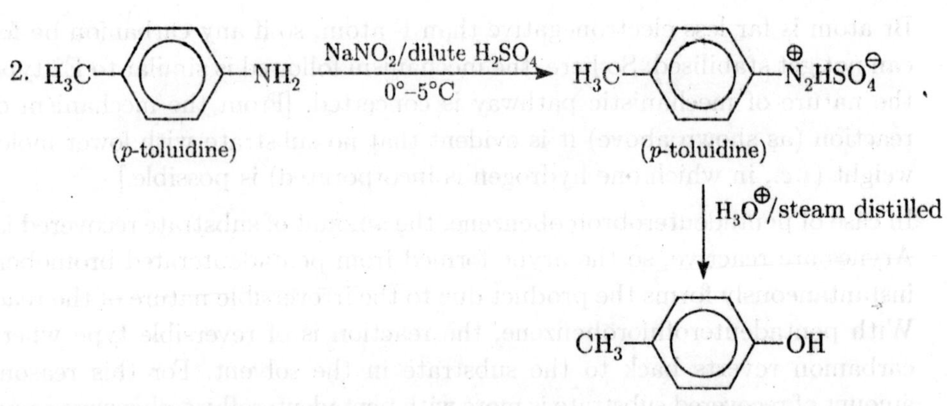

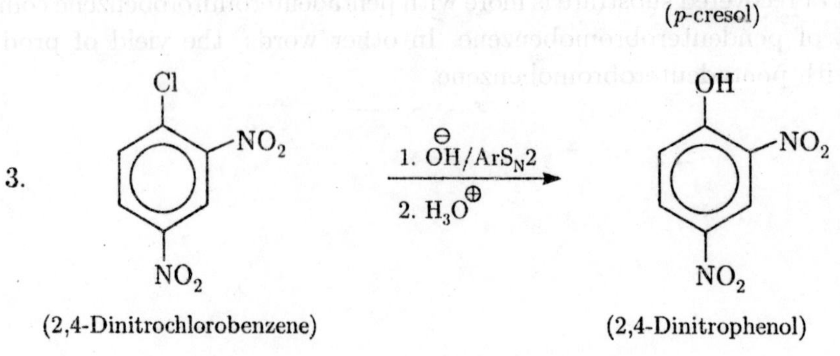

(2,4-Dinitrochlorobenzene) (2,4-Dinitrophenol)

4. 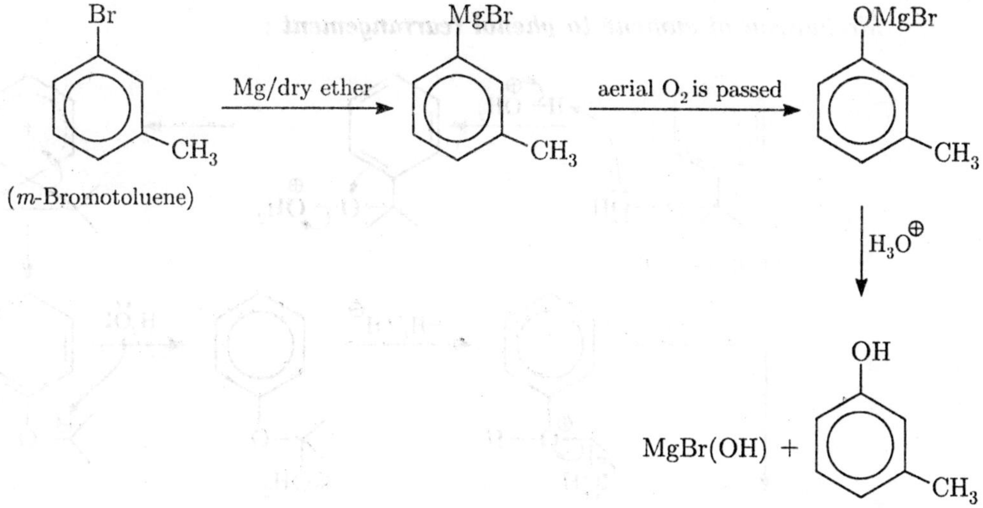

(*m*-Bromotoluene) (*meta*-cresol)

5. From cumene by cumene to phenol rearrangement. This is the most important method of preparation of phenols where acetone is produced as by product which is also a synthetically important molecule.

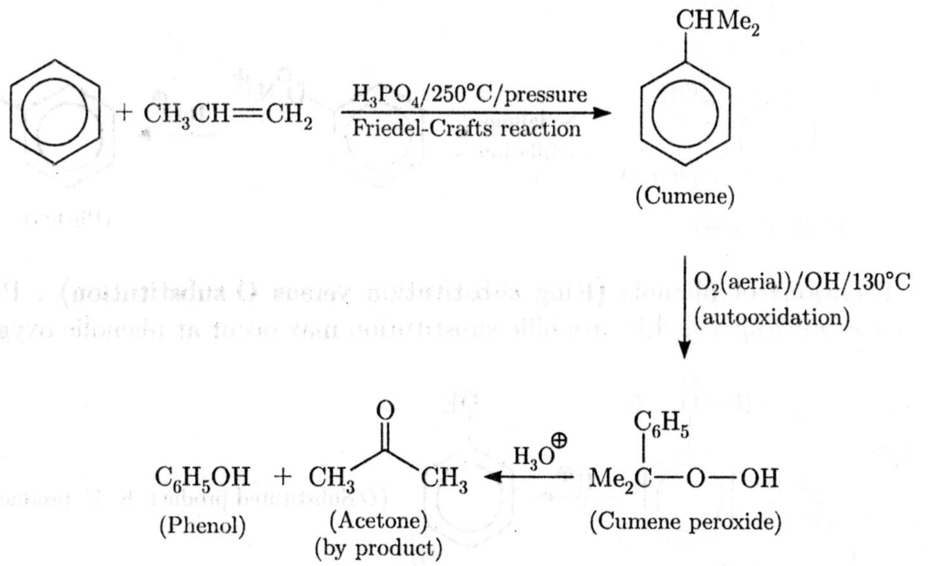

(Phenol) (Acetone) (by product) (Cumene peroxide)

Mechanism of cumene to phenol ***rearrangement*** :

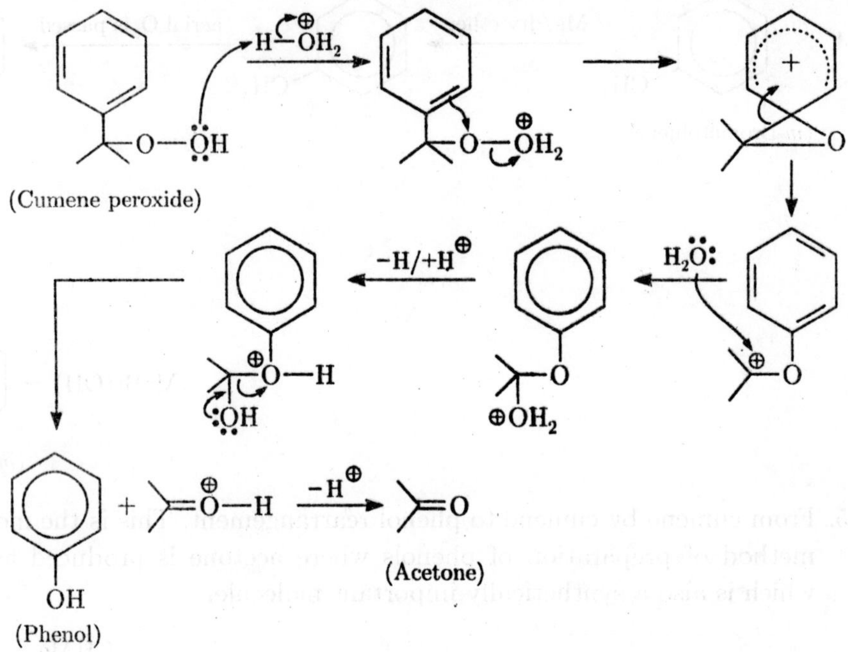

6.

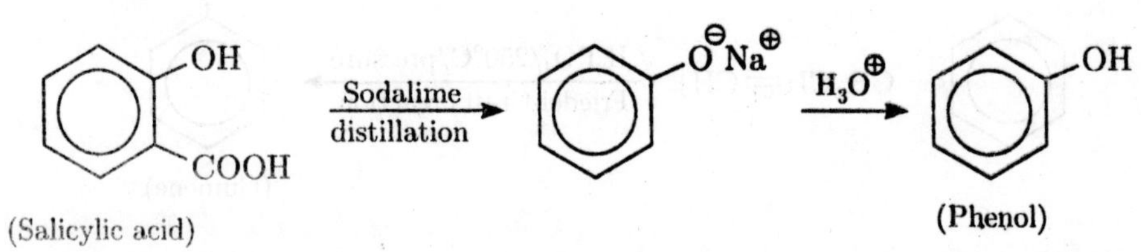

Reactions of phenols (Ring substitution versus O-substitution) : Phenols are *ambident nucleophiles.* Electrophilic substitution may occur at phenolic oxygen and

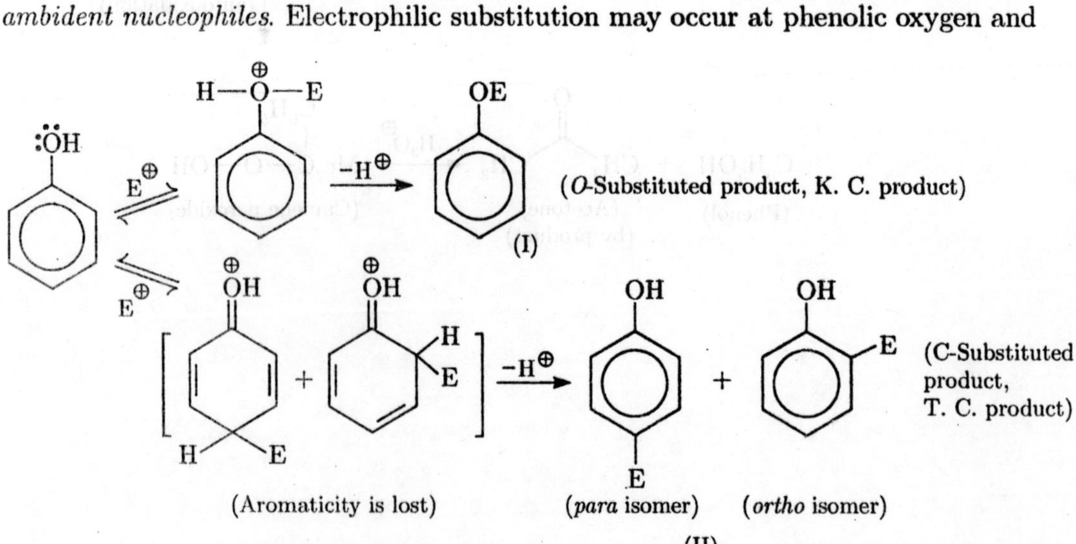

at the carbon atoms, ***ortho*** and ***para*** positions with respect to phenolic –OH group. (+R) effect of phenolic –OH group makes the benzene ring *highly activated* towards aromatic electrophilic (ArS_E2) substitution reactions.

The $\Delta G^{\neq}$ to achieve the transition state to lead the product I (O-substituted product) is *less* as the transition state does not lose any aromatic stability. On the other hand, $\Delta G^{\neq}$ to attain the transition state to have the products II (C-substituted products) is more as the transition state (transition state is σ-complex like where aromatic stability is lost) is no longer an aromatic compound. So the product (I) is produced at a faster rate (K.C. product) compared to products (II) which are thermodynamically controlled products. But regarding the stability of products, products (II) are more stable so they are T.C. products and as the product stability of (I) is poor (due to *ortho* effect etc.), it is the K.C. product although formed at a faster rate. In general the T.C. products *i.e.*, ring-substituted products are predominant, but if the stability of O-substituted product (*i.e.*, K.C. product) becomes considerable, it is formed at a reasonable rate. With increase in temperature of the reaction, the extent of ring-substituted product formation increases (T.C. product). If the O-substituted product (K.C. product) is heated, then also it gets converted to T.C. product (C-substitutd products). Steric factor also plays an important role. For example,

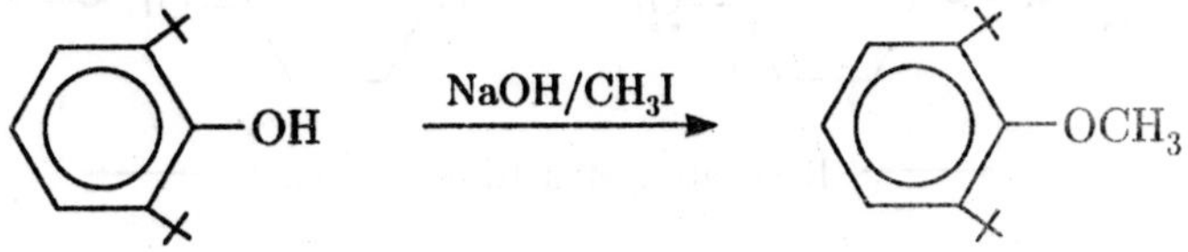

(2,6-Ditertiaryphenol) (88%) (K.C. product)

but,

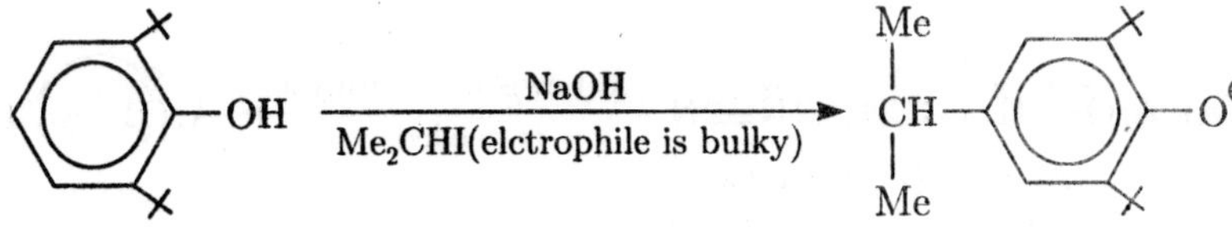

(~100%) (T.C. product)

Reactions of Phenols (Reactions involving O-substitution) :

1. 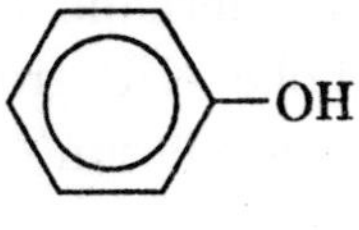 (Aqueous or alcoholic solution) + $\overset{III}{Fe}Cl_3$ (neutral) ⟶ $[Fe(OC_6H_5)_6]^{3+}$

(Phenol) (Blue or green or violet coloured complex)

2. 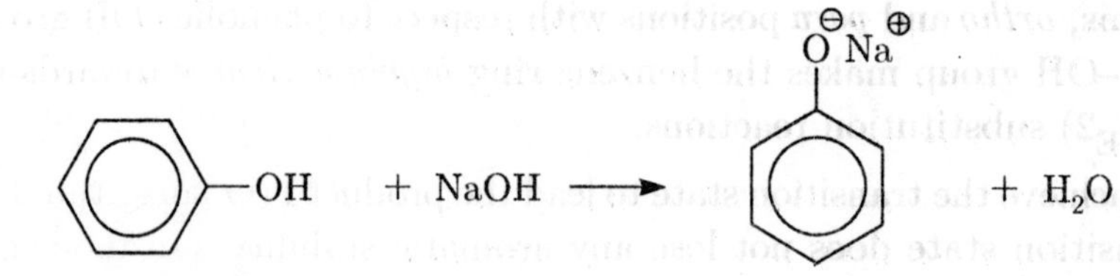

(pK$_a$≅10, weakly acidic) (Sodium phenoxide)
(Phenol)

3. 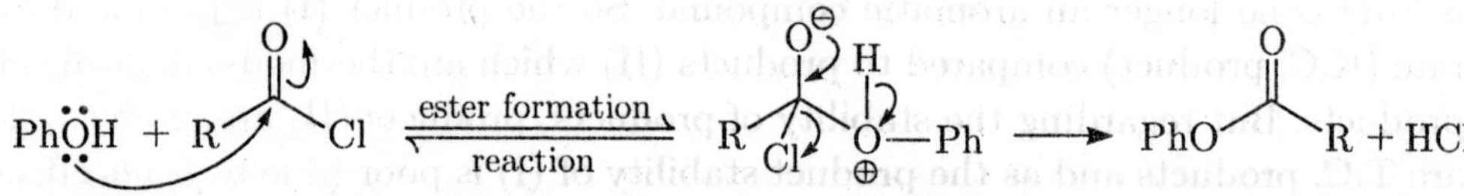

(Tetrahedral intermediate)

Esterification of phenols is slower than that compared to alcohols, as in the former case, the lone pair of electrons on the oxygen atom is involved with resonance into the benzene ring by making them less available for nucleophilic attack.

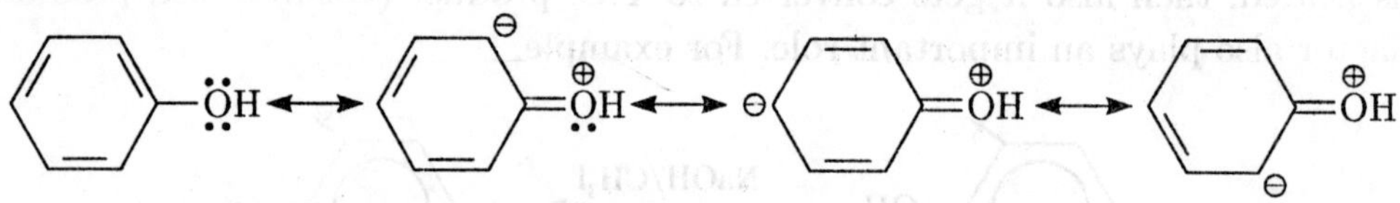

Resonating structures of phenol

4. 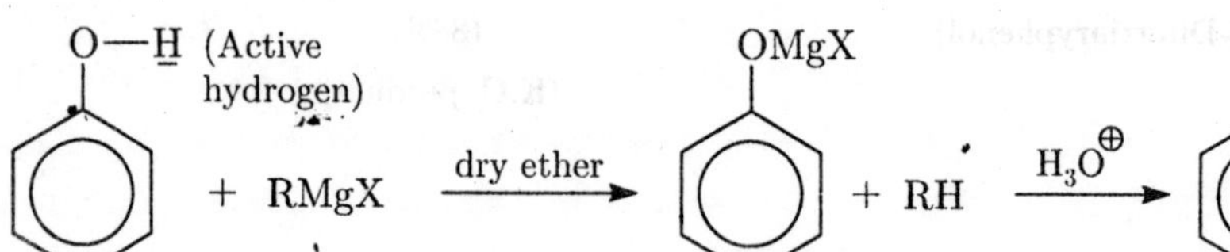

5. (a) 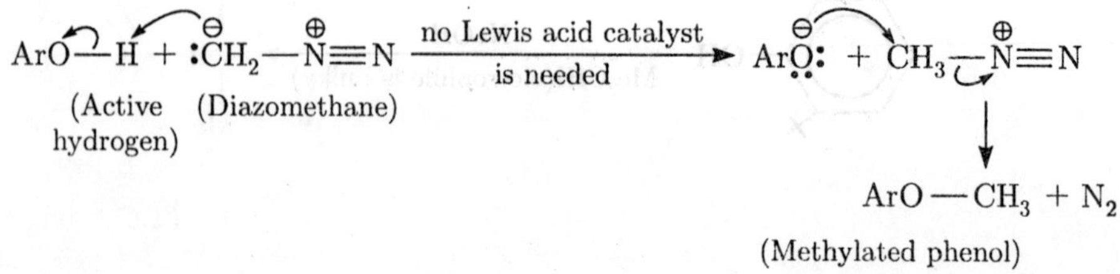

(Methylated phenol)

No Lewis acid catalyst is needed to methylate phenols, as the phenolic hydrogen group is sufficiently active to react with diazomethane. Lewis acid catalyst is needed to methylate alcohols where alcoholic –OH group is not sufficiently acidic and activation is needed prior to methylation.

(b) $ArO{-}H + Me_2SO_4 \xrightarrow{NaOH} ArO{-}Me + CH_3HSO_3^{\ominus}\,Na^{\oplus} + H_2O$

(Methylated phenol)

6. $ArOH \xrightarrow{NaOH} Ar\overset{\ominus}{O}\,\overset{\oplus}{Na} \xrightarrow{RI/(\text{williamson's synthesis of ether})} ArO{-}R + NaI$

7. 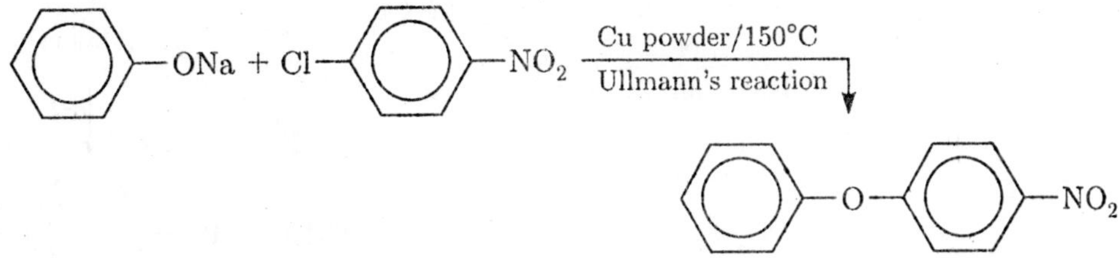

Reactions of phenols (Reactions involving C-substitution)

Hydroxyl (–OH) group and phenoxide ion (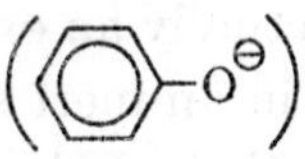) activate the benzene nucleus to a large extent regarding aromatic electrophilic substitution (ArS_E2) reactions and both $—\ddot{O}H$ and $—\ddot{O}:^{\ominus}$ groups are *ortho/para* directing.

Friedel-Crafts Reaction

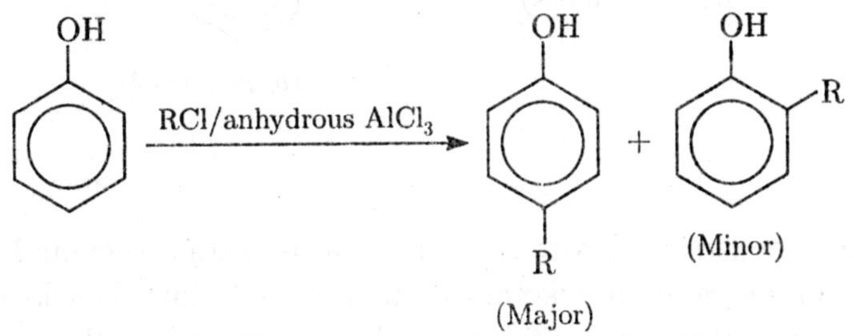

But a large amount of anhydrous $AlCl_3$ is needed as a side reaction occurs due to the acidic nature of hydrogen of phenolic –OH group which is as follows.

$$C_6H_5OH + AlCl_3 \longrightarrow C_6H_5OAlCl_2 + HCl$$

This problem is avoided when phenol is alkylated with an alkene or alcohol in the presence of hydrofluoric acid as follows

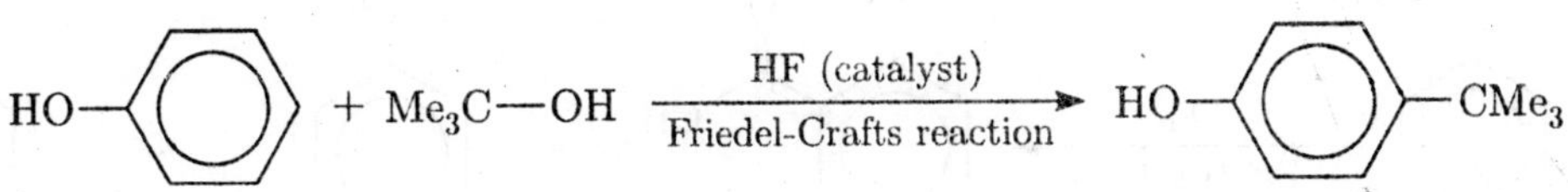

(*p*-tertiarybutylphenol)

or carrying out the alkylation by Friedel-Crafts reaction with corresponding methyl ether of phenol (anisole) and then hydrolyzing the alkyl substituted anisole by hydroiodic acid.

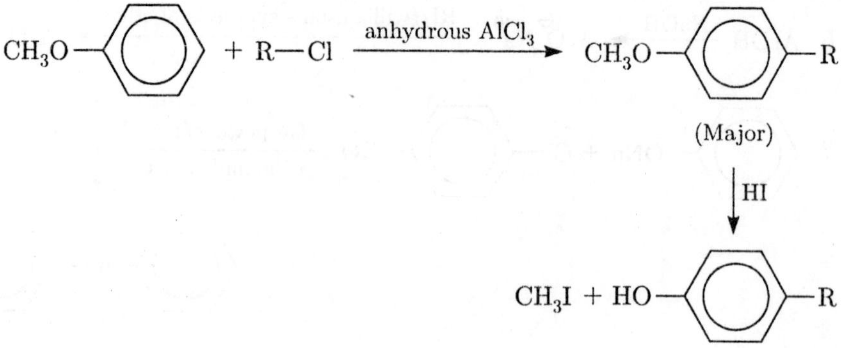

The Fries Rearrangement

This rearrangement reaction is actually an example of Friedel-Crafts acylation reaction. When a phenolic ester is heated in an inert solvent in the presence of a Lewis acid say $AlCl_3$ and the product is subsequently hydrolysed, a mixture of *ortho-* and *para-* acylphenols is obtained and the reaction is known as the *Fries Rearrangement.*

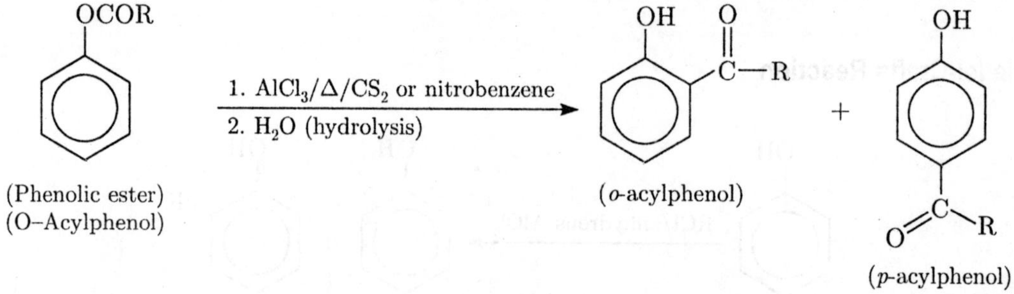

The *ortho* isomer (*ortho-* hydroxyketone) forms intramolecular hydrogen bonding which *para-* isomer (*para*-hydroxyketone) can not and thus, has lower boiling point, higher volatility and higher vapour preseure. As a result, the *ortho* isomer can be taken out by steam distillation from the mixture of *ortho-* and *para-* isomers as the *ortho* isomer is lower boiling where *para-* acylphenol remains in the flask (due to its higher boiling point).

The Fries rearrangement can also occur without any Lewis acid catalyst in the presence of UV light (source of hν) and the reaction is known as *photo Fries Rearrangement.*

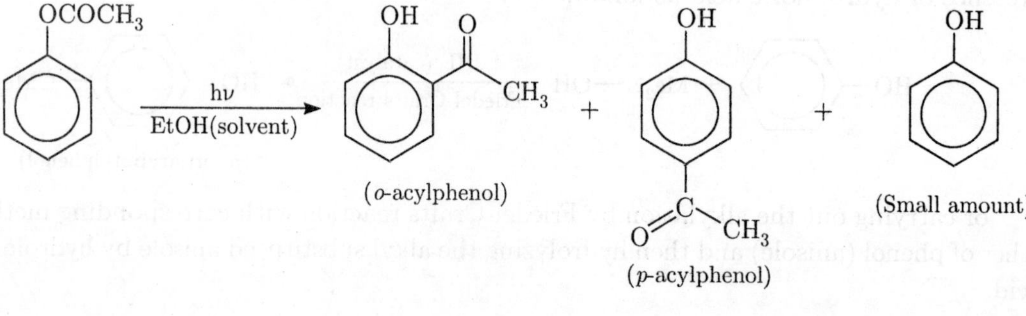

At lower temperature, Fries rearrangement produces *para* product as the major one while at a higher temperature, *ortho*-product predominates. Both solvent and catalyst have effects on product profile. The *para* product is a kinetically controlled product and the *ortho* product is a thermodynamically controlled product. *Ortho*- acylphenol gets extra stability through hydrogen bonding (intramolecular). Perhaps due to steric interaction, *ortho*-acylphenol is not formed in major amount at lower temperature.

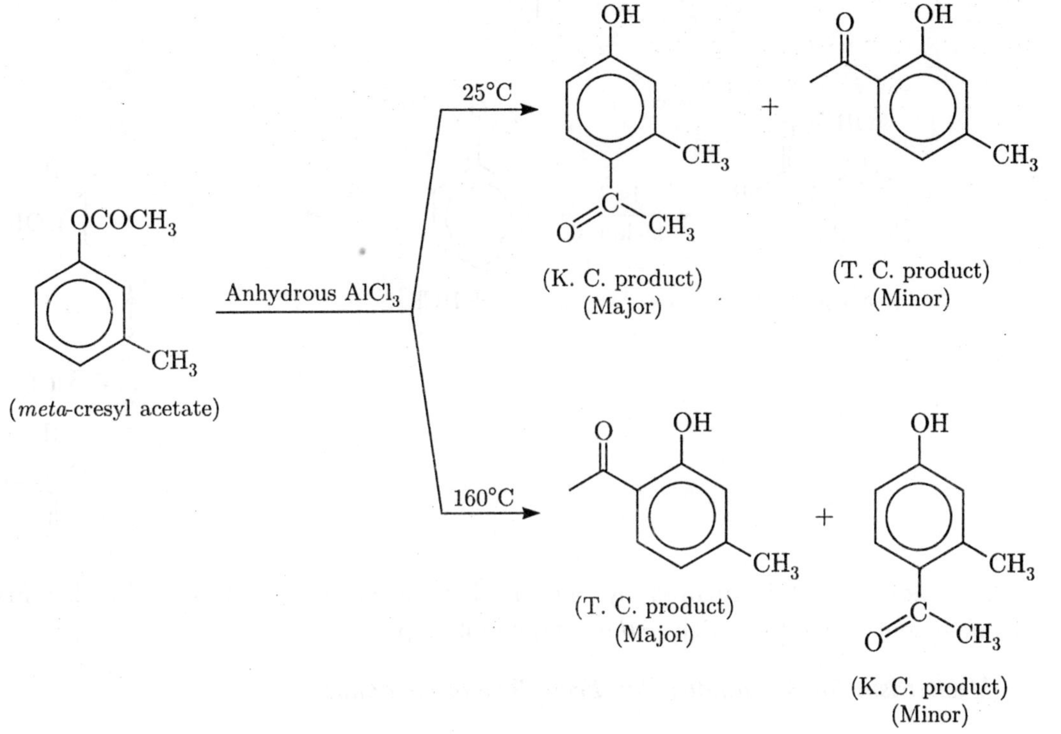

Presence of electron withdrawing groups in the substrate retard the reaction as is found in case of Friedel-Crafts reaction. Fries rearrangement is a good method for the preparation of acylphenols especially where Friedel-Crafts acylation of phenols give poor yield.

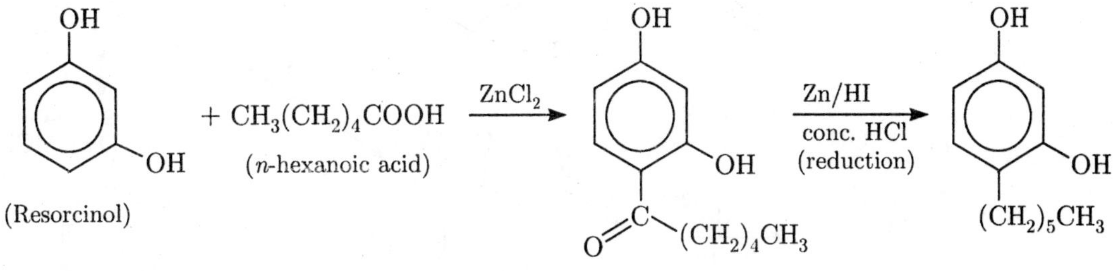

Mehanism of Fries Rearrangement : The mechanism of Fries Rearrangement is supposed to follow both *intramolecular* and *intermolecular pathways.*

Mechanism for Intermolecular Fries rearrangement :

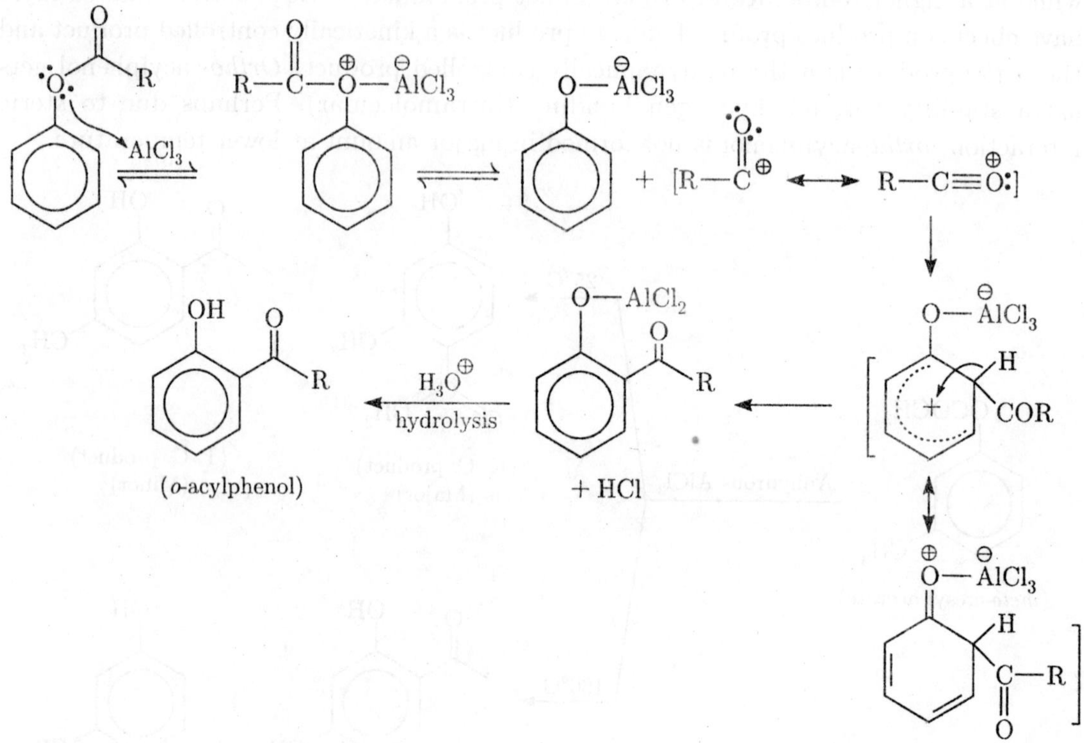

Para-acylphenol is formed by the similar mechanism in intermolecular Fries rearrangement as we find with *ortho*-acylphenol as product.

Mechanism for Intramolecular Fries Rearrangement :

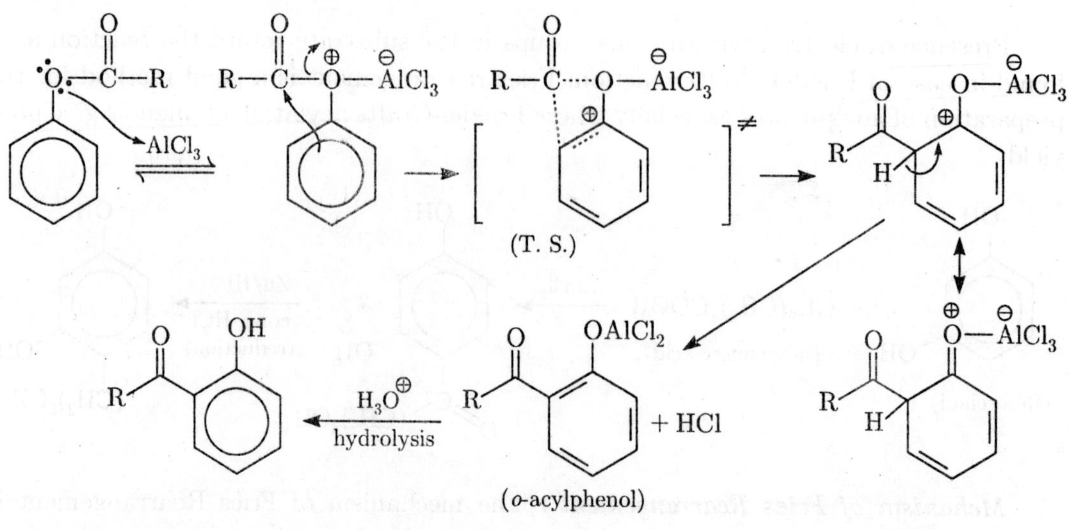

Similarly, *p*-acylphenol is formed through intramolecular pathway.

Photo Fries rearrangement follows *free radical pathway.*

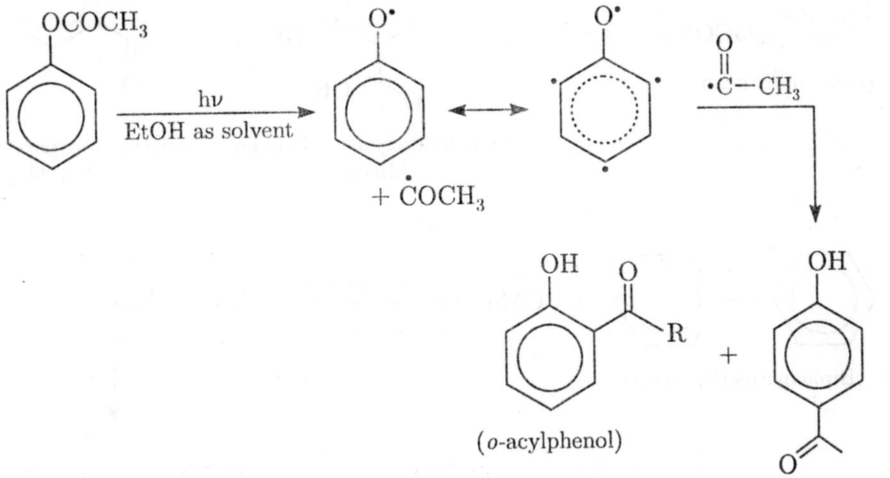

(*o*-acylphenol)

(*p*-acylphenol)

Applications of Fries Rearrangement :

1. *Preparation of aromatic hydroxyketones*

(a) 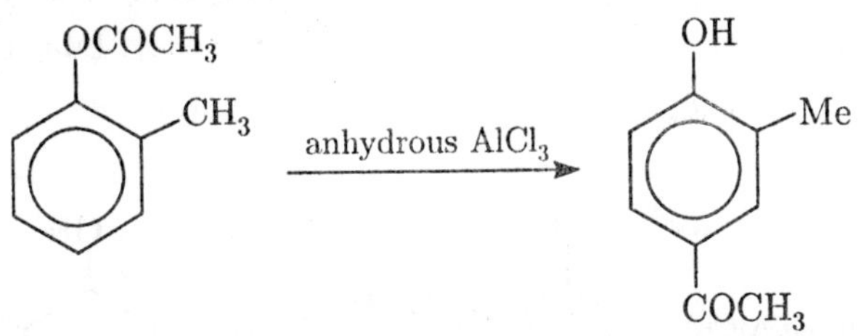

(Major)

(b) 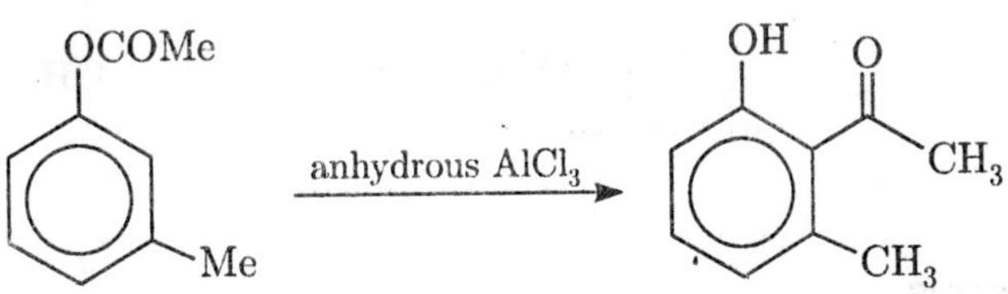

(Major)

(c) 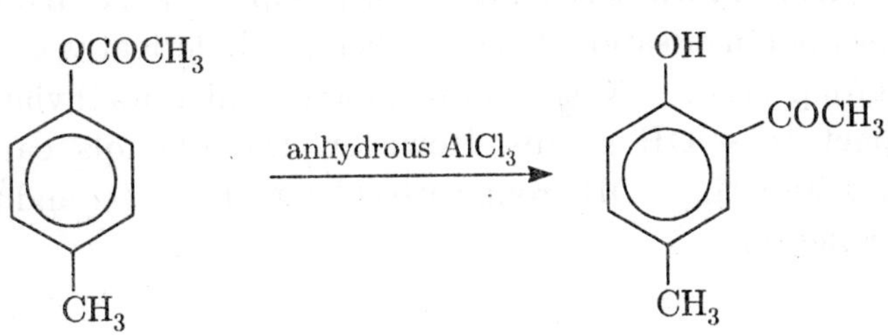

(100%)

2. 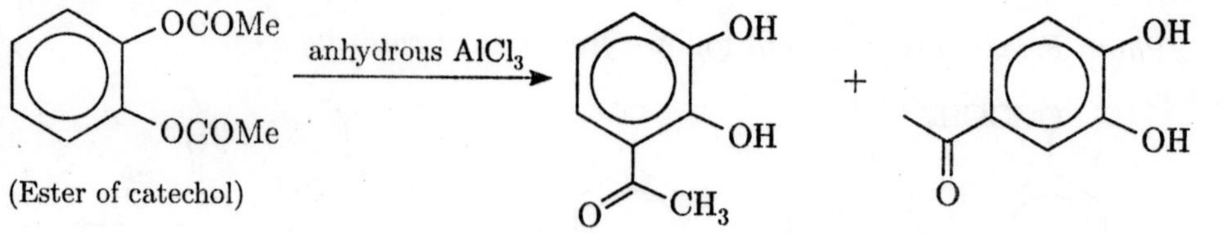

(Ester of catechol) (2,3-Dihydroxyacetophenone) (Minor) (3,4-Dihydroxyacetophenone) (~100%)

3. 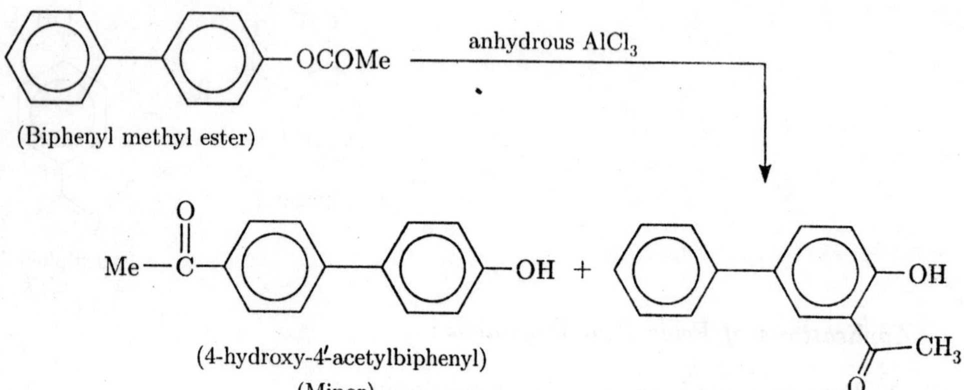

(Biphenyl methyl ester)

(4-hydroxy-4′-acetylbiphenyl) (Minor)

(4-hydroxy-3-acetylbiphenyl) (Major)

4. 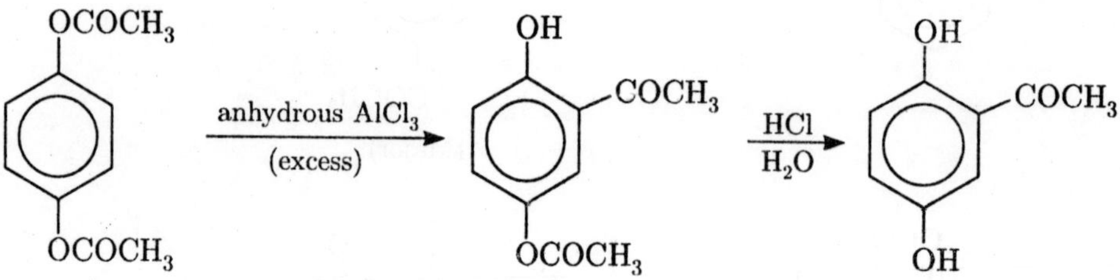

(Major)

Chloromethylation of Phenols

Phenols and substituted phenols with electron releasing groups undergo chloromethylation reaction followed by quick polymerisation. On the other hand, derivatives of phenol with electron withdrawing group (*e.g.*, —NO_2 group) undergo chloromethylation at *o*-and *p*-positions with respect to —OH group. However, the phenols can be readily chloromethylated by protecting the —OH group with chloroformic ester and then carrying out chloromethylation reaction.

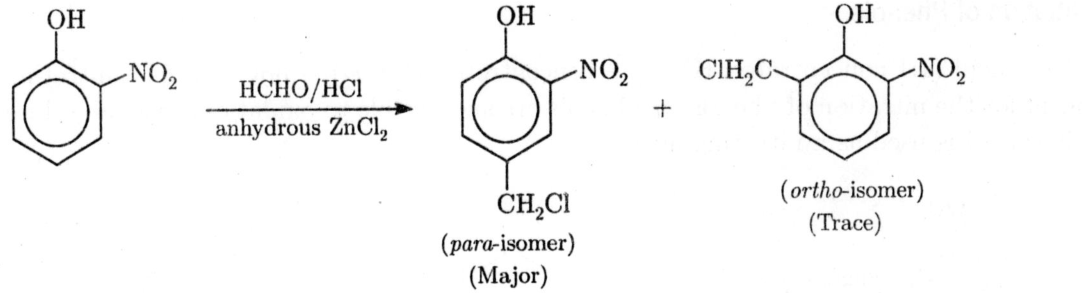

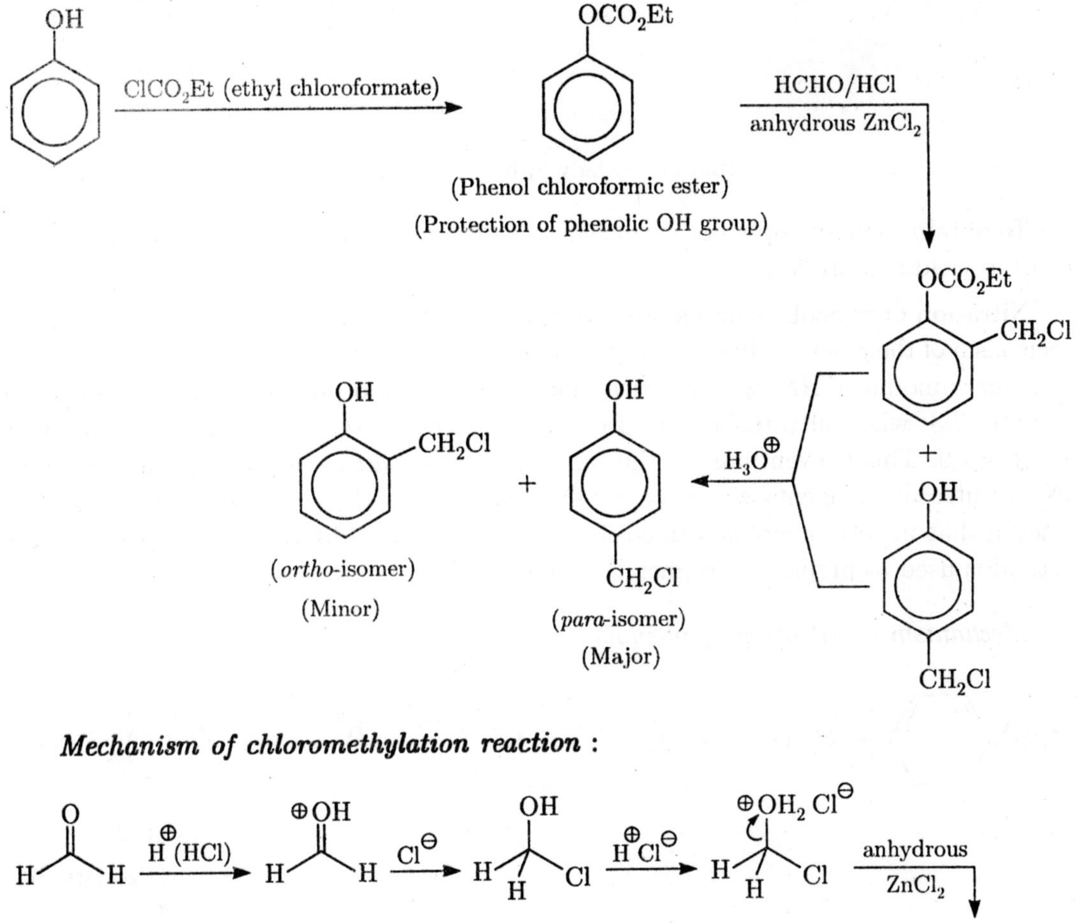

Mechanism of chloromethylation reaction :

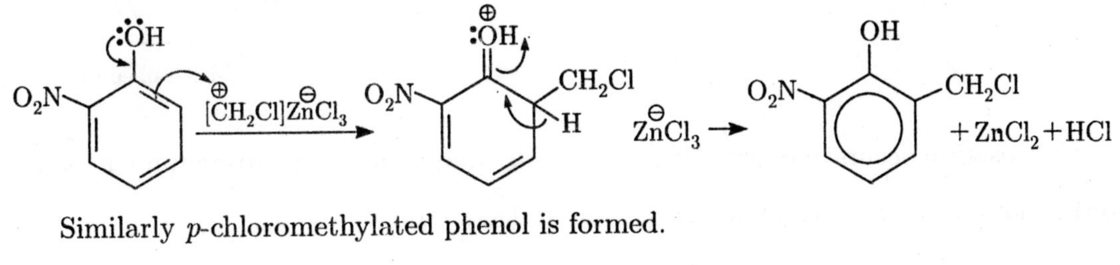

Similarly *p*-chloromethylated phenol is formed.

Nitration of Phenols

Mixed acid (1:1 concentrated HNO_3 + concentrated H_2SO_4) is not used as a nitrating agent for the nitration of phenols as phenols are succeptible to oxidation. Instead, dilute nitric acid is used as a nitrating agent.

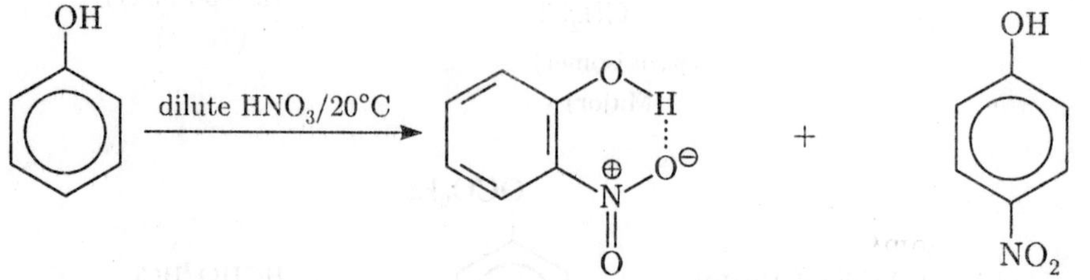

(*ortho*-nitrophenol) (Major) (Intramolecularly hydrogen bonded) (*para*-nitrophenol) (Minor)

To obtain mononitrophenol exclusively, the reaction temperature is kept low, even then the yield is quite low.

Nitration of phenols is accelerated in the presence of nitrous acid (HNO_2) and the mechanism of the reaction differs from that of ordinary nitration. When phenol is nitrated with *trace* amount of HNO_2 along with dilute HNO_3, *o*-and *p*-nitrophenol are formed in the ratio 7:3; when nitrated in the presence of excess HNO_2 the ratio of *o*:*p* product becomes 1:9. This is eventually is the same ratio when *nitrosophenols* are formed with HNO_2 (nitrosating agent) where no HNO_3 is present in the reaction mixture. So it is believed that nitrosophenol is formed first which is then oxidised to a nitrophenol. This method is used to prepare nitrophenols in good yield.

***Mechanism of nitration of phenols* :**

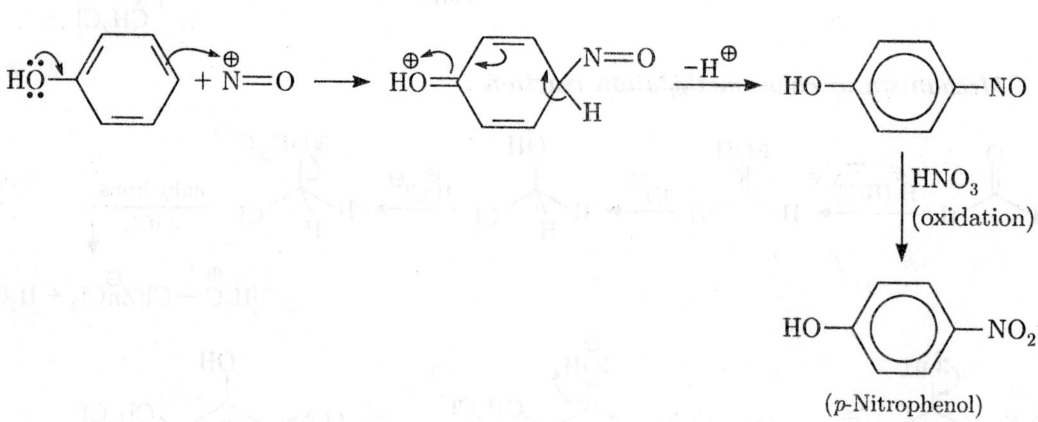

(*p*-Nitrophenol)

Nitrosation occurs only with active aromatic compounds, as nitrosonium ion ($\overset{\oplus}{N}=O$ ion) is not a strong electrophile like nitronium ($\overset{\oplus}{N}O_2$) ion.

Examples :

1. 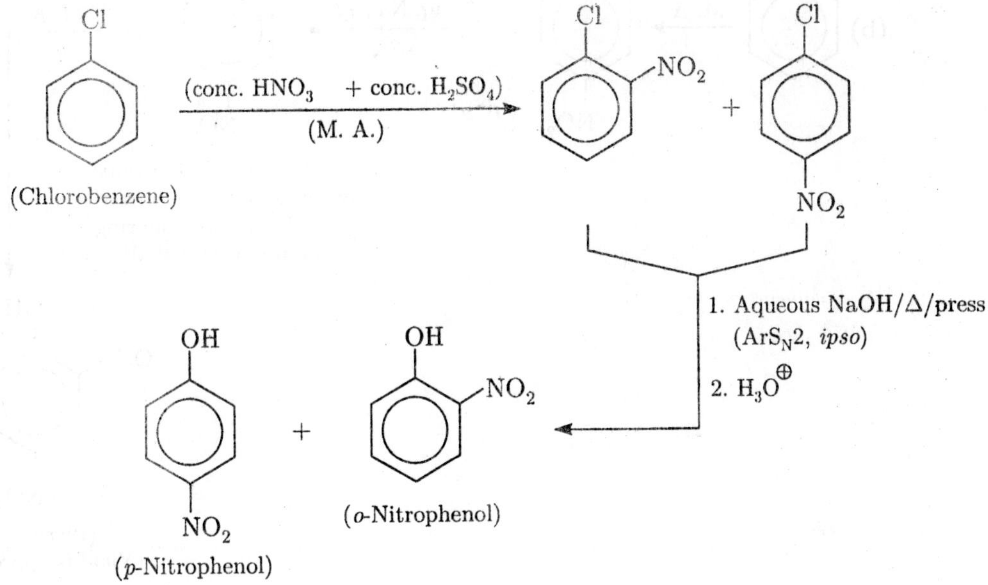

2. 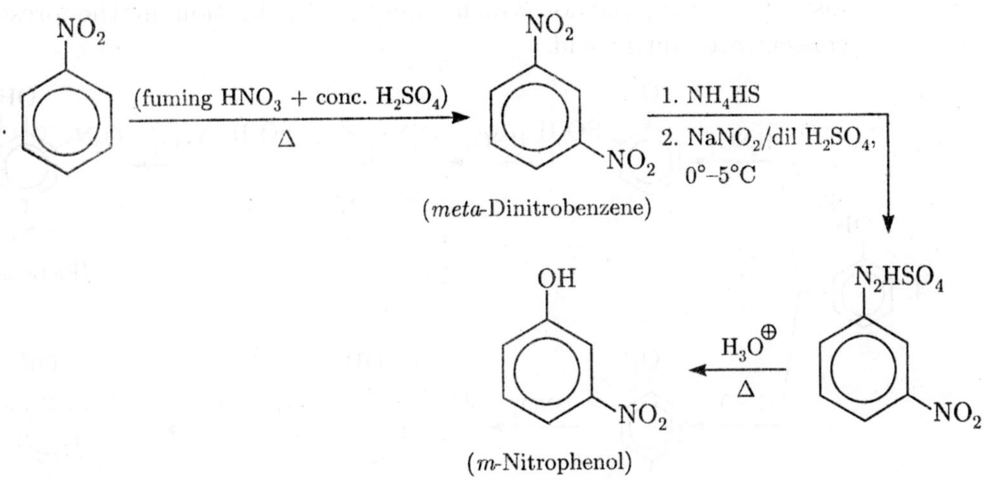

3. (a) 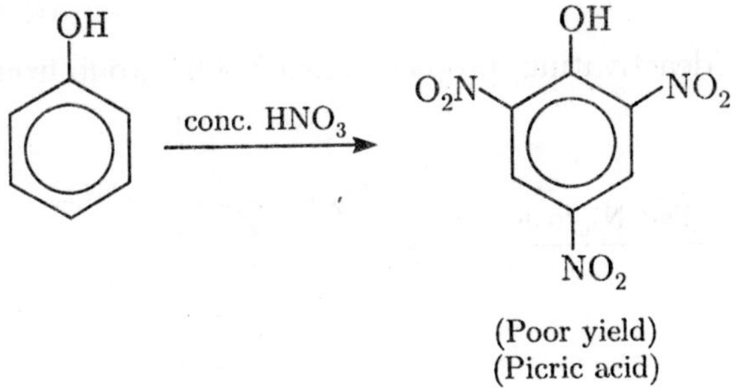

(Poor yield)
(Picric acid)

(b) 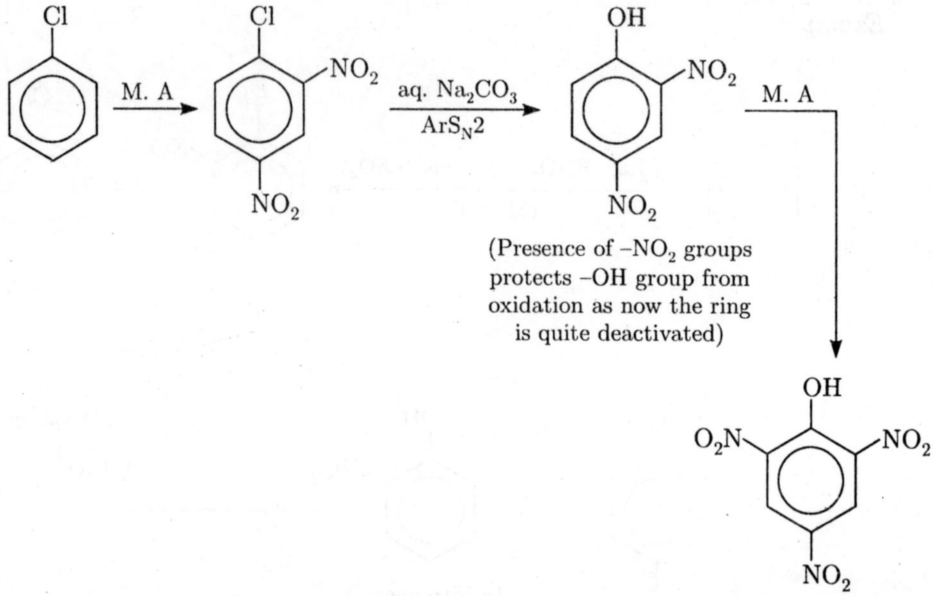

(Presence of $-NO_2$ groups protects $-OH$ group from oxidation as now the ring is quite deactivated)

(Picric acid)
(Yield is appreciable)

In the former method, the yield of picric acid is very poor as there is a huge loss of starting phenol which undergoes oxidation in the presence of concentrated nitric acid.

4. 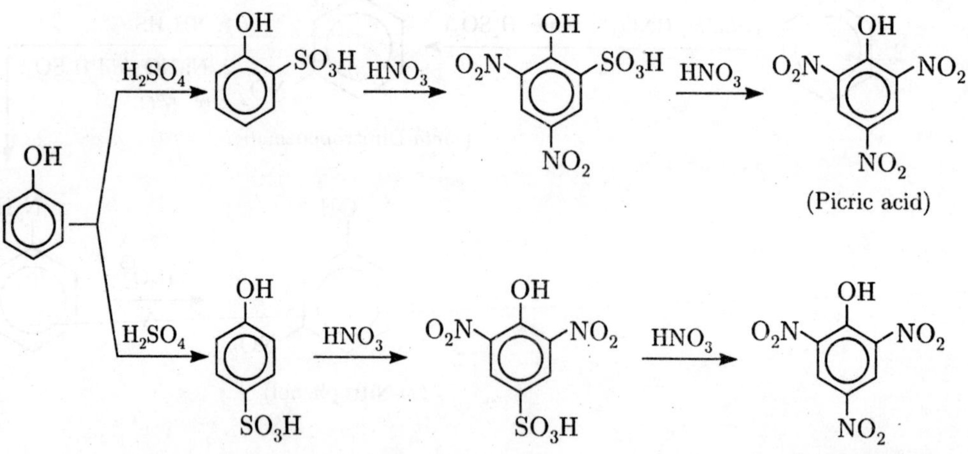

(Picric acid)

(Picric acid)

Presence of SO_3H group (deactivating) protects phenolic OH group from oxidation.

5. 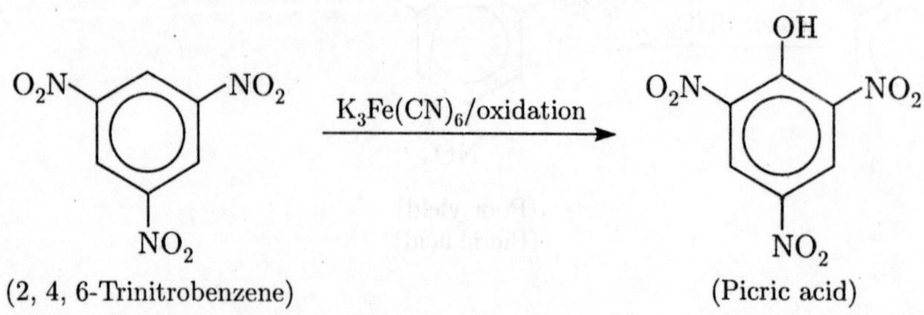

(2, 4, 6-Trinitrobenzene) (Picric acid)

6. 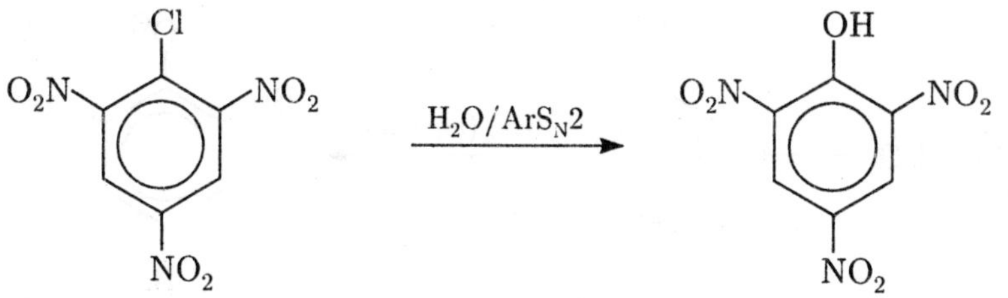

(2,4,6-Trinitrochlorobenzene) (Picric acid)

Picric acid (yellow coloured with bitter taste) is a strong acid which forms charge transfer complexes with aromatic hydrocarbons and phenols called *picrates*. Picrates are often used to detect the presence of aromatic hydrocarbons and activated molecules like phenols.

7. 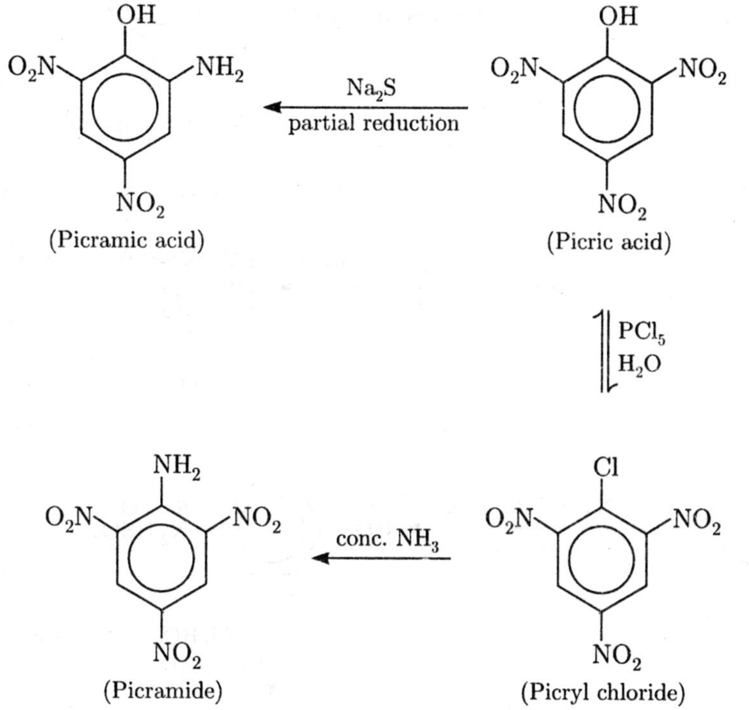

Halogenation of Phenols

Chlorine and bromine form precipitates of 2,4,6-trihalophenol immediately when they are treated with phenol in the aqueous medium. $PhO^{\ominus}$ ion has a strong (+R) effect and the benzene nucleus gets highly activated and can undergo electrophilic substitution very readily than the phenol itself. When chlorination or bromination is carried out in non-aqueous solvents, *e.g.*, in carbon disulphide (CS_2), the ring being less activated than the phenoxide ring, monohalogenation takes place.

1.
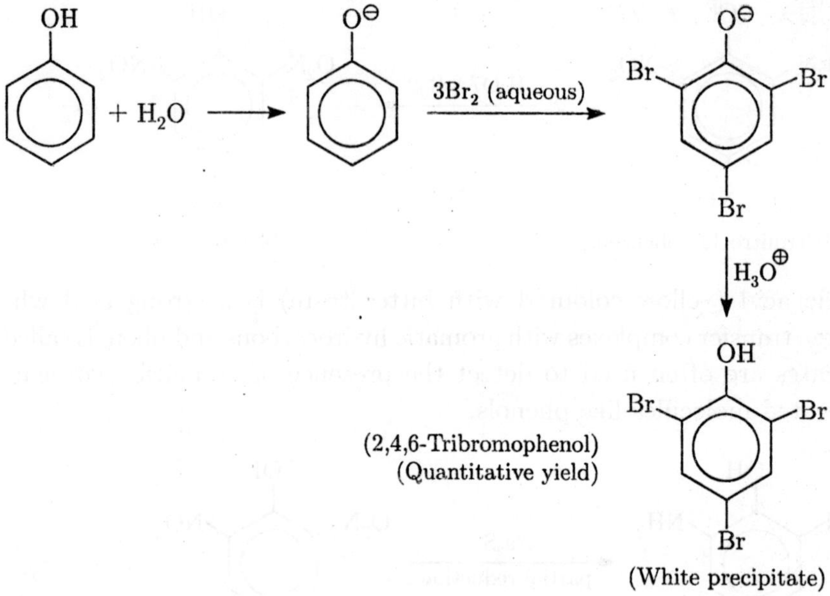
OH
$+ H_2O$
$O^{\ominus}$
$3Br_2$ (aqueous)
Br
$H_3O^{\oplus}$
(2,4,6-Tribromophenol)
(Quantitative yield)
(White precipitate)

2.
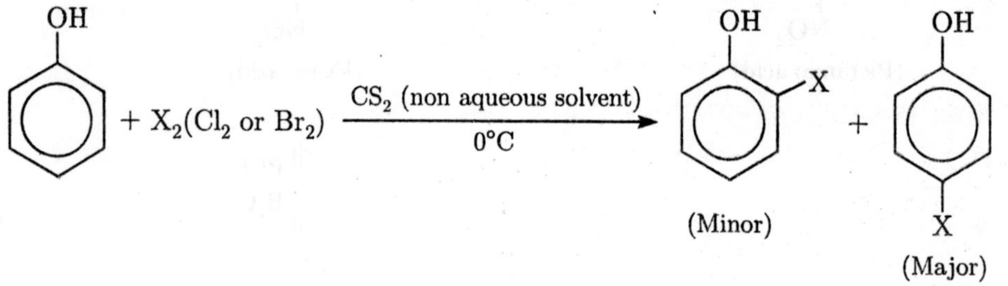
OH
$+ X_2(Cl_2$ or $Br_2)$
CS_2 (non aqueous solvent)
0°C
X
(Minor)
(Major)

3.
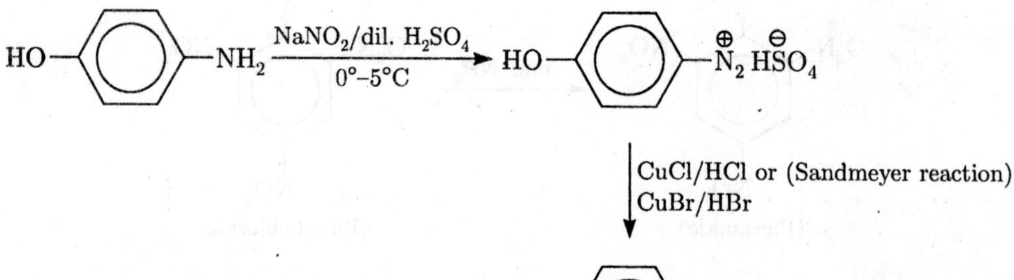
HO
NH_2
$NaNO_2$/dil. H_2SO_4
0°–5°C
$\overset{\oplus}{N_2}\,H\overset{\ominus}{S}O_4$
CuCl/HCl or (Sandmeyer reaction)
CuBr/HBr
Cl/Br

4.
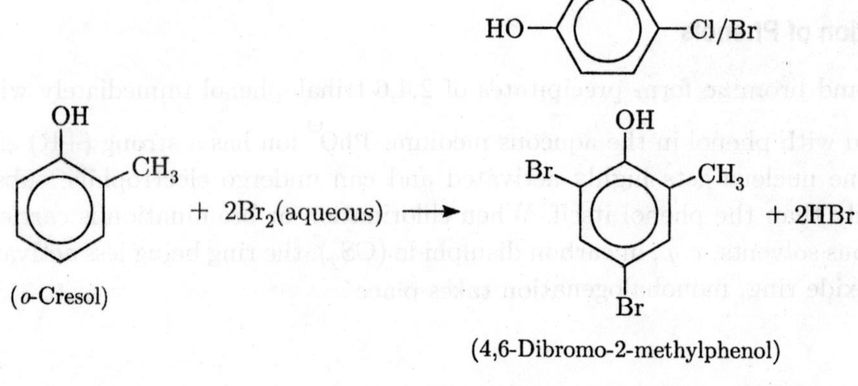
OH
CH_3
$+ 2Br_2$(aqueous)
Br
$+ 2HBr$
(o-Cresol)
(4,6-Dibromo-2-methylphenol)

5. 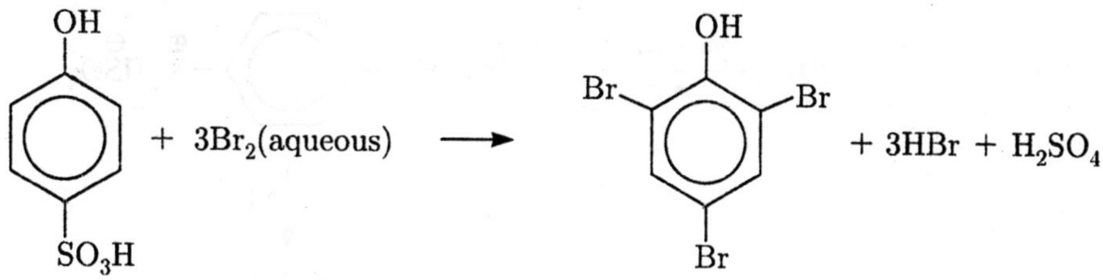

6. 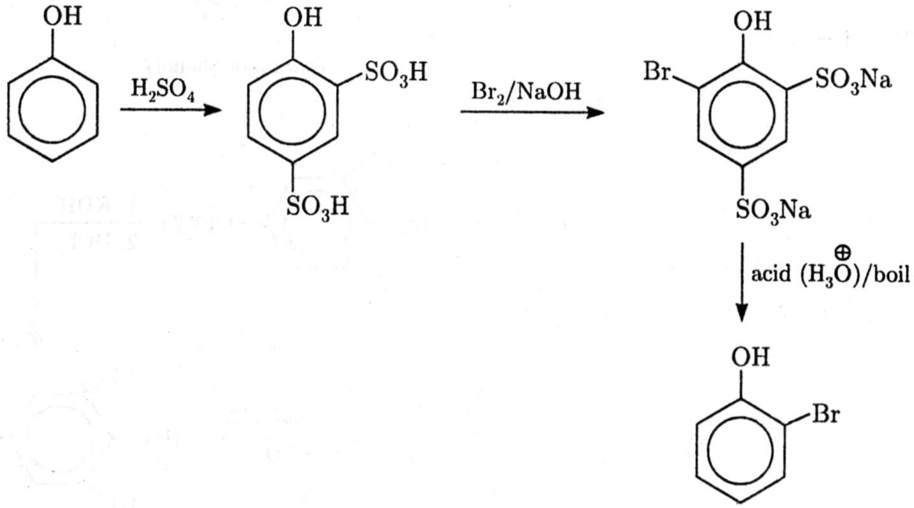

(*ortho*-bromophenol)
(43%)

7. 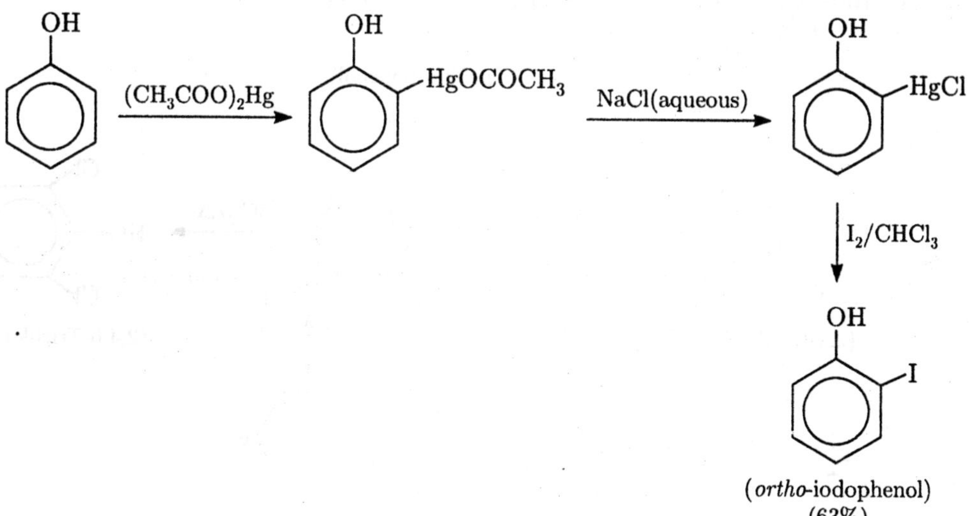

(*ortho*-iodophenol)
(63%)

8. 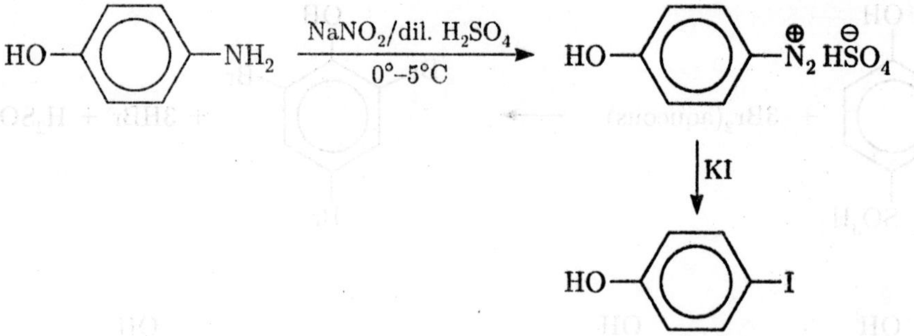

(*para*-iodophenol)

9. 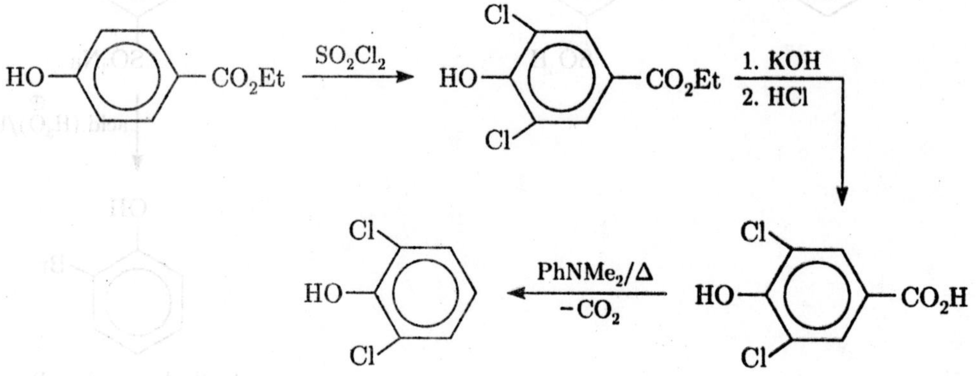

10. 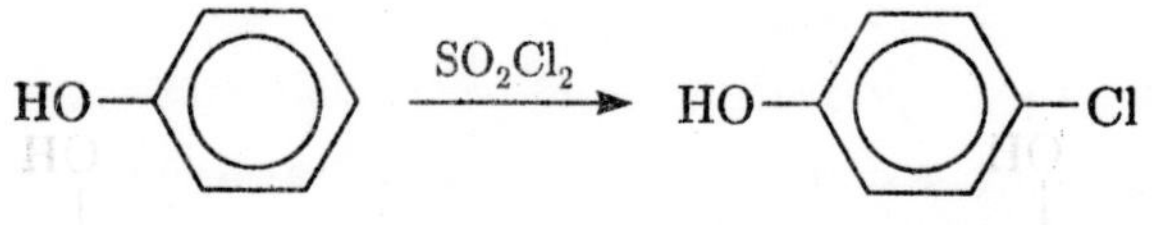

(p-Chlorophenol)

11. 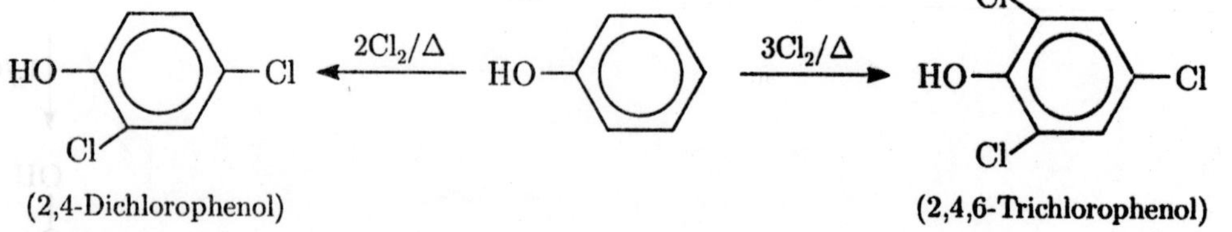

(2,4-Dichlorophenol) (2,4,6-Trichlorophenol)

Sulphonation of Phenols

1. 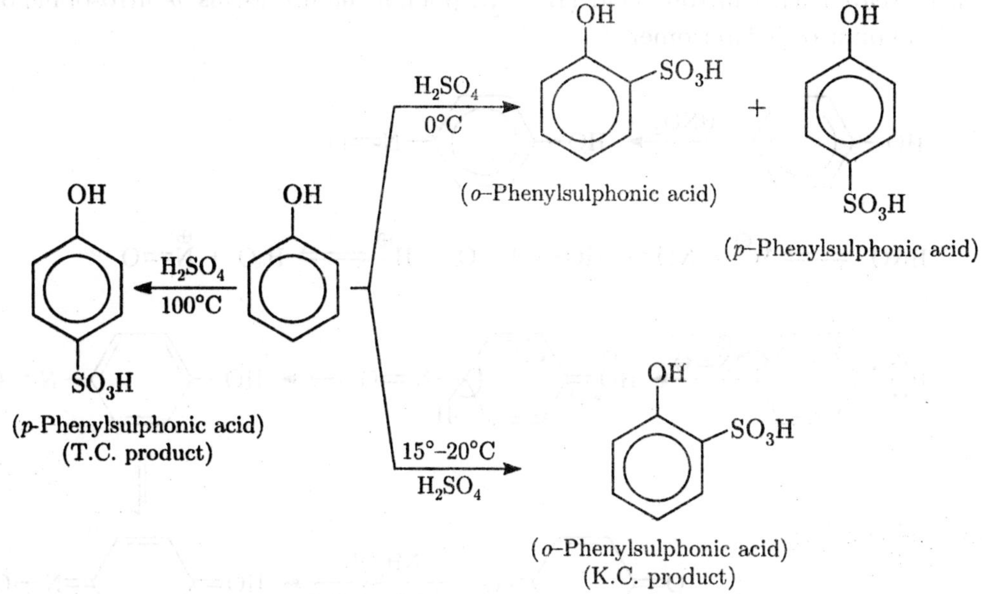

The kinetically controlled product (*ortho*-phenylsulphonic acid) rearranges to the *para*-isomer on heating, *i.e.*, to thermodynamically controlled product.

2. 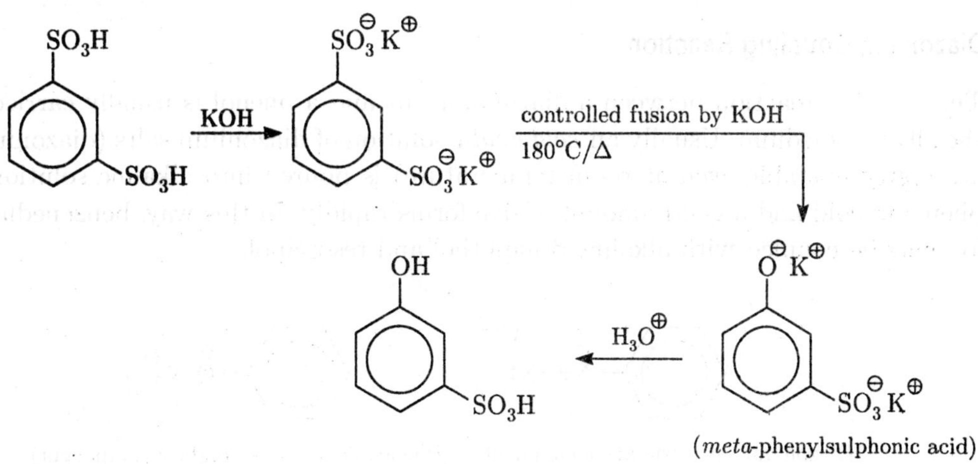

3. 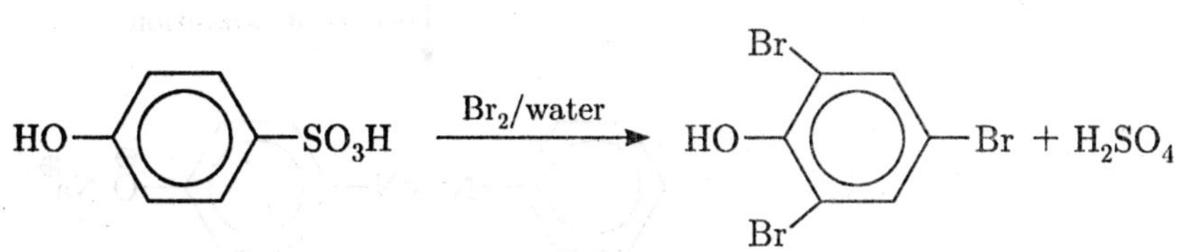

Nitrosation of phenols

When treated with nitrous acid (HNO_2), phenol mainly forms *p*-nitrosophenol and a small amount of *ortho* isomer.

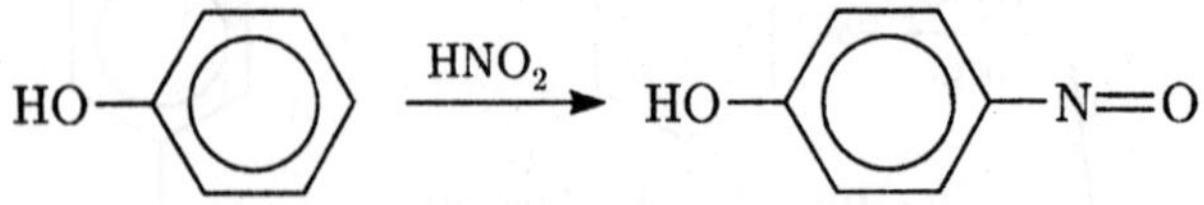

$$HNO_2 \rightleftharpoons H^{\oplus} + NO_2^{\ominus};\quad HO—N=O + H^{\oplus} \rightleftharpoons H_2O + \overset{\oplus}{N}=O$$

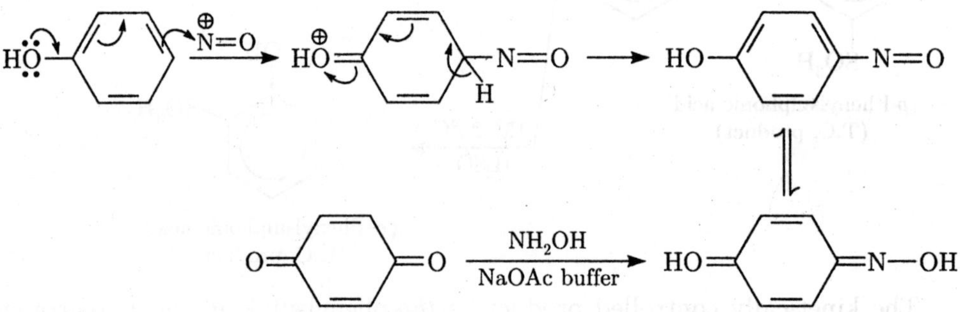

(*p*-Benzoquinone)

Diazonium Coupling Reaction

The coupling reaction between a diazonium salt and a phenol is usually carried out in the alkaline medium. Usually an *cold acidic* solution of diazonium salts (diazonium salts are pretty unstable even at room temperature) is poured into alkaline solution of the phenol in cold and a good amount of dye forms rapidly. In this way, benzenediazonium ion may be coupled with alkaline β-naphthol and resorcinol.

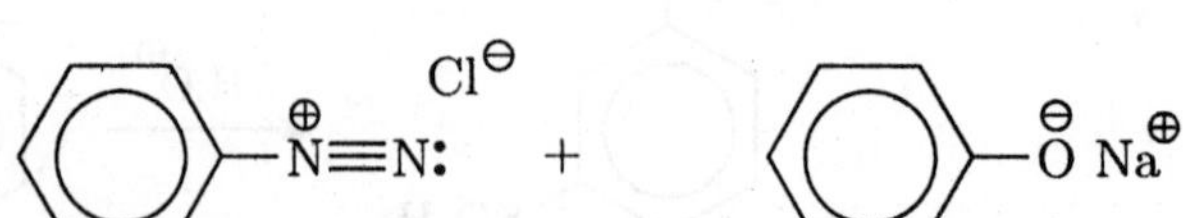

(Diazonium salt; Primary component) (Phenoxide anion; secondary component)

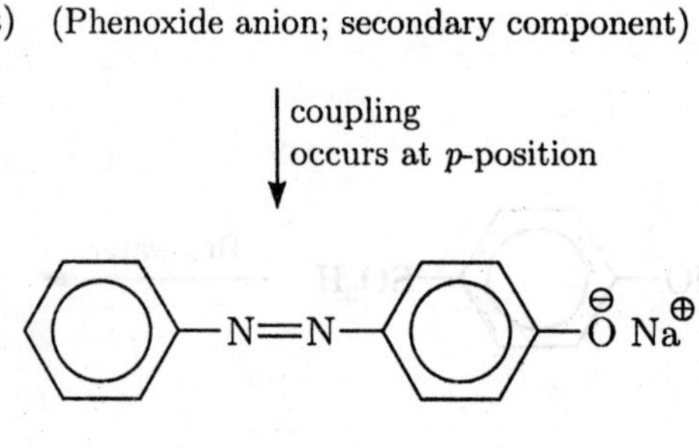

(Red azo dye)

Coupling occurs generally at the *para*-position. If the *para* position is not free, then coupling occurs at the *ortho* position. If both *para* and *ortho* positions are occupied, coupling does not occur.

Coupling involves competing with reaction like formation of phenol with water. Under unfavourable conditions formation of phenol is the major reaction over the coupling reaction. Side reactions take place in concentrated alkali as follows.

$$\underset{\text{(Couples)}}{Ar-\overset{\oplus}{N}\equiv N\ \overset{\ominus}{O}H} \underset{H^{\oplus}}{\overset{NaOH}{\rightleftharpoons}} \underset{\substack{\text{(Does not couple)}\\ \text{(aryldiazonium hydroxide)}}}{Ar-N=N-OH} \underset{H^{\oplus}}{\overset{NaOH}{\rightleftharpoons}} \underset{\substack{\text{(Does not couple)}\\ \text{(sodio salt of diazonium hydroxide)}}}{Ar-N=N-\overset{\ominus}{O}\ \overset{\oplus}{Na}}$$

The electrophilic reagent is the diazonium ion ($ArN_2^{\oplus}$) and coupling occurs at a low concentration of acid, where enough amine is present to get converted to diazonium salt.

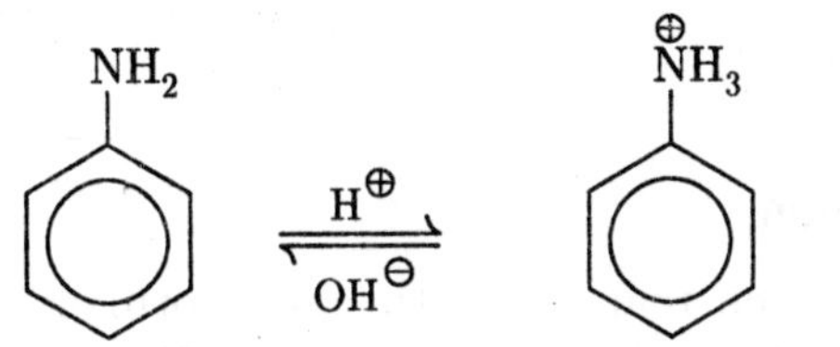

(Couples) (Does not couple)

Analogous situation exists for phenol. A phenol is appreciably acidic in aqueous solution; it exists in equilibrium with phenoxide ion.

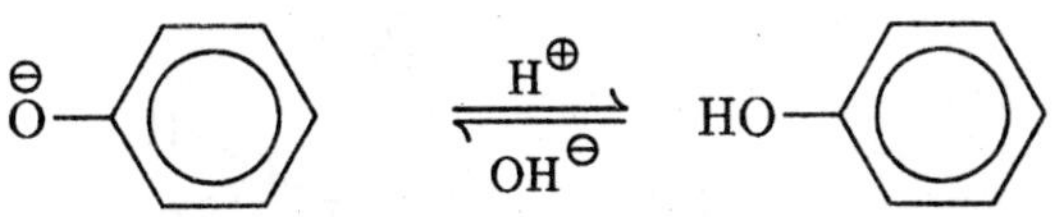

(Couples readily phenoxide ion) (Couples slowly) (phenol)

The fully developed negative charge makes $\overset{\ominus}{O}$ more powerfully electron releasing than OH and phenoxide ion is more reactive towards aromatic electrophilic substitution than the undissociated phenols. The higher the acidity of the medium, higher is the proportion of unionised phenol and lower is the rate of coupling. But the solution *must not be too alkaline* so that the concentration of diazonium salt becomes low, *i.e.*, ($ArN_2^{\oplus} \xrightarrow{OH^{\ominus}} ArN_2OH$ is not formed). It turns out that, *amines couple* fastest in *mildly acidic solutions* and *phenols couple* fastest in *mildly alkaline solutions.*

The Mannich Reaction

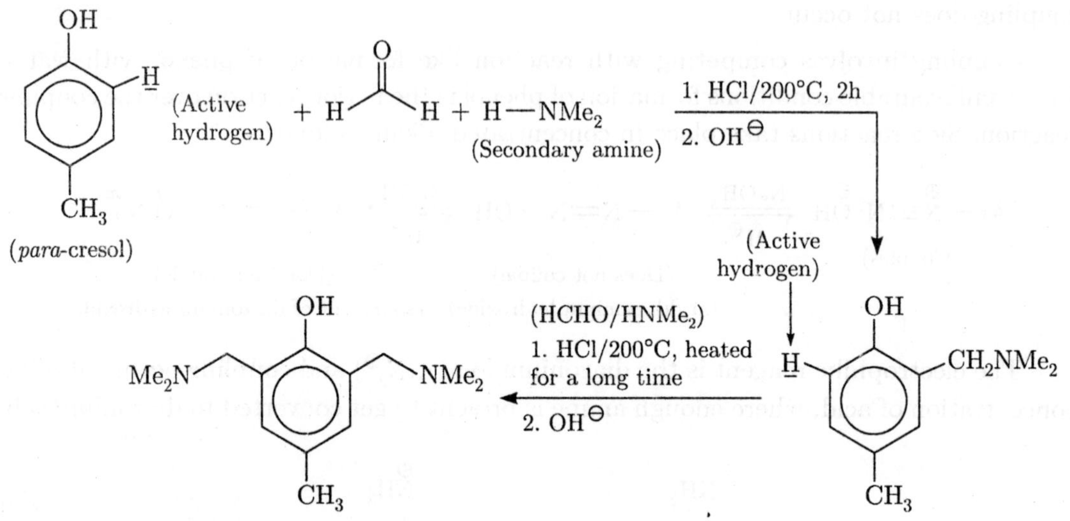

The Reimer-Tiemann Reaction

Formylation of phenols by the reaction with chloroform in strong sodium hydroxide solution is known as the Reimer-Tiemann reaction. When phenol is subjected to this reaction sodio salt of *ortho*-hydroxybenzaldehyde and *para*-hydroxybenzaldehyde are formed in the ratio 4:1. The hydroxyaldehydes are obtained on acidfication of the sodio salts.

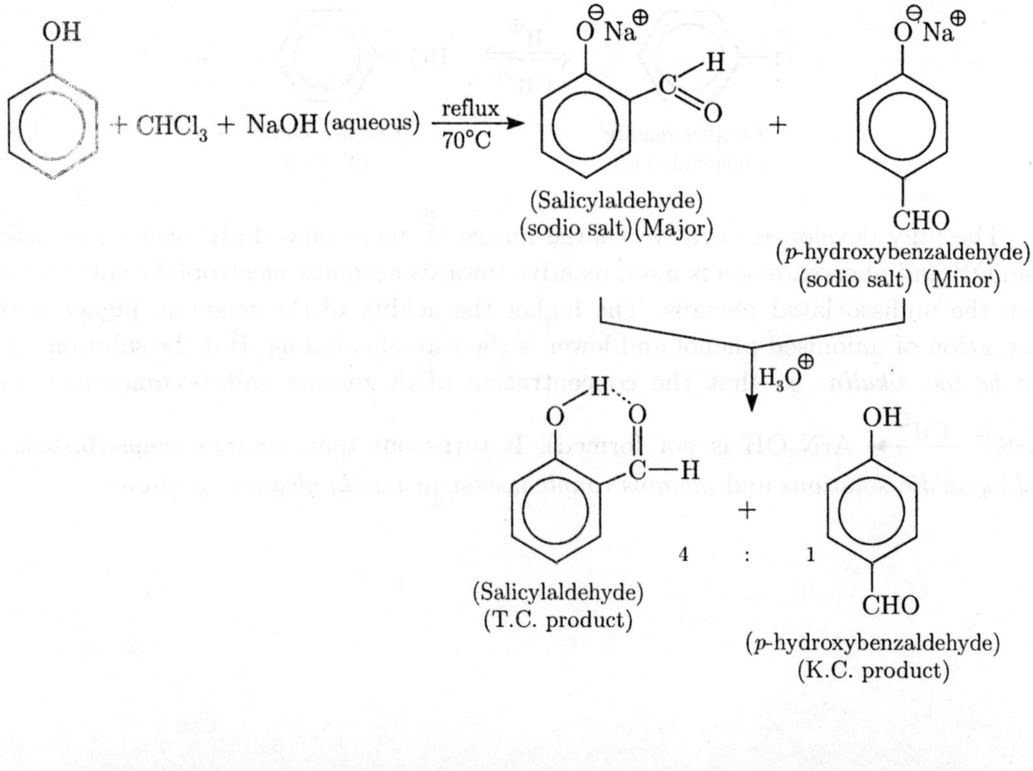

The reaction involves refluxing a mixture of phenol, chloroform and aqueous sodium hydroxide at 70°C followed by distilling off excess chloroform. The mixture on acidification forms hydroxybenzaldehydes. *Ortho*-hydroxybenzaldehyde can form intramolecular hydrogen bonding (six-membered chelate is formed) and can be distilled out by steam distillation from the *para*-isomer. The *ortho*-isomer can further be separated from unreacted phenol through the formation of aldehyde-bisulphite adduct. In Reimer-Tiemann reaction, generally the *o*-isomer predominates. Perhaps the internal hydrogen bonding yields the thermodynamically stable *ortho* product. When one *ortho* position is blocked, *p*-isomer is obtained. With KOH as a base, the predominant product is the *para* isomer. Most probably, the large size of $K^{\oplus}$ ion does not allow the formation of six-membered chelate as is formed with $Na^{\oplus}$ ion when NaOH is used as a base.

***Mechanism of Reimer-Tiemann Reaction* :**

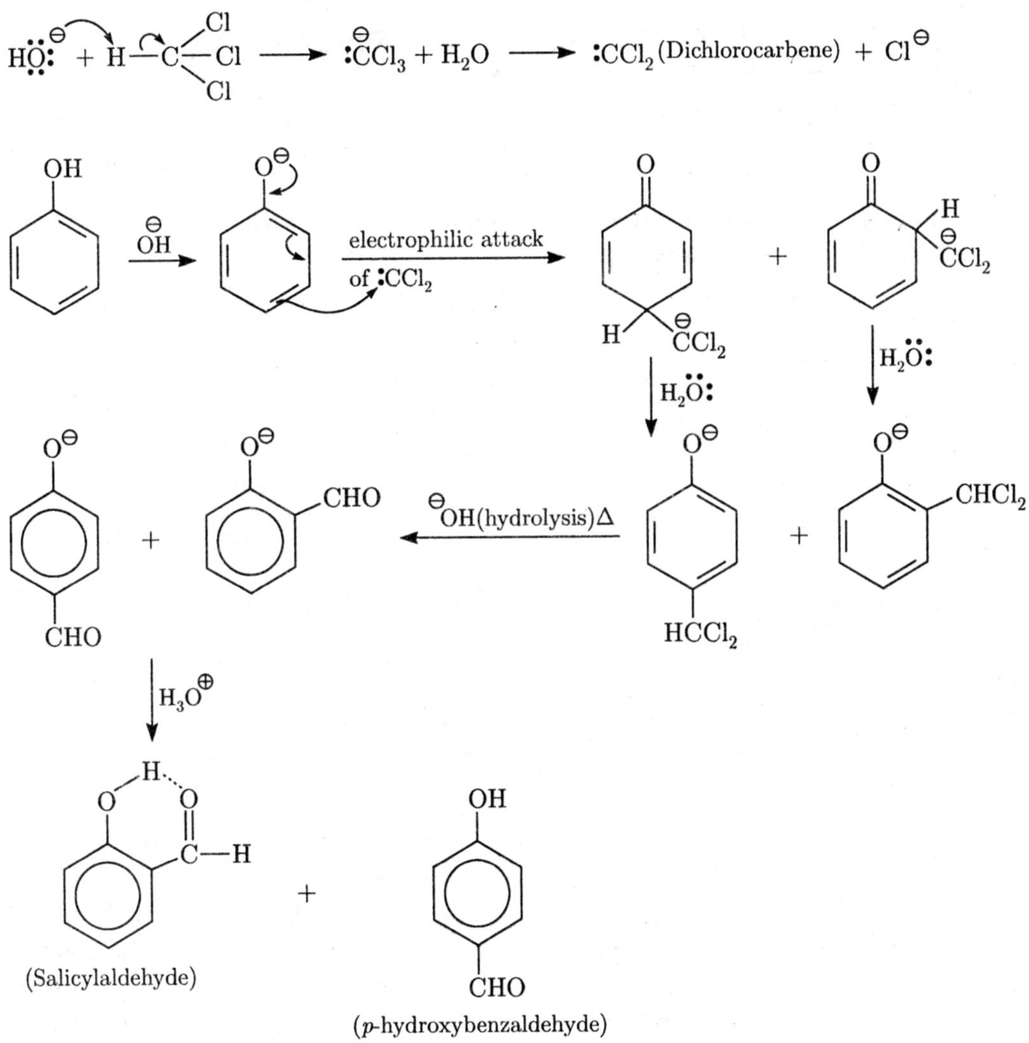

Dichlorocarbene is the attacking electrophile is supported by the following evidences :

1. Dichlorocarbene causes ring expansion which is observed in the reaction of pyrrole with chloroform and alkali.

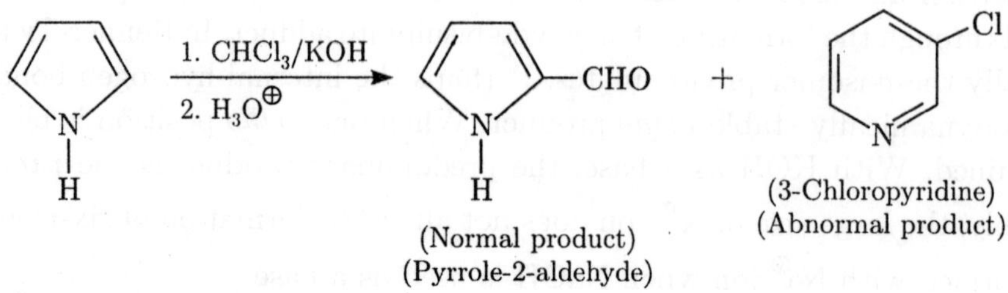

Mechanism for the formation of abnormal product :

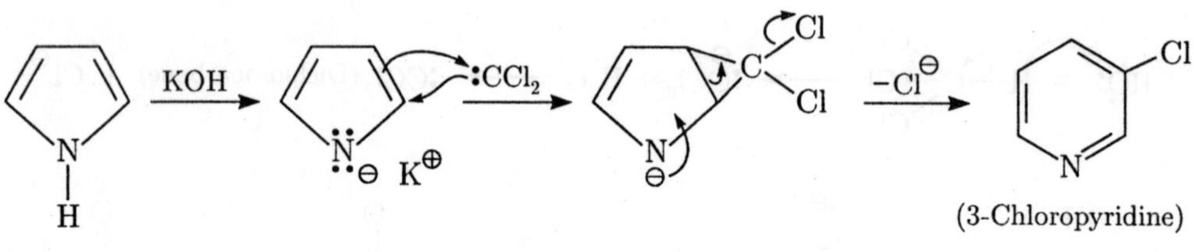

2. When *p*-cresol is used instead of a phenol, a dienone with dichloromethyl group is obtained as a by product.

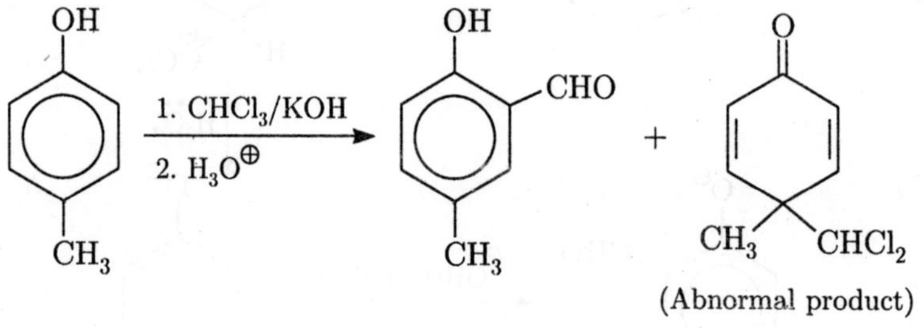

Mechanism :

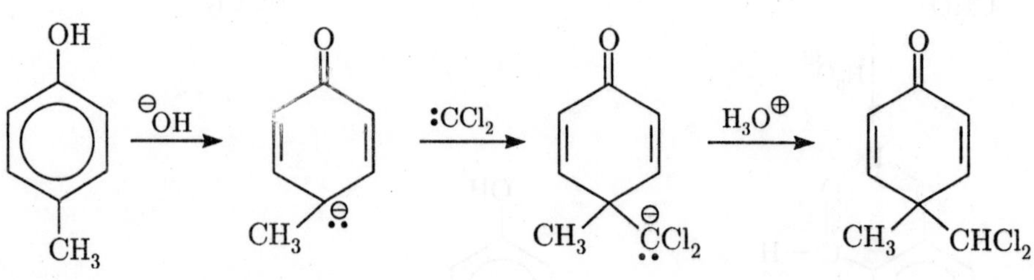

The presence of electron withdrawing substituents like CN, CO_2H, NO_2, SO_3H etc. decrease the yield of Reimer-Tiemann reaction. The yield of the reaction is maximum 50% and a large amount of phenol (reactant) remains unreacted. This may be due to the formation of diphenylacetal derivative as follows.

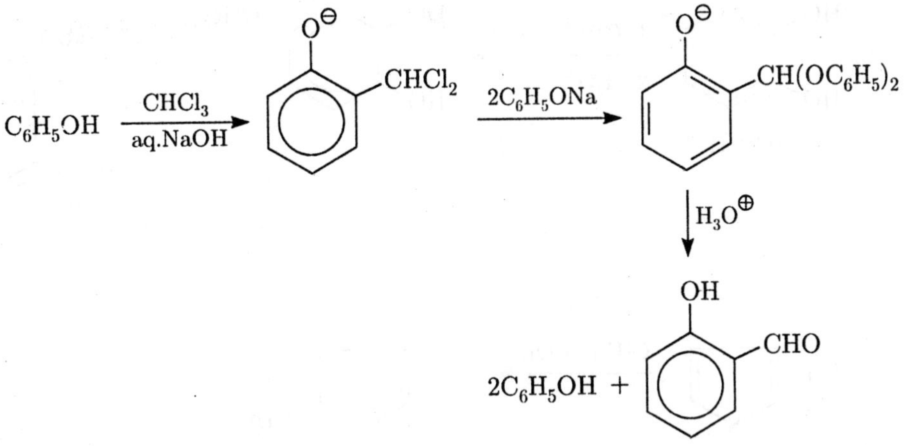

Carbon tetrachloride may be used in place of chloroform in Reimer-Tiemann reaction and in that case salicylic acid is obtained instead of salicylaldehyde from phenol.

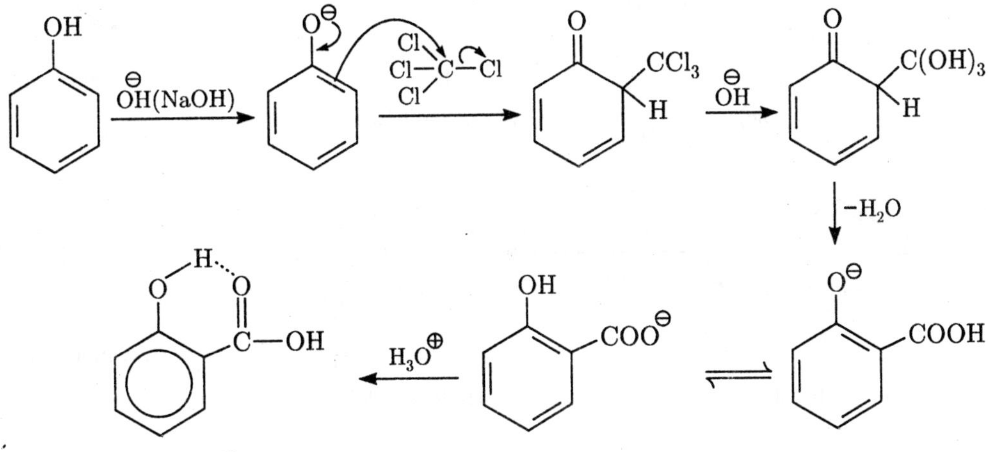

(Salicylic acid)

Applications of Reimer-Tiemann Reaction :

1.

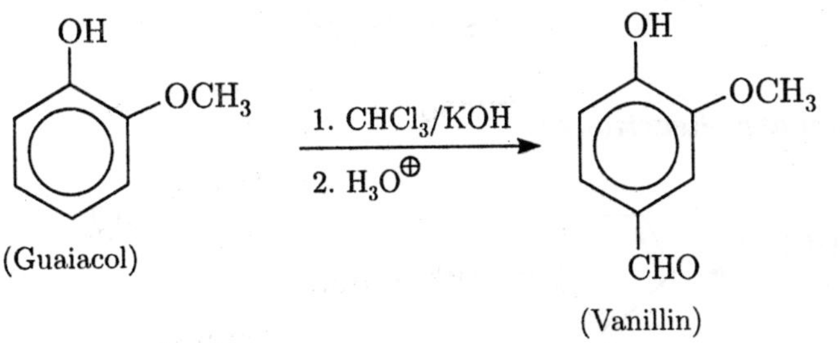

(Guaiacol) (Vanillin)

2. 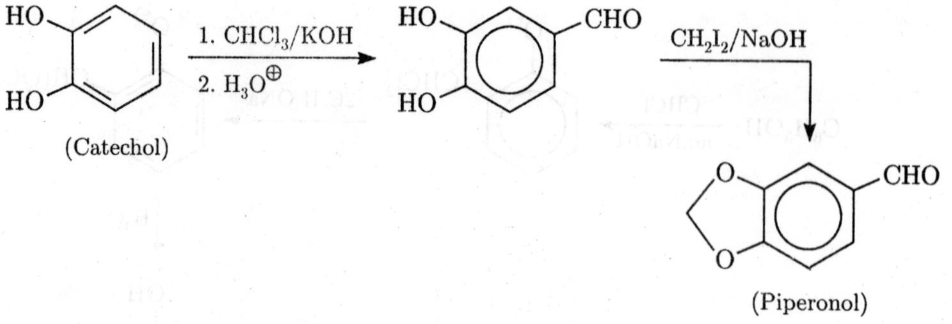

3. (a) 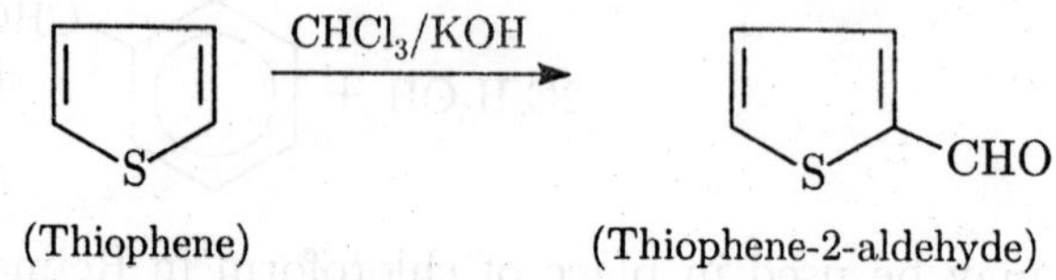

(b) 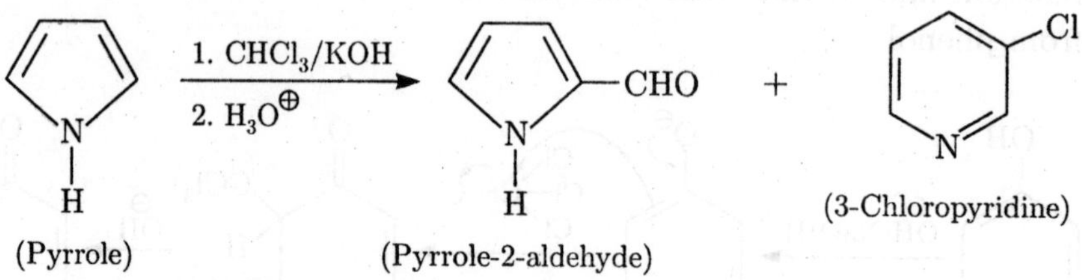

4. 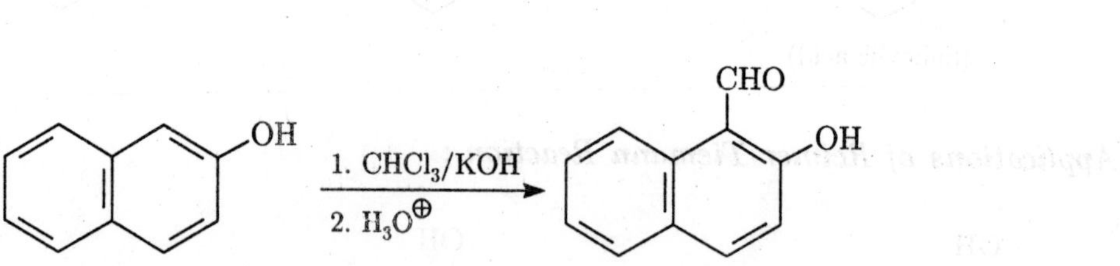

5. 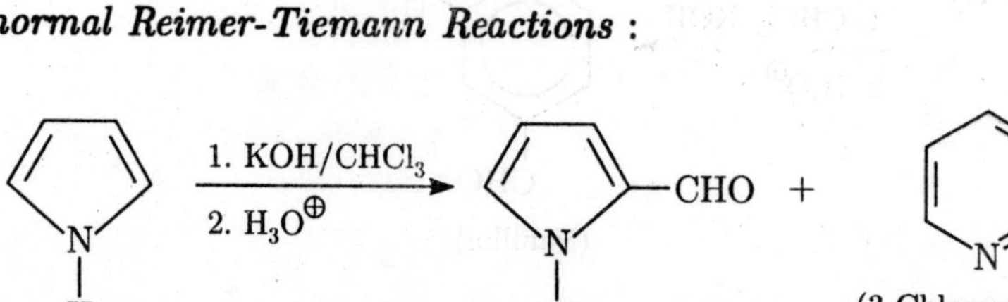

***Abnormal Reimer-Tiemann Reactions* :**

1.

2. 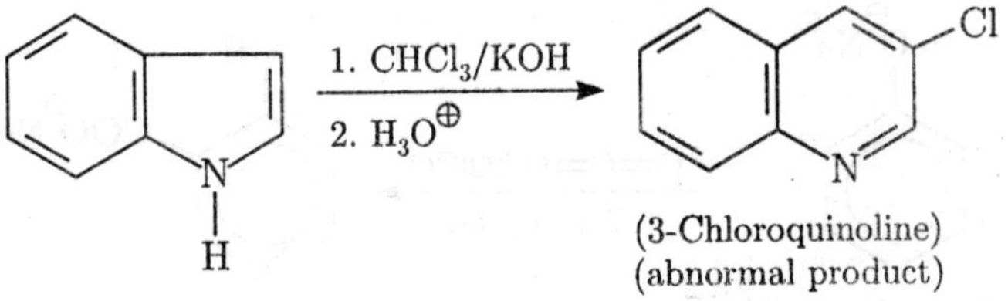

(3-Chloroquinoline)
(abnormal product)

3. 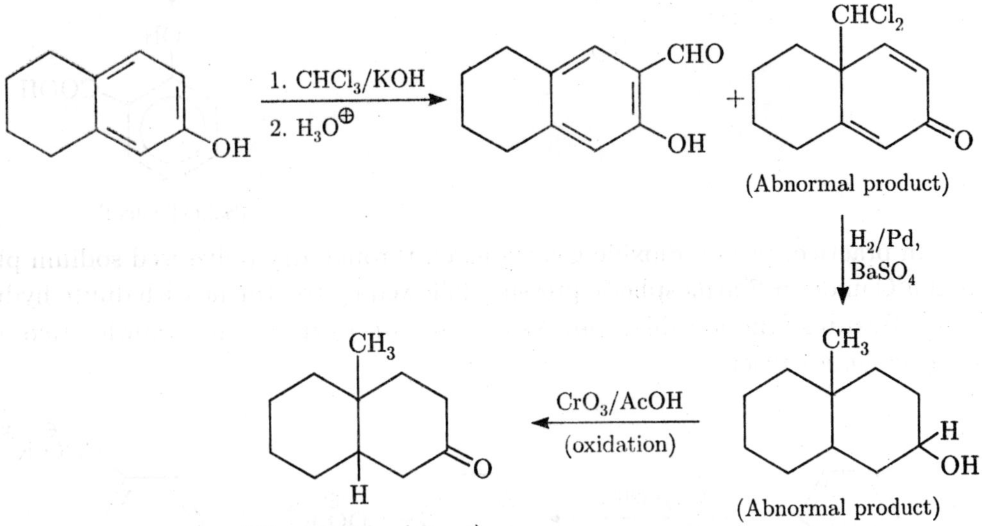

(10-methyl-decal-2-one)

Mechanism for the formation of abnormal product :

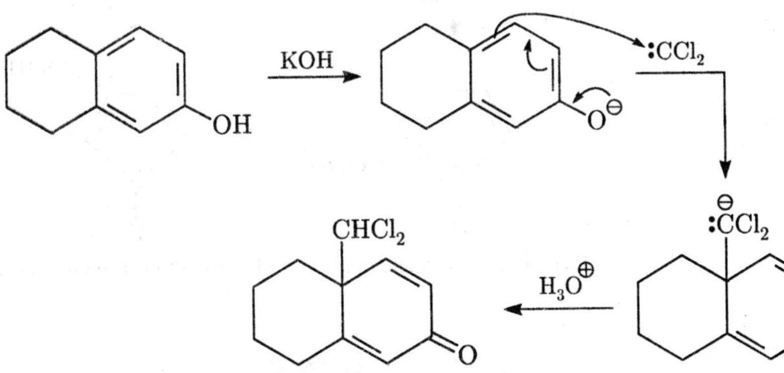

(Abnormal product)

The Kolbe-Schmidt Reaction

Carboxylation of phenoxide ions by carbon dioxide at an elevated temperature under pressure is known as Kolbe-Schmidt reaction. Salicylic acid is formed commercially along with a trace amount of *p*-hydroxybenzoic acid by this method.

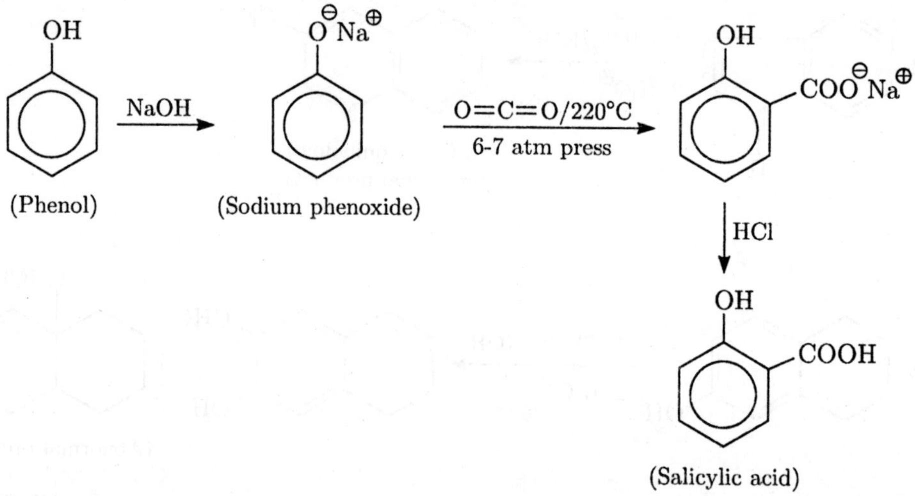

In practice, carbon dioxide gas is passed through dry pulverised sodium phenoxide at 200°C under 6–7 atmospheric pressure followed by treatment with dilute hydrochloric acid. Besides phenoxides, potassio salts of pyrrole and indole also undergo Kolbe-Schmidt reaction.

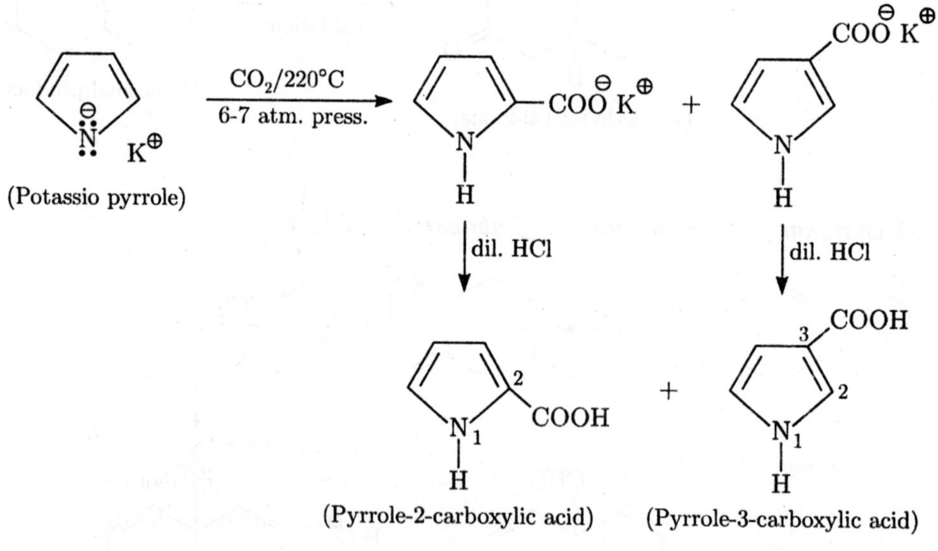

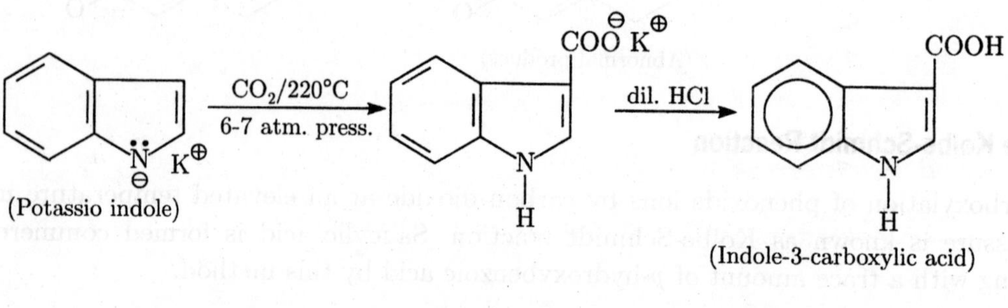

In case of sodium phenoxide, *o*-hydroxyacid is the major product, whereas with potassium phenoxide, *p*-hydroxybenzoic acid forms as the major product.

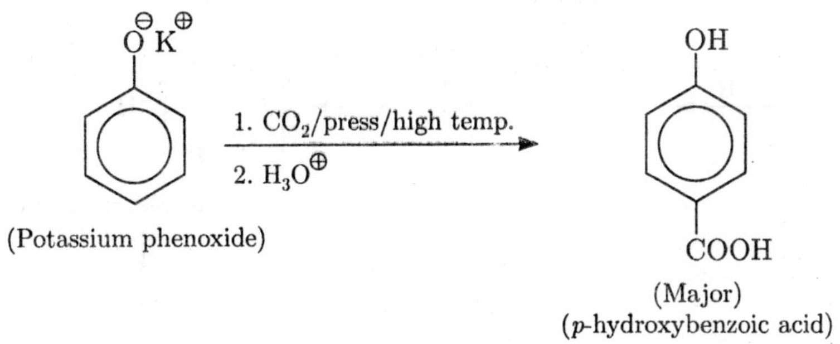

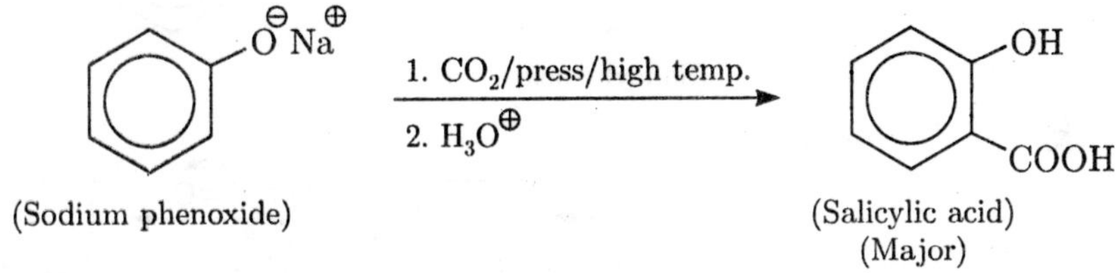

The reaction is essentially an aromatic electrophilic substitution reaction when potassio salt of phenol is used, perhaps chelation does not occur because of high volume and low positive charge density on the metal ion. On the other hand, the reaction of sodium phenoxide with CO_2 (a very weak electrophile) is the electrophilic attack of CO_2 *exclusively* at the *orthohydroxybenzoate (salicylate)*; Only traces of *para* isomer is obtained. It has been suggested that the preferential *ortho* attack with sodium phenoxide may result from stabilisation of the transition state through chelation by $Na^{\oplus}$ ion in the ion pair.

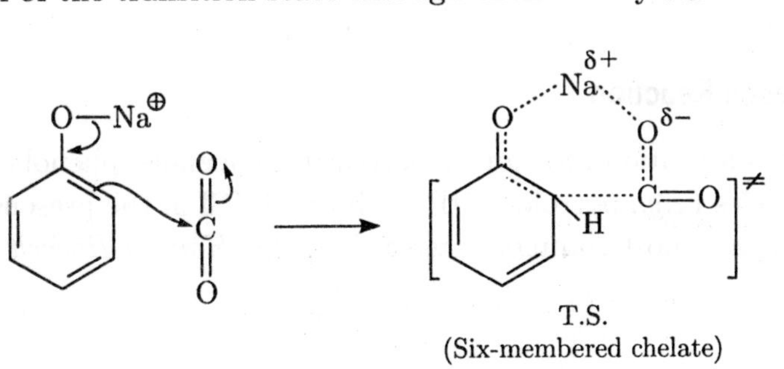

The size of $K^{\oplus}$ cation is larger and hence is likely to be *less effective* regarding the formation of chelate ring. So the attack of CO_2 at the *p*-position with the potassium phenoxide becomes more competitive.

***Mechanism of Kolbe-Schmidt Reaction* :**

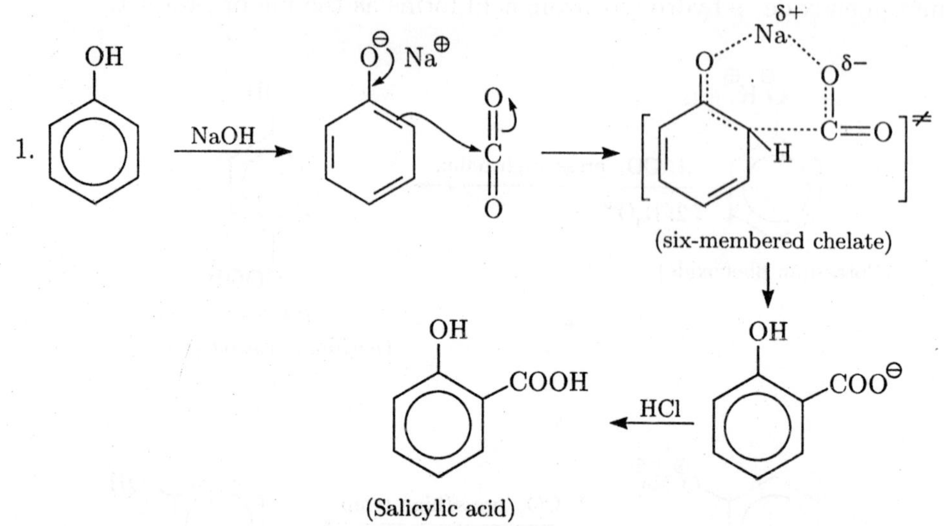

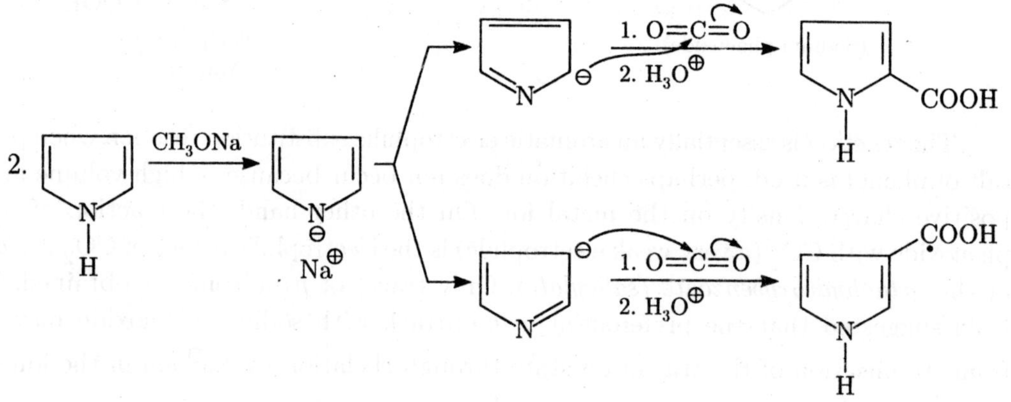

The Houben-Hoesch Reaction

The Friedel-Crafts acylation reaction of polyhydroxyphenols, phenolic ethers, and some reactive heterocycles (*e.g.*, pyrrole) with nitrile and HCl in the presence of a Lewis acid ($ZnCl_2$ and $AlCl_3$ are most commonly used) is called *Houben-Hoesch reaction.*

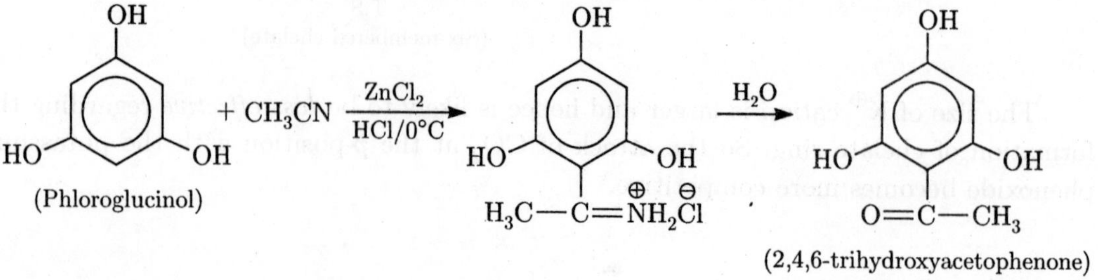

Houben-Hoesch reaction however is not successful with phenol, is due to

(a) Phenol is not activated enough with only one OH group while phloroglucinol contains three OH groups and so is activated much.

(b) Phenol forms an imino ether derivative as shown below.

$$C_6H_5OH + RCN \xrightarrow{ZnCl_2/HCl} \underset{\text{(Imino ether hydrochloride)}}{C_6H_5O-\overset{R}{\overset{|}{C}}=\overset{\oplus}{N}H_2\overset{\ominus}{Cl}} \xrightarrow{H_3O^{\oplus}} \underset{\substack{\text{(Phenyl ester)}\\ \text{(unwanted product)}}}{C_6H_5O-\overset{R}{\overset{|}{C}}=O}$$

***Mechanism of Houben-Hoesch Reaction* :**

$$R-C\equiv N + HCl + ZnCl_2 \rightleftharpoons [R-C\equiv\overset{\oplus}{N}H] + \overset{\ominus}{Z}nCl_3 \rightleftharpoons R-C\equiv\overset{\oplus}{N}H\ \overset{\ominus}{ZnCl_3}$$

$$\updownarrow$$

$$[R-\overset{\oplus}{C}=NH]\ \overset{\ominus}{ZnCl_3}$$

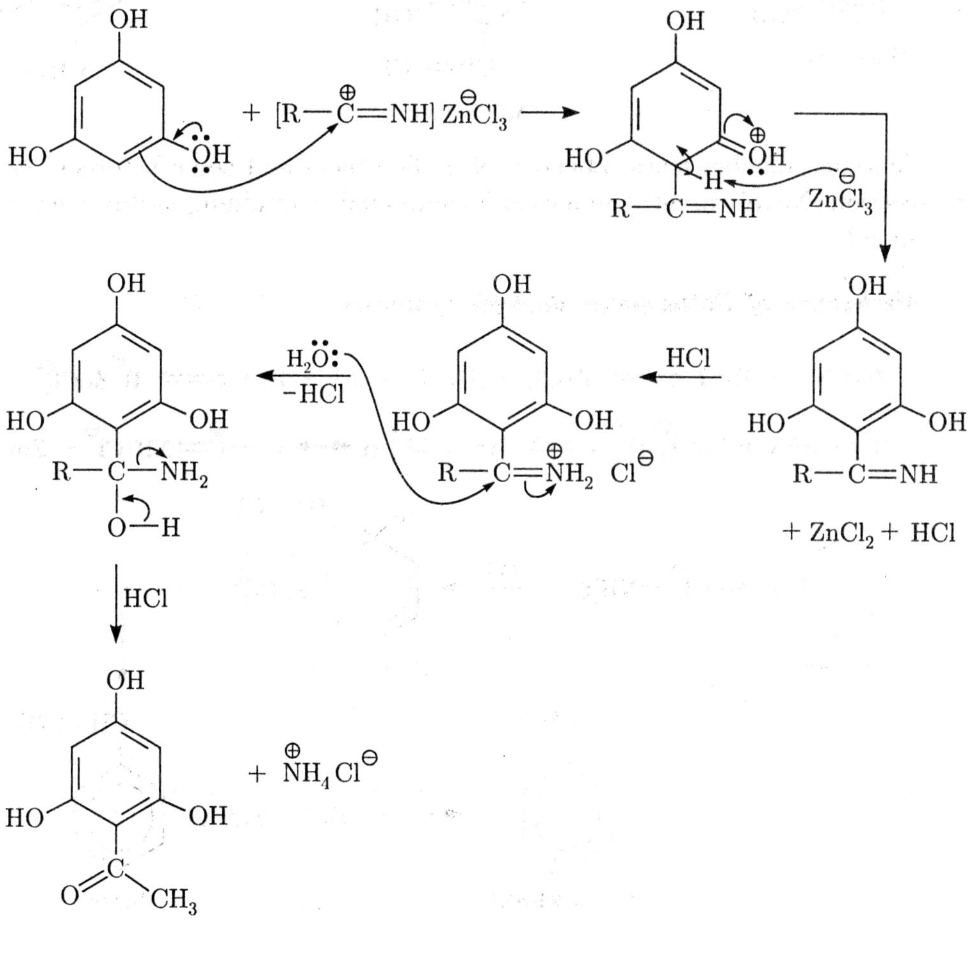

When HCN is used instead of nitriles, aromatic aldehydes are obtained. This is known as Gattermann aldehyde synthesis. Formylation of some organic compounds with HCN and HCl in the presence of $AlCl_3$ (Lewis acid catalyst) is called the *Gattermann aldehyde synthesis.*

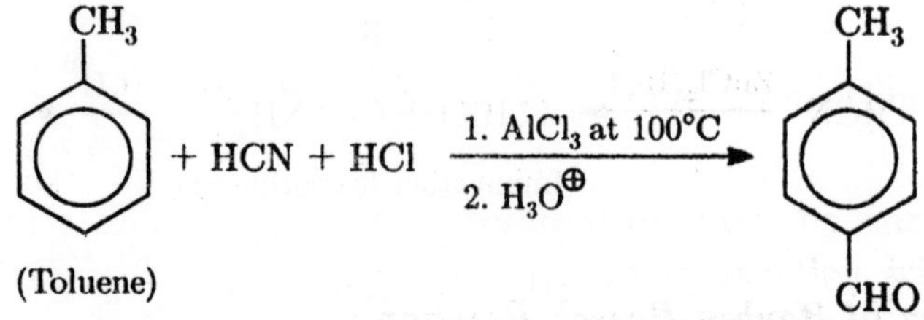

(Toluene)

Alternatively, the reaction may be carried out with the substrate and $Zn(CN)_2$ and HCl whereby $ZnCl_2$ and HCN are formed *in situ.* Nitrobenzene is used as a solvent.

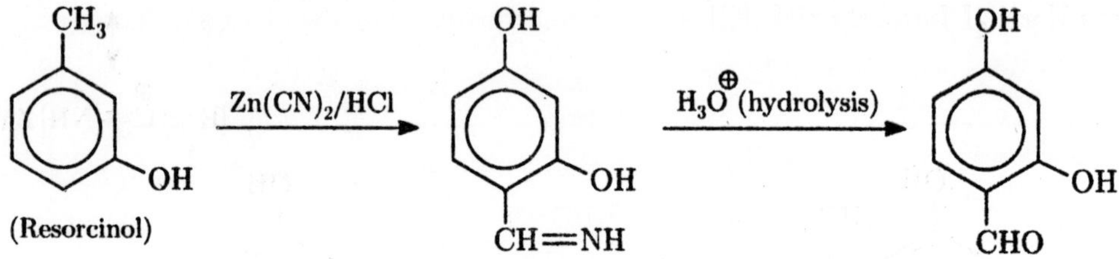

(Resorcinol) (Aryl imine)

Benzene, alkylbenzenes, phenols, phenolic ethers and some heterocycles undergo the reaction. Nitrobenzenes, amines and compounds containing *m*-directing groups fail to respond.

Mechanism of Gattermann aldehyde synthesis :

$$Zn(CN)_2 + 2HCl \rightleftharpoons ZnCl_2 + 2HCN; \quad ZnCl_2 + HCl \rightleftharpoons \overset{\oplus}{H}\,ZnCl_3^{\ominus}$$

$$H-C\equiv N + ZnCl_3^{\ominus}\,H^{\oplus} \rightleftharpoons [H-C\equiv\overset{\oplus}{N}H \longleftrightarrow H-\overset{\oplus}{C}=NH]\,Cl^{\ominus} + ZnCl_2$$

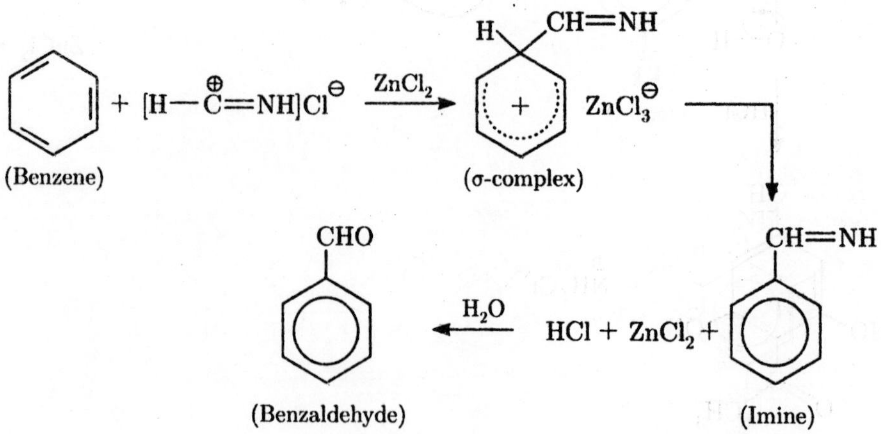

(Benzene) (σ-complex) (Benzaldehyde) (Imine)

Applications of Houben-Hoesch Reaction :

1. 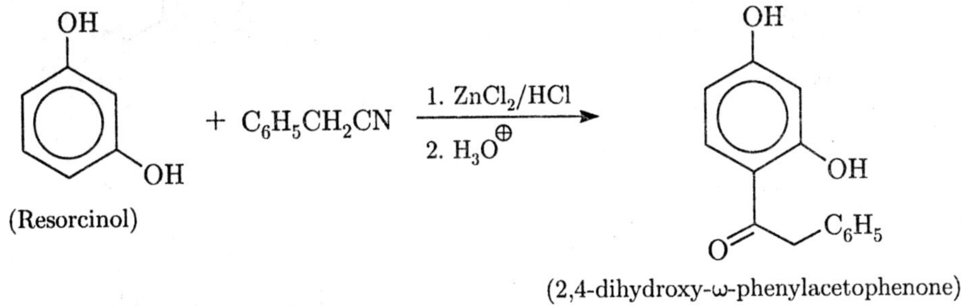

2. 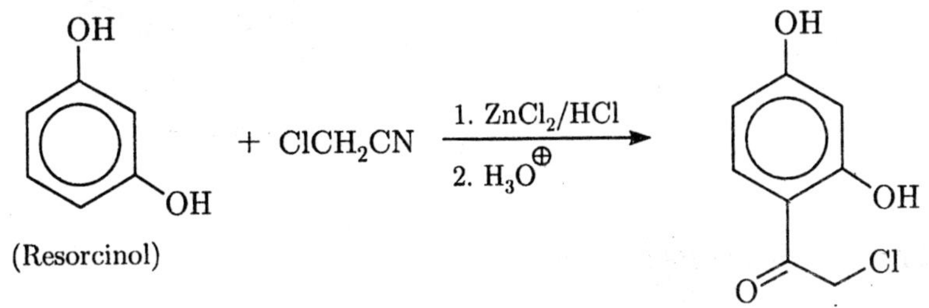

3. 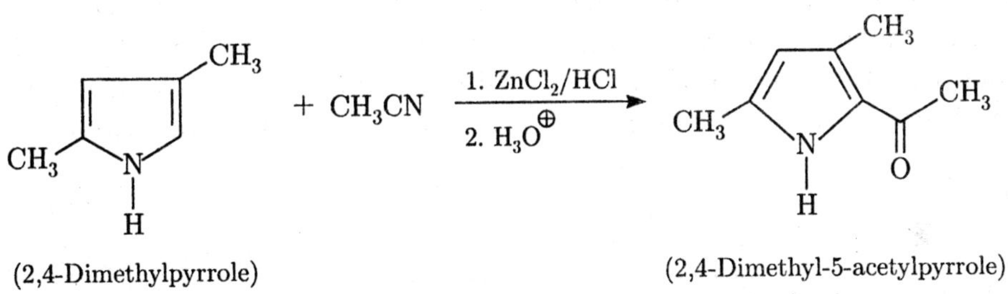

4. 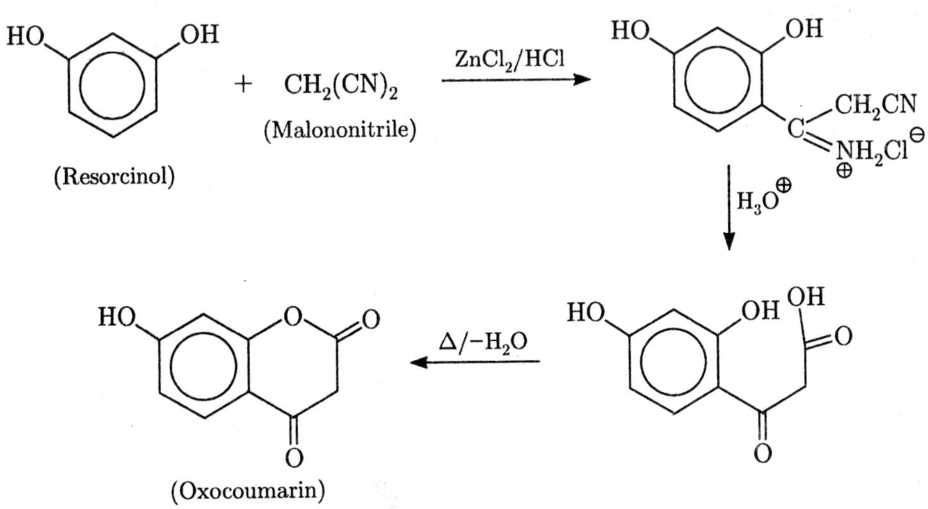

5.

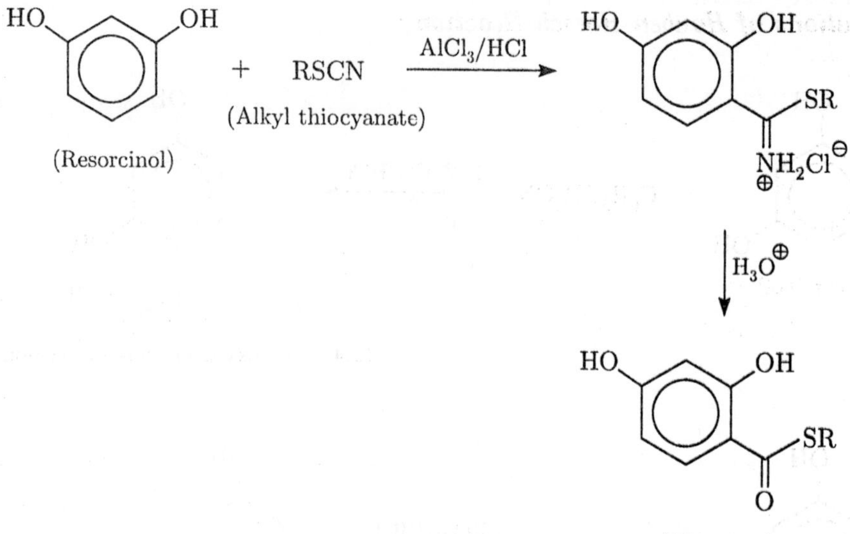

(Thioester)

The Lederer–Manasse Reaction

Phenols condense with aliphatic and aromatic aldehydes in the *ortho*- and *para* positions, the most important example being the condensation with *formaldehyde.* At low temperature, in the presence of dilute acid or alkali and using formalin (40% aqueous formaldehyde), the main product is *p*- hydroxybenzyl alcohol together with a small amount of *ortho* isomer. The reaction is known as *Lederer-Manasse reaction.*

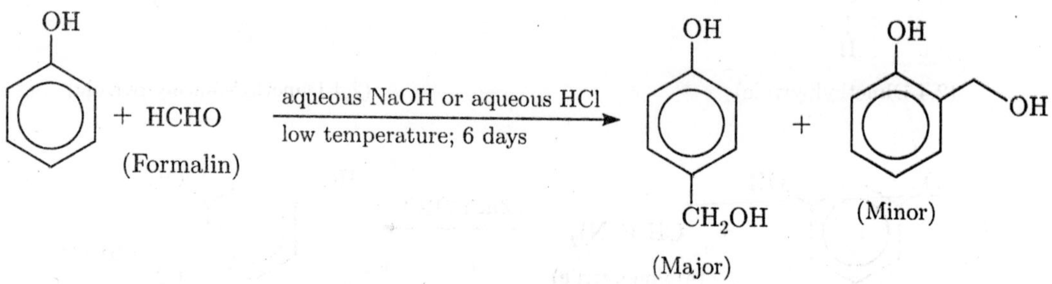

Mechanism of Lederer–Manasse reaction :

1. ***Acid catalysed Pathway*** :

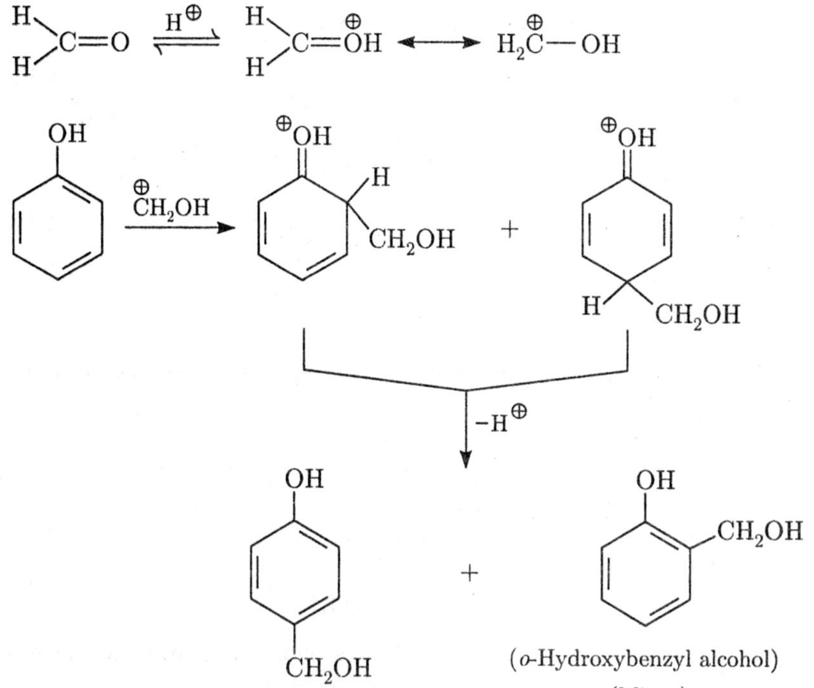

(p-Hydroxybenzyl alcohol) (Major)

(o-Hydroxybenzyl alcohol) (Minor)

2. ***Base catalysed Pathway*** :

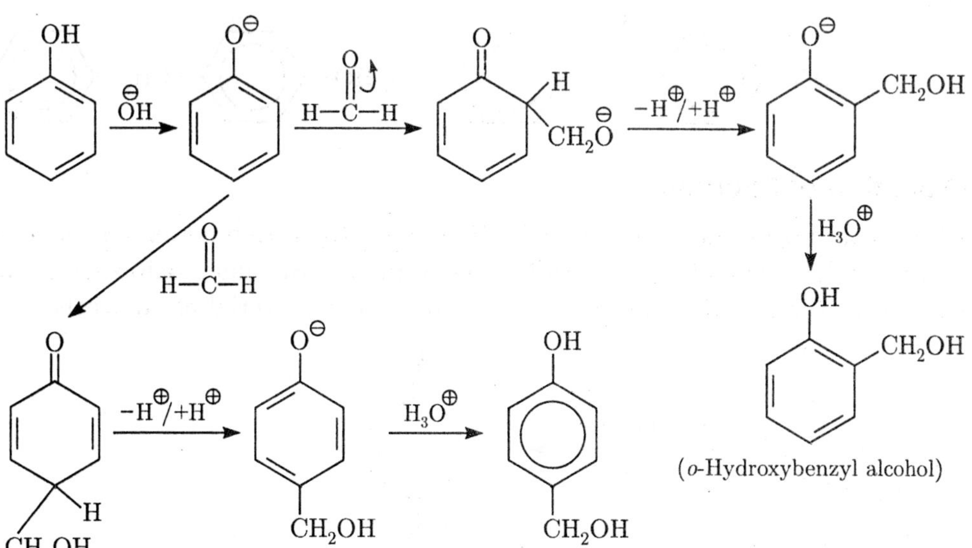

(o-Hydroxybenzyl alcohol)

(p-Hydroxybenzyl alcohol)

These condensation reactions are the basis of the preparation of *phenol-formaldehyde resins (bakelites).* Phenol and excess of formaldehyde in the presence of dilute NaOH, slowly forms a three dimensional polymer, the structure of which is uncertain. One possibility is as follows.

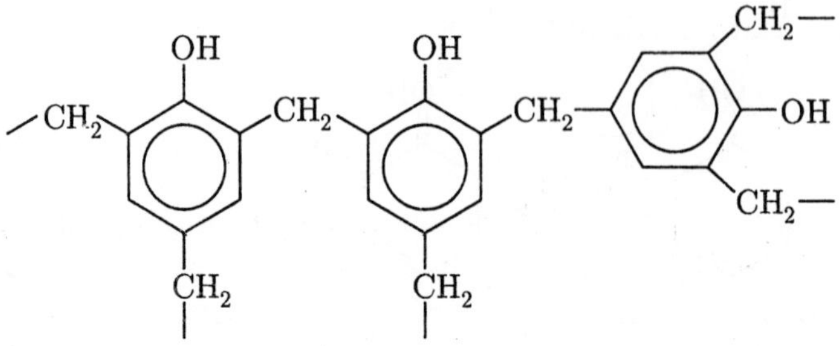

When a large excess of formalin is used, bishydroxymethylphenol is formed.

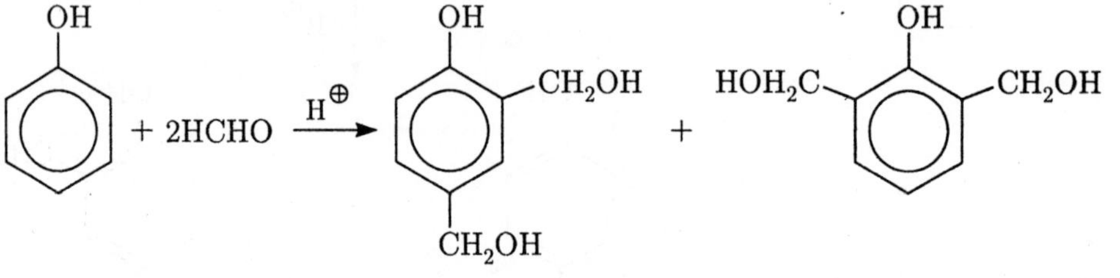

Formaldehyde and other aldehydes usually condense with phenols to give *p*–*p*′-dihydroxydiphenylmethane derivative.

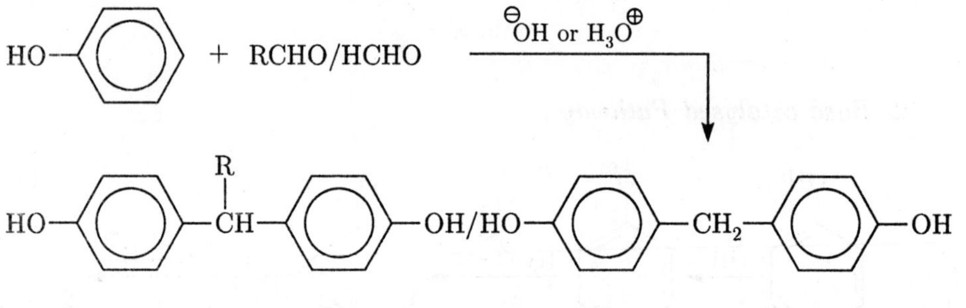

Oxidation of Phenols

Phenols are highly succeptible to oxidation. H_2O_2 (hydrogen peroxide) converts phenols to catechol, hydroquinol, pyrogallol and quinone. Stronger oxidising agents either decompose the ring or bring polymerisation to tarry material of no synthetic use.

1.

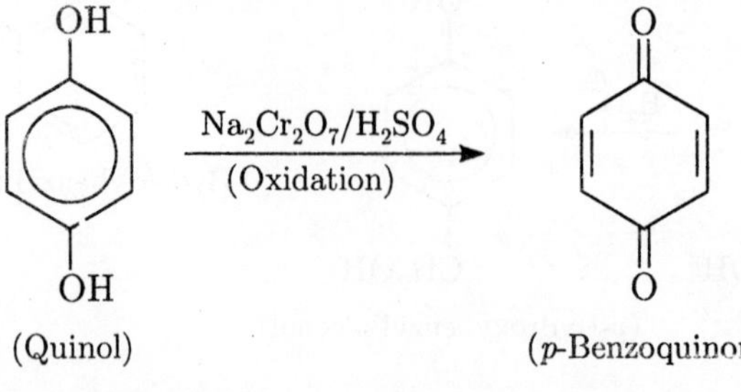

(Quinol) (*p*-Benzoquinone)

2. 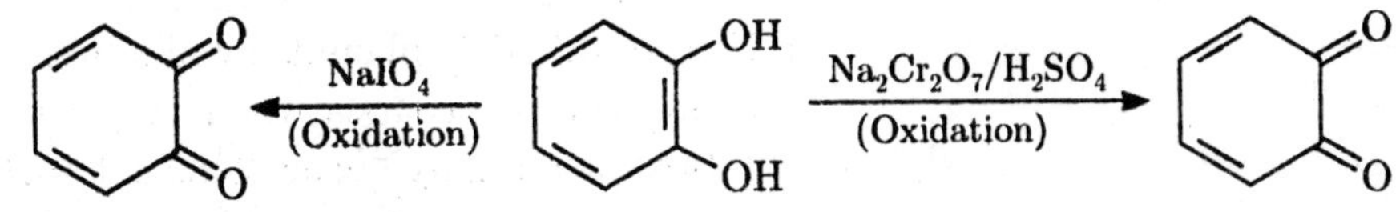

(o-Benzoquinone) (Catechol) (o-Benzoquinone)

3. ***Side chain oxidation of phenols***

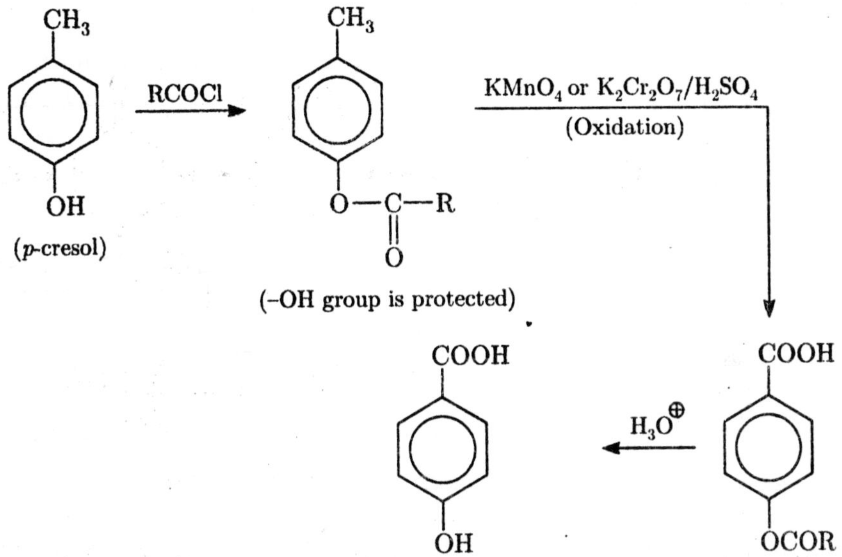

(p-cresol) (–OH group is protected) (p-Hydroxybenzoic acid)

4. ***Elbs persulphate oxidation***

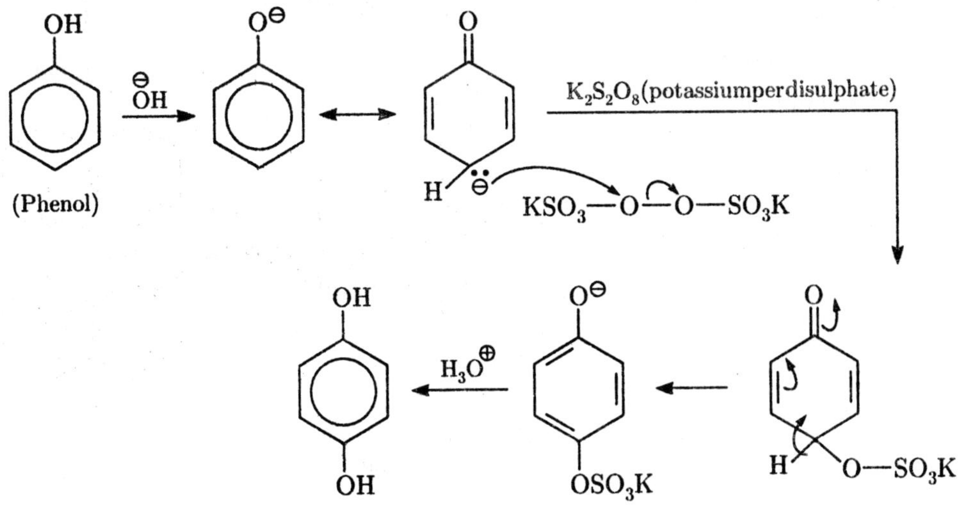

(Phenol) (Quinol)

Monohydric phenols may be oxidised to dihydric phenols by alkaline potassium perdisulphate ($K_2S_2O_8$). Usually hydroxylation occurs at the *para* position. When the *p*-position is blocked, *ortho* hydroxylation may occur. This is known as *Elbs persulphate oxidation* reaction.

5. ***Oxidative Coupling by Fe^{3+}*** : The aromatic ring or phenols are very succeptible to *oxidation by one electron oxidants*, for the removal of a hydrogen atom gives a delocalised aryloxy radical.

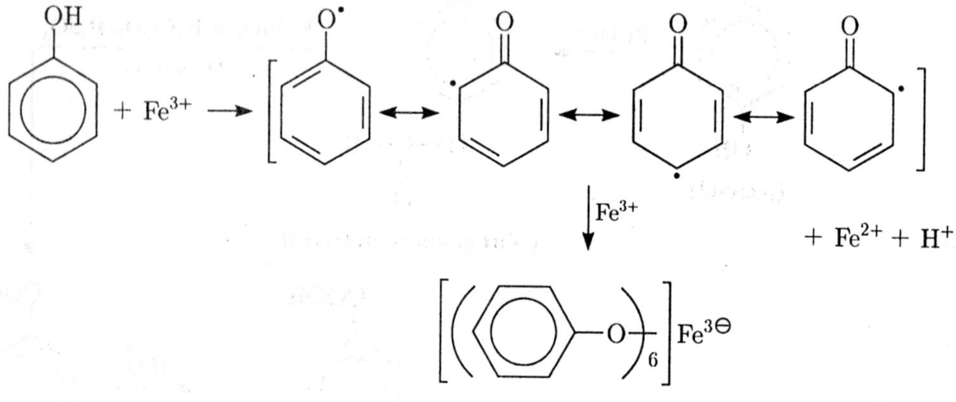

(Violet colour)

One electron oxidants are generally either $\overset{III}{FeCl_3}$ or $K_3Fe(CN)_6$. The fate of the radical depends upon the structure of the phenol taken.

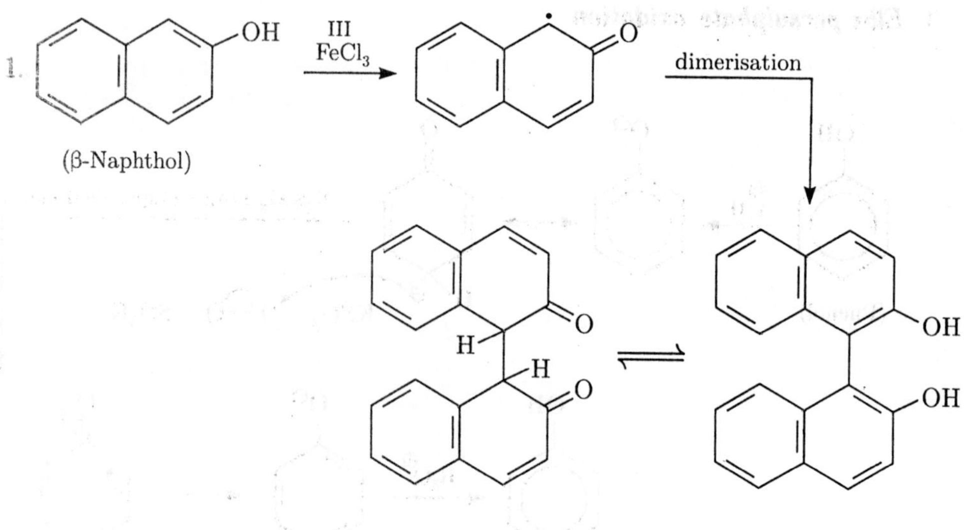

(Product)
(Green precipitate)

2. ***Further oxidation to quinones may occur***

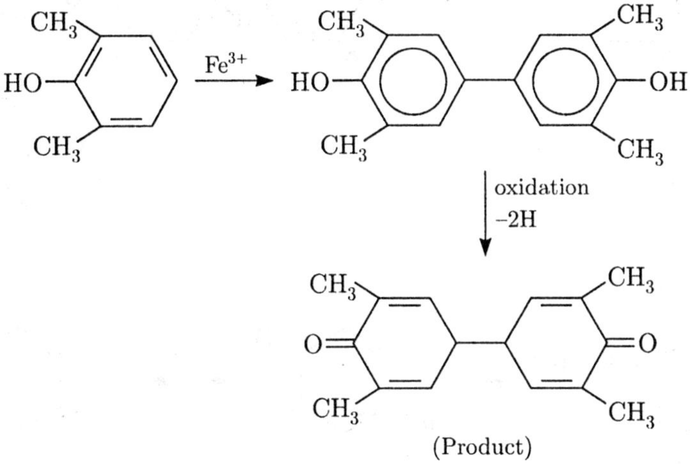

The phenoxy radical, because of its high reactivity, quickly disappears mainly by coupling (dimerisation), which is predominantly of C—C type (*ortho– ortho*, *para–para* or *ortho–para* type). The other possible modes of coupling, C—O and O—O occur less frequently particularly the latter.

Coupling between aroxyl radicals is sterically hindered by the presence of large substituents, *e.g.*, 2,4,6-tritertiarybutylphenol forms a stable free radical when oxidised in bezene solution (the solution is dark blue). This radical has been isolated as a dark blue solid (m. p. 96°C). In the presence of oxygen, the colour of the solution becomes light yellow due to the formation of peroxide.

3. 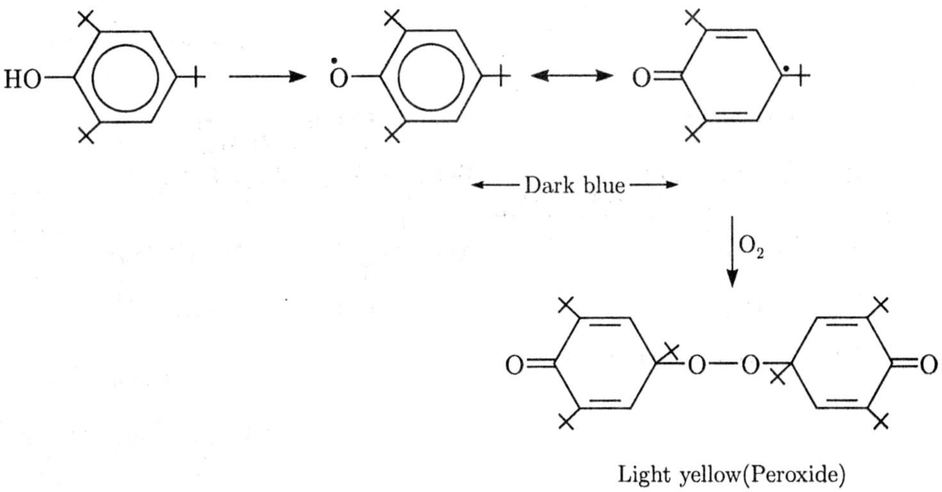

On the other, hand, if *p*- tertiarybutyl group is absent, *p*-coupling occurs and the dimer is then oxidised to a red compound.

4. 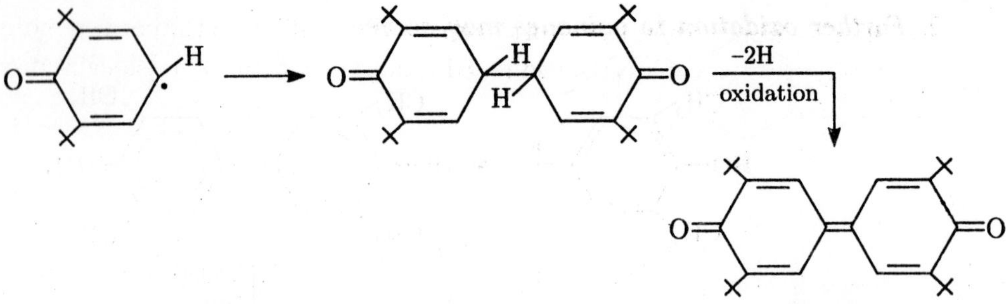

(Product)

5. 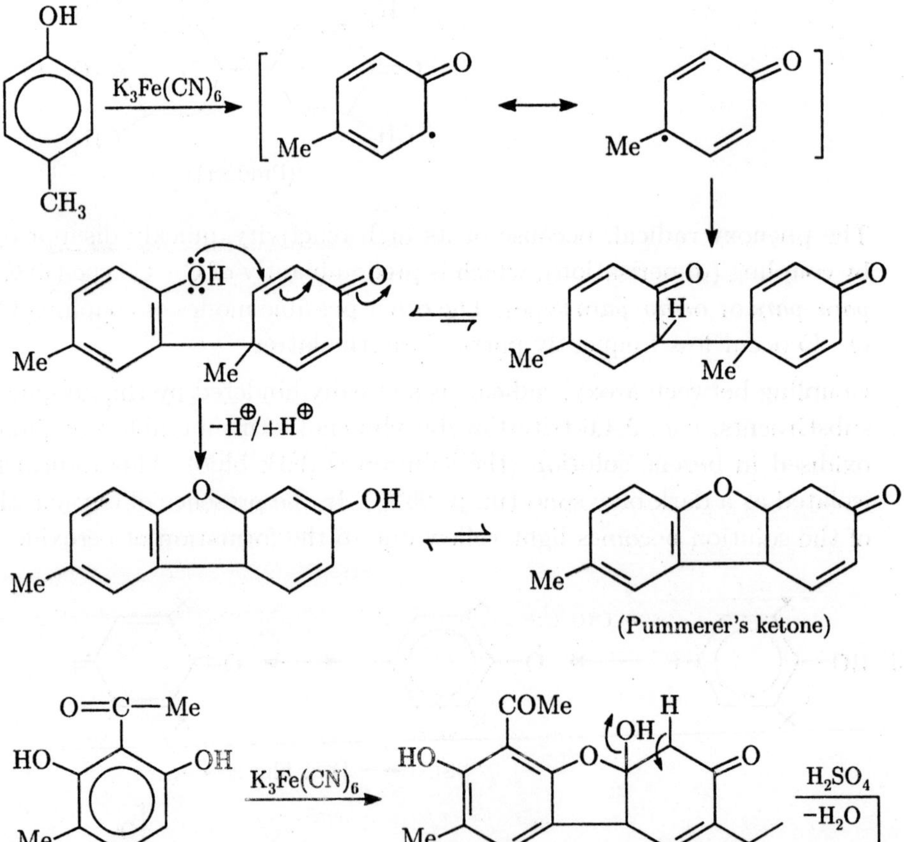

(Pummerer's ketone)

6. 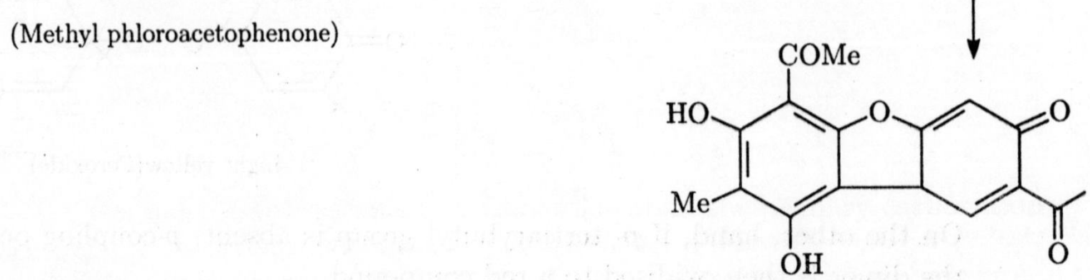

(Methyl phloroacetophenone)

(±)Usonic acid

7. *Ortho* and *para* dihydric phenols are readily oxidised to the corresponding quinones by one electron oxidising agents. Reactions occur through delocalised semiquinone radicals.

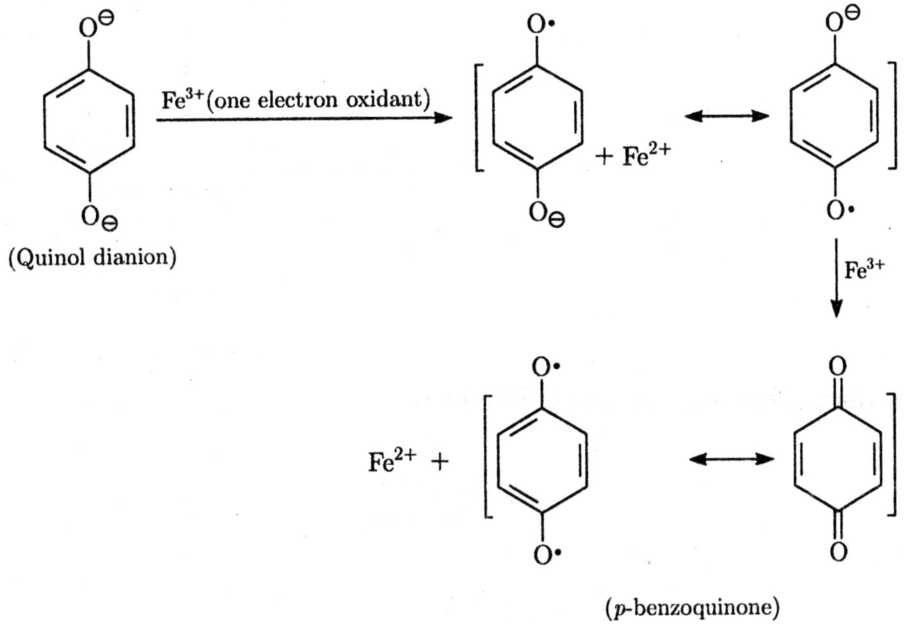

Similarly, *ortho* benzoquinone is formed from catechol.

8. ***Aerial oxidation of phenols*** : The reactions of organic compounds with elemental oxygen under mild conditions are generally referred to a *autooxidations*, for such oxidations often take place by themselves when the substrate (slightly impure) is exposed to the atmosphere. Compounds like phenols, amines, enols, alcohols, ethers etc. may undergo autooxidation.

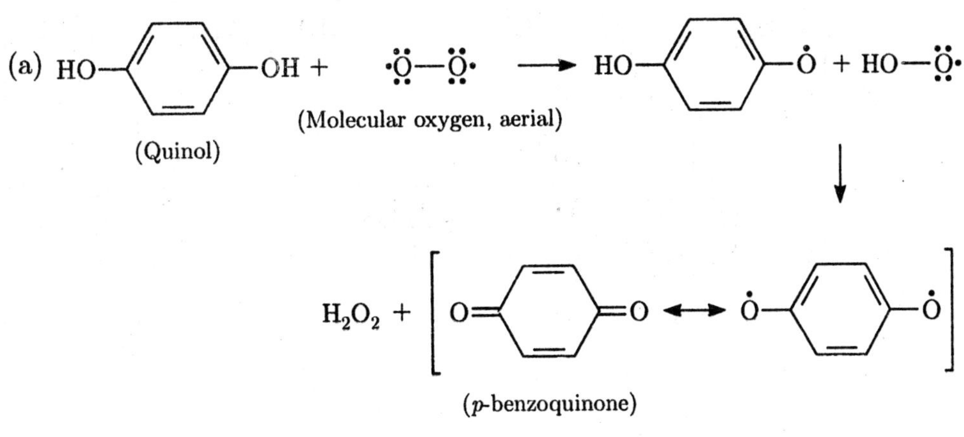

(b) 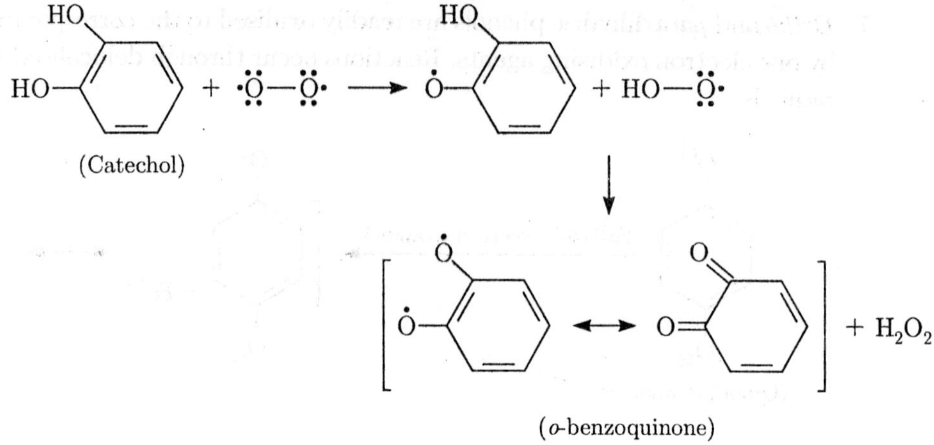

Condensation reactions of Phenols

1. 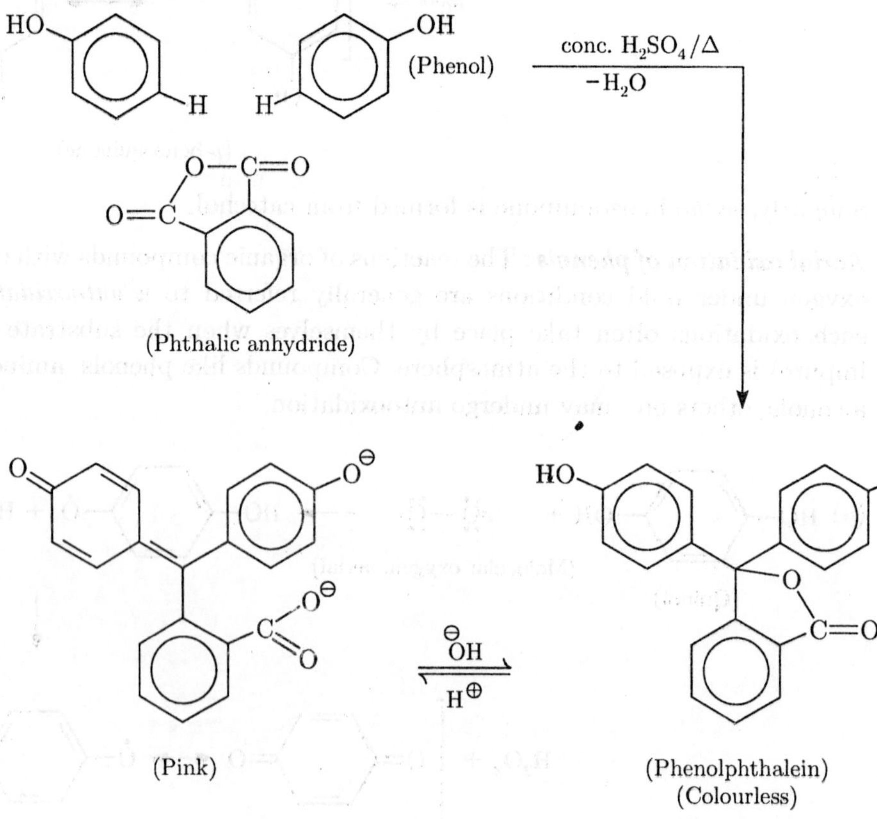

2. 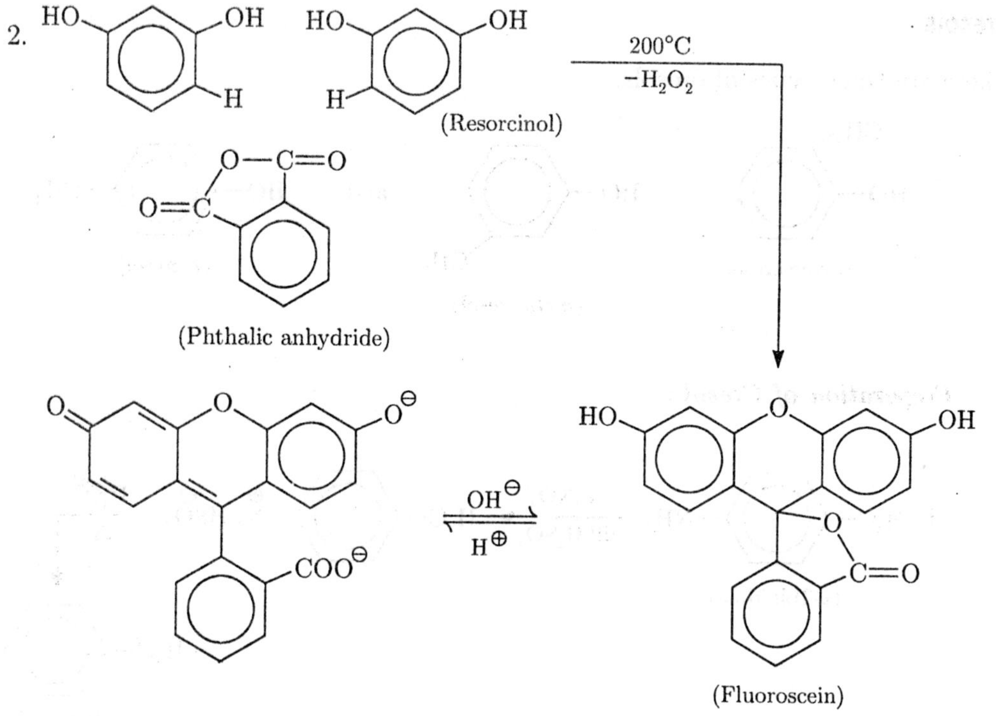

3. β–ketoesters condense with phenols to form coumarins.

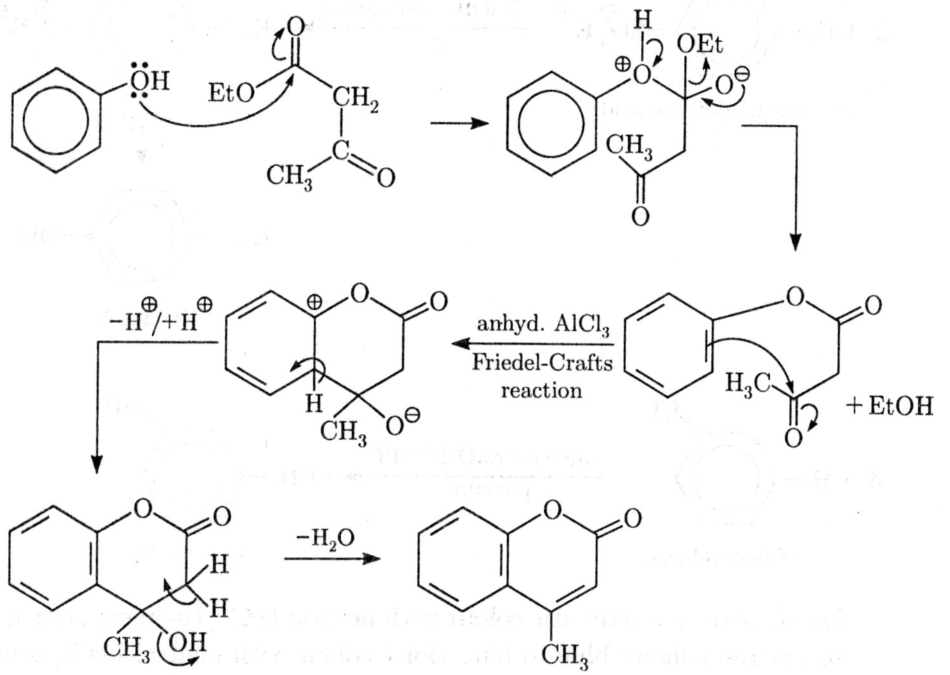

(Coumarin derivative)

Cresols

There are three types of cresols.

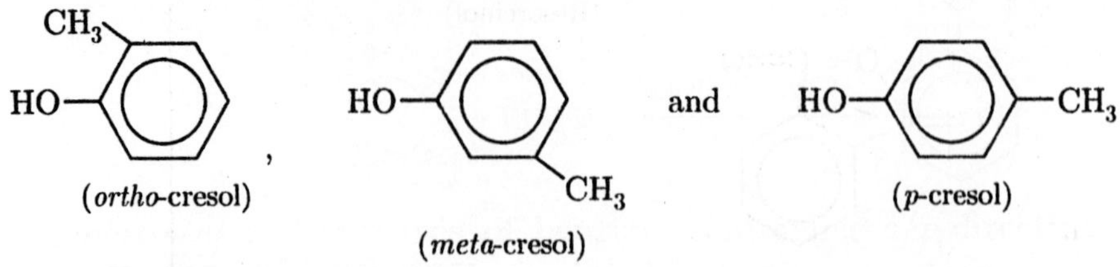

Preparation of Cresol :

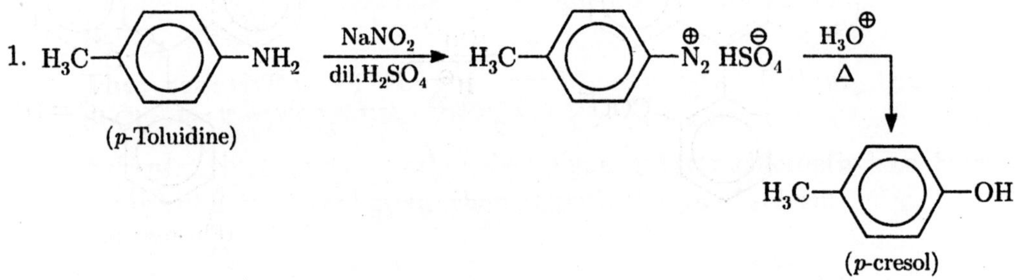

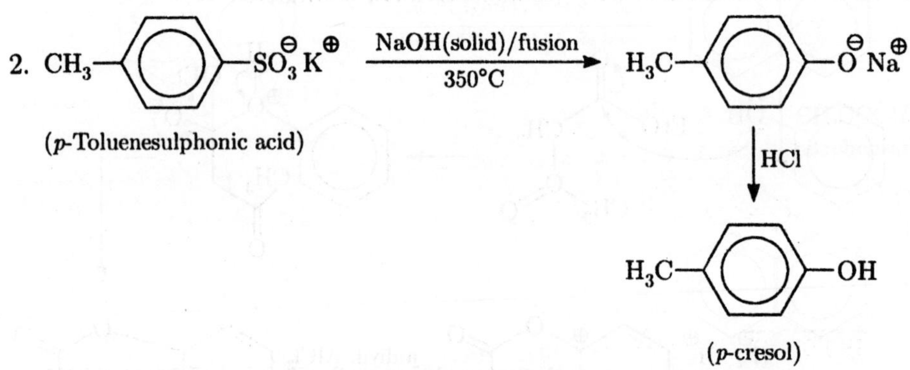

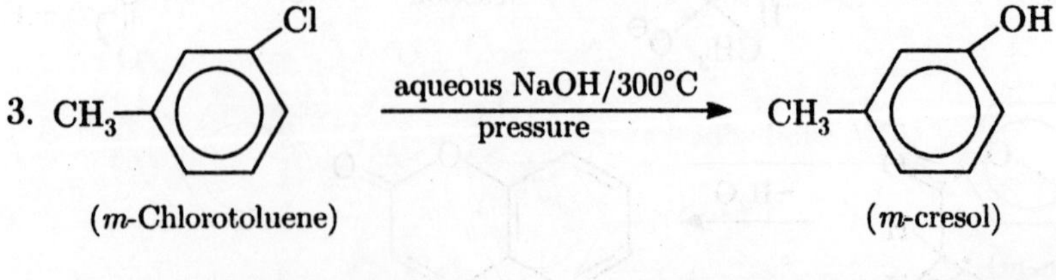

Cresols give characteristic colour with neutral $FeCl_3$ (*o*-cresol gives green colour and *p*-cresol shows blue to blue violet colour with neutral $FeCl_3$ solution).

Chemical Reactions given by Cresols :

1. 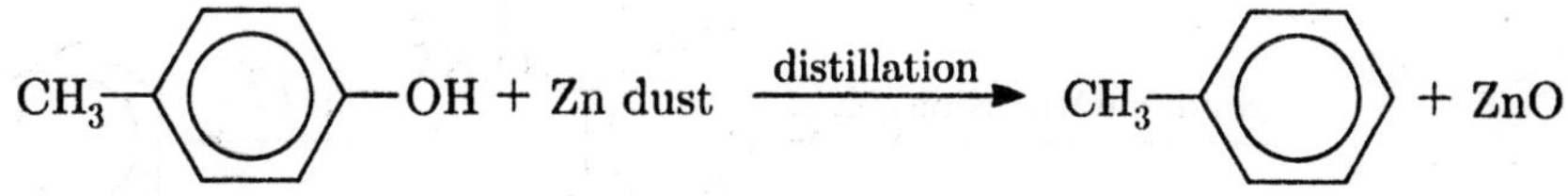

(*p*-cresol) (Toluene)

2. 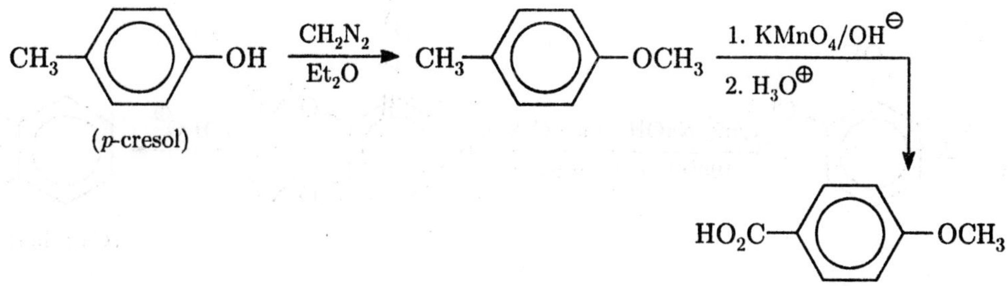

(*p*-cresol)

(*p*-Methoxybenzoic acid)

3. 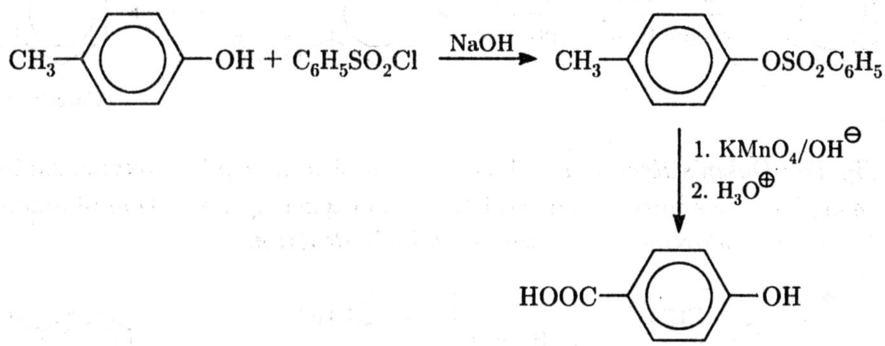

(*p*-Hydroxybenzoic acid)

Dihydric Phenols

There are three types of dihydric phenols as shown below.

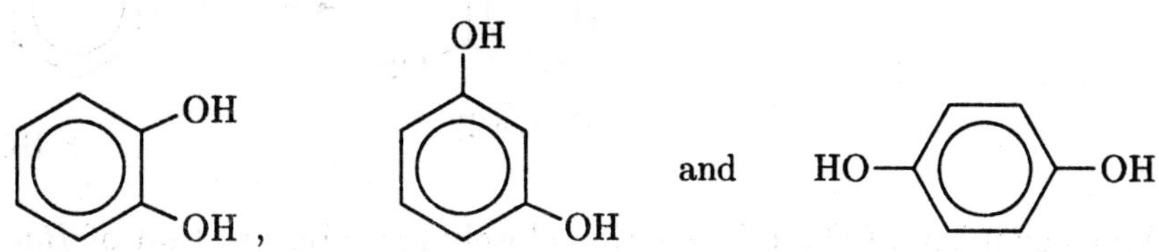

(Catechol) (Resorcinol) (Quinol)

Methods of preparation of catechol :

1. 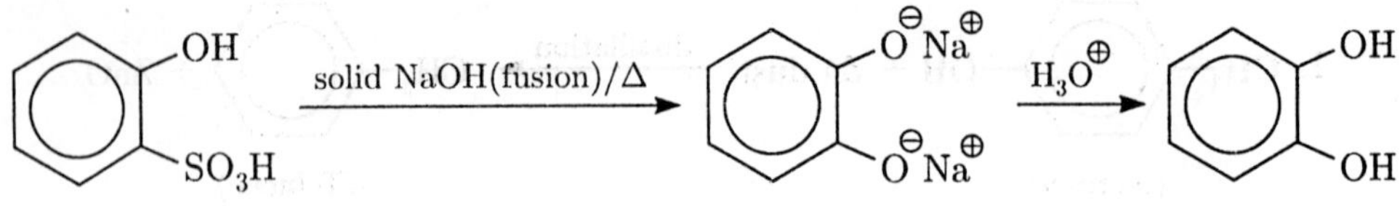

(Catechol)

2. 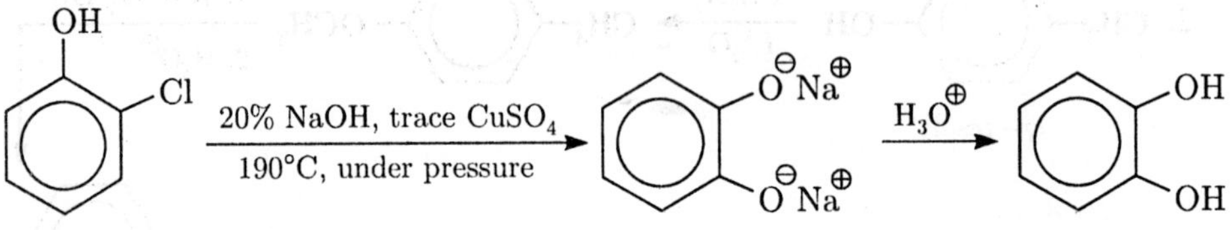

(Catechol)

3. 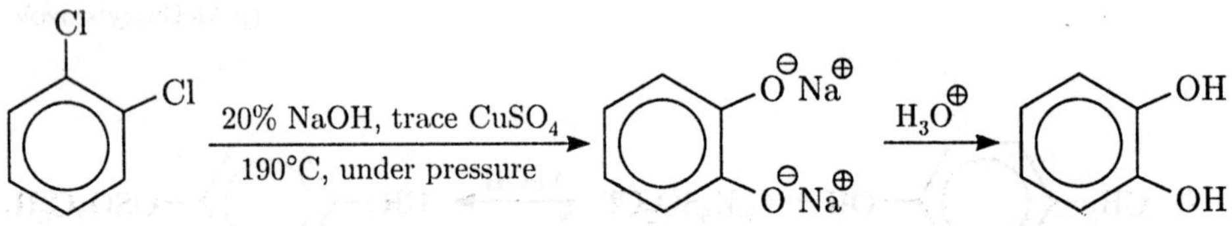

(Catechol)

4. ***By The Dakin's Reaction*** : The oxidation of *o*- and *p*-hydroxybenzaldehydes or phenyl ketones into *o*- and *p*-dihydroxybenzenes by the action of alkaline H_2O_2 (hydrogen peroxide) is known as ***Dakin's Reaction***.

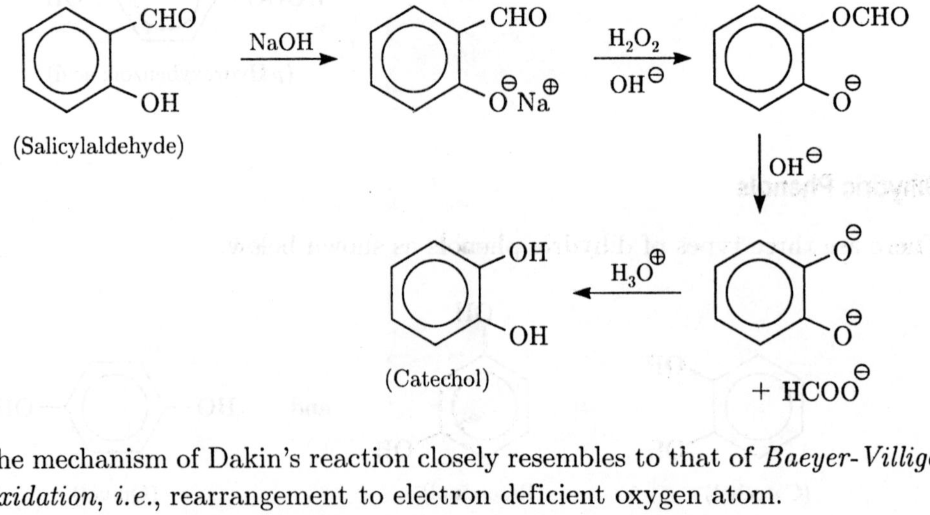

The mechanism of Dakin's reaction closely resembles to that of *Baeyer-Villiger Oxidation*, *i.e.*, rearrangement to electron deficient oxygen atom.

Mechanism of Dakin's reaction :

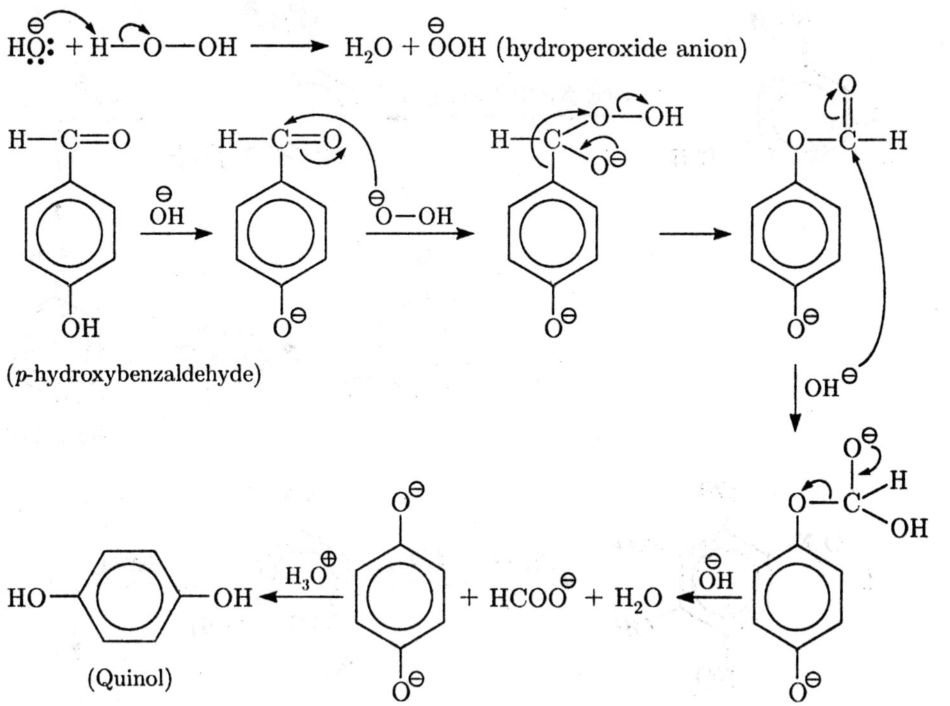

Similarly, catechol is formed from salicylaldehyde.

Properties of catechol :

1. 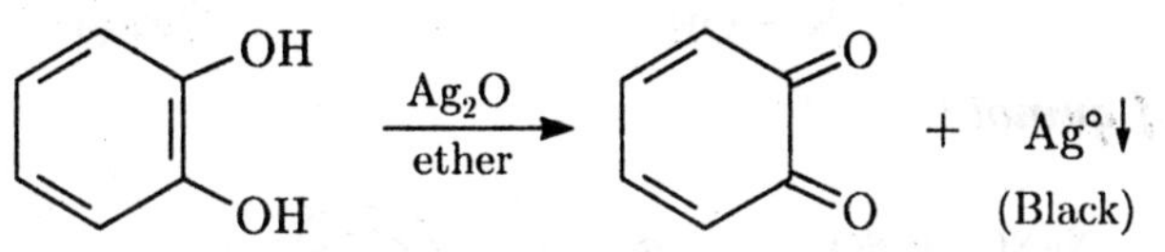

2. 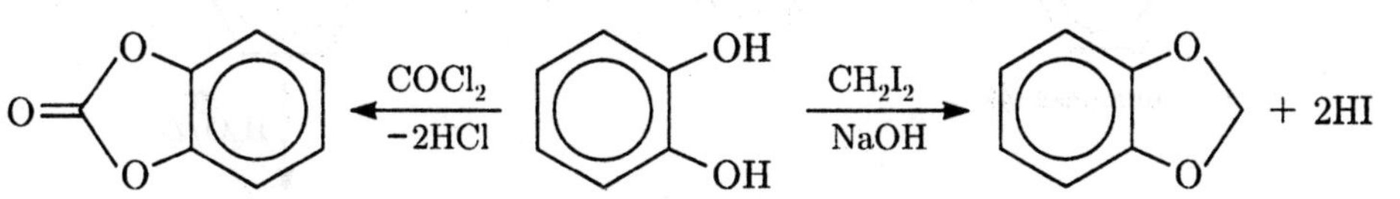

Catechol reduces cold $AgNO_3$ solution and warm Fehling's solution. With neutral $FeCl_3$ solution, catechol produces a green colour.

Methods of preparation of resorcinol :

1. 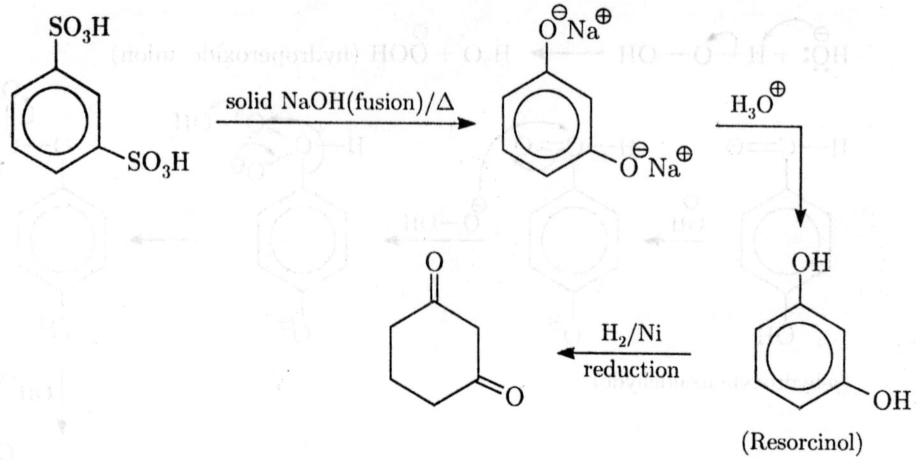

2. 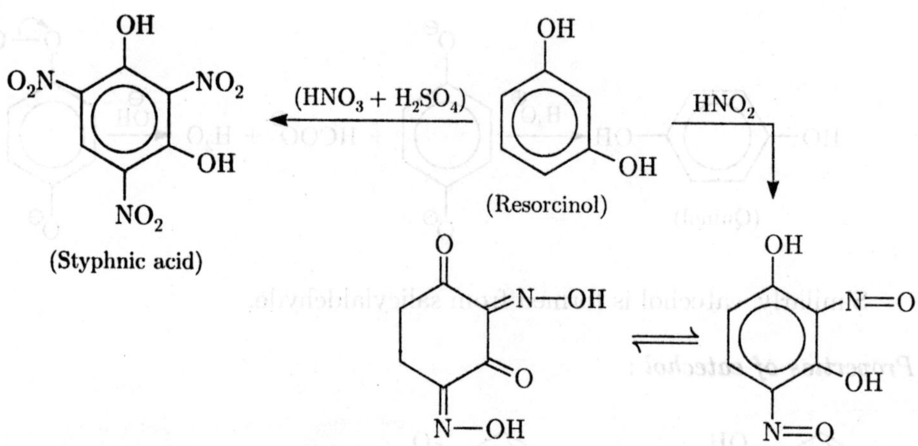

Methods of preparation of quinol :

1. 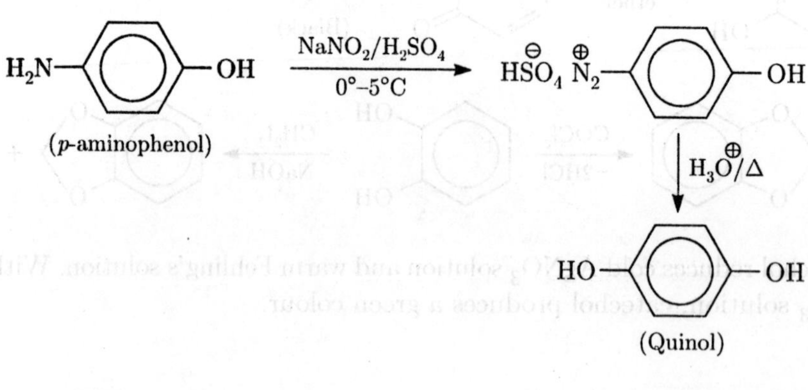

2. 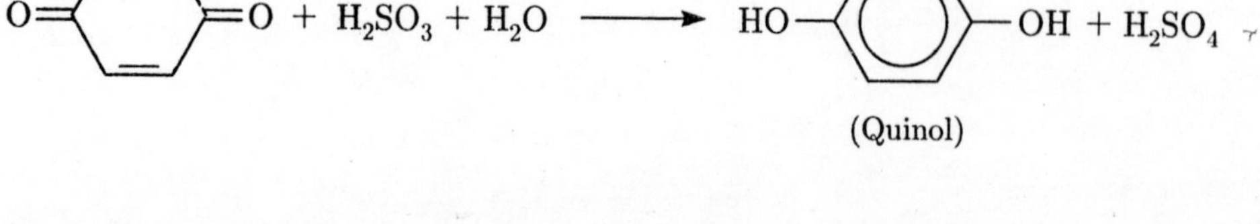

3. 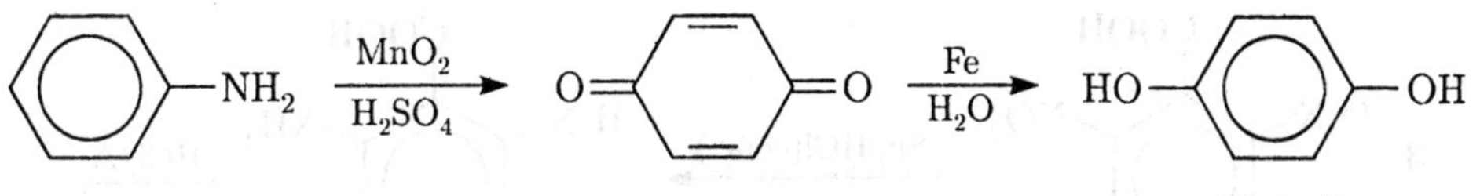

(Quinol)

Properties of Quinol :

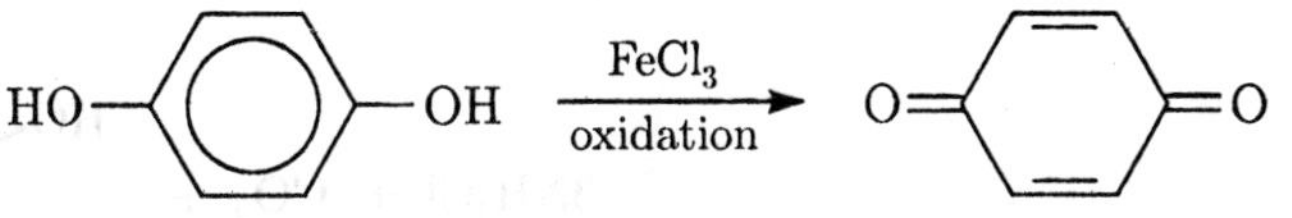

(*p*-benzoquinone)

Trihydric Phenols

There are three types of trihydric phenols.

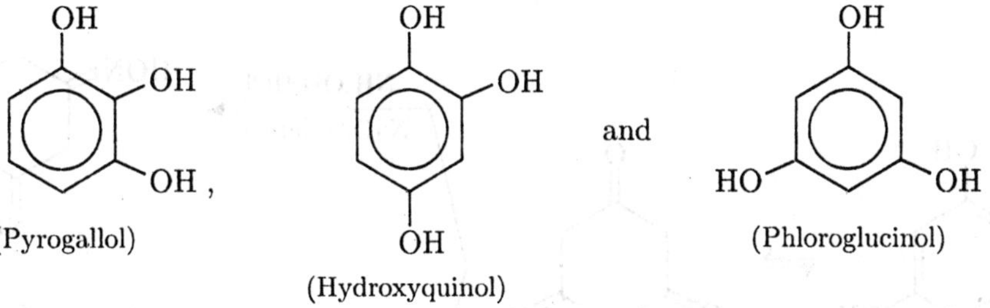

(Pyrogallol) (Hydroxyquinol) and (Phloroglucinol)

Methods of Preparation :

1. 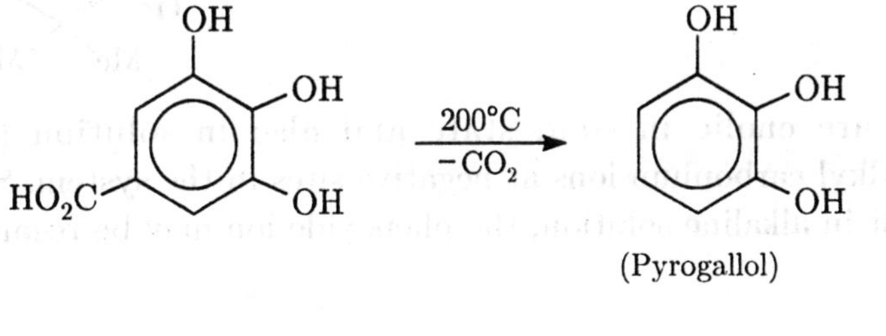

(Pyrogallol)

2. 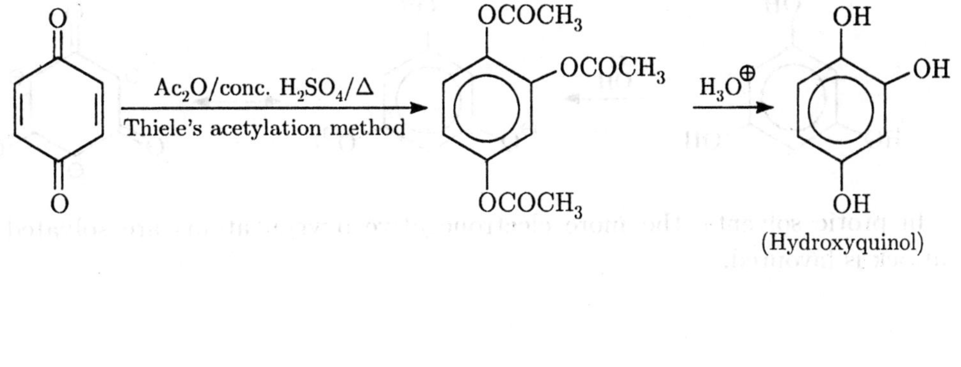

(Hydroxyquinol)

3. 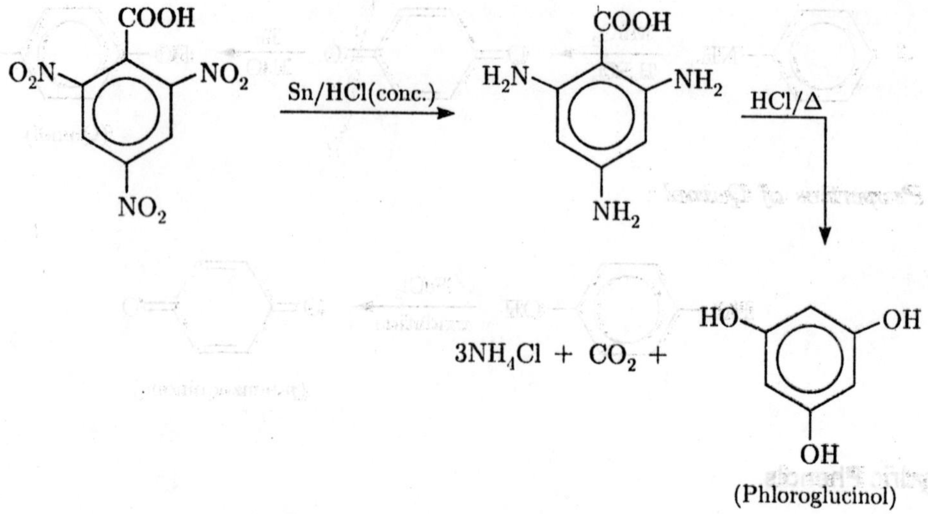

Phloroglucinol is a tautomeric compound as follows.

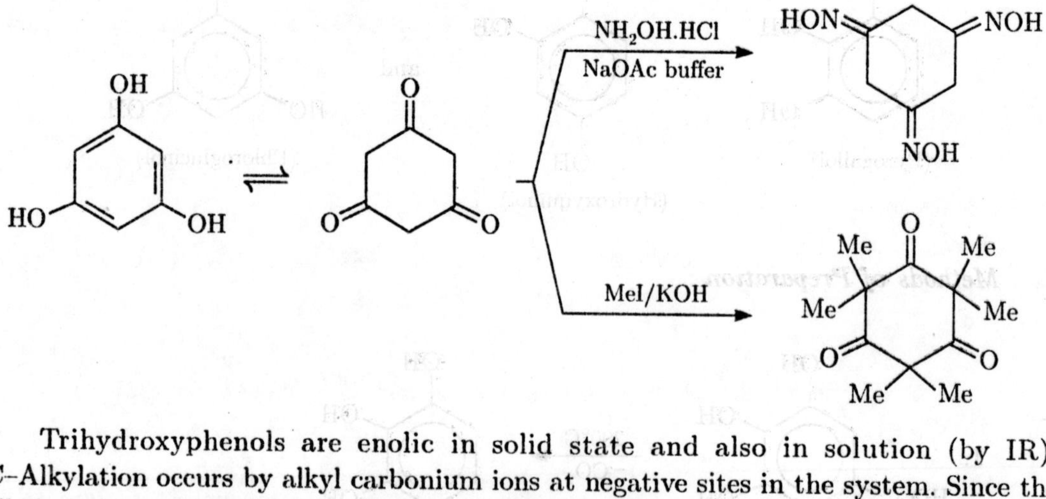

Trihydroxyphenols are enolic in solid state and also in solution (by IR). C–Alkylation occurs by alkyl carbonium ions at negative sites in the system. Since the alkylations are carried out in alkaline solution, the phenoxide ion may be regarded as a resonance hybrid.

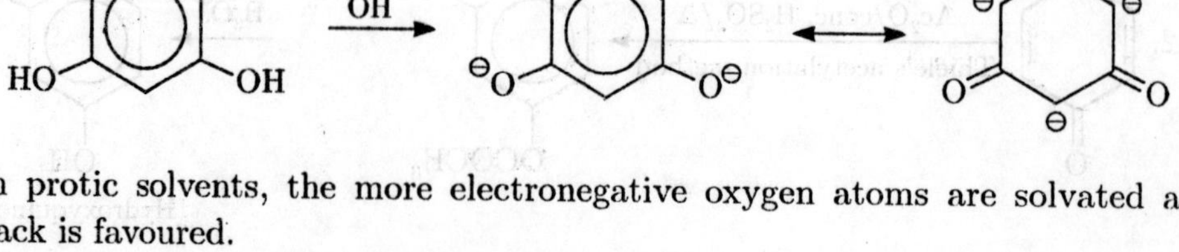

In protic solvents, the more electronegative oxygen atoms are solvated and so C–attack is favoured.

Aminophenols

Methods of preparation of amino phenols :

1. 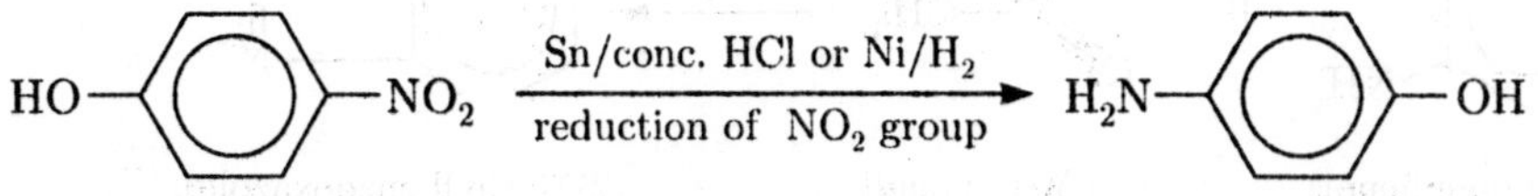

(p-nitrophenol) (p-aminophenol)

2. 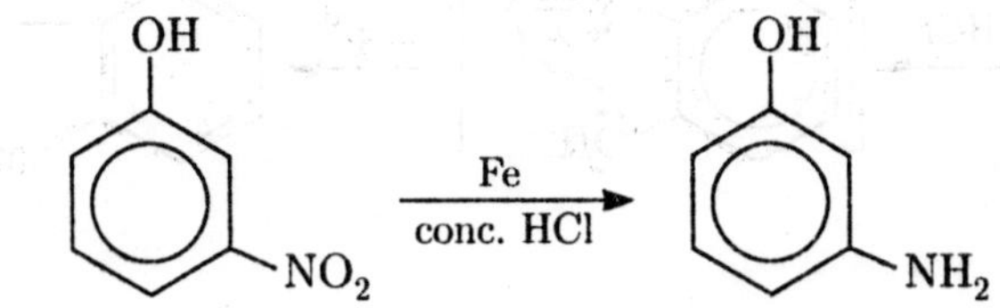

(m-nitrophenol) (m-aminophenol)

3. 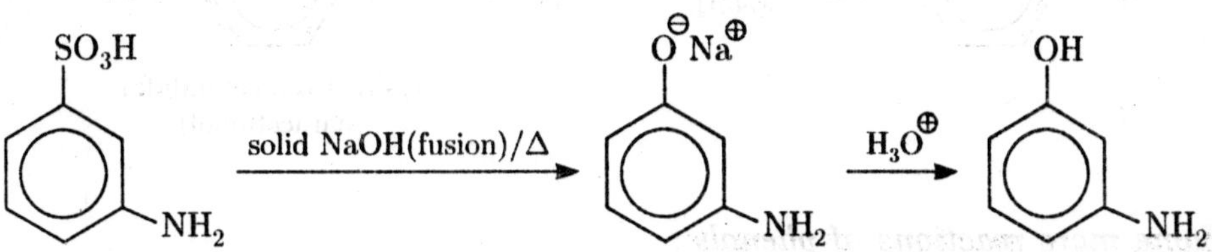

(m-aminophenol)

4. 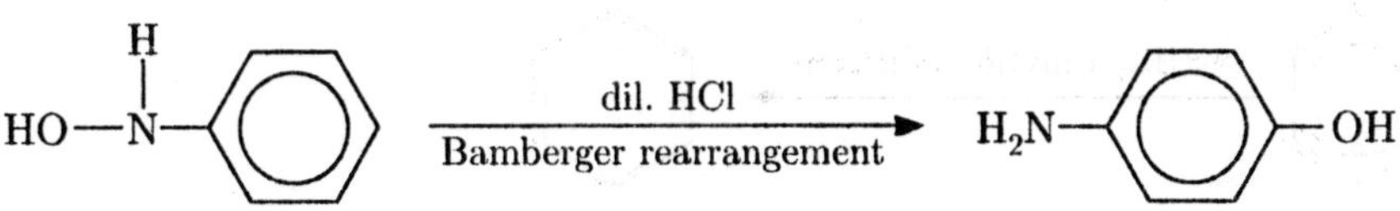

(Phenylhydroxylamine) (p-aminophenol)

5. 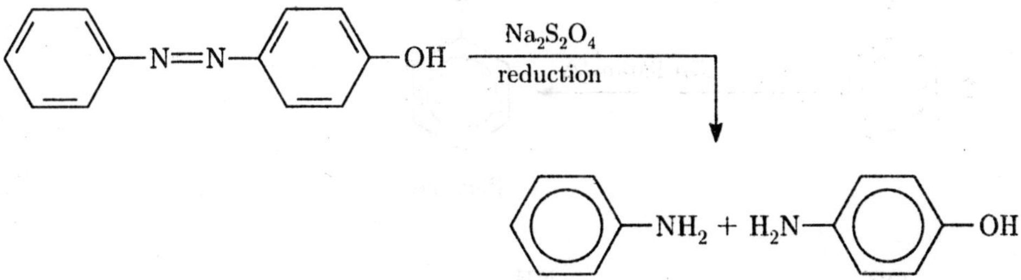

(p-aminophenol)

Ortho– and *para*-aminophenols are weaker acids compared to phenol due to electron donating +R effect of NH_2 group. *Meta* isomer is comparatively stronger acid. *Ortho*- and *para* isomers are readily oxidised to corresponding quinones but m-aminophenol does not get oxidised to give a quinone.

Properties of aminophenols :

1. 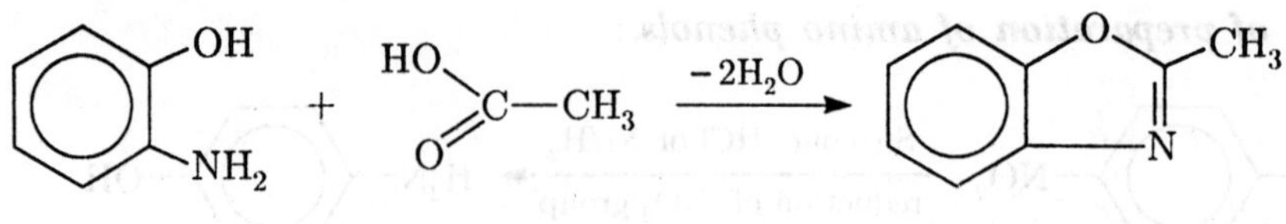

(*o*-aminophenol) (Acetic acid) (2-Methylbenzooxazole)

2. 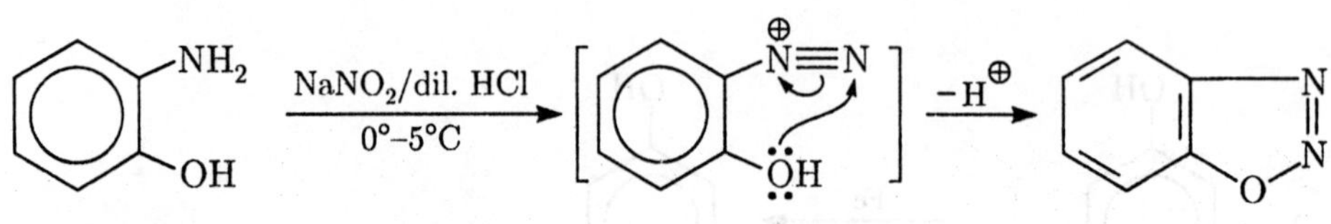

(*o*-aminophenol)

3. 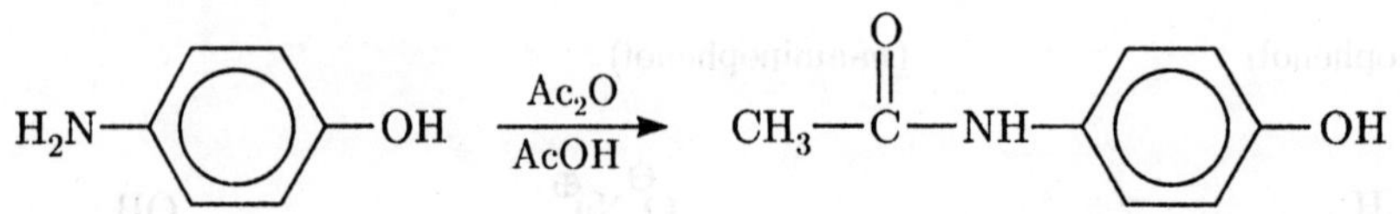

(*p*-hydroxyacetanilide)
(paracetamol)

Some more reactions of phenols :

1. 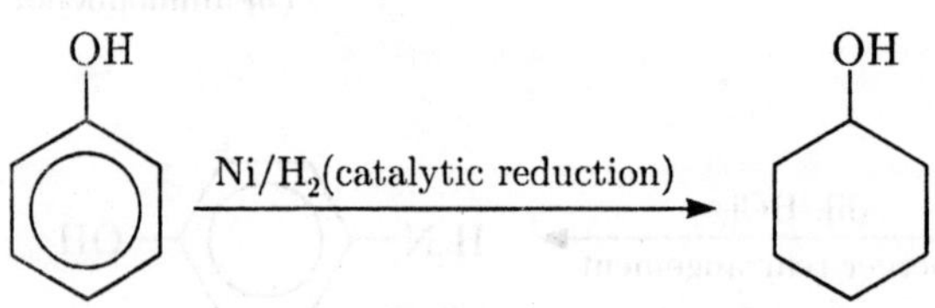

(Cyclohexanol)

2. 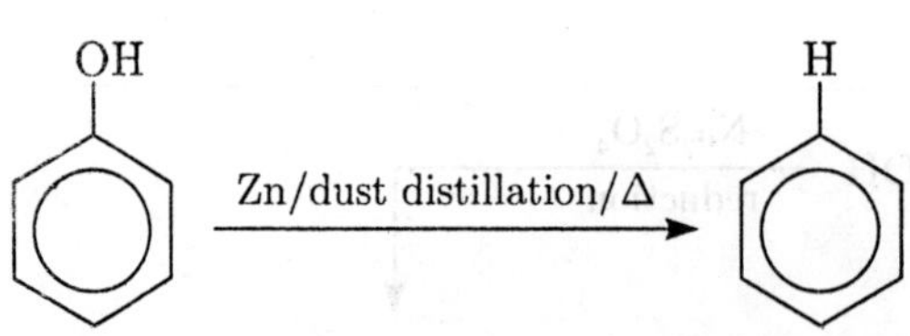

(Benzene)

3. 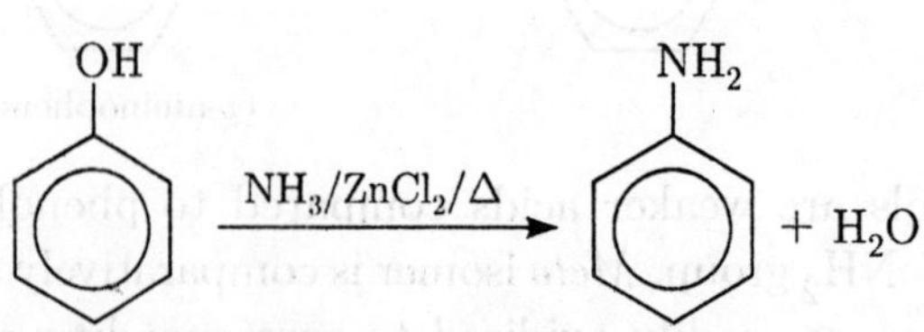

(Aniline)

The Vilsmeyer–Haack Reaction

Formylation of phenols, phenolic ethers, aromatic amines etc. by disubstituted formamides and phosphorus oxychloride ($POCl_3$) is called *Vilsmeyer–Haack* reaction. This is by for the best method of formylating activated aromatic compound.

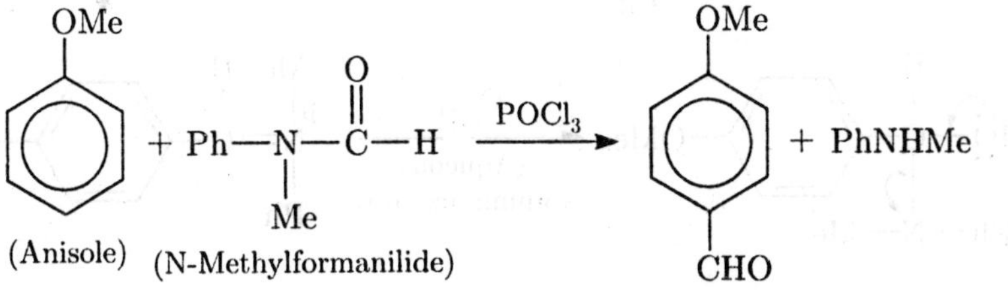

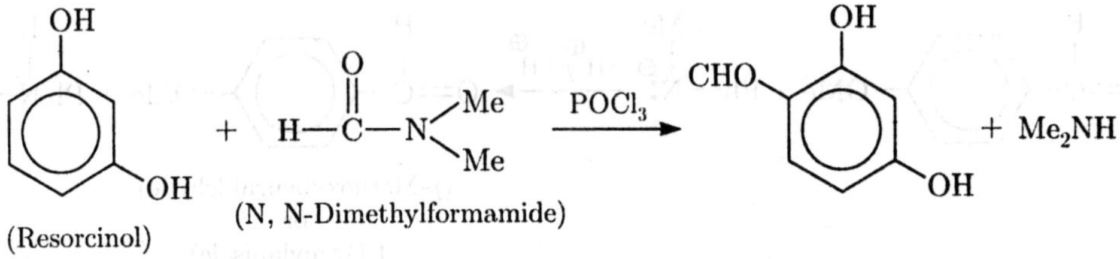

The method works well for the *o*- and *p*- positions of phenols, phenolic ethers and dialkylanilines; it does not work with hydrocarbons like benzene or naphthalene, but anthracene gives 9–aldehyde. The formylation is carried out by treating the compound with N,N-dimethylformamide and $POCl_3$ and when the reaction is complete, adding aqueous sodium acetate and steam distilling. N,N-dimethylaniline gives *p*-dimethylaminobenzaldehyde (yield 80%) and thiophene gives 2-aldehyde. This method is particularly effective for compounds such as pyrroles which are not formylated by other procedures. Pyrrole gives 2-aldehyde (yield 85%) and indole gives 3-aldehyde in 97% yield. The latter two are formylated in presence of N,N-dimethylfarmanide instead of N–methylformanilide. However, other aryl, alkyl and dialkyl amides are also used. Carbonyl chloride ($COCl_2$, phosgene) can also be used instead of phosphorus oxychloride ($POCl_3$) in some cases.

***Mechanism of Vilsmeyer–Haack reaction with phenolic ether* :**

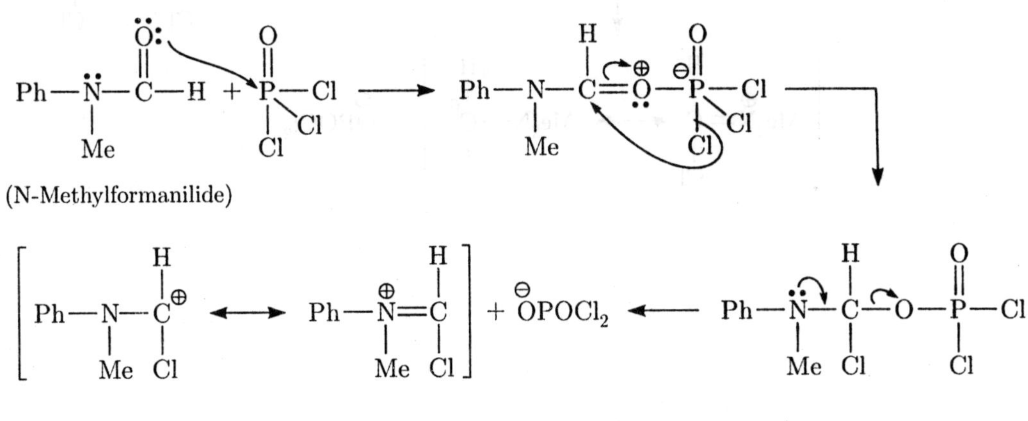

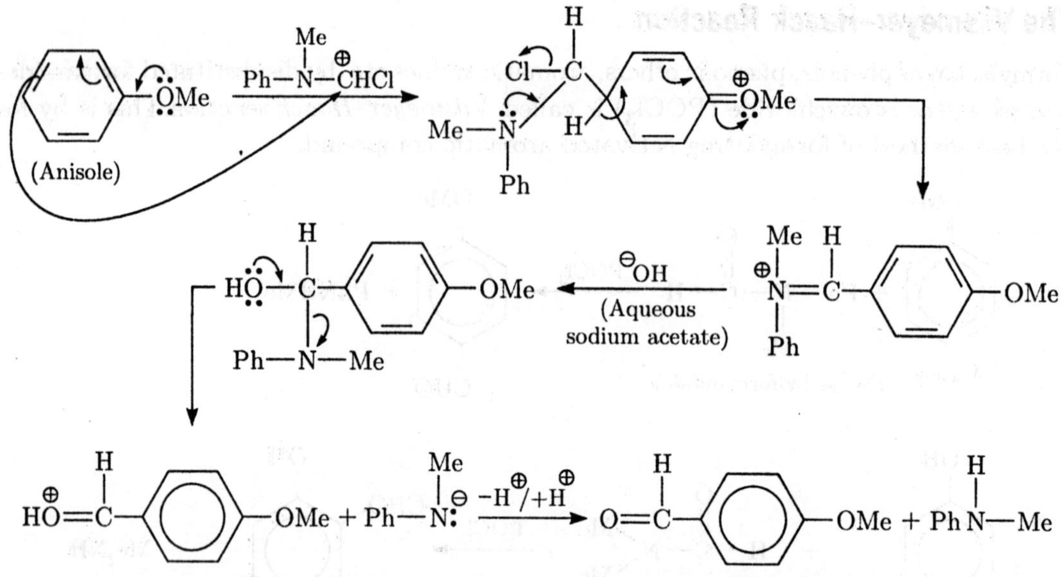

(*p*-Methoxybenzaldehyde)
or
(4-Formylanisole)

Similarly, 2-formylanisole can be prepared by the same mechanism.

Mechanism of Vilsmeyer–Haack reaction with phenol **:**

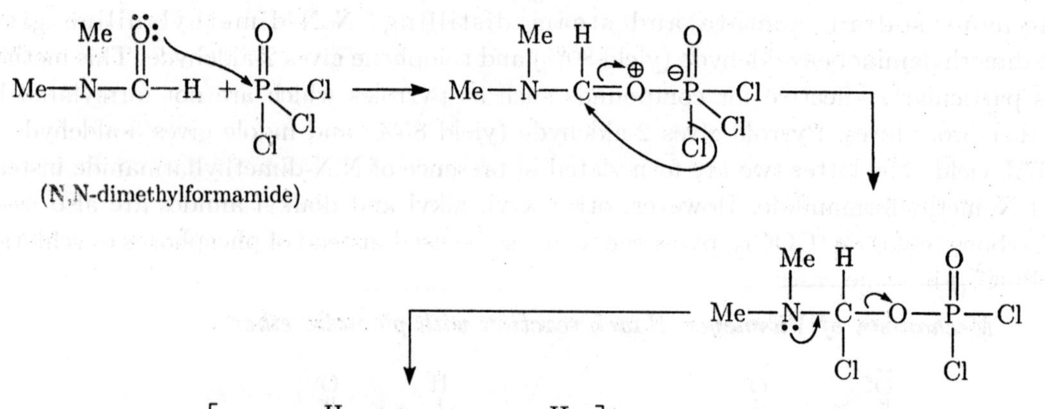

(N,N-dimethylformamide)

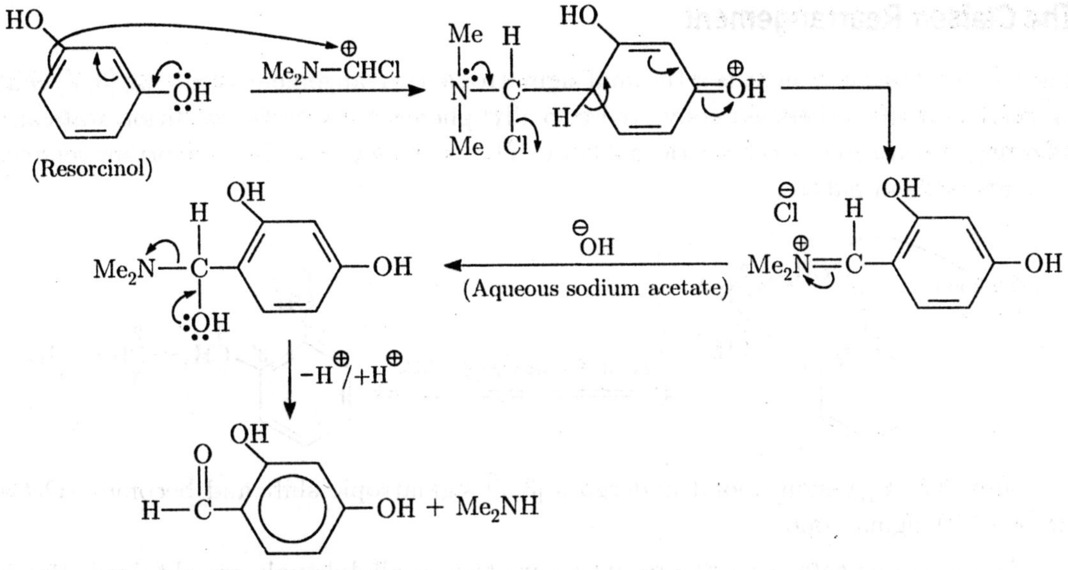

(4-Formylresorcinol)

***Mechanism of Vilsmeyer–Haack Reaction with secondary amine and formic acid* :**

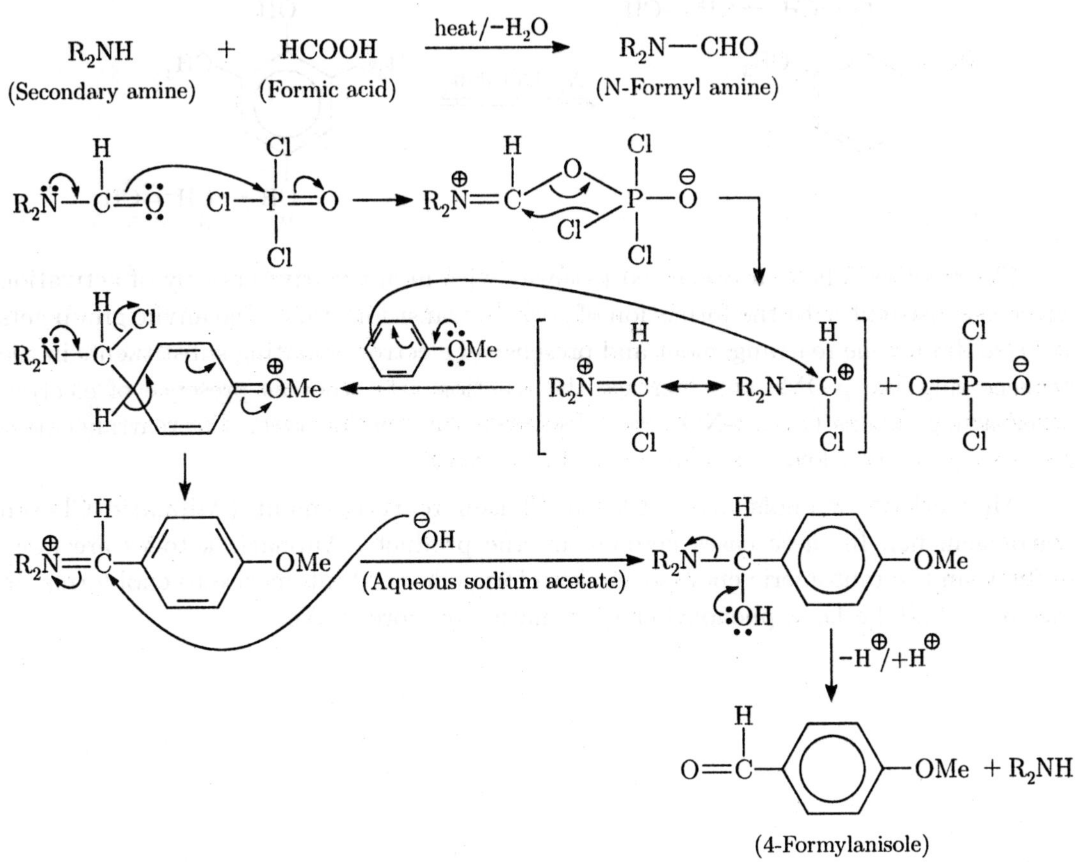

(4-Formylanisole)

The Claisen Rearrangement

The Claisen rearrangement is a thermal sigmatropic rearrangement involving [3,3′] shift in which aryl allyl ethers get converted into allyl phenol *via* a cyclic transition state and following a concerted mechanistic pathway. The rearrangement is equilibrium related, *i.e.*, reversible in nature.

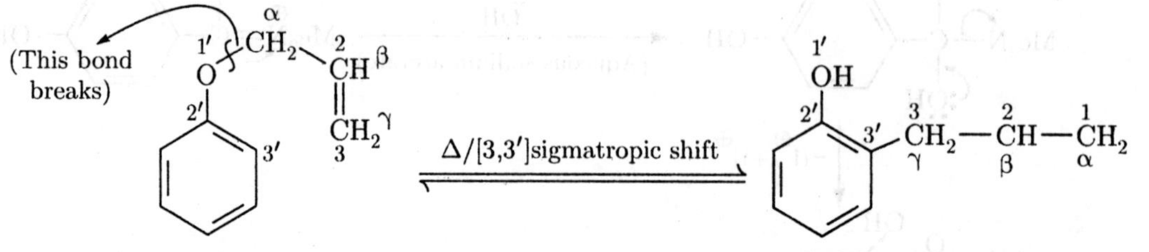

Here (O—C_α) sigma bond undergoes [3,3′] sigmatropic shift and becomes (*Ortho* carbon–Cγ) sigma bond.

When *one or both the ortho* positions are free, *o*–allylphenols are obtained. But if both the *ortho* positions are blocked, *p*-allylphenol is formed.

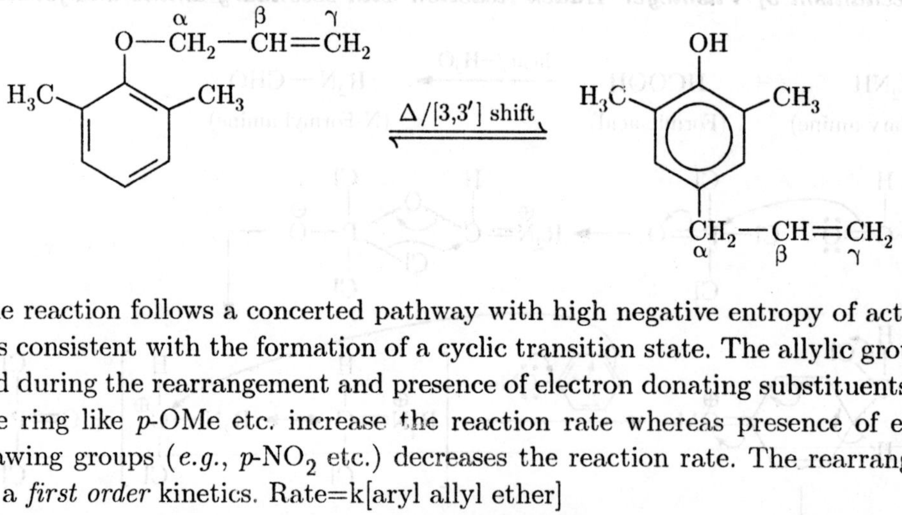

The reaction follows a concerted pathway with high negative entropy of activation which is consistent with the formation of a cyclic transition state. The allylic group gets inverted during the rearrangement and presence of electron donating substituents in the benzene ring like *p*-OMe etc. increase the reaction rate whereas presence of electron withdrawing groups (*e.g.*, *p*-NO_2 etc.) decreases the reaction rate. The rearrangement follows a *first order* kinetics. Rate=k[aryl allyl ether]

Allyl ethers of enols also undergo Claisen rearrangement (Aliphatic Claisen rearrangement). In these cases ketones are the products. Aliphatic ketones are more stable than the tautomeric enols so the keto forms do not tautomerise to enol forms. In case of aryl allyl ethers, phenols being aromatic are more stable.

***Aliphatic Claisen Rearrangements* :**

1. 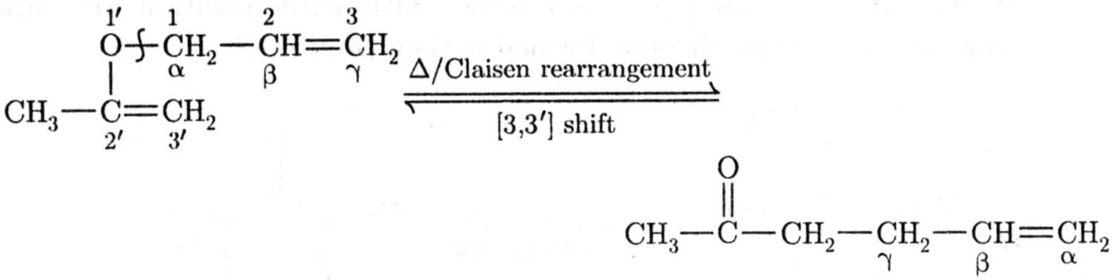

(No enalisation of the ketone formed)

but 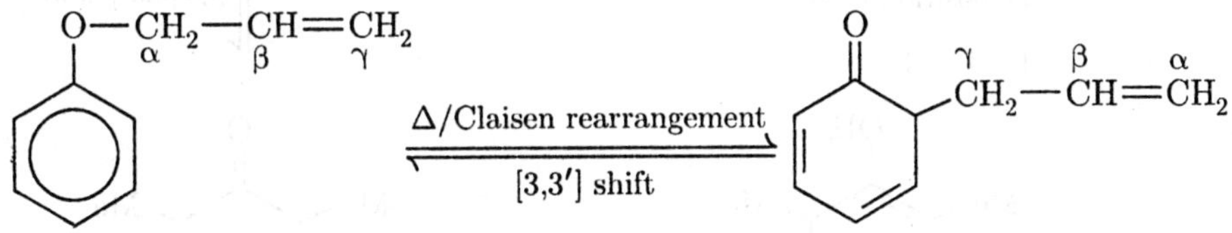

(Keto form, non-aromatic)

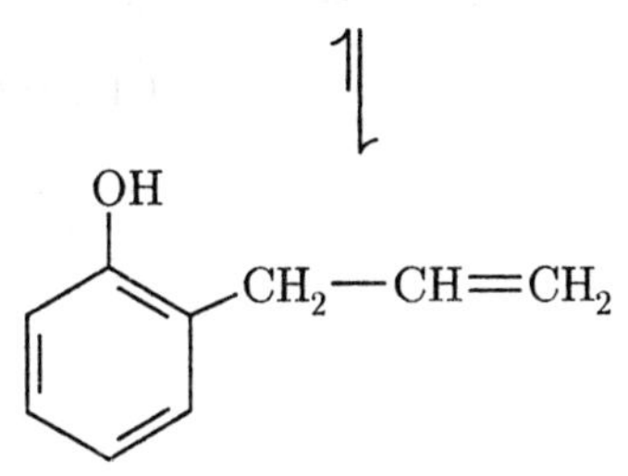

(Phenol form, aromatic, more stable)

2. Although Claisen rearrangement occurs in equilibrium, the energy difference between the starting material and the product drives the reaction to one side.

(a) 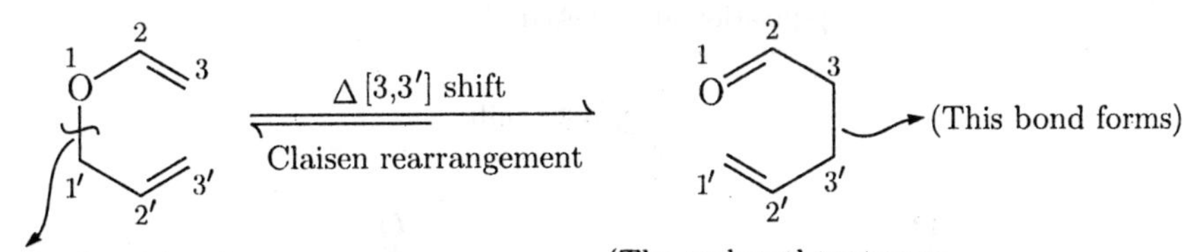

(The carbonyl tautomer predominates)

(b) 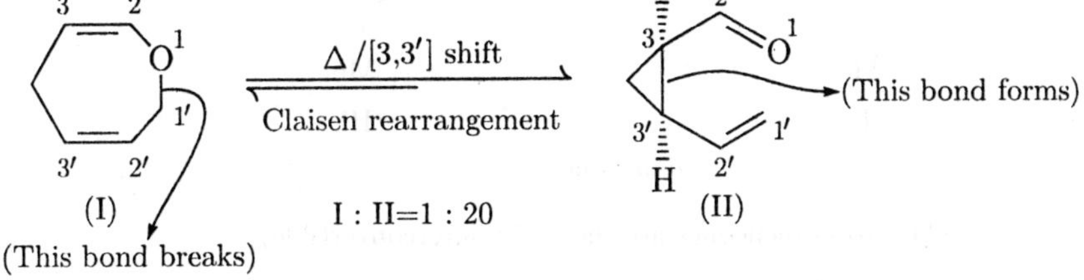

Carbonyl tautomer predominates although it contains a cyclopropyl ring in it.

When both the *ortho* positions along with *para*- position are substituted, enolisation of *ortho*- dienone formed is then prevented.

(a)

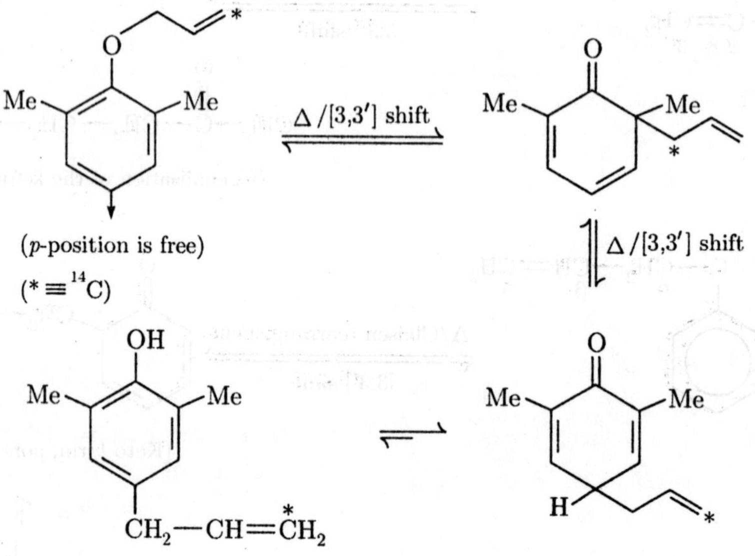

(b)

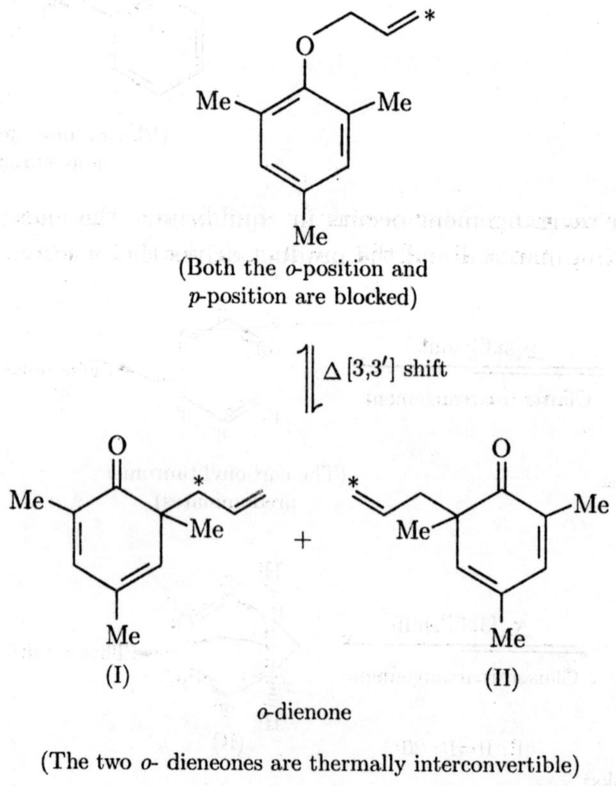

(The two *o*- dieneones are thermally interconvertible)

Mechanism of Claisen Rearrangement **:**

1.

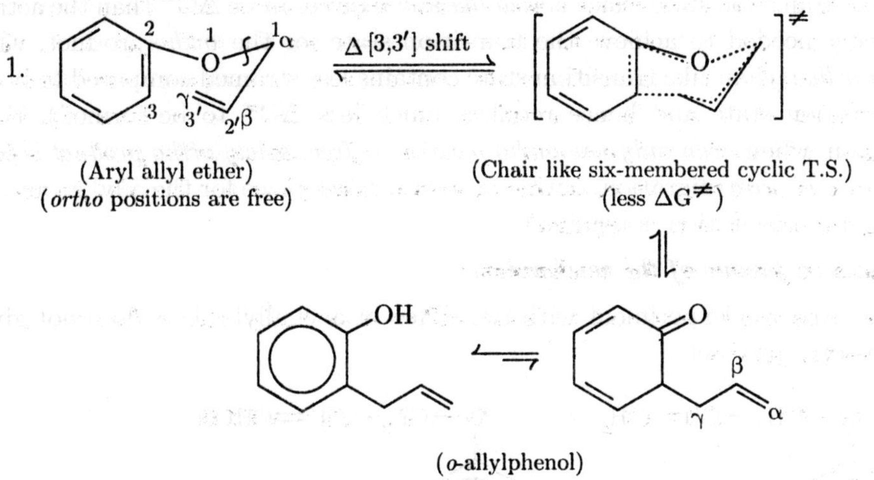

2.

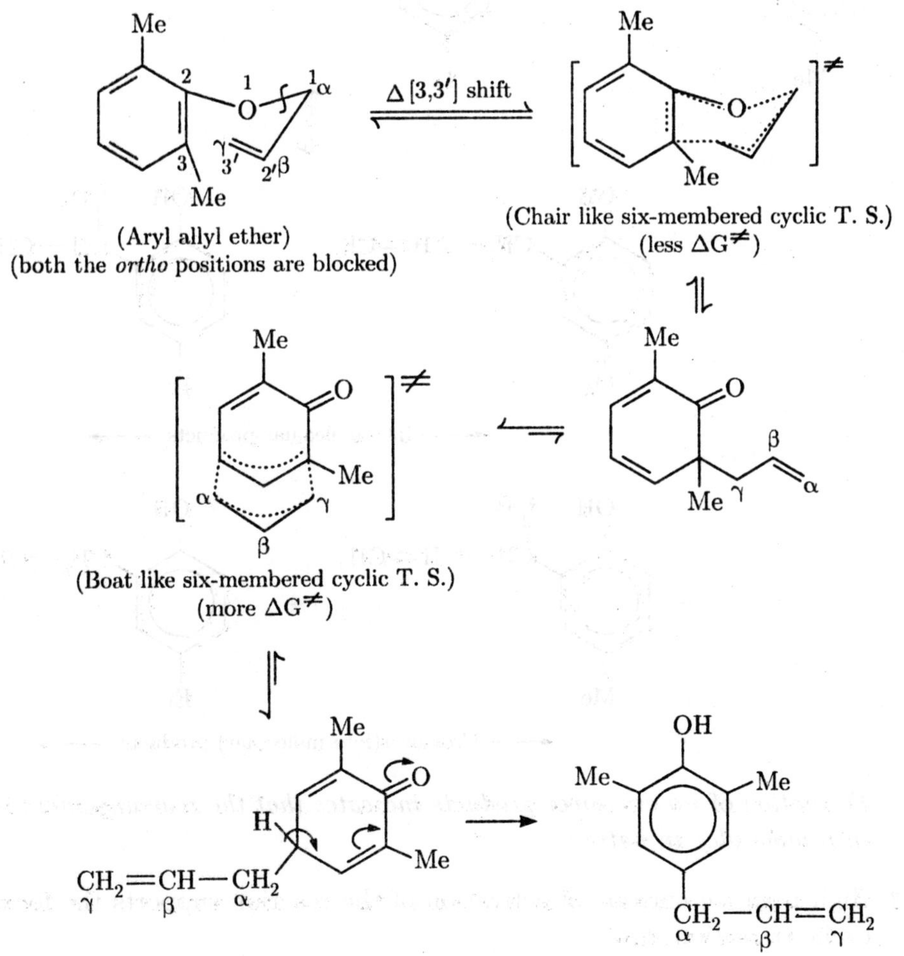

The second migration of allyl group takes place to the *p*-position *via* a deformed cyclic transition state which is *boat like* and requires more $\Delta G^{\neq}$ than the activation energy needed to achieve the transition state for the *ortho*-product, which is *chair like* (chair like transition state contains less strained compared to boat like transition state and hence requires much less $\Delta G^{\neq}$ to be formed). For this reason, when *even only one ortho position is free, solely ortho product is formed.* In case of *para* migration, double inversion takes place for the allyl group, so the original orientation is regained.

Evidences in favour of the mechanism :

1. The corssover experiment with two different aryl allyl ethers does not give any crossover product.

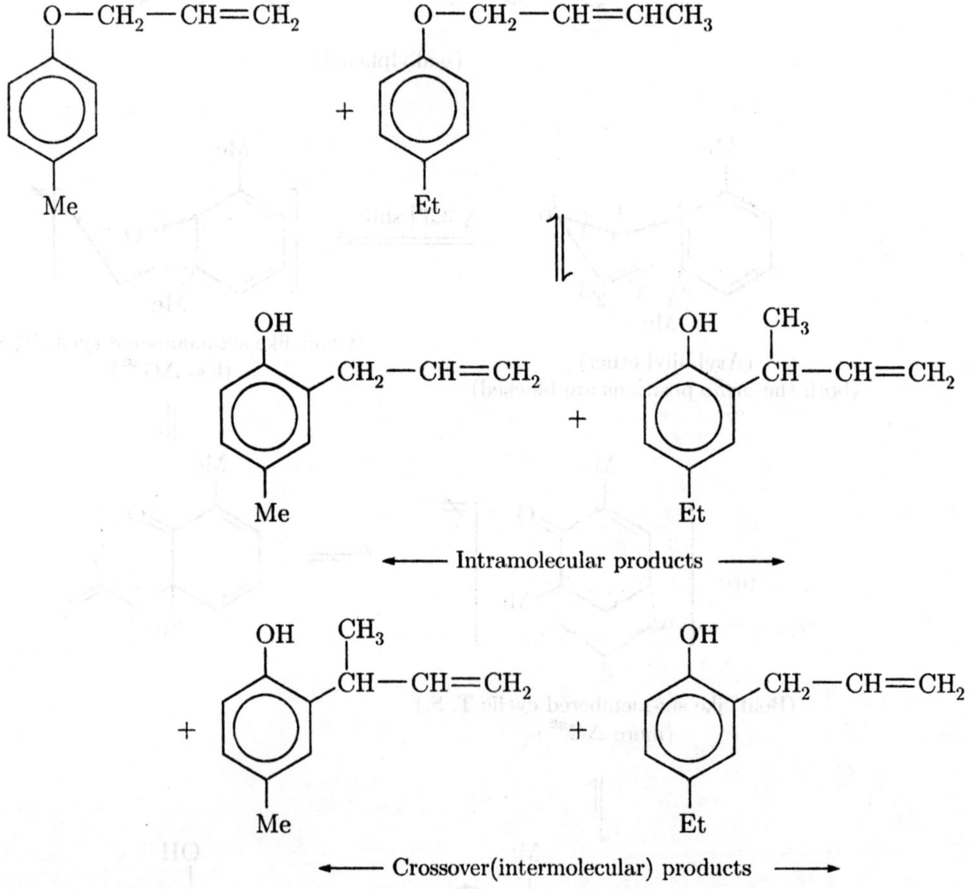

Formation of *no crossover products indicates that the rearrangement is strictly intramolecular in nature.*

2. High negative entropy of activation of the reaction supports the formation of cyclic transition state.

3. When an aryl allyl ether labelled with ^{14}C at γ-position is subjected to Claisen rearrangemement, the radioactivity gets associated with the carbon attached to the carbon which is *ortho* to phenolic –OH group.

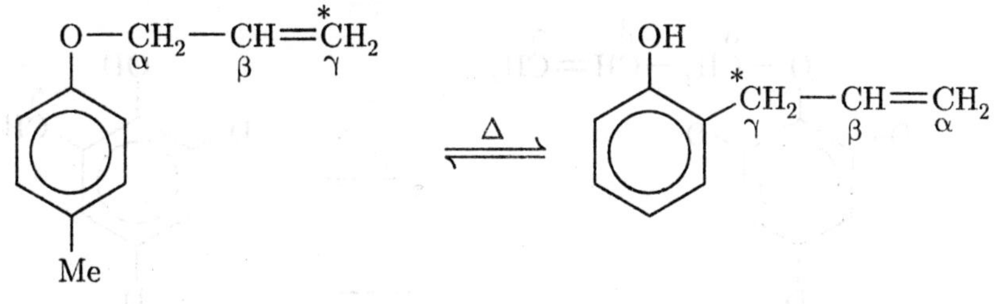

(*≡^{14}C)

This proves that, γ-carbon forms σ-bond with the *ortho* carbon (*ortho* to phenolic –OH group) in the *o*-allylphenol as product. By the same logic we see that double migration of allyl group takes place when both the *ortho* positions are blocked by substituents.

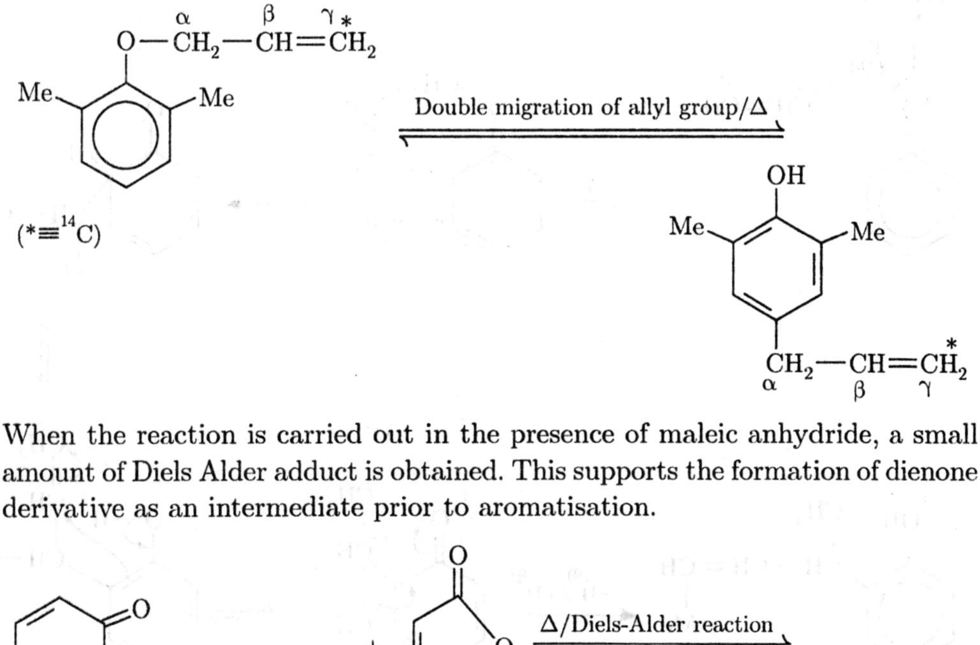

(*≡^{14}C)

4. When the reaction is carried out in the presence of maleic anhydride, a small amount of Diels Alder adduct is obtained. This supports the formation of dienone derivative as an intermediate prior to aromatisation.

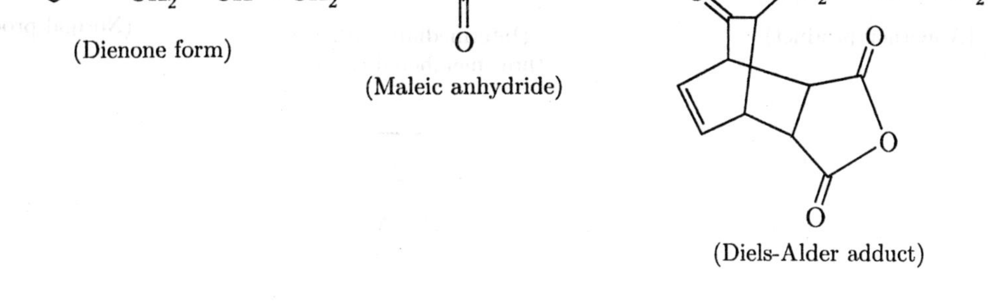

5. When 2,4,6-trideuterophenyl allyl ether is heated, O-allylphenol–D is obtained. This proves that either *ortho*– or *para*-hydrogen migrates during dienone-phenol rearrangement.

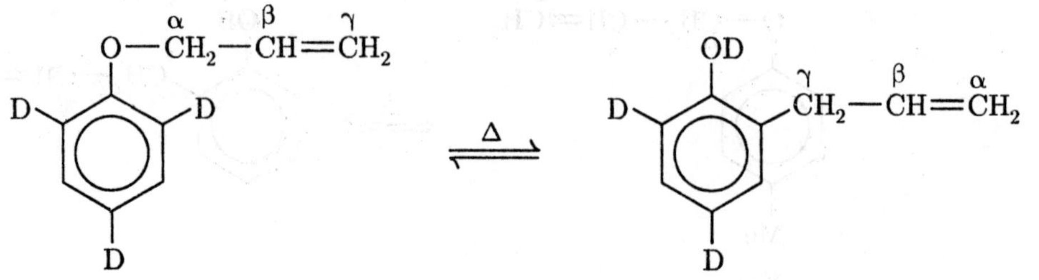

(2,4,6-trideuteroallyl ether) (Product)

Abnormal Claisen Rearrangement : Abnormal Claisen product is formed by the rearrangement of the normal product as follows.

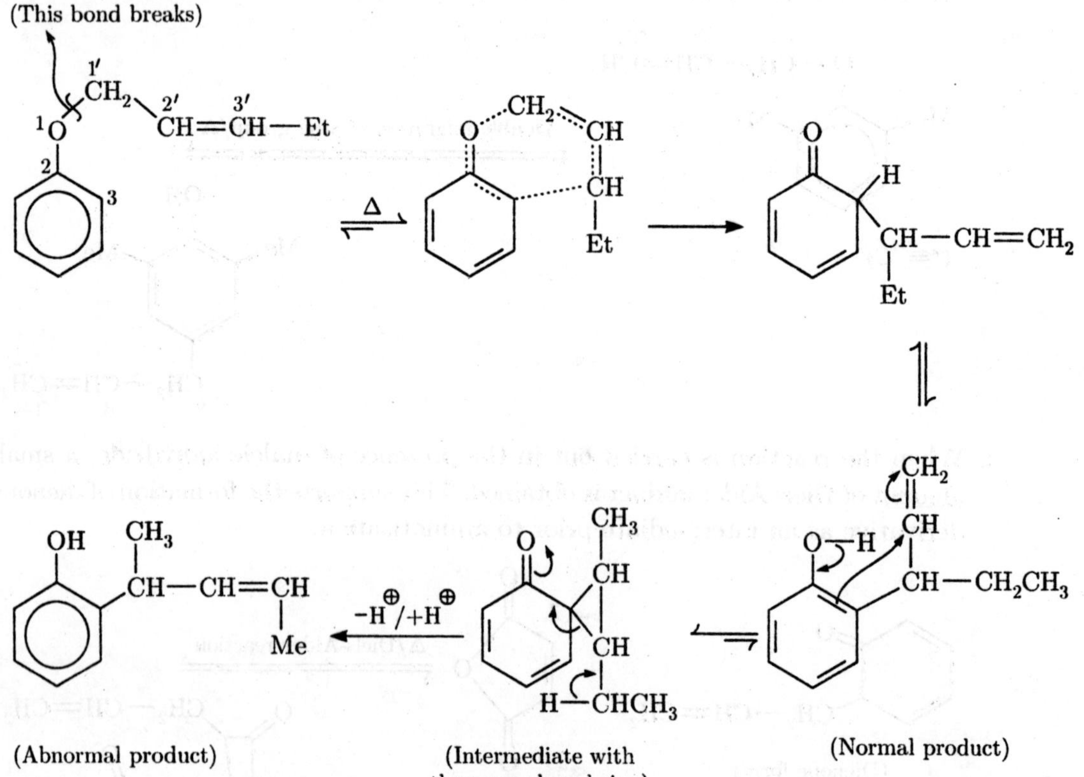

(Abnormal product) (Intermediate with three-membered ring) (Normal product)

Amines

Hydrocarbon derivatives of ammonia are called amines. When the hydrocarbon part is aliphatic (alkyl, cycloalkyl, allyl, alkenyl etc.), it is aliphatic amine and when the hydrocarbon part is aryl, the amine is called aryl amine. There are three classes of amines; $R\ddot{N}H_2$ or $Ar\ddot{N}H_2$ belongs to primary amine, $R_2\ddot{N}H$ or $R_1R_2\ddot{N}H$ or $ArR\ddot{N}H_2$ belongs to secondary amine and $R_3\ddot{N}$, $R_1R_2R_3\ddot{N}$ or $Ar\ddot{N}R_1R_2$ etc. belongs to tertiary amine.

Preparation of Amines

1. Ammonolysis Reaction

When a mixture of an alkyl halide and an ethanolic solution of ammonia is heated in a sealed tube, a mixture of primary, secondary, tertiary and quaternary amine salts is obtained. These amine salts are converted to amines by distilling with strong alkali.

$$RX + NH_3 \longrightarrow RNH_2 + HX \longrightarrow R\overset{\oplus}{N}H_3\overset{\ominus}{X}$$

$$RNH_2 + RX \longrightarrow R_2NH + HX \longrightarrow R_2\overset{\oplus}{N}H_2\overset{\ominus}{X}$$

$$R_2NH + RX \longrightarrow R_3N + HX \longrightarrow R_3\overset{\oplus}{N}H\overset{\ominus}{X}$$

$$R_3N + RX \longrightarrow R_4\overset{\oplus}{N}\,\overset{\ominus}{X}$$

The method is of very limited synthetic application because multiple alkylations occurs.

If a large excess of ammonia is allowed to react with a small amount of alkyl halide, a primary amine is formed predominantly. The reactivity order of alkyl groups and halides are as follows :

methyl>primary alkyl>secondary>tertiary alkyl

and $\overset{\ominus}{I} > \overset{\ominus}{Br} > \overset{\ominus}{Cl}$

with *tertiary halides*, alkenes are formed on ammonolysis reaction.

$$H_3\ddot{N}\quad H{-}CH_2{-}CMe_2{-}Cl \xrightarrow{E2} CH_2{=}CMe_2 + NH_4Cl$$

t-butyl chloride

When a haloarene (chloro and bromo) is heated with sedamide or potassamide ($NaNH_2$ or KNH_2) in liquid ammonia, a primary aromatic amine is formed, *via* an aryne.

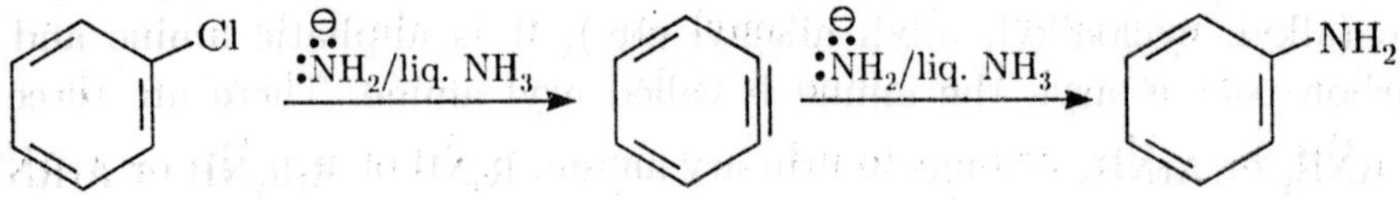

Aryne (benzene)

2. Reductive amination of carbonyl compounds

When a mixture of an aldehyde or a ketone and a large excess of ammonia and hydrogen is passed over Raney Ni at 40°–50°C under a high pressure (20–150 atm), a primary amine is formed. If ammonia is not taken in excess, a mixture of primary and secondary amines is formed. The reduction may also be carried out in the presence of excess of NH_4Cl and Adam's catalyst (Pt or Pd catalyst) under 3 atm pressure.

$$R_2C{=}O + NH_3 + H_2 \xrightarrow{Ni} R_2CHNH_2 \xrightarrow{R_2C=O} (R_2CH)_2NH \xrightarrow{R_2C=O} (R_2CH)_3N$$

3. Alkylation of azide ion and reduction

A much better method for preparing a primary amine from an alkyl halide is first to convert the alkyl halide to an alkyl azide (RN_3) by an S_N2 reaction.

$$R{-}X + \overset{\ominus}{:N}{=}\overset{\oplus}{N}{=}\overset{\ominus}{N}: \xrightarrow{S_N2} R{-}N{=}\overset{\oplus}{N}{=}\overset{\ominus}{N}: \xrightarrow[\text{or } LiAlH_4]{\text{Na/alcohol}} RNH_2$$

(Azide ion, a good nucleophile)

4. Reduction

(a) $RNO_2(ArNO_2) \xrightarrow{\text{Sn or Fe/HCl, } LiAlH_4} RNH_2(ArNH_2)$

(b) $ArNO_2 \xrightarrow{SnCl_2/HCl \text{ or } TiCl_2/\ HCl} ArNH_2$

(c) $ArNO_2\ (RNO_2) \xrightarrow{\text{Pd/Pt, Raney Ni/}H_2 \text{ or Raney Ni/}H_2N{-}NH_2} ArNH_2\ (RNH_2)$

(d) $O_2N\ ArNO_2 \xrightarrow{NH_4/ \text{ or } Na_2S} H_2N\ ArNO_2$(Partial reduction)

(e) $RCN\ (ArCN) \xrightarrow{\text{Pd/Pt, Raney Ni/}H_2 \text{ or Raney Ni/}H_2N{-}NH_2} RCH_2NH_2\ (ArCH_2NH_2)$

(f) $R{-}C{\equiv}N \xrightarrow{H_2/Pt} RCH_2NH_2$

(g) $CH_3CONH_2 \xrightarrow{LiAlH_4/\text{dry ether}} CH_3CH_2NH_2$

(h) $PhCONH_2 \xrightarrow{Na/EtOH} PhCH_2NH_2$

(i) $CH_3CH{=}NOH \xrightarrow{Na/EtOH \text{ or } LiAlH_4/Et_2O \text{ or } Pt/H_2} CH_3CH_2NH_2$

5. The Gabriel Phthalimide Synthesis (Synthesis of Primary Amines)

The method consists of

(a) Conversion of phthalimide to its potassio salt by ethanolic potassium hydroxide.

(b) Heating the salt with alkyl halide to form N-alkylphthalimide.

(c) Hydrolysis of N-alkyl derivative to phthalic acid and a primary amine corresponding to alkyl halide.

Phthalimide is quite acidic (pK_a=9); it can be converted to potassium phthalimide by KOH. The phthalimide anion is a strong nucleophile and it reacts with an alkyl halide by an S_N2 mechanism to give an N-alkylphthalimide. At this point, N-alkylphthalimide can be hydrolyzed with aqueous acid or base, but the hydrolysis is often difficult. It is more convenient to treat the N-alkylphthalimide with hydrazine (H_2N–NH_2) in refluxing ethanol to give a primary amine and phthalazine-1,4-dione.

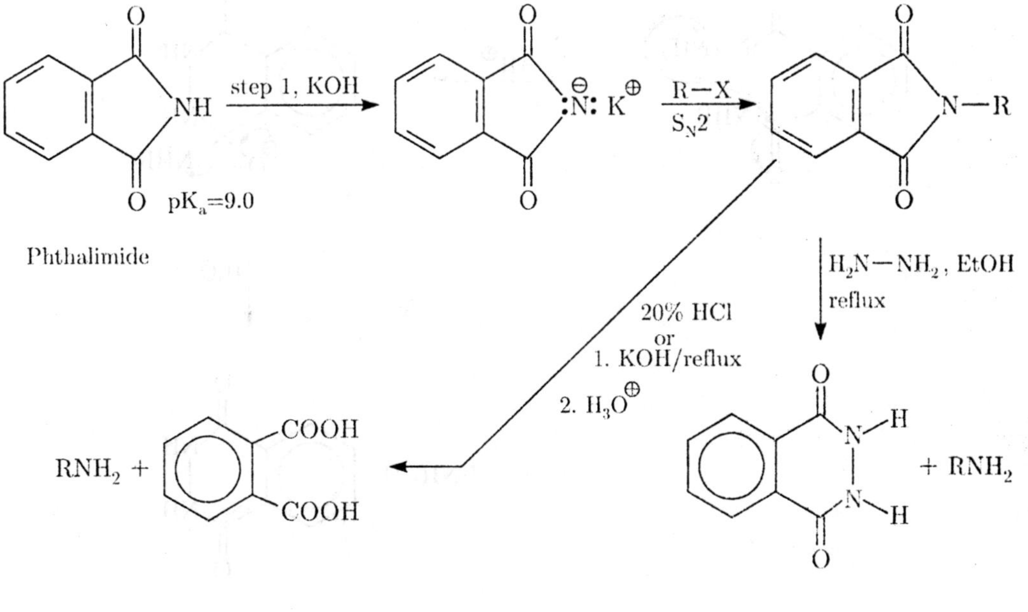

Mechanism of the reaction :

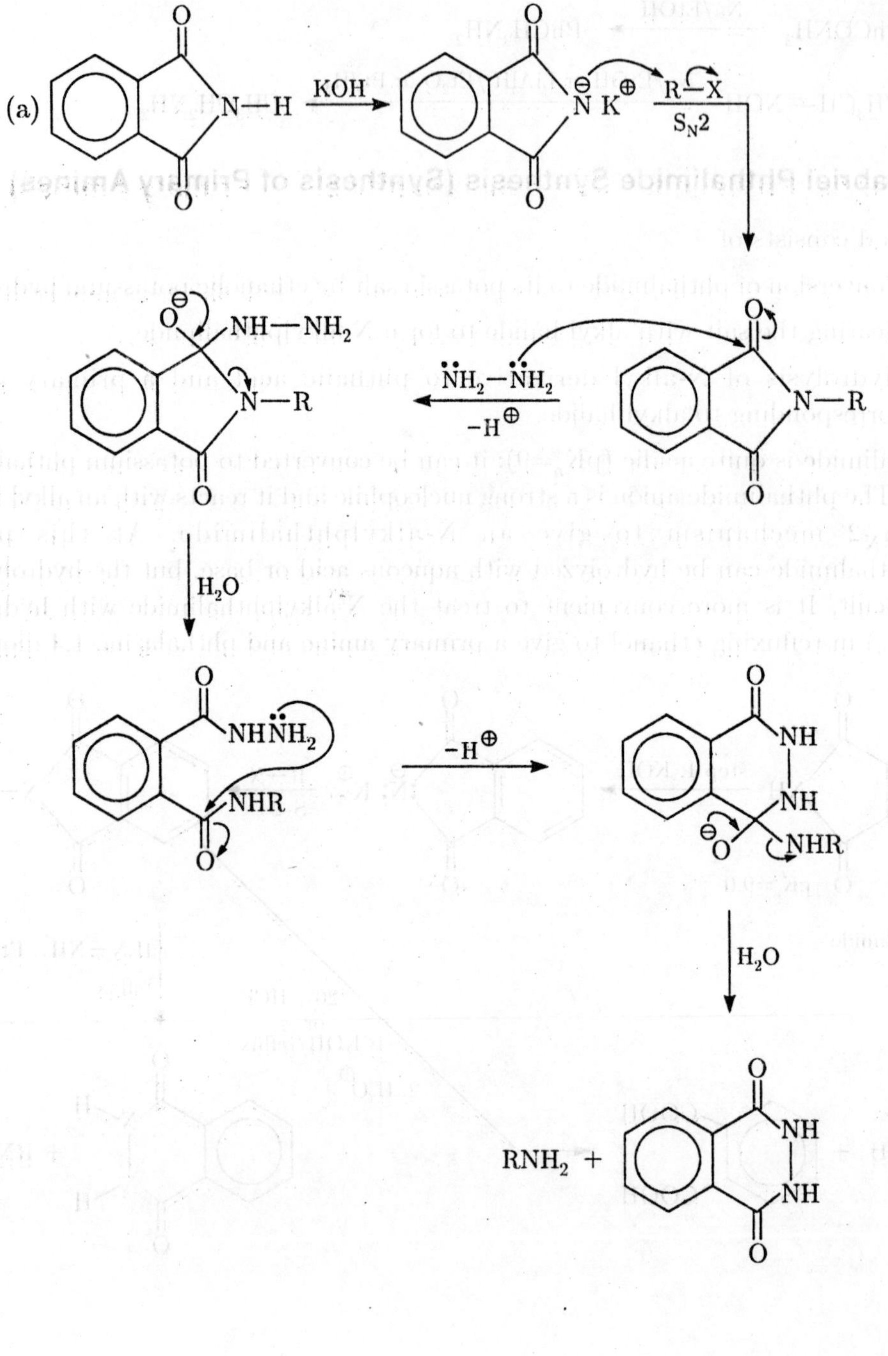

(b) ***Acid catalysed hydrolysis*** :

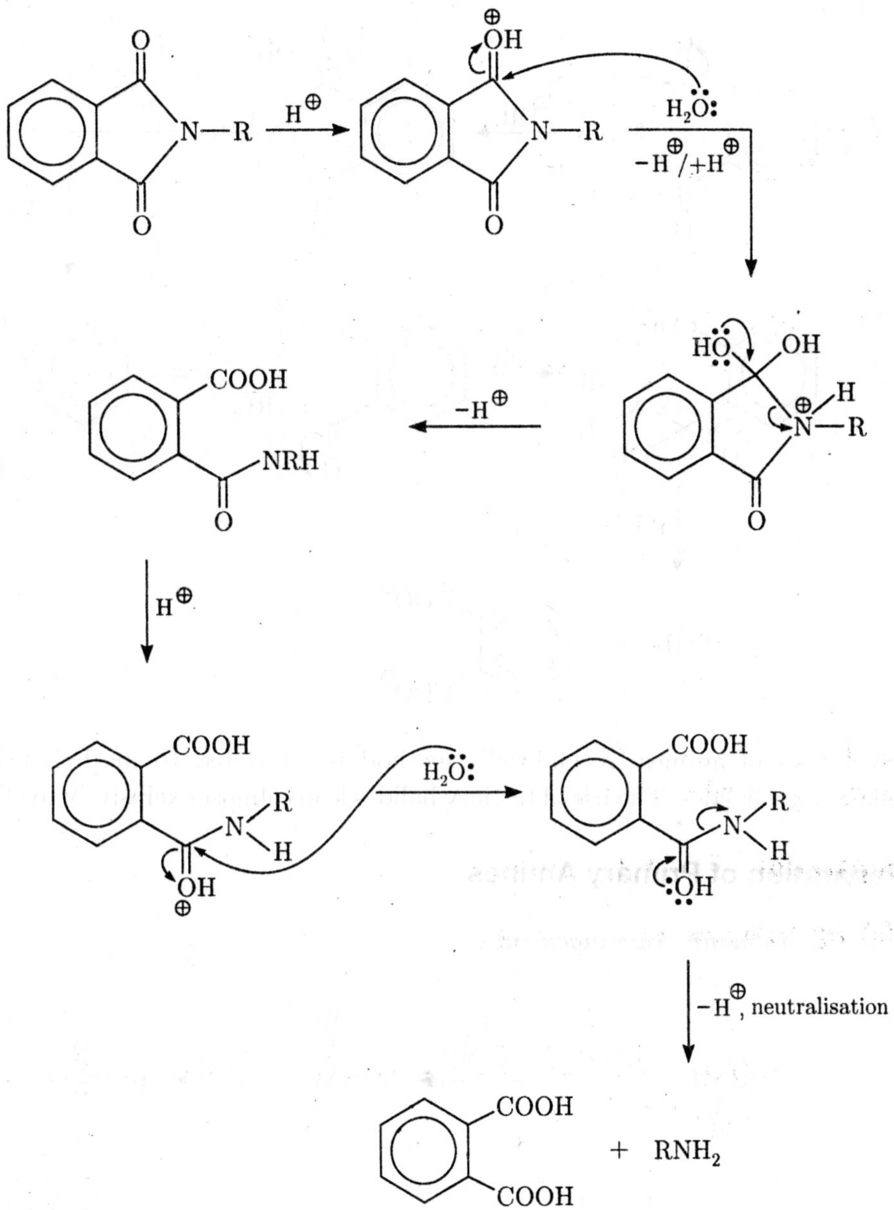

(c) ***Base-catalysed hydrolysis*** :

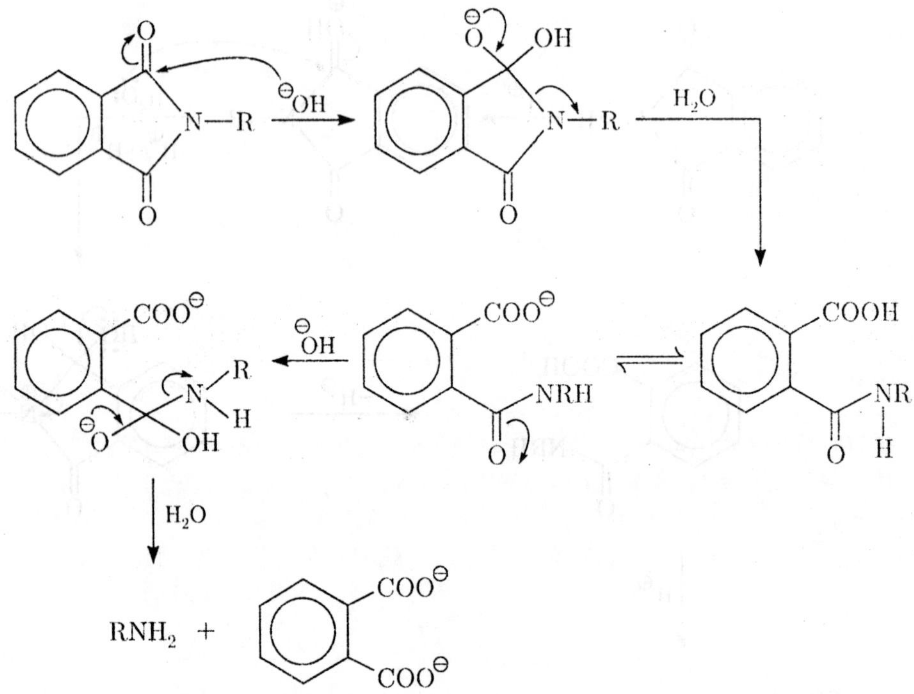

Syntheses of amines by Gabriel's method is restricted to methyl, primary and secondary alkyl halides. The use of tertiary halides leads almost exclusively to eliminations.

4. Preparation of Primary Amines

(a) ***By Hofmann rearrangement*** :

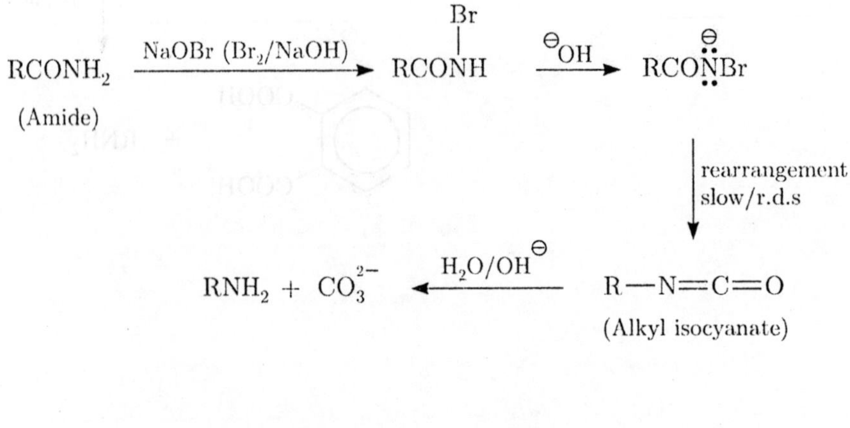

(b) ***By Lossen rearrangement*** :

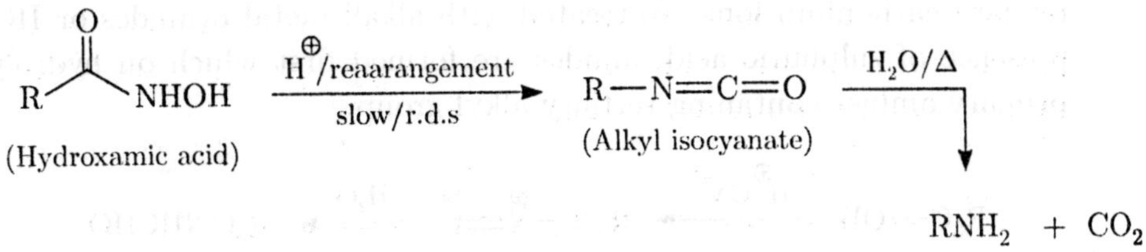

(c) ***By Curtius rearrangement***

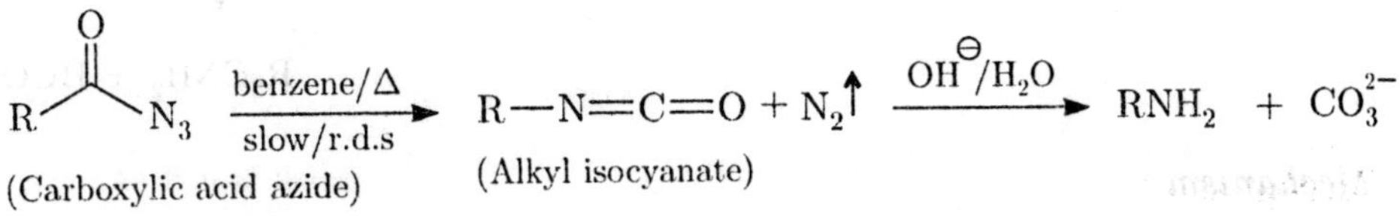

(d) ***By the Grignard Reagent***

$$RMgX + ClNH_2 \longrightarrow RNH_2 + MgX(Cl)$$

(e) ***By the Leuckart reaction*** : The reductive amination of high boiling ketones and aldehydes by ammonium formate or formamide is known as Leuckart reaction.

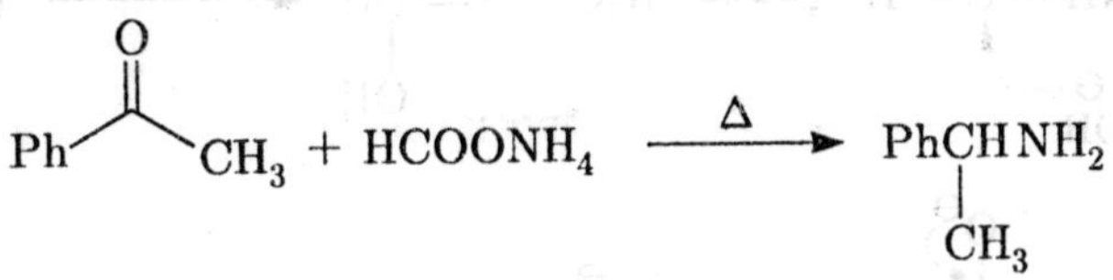

Mechanism :

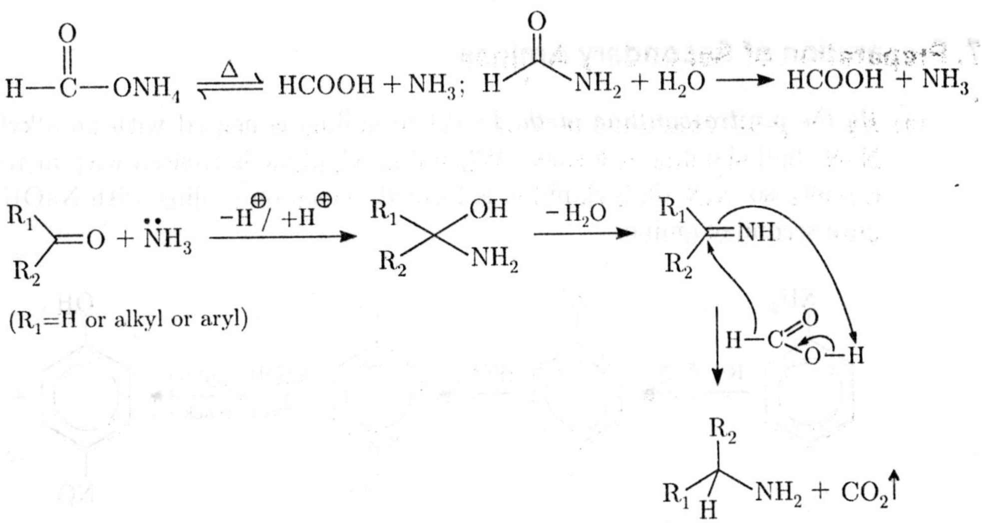

(f) ***By the Ritter reaction*** : When tertiary alcohols or alkenes capable of producing tertiary carbonium ions are treated with alkali metal cyanides or HCN in the presence of sulphuric acid, amides are formed first which on hydrolysis gives primary amines contaning tertiary alkyl group.

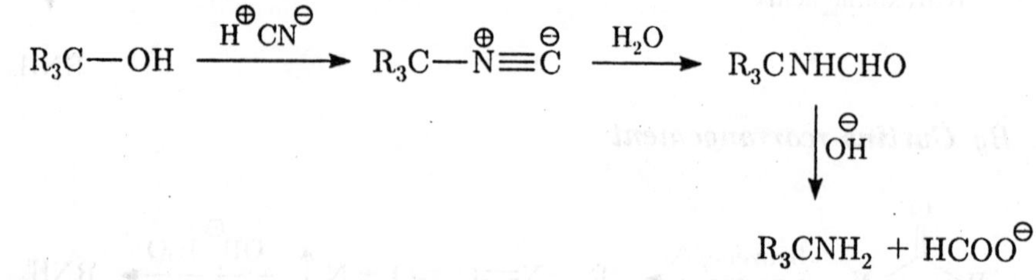

Mechanism :

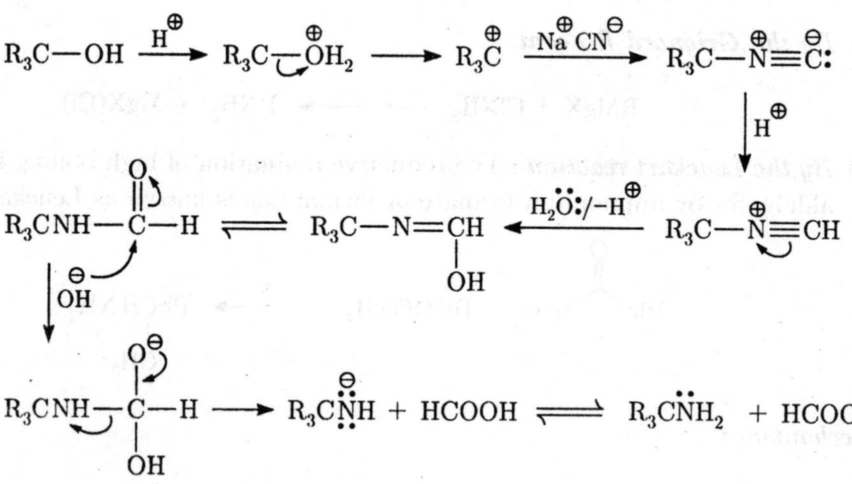

7. Preparation of Secondary Amines

(a) ***By the p-nitrosoaniline method*** : When aniline is heated with an alkyl halide, N–N–dialkylaniline is formed. When dialkylaniline is treated with nitrous acid, a *p*-nitroso–N,N–dialkylaniline is formed, which on boiling with NaOH gives a pure seconday amine.

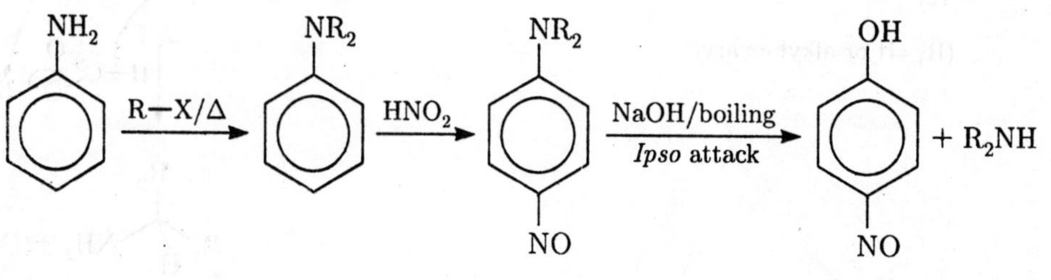

Mechanism :

$$PhNH_2 + RX \xrightarrow{S_N2} \underset{+\,HX}{PhNHR} \xrightarrow{RX/S_N2} PhNR_2$$

$$HO{-}NO \xrightarrow{H^{\oplus}} H_2\overset{\oplus}{O}{-}N{=}O \longrightarrow H_2O + \overset{\oplus}{N}{=}O$$

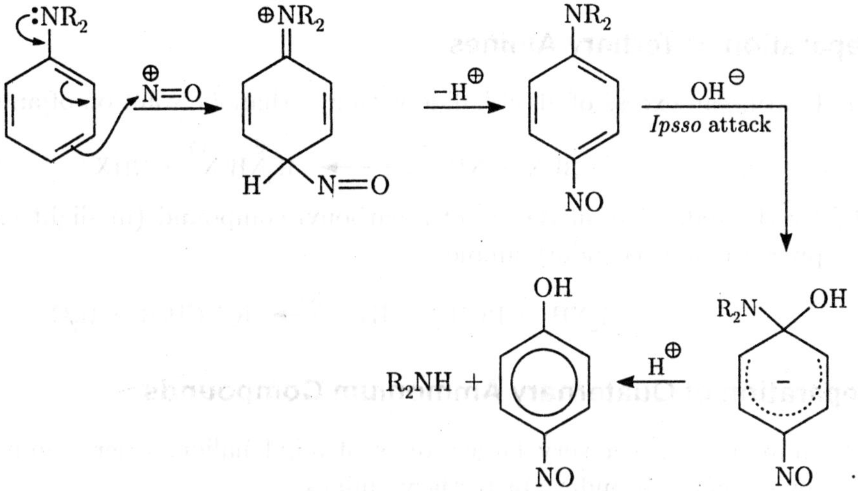

(b) ***By the p-toluenesulphonyl chloride method*** : When a primary amine is treated with *p*-toluenesulphonyl chloride, an N–alkyl-*p*-toluenesulphonamide is formed. This on successive treatment with an alkyl halide, aqueous alkali and excess of acid or water forms a secondary amine salt which is converted to a secondary amine by distilling the salt with aqueous alkali.

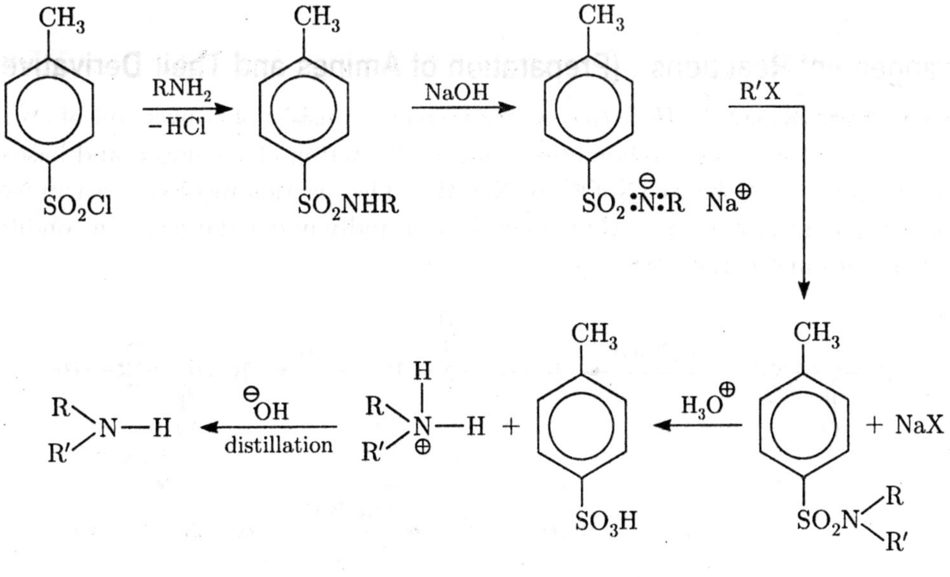

(c) *From calcium cyanamide* :

$$CaNCN \xrightarrow{NaOH} Na_2NCN \xrightarrow{2RX} R_2NCN \xrightarrow[\text{1. } OH^{\ominus} \text{ 2. } H_3O^{\oplus}]{H_3O^{\oplus} \text{ or}} R_2N{-}COOH \xrightarrow{\Delta/-CO_2} R_2NH$$

8. Preparation of Tertiary Amines

(a) Heating an excess of alkyl halide with an ethanolic solution of ammonia.

$$3RX + NH_3 \longrightarrow R_3\overset{\oplus}{N}H\ \overset{\ominus}{X} + 2HX$$

(b) By the reductive alkylation of a carbonyl compound (in slight excess) in the presence of a secondary amine.

$$R'_2NH + RCHO + H_2 \xrightarrow{Ni} R'_2NCH_2R + H_2O$$

9. Preparation of Quaternary Ammonium Compounds

Heating ammonia with a very large excess of alkyl halide, where ammonia may be replaced by primary, secondary or tertiary amines.

$$R_3N \text{ (tertiary amine)} + RX \xrightarrow{\Delta} R_4\overset{\oplus}{N}\ \overset{\ominus}{X}$$

$$R_4\overset{\oplus}{N}\ \overset{\ominus}{X} + NaOH \longrightarrow R_4\overset{\oplus}{N}\ \overset{\ominus}{O}H + NaX$$

$$R_4\overset{\oplus}{N}\ \overset{\ominus}{X} + AgOH \longrightarrow R_4\overset{\oplus}{N}\ \overset{\ominus}{O}H + AgI\downarrow$$

Preparation of quaternary ammonium hydroxide

Rearrangement Reactions : (Preparation of Amines and Their Derivatives)

Hofmann Rearrangement : Hofmann rearrangement consists of conversion of an amide to primary amine with one carbon atom less, by the action of a halogen and base (Br_2/ KOH or NaOH) or hypohalite (NaOCl or NaOBr). The reaction involves a rearrangement of N-haloamide into isocyanate which hydrolyses rapidly under the reaction condition to primary amines and carbonates.

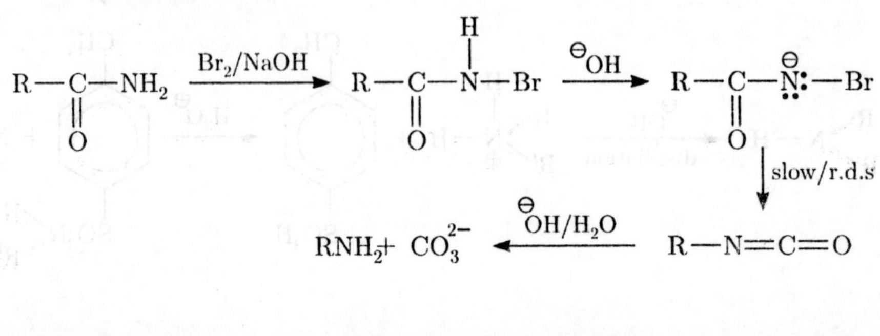

Overall reactions may be represented by

$$RCONH_2 + Br_2 + 4KOH \longrightarrow RNH_2 + 2KBr + K_2CO_3 + 2H_2O$$

Examples :

1. $CH_3-\underset{\underset{O}{\|}}{C}-NH_2 \xrightarrow{Br_2/KOH} CH_3NH_2$

2. $H_2N-\underset{\underset{O}{\|}}{C}-NH_2 \xrightarrow{NaOCl} H_2N-NH_2$

3. 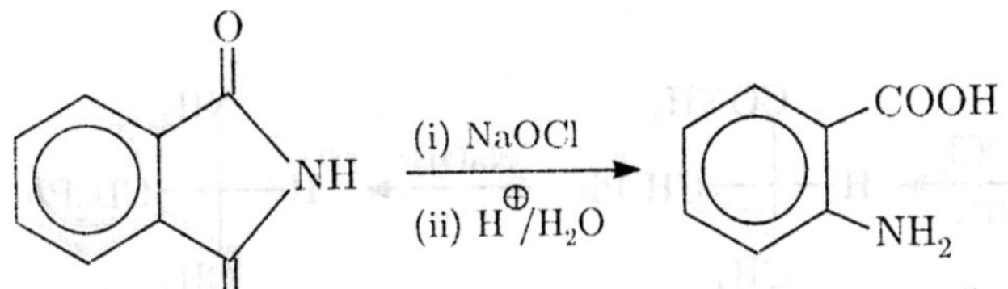

(Anthranilic acid)

Mechanism : Hofmann rearrangement is an intramolecular anionotropic 1,2-shift, involving migration of an alkyl or aryl group from a carbon atom to an electron deficient nitrogen atom with retention of configuration. The reaction follows a first order kinetics : rate $\propto$ [$RCONH_2$]. In the first step, nucleophilic attack by amide nitrogen non bonding pair to halogen converts it into N-haloamide. As halogen is introduced, the acidity of amide hydrogen is further increased and subsequently abstracted by base. The loss of halogen from nitrogen and subsequent migration of alkyl or aryl group completes the reaction forming isocyanate.

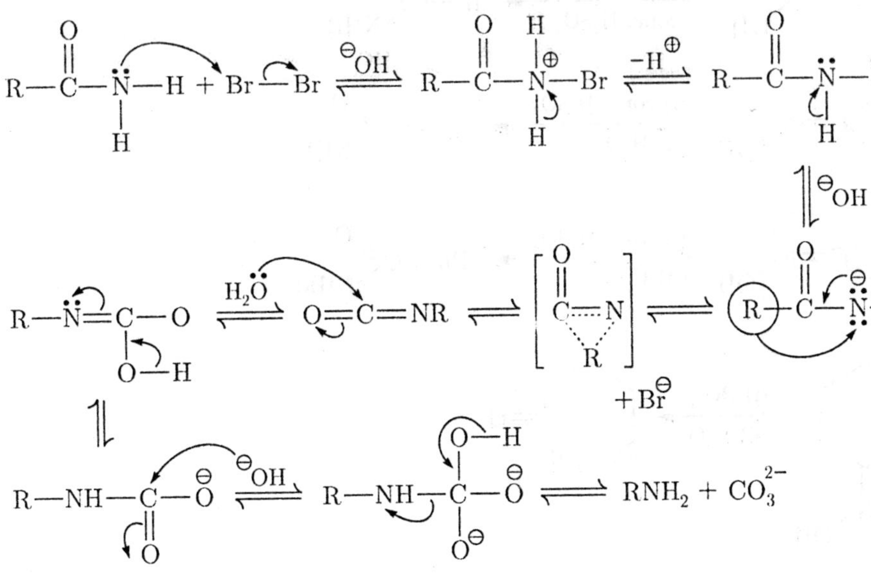

The reaction is totally **intramolecular**. It has been proved by crossover experiments. When two diferent amides are used, no crossover products are obtained. Using ^{14}C and ^{15}N isotope studies it has been proved that the rearrangement does not involve any nitrene intermediate and a concerted elimination of halide and migration of alkyl or aryl has been proposed and this step is rate determining step here. The presence of an electron releasing group like $-\ddot{N}H_2$, $-\ddot{\underset{\cdot\cdot}{O}}H$, $-\ddot{N}Me_2$ etc. at *p*–position of the aromatic amide accelerate the reaction, and electron withdrawing groups like $-NO_2$, –CHO, –COOH etc. retards the same.

Stereochemistry : If the migrating group of the amide is chiral, the primary amine is also chiral, with retention of configuration, *e.g.*, 2-(S)-benzylpropanoic acid forms 1-(S)-benzylethanamine which also proves the intramolecularity showing that the migrating group never be free to racemise.

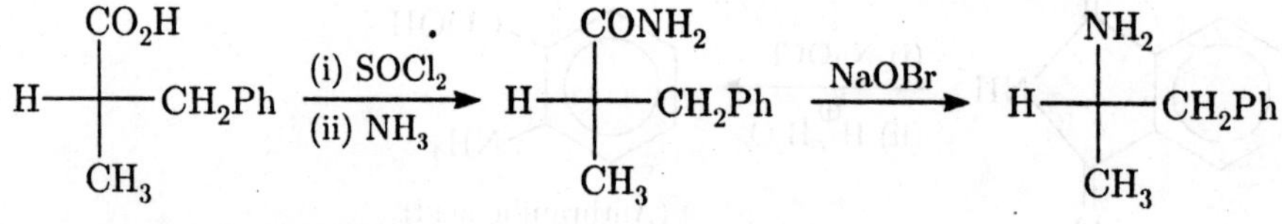

2-(S)-benzylpropanoic acid

Beckmann rearrangement : The acid catalysed transformation of ketoximes to substituted amides is known as Beckmann rearrangement. Acidic catalysts used are of wide types, both protonic and Lewis acids, *e.g.*, concentrated H_2SO_4, HCl, PCl_5, $PhSO_2Cl$, $SOCl_2$, SO_3, BF_3 or P.P.A etc.

Example :

(a) 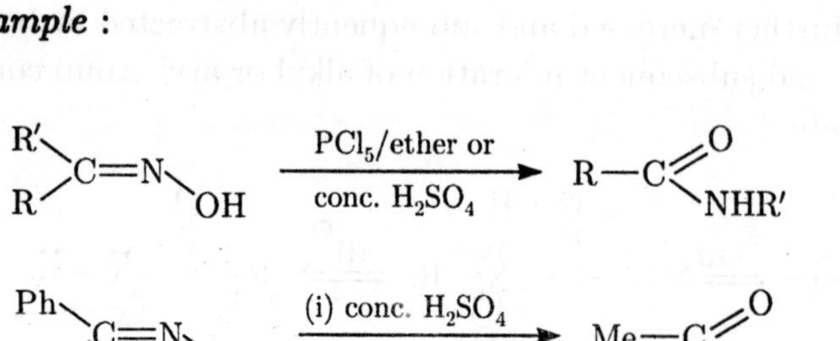

(b) 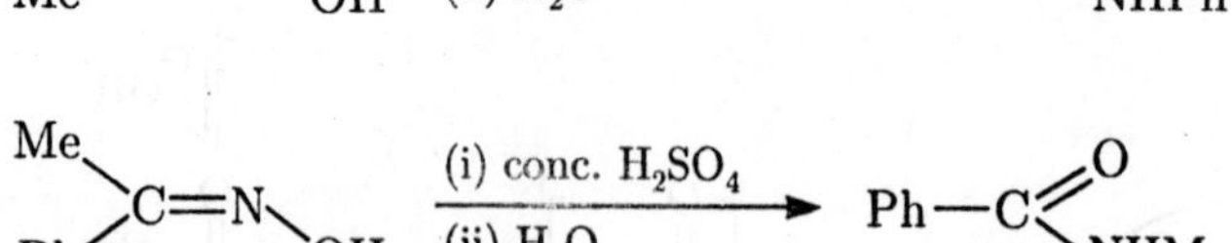

(c) 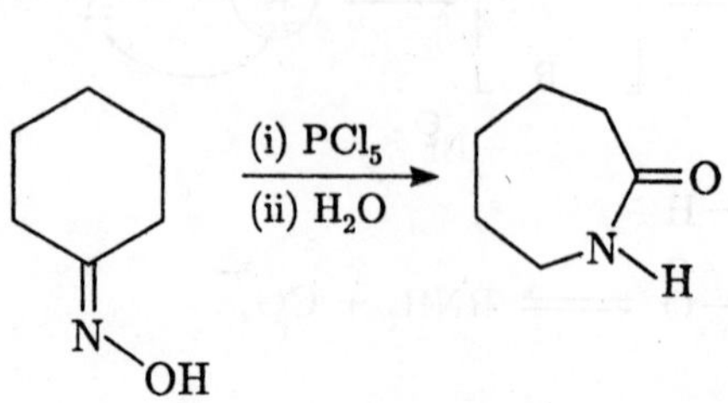

(d) 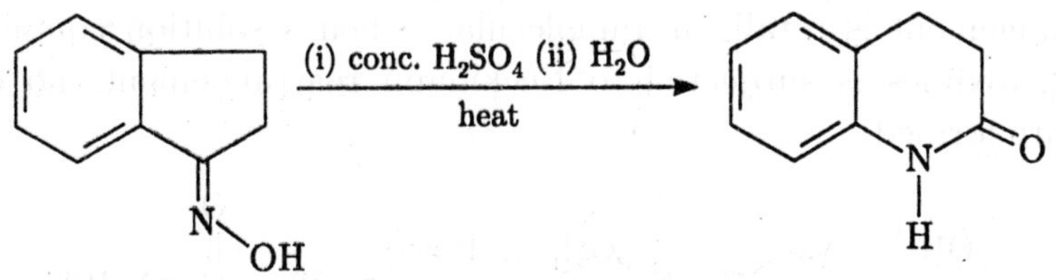

Mechanism : The mechanism involves an intramolecular anionotropic 1,2-shift, first by protonation with inorganic protonic acids, or formation of O-esters with Lewis acids, followed by elimination of water or oxyanions with synchronous migration of alkyl or aryl group to generate isocyanate. The hydrolysis of the isocyanate generates the primary amine.

The rearrangement is highly stereospecific. The migrating group always migrates from *anti* position to the leaving group.

(a) ***With protonic acids*** :

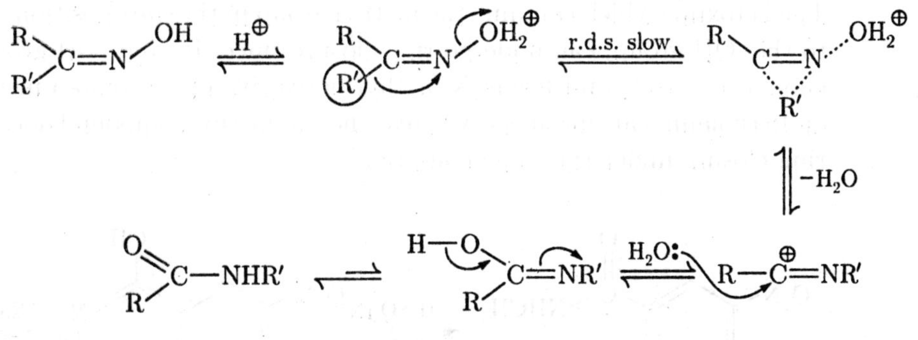

(b) ***With PCl_5*** :

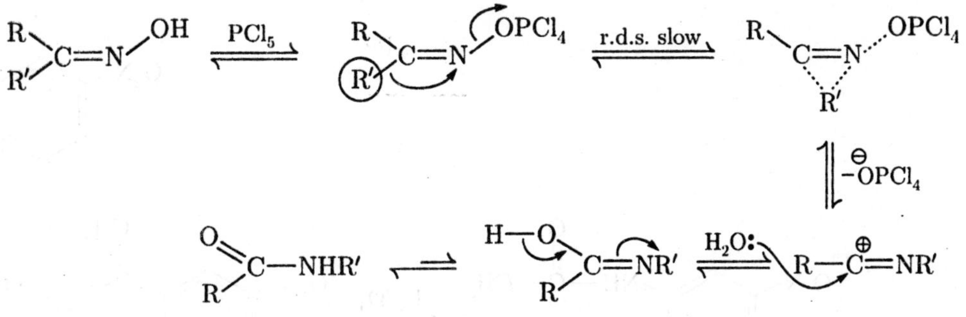

(i) The rearrangement is totally intramolecular, when a solution containing two different ketoximes is subjected to Beckmann rearrangement, no crossover products are formed.

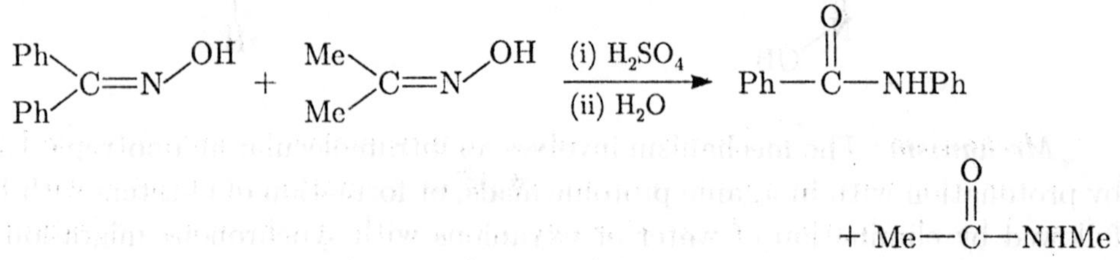

(ii) When the rearrangement is carried out in solvents of different polarities, the rate of rearrangement increases with increasing polarity. This proves that the step of ionization and migration is the rate determing step.

(iii) The rearrangement is highly stereospecific and the *anti* migration always takes place. The exclusive migration of the *anti* group has been confirmed in the conversion of 2-bromo-5-nitrobenzophenonoxime by Beckmann rearrangement. The ketoxime which contains the methyl group in the *anti*-position, with respect to the OH group, can undergo ring closure since Br and OH groups are close enough to react, and forms N-methyl derivative of 2-bromo-5-nitrobenzamide on Beckmann rearrangement, whereas the *syn*-methyl compound does not undergo ring closure under the same condition.

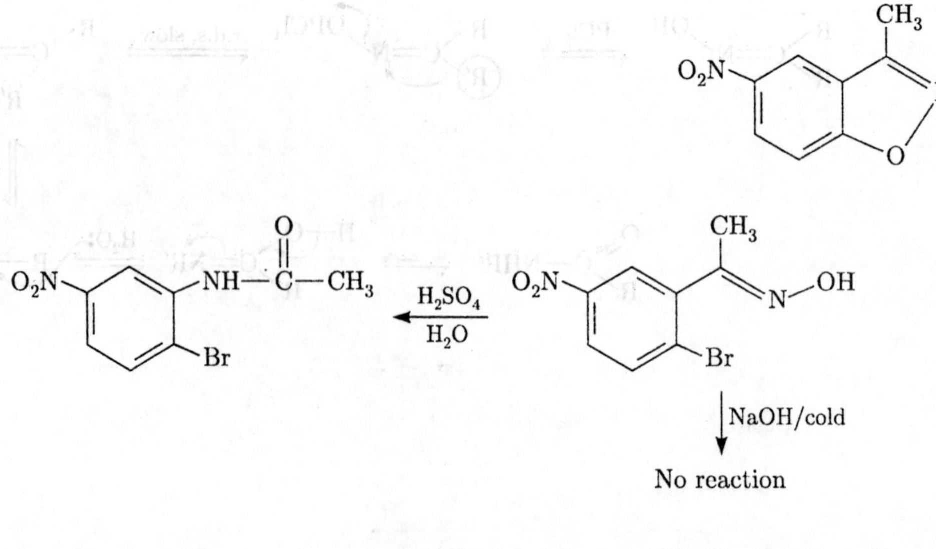

(iv) If the migrating group is asymmetric, it migrates with retention of configuration, *e.g.*, 3-(R)-heptyl methylketoxime on rearrangement forms 3-(R)-heptylamine.

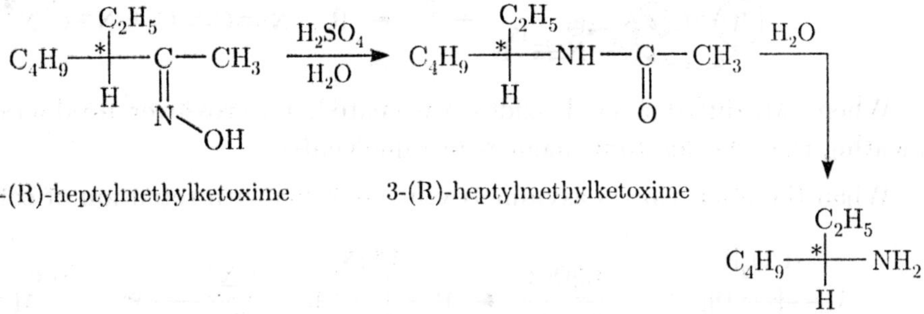

3-(R)-heptylmethylketoxime 3-(R)-heptylmethylketoxime

3-(R)-heptylamine

Curtius Rearrangement : Thermal decomposition of carboxylic acid azide to generate isocyanate in benzene or chloroform solution, is known as Curtius rearrangement. For example,

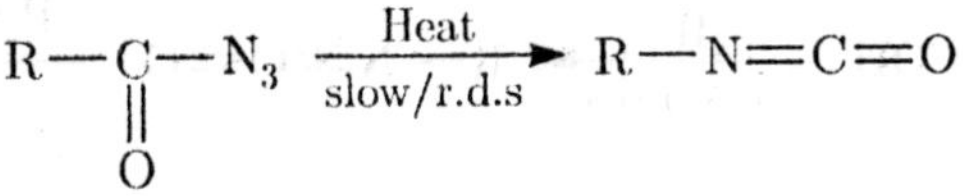

This reaction can be used to all sorts of acid azides *viz.*, acyclic, cyclic, aromatic, heterocyclic and unsaturated ones. The isocyanate formed can be hydrolysed to primary amine in a pure state.

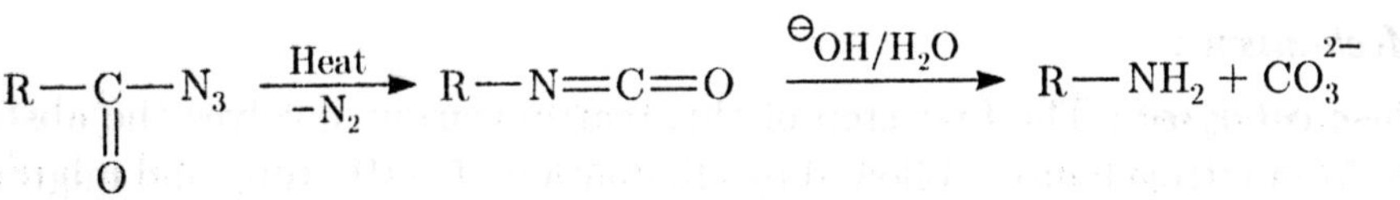

When the rearrangement is carried out in presence of an alcohol, urethan is the product.

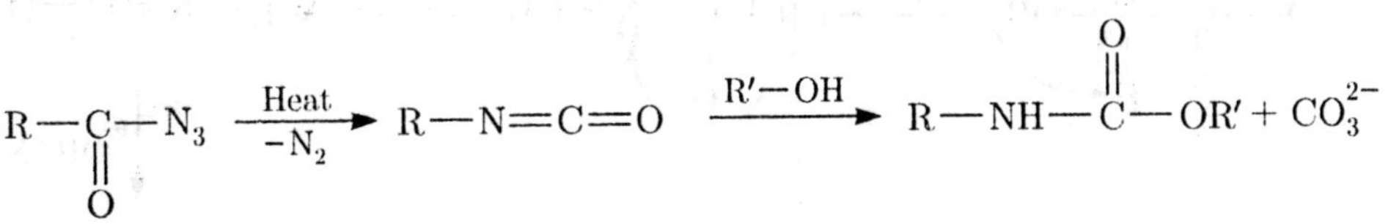

Mechanism : The Curtius rearrangement involves an intramolecular 1,2-anionotropic shift in which molecular nitrogen is eliminated followed by migration of alkyl or aryl group with bonding electrons which takes place in a concerted step.

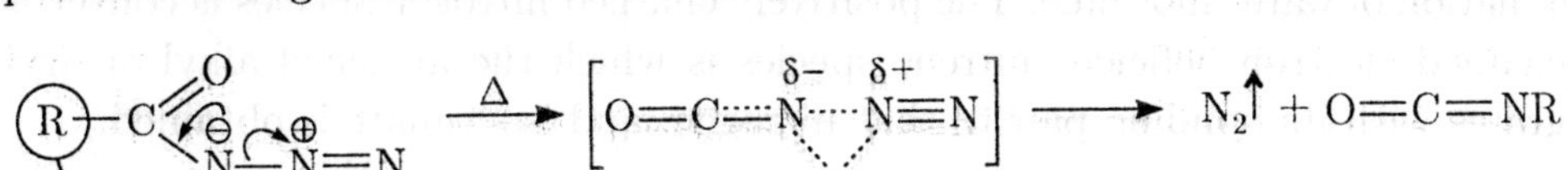

Isotope labeling experiments indicate that the terminal nitrogen is eliminated during pyrolysis.

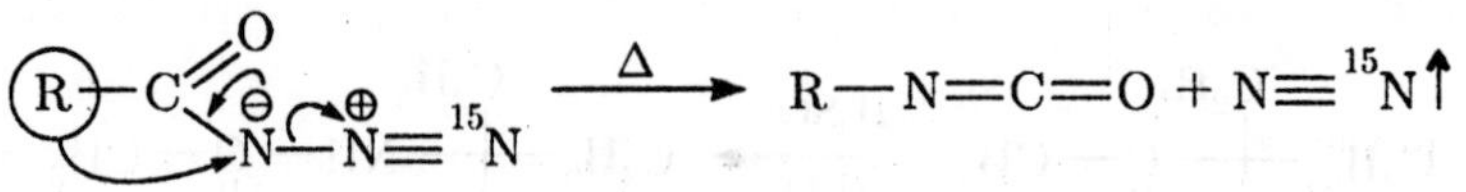

When two different acid azides are heated, no crossover products are obtained, indicating that the rearrangement is intramolecular.

When the migrating is asymmetric, it migrates with retention of configuration.

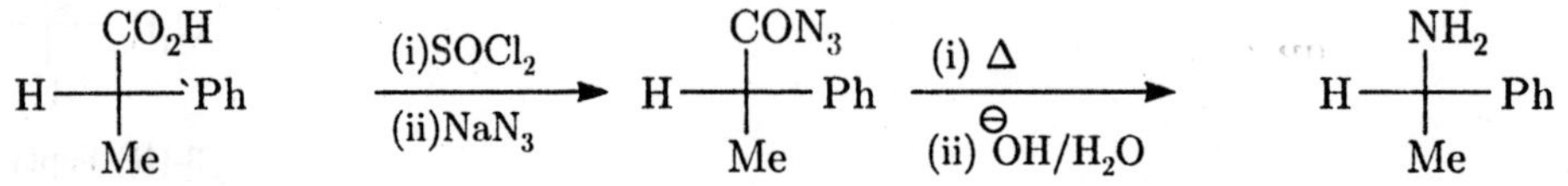

2-(S)-Phenylpropanoic acid 1-(S)-Phenylethanamine

Lossen rearrangement : The acid or base catalysed conversion of hydroxamic acid or their acyl or aryl derivatives to isocyanate is known as Lossen rearrangement.

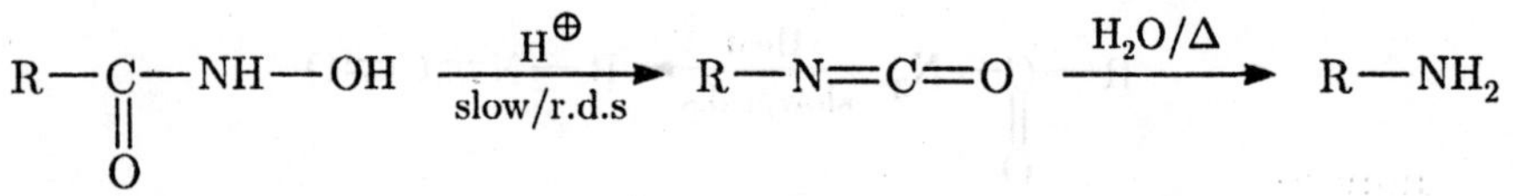

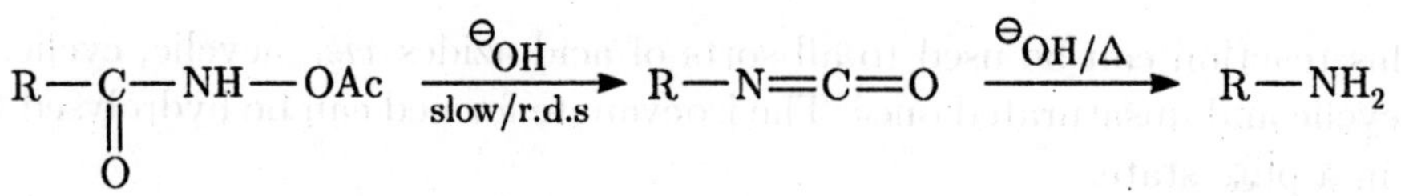

Mechanism :

Base catalysed : The first step of this rearrangement involves the abstraction of a proton, from nitrogen atom followed by elimination of –OH group and migration of alkyl group with bonding electron to electron deficient nitrogen.

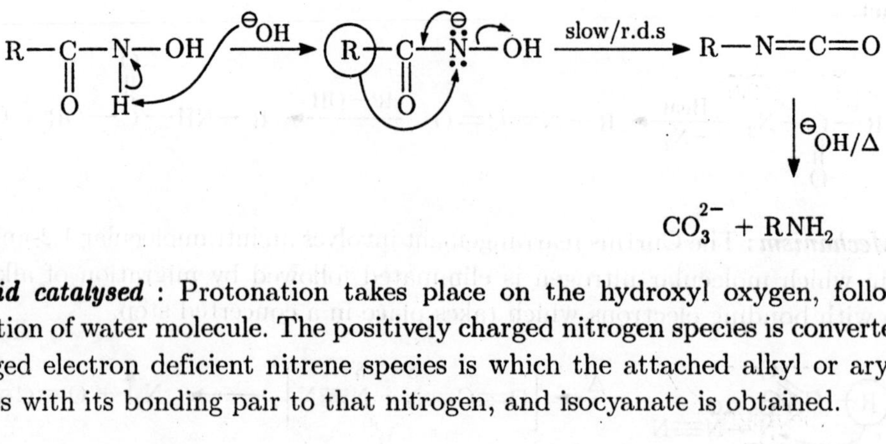

Acid catalysed : Protonation takes place on the hydroxyl oxygen, followed by elimination of water molecule. The positively charged nitrogen species is converted to an uncharged electron deficient nitrene species is which the attached alkyl or aryl group migrates with its bonding pair to that nitrogen, and isocyanate is obtained.

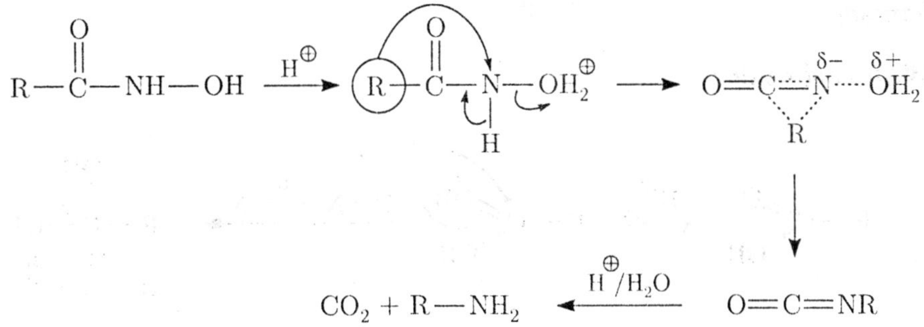

***Lossen rearrangement is intramolecular*:** The crossover experiments with two different hydroxamic acids in a mixture do not form any crossover products, thus it is totally intramolecular and the migrating group never leaves the substrate.

When the migrating group is aryl, electron donating group at *p*-position accelerate the rate, while, electron withdrawing groups retard the reaction. If the migrating group is asymmetric, migration takes place with retention of configuration.

Schmidt Rearrangement : It is the intramolecular conversion of acid azide to isocyanates by catalytic action of sulphuric acid or Lewis acids. In this reaction, the acyl azide is prepared by condensing a carboxylic acid and hydrazoic acid (N_3H) in presence of sulphuric acid. The acyl azide is normally not isolated, instead, allowed to decompose and rearrange in the reaction mixture itself.

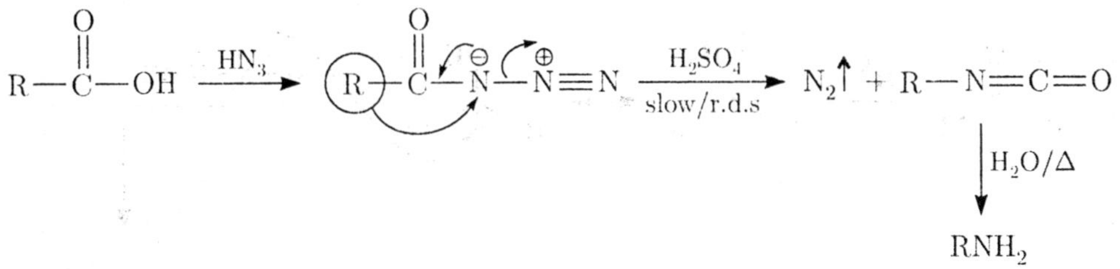

Carbonyl compounds also undergo Schmidt rearrangement, when treated with HN_3 in sulphuric acid (H_2SO_4). Ketones produce amides, while aldehydes yield mixture of nitrile and N-phenyl derivative of amine.

$$R{-}CHO + HN_3 \xrightarrow{\text{conc. } H_2SO_4} RCN + RNHCHO + N_2\uparrow$$

$$R{-}CO{-}R + HN_3 \xrightarrow{\text{conc. } H_2SO_4} RCONHR + N_2\uparrow$$

Mechanism :

(i) ***With acyl azide*** :

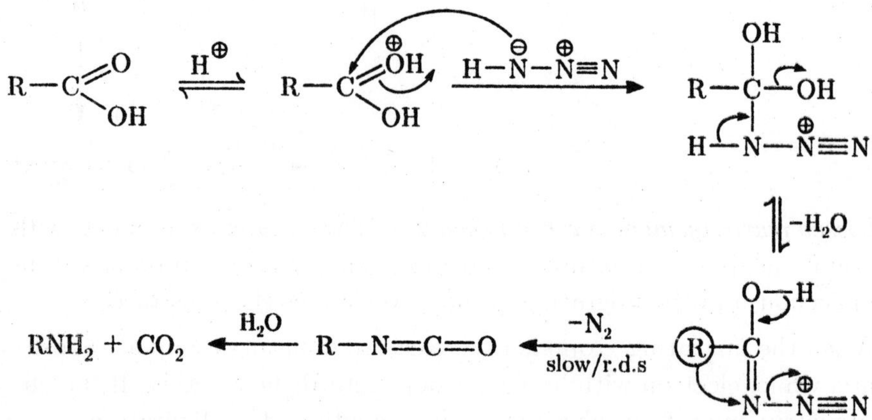

(ii) ***With Carbonyl compounds*** : The carbonyl compounds increase the electrophilicity of carbonyl carbon, by protonation on oxygen and is subsequently attacked by hydrazoic acid (HN_3). This intermediate loses a nitrogen molecule to generate an electron deficient nitrogen to which an alkyl or aryl group migrates followd by hydrolysis and tautomerism.

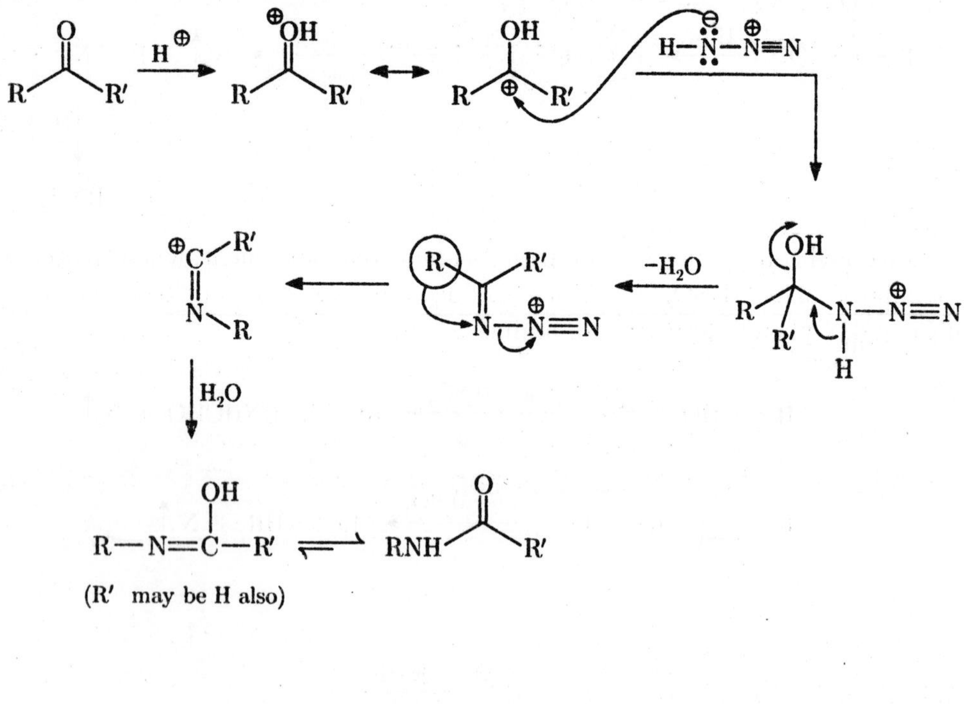

(R′ may be H also)

Structure, Reactivity and Physical Properties of Amines

Aliphatic amines possess an sp^3 hybridised nitrogen atom and the lone pair of electrons reside in one of the four sp^3 hybrid orbitals. As a result, aliphatic amines bear a pyramidal shape.

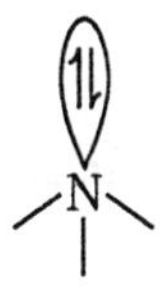

Aromatic amines also have a lone pair of electrons on nitrogen but these electrons are brought into resonance with the π-electrons of the benzene nucleus. As a result, an aromatic amine bears a partial positive charge on nitrogen and the basicity becomes less.

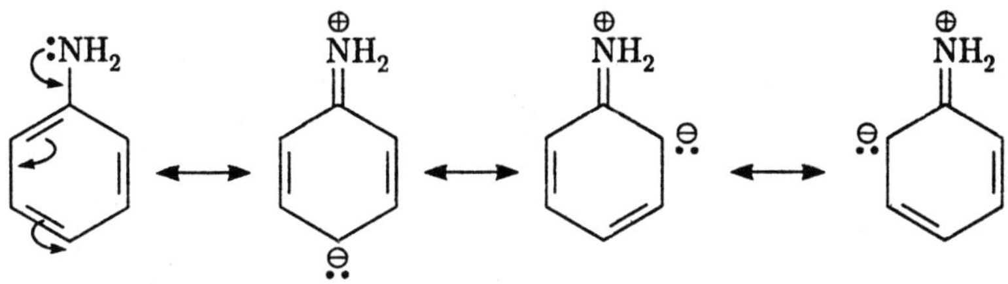

The properties of amines are due to the presence or availability of the lone pair of electrons and also due to the presence of active hydrogen(s) attached to nitrogen.

Amines can form intermolecular hydrogen bonding but the strength of the bond is not found that strong which is present with alcohols. So amines boil at lower temperature compared to corresponding alcohols. Primary and secondary amines can form intramolecular hydrogen bonding through the active hydrogen atoms but tertiary amines can not. So the tertiary amines are lower boiling than primary and secondary ones. Lower amines can form hydrogen bonding with water and hence they become soluble in it. Solubility decreases with increasing molecular weight.

Aromatic amines are practically insoluble in water. $-NH_2$ group has –I and +R effect, where + R effect predominates over –I effect. Ring substituted $-NH_2$, –NHR and $-NR_2$ groups activate the benzene nucleus towards electrophilic substitution faster than benzene. For this reason, aromatic amines do not undergo nucleophilic substitution reactions.

Separation of Primary, Secondary and Tertiary Amines from their Mixture

A mixture of amine salts and quaternary ammonium salts may be separated out as follows.

$$R\overset{\oplus}{N}H_3\overset{\ominus}{X} + R_2\overset{\oplus}{N}H_2\overset{\ominus}{X} + R_3\overset{\oplus}{N}H\overset{\ominus}{X} + R_4\overset{\oplus}{N}\overset{\ominus}{X} \xrightarrow[\text{distillation}]{\text{NaOH}} \begin{cases} \xrightarrow{\text{residue}} R_4\overset{\oplus}{N}\overset{\ominus}{O}H \\ \xrightarrow{\text{distillate}} RNH_2 + R_2NH + R_3N \end{cases}$$

Then the three types of amines may be separated by any one of the following processes.

1. Hofmann's Method

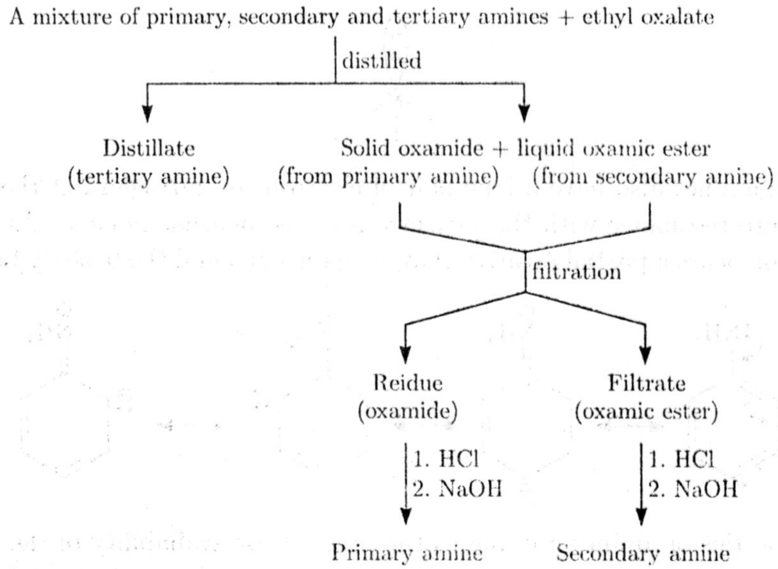

Reactions involved :

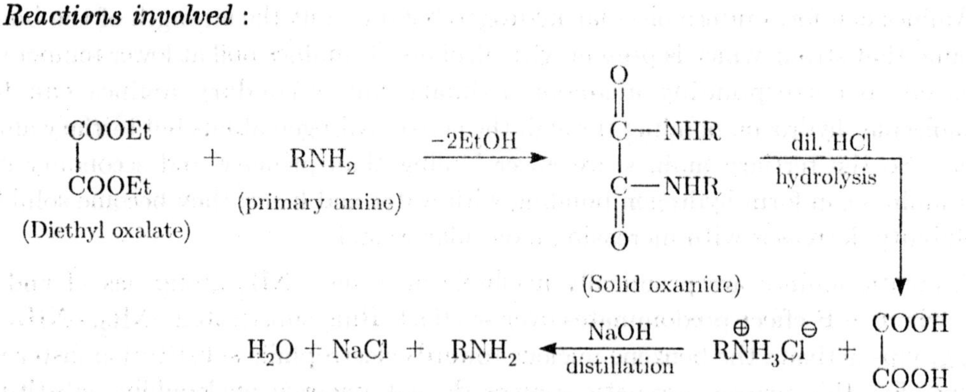

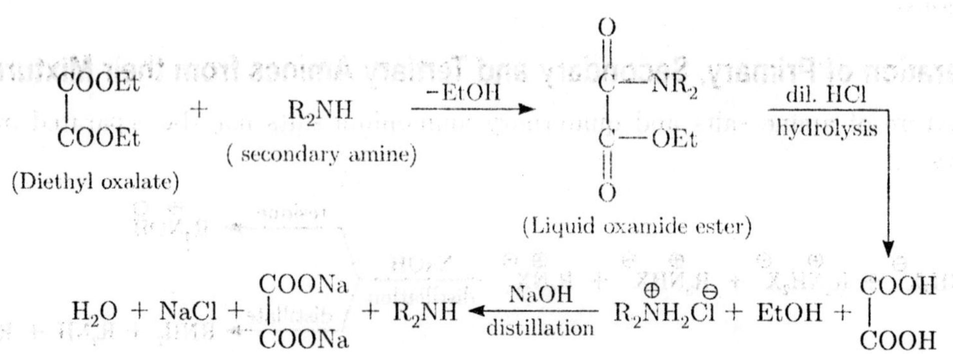

2. Hinsberg's Method by *p*-toluenesulphonyl Chloride

$$R_3N + R_2NH + RNH_2$$

$\downarrow$ $p\text{-}CH_3C_6H_4SO_2Cl$

$$R_3N + p\text{-}CH_3C_6H_4SO_2NHR + p\text{-}CH_3C_6H_4SO_2NR_2$$

$\downarrow$ Distilled

$$(p\text{-}CH_3C_6H_4SO_2NHR + p\text{-}CH_3C_6H_4SO_2NR_2) + R_3N$$

(In the distilling flask) Distillate (distils over)

$\downarrow$ Aqueous KOH

$$(p\text{-}CH_3C_6H_4SO_2\ddot{N}R_2 + p\text{-}CH_3C_6H_4SO_2\ddot{\overset{\ominus}{N}}R\ K^{\oplus})$$

(Solid) Potassium salt (Soluble)

$\downarrow$ filtered

$(p\text{-}CH_3C_6H_4SO_2NR_2$(residue)	$p\text{-}CH_3C_6H_4SO_2\ddot{\overset{\ominus}{N}}R\ K^{\oplus}$ (filtrate)
$\downarrow$ 25% HCl, H_2O	$\downarrow$ 25% HCl, H_2O
$R_2\overset{\oplus}{N}H_2\overset{\ominus}{Cl}$	$R\overset{\oplus}{N}H_3\overset{\ominus}{Cl}$
$\downarrow$ Aqueous NaOH/distilled	$\downarrow$ Aqueous NaOH/distilled
R_2NH	RNH_2
(Secondary amine)	(Primary amine)

Distinction Between Primary, Secondary and Tertiary Amines

1. ***Reaction with Nitrous Acid*** :

A. ***Aliphatic primary amines*** on reaction with nitrous acid gives alcohols and nitrogen is evolved.

$$NaNO_2 + \text{dilute } HCl \longrightarrow NaCl + HNO_2 \quad (\text{generated } \textit{in situ})$$

$$CH_3CH_2CH_2NH_2 + HNO_2 \longrightarrow CH_3CH_2CH_2OH + N_2\uparrow + H_2O$$

Mechanism :

$$HO{-}N{=}O \xrightarrow{H^{\oplus}} H_2\overset{\oplus}{O}{-}N{=}O \longrightarrow \overset{\oplus}{N}{=}O \text{ (Nitrosonium cation)} + H_2O$$

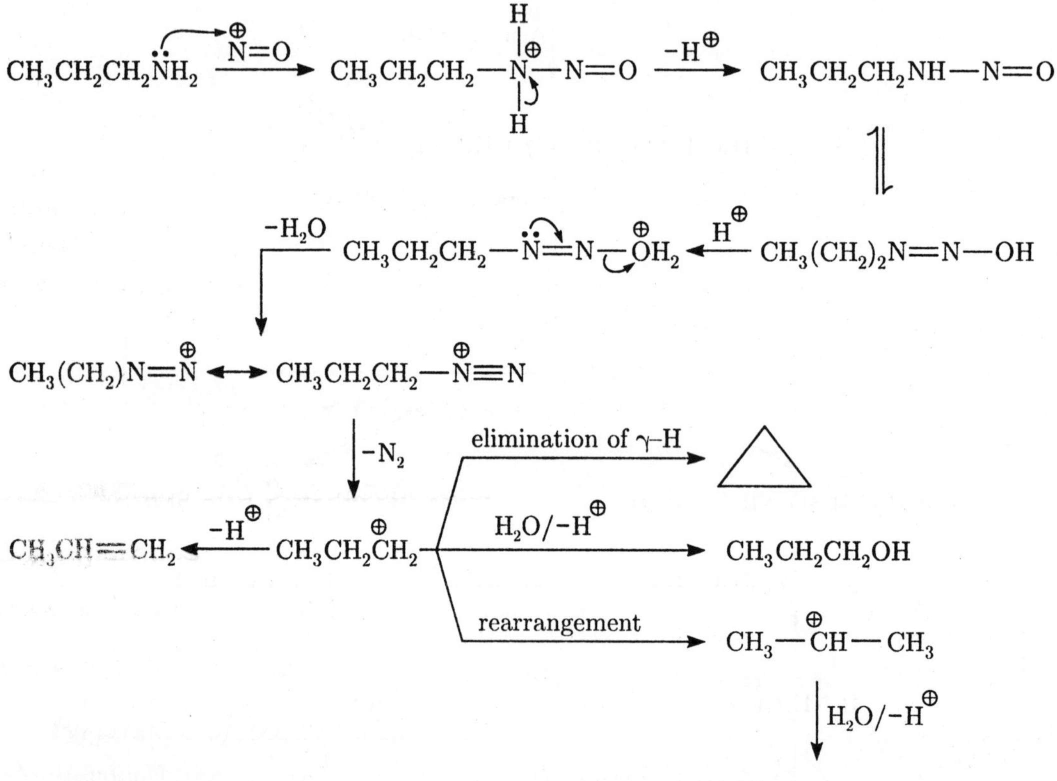

B. ***An aromatic primary amine*** forms arenediazonium salt on treatment with nitrous acid. The general features for arenediazonium salts are as follows.

(a) Arenediazonium salts at low temperatures (0°-5°C) are more stable than aliphatic diazonium salts as the former is resonance stabilised.

$$Ph{-}\overset{\oplus}{N}{\equiv}\ddot{N} \longleftrightarrow Ph{-}N{=}\overset{\oplus}{N}$$

(b) Phenyl cation is not formed like corresponding aliphatic carbocation on treatment with nitrous acid. Phenyl cation is unstable as the electron lost from the unhybridised *p*-orbital lies perpendicular to the benzene ring. As a result, π-electrons from the ring can not stabilise the positive charge by delocalisation.

Mechanism of diazotization reaction :

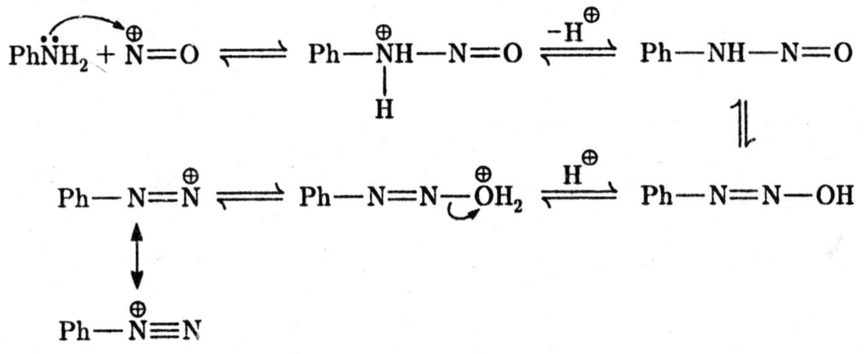

2. *A secondary amine, aliphatic or aromatic* forms an N-nitrosoamines usually separate from the reaction mixture as *oily yellow liquids.* N-nitrosoamines can be identified by Libermann's nitrosoamine test (mixture of nitrosoamines + few crystals of phenol + conc. H_2SO_4 → green solution + NaOH solution → deep blue colouration). Therefore, treatment of secondary amine with nitrous acid followd by Libermann's test is a confirmatory test for secondary amines.

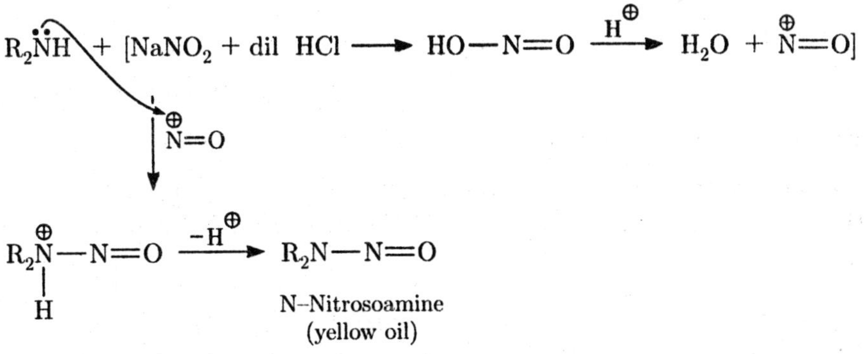

Libermann's test for secondary amines

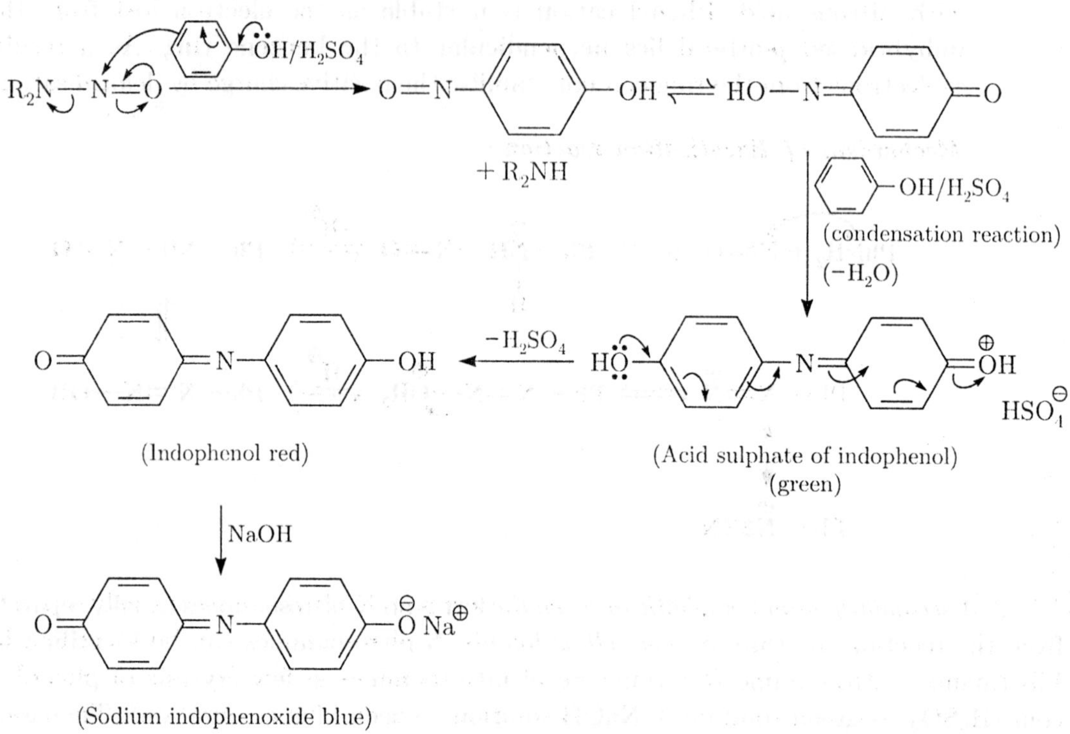

3. When a *tertiary aliphatic amine* is mixed with nitrous acid, an equilibrium is established among the tertiary amine, its salt and N-nitrosoammonium compound.

$$2R_3N\text{:} + HX + NaNO_2 \rightleftharpoons \underset{\text{(Amine salt)}}{R_3\overset{\oplus}{N}H\overset{\ominus}{X}} + \underset{\text{(N-nitrosoammonium compound)}}{R_3\overset{\oplus}{N}-N=O\ \overset{\ominus}{X}}$$

N-nitrosoammonium compounds are stable at low temperatures.

Tertiary arylamines react with nitrous acid to form C-nitroso aromatic compounds. Nitrosation takes place almost exclusively at the *p*-position if it is open and if not at the *o*-position.

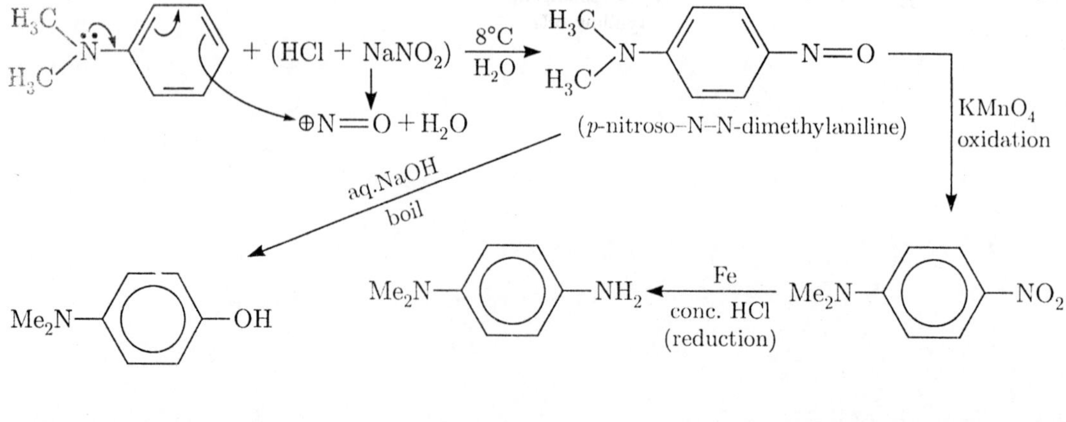

2. Reaction with Carbon Disulphide (Hofmann's Mustard oil Reaction)

This is a differential reaction for the three classes of aliphatic amines.

(a) 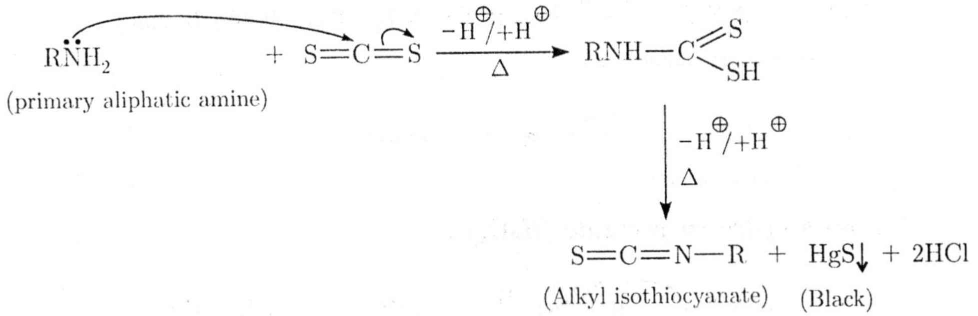

(b) $$\underset{\text{(Secondary aliphatic amine)}}{R_2NH} + S{=}C{=}S \xrightarrow[-\overset{\oplus}{H}/+\overset{\oplus}{H}]{\Delta} S{=}C{-}C\begin{smallmatrix}NR_2\\SH\end{smallmatrix} \xrightarrow{HgCl_2/\Delta} \text{No reaction}$$

(c) $$\underset{\text{(tertiary aliphatic amine)}}{R_3N} + S{=}C{=}S \xrightarrow{\Delta} \text{No reaction}$$

(d) $$CS_2 + 2PhNH_2 + 2KOH \longrightarrow S{=}C(NHPh)_2 + K_2S + H_2O \xrightarrow{\text{conc. HCl}} \underset{\text{(Phenyl isothiocyanate)}}{Ph{-}N{=}C{=}S}$$

3. Oxidation of Primary, Secondary and tertiary Amines

(a) ***With potassium permanganate ($KMnO_4$)*** :

(i) 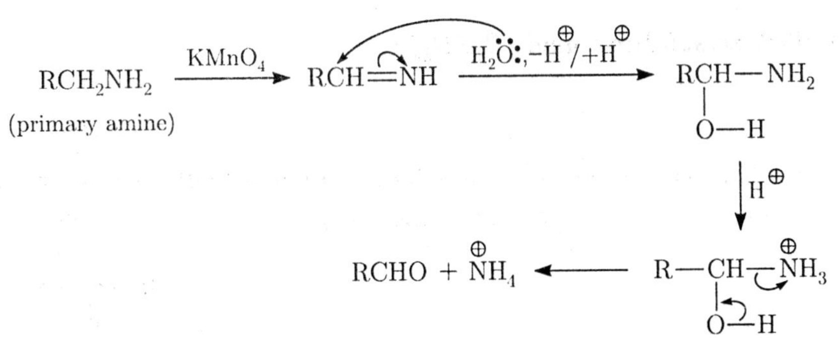

(ii) $$\underset{\text{(primary amine)}}{R_2CHNH_2} \xrightarrow{KMnO_4} R_2CH{=}NH \xrightarrow{H_2O/\overset{\oplus}{H}} R_2C{=}O + \overset{\oplus}{N}H_4$$

(iii) $R_2CNH_2 \xrightarrow{KMnO_4} R_2CNO_2$

(primary amine with tertiary alkyl group)

(iv) $R_2NH \xrightarrow{KMnO_4} R_2N{-}NR_2$ (Tetraalkylhydrazine)

(secondary amine)

(v) $R_3N \xrightarrow{KMnO_4}$ No reaction

(tertiary amine)

(b) ***With hydrogen peroxide (H_2O_2) :***

(i) 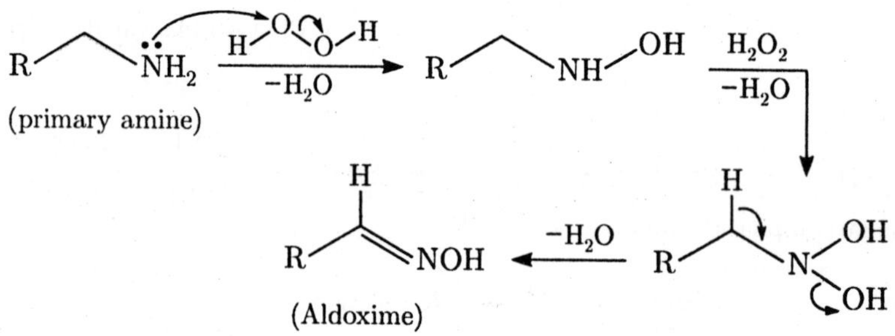

(ii) 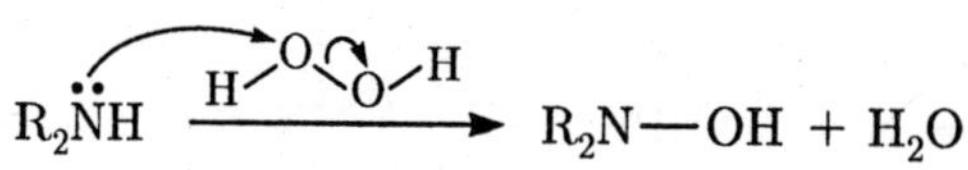

(secondary amine)

(iii) 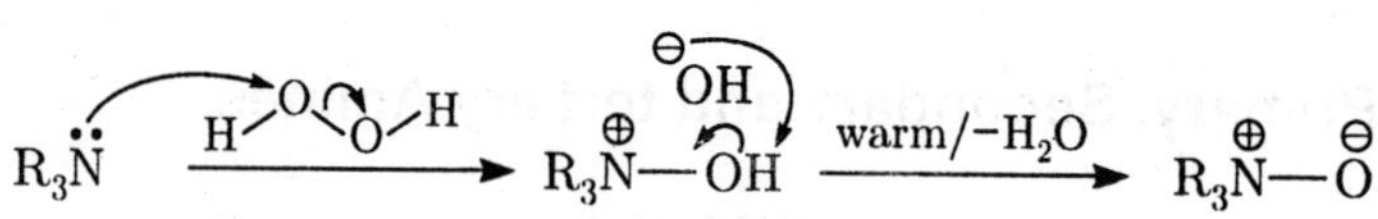

(tertiary amine)

(amine-N-oxide)

(c) ***With persulphuric acid (H_2SO_5) :***

(i) 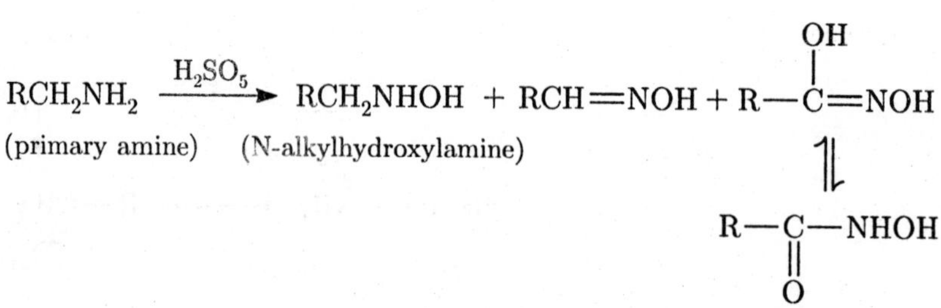

(Hydroxamic acid)

(ii) $R_2CHNH_2 \xrightarrow{H_2SO_5} R_2C{=}NOH$

(primary amine)

(iii) $R_3CNH_2 \xrightarrow{H_2SO_5} R_3CNO$ (Tertiary nitrosoalkane)

(primary amine with tertiary alkyl group)

(iv) $R_2NH \xrightarrow{H_2SO_5} R_2N—OH$ (N-N-dialkylhydroxylamine)

(secondary amine)

(v) $R_3N \xrightarrow{H_2SO_5 \text{ or } H_2O_2 \text{ or } O_3} R_3\overset{\oplus}{N}—\overset{\ominus}{O} \xrightarrow{\Delta}$ Cope reaction

(tertiary amine)

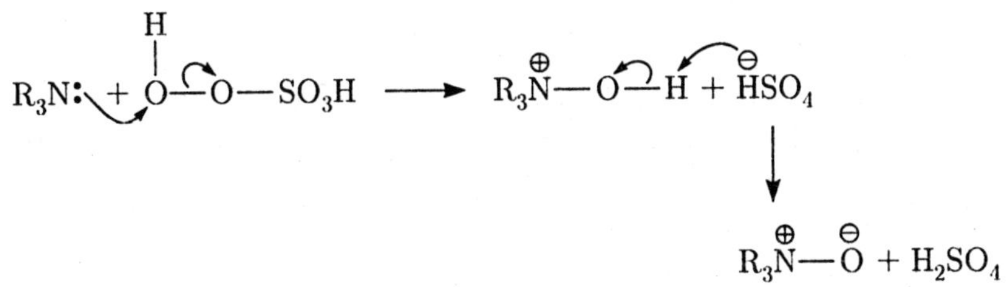

(d) ***Different oxidation products of aniline***

(i) $PhNH_2 \xrightarrow{(NH_4)S_2O_8/H_2SO_4} Ph—N{=}O$

(ii) $PhNH_2 \xrightarrow{H_2CrO_4}$ 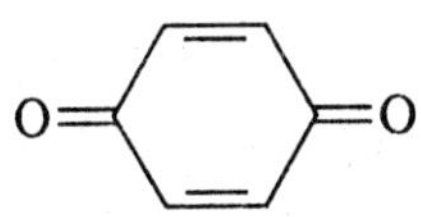

(iii) $PhNH_2 \xrightarrow{NaOCl}$ 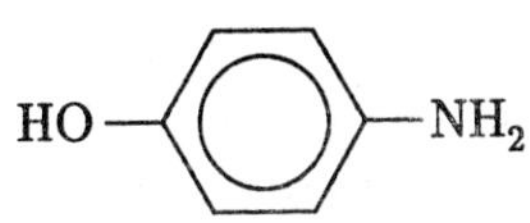

(iv) $PhNH_2 \xrightarrow{H_2SO_5} Ph—N{=}O + H_2SO_4$

Reactions Given by Amines

1. Amines being basic (contains lone pair of electrons on nitrogen) in nature, they form salts with acids.

$$RNH_2 + HA \longrightarrow R\overset{\oplus}{N}H_3\,\overset{\ominus}{A}$$

$$R_2NH + HA \longrightarrow R_2\overset{\oplus}{N}H_2\,\overset{\ominus}{A}$$

$$R_3N + HA \longrightarrow R_3\overset{\oplus}{N}H\,\overset{\ominus}{A}$$

2. ***Pyrolysis of ammonium salt*** : When tertiary ammonium salts are heated, secondary amines are formed, whereas on heating secondary ammonium salts, a primary amine is formed.

$$R_3\overset{\oplus}{N}H\ \overset{\ominus}{X} \xrightarrow{\Delta} R_2NH + HX$$

$$R_2NH + HCl \longrightarrow R_2\overset{\oplus}{N}H_2\overset{\ominus}{Cl} \xrightarrow{\Delta} RNH_2 + RCl \xrightarrow{HCl} R\overset{\oplus}{N}H_3\overset{\ominus}{Cl}$$

$$R\overset{\oplus}{N}H_3\overset{\ominus}{Cl} \xrightarrow{\Delta} NH_3 + RCl$$

$$NH_3 + RCl \xrightarrow{HCl} NH_4Cl$$

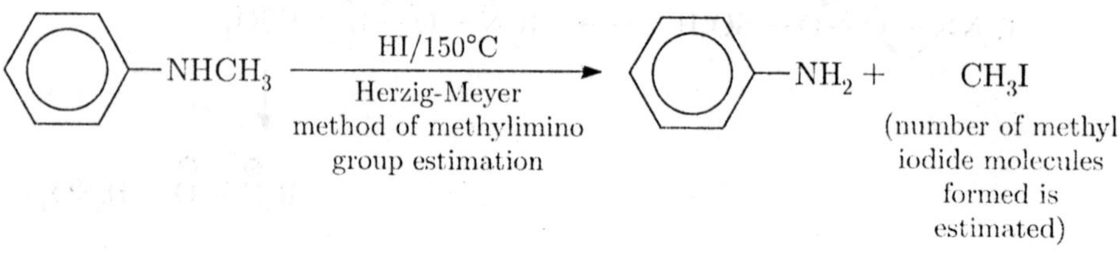

3. ***The Hofmann Exhaustive Methylation Reaction*** : The process involves converting amines *viz* primary, secondary or tertiary to an unsaturated compound by pyrolytic decomposition of quaternary ammonium hydroxides of the amines. The quaternary ammonium hydroxides are obtained by treating the amines with excess of methyl iodide (MeI), followed by the hydrolysis of the resulting quaternary ammonium iodide with moist Ag_2O (AgOH is generated *in situ*). Silver halide precipitates from the solution and can be removed by filtration. Although most eliminations involving neutral substrates tend to follow saytreff rule, eliminations with charged substrates tend to follow what is called the Hofmann rule and *yield mainly the least substituted alkene.* The products are identified after the pyrolysis of corresponding ammonium hydroxides and the process is known as Hofmann's exhaustive methylation.

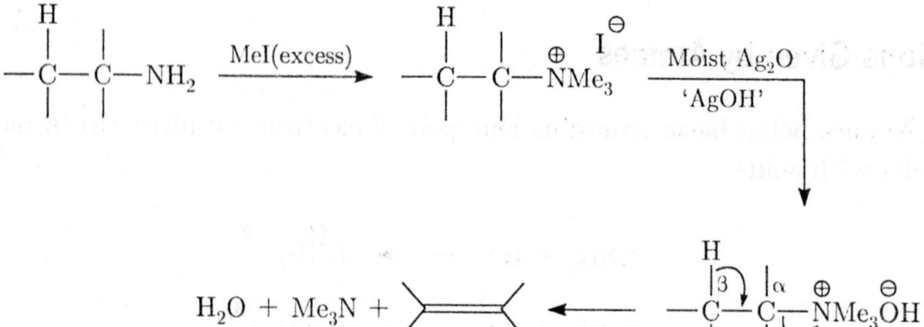

Thus, the process consists of following steps :

1. The exhaustive methylation of the amine; this step involves the treatment of the amine with a large excess of MeI, a quaternary ammonium iodide is formed.

$$CH_3CH_2NH_2 \xrightarrow{3MeI} CH_3CH_2\overset{\oplus}{N}Me_3\overset{\ominus}{I}$$

2. Formation of the quaternary ammonium hydroxide

$$CH_3CH_2\overset{\oplus}{N}Me_3\overset{\ominus}{I} \xrightarrow{\text{Moist } Ag_2O \text{ ('AgOH')}} CH_3CH_2\overset{\oplus}{N}Me_3\,\overset{\ominus}{OH} + AgI\downarrow$$

3. The pyrolysis of quaternary ammonium hydroxide.

$$CH_3CH_2\overset{\oplus}{N}Me_3\,\overset{\ominus}{OH} \xrightarrow{\text{aqueous or alcoholic solution}/\Delta/100°C} CH_2{=}CH_2 + Me_3N + H_2O$$

4. Identification of the products after pyrolysis. This method is exclusively used to elucidate the structure of the alkaloids.

Mechanism of Hofmann's exhaustive methylation reaction :

Step 1 : $R\ddot{N}H_2 + CH_3{-}I \xrightarrow{S_N2} RNHCH_3 + HI \xrightarrow{CH_3I/S_N2} RN(CH_3)_2 + HI \xrightarrow{CH_3I/S_N2} R\overset{\oplus}{N}Me_3\overset{\ominus}{I}$

Step 2 : $R\overset{\oplus}{N}Me_3\,\overset{\ominus}{I} \xrightarrow[\text{exchange}]{\text{'AgOH'}} R\overset{\oplus}{N}Me_3\,\overset{\ominus}{OH} + AgI\downarrow$

Step 3 :

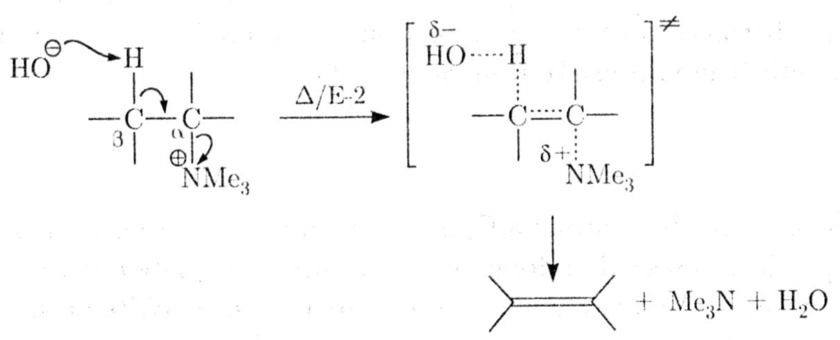

For the elimination to occur, both the eliminating groups acquire antiperiplanar conformation. The most acidic hydrogen from the less sterically hindered β-carbon gets eliminated. The leaving group ($Me_3\overset{\oplus}{N}$– or L) is positively charged and so with strong –I effect increases the acidity of C_β–H and the polarisability of C_β–H bond also increases.

As a result, C–H bond breaks before the C–L bond cleavage, and transition state formed has considerable *carbanionic character.* If the β-carbon contains any group with +I effect, the stability of carbanion decreases and in the presence of groups containing –I effect, the stability of carbanion increases. So with quaternary ammonium salt, proton is eliminated from that β-carbon which has least number of alkyl groups (+I effect), or in other words, β–H is abstracted from least substituted β-carbon atom.

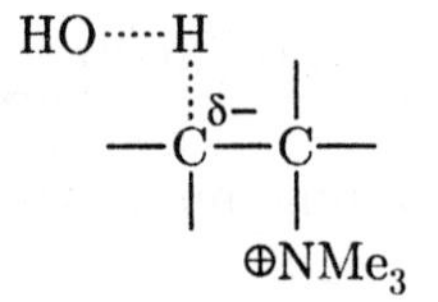

(Carbanion like T.S. in Hofmann elimination)

The stereoelectronic factor of E-2 elimination is that the eliminating group and β–H should be antiperiplanar to each other. So gauche interactions are present between L and other group joined to β-carbon atom. If the size of groups joined to β–C increases, then the extent of gauche interactions increase and the $\Delta G^{\neq}$ for the formation of transition state increases as steric strain increases. For this reason, β–H is abstracted from that carbon atom which contains comparatively smaller groups and we get less substituted alkene.

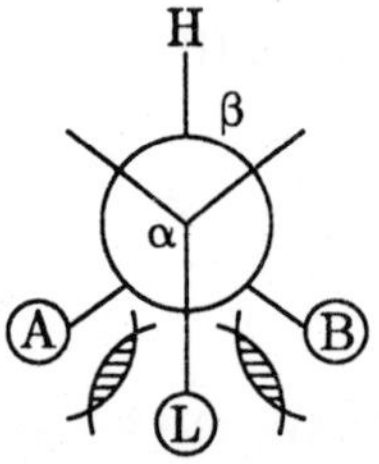

With increasing sizes of A and B, the extent of gauche interaction increases and the transition state becomes unstable. Elimination is favoured if A and B are small or preferably not substituted (only H atom is present).

Problems

1. A nitrogeneous base formula C_4H_5N, on complete hydrogenation give C_4H_9N. C_4H_9N when subjected to Hofmann's exhaustive methylation twice; 1,3-butadiene, trimethylamine and two moles of water are obtained. Write down the structure of the organic base.

   Ans. : Since the compound absorbs two moles of hydrogen (H_2), it is expected to contain either two double bonds or one triple bond. C:H ratio shows that C_4H_9N is fully saturated and cyclic, and contains only one N atom as one mole of Me_3N is produced.

Ans. :

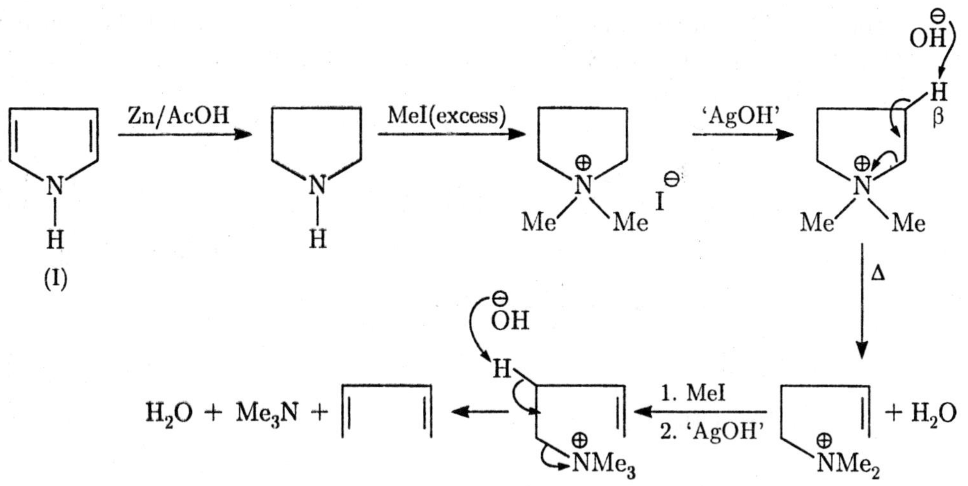

So pyrrole(I) is the original base.

2. Synthesise 1, 4-pentadiene from pyridine.

Ans. :

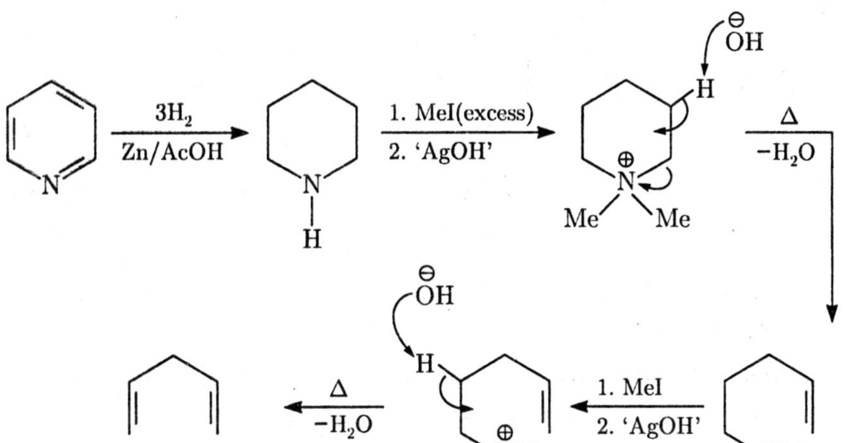

(1,4-pentadiene)

3. Predict the major alkene for the following reaction :

$$CH_3CH_2CH_2\overset{\oplus}{N}(CH_3)_2C_2H_5\overset{\ominus}{O}H \xrightarrow{\Delta}$$

Ans. :

$$\underset{(+I)}{CH_3}-\overset{H}{\underset{\beta'}{C}}H-CH_2-\overset{\oplus}{\underset{CH_3\ \ CH_3}{N}}-\underset{\alpha}{C}H_2-\overset{H}{\underset{\beta}{C}}H_2 \ \ \overset{\ominus}{O}H \xrightarrow{\Delta} CH_3CH_2CH_2NMe_2 + \underset{(Major)}{CH_2{=}CH_2}$$

Terminal CH_3 at the other β-carbon being +I in nature, destabilises the carbanion like trnsition state and the alternate β-elimination occurs when $CH_2{=}CH_2$ is the major alkene formed.

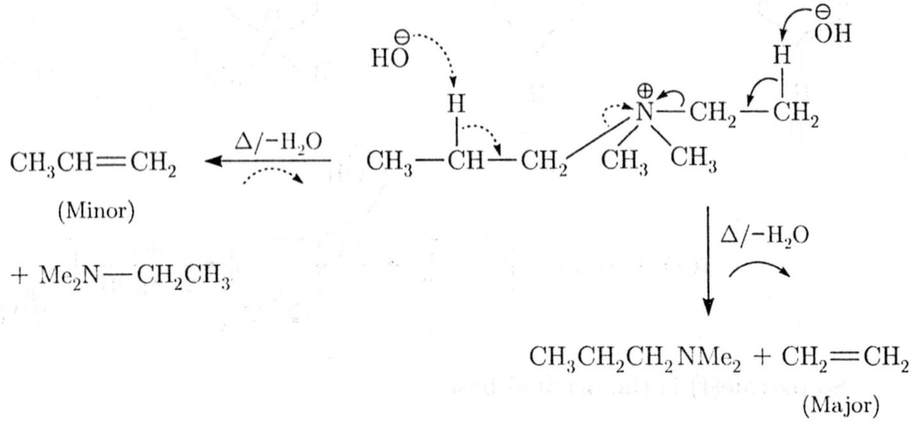

4. Give an example when no alkene is obtained by Hofmann reaction with a quarternary ammonium hydroxide.

Ans. :

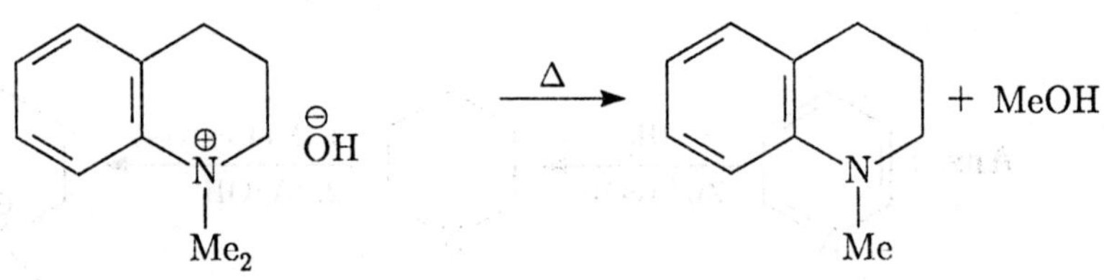

(Quaternised tetrahydroquinoline))

5. Give an example where Hofmann's rule is not followed by heating a quarternary ammonium hydroxide.

Ans. : In some cases, Hofmann's rule is not followed, *e.g.*, styrene and not ethylene is formed in the following elimination.

$$PhCH_2CH_2\overset{\oplus}{N}Me_2Et \xrightarrow{\overset{\ominus}{O}H/\Delta} PhCH{=}CH_2 + Me_2NHEt + H_2O$$

Ans. : This may be explained on the basis that, β–H adjacent to the benzene ring (benzylic hydrogen) is more acidic than the β-hydrogen of ethyl group.

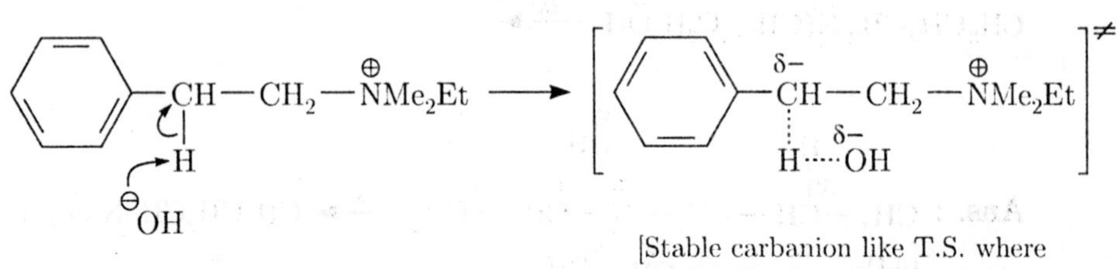

[Stable carbanion like T.S. where delocalisation of the negative occurs over the phenyl ring]

The Cope Elimination

Tertiary amine oxides undergo the elimination of a dialkylhydroxylamine when they are heated. This reaction is called the Cope elimination.

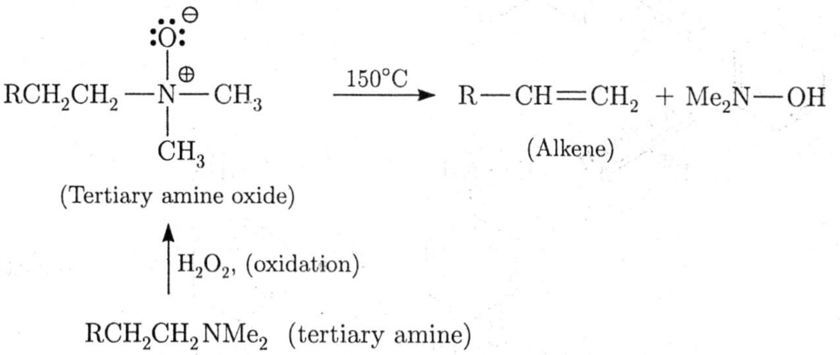

Cope elimination is a *syn* elimination and proceeds through a cyclic transition state.

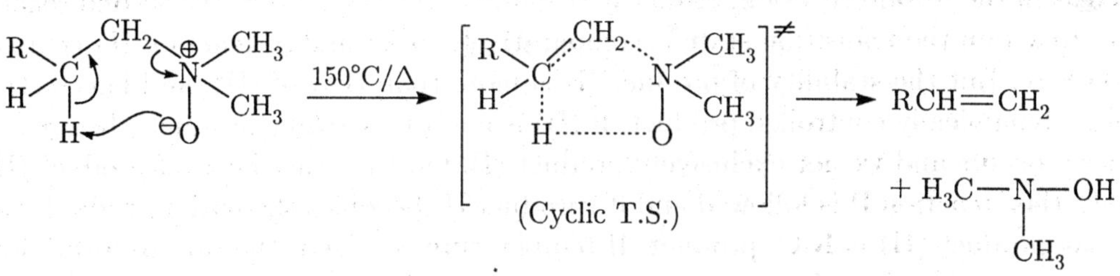

Example :

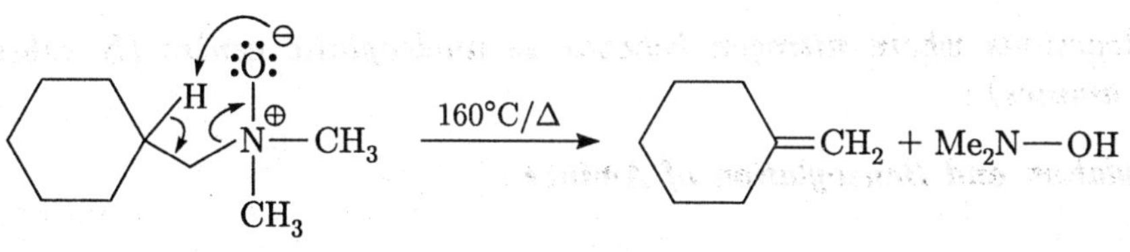

Aromatic Amine – An Ambident Nucleophile

When a benzene ring contains substituents like $-\ddot{N}H_2$ or $-\ddot{O}H$, *i.e.*, heteroatom belonging to second period of the periodic table having lone pair of electron(s), it can act as an ambident nucleophile, as these group themselves can behave as nucleophiles. For this reason, two parallel *reactions* may occur. In one reaction, electrophile gives rise to the ring substitution and in another case electrophilic addition occurs to $-\ddot{N}H_2$ (or $-\ddot{O}H$) group.

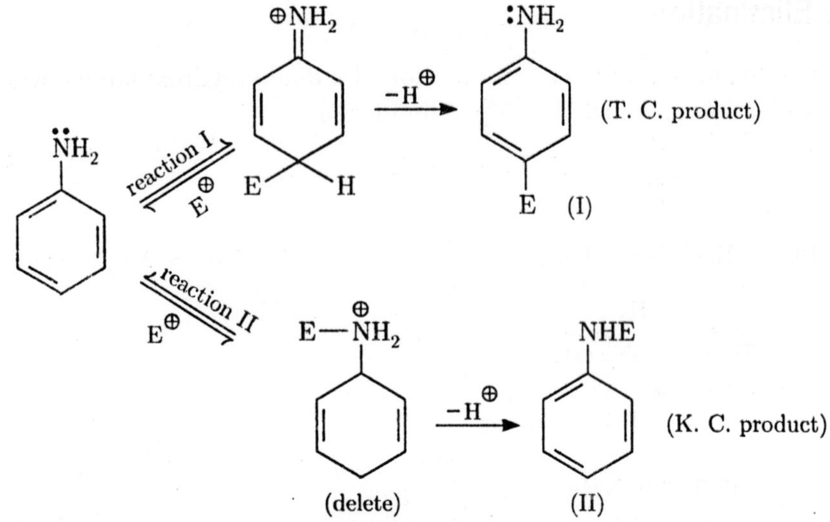

In the first reaction, the transition state is formed where aromatic stability is lost, whereas in the second reaction, aromatic stability is retained. So in the second reaction, $\Delta G^{\neq}$ to attain the transition state is comparatively lower and so reaction II occurs at a faster rate. But the stability of product (I) is more than that of (II), and hence (I) is a thermodynamically controlled product. If (II) is not a very stable product, then reaction II never occurs and we get exclusively product (I). On the other head, if product (II) is stable, then reaction II is followed and it (product II) becomes the major product. So we can say product (II) is K.C. product. If temperature is raised, the rate of formation of T.C. product (product I) increases and if product II (K.C. product) is heated for a prolonged time, it gets converted to product I, *i.e.*, T.C. product. So aromatic amines behave as ambident nucleophiles where we get both N-substituted product and C–substituted product upon electrophilic substitution.

A. ***Reactions where nitrogen behaves as nucleophilic centre (N–substitution of aromatic amines)*** :

Acetylation and Benzoylation of Amines :

(a) $R\ddot{N}H_2 \xrightarrow[\text{pyridine}]{CH_3COCl \text{ or } CH_3-\overset{O}{\overset{\|}{C}}-O-\overset{O}{\overset{\|}{C}}-CH_3} RNH-\overset{O}{\overset{\|}{C}}-CH_3$ (Monoacetyl amine) $\xrightarrow[\text{pyridine}]{CH_3COCl \text{ or } Ac_2O}$ $RN(COCH_3)_2$ (Diacetylamine)

(b) $RNH_2 \xrightarrow[\text{pyridine}]{PhCOCl} RNHCOPh \xrightarrow[\text{pyridine}]{PhCOCl} RN(COPh)_2$

(c) $R_2NH \xrightarrow[\text{pyridine}]{\text{PhCOCl or } Ac_2O} R_2NCOCH_3/R_2NCOPh$

(d) $PhNH_2 \xrightarrow[\text{pyridine}]{CH_3COCl \text{ or } Ac_2O} Ph\overset{H}{N}COCH_3 \xrightarrow[\text{pyridine}]{CH_3COCl \text{ or } Ac_2O} PhN(COCH_3)_2$

(e) $PhNH_2 \xrightarrow[\text{pyridine}]{PhCOCl} PhNHCOPh$

Mechanism of the reaction :

The reaction follows a tetrahedral pathway.

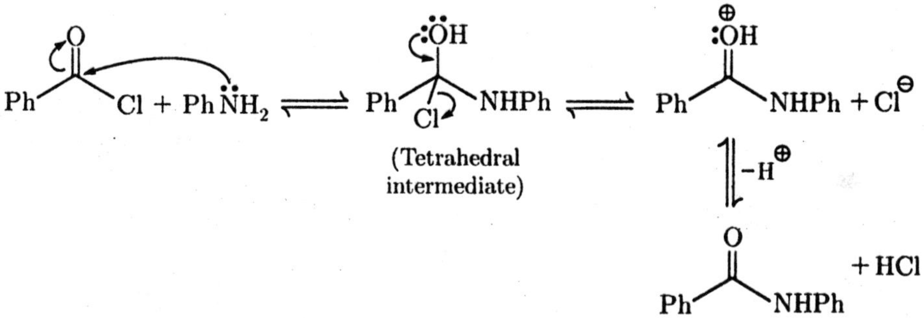

Acylation and benzoylation reactions are reversible and can revert to original amines in the presence of acids formed during the reaction. To avoid hydrolysis, the acid formed is removed by pyridine as pyridinium salts. Acetyl and benzoyl derivatives have sharp melting points. Phenols and amines can be identified from their corresponding acetyl and benzoyl derivatives.

B. ***Reactions where carbon behaves as nucleophilic centre (C–substitution or ring substitution of aromatic amines).***

Phenols and aromatic amines activate the aromatic ring and produce polysubstituted derivatives through aromatic electrophilic substitution. This high reactivity decreases when phenolic –OH or aromatic $-NH_2$ are acetylated or benzoylated. Generally monosubstituted product is formed.

Examples :

1. ***Bromination of aniline***

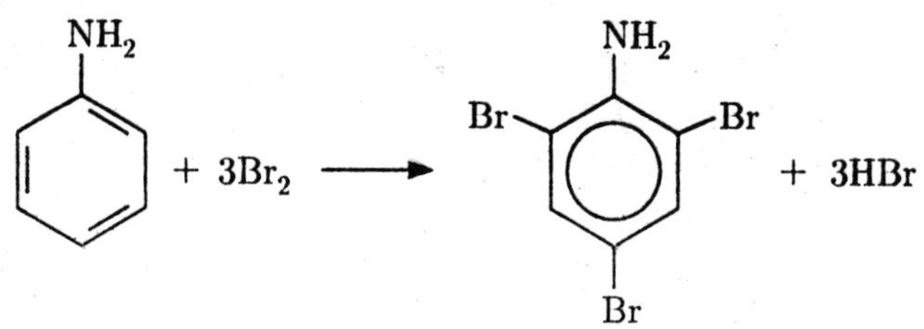

(1,3,5-tribromoaniline)

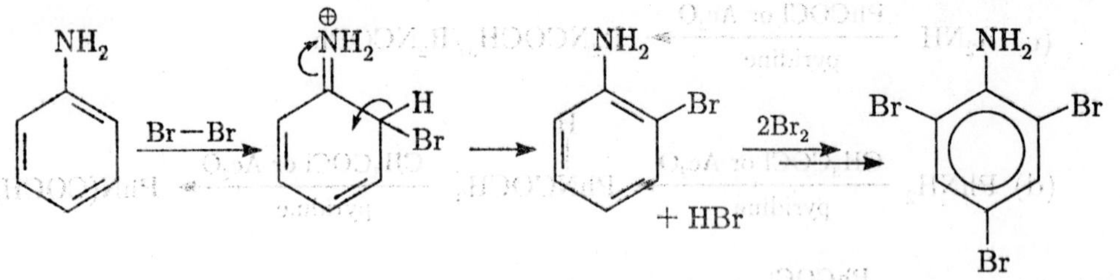

2.

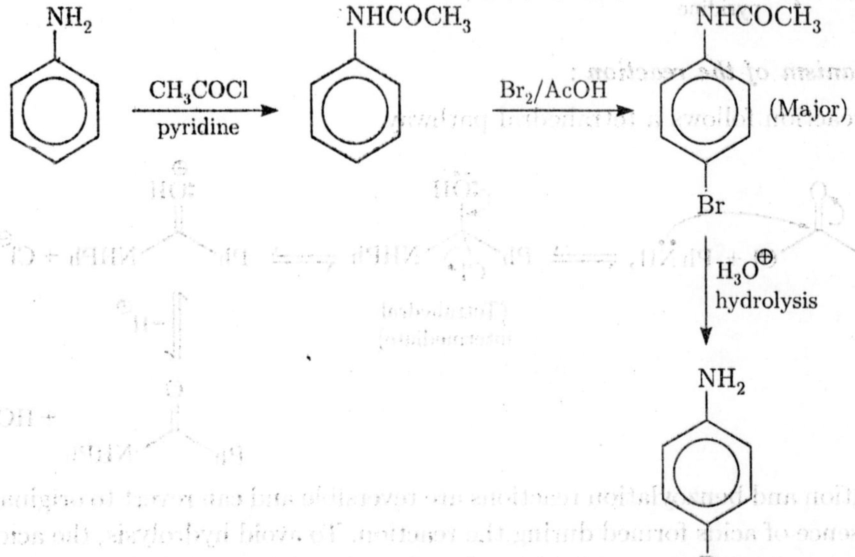

3. ***Synthesis of p-nitroaniline***

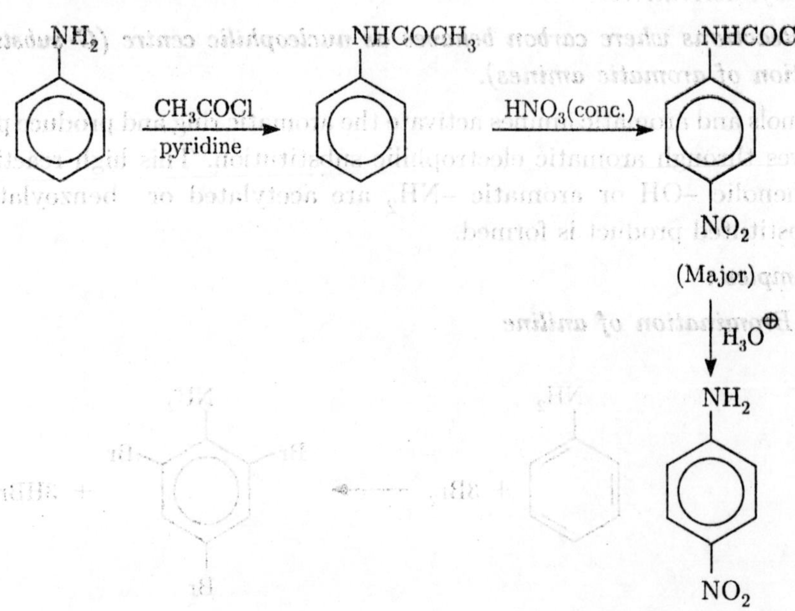

(*p*-nitroaniline)

4. ***Synthesis of sulphanilic acid***

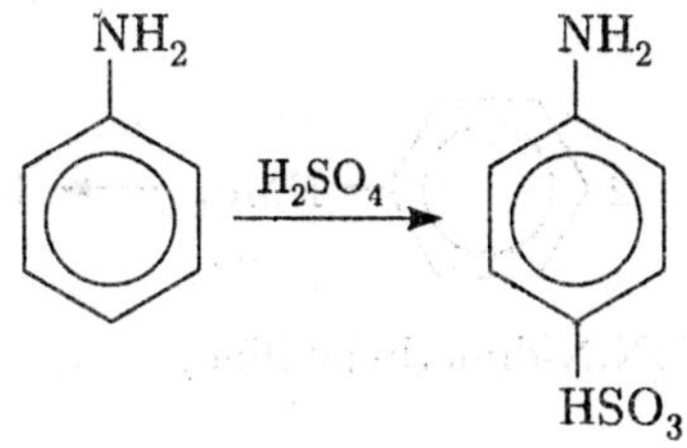

(Sulphanilic acid)

Mechanism :

$$H_2SO_4 \rightleftharpoons H^{\oplus} + HSO_4^{\ominus}$$

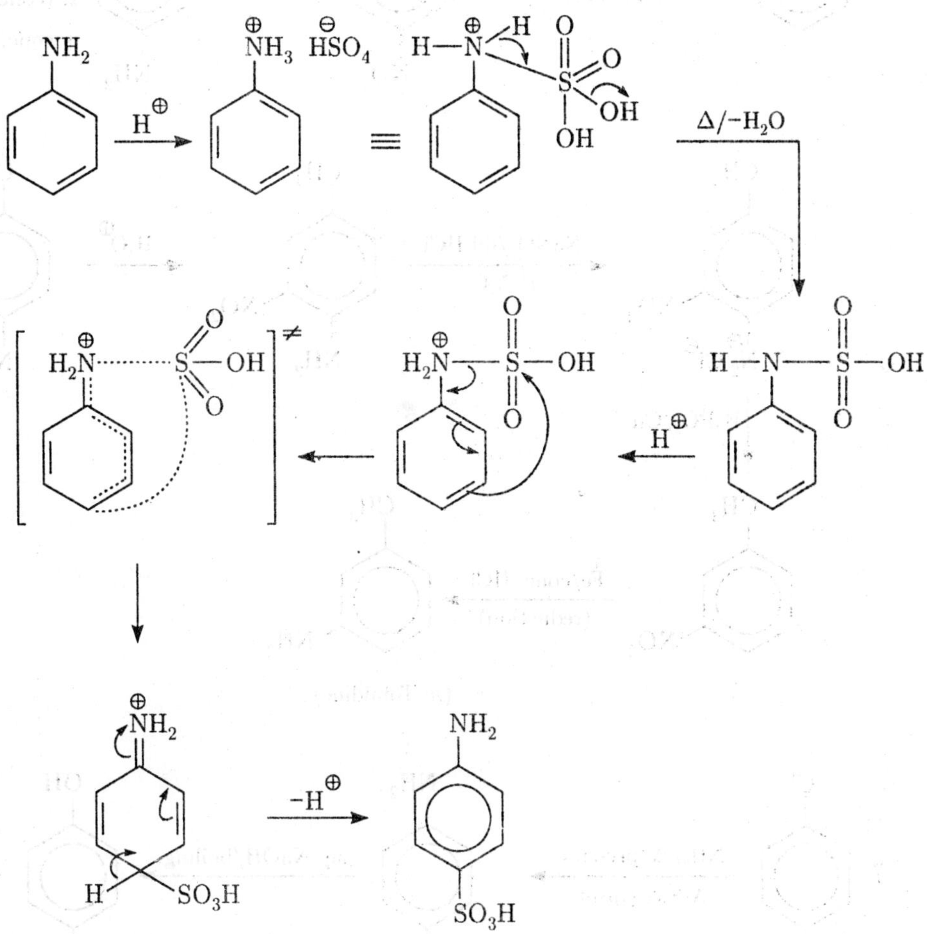

(Sulphanilic acid)

5. ***Preparation of Michler's ketone***

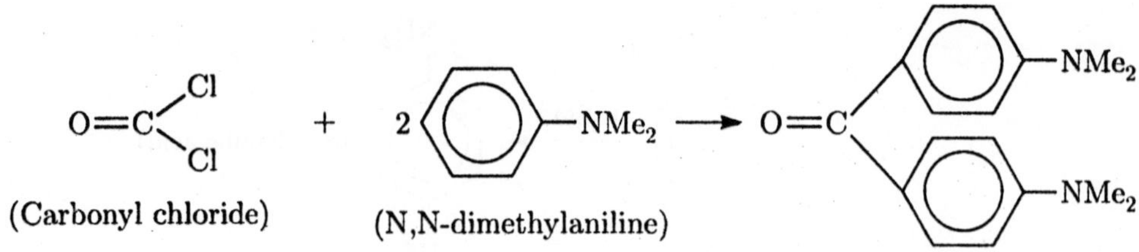

(Mischler's ketone)

6. ***Preparation of m-toluidine***

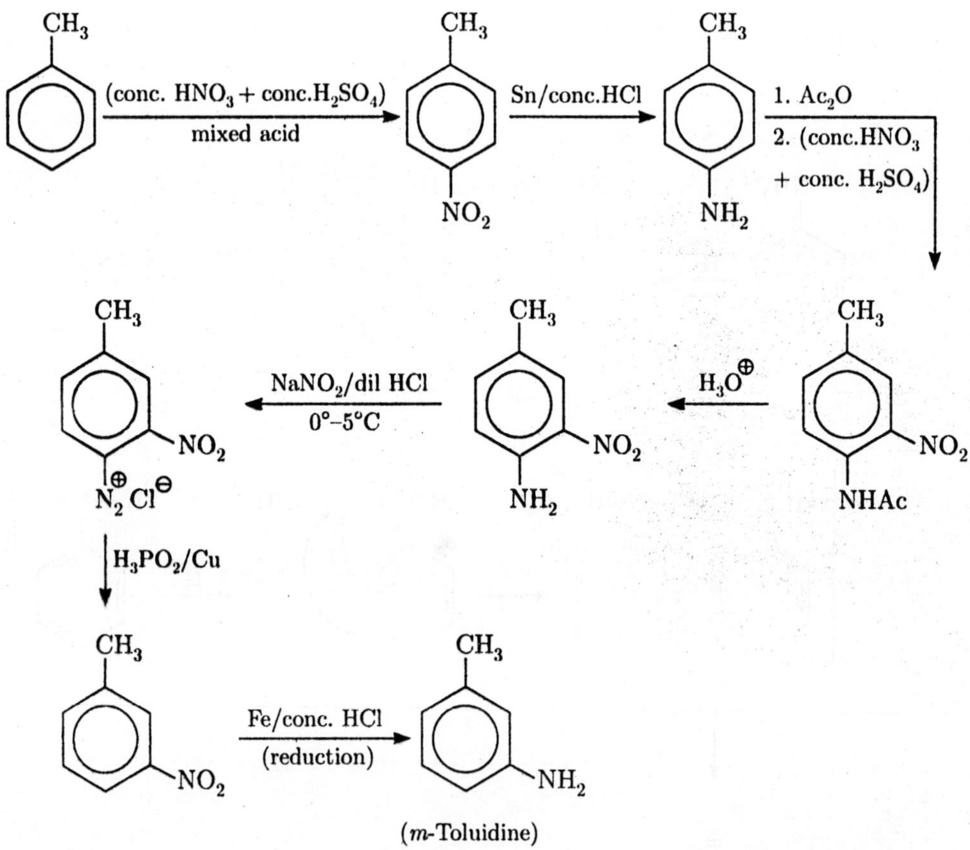

(*m*-Toluidine)

7. 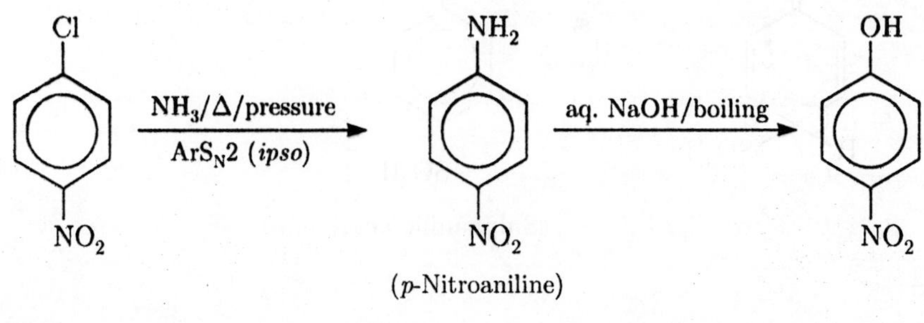

(*p*-Nitroaniline)

Other important reactions given by amines :

1. ***The Mannich reaction***

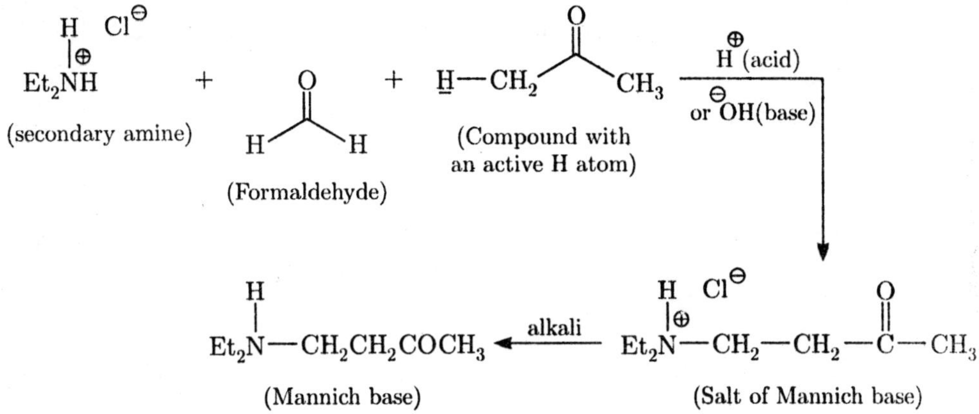

2. ***Formation of isocyanides***

$$R\ddot{N}H_2 + CHCl_3 + 3KOH \xrightarrow{\Delta} R{-}NC + 3KCl + 3H_2O$$

(primary alkyl or arylamine) (Alkyl or arylisocyanide) (carbylamine)

3. ***Formation of N-alkyl or arylaldimine***

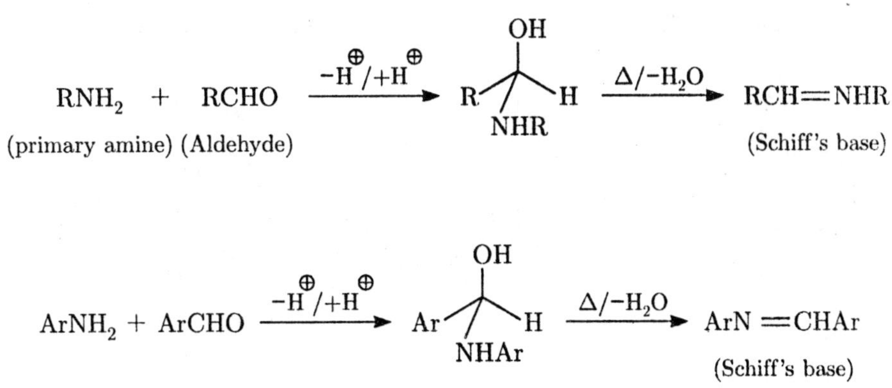

4. ***Hofmann-Martius Rearrangement*** : The thermal rearrangement of tri- and dialkylanilines as their hydrochlorides to salts of C- alkylanilines where an alkyl group migrating from the nitrogen and preferably entering to *para* position, or if the *para* position is occupied, to the *ortho*- position, is called Hofmann-Martius rearrangement.

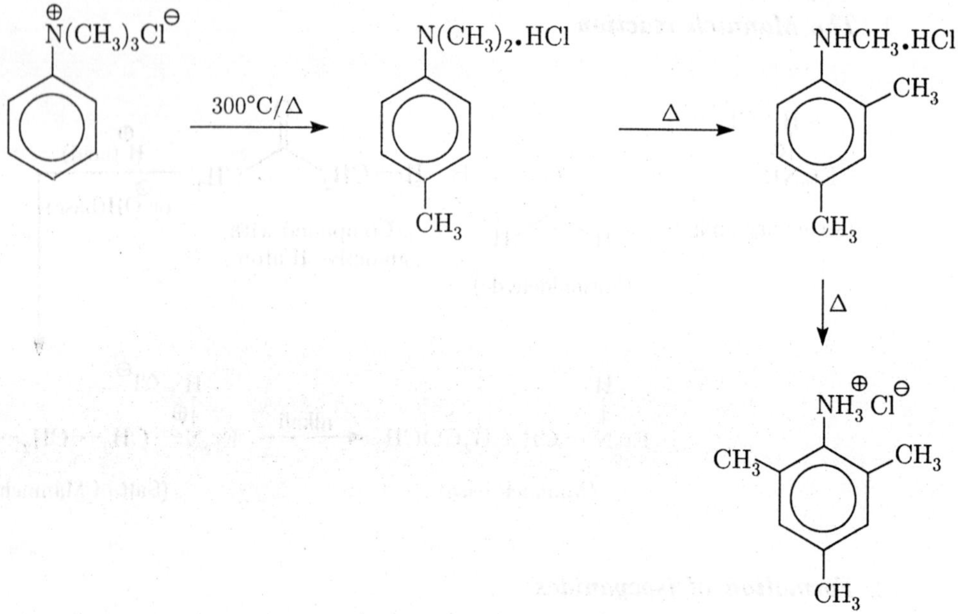

The reaction is usually carried out by heating the salt of alkylaryl amine under pressure, when usually the *para* product predominates.

Mechanism : Firstly, the salt decomposes into aniline and alkyl chloride followed by electrophilic attack at the activated *para* or *ortho* position with respect to the NH_2 group by positive pole of the alkyl chloride separated earlier, to form a σ-complex. Finally fast aromatisation takes place with the loss of a proton.

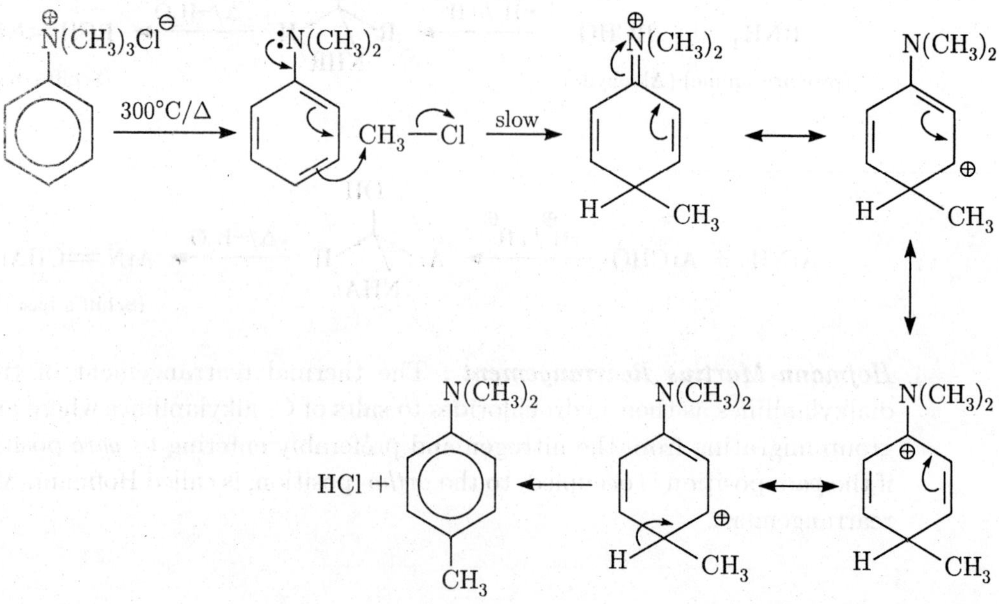

The reaction is totally **intermolecular**, it may be proved by the fact that alkyl halide can be isolated from this reaction. This reaction provides a good means for preparing homologues of aniline.

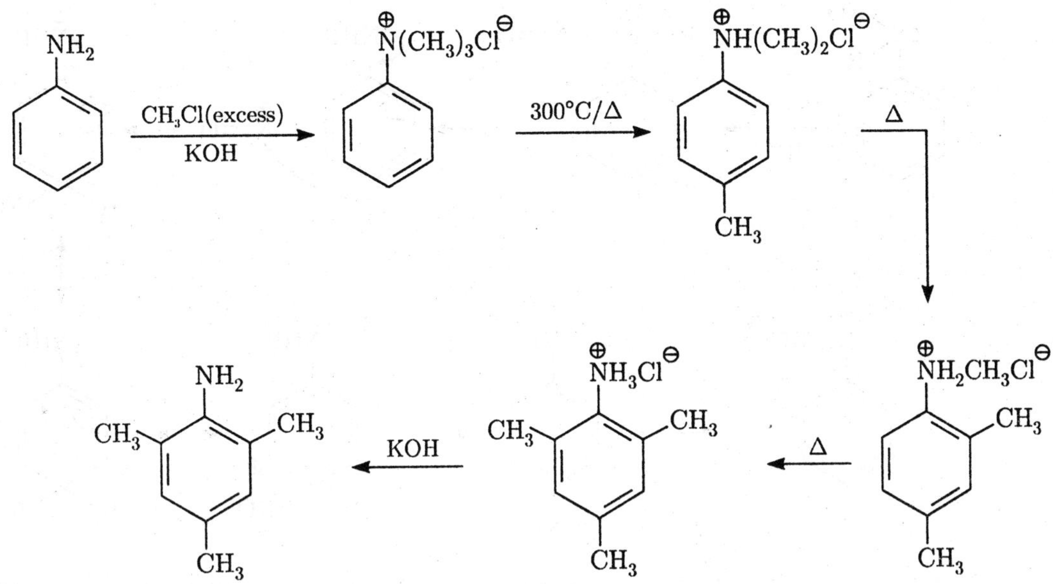

Hofmann-Martius rearrangements have been found to take place with aniline derivatives of the type as follows.

$$C_6H_5—\underset{|}{N}—Z$$

(Z=R, NH_2, NO or NO_2)

5. ***Fischer-Hepp Rearrangement*** : The acid catalysed rearrangement of N-alkyl-N-nitroso derivative of anilines to N-alkyl-*p*-nitrosoanilines is called Fischer-Hepp rearrangement.

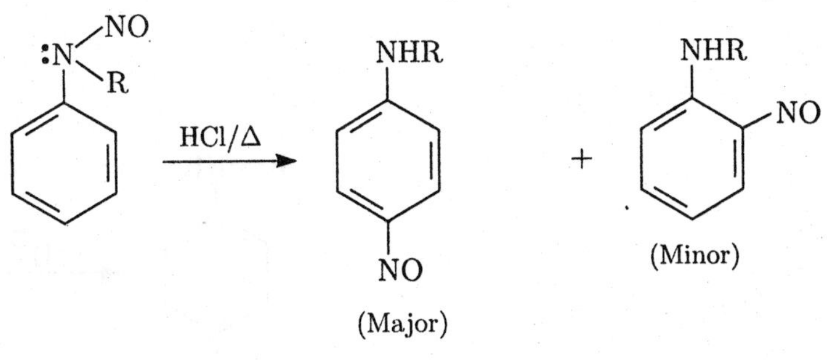

Mechanism : In acid, protonation takes place on amino nitrogen atom which leaves out the nitrosonium ion ($\overset{\oplus}{N}O$). Aromatic electrophilic substitution involving the nitrosonium ion follows at the *p*-position *via* σ-complex.

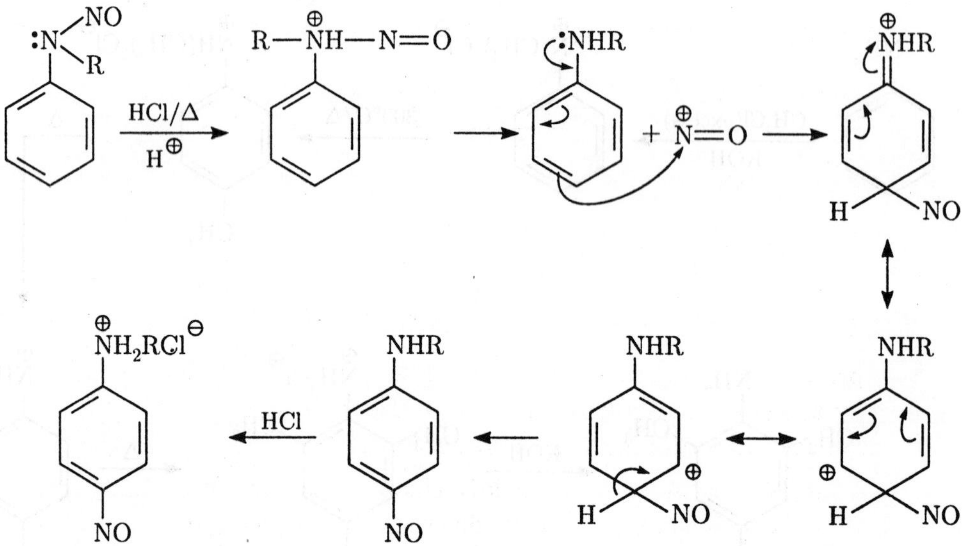

The reaction has been proposed to be intermolecular, which is supported by spectroscopy and also by the formation of *para* product predominantly.

However, Williams proposed the mechanism to be intramolecular. By carrying out the reaction with $Na^{15}NO_2$ and H_2SO_4 no ^{15}NO is incorporated in the product, indicating an intramolecular process *via* the following boat type configuration of the ring.

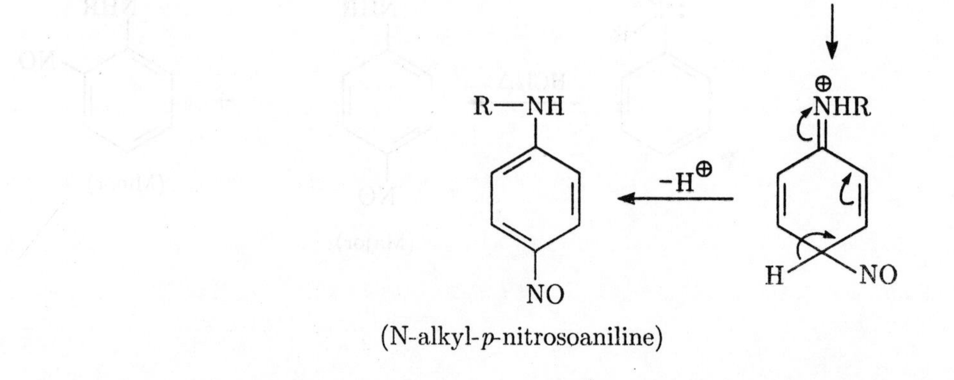

(N-alkyl-*p*-nitrosoaniline)

6. ***Orton or Chloramine Rearrangement*** : The mineral acid catalysed intermolecular rearrangement of N–haloacetanilide to *o*-and *p* haloacetanilides is called Orton rearrangement. For example, N-chloroacetanilide and hydrochloric acid give a mixture of *o*-and *p*-chloroacetanilide.

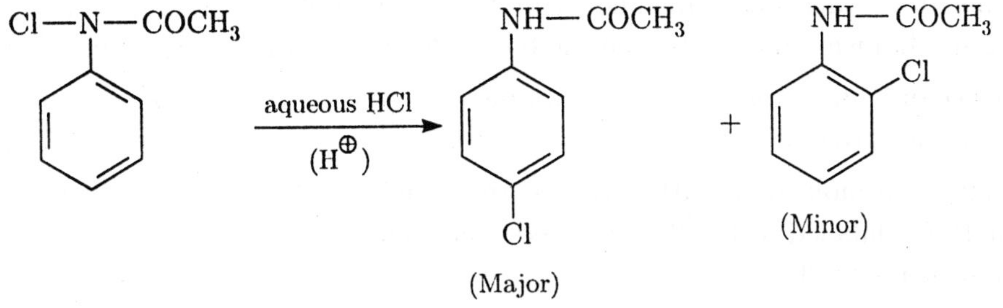

Mechanism : On treatment with acid, the nitrogen of N-chloroacetanilide gets protonated through a fast reversible step. Abstraction of chloronium ion ($Cl^{\oplus}$) by the chloride ion from H–Cl used, forming molecular chlorine is the slowest and rate determining step is proved by the fact that the reaction follows a **third** order kinetics and the rate = k[N–chloroacetanilide] [$H^{\oplus}$] [$Cl^{\ominus}$]. The final step is the fast bimolecular electrophilic substitution either at *para-* or *ortho-* position *via* a σ-complex.

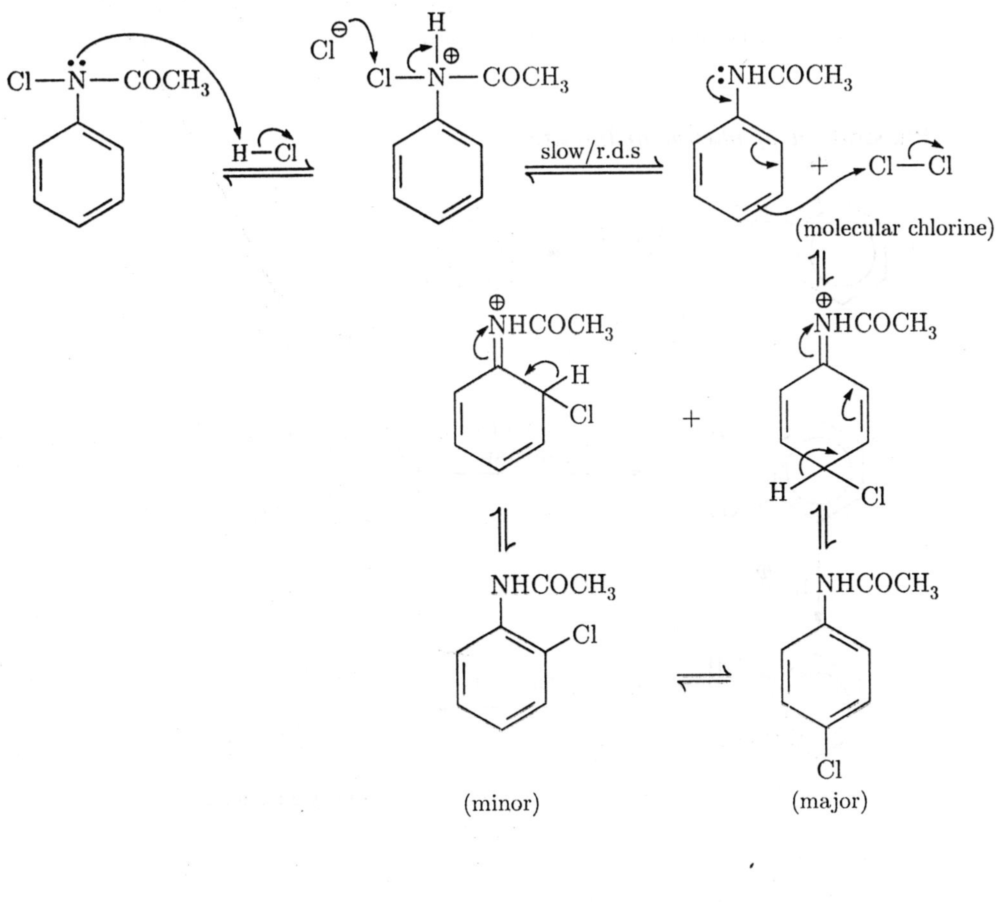

When N-chloroacetanilide is heated with hydroiodic acid (HI), the *p*- iodoacetanilide is the sole product, because of the bulk of the iodine atom which does not permit the iodine to enter into the ortho position.

The intermoleculerity of this reaction has been established by the isolation of molecular chlorine from this reaction. The formation of monohaloacetanilide also supports the above mechanism since only one mole of chlorine is formed per mole of the substrate, and since only one mole of $Cl^{\oplus}$ is available per mole of chlorine, the monohaloacetanilide can only be formed.

The intermolecular nature of the reaction is further established by the fact that when H–Cl labeled with ^{37}Cl is used, the *p*-chloro- or *o*-chloroacetanilide produced contains some ^{37}Cl.

Phenylenediamines

There are three types of phenylenediamines, namely *o*-, *m*- and *p*-.

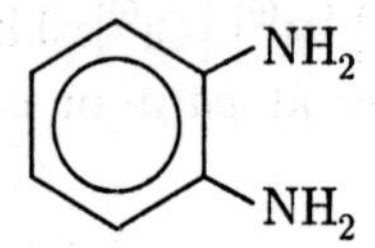

(*o*-phenylenediamine)

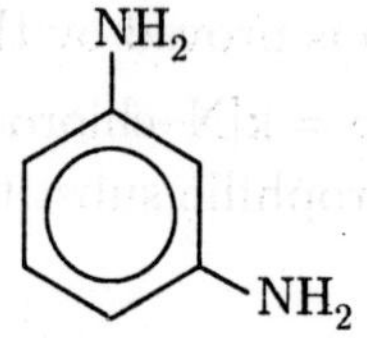

(*m*-phenylenediamine)

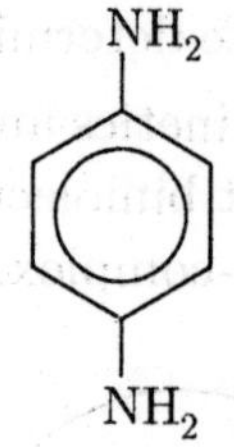

(*p*-phenylenediamine)

Preparation of phenylenediamines :

1.

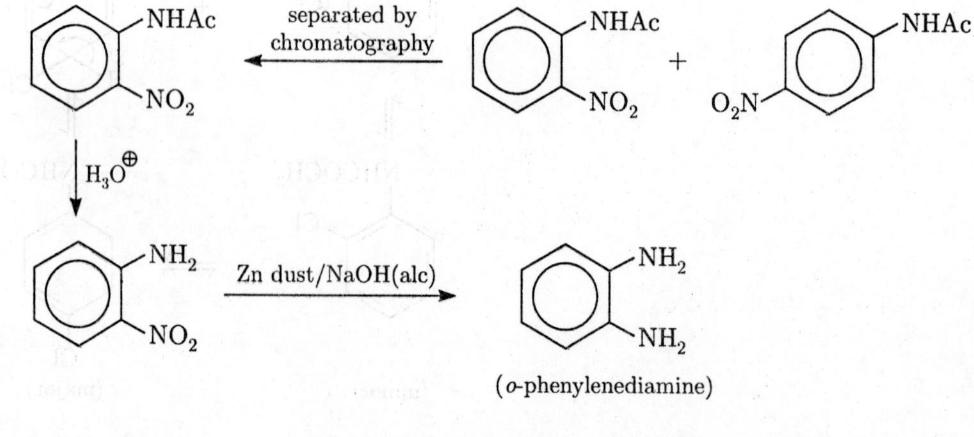

(*o*-phenylenediamine)

2.

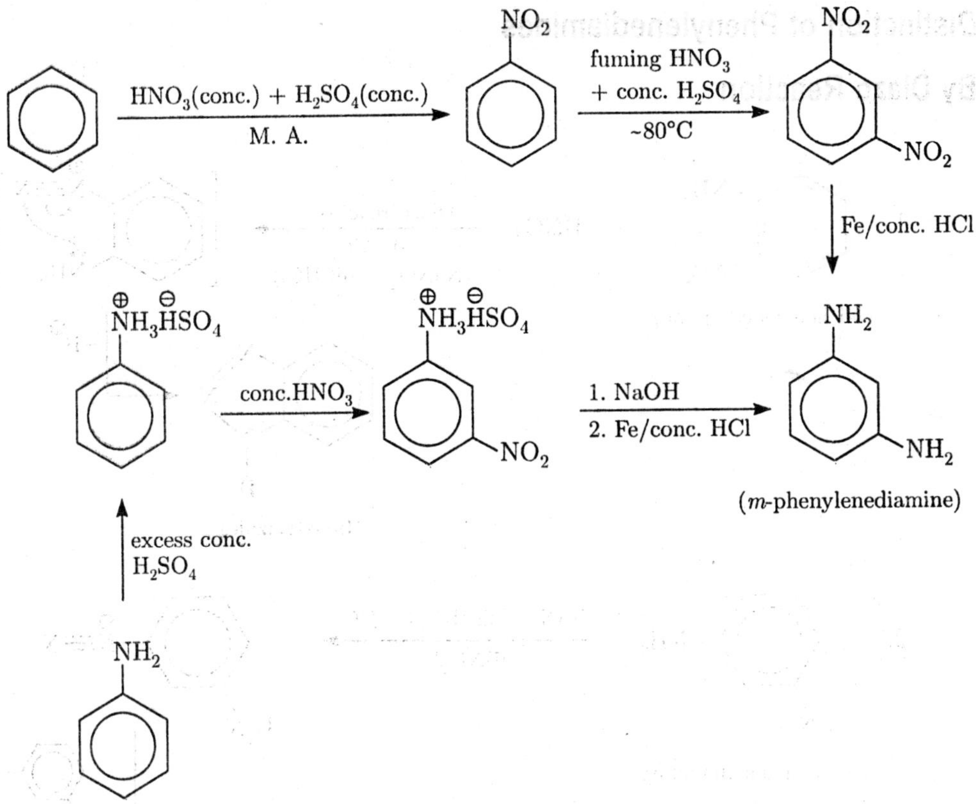
NO_2
HNO_3(conc.) + H_2SO_4(conc.)
M. A.
NO_2
fuming HNO_3
+ conc. H_2SO_4
~80°C
NO_2
Fe/conc. HCl
NH_2
NH_2
(m-phenylenediamine)
1. NaOH
2. Fe/conc. HCl
$\overset{\oplus}{N}H_3\overset{\ominus}{H}SO_4$
NO_2
conc.HNO_3
$\overset{\oplus}{N}H_3\overset{\ominus}{H}SO_4$
excess conc. H_2SO_4
NH_2

3.

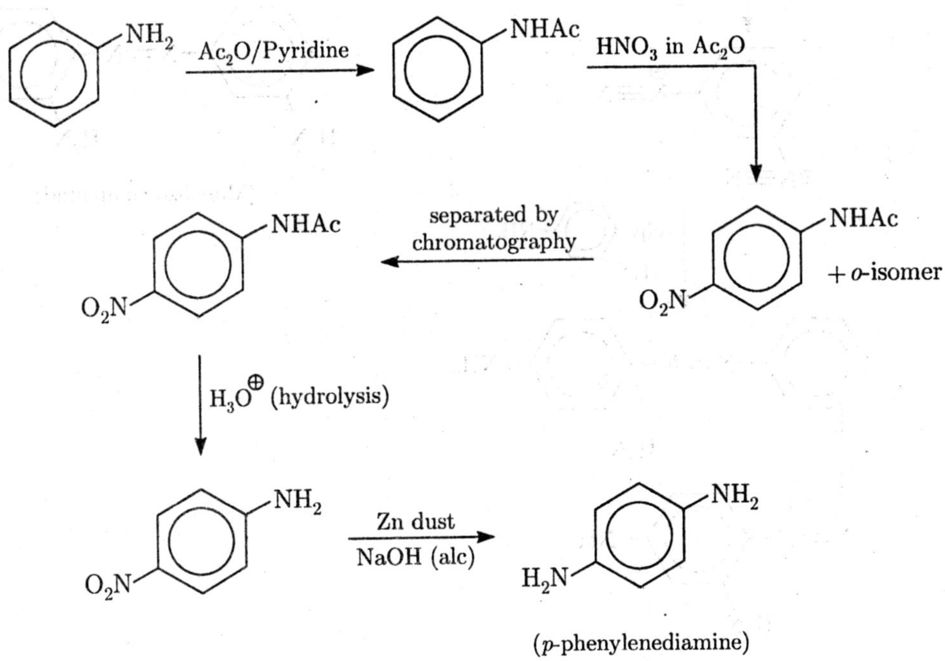
NH_2
Ac_2O/Pyridine
NHAc
HNO_3 in Ac_2O
NHAc
+ o-isomer
O_2N
separated by chromatography
NHAc
O_2N
$H_3O^{\oplus}$ (hydrolysis)
NH_2
O_2N
Zn dust
NaOH (alc)
NH_2
H_2N
(p-phenylenediamine)

Distinction of Phenylenediamines

By Diazo Reaction

1.

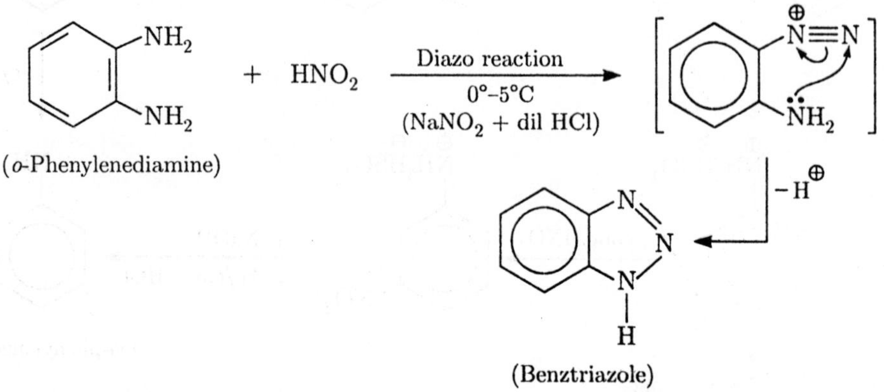

2.

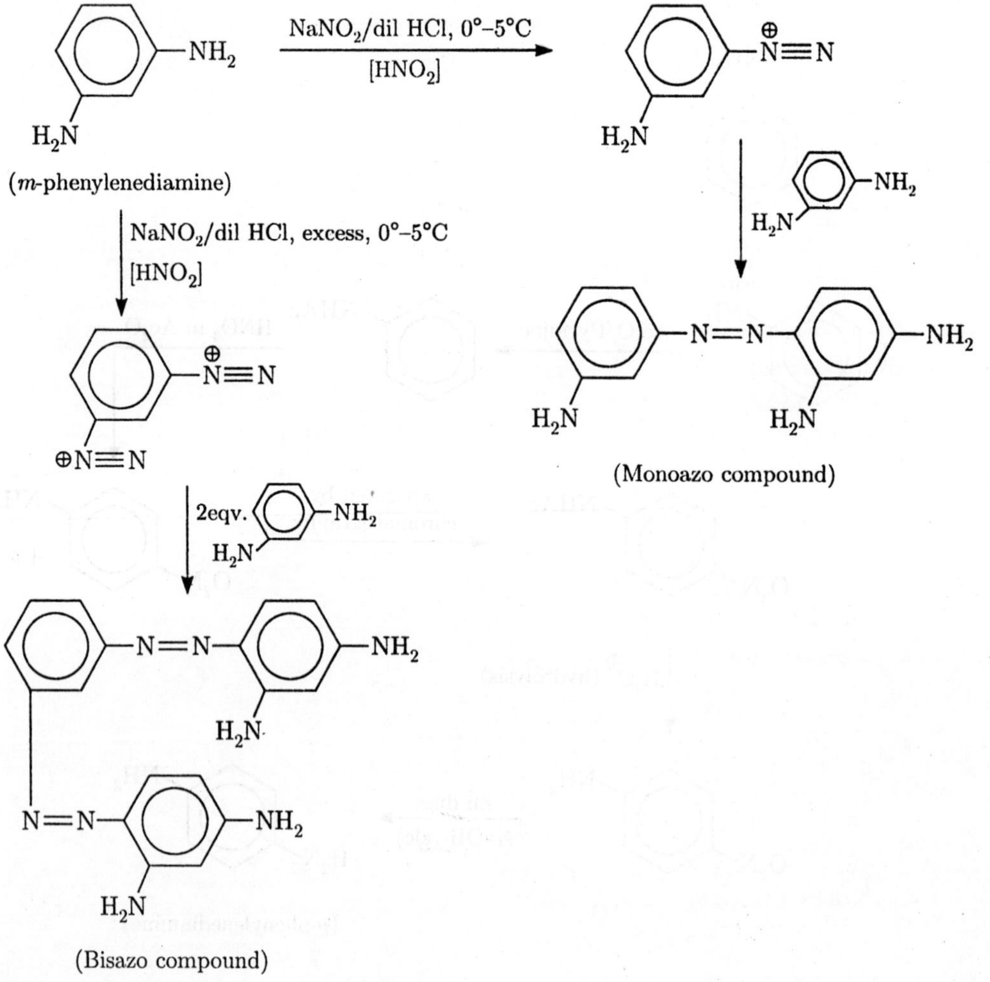

Combination of monoazo- and bisazo compounds produces a brown dye called **Bismarck Brown.**

3. 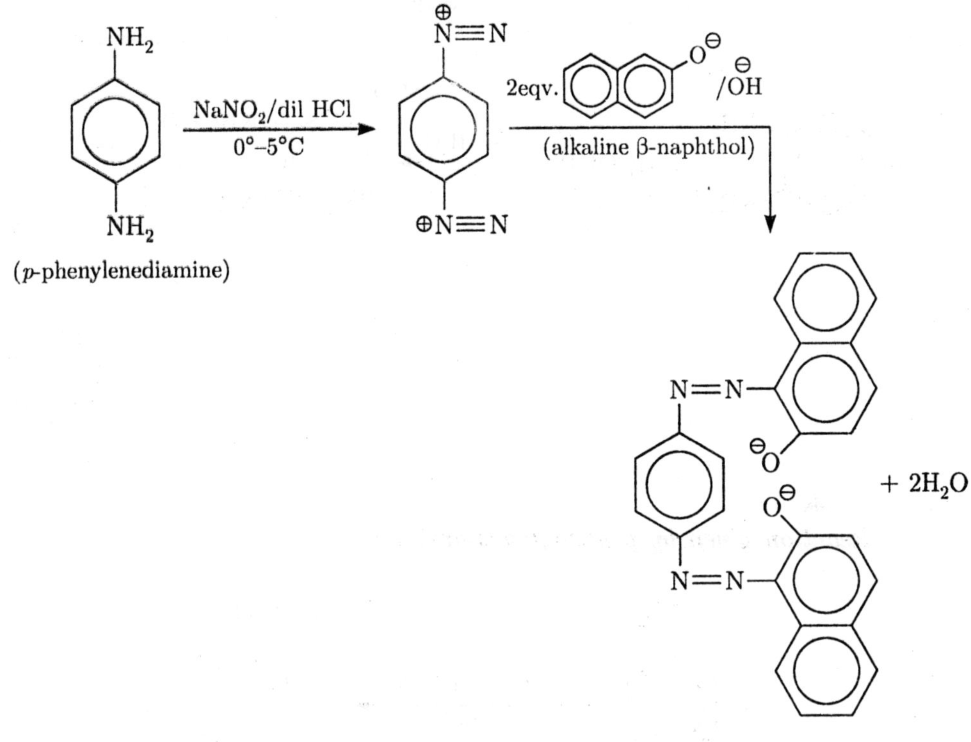

(Brilliant red azo dye)

Reactions given by o-phenylenediamine :

1. 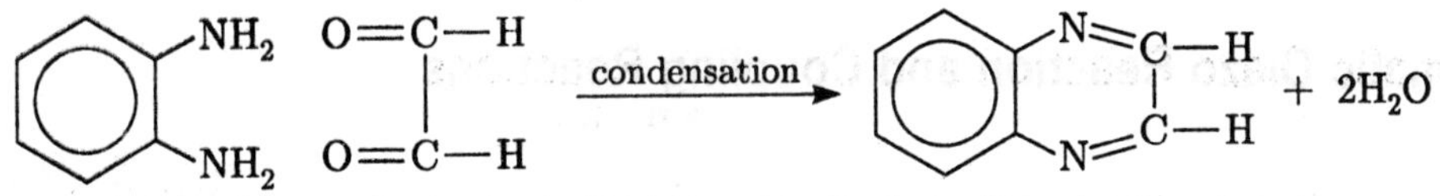

(Quinoxaline)

2. 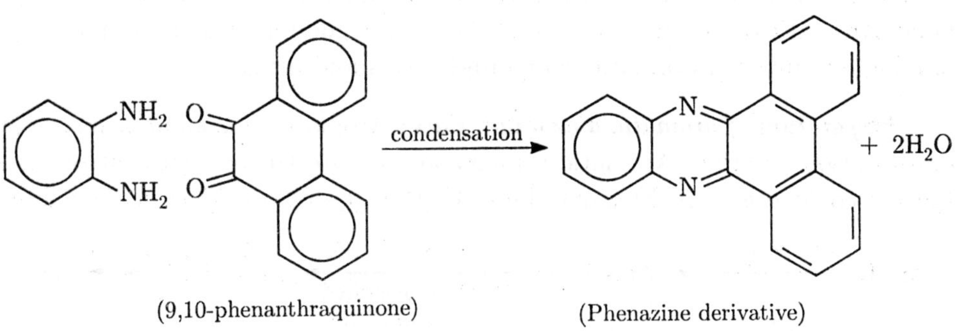

(9,10-phenanthraquinone) (Phenazine derivative)

3. 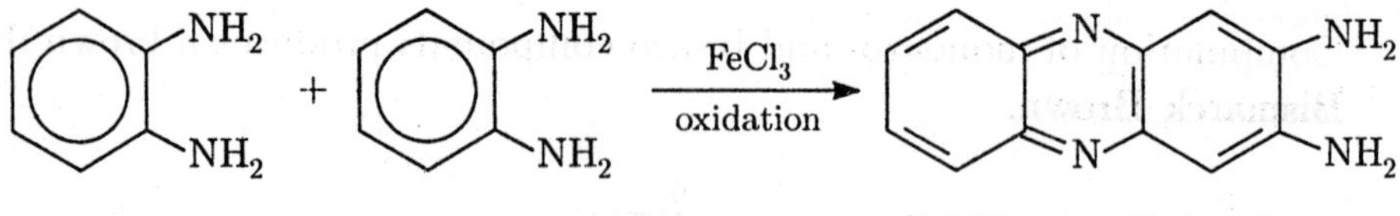

(2,3-Diaminophenazine)

4. 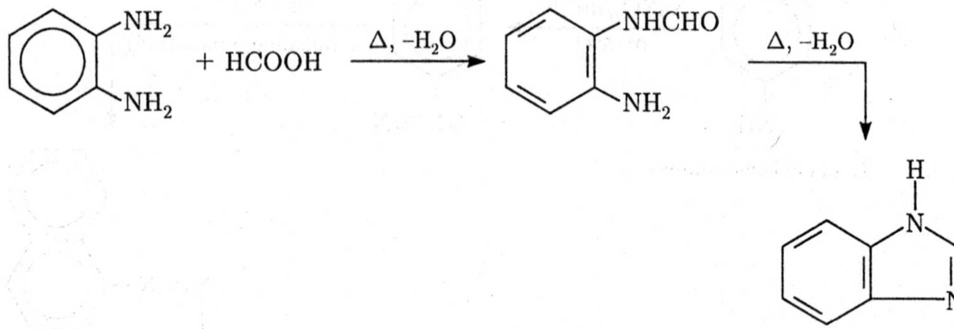

(Benzimidazole)

Reaction given by p-phenylenediamine :

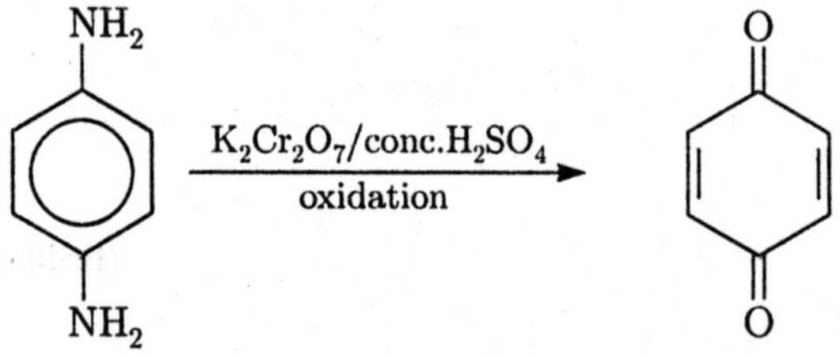

(*p*-benzoquinone)

Aromatic Diazo Reaction and Coupling Reactions

Aromatic diazoniums compounds are usually represented by $Ar—\ddot{N}{=}\overset{\oplus}{N}\ \overset{\ominus}{X}$ (X=Cl, Br, HSO_4 etc.) They contain two nitrogen (azo) atoms, of which one is directly bonded to the nuclear carbon and the other nitrogen is bonded to the former nitrogen by a multiple bond. Aromatic diazonium compounds (salts) are good intermediates for the preparation of a large number of aromatic compounds, dyes and drugs.

Preparation of aromatic diazonium slats : Aromatic diazonium salts are prepared by diazotization reaction. Aromatic primary amines are treated with nitrous acid (HNO_2) (generated *in situ* by $NaNO_2$ and dilute HCl) at 0°–5°C in *dilute acid* medium, and the

$$ArNH_2 \xrightarrow{H—X,\ 0°–5°C} ArNH_2.HX \xrightarrow[\text{HNO}_2 \text{ is generated } \textit{in situ}]{(\text{aq. NaNO}_2 + \text{HX})} Ar\overset{\oplus}{N}{\equiv}\ddot{N}\ \overset{\ominus}{X} \longleftrightarrow Ar—N{=}\overset{\oplus}{N}\ \overset{\ominus}{X}$$

reaction is known as aromatic diazotization reaction as a two-azo (French synonym for nitro is azoate) system is bonded to the nuclear carbon by this process.

The equation shows that *2 moles of mineral acid* is required to diazotize *one mole of an aromatic primary amine.* In practice, however, one equivalent of the amine is dissolved in *2.5–3.0 equivalent* of dilute HCl or H_2SO_4 cooled to 0°–5°C. To the cold solution, an aqueous dilute solution of sodium nitrite ($NaNO_2$) is added gradually, during the course of about five minutes and the mixture is allowed to stand for additional 5–10 minutes. Throughout the process, the temperature is kept preferably above 0°C and below 5°C at which the rate of the reaction is optimum and the diazonium ion is fairly stable. The diazonium salt so formed remains in the solution and used as such *in situ.*

Mechanism of Diazotization Reaction :

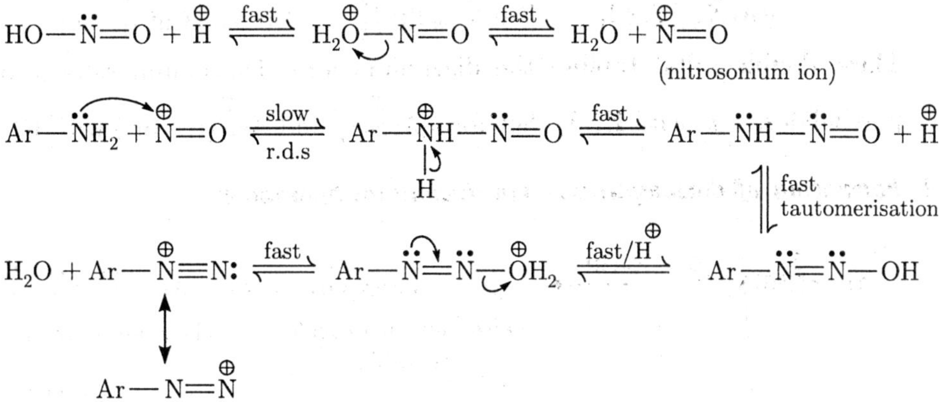

The rate determining step (slow) is the nitrosation of the free amine as shown above, which is consistent with the kinetic studies.

Some derivatives of primary aromatic amines give *anomalous results* which exist as dipolar ions as follows :

1. 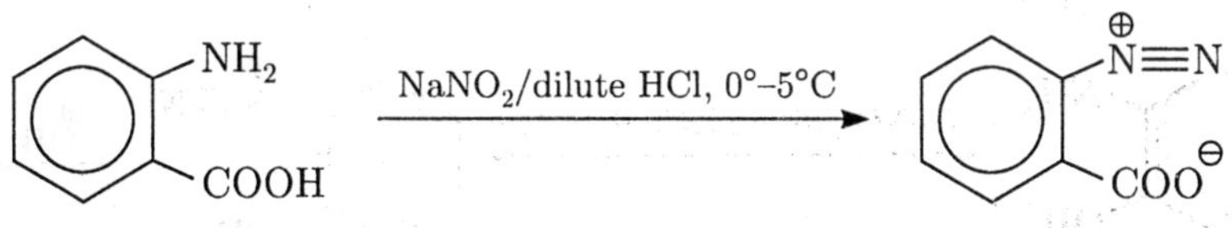

(Anthranilic acid)

2. 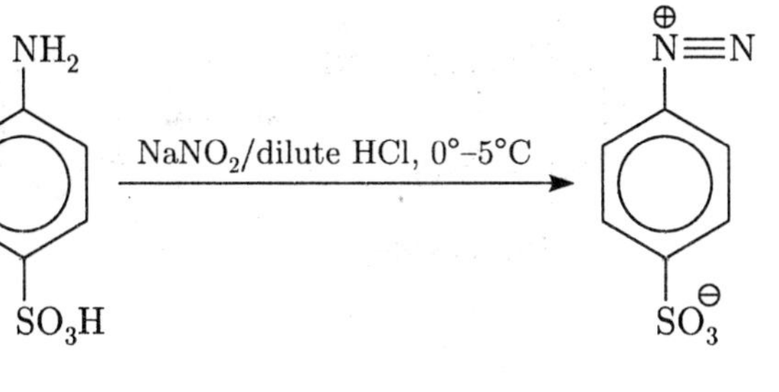

Solid diazonium salts may be prepared by dissolving the amine salt in an acidic solution of alcohol and adding an alkyl nitrite, ethyl or isoamyl nitrite. The diazonium salt is then precipitated by the addition of ether and placing the reaction vessel in a freezing mixture. The salt is separated by filtration.

$$ArNH_2.HCl + EtO{-}N{=}O \longrightarrow Ar\overset{\oplus}{N}{\equiv}N\overset{\ominus}{Cl} + EtOH + H_2O$$

The stability of diazonium salt varies from salt to salt.

Reactions and Applications of Diazonium Salts

1. ***Formation of double salts and polyhalides*** : Diazonium salts form double salts with $ZnCl_2$, $PtCl_4$, $CuCl_2$ etc.

$$[(Ar\overset{\oplus}{N_2})_2]\,ZnCl_4^{2-},\quad [(Ar\overset{\oplus}{N_2})_2]\,PtCl_6^{2-},\quad [(Ar\overset{\oplus}{N_2})_2]\,CuCl_3^{2-}\ \text{etc.}$$

These double salts stabilise the diazonium ions. Diazonium salts also form polyhalides, *e.g.*, with KI/I_2 they form $Ar\overset{\oplus}{N_2}\overset{\ominus}{I_3}$ and $Ar\overset{\oplus}{N_2}(Cl\,\overset{\ominus}{Br_2})$ with KCl/Br_2.

2. ***Formation of diazohydroxide via diazonium hydroxide*** :

$$[Ar{-}\overset{\oplus}{N}{\equiv}N]\overset{\ominus}{Cl} \xrightarrow{NaOH} \underset{\substack{\text{(Diazonium hydroxide)}\\\text{(unstable)}}}{[Ar{-}\overset{\oplus}{N}{\equiv}N]\overset{\ominus}{O}H} \rightleftharpoons \underset{\text{(Diazonium hydroxide)}}{Ar{-}\ddot{N}{=}\ddot{N}{-}OH}$$

$$Ar{-}\ddot{N}{=}\ddot{N}{-}OH \xrightarrow{NaOH} \underset{\text{(Sodium diazoate)}}{Ar{-}N{=}N{-}\overset{\ominus}{O}\overset{\oplus}{Na}}$$

3. ***Formation of diazophenol***

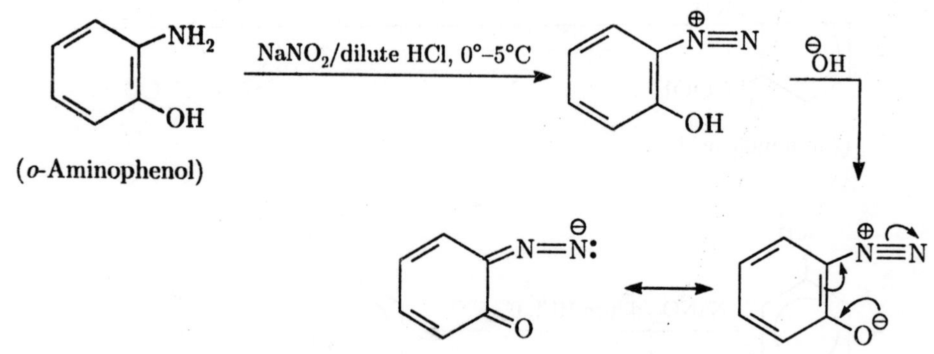

(Diazooxide)

4. ***Formation of hydrazines***

$$C_6H_5\overset{\oplus}{N}_2Cl^{\ominus} \xrightarrow{SnCl_2/HCl} C_6H_5NHNH_2.HCl$$

The reduction is commercially carried out with sodium sulphite.

Mechanism :

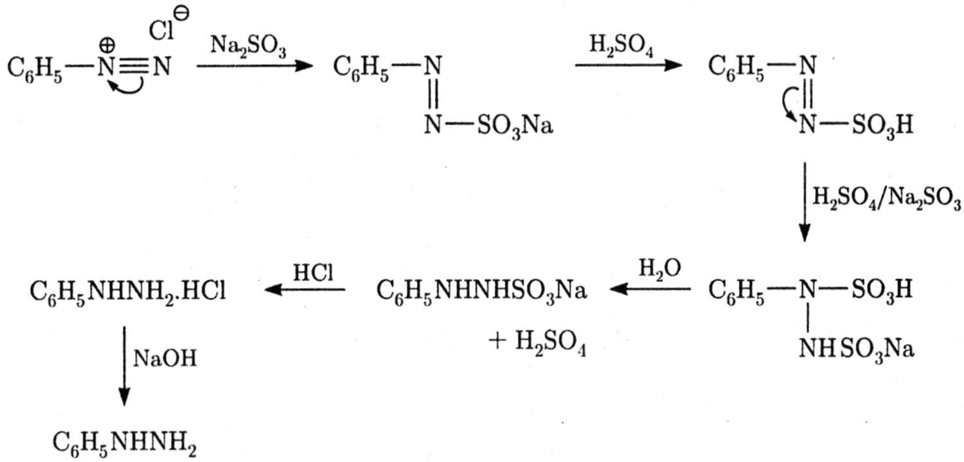

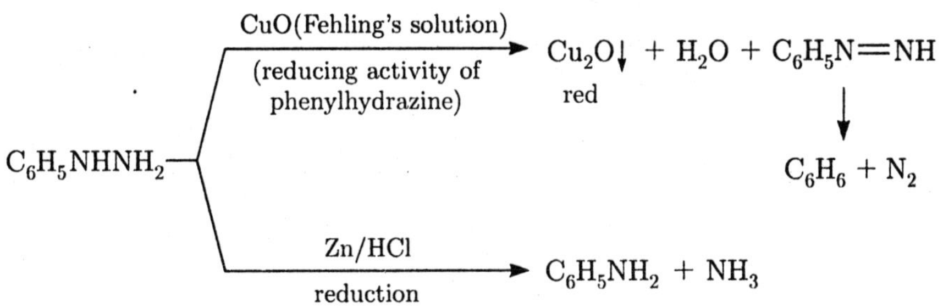

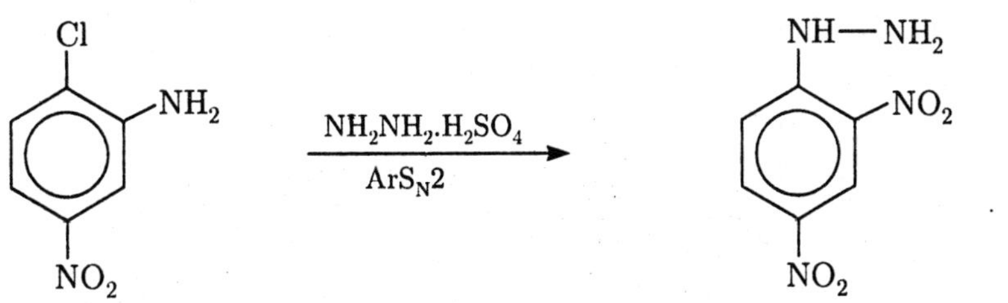

(2,4-dinitrophenylhydrazine)
(red, crystalline)

5. ***The diazonium coupling reaction*** : Aromatic diazonium ions combine with phenoxide ions and aromatic tertiary amines to form a large number of azo dyes

and this sort of reactions are known as the diazonium coupling reaction. The diazonium salt is called the **primary component** and the compound with which diazonium ion couples is called the **secondary component**.

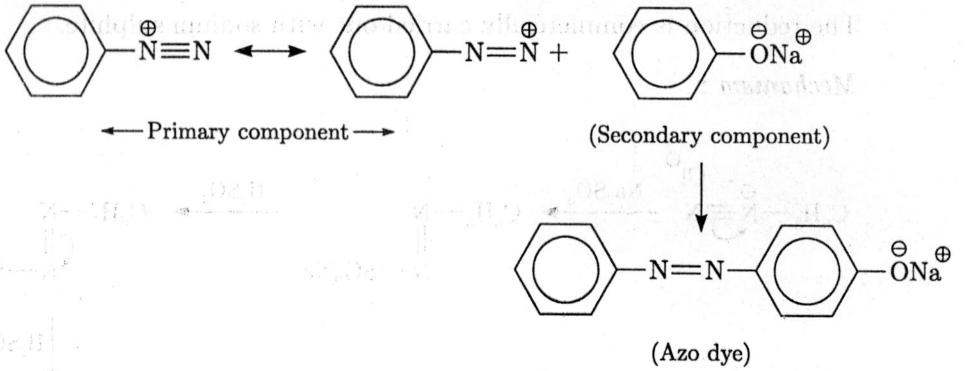

Depending on the nature of the secondary component, the coupling reaction is carried out either in alkaline or in a neutral or in a slightly acidic medium. The coupling reactions are generally done in cold, as diazonium salts are not very stable at higher temperatures.

Case A : Coupling between arenediazonium cations and amines take place most rapidly in slightly acidic solutions (pH 5-7). Under these conditions, the concentration of arene diazonium cation is at a maximum; at the same time, an excessive amount of the amine has not been converted to an unreactive aminium salt. If the pH of the solution is lower than 5, the rate of amine coupling is low.

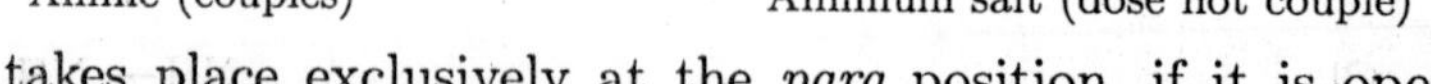

Coupling takes place exclusively at the *para* position, if it is open. If it is not, coupling takes place at the *ortho* position.

1. 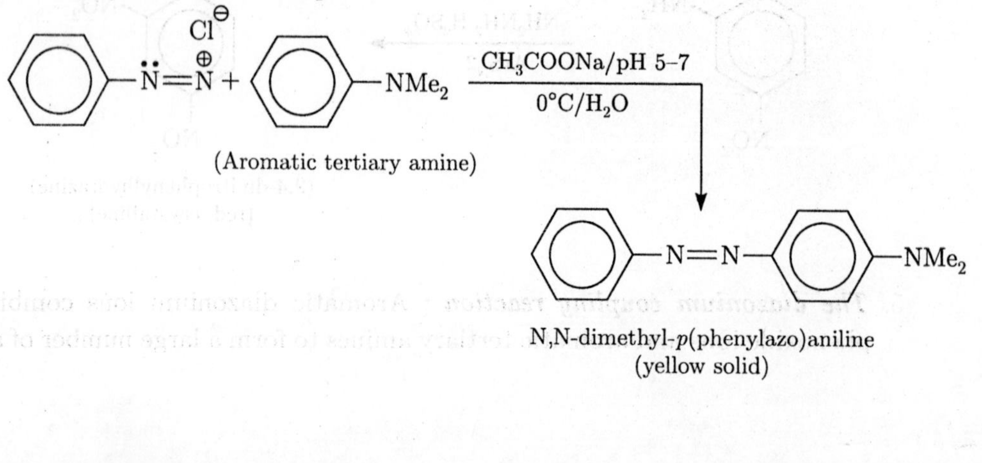

2. 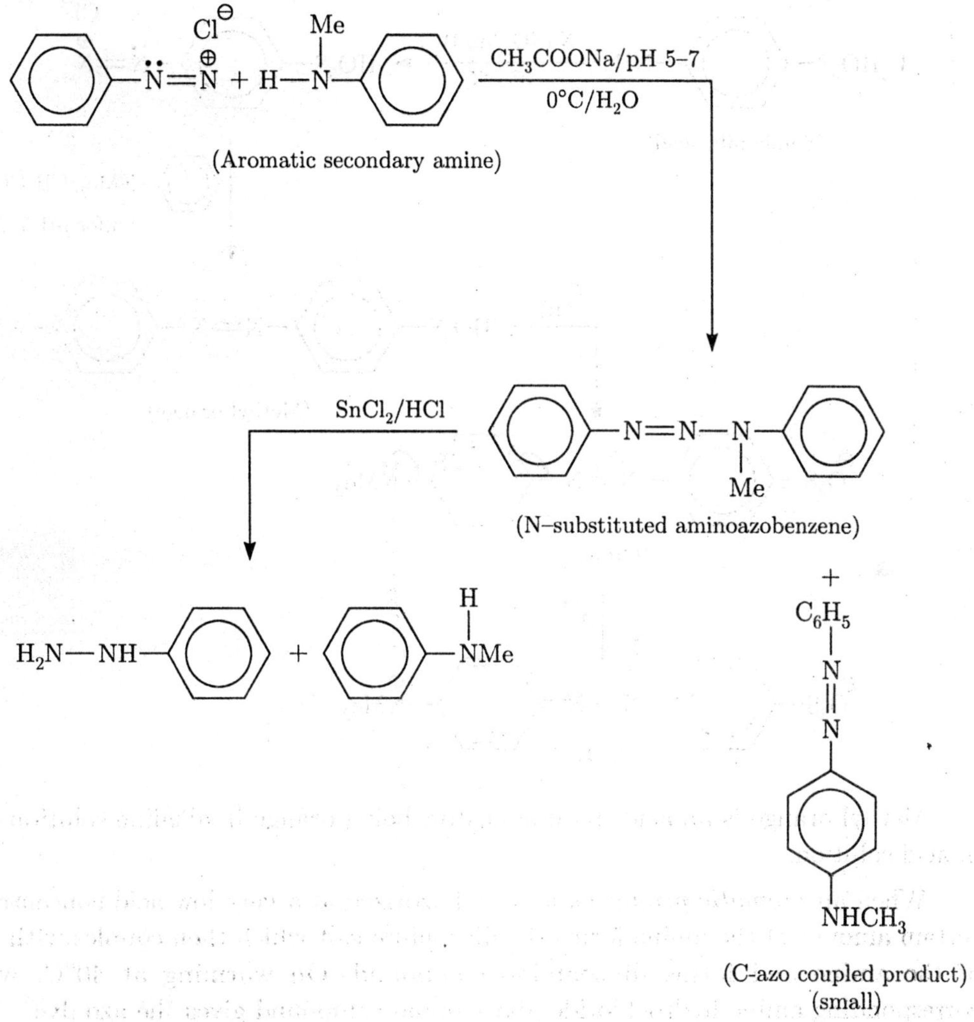
Cl⊖
Me
N=N⊕ + H—N
CH3COONa/pH 5–7
0°C/H2O
(Aromatic secondary amine)
SnCl2/HCl
N=N—N
Me
(N–substituted aminoazobenzene)
+
C6H5
N
N
NHCH3
(C-azo coupled product)
(small)
H2N—NH
+
H
NMe

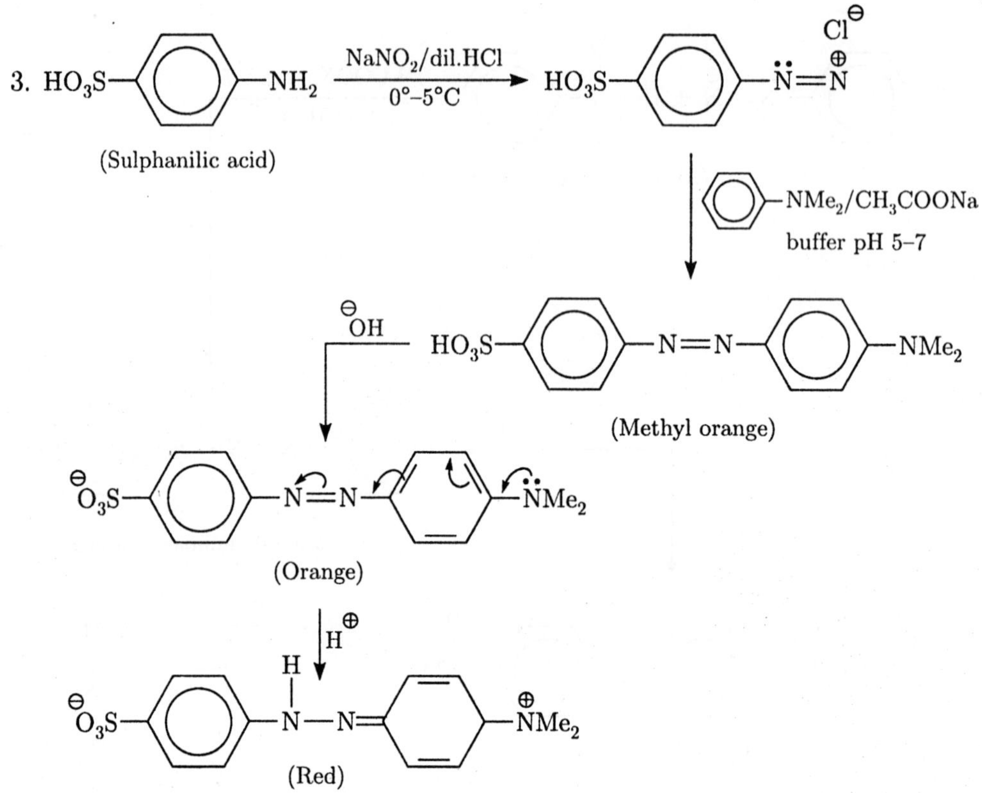

Methyl orange is an acid- base indicator, being orange in alkaline solution and red in acid solution.

When an *aromatic primary amine* is diazotized at a very low acid concentration, a certain amount of the amine forms the diazonium salt which then couples with the rest of the amine and forms diazoamino compound. On warming at 40°C, with the corresponding amine hydrochloride, diazoamino compound gives the azo dye.

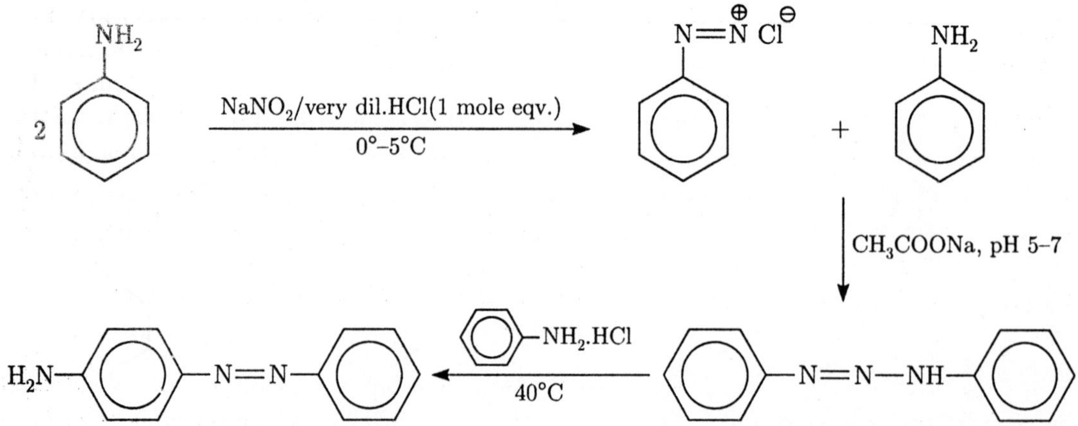

(Azo dye)

(Diazoamino compound)
(yellow solid)

So diazotization of primary amine is done under *sufficiently acidic* condition in order to avoid coupling with undiazotized amine.

Contributory structure of diazonium cation in diazo coupling :

$$\underset{\text{(I)}}{C_6H_5-\overset{\oplus}{N}\equiv N} \longleftrightarrow \underset{\text{(II)}}{C_6H_5-N=\overset{\oplus}{N}}$$

Since (II) is the reactive contributing resonating structure, any factor that increases its contribution will increase the reactivity of that diazonium cation. It can be anticipated that electron-withdrawing groups would favour (II) and electron releasing group would favour (I). This has been found so to be in practice. For example, *p*-nitrobenzenediazonium cation is more than 10,000 times as reactive as the *p*-methoxy ion under the same conditions. The 2,4,6-trinitrobenzenediazonium cation is so reactive that it couples with certain hydrocarbons, *e.g.*, mesitylene.

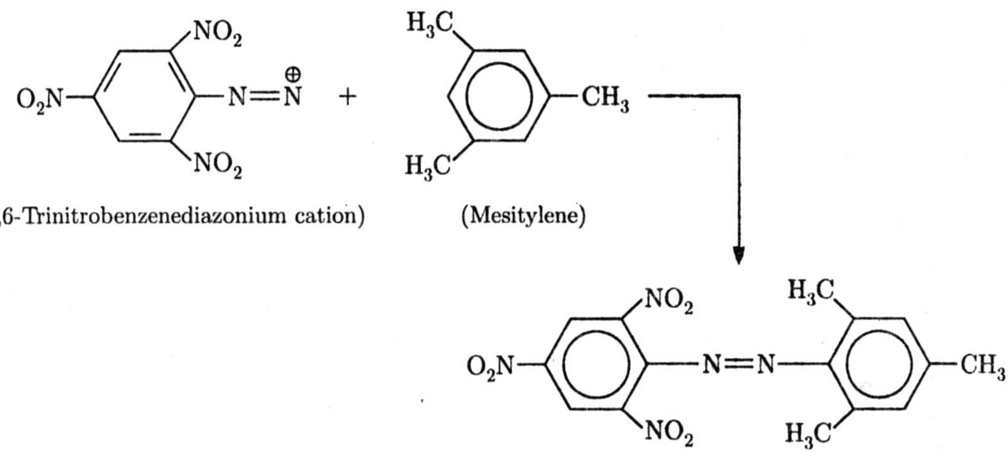

(2,4,6-Trinitrobenzenediazonium cation) (Mesitylene)

Whether C–N or N–N coupling will occur, it depends upon two factors.

1. The electron density on the carbon or nitrogen of the secondary component.
2. Stability of the bond formed through coupling.

In a primary amine, the $-\ddot{N}H_2$ group (in sp^3 orientation) has got sufficient electron density on nitrogen to couple with diazonium cation. So N–N coupling occurs at first. However, N–N bond is weak (due to repulsion between the lone pairs of electrons on two nitrogen atoms). At 40°C, the N–N bond breaks and thermodynamically more stable C–N bond is formed through C–N coupling. For aromatic tertiary amines, the *para* carbon has enough electron density for C–N coupling and a C–N bond is formed through both kinetically controlled and thermodynamically controlled reactions.

Case B : Couplings between arenediazonium cations and phenols take place most rapidly in *slightly* alkaline solution. Under these conditions, an appreciable amount of phenol is present as phenoxide ion; $ArO^{\ominus}$ and the phenoxide ions are even more reactive toward electrophilic substitution than are phenols themselves. If the solution is too alkaline (pH>10), however, the arenediazonium salt itself reacts with hydroxide ion to form a relatively unreactive diazohydroxide or diazotate ion.

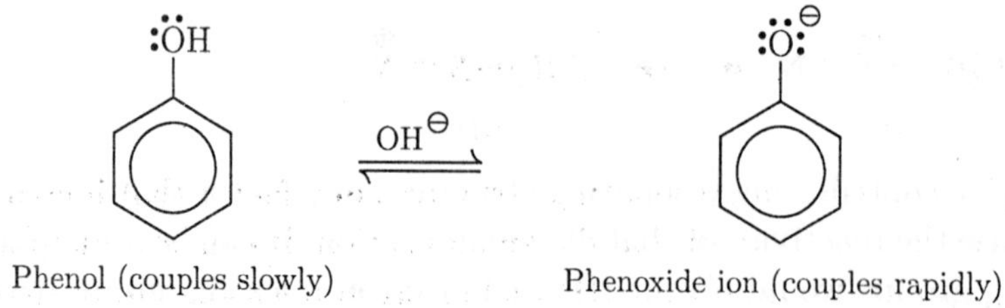

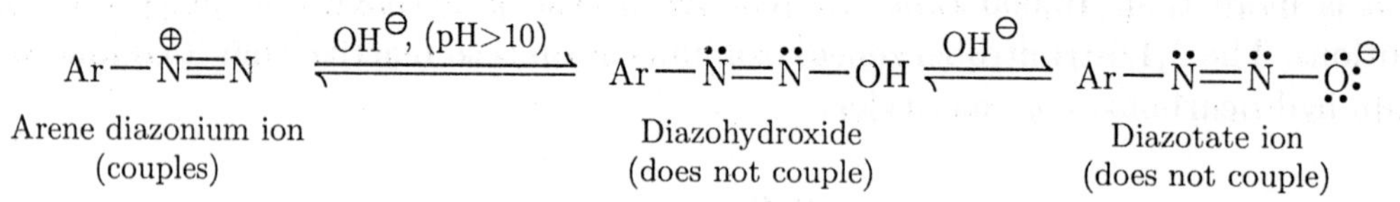

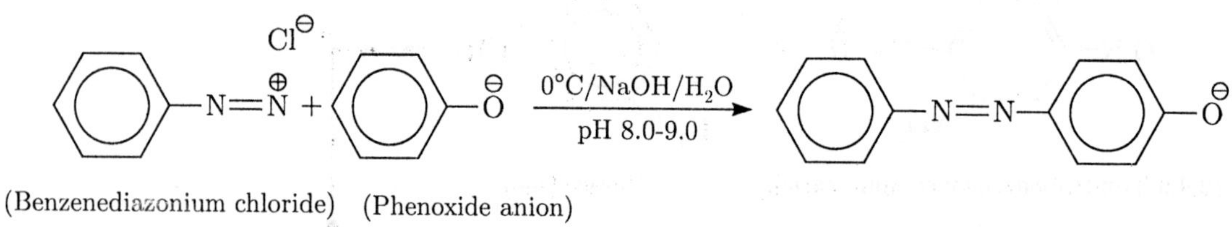

The presence of another activating group in the *meta*-position of the phenol or amine accelerates coupling. Resorcinol forms mono-, bis- and trisazo compounds more readily than does phenol.

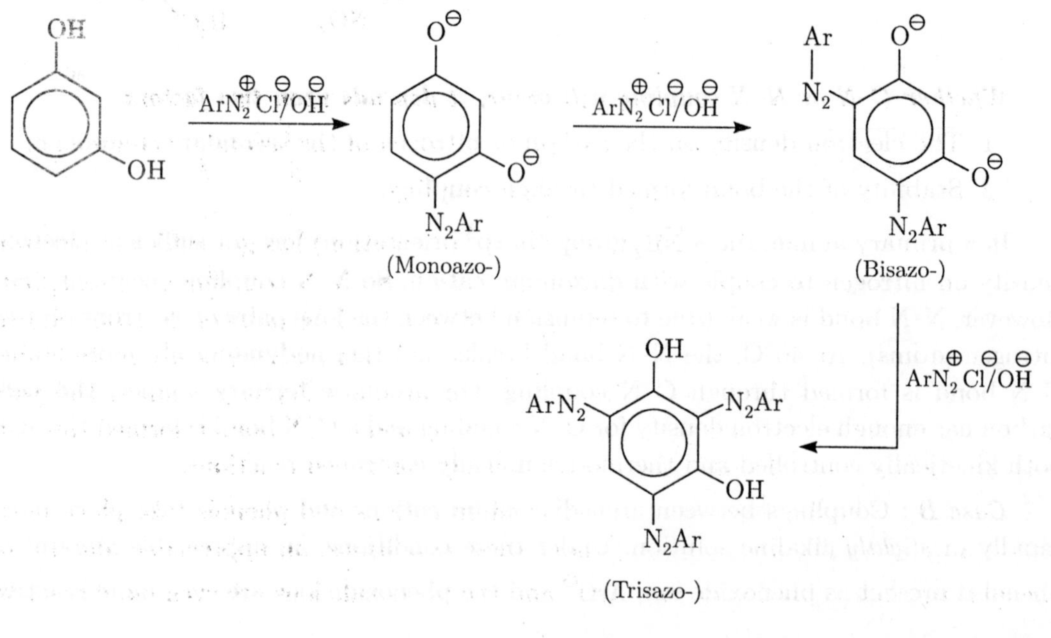

1- and 2- Naphthols in alkaline solution couple with diazonium salts respectively in the 4- and 1- positions. The formation of the azo-2-naphthol is used as a test for primary aromatic amines.

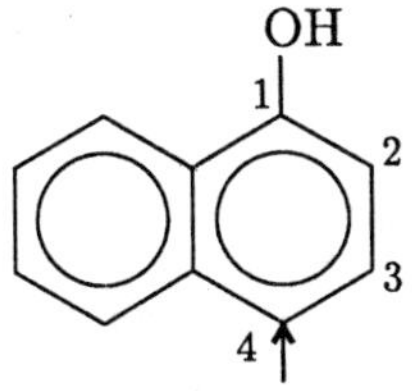

(1-naphthol)

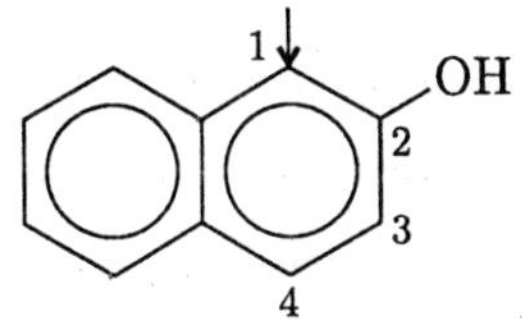

(2-naphthol)

Mechanism of diazo coupling reaction :

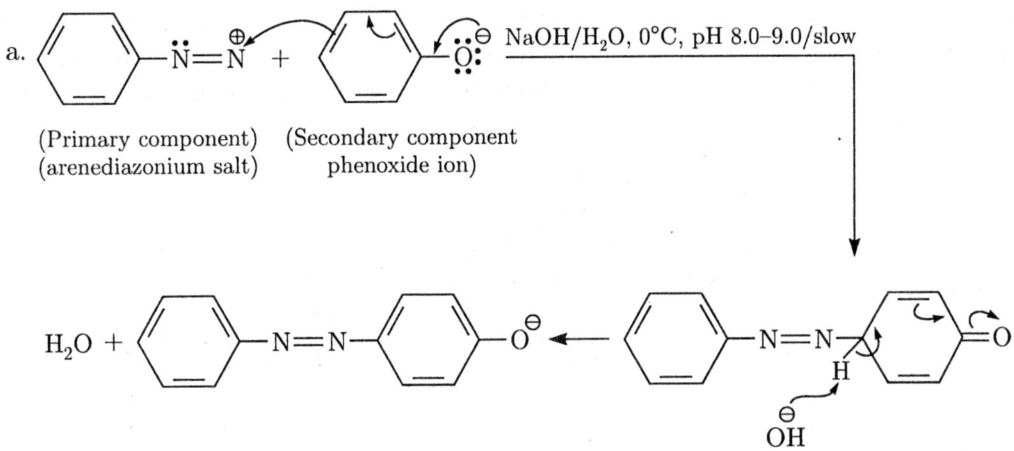

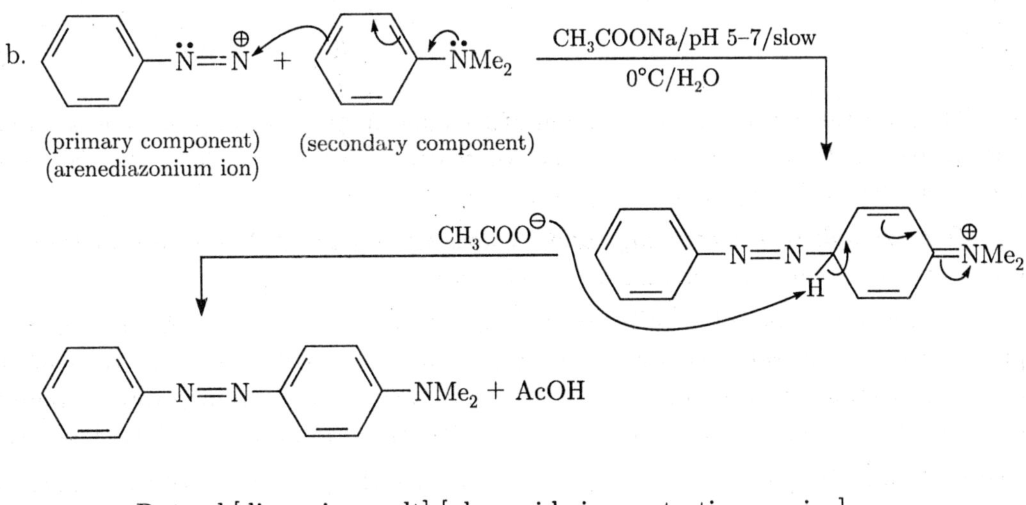

Rate=k[diazonium salt] [phenoxide ion or tertiary amine]

Coupling reaction generally occurs at the *p*- position if it is open and if not to the *o*- position. When both *o*- and *p*- positions are blocked, coupling does not occur. There are some instances where coupling occurs even if the *p*- position is blocked. In this case the original substituent present at the *p*- position is ejected.

The diazonium coupling may occur between–

(a) A strong electrophile and a strong nucleophile

(b) A strong electrophile and a weak nucleophile

(c) A weak electrophile and a strong nucleophile

No coupling occurs between a weak electrophile and a weak nucleophile. Benzene diazonium chloride, being a weak electrophile can not couple with anisole which is a weak nucleophile. 2,4-dinitrobenzenediazonium chloride is a strong electrophile (due to the presence of two $-NO_2$ groups containing –I and –R effects) can couple with anisole and 2,4,6-trinitrobenzene can couple with mesitylene, a very weak nucleophile. Resorcinol, a good nucleophile couples with benzenediazonium chloride but *phenol itself* being a weak nucleophile can not combine with benzenediazonium chloride. To increase the nucleophillicity of phenol, coupling is done in slightly alkaline condition (pH 8.0–9.0) where phenoxide ion, a strong a nucleophile is produced.

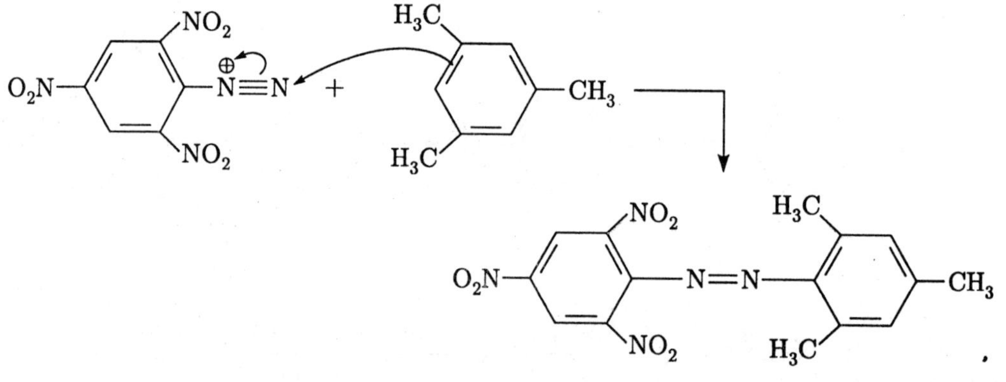

The increased electrophilic character of such diazonium ion compels the less activated nucleus to couple by drawing the π-electron density from the nucleus, thereby forming the σ-complex easier followed by fast aromatization.

One example where coupling reaction does not occur : N,N,2,6-Tetramethylaniline does not couple with benzenediazonium chloride.

The non occurance of coupling in this case is due to steric factor. As the four methyl groups are very closely oriented with respect to one another, a great deal of steric crowding occurs. In order to avoid steric hindrance, NMe_2 group rotates around the C–N bond axis and becomes out of plane with the aromatic ring. The lone pair of electrons on $\ddot{N}Me_2$ can not come into resonance with the π-electrons of the benzene ring and as a result, the *p*-position is *not electron-dense* (by +R effect of $\ddot{N}Me_2$ group). This makes N, N, 2,6-tetramethylaniline a very weak nucleophile and hence it can not couple with benzenediazonium chloride, a weak electrophile.

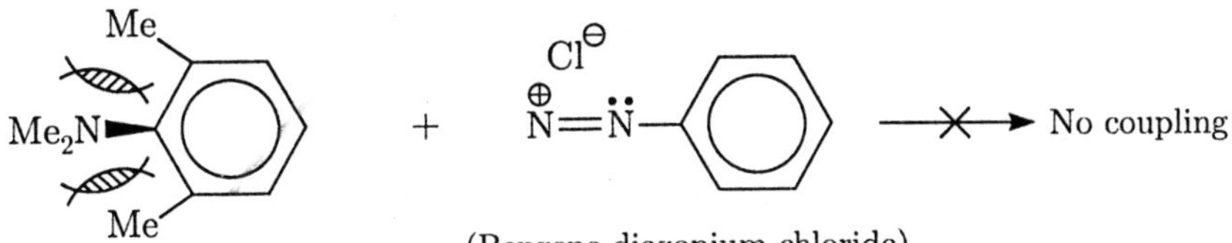

(Benzene diazonium chloride)

(N,N,2,6-Tetramethylaniline)

Coupling with Phenols : The coupling of diazonium salt with phenols occurs in alkaline solution, *via* phenoxide ions, which are strongly activated to electrophiles than phenol itself. Precautions must be taken so that in alkaline solution, the diazonium salt is not converted to diazohydroxide. The optimum pH for such coupling is 9-10. It is convenient to add an acidic solution of diazonium salt to a solution of phenol in sufficient alkali so that excess acid is neutralized and the alkali maintains the required pH.

$$\mathrm{Ph{-}O{-}H} + \overset{\ominus}{\mathrm{O}}\mathrm{H} \rightleftharpoons \mathrm{Ph{-}}\overset{\ominus}{\mathrm{O}} + \mathrm{H_2O}$$

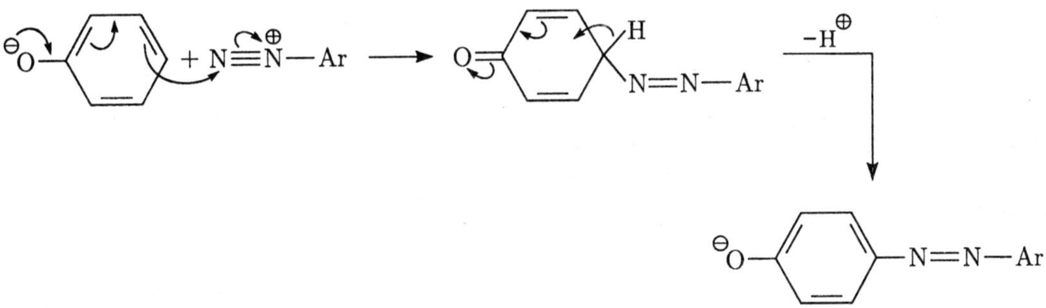

When *para* position is blocked, *ortho* coupling occurs. *e.g.*, *p*-cresol couples with benzenediazonium ion to form 2-hydroxy-5-methylphenylazoarene.

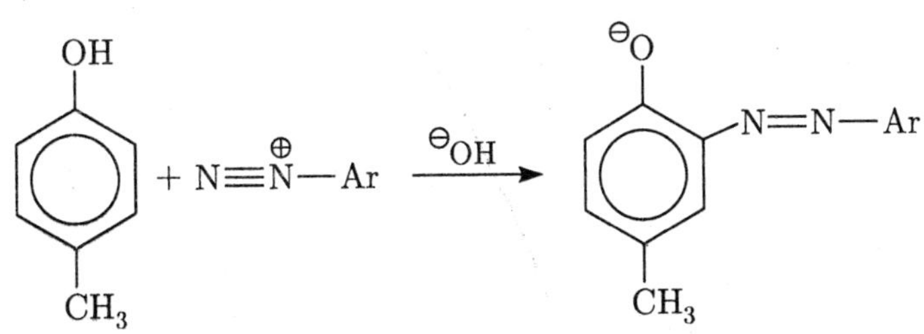

This *o*-azophenols are much weaker acids than their *p*-isomers, because the unionized forms become stabilized *via* chelation involving the hydroxylic proton. Use of this property is made in detecting aromatic primary amines. In practice, the amine is treated with $NaNO_2$ and dilute HCl and the resulting solution is poured into an alkaline solution of β-naphthol. Coupling with diazonium ion takes place at α-position of β-naphtholate ion to give a brilliant precipitate of azonaphthol which becomes insoluble by intramolecular hydrogen bonding, using the hydroxylic proton in alkaline medium.

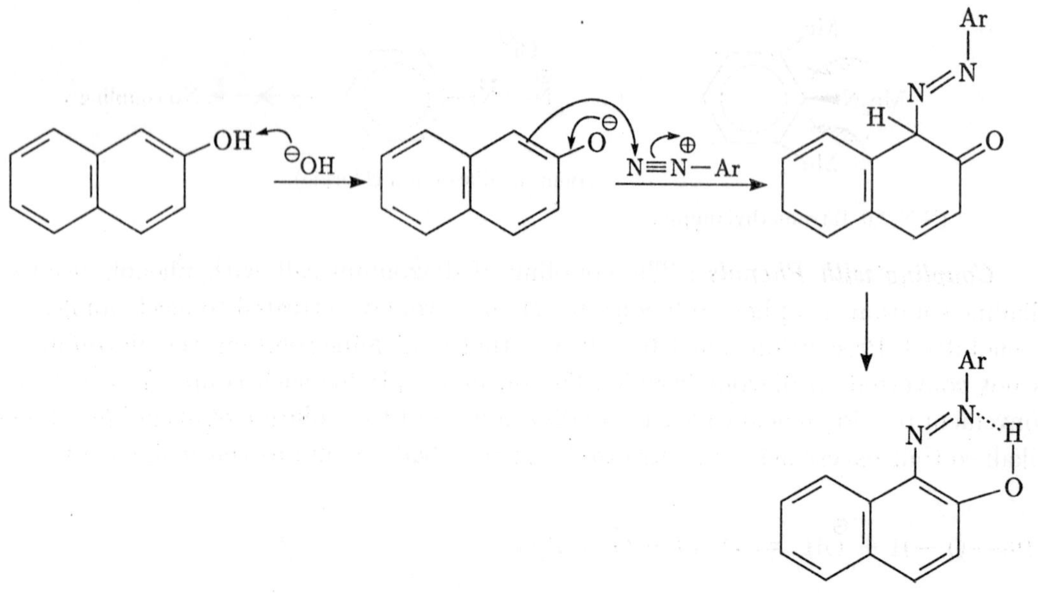

(Red precipitate)

For identification of amines, α-naphthol is not used, because it couples at 4-position and gives the dye in its ionized form, which remains in solution, and gives no precipitate of red dye. Here the unionized form cannot form because, it fails to form any chelate through intramolecular hydrogen bonding to be separated out from the medium as precipitate.

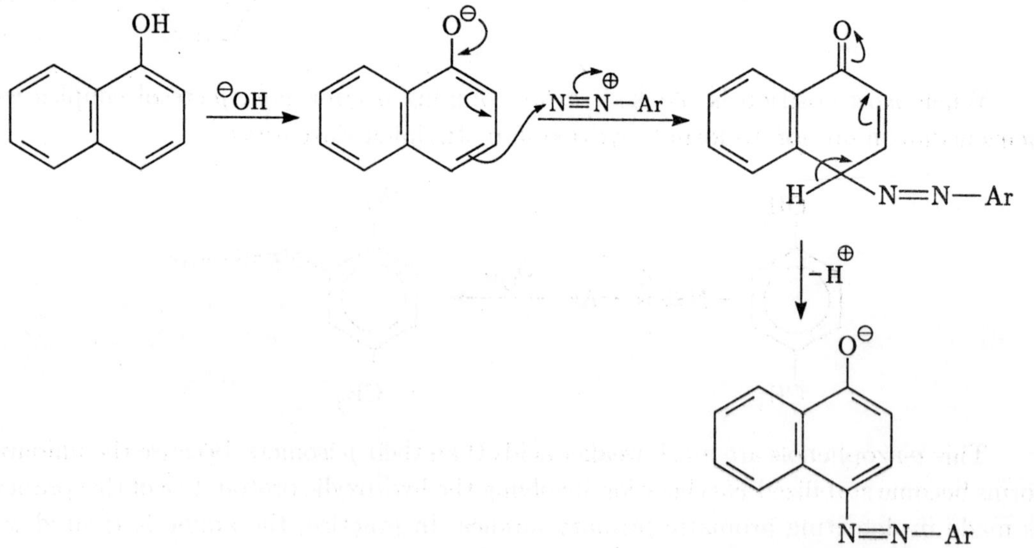

(Red coloured solution,
but no precipitate)

Coupling with enols : Although enols do not couple with diazonium ions, enolates, in which the hydroxylic oxygen activates the double bond to electrophiles do so. Reactions occur is alkaline conditions since enolate ion is more reactive than enol itself, *e.g.*, acetoacetic ester reacts with benzenediazonium chloride in sodium acetate buffer, giving α,β-dioxobutyrate-α-phenylhydrazone. Reaction differs from those with phenols in that the azo compounds undergo a tautomeric shift to give arylhydrazone.

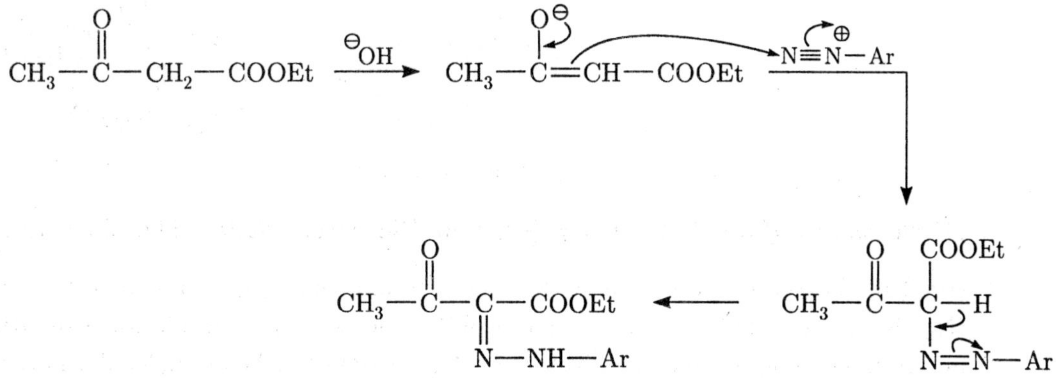

Japp-Klingemann reaction : While coupling between benzenediazonium ion and enol occurs, if the carbon atom at which coupling takes place, does not possess any α-H atom so that the final prototropic shift cannot take place, the initial product readily undergoes C–C bond fission on subsequent attack by $OH^{\ominus}$ to give arylhydrazone.

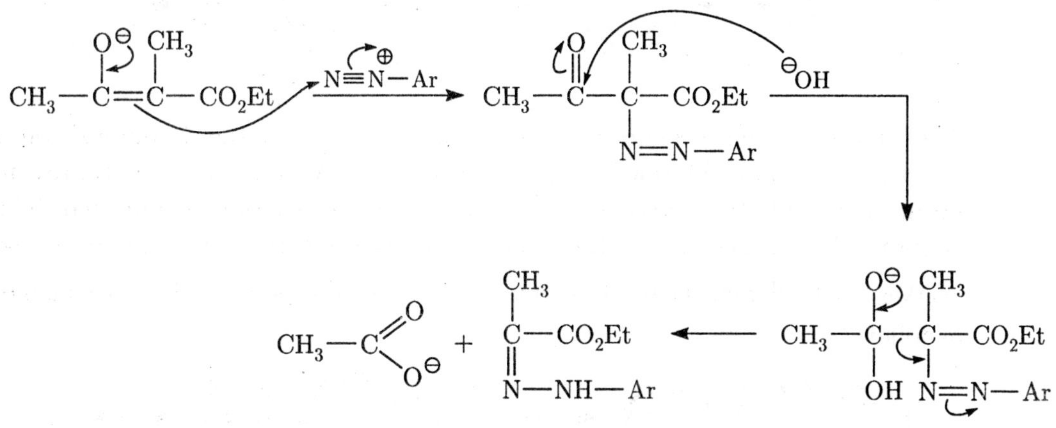

Compounds with decreasing enol content react with benzenediazonium chloride with decreasing ease. *e.g.*, acetophenone and its derivatives do not couple with benzenediazonium ion, but if stereochemistry is suitable, intramolecular coupling occurs more readily than intermolecular coupling *e.g.*, diazotization of *o*-aminoacetophenone leads to formation of 4-hydroxycinnoline.

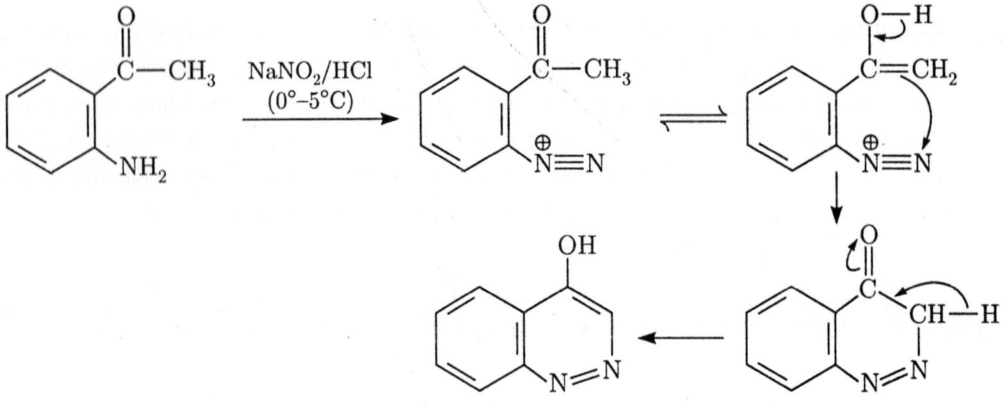

(4-Hydroxycinnoline)

6. ***Displacement of the Diazo group*** ($-\overset{\oplus}{N}_2$) ***In Diazonium Salts*** : The diazogroup ($-\overset{\oplus}{N}_2$) of diazonium salts can be replaced by another group and nitrogen gas (N_2) is evolved. The reaction is nucleophilic and sets an example for aromatic nucleophilic unimolecular substitution (ArS_N1) reaction. The unimolecular nature of the reaction is due to the fact that molecular nitrogen (N_2) is a good leaving group.

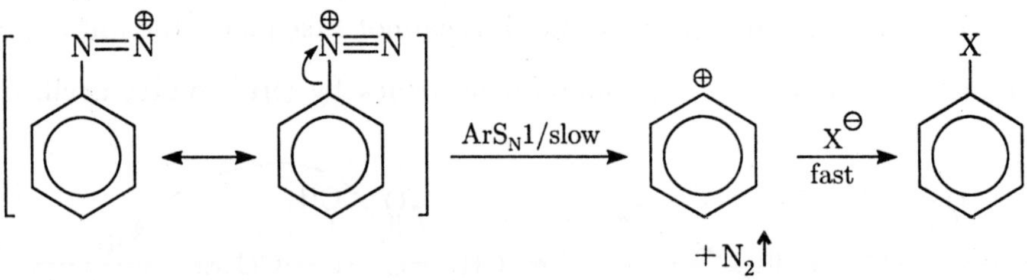

The support of the mechanism comes from the fact that the decomposition of benzene diazonium chloride is a first order reaction. When electron withdrawing group like –COOH is present at the *p*-position the reaction is inhibited. This supports ArS_N1 mechanism. So it is expected that electron releasing group like $-\ddot{\underset{\cdot\cdot}{O}}Me$ will accelerate the reaction but *reverse* is found is practice. This is explained as follows.

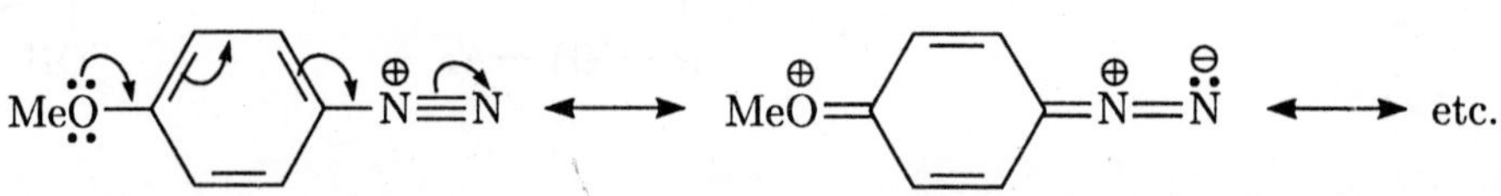

Resonance gives $Ar-\overset{\oplus}{N}_2$ bond some double bond character with consequent increase in strength. Since the breaking of this bond is involved in the rate determining step, activation energy of this step is raised and the reaction is retarded. This retardation is observed for groups which are electron releasing by +R or hyperconjugative effect. Electron releasing group at the *m*-position accelerates the reaction due to its +I effect.

$$ArNH_2 \xrightarrow[0^\circ\text{–}5^\circ C]{HO\text{–}NO} Ar-\overset{\oplus}{N}\equiv N$$ (Arenediazonium salt)

1. 1. Cu_2O/Cu^+, H_2O or 2. boiled with water ⟶ $ArOH + N_2\uparrow$ (replacement by –OH)
2. 1. H_3PO_2/Cu^{2+} or Mn^{2+} or Fe^{2+} or 2. C_2H_5OH/Cu or 3. Sodium arsenite/$OH^{\ominus}$ or 4. $NaBH_4/EtOH$ ⟶ $ArH + N_2\uparrow$ (replacement by H)
3. $CuCl/HCl$, 15–60°C, Sandmeyer's reaction ⟶ $ArCl + N_2\uparrow$ (replacement by Cl)
4. $CuBr/HBr$, 15–60°C, Sandmeyer's reaction ⟶ $ArBr + N_2\uparrow$ (replacement by Br)
5. $CuCN/KCN$ or HCN/Cu powder ⟶ $ArCN + N_2\uparrow$ (replacement by CN)
6. aqeous KI ⟶ $ArI + N_2\uparrow$ (replacement by I)
7. Cu powder/Δ/HBr, Gattermann reaction ⟶ $ArBr + N_2\uparrow$ (replacement by Br)
8. 1. HBF_4, 2. Δ ⟶ $ArF + N_2\uparrow$ (replacement by F)
9. Diazonium fluobrorate $(Ar\overset{\oplus}{N_2}\overset{\ominus}{BF_4})$ $\xrightarrow{NaNO_2/Cu}$ $ArNO_2 + N_2\uparrow + NaBF_4$ (replacement by $-NO_2$)
10. EtOH/Cu powder ⟶ $Ar\text{–}Ar + N_2\uparrow$ (replacement by an aryl group)
11. NaOH/NaOH, Gomberg reaction ⟶ $Ar\text{–}Ar + N_2\uparrow$ (replacement by Br)
12. CuSCN ⟶ $ArSCN + N_2\uparrow$
13. KNCO/Cu ⟶ $ArN{=}C{=}O + N_2\uparrow$
14. $(NH_4)_2S$ ⟶ $Ar_2S + N_2\uparrow$
15. NaSH ⟶ $ArSH + N_2\uparrow$

Explanation of displacement reactions

2. ***Displacement by hydrogen*** :

$$Ar\overset{\oplus}{N_2}\overset{\ominus}{Cl} \xrightarrow[2.\ H_2O]{1.\ H_3PO_2/Cu^{2+}} Ar-H + N_2\uparrow + H_3PO_3$$

The reaction proceeds through free radical mechanism.

Chain Initiation :

$$ArN_2^{\oplus}Cl^{\ominus} + \underset{(H_3PO_2)}{H_2P(O)OH} \longrightarrow HCl + Ar{-}N{=}N{-}PH(O)OH$$

$$Ar{-}N{=}N{-}PH(O)OH \longrightarrow \dot{A}r + N_2\uparrow + \dot{P}H(O)OH$$

Chain Propagation :

$$\dot{A}r + H_2P(O)OH \longrightarrow ArH + \dot{P}H(O)OH$$

$$ArN_2^{\oplus} + \dot{P}H(O)OH \longrightarrow Ar\dot{N}_2 + {}^{\oplus}PH(O)OH$$

$$Ar\dot{N}_2 \longrightarrow \dot{A}r + N_2\uparrow \qquad {}^{\oplus}PH(O)OH \xrightarrow{H_2O} H_3PO_3 + H^{\oplus}$$

In method 2, two reactions may occur

$$ArOMe \xleftarrow{MeOH} ArN_2^{\oplus} \xrightarrow{EtOH/Cu/\Delta} ArH + CH_3CHO$$

If –I containing group is present in the nucleus and ethanol is used, replacement of diazo group by hydrogen predominates. On the other hand, if methanol is used, the predominant product is aryl methyl ether.

3. ***Sandmeyer reaction*** :

$$ArN_2^{\oplus}Cl^{\ominus} \xrightarrow[\text{or } CuBr/HBr]{CuCl/HCl} ArCl \text{ or } ArBr + N_2\uparrow$$

Mechanism of the reaction

$$CuCl + Cl^{\ominus} \longrightarrow CuCl_2^{\ominus}$$

$$ArN_2^{\oplus} + Cl{-}Cu{-}Cl^{\ominus} \xrightarrow{slow} ArN_2^{\oplus}[CuCl_2]^{\ominus} \longrightarrow Ar{-}\overset{\oplus}{N}{\equiv}N\cdots\overset{\ominus}{Cl}{-}Cu{-}Cl$$

(Chloride bridge)

$$CuCl + ArCl \longleftarrow Cl{-}\overset{+II}{Cu}{-}Cl + \dot{A}r + N_2$$

$$Rate = k[ArN_2^{\oplus}][CuCl_2^{\ominus}]$$

12. ***Replacement by an aryl group (Gomberg reaction)*** :

$$ArN_2^{\oplus} + ArH \xrightarrow{NaOH} Ar{-}Ar + N_2\uparrow$$

The reaction takes place by a *free radical* mechanism *via* a complex type of electron transfer.

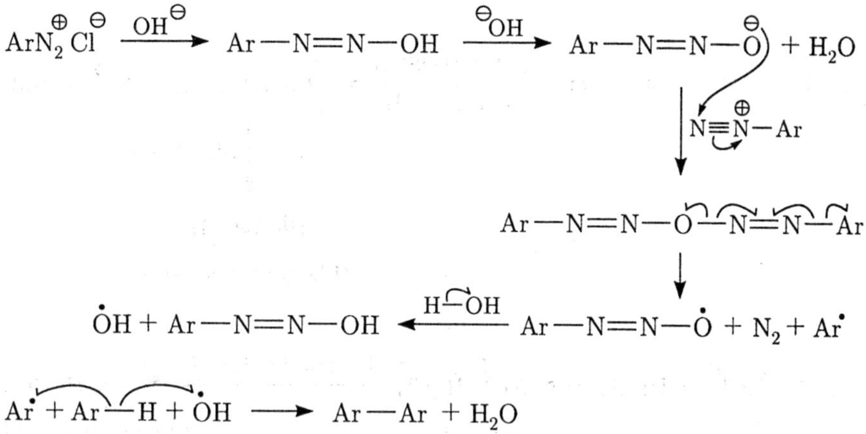

4. ***Meerwin Reaction*** : This is a reaction between diazonium salts and compounds containing an activated ethylenic bond to give arylated products. The reaction is carried out in acetone solution in the presence of Cu^{2+} (cupric) salt.

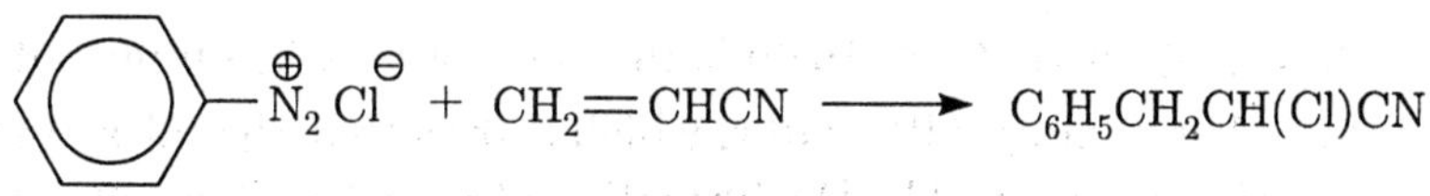

Mechanism : Follows free radical pathway.

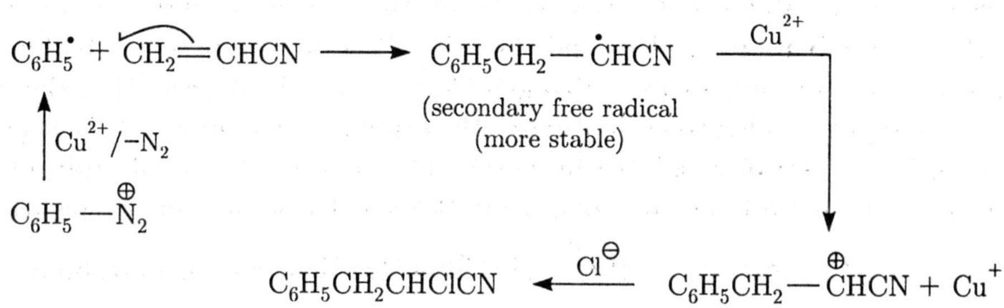

When the alkene is an α,β-unsaturated acid, then arylation may occur with decarboxylation.

$$C_6H_5\overset{\oplus}{N}_2\overset{\ominus}{Cl} + \underset{\text{(Cinnamic acid)}}{C_6H_5CH{=}CHCOOH} \longrightarrow \underset{\text{(Stilbene)}}{C_6H_5CH{=}CHC_6H_5} + N_2\uparrow + CO_2\uparrow + HCl$$

Some other reactions given by diazonium salts :

1. $$Ar\overset{\oplus}{N}_2\overset{\ominus}{Cl} + \underset{\text{(Formaldoxime)}}{RCH{=}NOH} \xrightarrow{NaOH} Ar\overset{R}{\overset{|}{C}}{=}NOH \xrightarrow{NaOH} \underset{\text{(Alkyl aryl ketone)}}{ArCOR}$$

2. $Ar\overset{\oplus}{N}_2 + HS\overset{\ominus}{O_4} + SO_2 + Cu \longrightarrow \underset{\text{(Arylsulphonic acid)}}{ArSO_3H} + N_2\uparrow + CuSO_4$

3. $Ph\overset{\oplus}{N}_2\overset{\ominus}{Cl} + Na_3AsO_3 \xrightarrow[\text{Bart's reaction}]{Cu^{II}(CuSO_4)} PhAsO_3Na_2 + N_2\uparrow + NaCl$

$$PhAsO_3Na_2 \xrightarrow{HCl(dilute)} \underset{\text{(Phenylarsonic acid)}}{PhAsO_3H}$$

4. $Ar\overset{\oplus}{N}_2\overset{\ominus}{Cl} + HgCl_2 \longrightarrow \underset{\text{(Complex)}}{Ar\overset{\oplus}{N}_2Hg\overset{\ominus}{Cl_3}} \xrightarrow{\text{Cu powder/EtOH/}\Delta} \underset{\text{(Aryl mercuric chloride)}}{ArHgCl} + N_2\uparrow + CuCl$

Elucidation of the Structure of Benzenediazonium Salt

Analytical data suggest that the formula unit of benzenediazonium salt is $C_6H_5\overset{\oplus}{N}_2$. These salts form phenol on boiling with water, which proves that the salts are mono substituted benzene. This is further proved by the formation of monohalobenzene under S_N1 condition. Langfurth (1878) prepared diazonium salt from tetrabromosulphonic acid of aniline in which the four Br atoms and SO_3H group are still present. So only *one N atom* is directly attached to the benzene nucleus and the other N atom is bonded to the former N atom. Benzenediazonium salts evolves nitrogen (N_2) gas which suggests that the two nitrogen atoms are triply bonded to each other in the original diazonium salt. Benzenediazonium salts conduct electricity, soluble in water but insoluble in organic solvents like ether, which suggests that it is an ionic compound. Benzenediazonium salts couple with phenoxide ion to form $C_6H_5—N{=}N—C_6H_4\overset{\ominus}{O}$. This indicates that benzenediazonium salt contains $C_6H_5—N{=}\overset{\oplus}{N}$ unit. Spectral analyses indicate that the C—N and N—N bond length in benzenediazonium salts have some C=N and N≡N character. In order to explain it, benzenediazonium salt is represented as a resonance hybrid as follows.

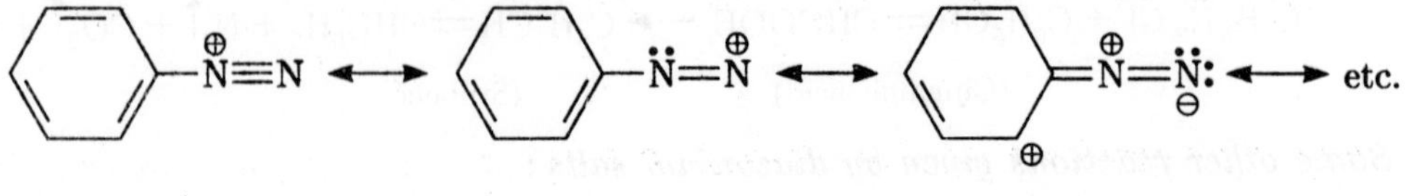

The positive charge of the benzenediazonium ion gets delocalised through π-molecular orbitals involving all the six carbon atoms and two nitrogen atoms.

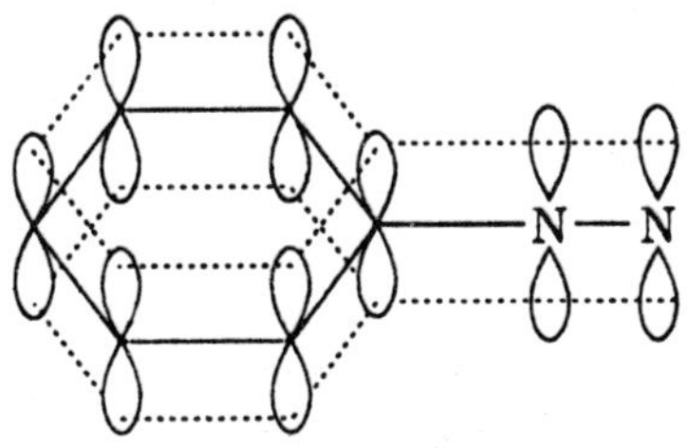

Diazoamino and Aminoazo Compounds

Diazoaminobenzene may be prepared by treating aniline hydrochloride solution with sodium nitrite just suficient *to diazotise half* of the aniline, and then adding sodium acetate.

$$C_6H_5\overset{\oplus}{N}_2\overset{\ominus}{Cl} + C_6H_5NH_2 + CH_3COONa \longrightarrow \underset{\text{(Diazoaminobenzene)}}{C_6H_5N{=}NNH\,C_6H_5} + NaCl + CH_3COOH$$

Diazoaminobenzene is often formed during the diazotisation of aniline, especially when the solution is *only weakly acidic.*

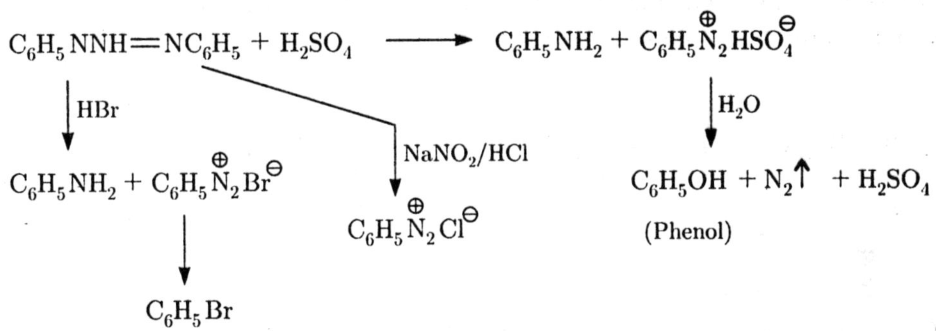

Diazoaminobenzene has a tendency to rearrange to aminoazobenzene. This is illustrated as follows.

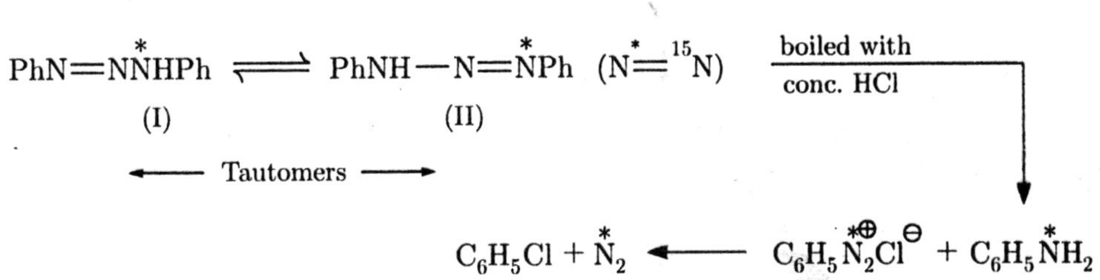

When (I) is boiled with concentrated hydrochloric acid, aniline, chlorobenzene and nitrogen are produced. If the structure were (I) then all the labelled nitrogen would be in the aniline. But in fact, the isotopic nitrogen was found to be distributed between the aniline and the nitrogen liberated. This is consistent with diazoaminobenzene being a tautomeric compound of forms (I) and (II). This tautomeric system is known as the *diazoamino triad system*, or the *three nitrogen system.* This type of tautomerism is also known as *mesohydric tautomerism.*

***p*-Aminoazobenzene** :

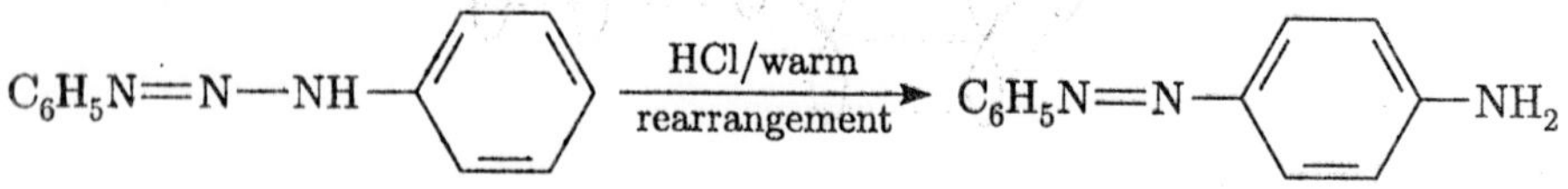

If the *p*-position in the anilino compound is occupied, then the isomeric change occurs slowly and the azo group takes up the *o*-position.

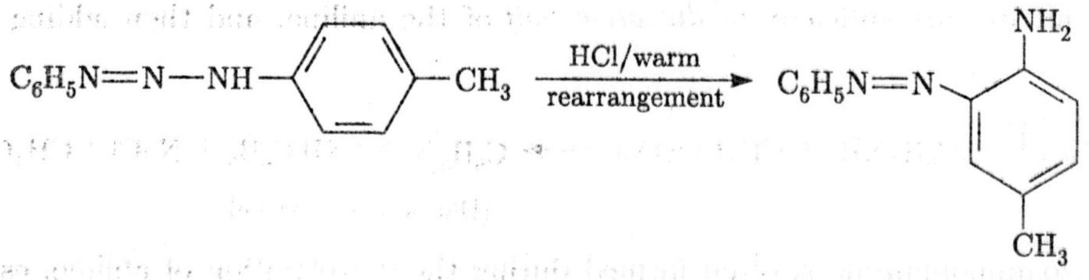

The rearrangement is better effected by $C_6H_5NH_2.HCl$ than by hydrochloric acid. This is shown by the following mechanism where aniline hydrochloride serves both as a proton donor and as a source of aniline.

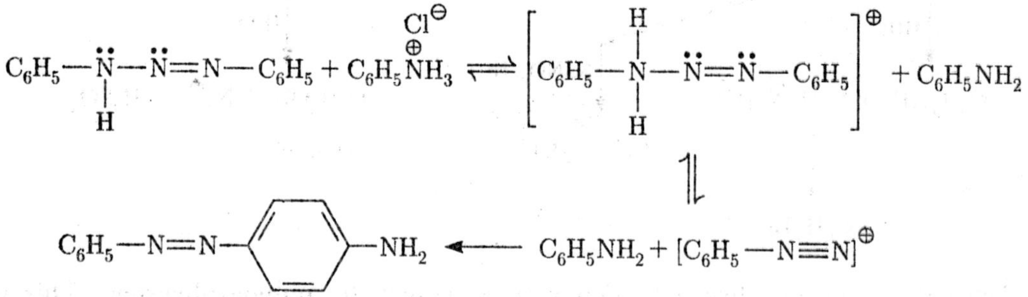

(*p*-aminoazobenzene)

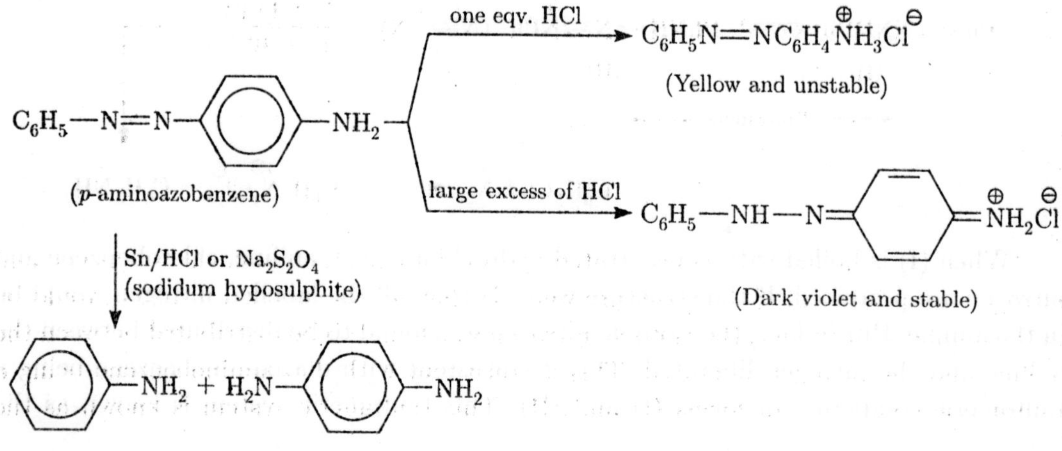

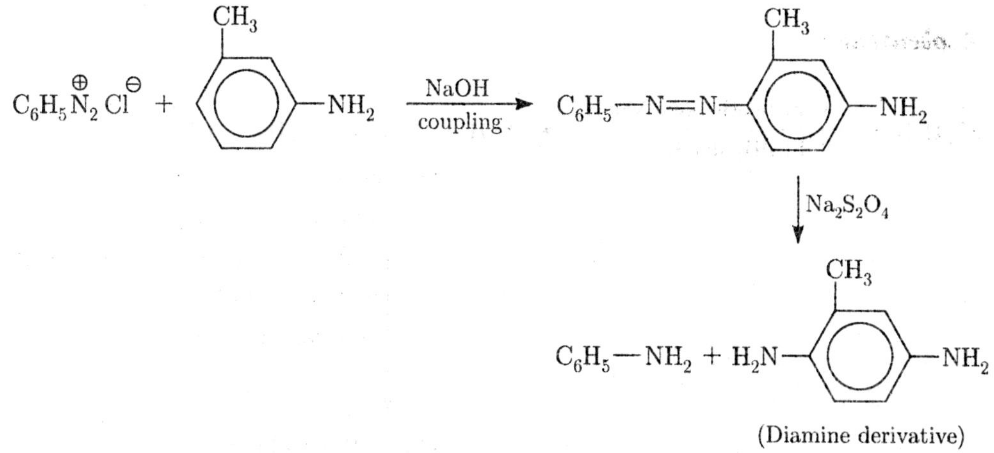

Azoxybenzene :

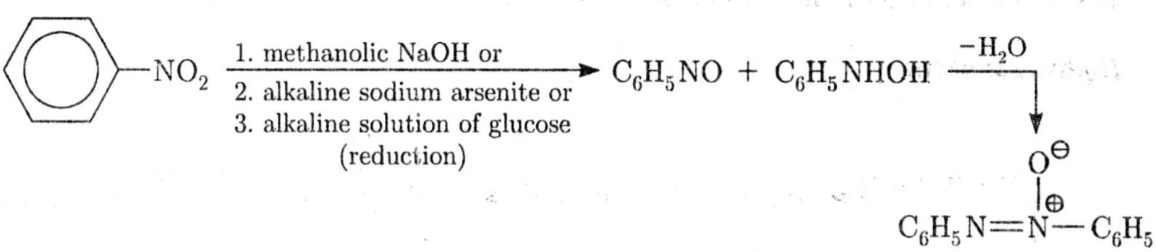

Two geometrical isomers of azoxybenzene :

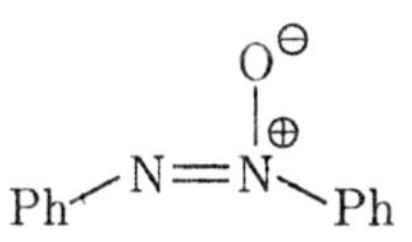

Cis-(m.p. 80°C)

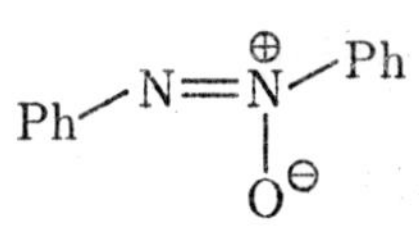

Trans-(m.p. 36°C)

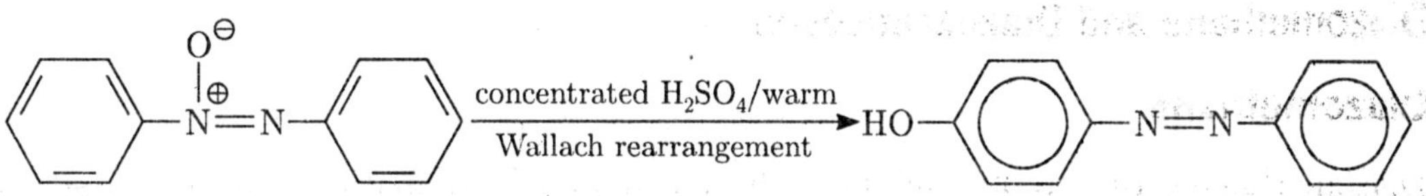

When irradiated with UV light, the product is exclusively the *o*-isomer.

Mechanism :

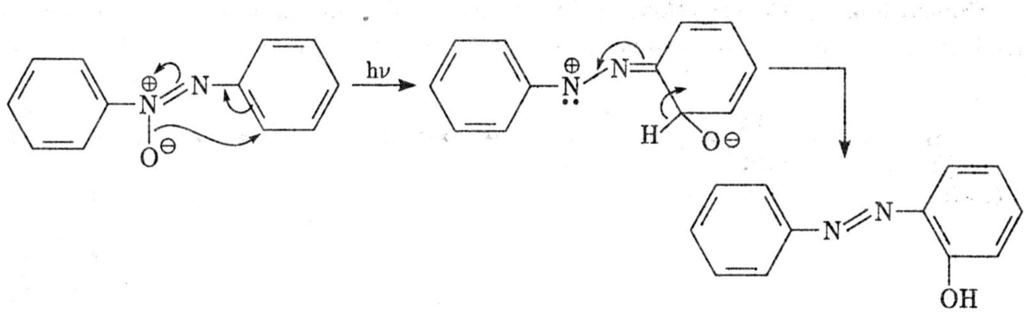

Azobenzene :

$$2C_6H_5NO_2 \xrightarrow[\text{2. LiAlH}_4\text{/dry Et}_2\text{O}]{\text{1. Zn/methanolic NaOH or}} C_6H_5{-}N{=}N{-}C_6H_5 + 4H_2O$$

(Azobenzene)

(reduction) ↓ 1. Zn dust/aq NaOH or 2. $NaBH_4/H_2O$ or $NaBH_4/MeOH$ or 3. $SnCl_2/HCl$ or 4. $Na_2S_2O_4/OH^{\ominus}$

$C_6H_5NH_2$ (Aniline)

The intermediate of the reduction is azoxybenzene.

Hydrazobenzene :

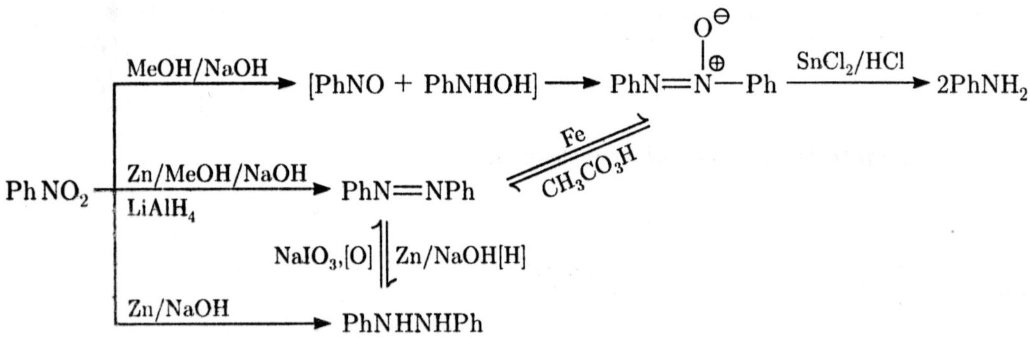

Diazomethane and Diazoaceticester

Diazomethane

Diazomethane is the simplest aliphatic diazo compound. Aliphatic diazo compounds are characterized by the presence of $-\overset{|}{C}N_2$ group.

Preparation of Diazomethane : Theoretically diazomethane can be prepared by withdrawing a proton from methyldiazonium ion by the action of a base as shown below.

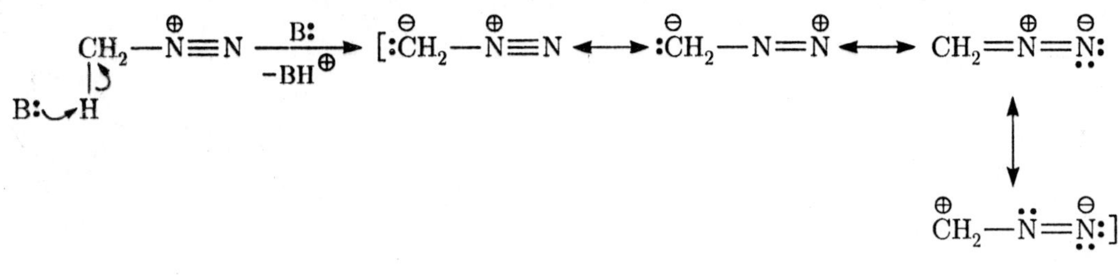

1. ***From N-methylurethan (Method of Von Pechmann)*** : When N-methylurethan is treated with nitrous acid in ether medium, N-methyl-N-nitrosourethan forms; the latter on warming with methanolic potassium hydroxide solution gives diazomethane which is collected in cold ether. N-methylurethan is prepared by the reaction between methylamine and ethyl chloroformate.

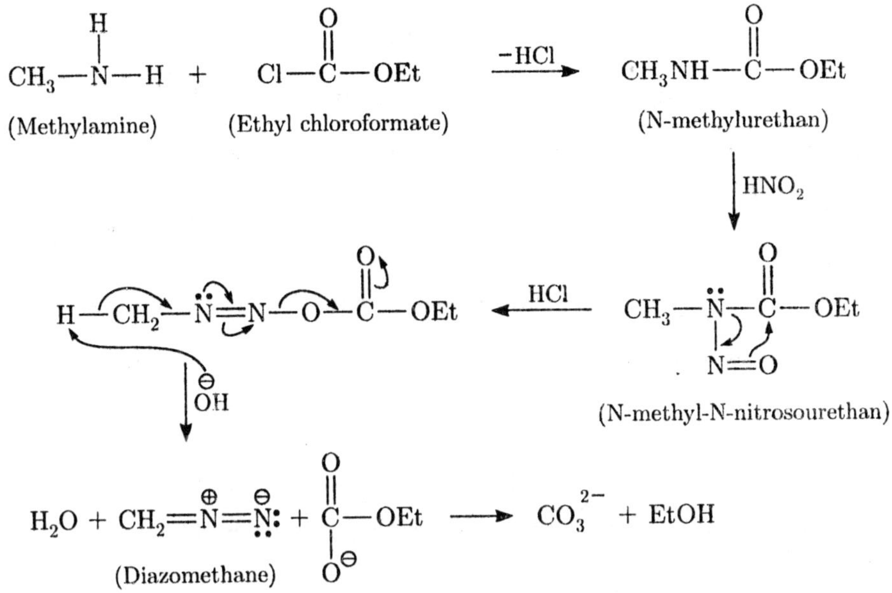

An **improved** method starts with methylurea.

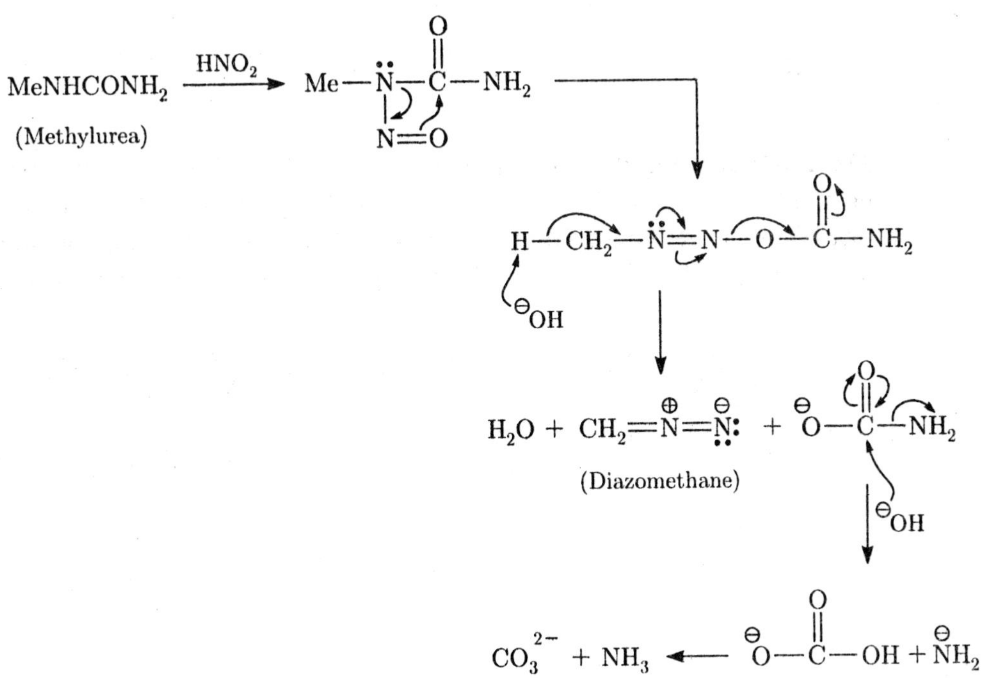

2. ***From N-methyl-N-nitroso-N′-nitroguanidine (Mckay's method)*** : Methylammonium chloride on reaction with nitroguanidine in potassium hydroxide solution forms N-methyl-N′-nitroguanidine. This on treatment with nitrous acid gives N-methyl-N-nitroso-N′-nitroguanidine which on warming with potassium hydroxide solution produces diazomethane.

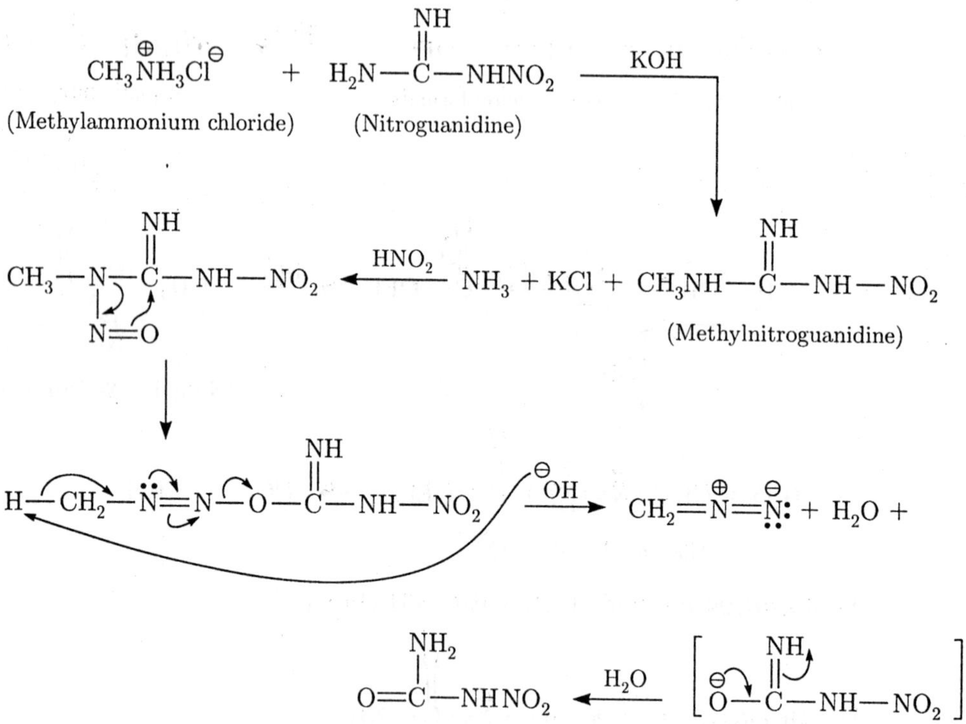

3. ***From p-toluenesulphonamide (Backer's method)*** : *p*-Toluenesulphonyl chloride on treatment with methylamine give N-methyl-*p*-toluenesulphonamide; this on nitrous acid treatment forms N-methyl-N-nitroso- *p*-toluenesulphonamide which on warming with ethanolic potassium hydroxide produces diazomethane.

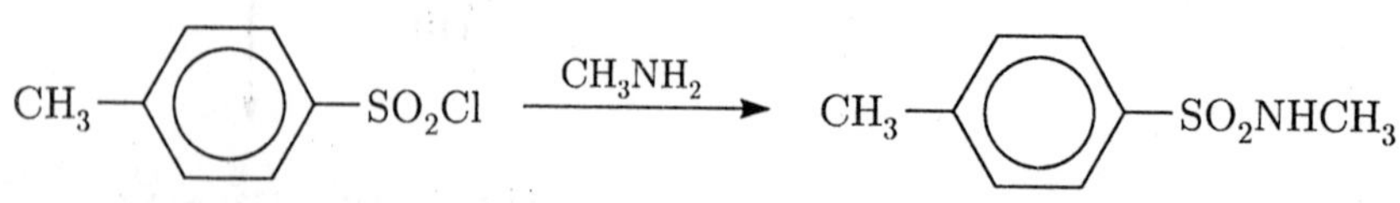

(N-methyl-*p*-tolueneslphonamide)

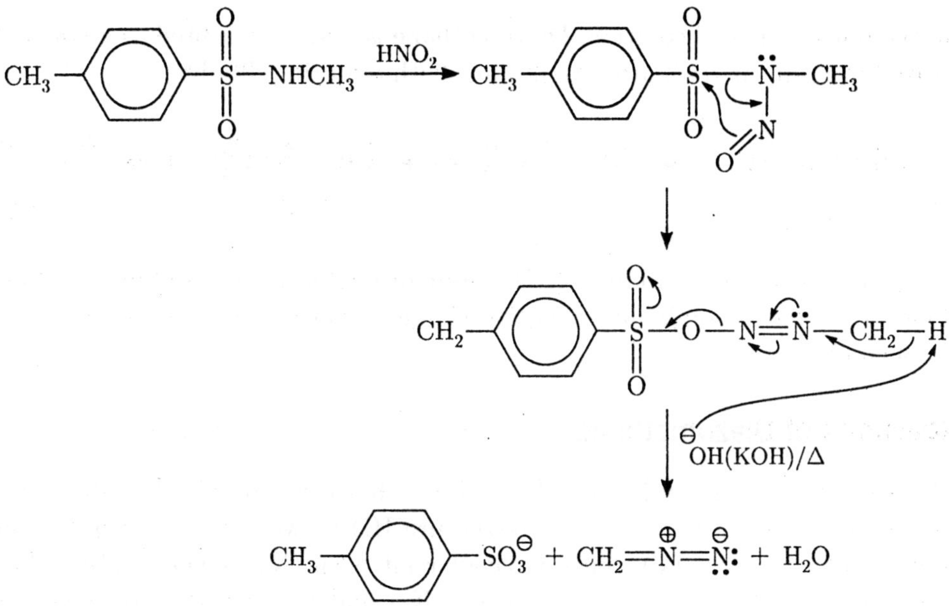

4. ***From N-N′-dimethyl-N-N′-dinitrosoterephthalamide (NTA)*** : N-N′-dimethyl-N-N′-dinitrosoterephthalamide (NTA) is commercially available and stable at room temperature. Diazomethane is best prepared from NTA.

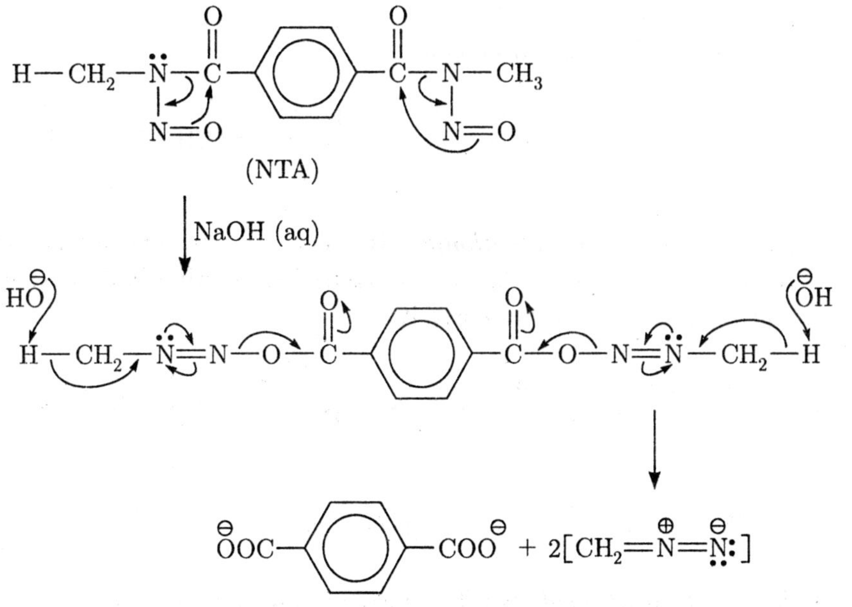

(Terephthalic acid dianion)

Physical properties and structure of diazomethane : Diazomethane is a yellow coloured gas at N.T.P. (b.p.–24°C) and is highly poisonous and explosive. So the reactions are carried out in ethereal solution. Diazomethane is best represented as a resonance hybrid derived from linear resonating structures with opposing dipoles.

$$\underset{\text{(I)}}{CH_2{=}\overset{\oplus}{N}{=}\overset{\ominus}{\ddot{N}}:} \longleftrightarrow \underset{\text{(II)}}{\overset{\ominus}{\ddot{C}}H_2{-}\overset{\oplus}{N}{\equiv}N} \longleftrightarrow \underset{\text{(III)}}{\overset{\oplus}{C}H_2{-}\ddot{N}{=}\overset{\ominus}{\ddot{N}}:} \longleftrightarrow \underset{\text{(IV)}}{\overset{\ominus}{\ddot{C}}H_2{-}\ddot{N}{=}\overset{\oplus}{N}:}$$

(I) is the most contributory to the resonance hybrid, as it contain maximum number (four) of covalent bonds and negative charge resides on one negative electronegative nitrogen atom.

Reactions of Diazomethane

The resonance hybrid of diazomethane shows that it is a dipolar ion; it can attack as an electrophile through carbon atom (structure III) as well as a nucleophile through the same atom (structure IV). Since molecular nitrogen (N_2) is very stable, diazomethane (structure II) explodes to give nitrogen (N_2) and carbene ($:CH_2$). This carbene can undergo addition and insertion reactions.

1. ***Generation of carbene*** :

$$:\overset{\ominus}{C}H_2{-}\overset{\oplus}{N}{\equiv}N \xrightarrow{\text{ultra violet light (hv) or heat}} :CH_2 + N_2\uparrow$$

2. ***Reduction by sodium amalgam*** :

$$CH_2{=}\overset{\oplus}{N}{=}\overset{\ominus}{\ddot{N}}: \xrightarrow{Na/Hg,\ H_2O} \underset{\text{(Methylhydrazine)}}{CH_3NH{-}NH_2}$$

3. ***Methylation by diazomethane*** : Haloacids, carboxylic acids, phenols etc. are readily methylated by diazomethane to form methyl halides, methyl esters, and methylphenyl esters respectively.

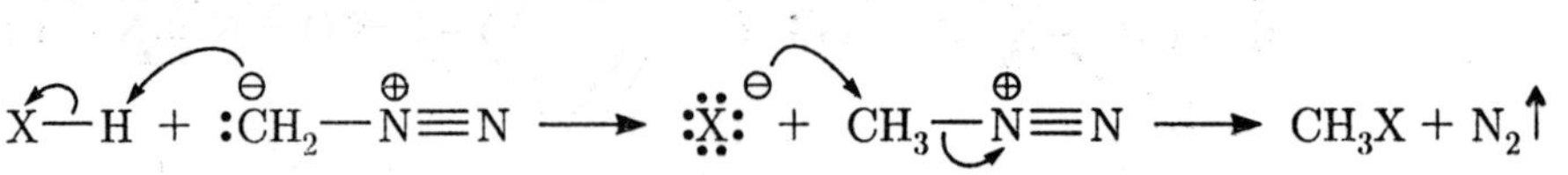

(X=Cl, $R{-}\overset{O}{\overset{\|}{C}}{-}O{-}$, $C_6H_5O{-}$ etc.)

4. ***Methylation of alcohols*** : The alcohols are not methylated easily because the hydrogen atom of an alcohol can not be displaced easily as the acidity of alcoholic hydrogen (–OH) is not much. In the presence of aluminium alkoxide, a Lewis acid, the methylation by diazomethane can be done.

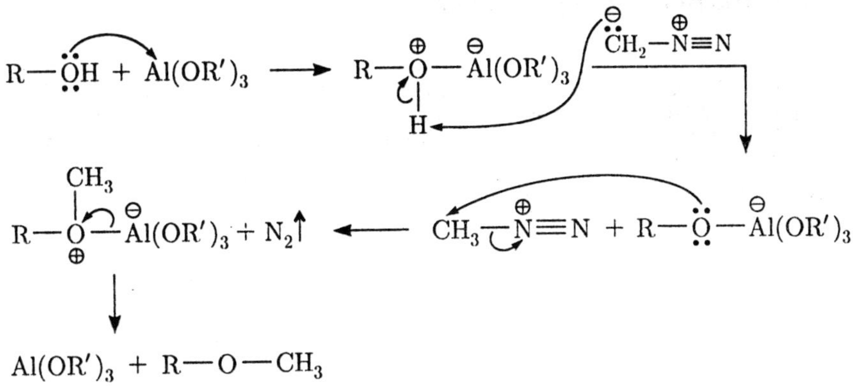

5. ***Methylation of amines*** :

$$CH_2N_2 + R_2NH \xrightarrow{BF_3} CH_3R_2N$$

(tertiary amine)

6. ***Reaction with carbonyl compounds*** : Diazomethane reacts with carbonyl compounds (aldehydes and ketones) to form methyl and higher ketones. Epoxides are also formed as by products.

(a) 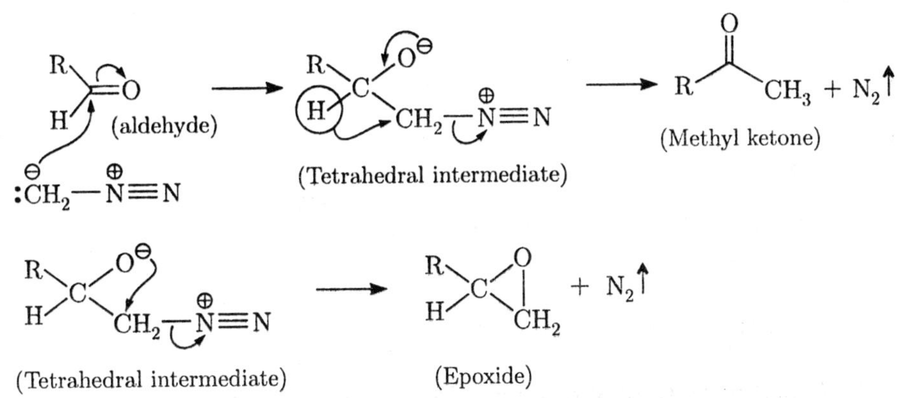

(b) 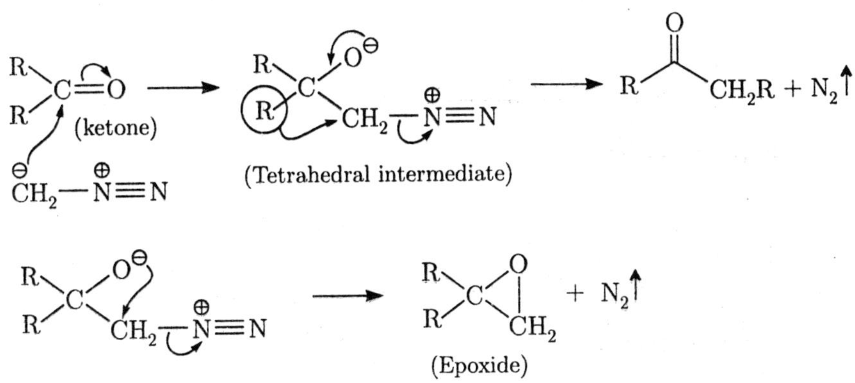

So aldehydes and ketones are converted into their next **higher homolgoue.**

(c) ***Reaction with cyclic ketones*** :

(i)

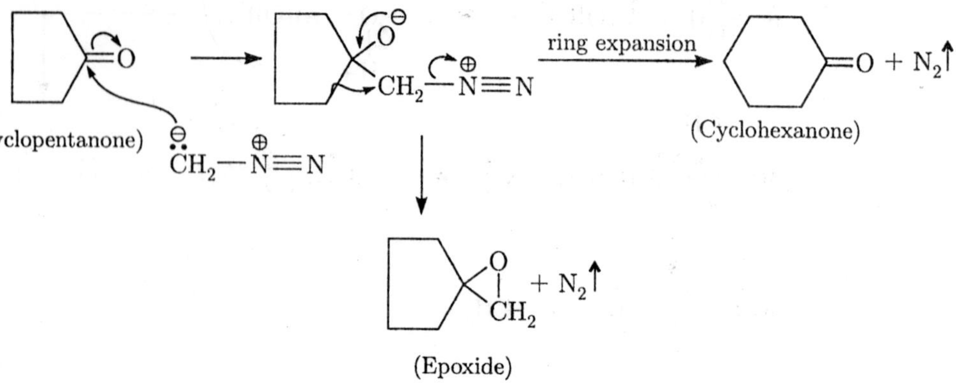

(ii)

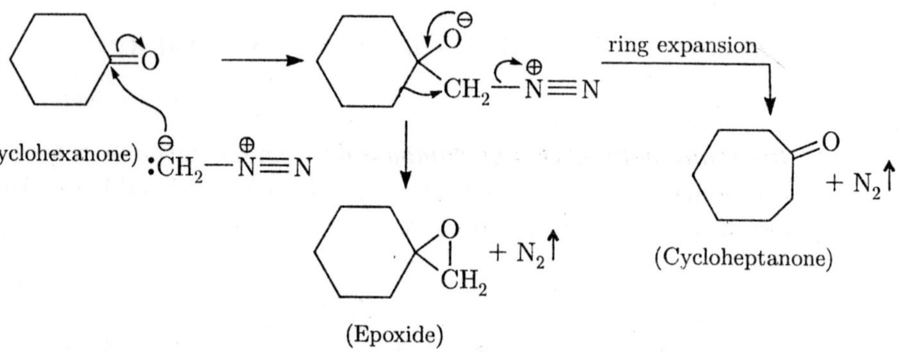

(d)

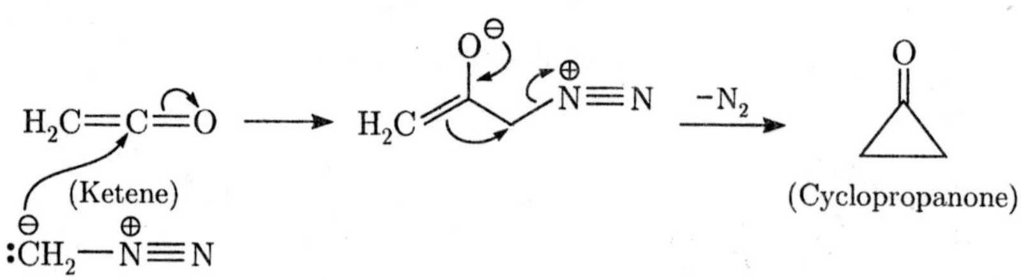

6. ***Reaction with olefinic double bond and triple bond*** :

(a)

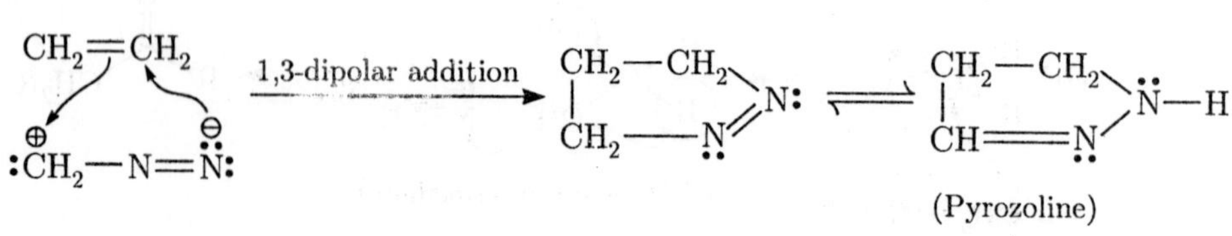

(b)

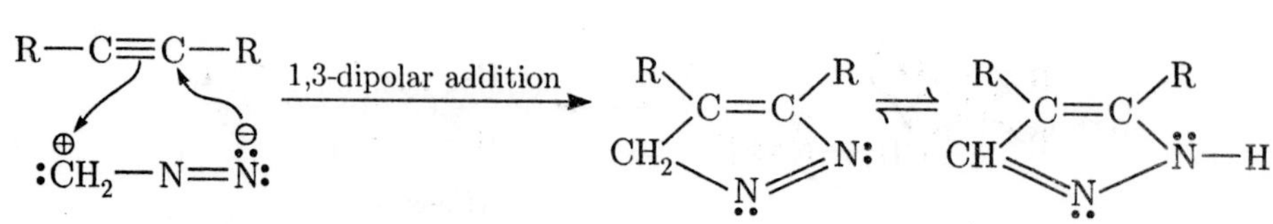

(c) 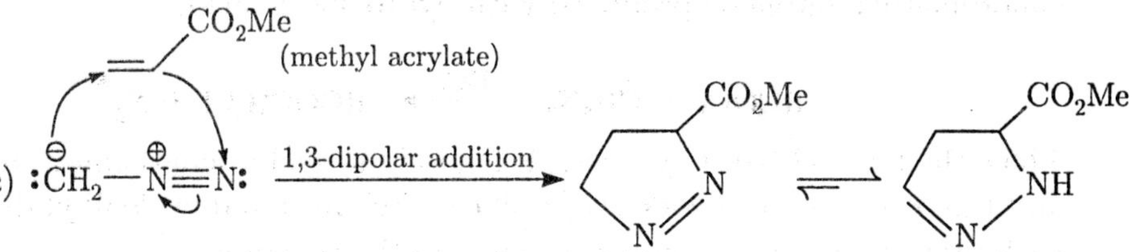

7. *Aromatic ring expansion*

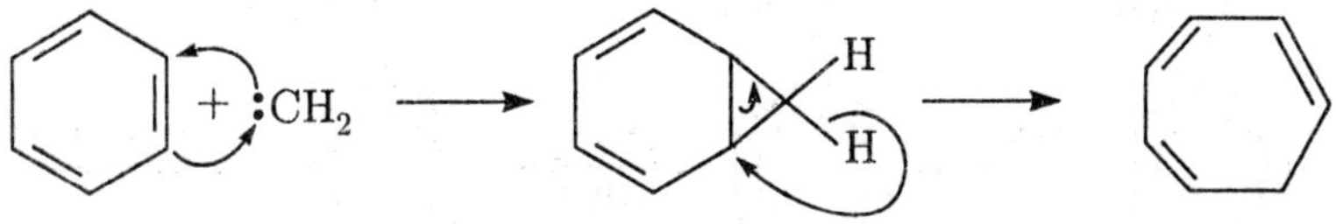

(Cycloheptatriene)

8. ***The Arndt-Eistert Synthesis and Wolff Rearrangement*** : The thermal or photochemical or catalytic conversion of a diazoketone to a ketene with the liberation of molecular nitrogen is known as the *Wolff rearrangement.* Usually diazoketones are prepared from acyl halides by the action of diazomethane.

$$\underset{\text{(R=alkyl or aryl)}}{RCOCl} + CH_2N_2 \longrightarrow \underset{\text{(Diazoketene)}}{RCOCHN_2} \xrightarrow{\text{rearrangement}} O{=}C{=}CHR + N_2\uparrow$$

However, the reaction is usually carried out in the presence of water and Ag_2O ("AgOH") and the ultimate product is a carboxylic acid having one carbon atom more than the starting acyl halide.

$$RCOCl + CH_2N_2 \xrightarrow{H_2O/Ag_2O} RCH_2COOH + N_2\uparrow + HCl$$

The overall reaction is known as *Arndt-Eistert synthesis*, where a carboxylic acid is converted into its higher homologue by reaction of its acyl halide with diazomethane in the presence of water and silver oxide (Ag_2O) as catalyst. If the reaction is carried out with an alcohol or ammonia, instead of water, the product will be a higher ester or amide respectively.

$$RCOCl + CH_2N_2 \xrightarrow{R'OH/Ag_2O} RCH_2COOR' + N_2\uparrow$$

$$RCOCl + CH_2N_2 \xrightarrow[Ag_2O]{NH_3/R'NH_2} RCH_2CONH_2/RCH_2CONHR' + N_2\uparrow$$

When the reaction is carried out in the presence of water and formic acid in the absence of any catalyst, hydroxymethyl ketones are formed.

$$RCOCl + CH_2N_2 \xrightarrow{H_2O/HCOOH} RCOCH_2OH + N_2\uparrow$$

Chloromethyl ketone is produced with hydrochloric acid.

$$RCOCl + CH_2N_2 \xrightarrow{HCl} RCOCH_2Cl + N_2\uparrow$$

Thus, the Erndt-Eistert synthesis is a good means for lengthening carbon chain and the reaction has a wide scope since alkyl, aryl and cycloalkyl diazoketones with other functional groups can undergo the reaction.

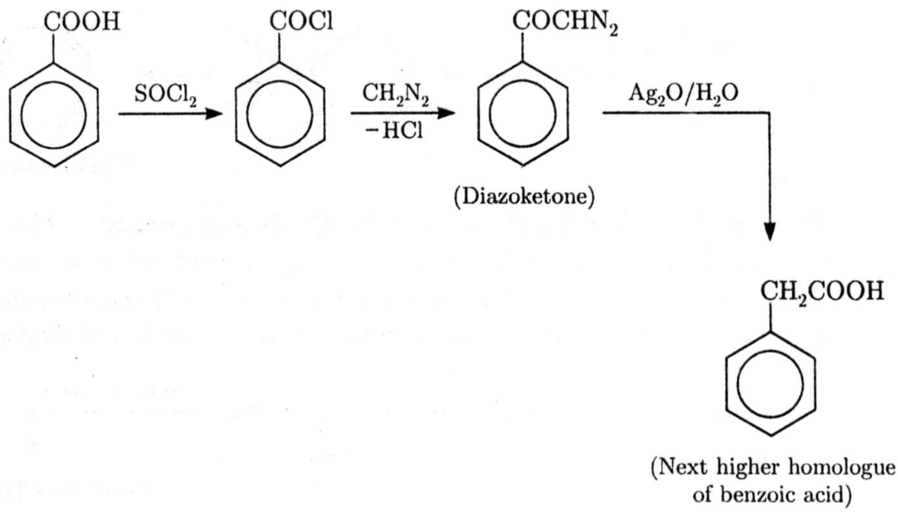

Mechanism of Erndt-Eistert synthesis :

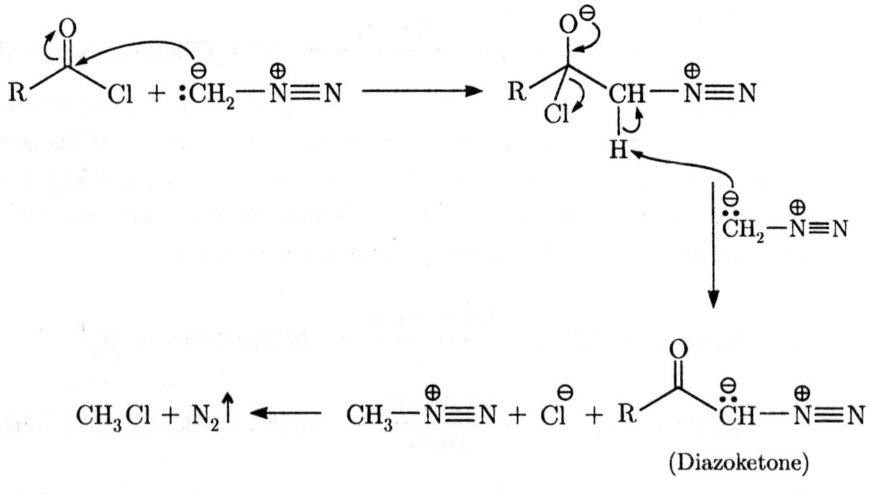

In the next step, molecular nitrogen is eliminated and R group migrates to the anionic carbon in an 1,2-shift and concerted manner.

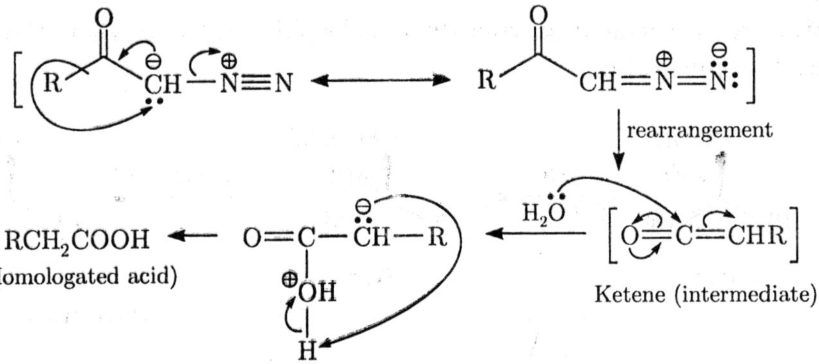

Excess of diazomethane per molecule of RCOCl is essential in Erndt-Eistert synthesis, and Wolff rearrangement. $RCOCH_2Cl$ will be formed instead of diazoketone if we do not use excess diazomethane.

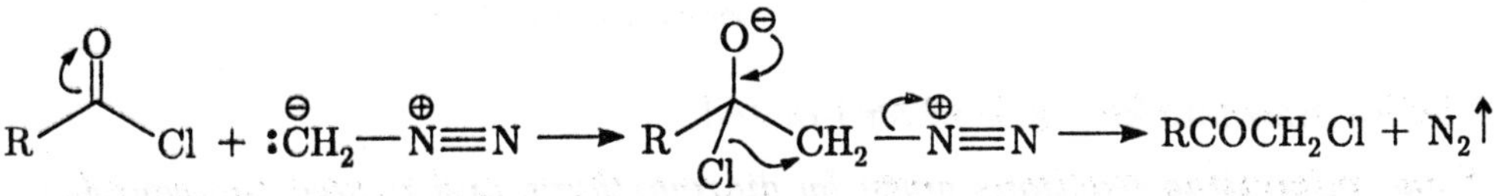

Evidence for 1,2-shift in Wolff rearrangement by radioisotope dating :

Preparation of phenylacetic acid from benzoic acid : The carboxyl carbon of benzoic acid is taken radioactive and the phenylacetic acid formed by Erndt-Eistert synthesis is oxidised with $CuO—Cr_2O_3$ and the carbon dioxide (CO_2) evolved contains radioactive carbon. If the phenyl group does not migrate from the carboxyl carbon to the α-carbon of diazoketone (Wolff rearrangement) this can not be the result.

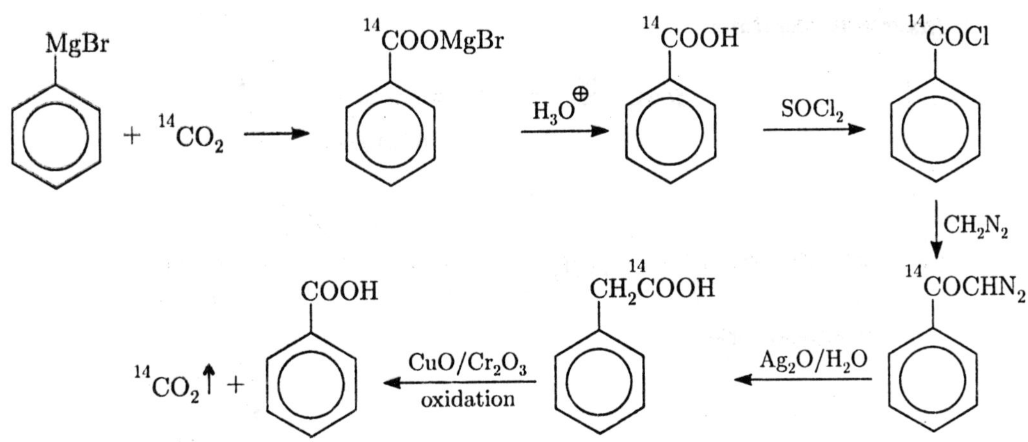

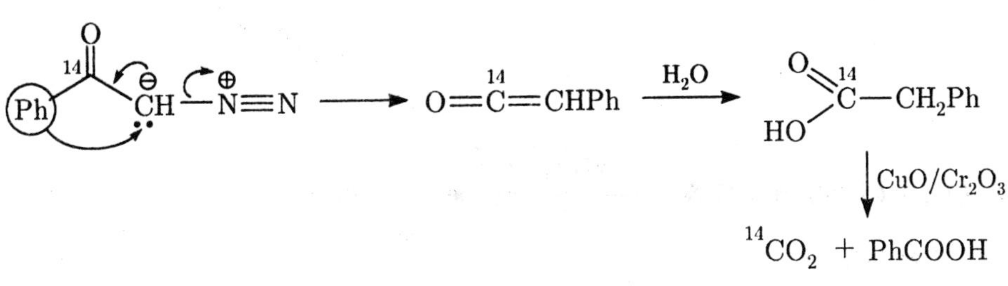

Wolff rearrangement is typically a nucleophilic 1,2-shift where the migrating group retains its configuration.

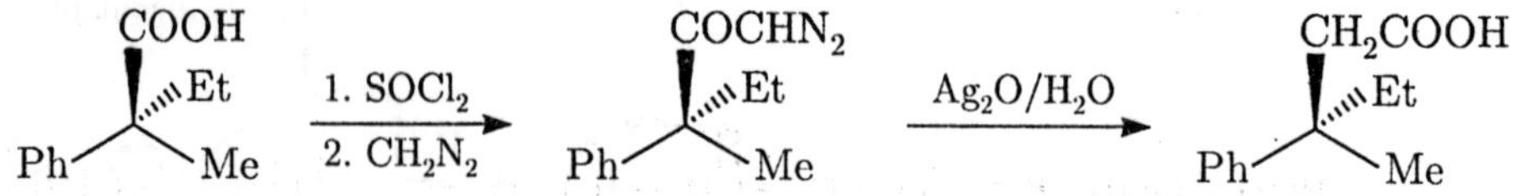

(R)- (R)- (R)-
(Retention of configuration)

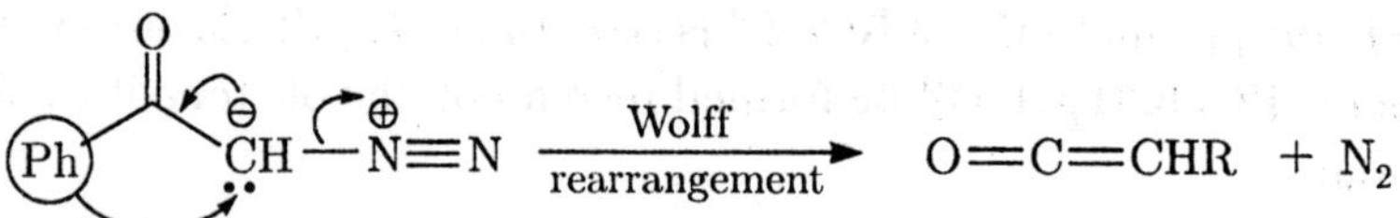

Ketene(intermediate)

The intermediate ketene is never isolated.

***Some interesting reactions given by diazomethane and related compounds* :**

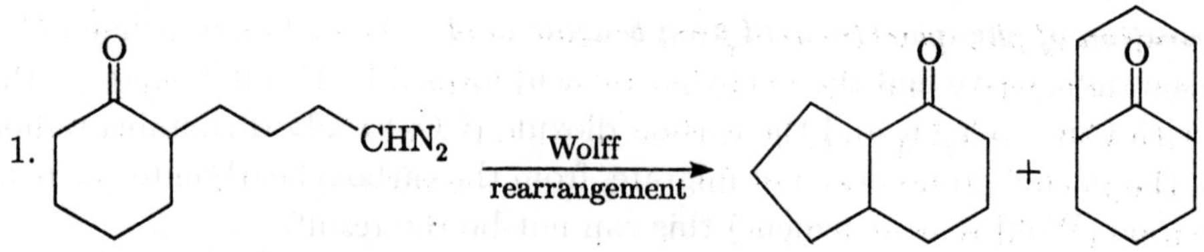

2. ***Insertion reactions* :**

$$:\overset{\ominus}{C}H_2-\overset{\oplus}{N}\equiv N \xrightarrow{h\nu} :CH_2 \ + N_2\uparrow$$

(Carbene)

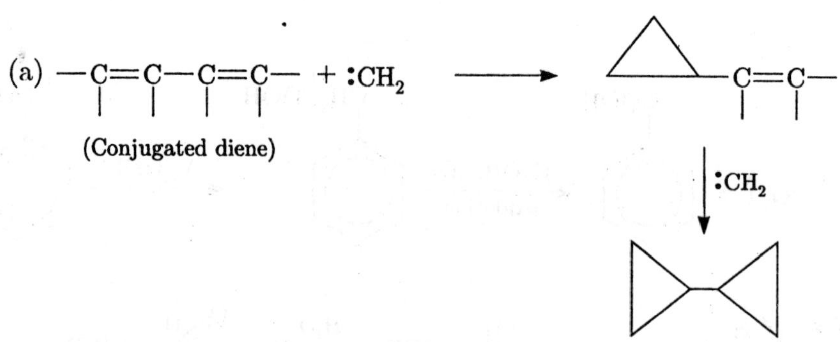

(Conjugated diene)

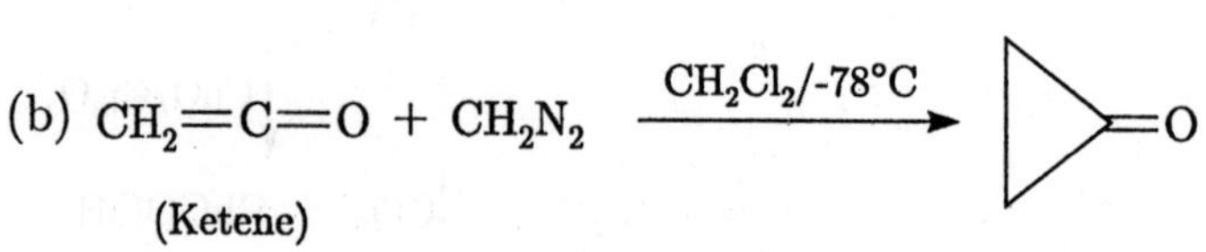

(Ketene)

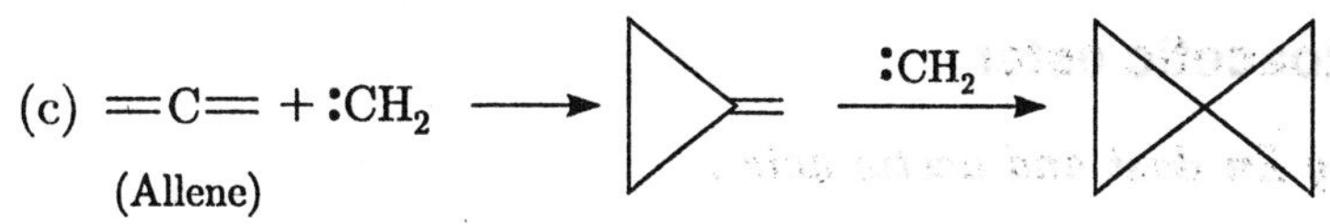

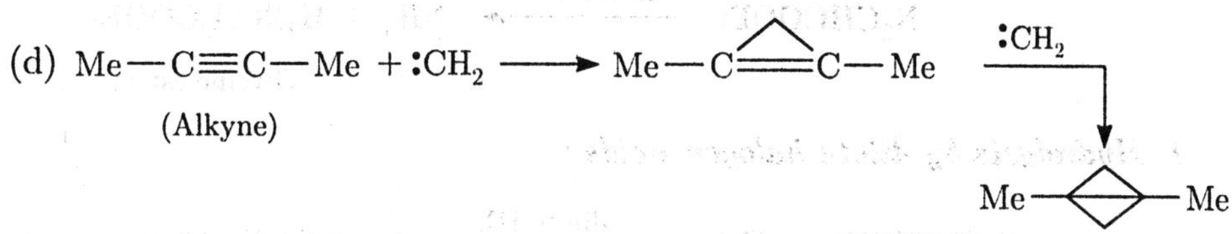

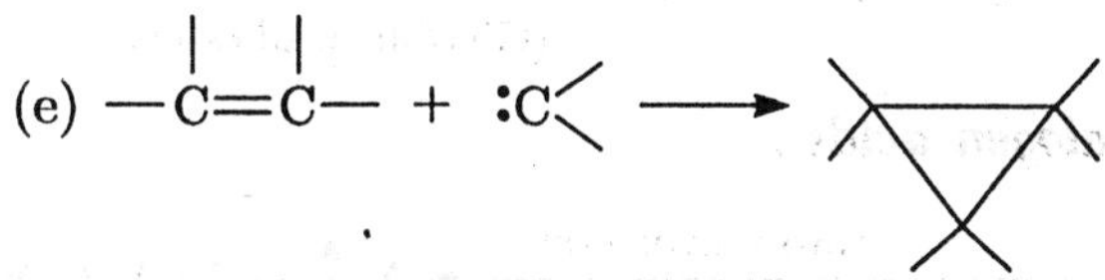

Diazoacetic Ester (Ethyl Diazoacetate, $N_2CHCOOEt$)

Ethyl diazoacetate ($N_2CHCOOEt$) is a fairly stable compound and has synthetic importance.

Preparation of Diazoacetic ester : When a cooled solution of hydrochloride of ethylglycine ester is treated with cold and dilute sodium nitrite solution in water, ethyl diazoacetate is formed.

$$CH_3COOH \xrightarrow{Cl_2/\text{sunlight}} ClCH_2COOH \xrightarrow{\text{conc.}H_2SO_4/EtOH} ClCH_2COOEt$$

$$ClCH_2COOEt \xrightarrow{\text{conc.}NH_4OH} H_2N{-}CH_2COOEt \xrightarrow{HCl} \overset{\ominus}{Cl}\ \overset{\oplus}{N}H_3CH_2COOEt$$

(Ethylglycine hydrochloride)

$$\xrightarrow{\text{cold aq. }NaNO_2} N_2CHCO_2Et + H_2O + NaCl$$

(Diazoacetic ester)

Physical properties and structure of diazoacetic ester : It is a yellow oil (b.p. 141°C at 720 mm), soluble in alcohol and ether, insoluble in water. Diazoacetic ester is a resonance hybrid of the following structures–

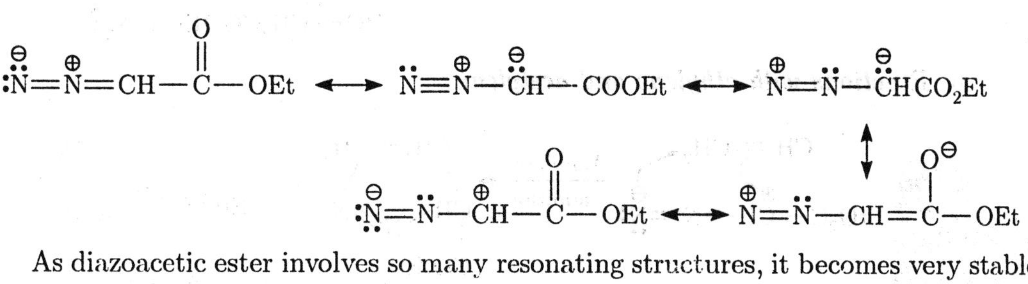

As diazoacetic ester involves so many resonating structures, it becomes very stable.

Reactions of Diazoacetic ester

1. ***Reduction by Zn dust and acetic acid*** :

$$N_2CHCOOEt \xrightarrow{Zn/AcOH} NH_3 + H_2NCH_2COOEt$$

(Glycine ester)

2. ***Hydrolysis by dilute halogen acids*** :

$$N_2CHCOOEt + H_2O \xrightarrow[\text{(nucleophile is } H_2O)]{\text{dilute HX}} HOCH_2COOEt + N_2\uparrow$$

(Glycollic acid ester)

3. ***Action of concentrated halogen acids*** :

$$N_2CHCOOEt + HX \text{ (conc.)} \xrightarrow[\text{(nucleophile is } :\ddot{X}:^{\ominus})]{\text{warm, hydrolysis}} N_2\uparrow + XCH_2COOEt$$

4. ***Reactions of diazoacetic ester on carboxylic acids, phenols and alcohols*** : Ethyl diazoacetate replaces active hydrogen of acids, phenols and alcohols to form derivatives of glycollic ester.

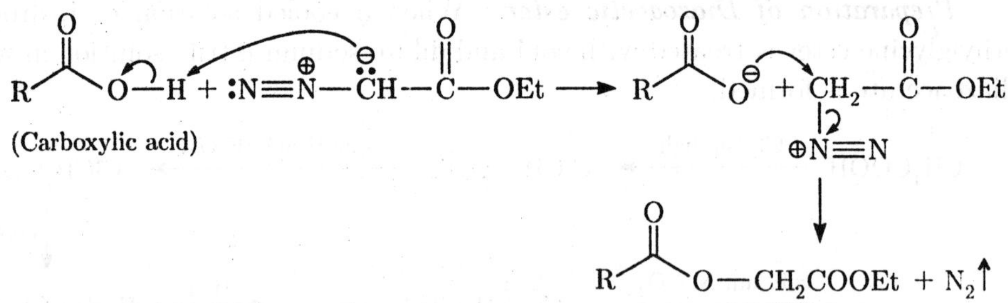

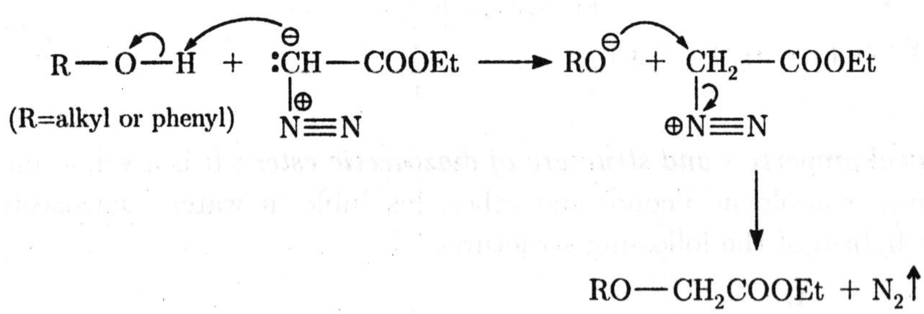

5. ***Reactions with ethylene and acetylene*** :

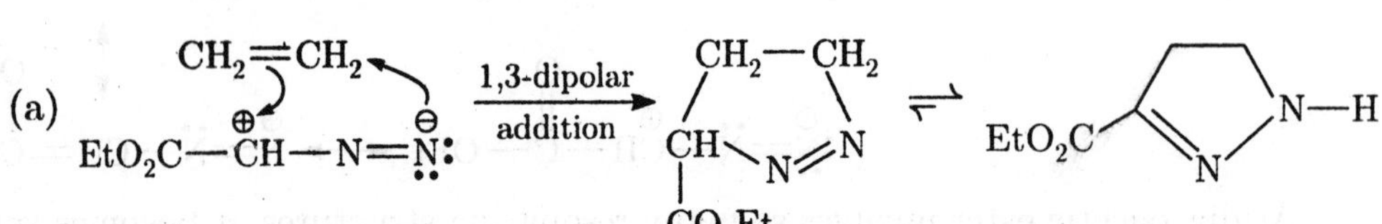

(Pyrazoline-3-carboxylic ester)

(b) 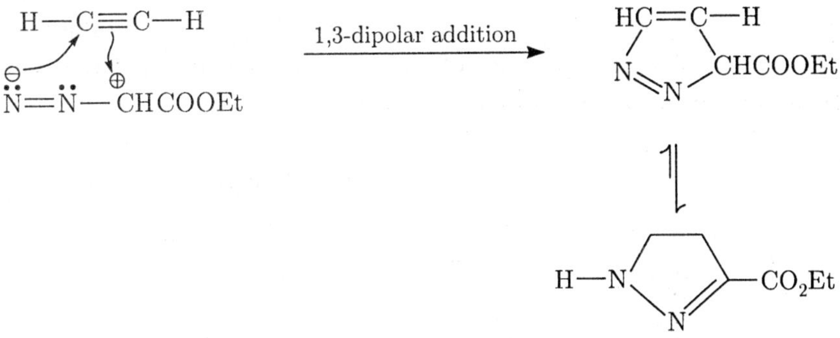

(Pyrazoline-3-carboxylic ester)

6. *Ring expansion reactions* :

$$N_2CHCOOEt \xrightarrow{h\nu} N_2\uparrow + :CHCOOEt$$

(a) 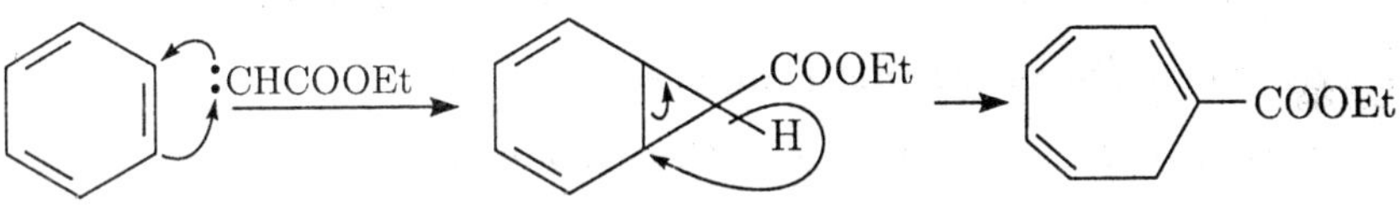

(b) 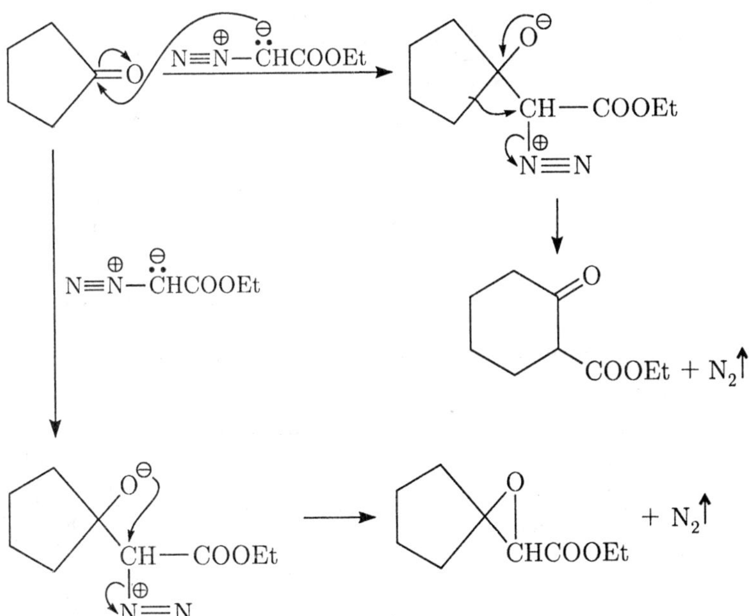

(Epoxide)

Diazoketones

Diazocarbonyl compounds (diazoketones) are important source for the generation of carbene (:C<), a very reactive reaction intermediate. Diazomethane or rather diazoalkanes also can produce carbene (:CR_2 or simple carbene :CH_2), but this is not a very practical way of generating carbenes, because of the explosive nature of diazoalkanes. However, *diazocarbonyl compounds* are a different matter.

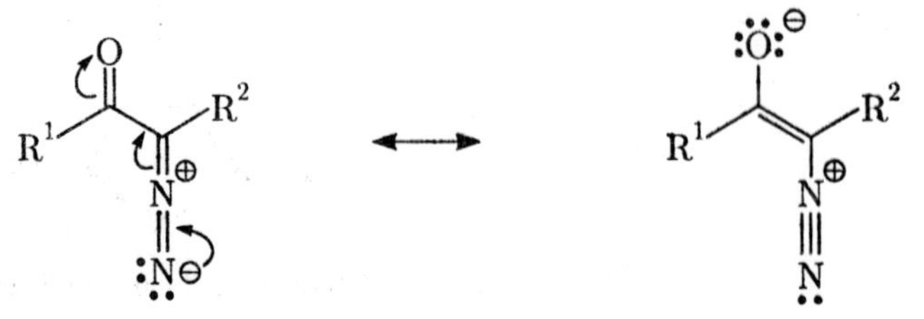

(Diazocarbonyl compound) (The diazo dipole is stabilised by the carbonyl group)

They are much more stable, because the electron withdrawing carbonyl group stabilises the diazo dipole, and are very useful sources of carbenes carrying a carbonyl substituent. There are two main ways of making diazocarbonyl compounds.

Preparation of Diazocarbonyl compounds **:**

1. By reacting an acyl chloride with diazomethane.

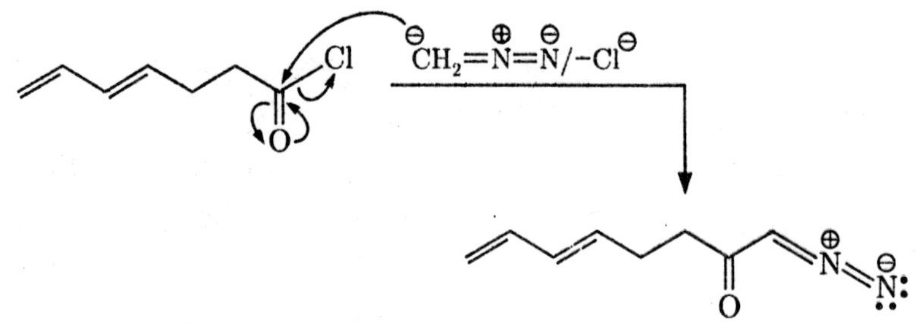

(Diazocarbonyl compound isolated in 100% yield)

2. By reacting the parent carbonyl compound with tosyl azide (TsN_3), in the presence of a base.

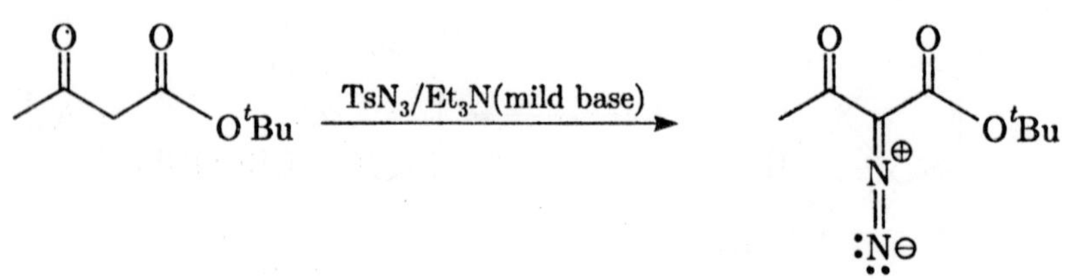

(Diazocarbonyl compound isolated in 95% yield)

The reaction of diazomethane with acyl chlorides starts as a simple acylation to give a diazonium compound. If there is an *excess* of diazomethane, a second molecule acts as a base to remove rather acidic proton between the carbonyl and diazonium groups to give the diazocarbonyl compound.

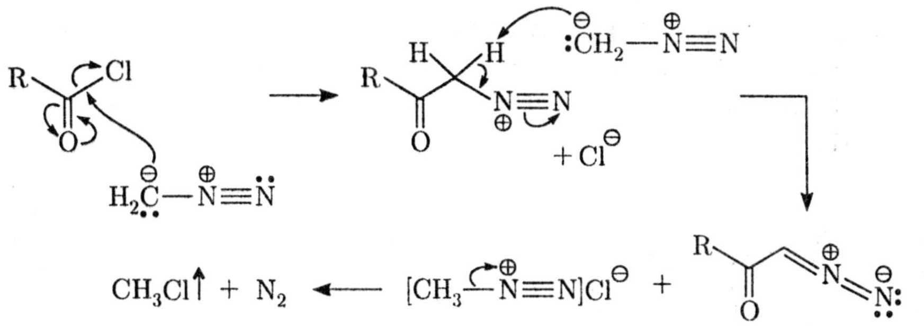

What happens to that second molecule of diazomethane? By collecting a proton it turns into the very reactive diazonium salt, which collects a chloride ion and methylchloride is given off as a gas.

The *second method* uses *tosylazide* which is known as a *Diazo transfer reagent.* It is just N_2 attached to a good leaving group.

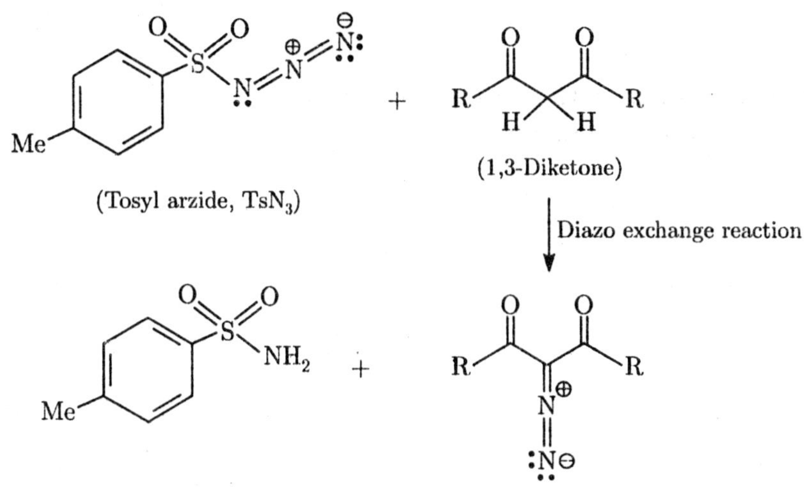

(Diazocarbonyl compound)

Diazocarbonyl compounds can be decomposed to *carbenes* by *heat* or *light.* The formation of very stable gaseous nitrogen compensates for the formation of the unstable carbene.

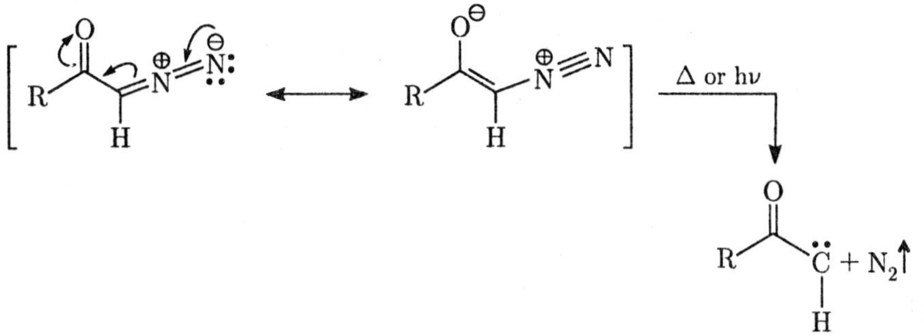

(Carbene)

3. The carbenes from α-diazoketones have the special property that they undergo rearrangement faster than they are trapped by, for example, alkenes. Rearrangement gives a ketene which can be trapped by an alkene and this forms the basis of a method for *synthesising four-membered rings*. For example,

(a) 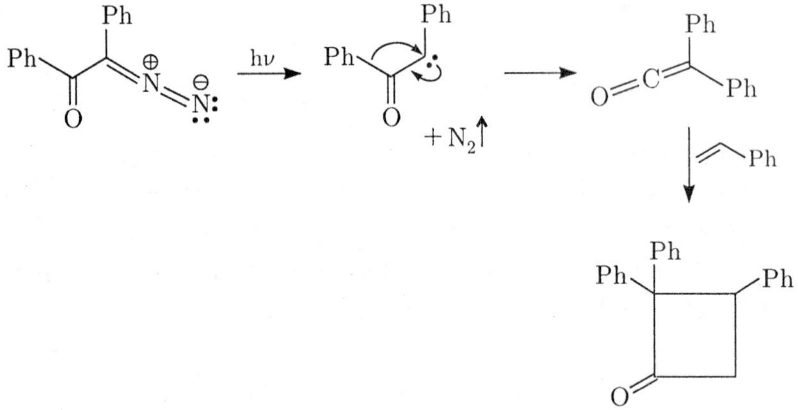

(b) A variant of this reaction is the ring contraction of carbenes from cyclic α-diazoketones. For example,

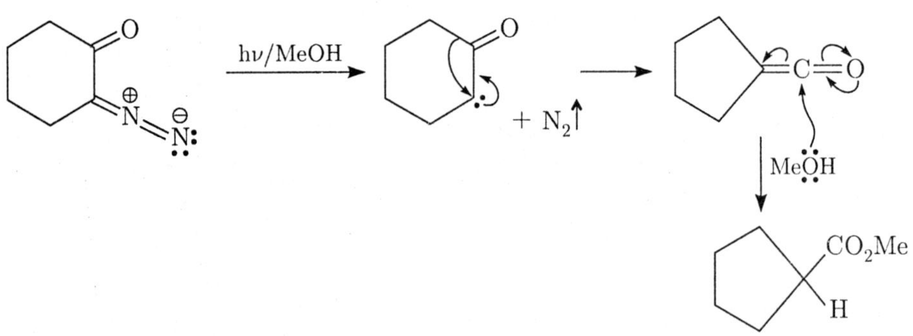

(c) Some highly strained small ring compounds have been made in this way. For example,

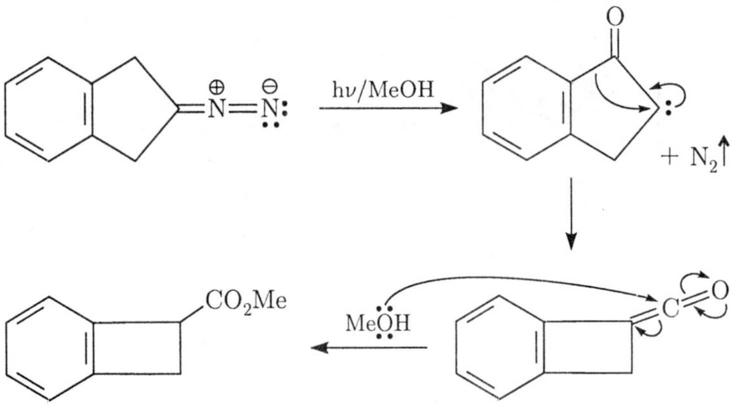

(d) 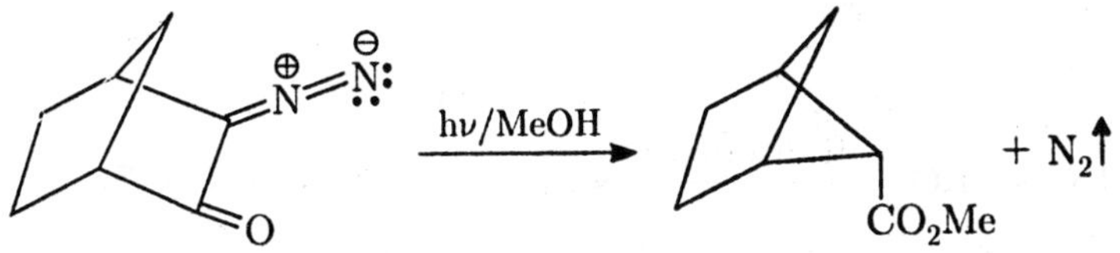

4. *The reaction* of *diazomethane with an acid chloride gives a diazoketone*, which on heating in the presence of Ag_2O, undergoes the *Wolff Rearrangement* to give a ketene.

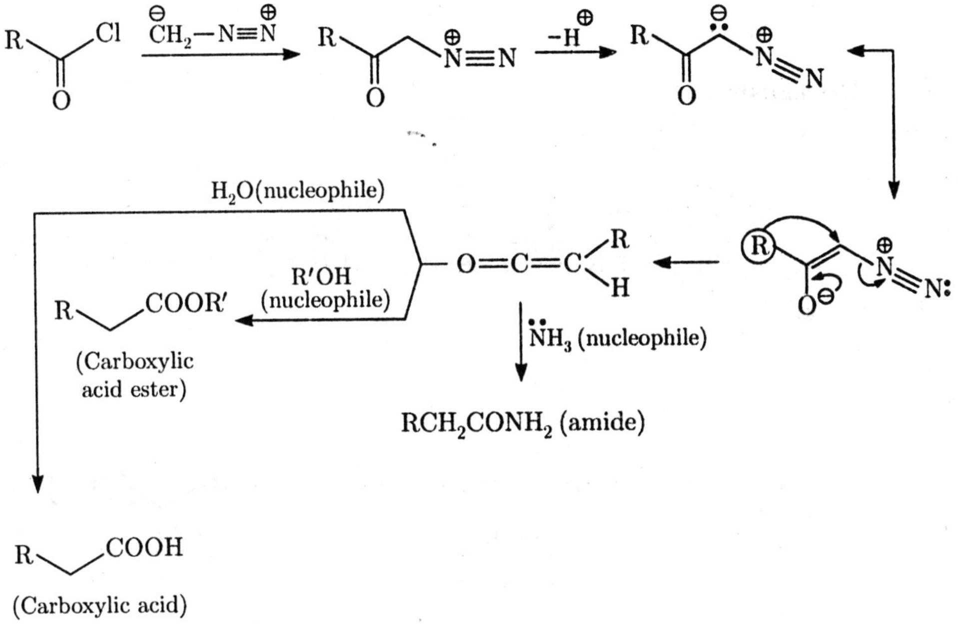

The overall process (Arndt Eistert Synthesis) provides a method for the conversion of an *acid RCOOH into the homologue RCH_2COOH* in three stages. Total yields are normally good (50-80%).

5. 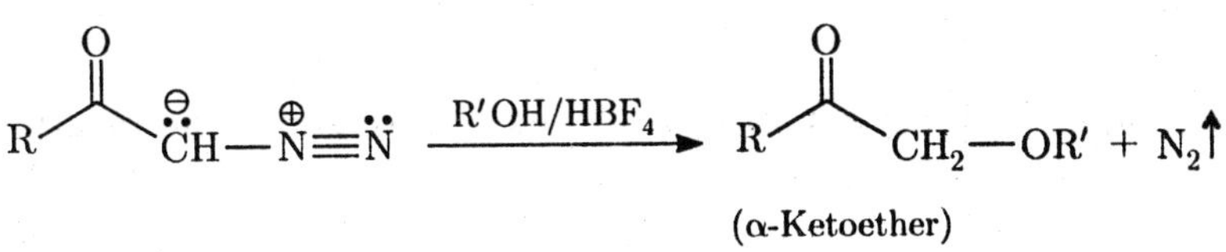

6. 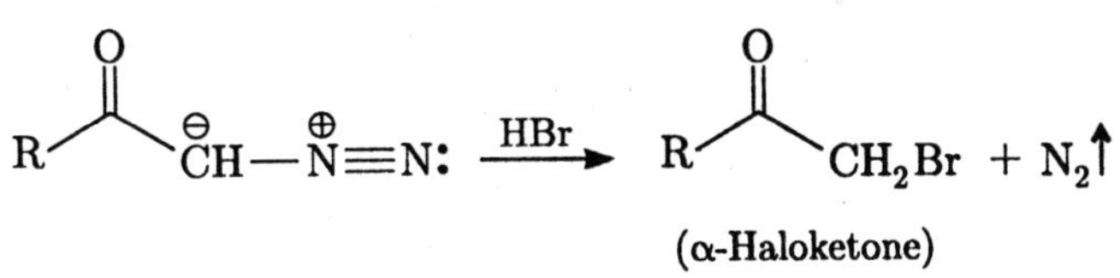

7. 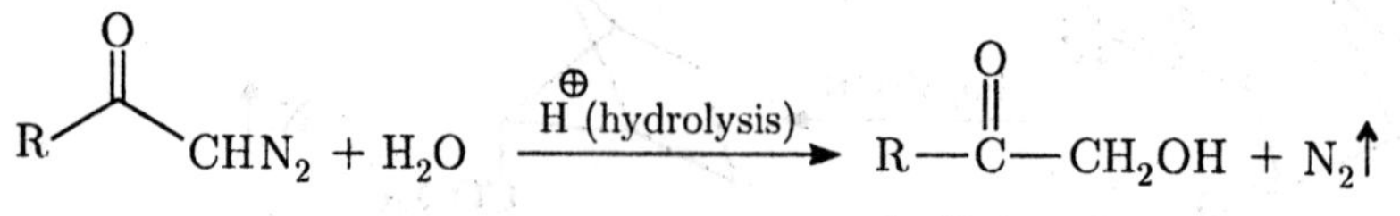

(α-Hydroxyketone)

8. 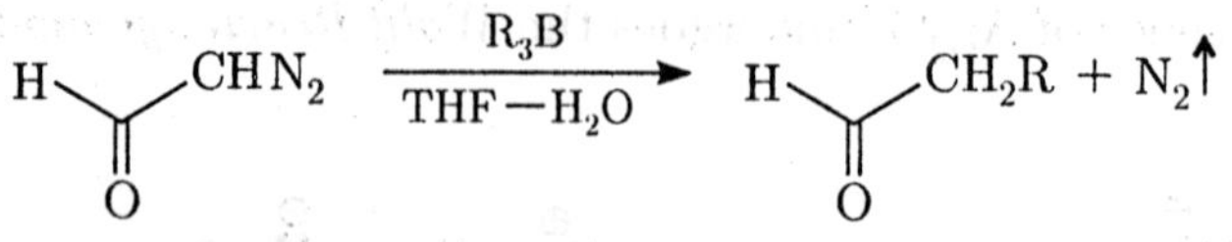

Mechanism :

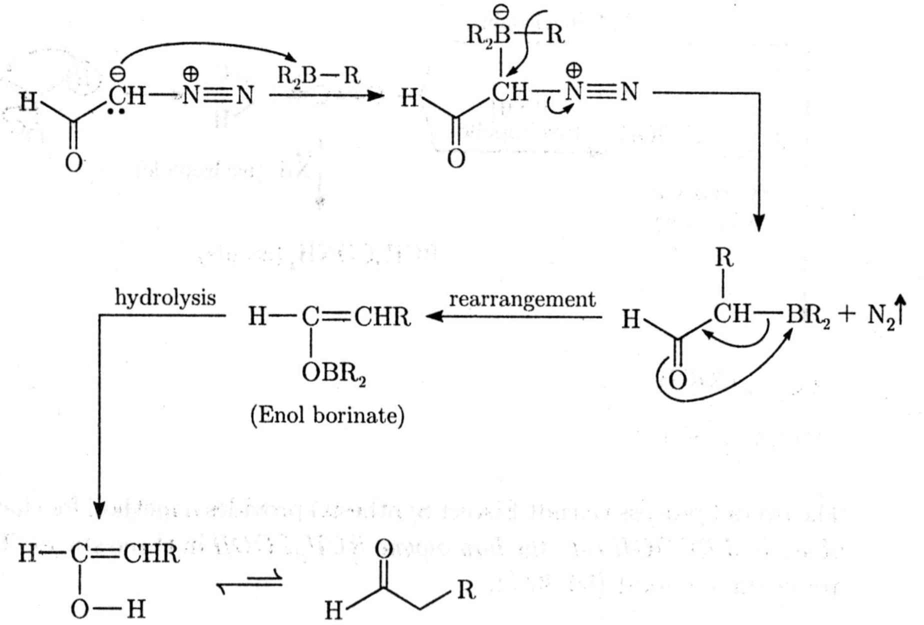

Configuration of R (if asymmetric) is retained throughout the reaction.

9. 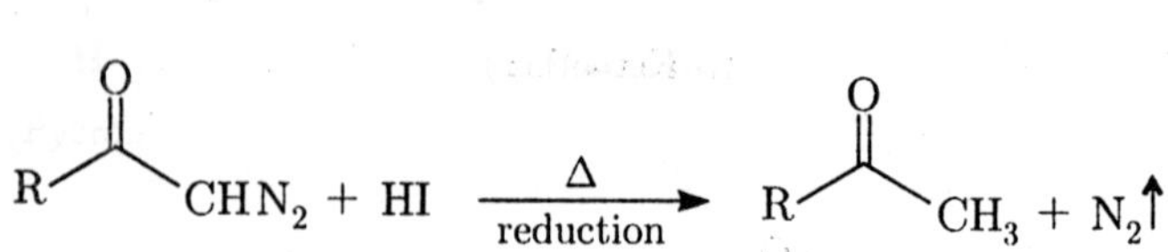

Organonitrogen Compounds

Nitroalkanes

Nitroalkanes contain nitro ($-\overset{\oplus}{N}\begin{smallmatrix}\nearrow O \\ \searrow O^{\ominus}\end{smallmatrix}$) group and are represented by the general formula R–NO_2. Nitroalkanes are isomeric with alkyl nitrites (R–O–N=O).

General Methods of Preparation of Nitroalkanes

1. $$\underset{\text{(Alkane)}}{R{-}H} \xrightarrow[\text{or vapour phase nitration at 400°C}]{\text{liquid phase nitration at 140°C}} \text{Mixture of nitroalkanes}$$

   Mechanism : The reaction proceeds through free radical mechanism.

   Step 1 : *Step Initiation* $HO{-}NO_2 \longrightarrow HO\cdot + \cdot NO_2$

   Step 2 : *Step Propagation* $R{-}H + HO\cdot \longrightarrow R\cdot + H_2O$

   $R\cdot + HO{-}NO_2 \longrightarrow RNO_2 + HO\cdot$

   Step 3 : *Step Termination* $R\cdot + O_2N{-}OH \longrightarrow ROH + \dot{N}O_2$

2. When alkyl iodides are treated with sodium nitrite ($NaNO_2$) and silver nitrite ($AgNO_2$) separately, mixture of alkyl nitrite and nitroalkanes are obtained. *Alkyl nitrite predominates with $AgNO_2$ while nitroalkane is the major product with $NaNO_2$.*

$$R{-}X \xrightarrow[\text{or } AgNO_2/DMF \text{ or } AgNO_2/DMSO]{\text{Aqueous ethanolic } AgNO_2} \underset{\text{(Minor)}}{R{-}\overset{\oplus}{N}\begin{smallmatrix}\nearrow O^{\ominus} \\ \searrow O\end{smallmatrix}} + \underset{\text{(Major)}}{R{-}O{-}N{=}O}$$

$$R{-}X + NaNO_2 \xrightarrow{\text{DMSO}} \underset{\text{(Major)}}{R{-}\overset{\oplus}{N}\begin{smallmatrix}\nearrow O \\ \searrow O^{\ominus}\end{smallmatrix}} + \underset{\text{(Minor)}}{R{-}O{-}N{=}O}$$

Nitrite ion reacts with R–X by S_N2 pathway, when the reagent is $NaNO_2$ and the pathway followed is S_N1 when nitrite ion attacks R–X with $AgNO_2$ as reagent.

Examples with mechanism

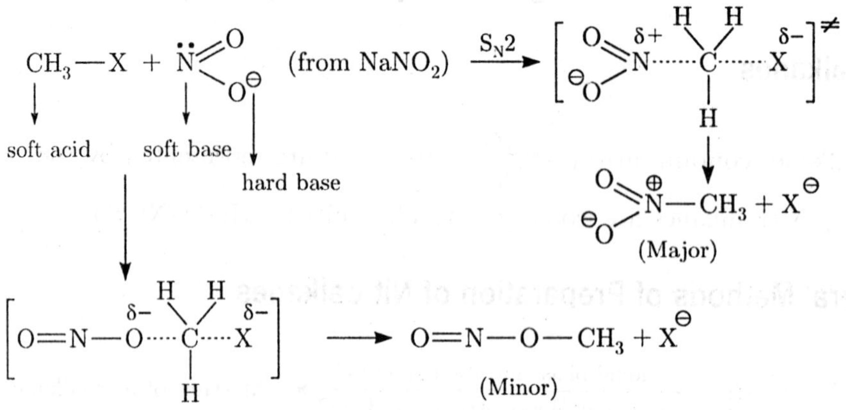

As soft/soft interaction is favoured over soft/hard interaction, *nitroalkane* becomes the major product here.

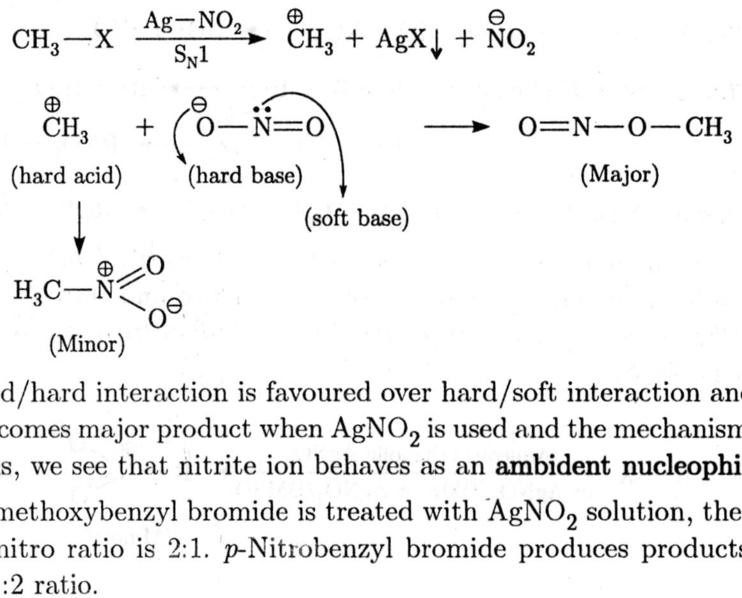

Here, hard/hard interaction is favoured over hard/soft interaction and so alkyl nitrite becomes major product when $AgNO_2$ is used and the mechanism becomes S_N1. Thus, we see that nitrite ion behaves as an **ambident nucleophile.**

2. When *p*-methoxybenzyl bromide is treated with $AgNO_2$ solution, the products nitrite : nitro ratio is 2:1. *p*-Nitrobenzyl bromide produces products nitrite : nitro in 1:2 ratio.

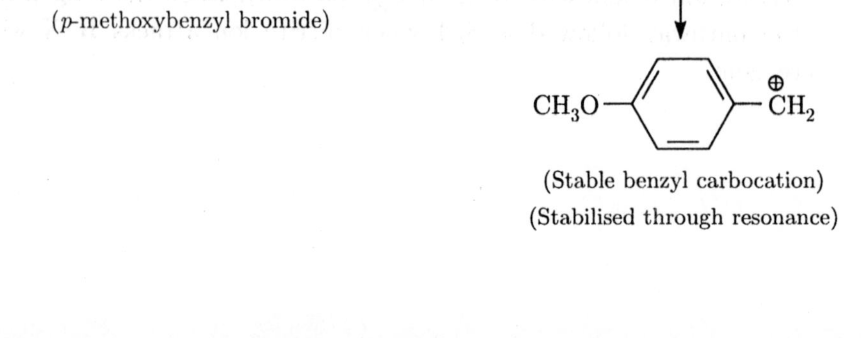

As nitrite formation reaction follows S_N1 pathway, alkyl nitrite becomes major product here.

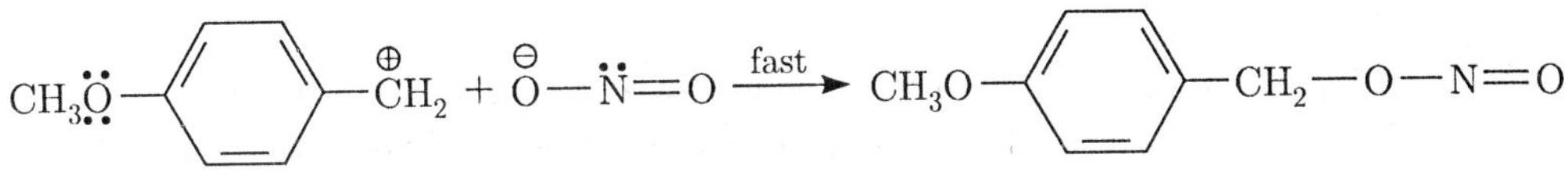

(+R effect of $-OCH_3$ group operates)

(Major)

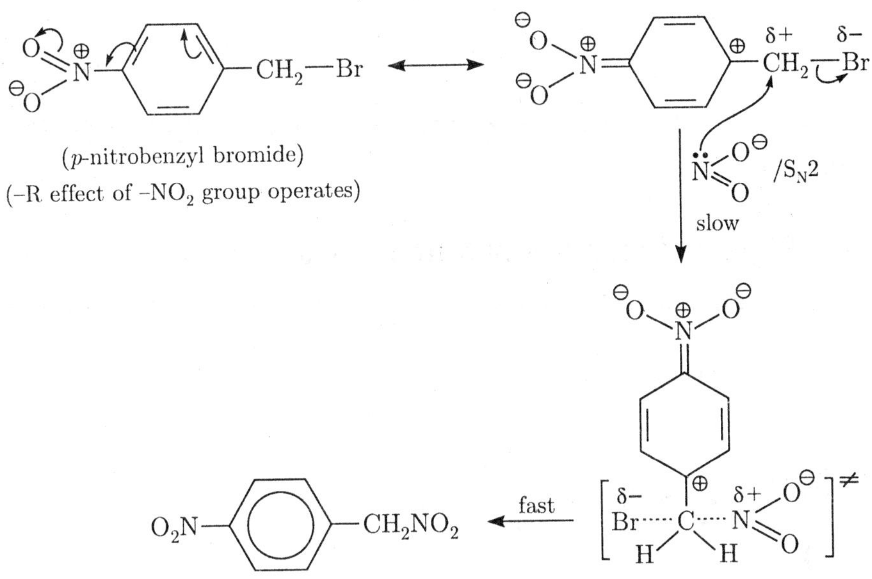

(p-nitrobenzyl bromide)

(–R effect of $-NO_2$ group operates)

(Major)

3. When an aqueous solution of sodium chloroacetate is boiled with an aqueous solution of $NaNO_2$, nitromethane is formed through S_N2 pathway.

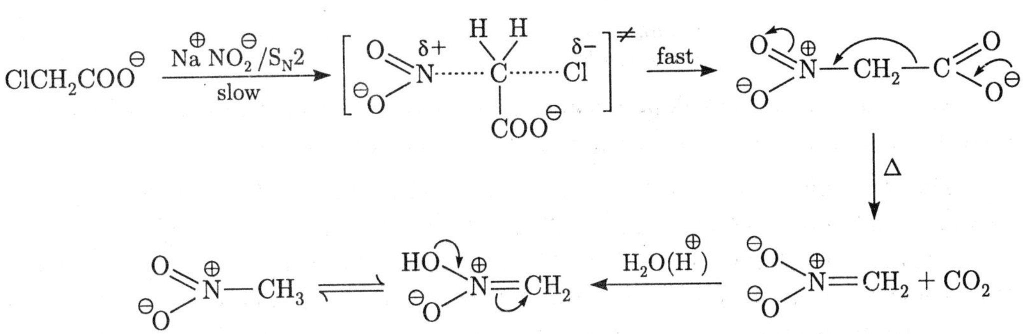

4. By the oxidation of tertiaryalkyl amines.

$$Me_3C—NH_2 \xrightarrow{KMnO_4.[O]} Me_3C—NO_2$$

(Tertiarynitroalkane)

5. *By the oxidation of oximes* : When aldoximes and ketoximes are oxidised by trifluoroacetic acid, primary and secondary nitroalkanes are formed.

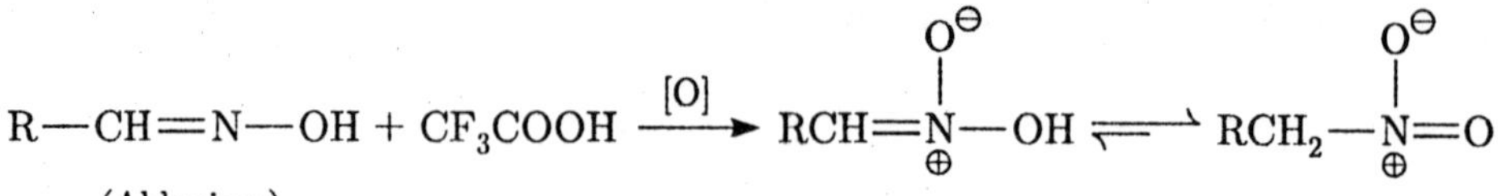

(Aldoxime)

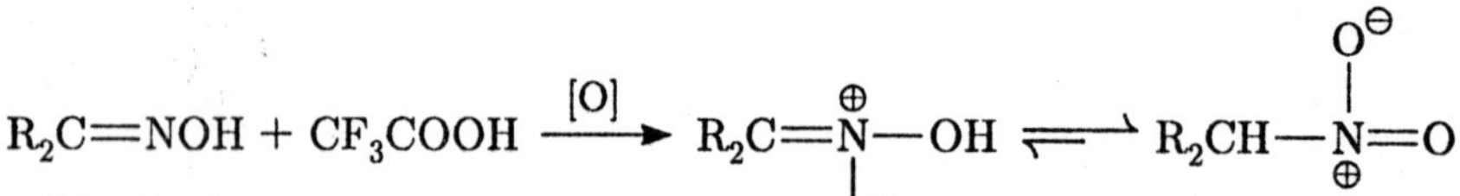

(Ketoxime)

Structure and Physical Properties of Nitroalkanes

Nitro compounds contain a C–N bond and two oxygen atoms bonded to the nitrogen atom and this nitrogen atom is sp^2 hybridised. Nitro group is a resonance hybrid of two equivalent resonating structures as shown below.

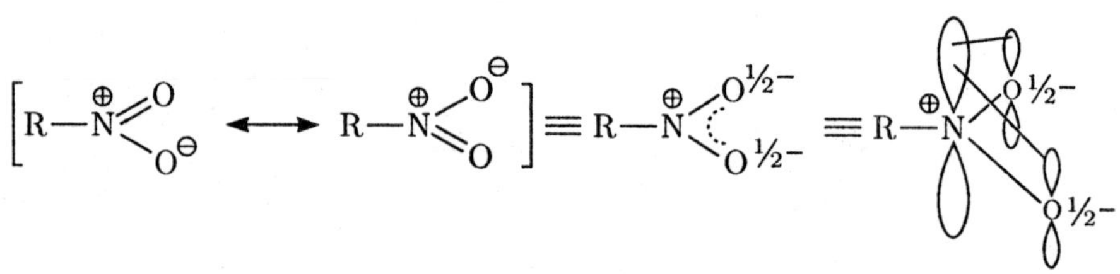

In the liquid state, or in solution, nitroalkanes tautomerise to acinitro form.

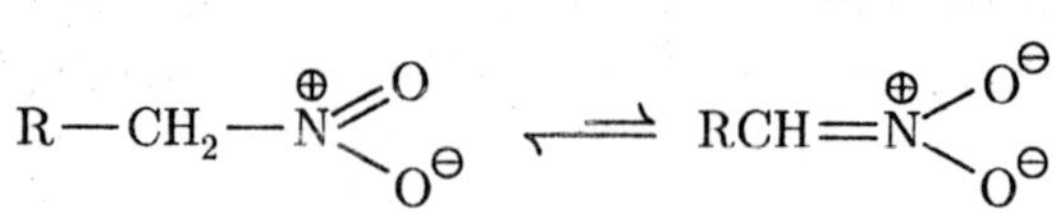

Nitro form(solid) (or pseudoaci form) Aci form(liquid)

Nitro form has equivalent resonating structures which the aci form lacks, so the nitro form is more stable and predominates in the equilibrium.

The semipolar nature of the nitro group and strong –I effect of two oxygen atoms develop a high dipole moment in nitroalkanes ($\mu \cong 3.6D$). Due to the high dipole-moments, nitroalkanes have high melting points. The two oxygen atoms bear partial negative charge and they can form hydrogen bond, lower nitroalkanes are water soluble. However, the solubility decreases with increasing R, *i.e.*, with increasing molecular weight. Nitroalkanes have high dielectric constant (ε=25-35) and so are used as solvents for dissolving polar compounds.

Acidity of α-H of Nitroalkanes

The nitrogroup in nitroalkanes has –I and –R effects. Because of these effects, the α-H atoms are acidic and can be abstracted by a base to form a carbanion. This carbanion can undergo condensation reactions.

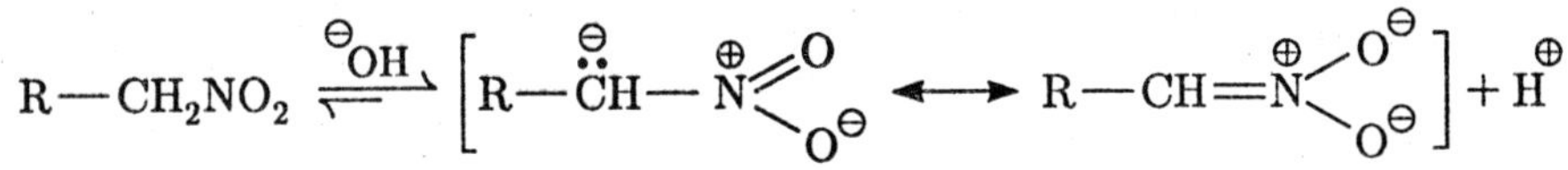

The equilibrium shifts towards right as the conjugate base is stabilised through resonance. Primary and secondary nitroalkanes are moderately acidic ($pK_a \cong 9$).

Substitution of α-H of Nitroalkanes

1. ***Salt formation reactions*** : Nitroalkanes are acidic due to the –I and –R effect of NO_2 group and when treated with a base, one α-hydrogen can be removed as a proton and the conjugate base thus, formed becomes resonance stabilised.

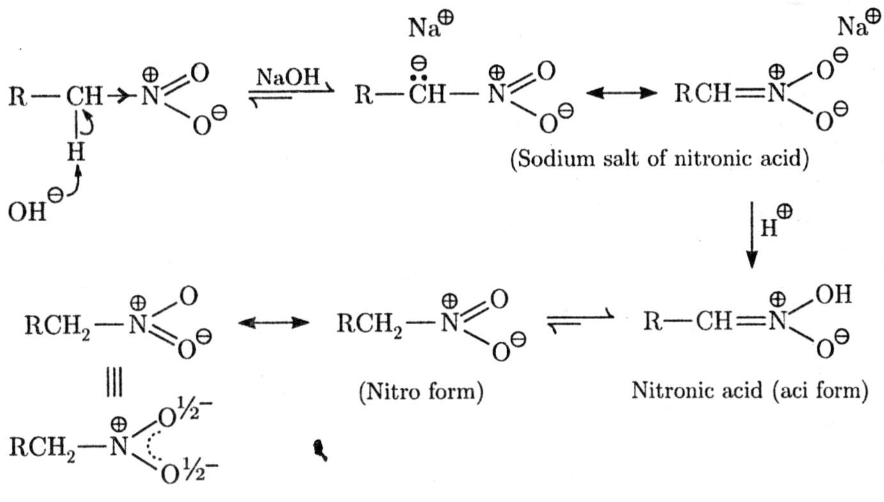

   When any acid stronger than nitroalkane (*e.g.*, HCl) is added to the salt of nitroalkane, nitronic acid or aci form of nitroalkane is formed first, which then tautomerises to nitro form. The acidity of aci-form is as great as carboxylic acids ($pK_a \cong 4\text{-}6$), but the contribution of aci-form is much lower than the nitro form, as the latter is resonance stabilised. As a result, nitroalkanes show slight acidity. Tertiaryalkyl nitrates have no α-H atom, so they can not form salts, with bases.

2. ***NEF carbonyl synthesis*** : When salts of primary and secondary nitroalkanes are treated with 50% sulphuric acid, aldehydes and ketones are formed respectively and the reaction is popularly known as **NEF carbonyl synthesis**. This is a good method of synthesising aldehydes and ketones.

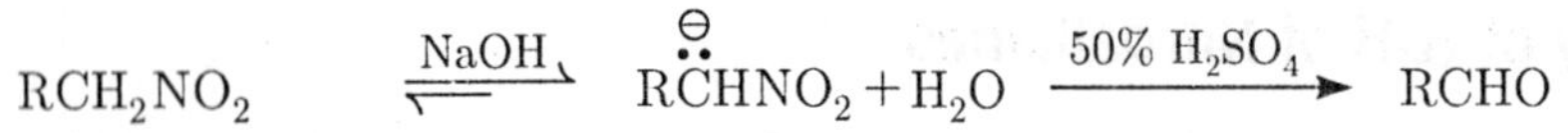

(Primary nitroalkane)

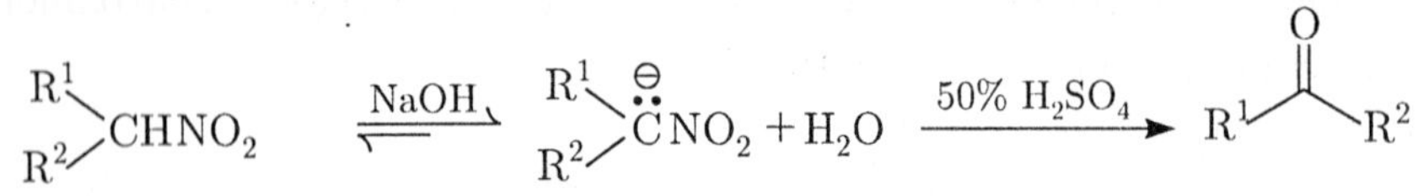

(Secondary nitroalkane)

NEF carbonyl synthesis fails with tertiary nitroalkenes as tertiary nitroalkanes do not have any α-hydrogen.

Mechanism of NEF carbonyl synthesis :

(Shown with secondary nitroalkanes)

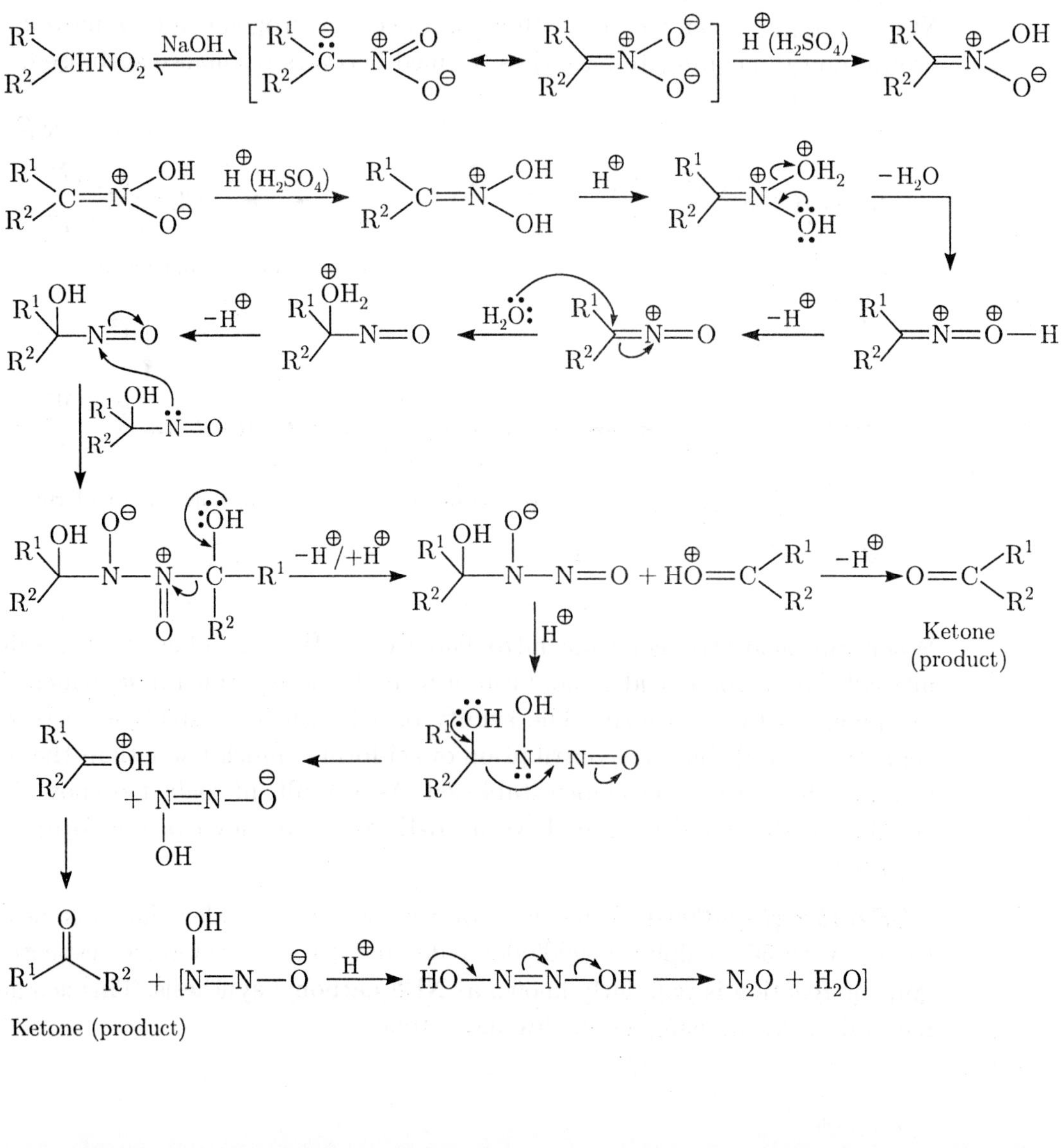

3. ***Bromination of nitroalkanes*** : In the alkaline medium, bromine undergoes electrophilic substitution reaction with primary and secondary nitroalkanes to form α,α-dibromo-and α-bromonitroalkene respectively. Tertiary nitroalkanes do not respeond as they do not have any α-hydrogen.

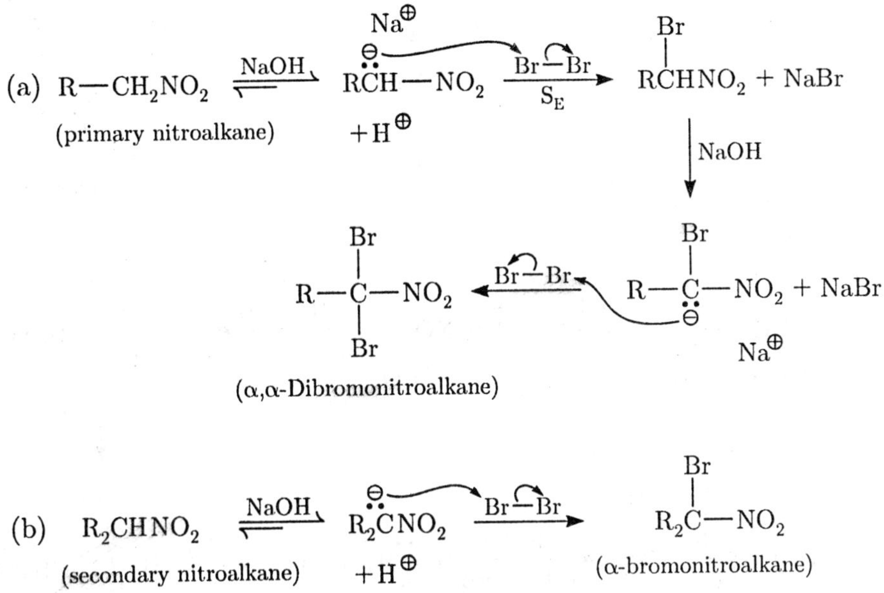

4. ***Condensation Reactions of Nitroalkanes*** :

I. ***Henry's Reaction*** : Aliphatic and aromatic aldehydes undergo condensation reaction with primary and secondary nitroalkanes in the presence of a base. This reaction is known as Henry's reaction.

$$RCH_2NO_2 \underset{}{\overset{^{\ominus}OH}{\rightleftharpoons}} R-\overset{\ominus}{\ddot{C}}HNO_2 + H_2O$$

(primary nitroalkane)

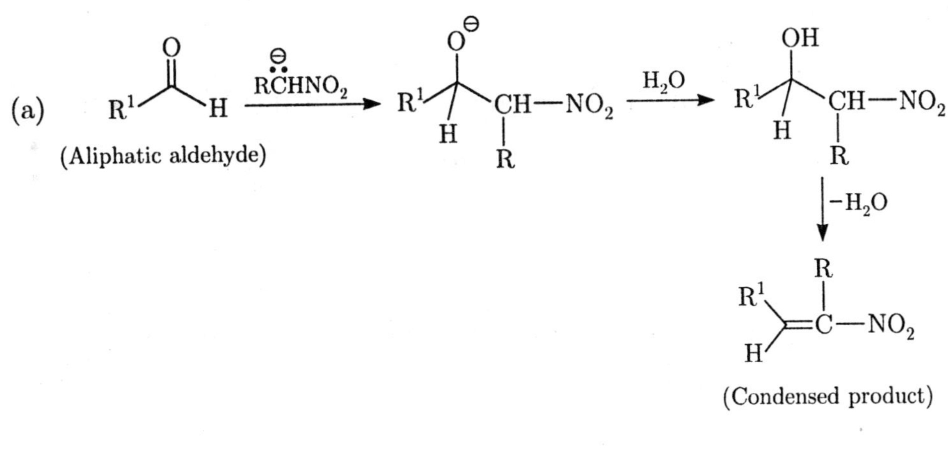

(b) 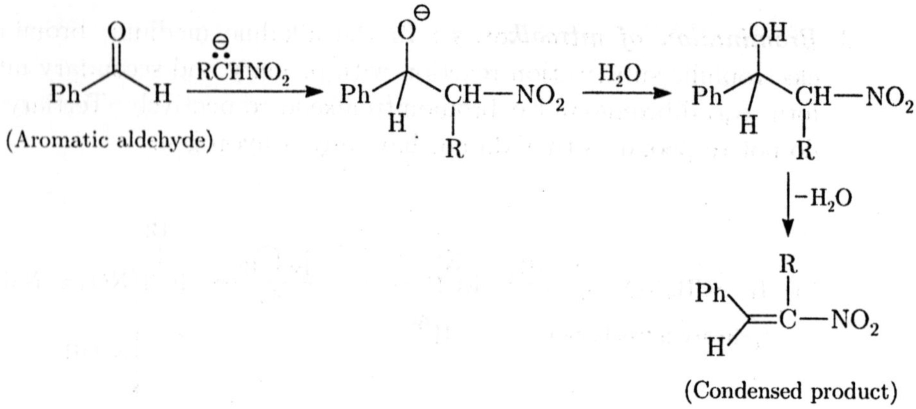

(c) 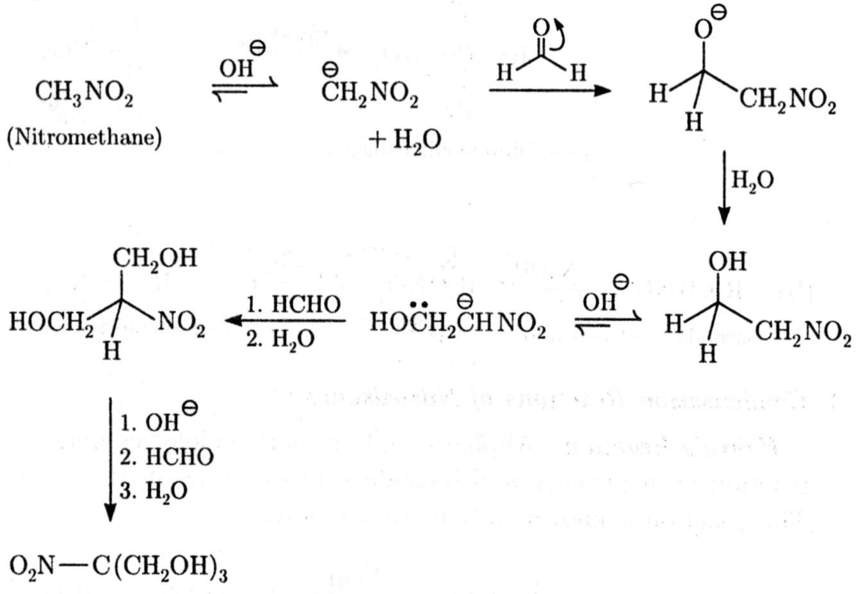

II. ***The Mannich Reaction*** : Primary and secondary nitroalkanes undergo the Mannich reaction with formaldehyde and secondary amine.

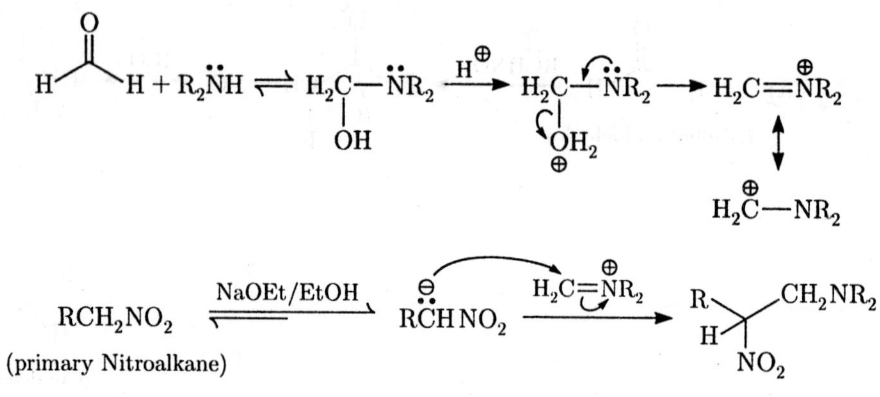

III. ***The Michael Reaction*** : In the presence of base, primary and secondary nitroalkanes undergo the Michael reaction with α, β-unsaturated compounds.

$$RCH_2NO_2 \xrightleftharpoons{NaOEt/EtOH} R\overset{\ominus}{C}HNO_2\,Na^{\oplus} \quad \text{(Sodium salt of primary nitroalkane)}$$

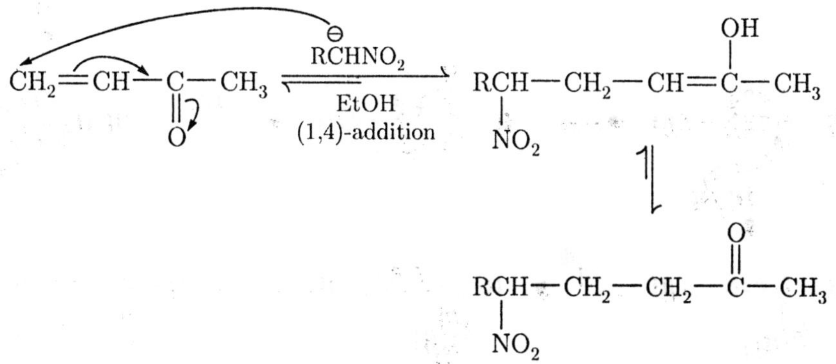

Hydrolysis of nitroalkanes : When a primary nitroalkane is boiled with concentrated aqueous HCl or 85% H_2SO_4, an alkane carboxylic acid and a salt of hydroxylamine are formed. The reaction involves reduction of the nitro group and oxidation of the methylene group to form hydroxamic acid which then hydrolyses to the products.

$$\underset{\text{(primary nitroalkane)}}{RCH_2NO_2} \xrightarrow{85\%\ H_2SO_4} RCOOH + \overset{\oplus}{N}H_3OH$$

***Mechanism of the reaction* :**

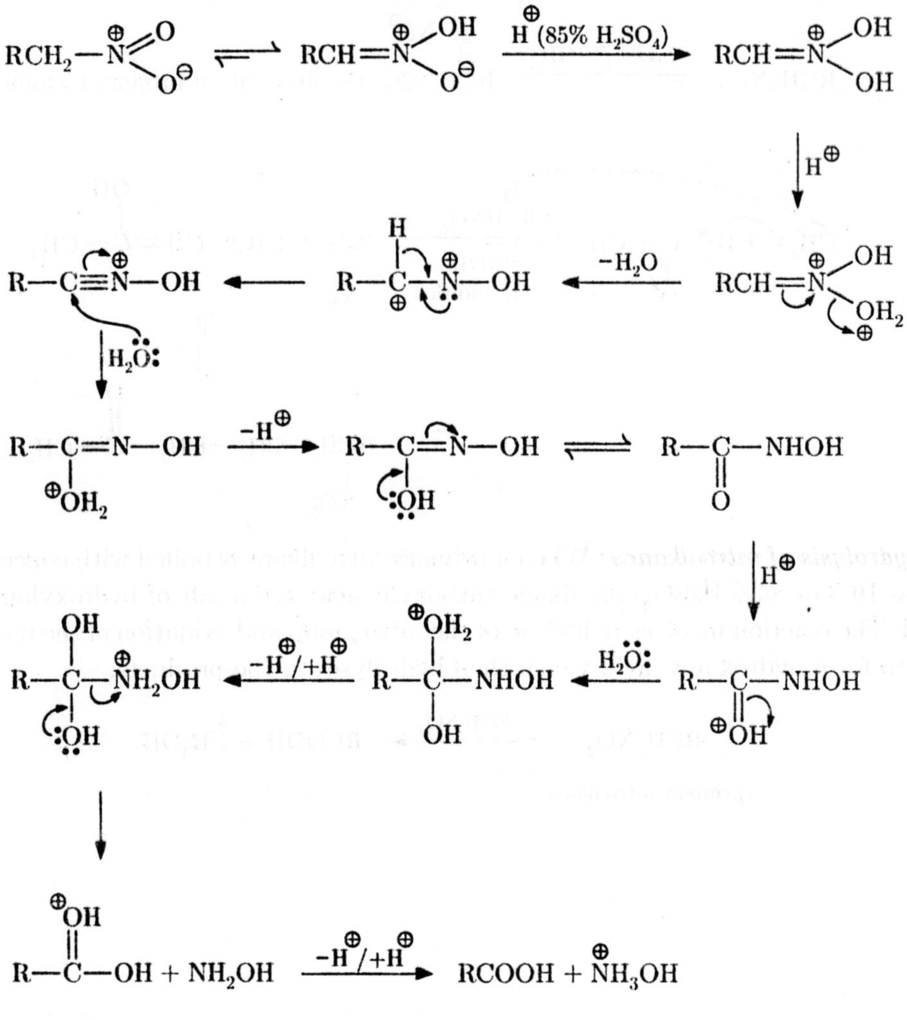

***Reduction of nitroalkanes* :**

1. ***Reduction by metal and acid or by $LiAlH_4$***

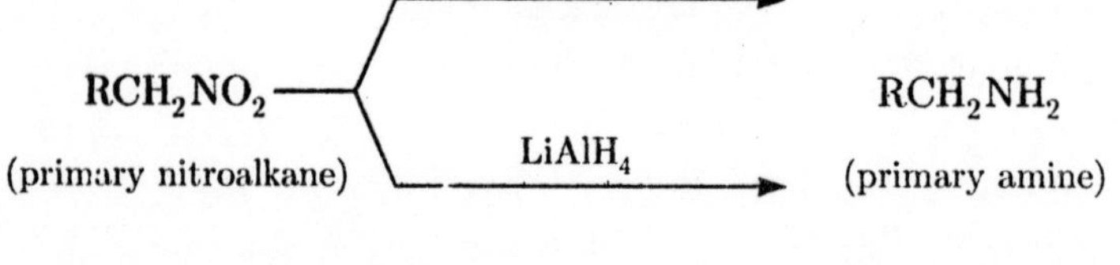

Mechanism of metal-acid reduction :

$$M \rightarrow M^{2+} + 2e^- \quad (M = \text{metal} = Zn, Sn, Fe)$$

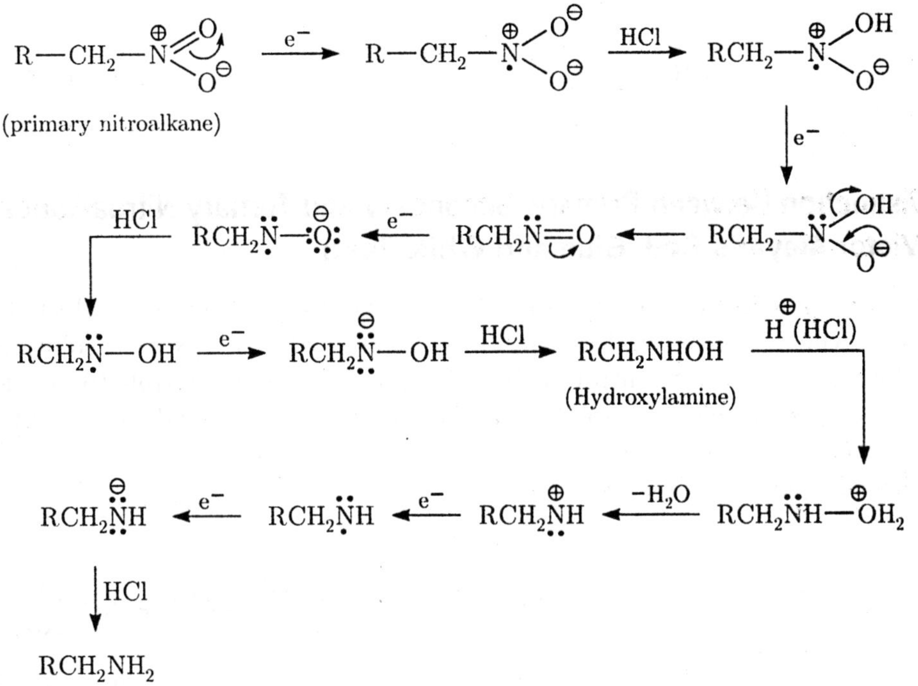

2. ***Reduction by $SnCl_2$ in hydrochloric acid*** : $SnCl_2$ in HCl reduces nitroalkanes to a mixture of hydroxylamine and oxime; whereas sodium salts of primary and secondary nitroalkanes form only oximes through $SnCl_2$ reduction.

$$\underset{\text{(primary nitroalkane)}}{RCH_2NO_2} \xrightarrow{SnCl_2/HCl} \underset{\text{(Alkyl hydroxylamine)}}{RCH_2NHOH} + \underset{\text{(Oxime)}}{RCH{=}NOH}$$

$$\underset{\text{(primary nitroalkane)}}{RCH_2NO_2} \xrightarrow{NaOH} RCH{=}\overset{\oplus}{N}(OH)\overset{\ominus}{O}\,\overset{\oplus}{Na} \xrightarrow{SnCl_2/HCl} RCH{=}N{-}OH$$

3. ***Reduction by neutral reducing agent***: When nitroalkanes are reduced by metallic zinc (Zn) and ammonium chloride (NH_4Cl) in aqueous or alcoholic suspension, hydroxylamines are formed.

$$\underset{\text{(primary nitroalkane)}}{RCH_2NO_2} \xrightarrow{Zn/NH_4Cl} \underset{\text{(Alkyl hydroxylamine)}}{RCH_2NHOH}$$

Metal and ammonium chloride reductions follow the same pathway the metal and acid follows, but here the reduction stops at the alkyl hydroxylamine stage.

4. ***Catalytic reduction*** :

$$\underset{\text{(primary nitroalkane)}}{CH_3CH_2NO_2} \xrightarrow{\text{Raney Ni/H}_2 \text{ or Pt/Pd/H}_2} \underset{\text{(Primary aliphatic amine)}}{CH_3CH_2NH_2}$$

Distinction Between Primary, Secondary and Tertiary Nitroalkanes (Victor-Meyer's Red, Blue and White Test)

A *primary nitroalkane* reacts with *nitrous acid* to form nitrolic acid, which develops a *red colour* when dissolved in dilute aqueous sodium hydroxide (NaOH) solution. *Secondary nitroalkanes* react with nitrous acid (HNO_2) to form pseudonitrole (*p*-nitrole), a neutral *blue compound* which is insoluble in dilute aqueous sodium hydroxide solution. *Tertiary nitroalkanes do not undergo any reaction with nitrous acid* (HNO_2). This is the basis of Victor-Meyer's red, blue and while test.

$$\underset{\text{(primary nitroalkane)}}{RCH_2NO_2} + HO{-}NO \xrightarrow{-H_2O} RC(=NOH)NO_2 \xrightarrow{NaOH} \underset{\text{(Red coloured salt)}}{RC(=N\overset{\ominus}{O}\,\overset{\oplus}{Na})NO_2}$$

$$\underset{\text{(secondary nitroalkane)}}{R_2CHNO_2} + HO{-}NO \xrightarrow{-H_2O} \underset{\text{(Blue)}}{R_2C(NO)NO_2} \xrightarrow{NaOH} \text{(Insoluble)}$$

$$\underset{\text{(Tertiary nitroalkane)}}{R_3CNO_2} + HO{-}NO \longrightarrow \text{No reaction}$$

Mechanism of the reaction :

$$HO-N=O \xrightleftharpoons{H^{\oplus}} H_2\overset{\oplus}{O}-N=O \rightleftharpoons H_2O + \overset{\oplus}{N}=O$$

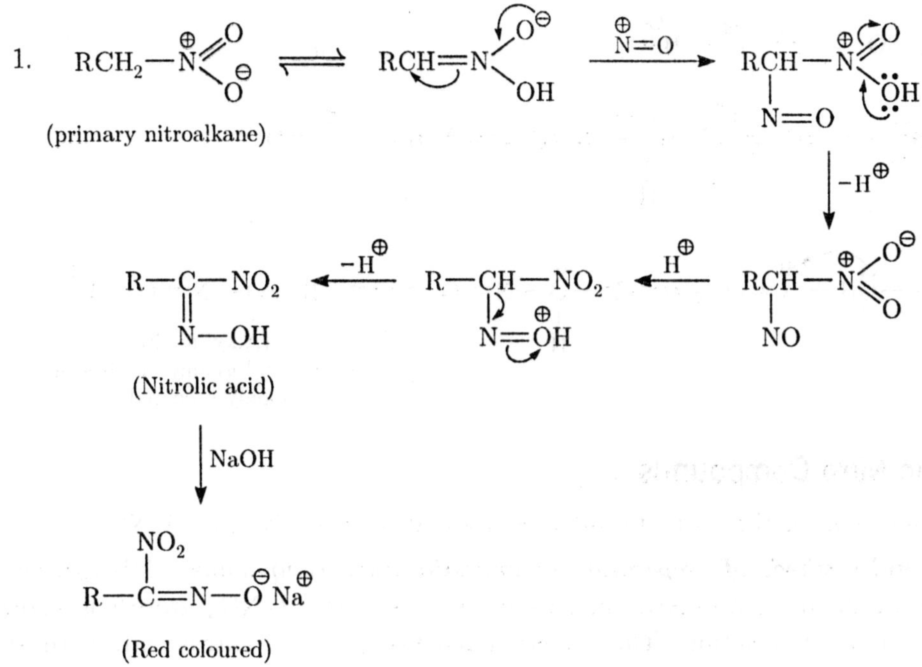

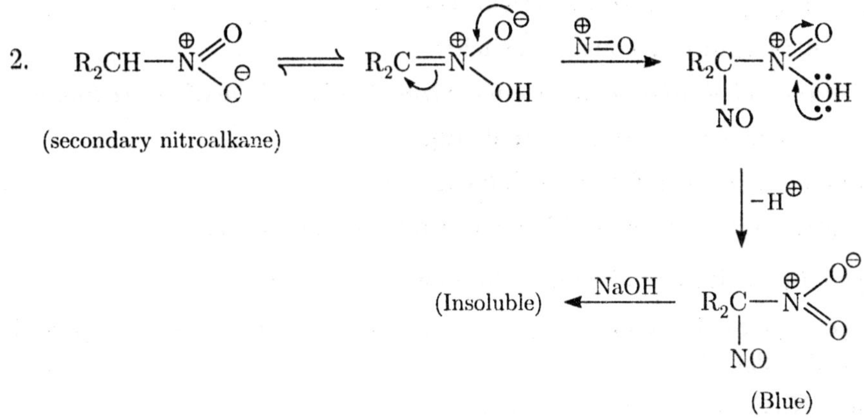

Alkyl Nitrites (R–O–N=O)

Preparation of alkyl nitrites :

$$\underset{\text{(Alcohol)}}{R-OH} \xrightarrow{NaNO_2/\text{conc. } H_2SO_4/\text{cold}} R-O-N=O$$

Mechanism :

$$NaNO_2 + H_2SO_4 \longrightarrow HNO_2 + Na_2SO_4$$

$$H_2SO_4 \rightleftharpoons \overset{\oplus}{H} + H\overset{\ominus}{SO_4}$$

$$H\ddot{\underset{..}{O}}-N=O \xrightleftharpoons{\overset{\oplus}{H}} H\overset{\oplus}{\underset{|}{\underset{H}{O}}}-N=O \rightleftharpoons H_2O + \overset{\oplus}{N}=O$$

$$R-\ddot{\underset{..}{O}}H + \overset{\oplus}{N}=O \rightleftharpoons R-\overset{\oplus}{\underset{|}{\underset{H}{O}}}-N=O \rightleftharpoons R-O-N=O + \overset{\oplus}{H}$$

(Alkyl nitrite)
(Amyl and isoamyl nitrites are commonly prepared ones)

Aromatic Nitro Compounds

General formula for the aromatic nitro compounds can be given be $ArNO_2$.

General methods of preparation of aromatic nitro compounds : Substitution of a hydrogen atom in an aromatic nucleus by a nitro group ($-NO_2$ group) is known as aromatic nitration reaction. The nitration reaction may be carried out with *several nitrating agents* as given below.

1. Concentrated nitric acid and glacial acetic acid.
2. Dilute nitric acid (aqueous nitric acid).
3. 1:1 *Concentrated nitric acid in concentrated sulphuric acid (mixed acid).*
4. Fuming nitric acid in concentrated sulphuric acid.
5. Fuming nitric acid in fuming sulphuric acid.
6. Acyl nitrates like acetyl and benzyl nitrate in organic solvents.
7. Nitrosonium salts like nitronium fluoborate.($NO_2^{\oplus} BF_4^{\ominus}$)
8. Nitrogen pentoxide (N_2O_5) in carbon tetrachloride in the presence of phosphorous pentoxide (P_2O_5).
9. Fuming Nitric acid in acetic anhydride.

Among the available nitrating agents, the most common nitrating agent is *mixed acid. (M.A.).*

A wide variety of aromatic compounds undergo nitration reaction, like

1. Aromatic hydrocarbons like benzene, toluene, naphthalene etc.
2. Halobenzenes, phenols, phenolic ethers, amines, amides.
3. Nitrobenzenes, carboxylic acids, sulphonic acids.
4. Heterocyclic compounds like furan, pyridine, thiophene, quinoline etc.

The nitrating agents and conditions for the reaction differ from substrate to substrate. Benzene nucleus containing activating groups require mild nitrating agents and mild conditions; while aromatic compounds containing deactivating groups demand strong nitrating agents and vigorous conditions. For example, alkyl groups activate the benzene ring, so alkylbenzenes require mild nitrating agent and mild conditions for nitration. On the other hand, $-NO_2$ group is deactivating, so nitrobenzene requires stronger nitrating agent and drastic conditions for further nitration.

Some examples of nitration reaction are given below :

1. 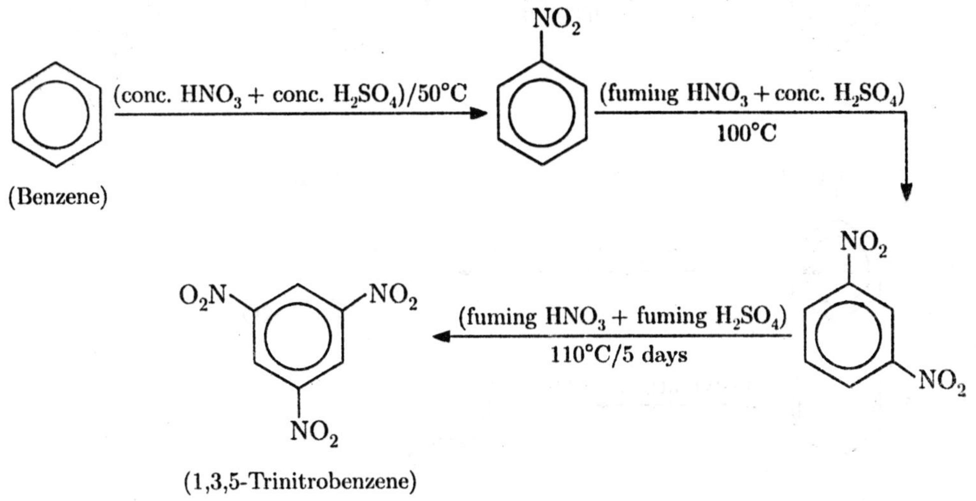

2. 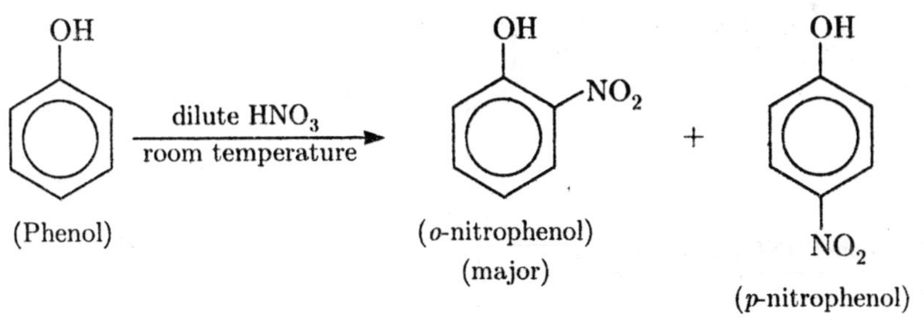

3. 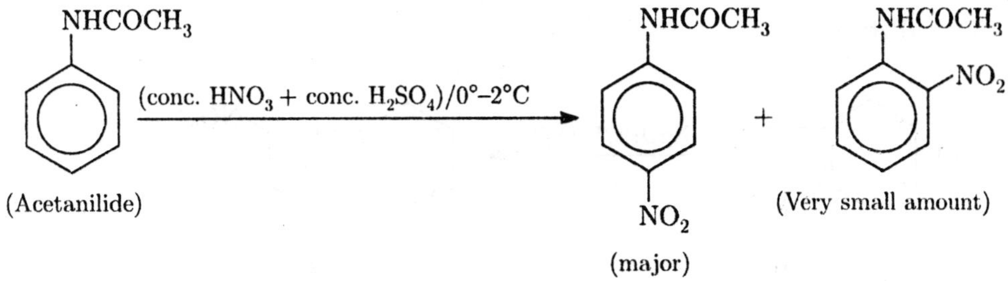

4. 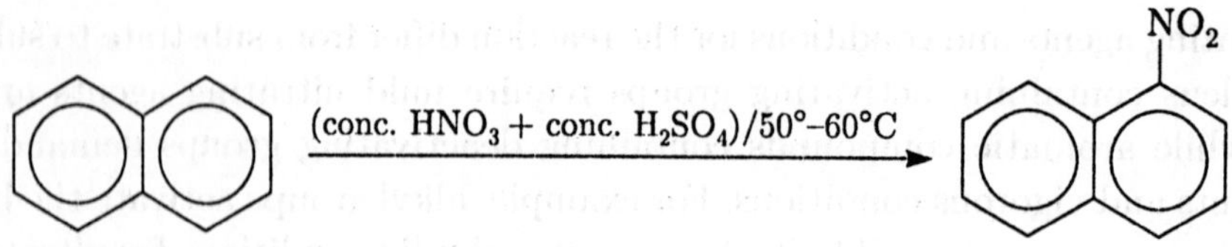

(Naphthalene)

5. 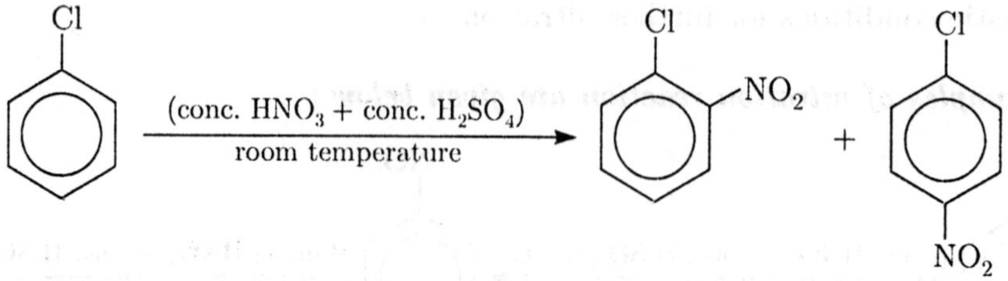

6. 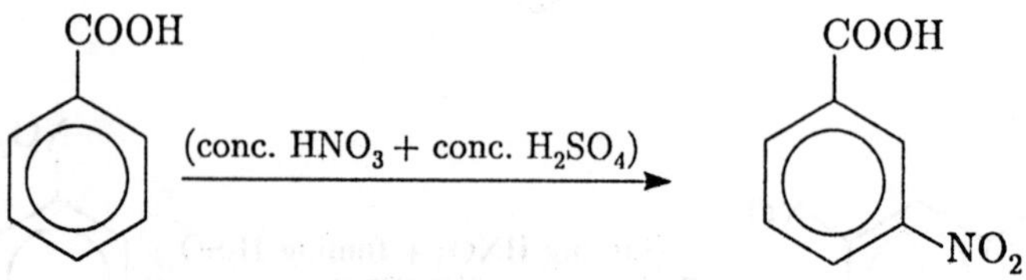

7. 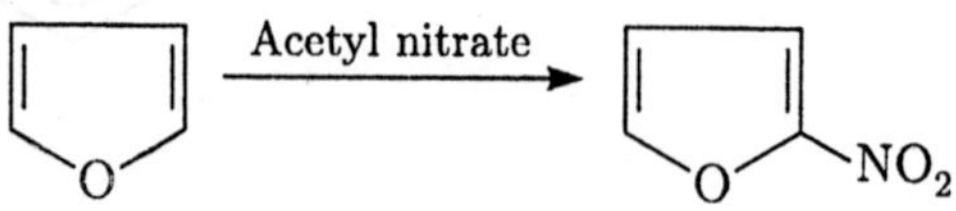

(Furan)

8. 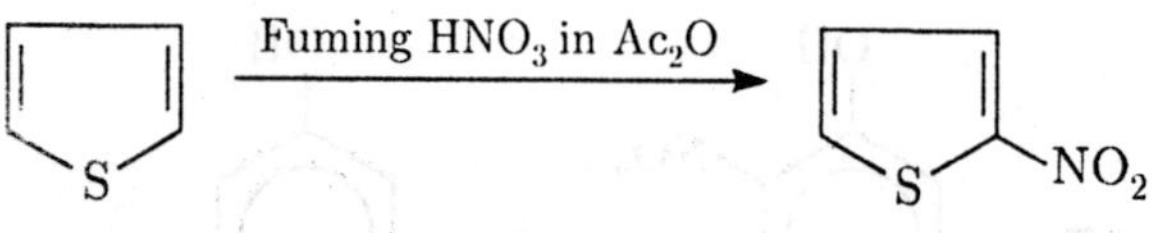

(Thiophene)

9. 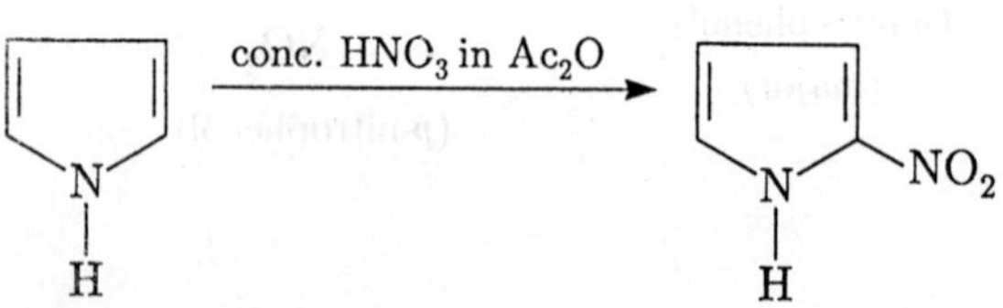

(Pyrrole)

10. 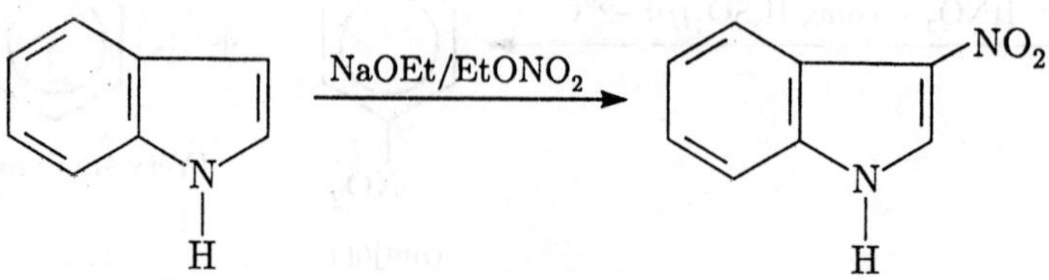

(Indole)

11. 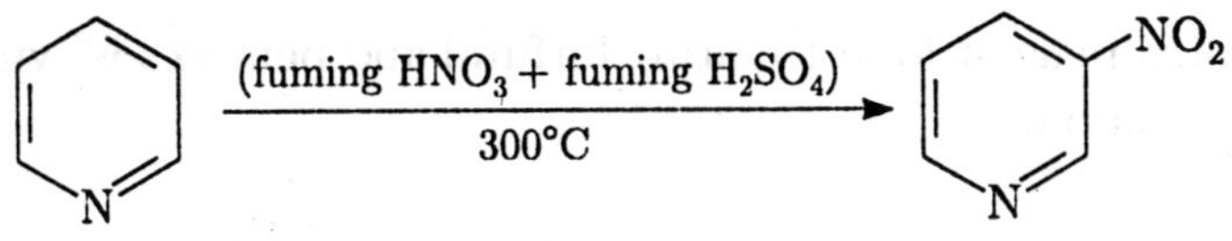

(Pyridine)

12. 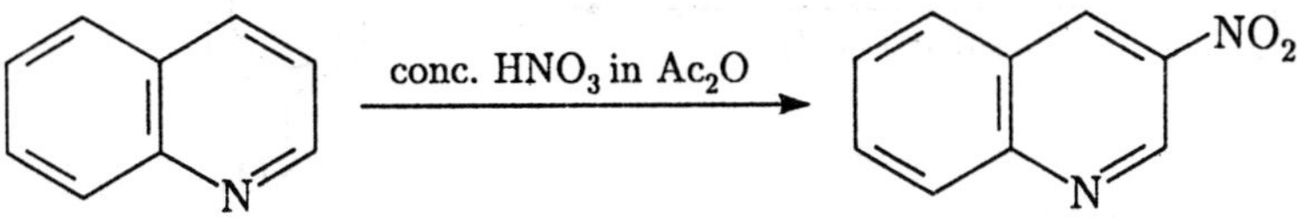

(Quinoline)

The orientation of the incoming nitro group in the nitration reaction is determined by the substituent already present in the benzene ring.

Importance of nitration reaction in aromatic compounds :

1. There is no simple and direct method of introducing $-NH_2$ group in the benzene nucleus. This can be done only by nitrating the compound first followed by the reduction of the $-NO_2$ group.

(a) 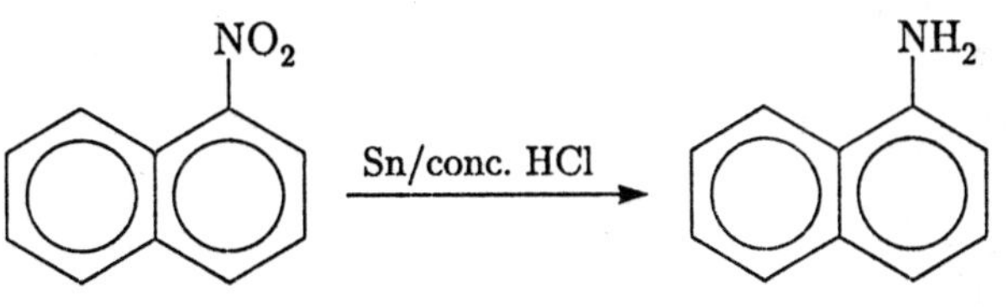

(b) 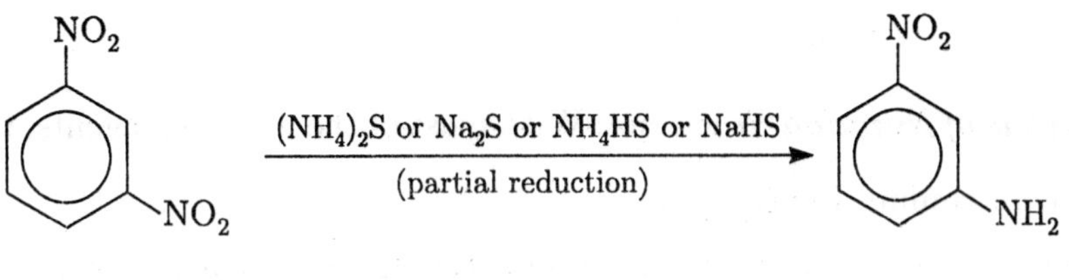

(c) Phloroglucinol, a reagent for estimating furfural and pentoses is synthesised *via* nitration reaction.

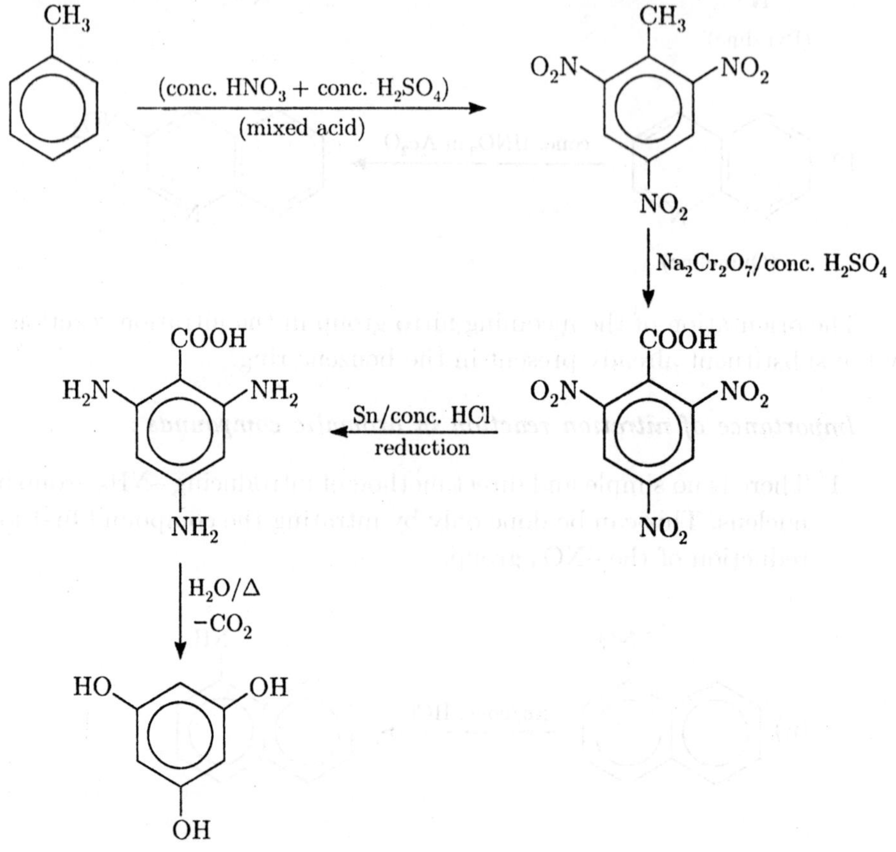

(Phloroglucinol)

Mechanisms of Nitration Reactions : With most of the nitrating agents, the attacking electrophile is nitronium ($-\overset{\oplus}{N}O_2$) ion.

1. In the case of concentrated nitric acid (HNO_3) as a nitrating agent, one molecule of the acid acts as an acid and one molecule acts as a base. Thus, through an acid-base reaction, nitronium ion ($-\overset{\oplus}{N}O_2$) is formed.

$$HNO_3 \rightleftharpoons \overset{\oplus}{H} + \overset{\ominus}{N}O_3$$

$$\overset{\oplus}{H} + HNO_3 \rightleftharpoons H_2O + \overset{\oplus}{N}O_2$$

$$2HNO_3 \rightleftharpoons \overset{\ominus}{N}O_3 + H_2O + \overset{\oplus}{N}O_2$$

The equilibrium generally lies to the left; however sufficient amount of $\overset{\oplus}{N}O_2$ ions remain in the equilibrium to carry on the nitration reaction smoothly.

2. With mixed acid (mixture of nitric and sulphuric acids), an acid-base reaction is found to occur. Here, sulphuric acid (H_2SO_4) acts as an acid and nitric acid (HNO_3) as a base. The ionisation in both the cases is essentially complete.

$$H_2SO_4 \rightleftharpoons \overset{\oplus}{H} + H\overset{\ominus}{SO_4}$$

$$HNO_3 + \overset{\oplus}{H} \rightleftharpoons H_2O + \overset{\oplus}{NO_2}$$

$$H_2O + H_2SO_4 \rightleftharpoons H_3\overset{\oplus}{O} + H\overset{\ominus}{SO_4}$$

$$HNO_3 + 2H_2SO_4 \rightleftharpoons H_3\overset{\oplus}{O} + \overset{\oplus}{NO_2} + 2H\overset{\ominus}{SO_4}$$

3. With dinitrogen pentoxide (N_2O_5) as nitrating agent, nitronium ($\overset{\oplus}{NO_2}$) ion is formed through spontaneous dissociation.

$$N_2O_5 \rightleftharpoons \overset{\oplus}{NO_2}\,\overset{\ominus}{NO_3} \rightleftharpoons \overset{\oplus}{NO_2} + \overset{\ominus}{NO_3}$$

4. With nitronium salts like nitronium hydrofluoborate ($\overset{\oplus}{NO_2}\,\overset{\ominus}{HBF_4}$), the salt itself contains $\overset{\oplus}{NO_2}$ ion.

$$\overset{\oplus}{NO_2}\,\overset{\ominus}{HBF_4} \rightleftharpoons \overset{\oplus}{NO_2} + \overset{\ominus}{HBF_4}$$

5. Nitration wih acyl nitrate (*e.g.*, acetyl nitrate) (HNO_3–Ac_2O), the mechanism of nitration involving acetyl nitrate appears to be an open question owing to the uncertainty of the nature of nitrating species. The following have been proposed like CH_3COONO_2, $CH_3COOH\,\overset{\oplus}{NO_2}$, N_2O_5, $\overset{\oplus}{NO}$ etc. An interesting feature of this reagent is the unusually high percentage of *o*-isomer that is obtained when the side chain contains a hetero atom. For example, anisole with mixed acid gives *o*-isomer 31% but with HNO_3–Ac_2O, *o*- isomer becomes 71% of the total product. One explanation is that the nitrating species is dinitrogen pentoxide (N_2O_5), which reacts *via* a six-centre rearrangement.

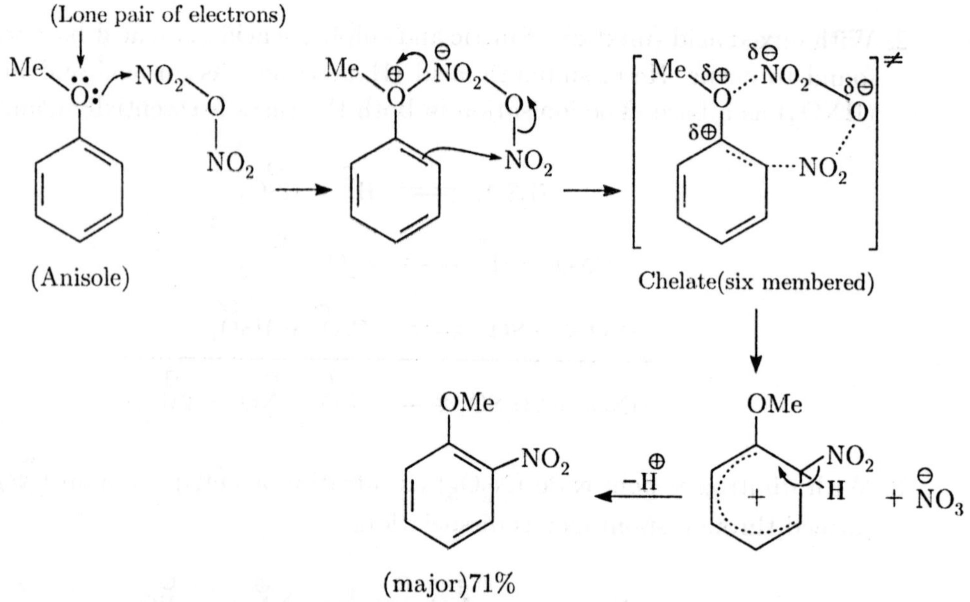

Formation of N_2O_5 :

$$HO—NO_2 + Ac—O—Ac \rightleftharpoons HO—Ac + AcONO_2$$

$$2AcONO_2 \rightleftharpoons AcOAc + O_2N—O—NO_2$$

6. When the reagent is dilute nitric acid (HNO_3), $\overset{\oplus}{N}O$ (nitrosonium ion) is formed instead of nitronium ion. Nitonium ion is then generated in the system through a minor redox reaction between the organic compound and nitric acid.

$$HNO_3 \rightleftharpoons \overset{\oplus}{H} + \overset{\ominus}{NO_3}$$

$$HNO_3 + \text{organic compound} \longrightarrow HNO_2 + \text{oxdised organic compound}$$

$$HO—N{=}O + \overset{\oplus}{H} \rightleftharpoons \overset{\oplus}{NO} \text{ (nitrosonium cation)} + H_2O$$

7. With more dilute nitric acid, probably nitracidium cation is involved in nitration reaction. Nitracidium cation is less reactive than nitronium cation.

$$2HNO_3 \rightleftharpoons H_2\overset{\oplus}{N}O_3 \text{ (nitracidium cation)} + \overset{\ominus}{NO_3}$$

Mechanistic Steps of Nitration Reaction in Benzene

***Step* 1 :**

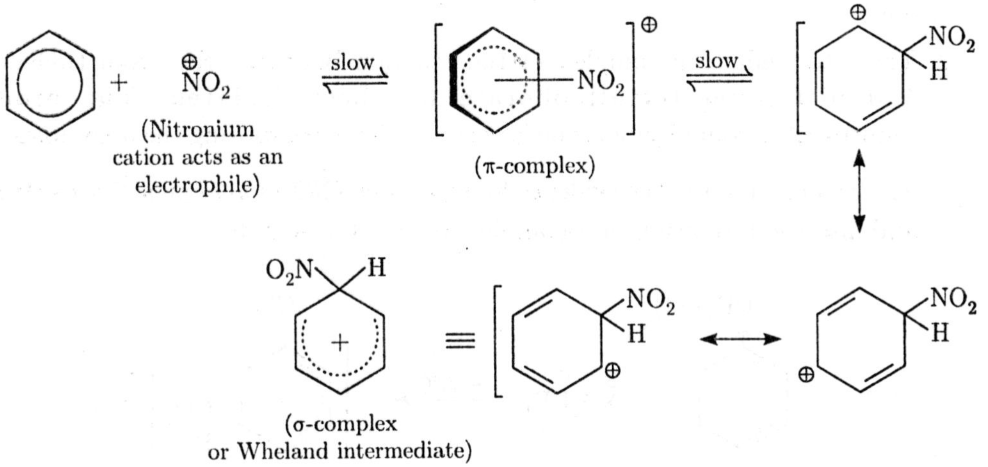

***Step* 2 :**

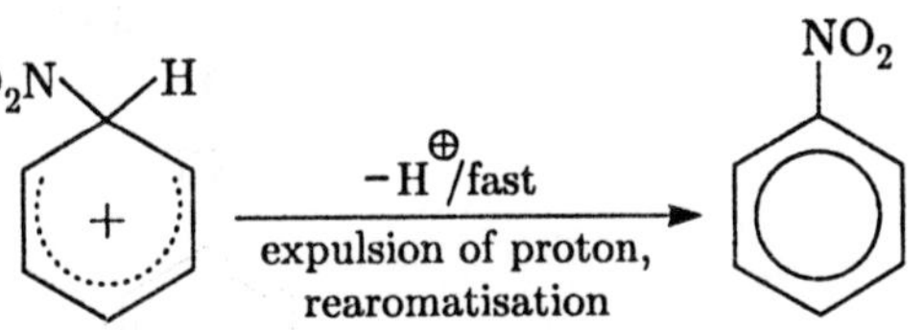

In aromatic electrophilic substitution reaction like nitration reaction as shown above, both the substrate and the electrophile take part in the slow (hence rate determining step) step and so is known as ArS_E2 (aromatic electrophilic substitution bimolecular).

Energy profile diagram of nitration of benzene :

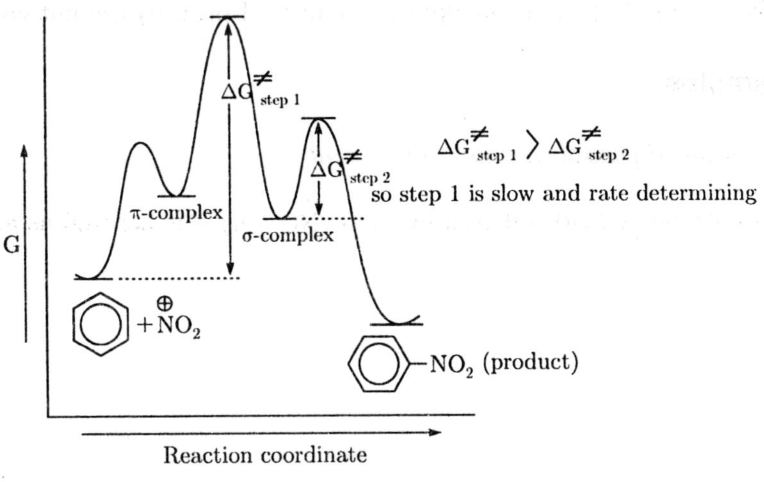

Fig. 3.8 :

Supports in the favour of nitronium cation as an attacking electrophile during nitration reaction :

1. X-ray crystallographic study of NO_2BF_4 shows the presence of $\overset{\oplus}{N}O_2$ (nitronium ion).
2. The intermediate σ-complex of the reaction between trifluoromethylbenzene and nitronium tetrafluoborate has been isolated. The product, *m*-nitrotrifluoromethylbenzene is prepared by decomposing the σ-complex. This experiment supports the evidence for nitronium ($\overset{\oplus}{N}O_2$) ion as an active electrophile and also the formation of σ-complex as an intermediate.

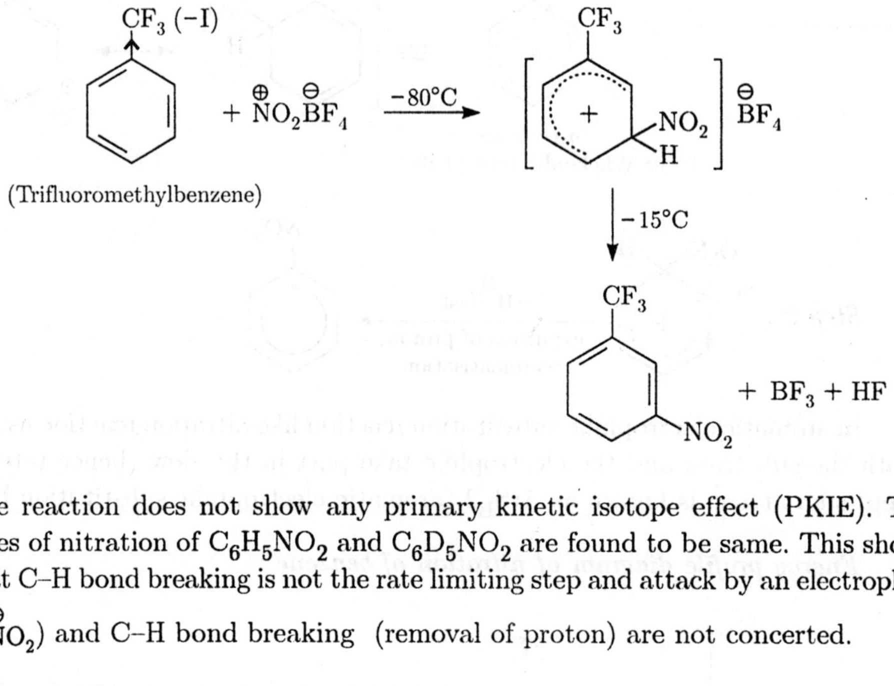

3. The reaction does not show any primary kinetic isotope effect (PKIE). The rates of nitration of $C_6H_5NO_2$ and $C_6D_5NO_2$ are found to be same. This shows that C–H bond breaking is not the rate limiting step and attack by an electrophile ($-\overset{\oplus}{N}O_2$) and C–H bond breaking (removal of proton) are not concerted.

Some Examples

1. *Nitration of phenol in dilute nitric acid* :

   In dilute nitric acid, nitrosonium ion ($\overset{\oplus}{N}O$ ion) is generated as an electrophile.

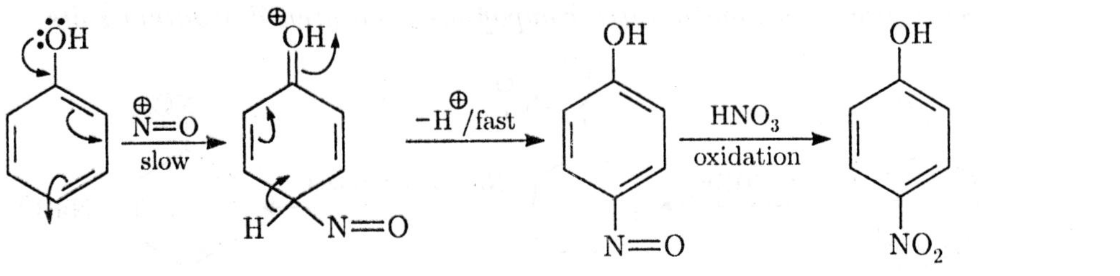

(p-Nitrophenol)

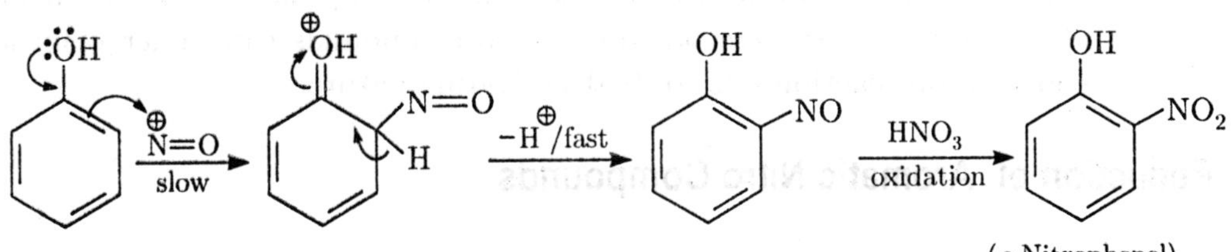

(o-Nitrophenol)

Generally dilute nitric acid contains very low percentage of nitrous acid (HNO_2).

2. *Nitration of pyridine-N-oxide by solid KNO_3 in fuming sulphuric acid* :

$$KNO_3 + H_2SO_4 \longrightarrow HNO_3 + KHSO_4$$

$$HNO_3 + 2H_2SO_4 \rightleftharpoons \overset{\oplus}{N}O_2 + 2H\overset{\ominus}{S}O_4 + H_3\overset{\oplus}{O}$$

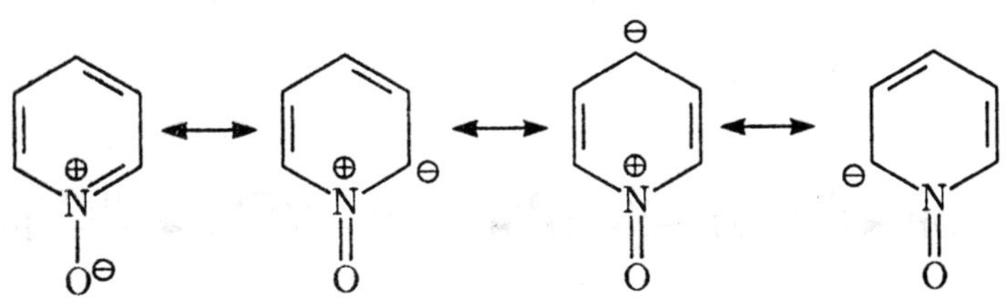

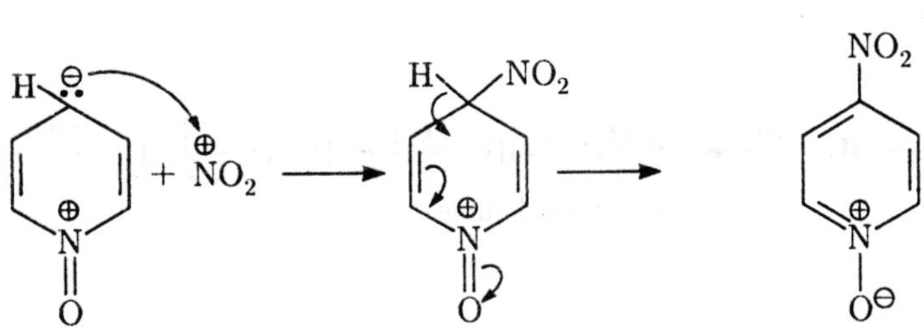

(4-Nitropyridine-N-oxide)

3. *Preparation* of *aromatic nitro compounds from arenediazonium salts* :

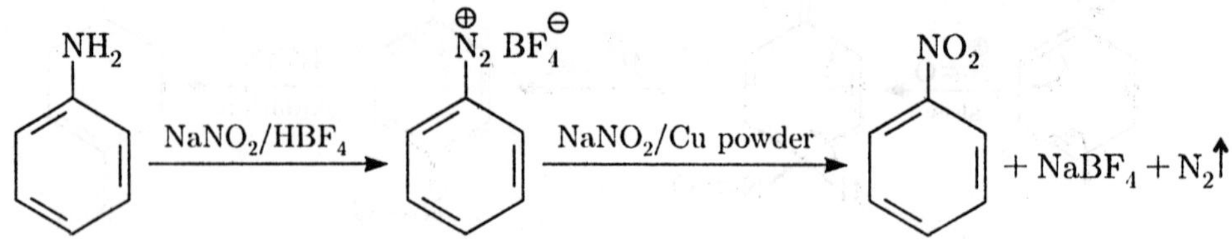

(Diazonium fuoborate)

Nitro ($-NO_2$) group deactivate the benzene ring and so directs an incoming electrophile to the *meta* position. Nitro compounds can undergo nucleophilic substitution reaction due to its deactivating nature.

Reduction of Aromatic Nitro Compounds

1. ***Reduction by metal and acid*** :

$$PhNO_2 \xrightarrow{\text{Zn or Sn or Fe/conc. HCl}} PhNH_2$$

Mechanism :

$$\text{M (metal=Sn or Zn or Fe)} \longrightarrow M^{2+} + 2e^-$$

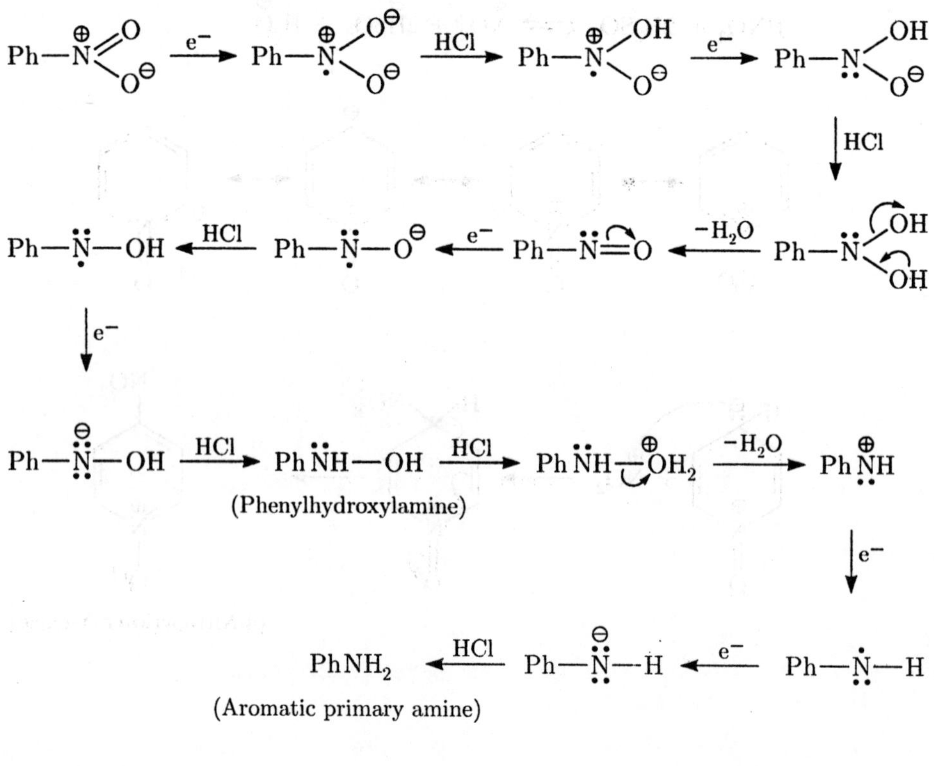

2. ***Reduction by $SnCl_2$ or $TiCl_2$ and concentrated HCl*** :

$$PhNO_2 \xrightarrow{SnCl_2 \text{ or } TiCl_2/\text{concentrated HCl}} \underset{\text{(Aromatic primary amine)}}{PhNH_2}$$

3. ***Catalytic reduction*** :

$$PhNO_2 \xrightarrow[\text{reduction}]{\text{Pt or Pd or Ni}/H_2} \underset{\text{(Aromatic primary amine)}}{PhNH_2}$$

Partial Reduction of Aromatic Nitro Compounds

1. ***Reduction by neutral reducing agent*** :

$$PhNO_2 \xrightarrow{Zn/NH_4Cl/\text{alcohol}} \underset{\text{(Phenylhydroxylamine)}}{PhNHOH}$$

   Mechanism of the reaction is the same as given by dissolving metal reduction, but it is limited upto the phenylhydroxylamine stage.

2. ***Selective reductions*** : When an aromatic nitro compound contains more than one nitro group, one of them may be selectively reduced to an amino group by the reducing action of sodium sulphide (Na_2S) or ammonium sulphide $(NH_4)_2S$ or NaHS (sodium bisulphide) or NH_4HS (ammonium bisulphide).

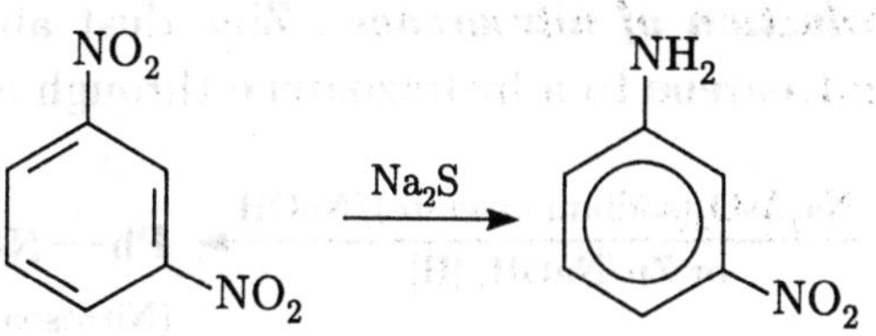

Na_2S or $(NH_4)_2S$ cannot reduce a $-NO_2$ group *o*-to an alkyl group, which is done satisfactorily by $SnCl_2$/conc. HCl.

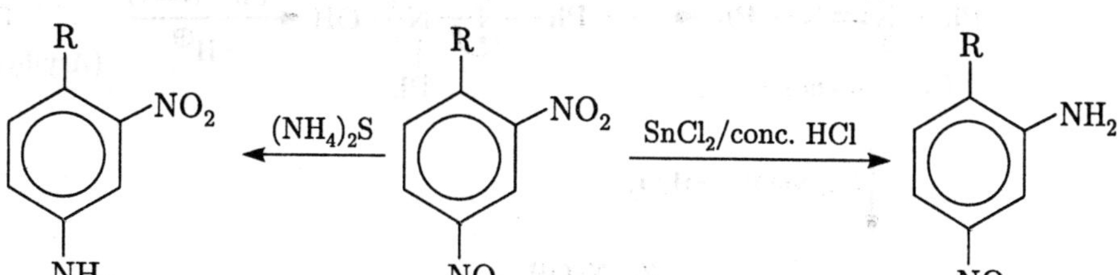

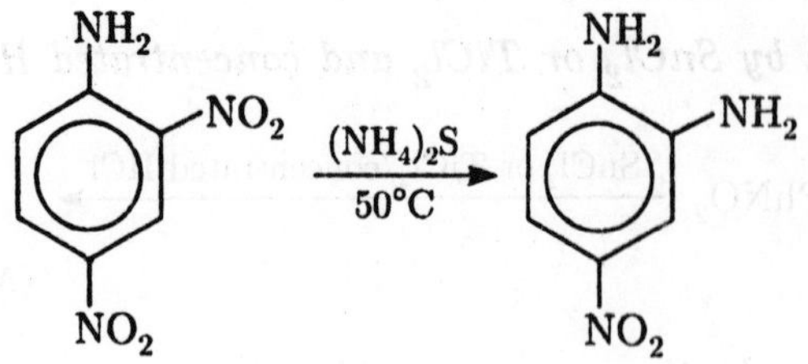

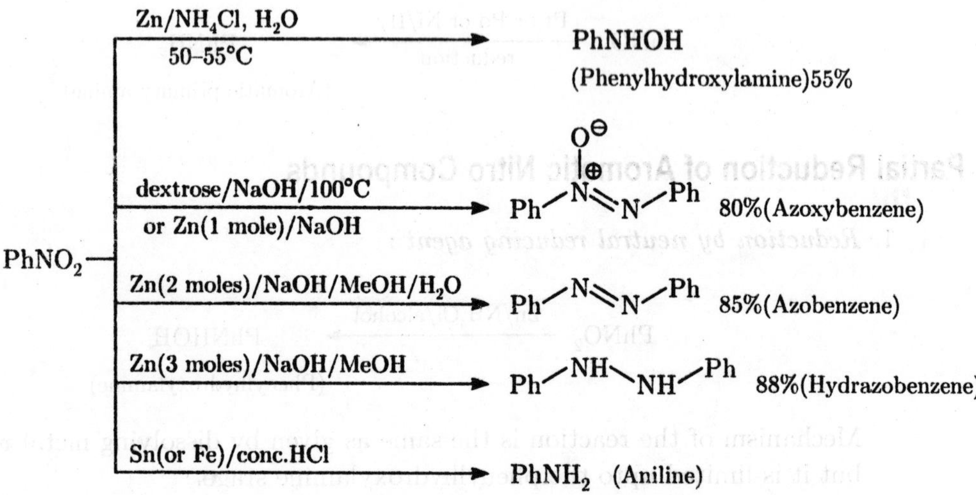

In basic solution, using a weak reducing agent such as dextrose or glucose, the intermediate nitrosobenzene reacts with phenylhydroxylamine to give azoxybenzene.

3. ***Alkaline reduction of nitroarenes*** : Zinc dust and aqueous sodium hydroxide reduces a nitroarene to a hydrazoarene through azoxyarene and azoarene.

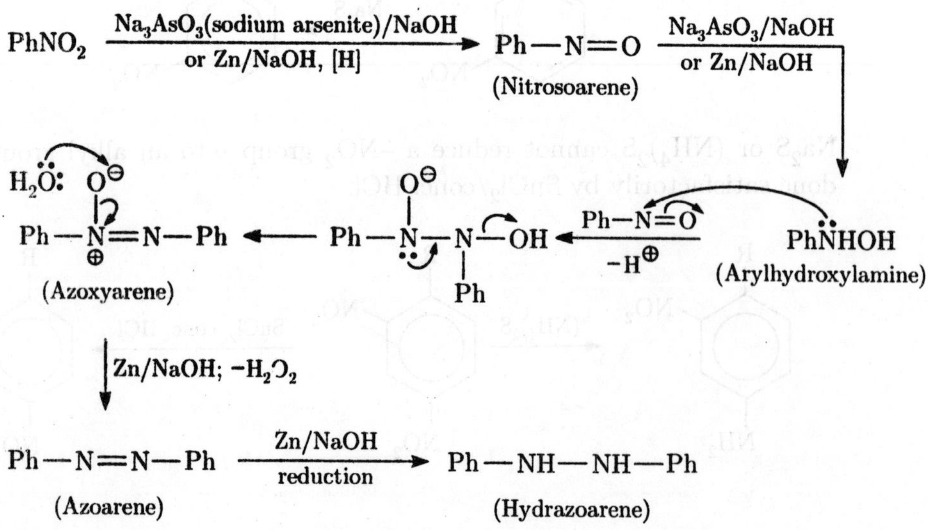

Sodium arsenite and aqueous sodium hydroxide however reduces a nitroarene to azoxyarene which may further be reduced to hydrazoarene. Hydrazoarene may be reduced to aryl amines by sodium and absolute ethanol.

Hydrazoarenes on treatment with warm and dilute hydrochloric acid, undergoes benzidine-semidine rearrangement.

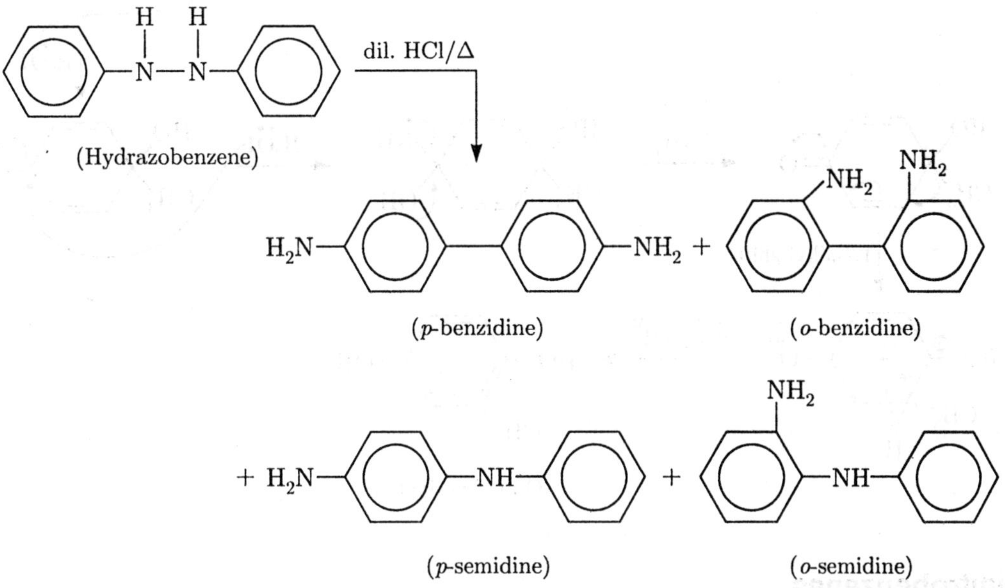

When nitrobenzene is reduced by Zn/NH_4Cl, phenylhydroxylamine is formed first, which then undergoes rearrangement to *p*-aminophenol.

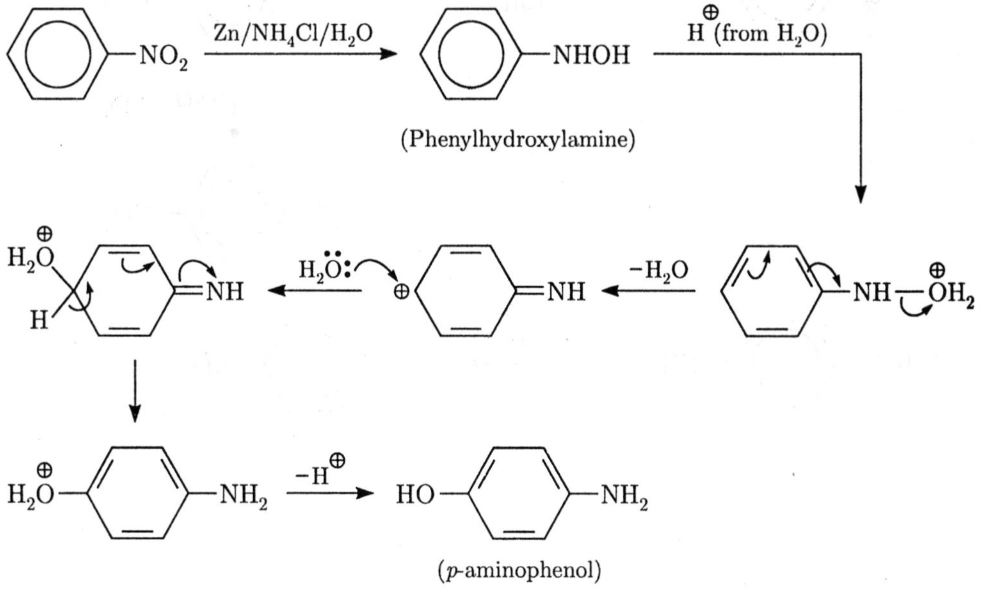

If the *para* position is occupied, NH_3 gets eliminated and the reaction is known as **Bamberger Reactions.**

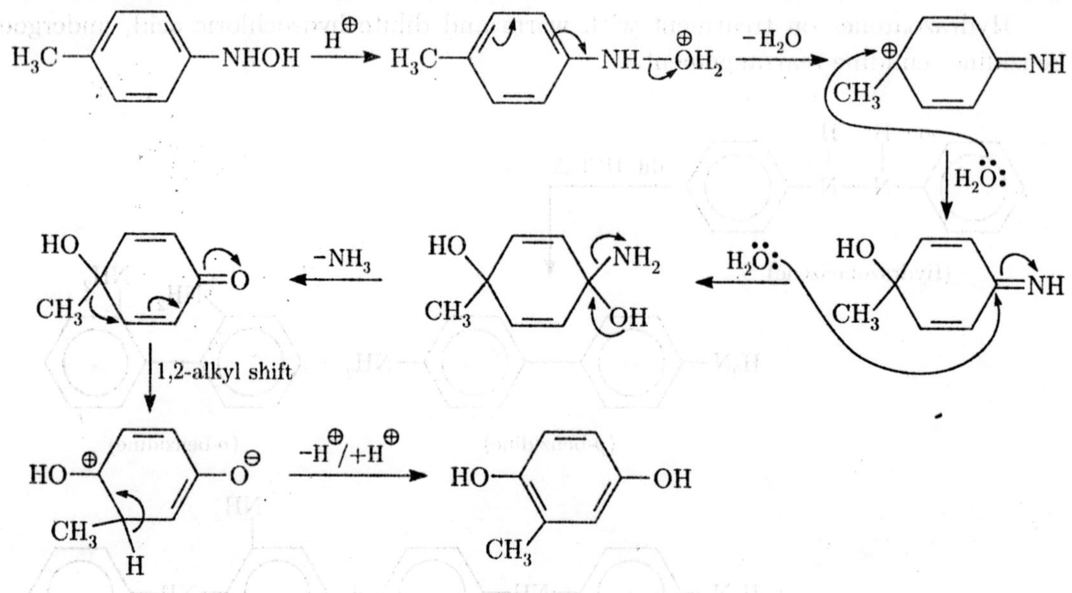

(Quinol derivative)

Dinitrobenzenes

1. 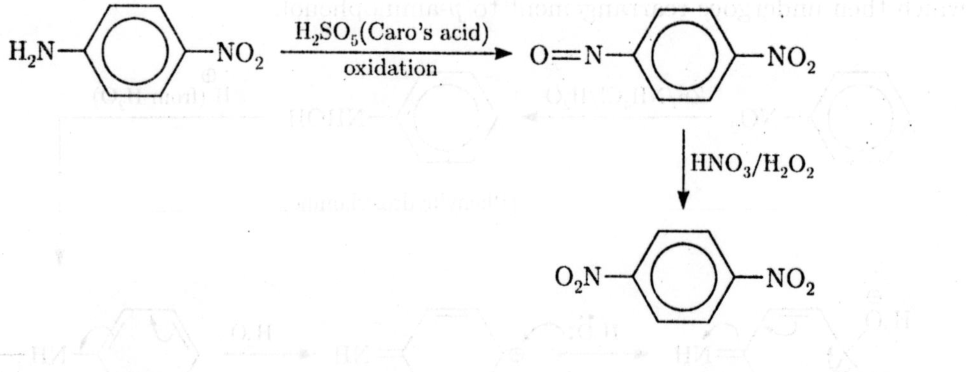

2. 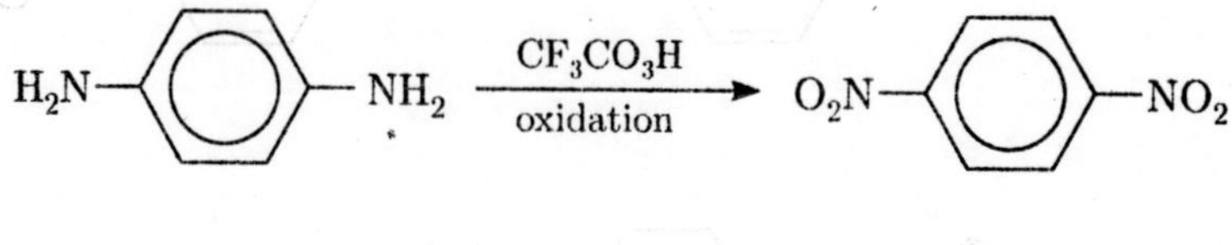

Salt formation reaction by aromatic nitro compounds : Owing to –I and –R effects of $-NO_2$ group in *o*-nitrotoluene, methyl group form a salt with NaOEt as shown below.

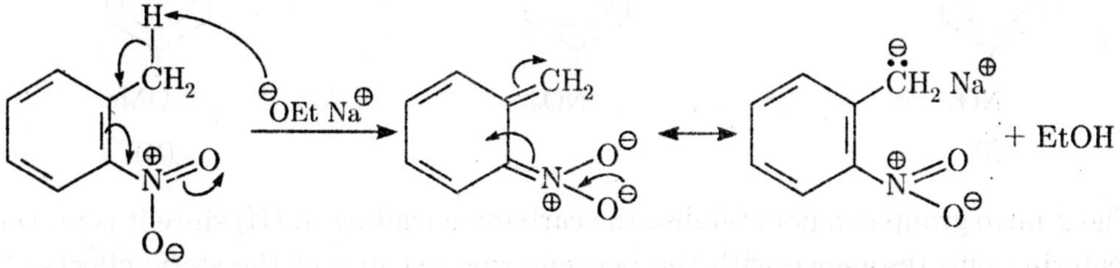

Aromatic nucleophilic substitution reactions of aromatic nitro compounds : Aromatic nitro compounds can undergo bimolecular nucleophilic substitution as nitro group deactivates the benzene nucleus by making it electron deficient.

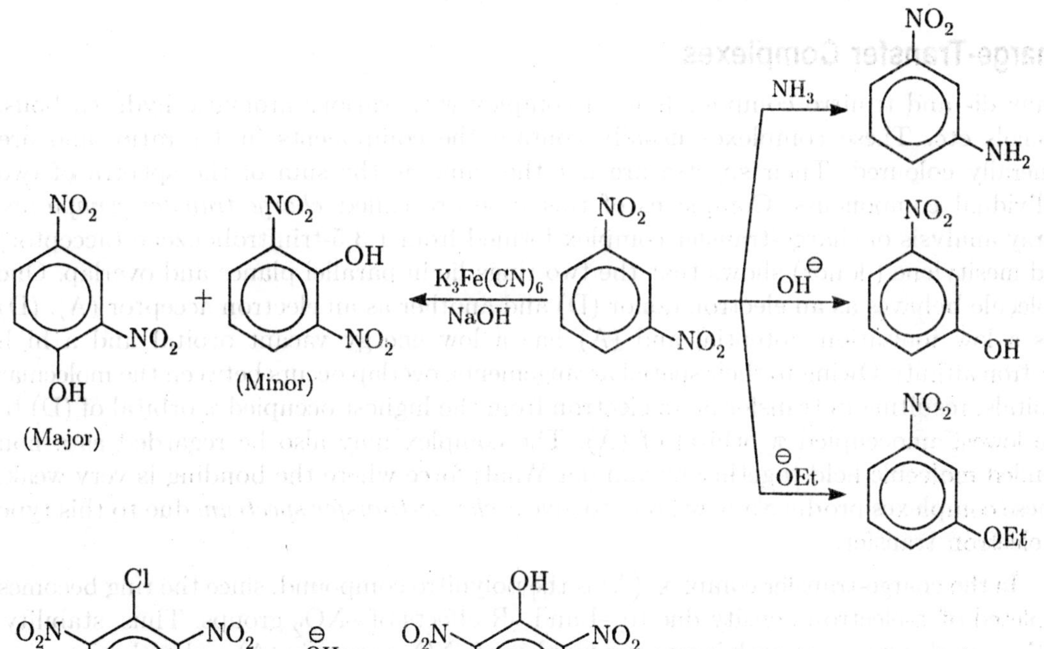

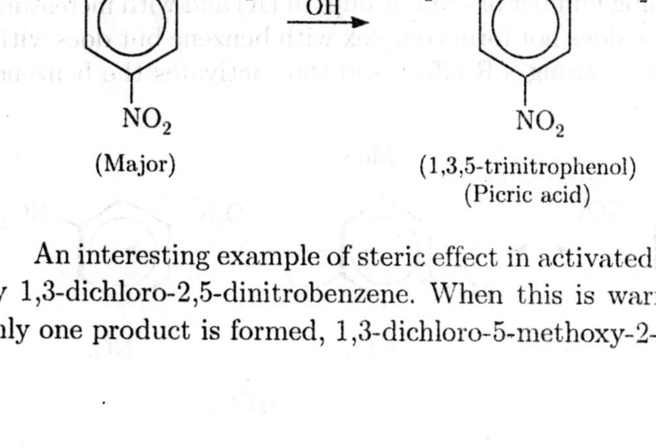

An interesting example of steric effect in activated nucleophilic substitution is shown by 1,3-dichloro-2,5-dinitrobenzene. When this is warmed with methanolic methoxide, only one product is formed, 1,3-dichloro-5-methoxy-2-nitrobenzene.

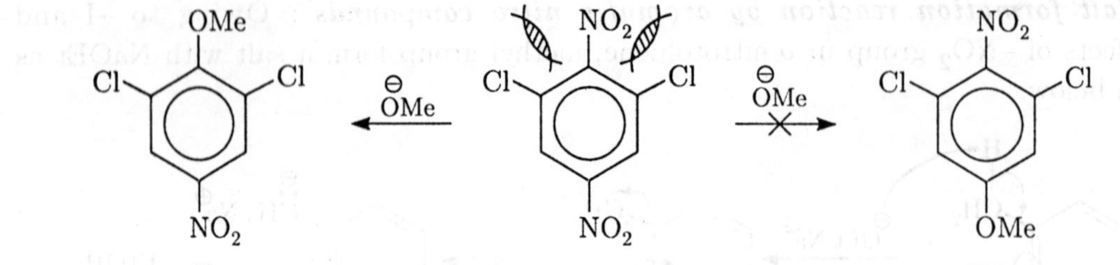

The 2-nitro group can not stabilise the carbanion leading to (II) since it is prevented from entering into resonance with the benzene ring because of the steric effects of the *ortho* chlorine atoms. On the other hand, this steric inhibition of resonance is absent in the carbanion leading to (I) (the entering OMe group and ejected NO_2 group are both perpendicular to the ring). Hence, the carbanion, leading to (I) has a lower energy of activation than (II). So only (I) is formed exclusively.

Charge-Transfer Complexes

Many di- and trinitro compounds form complex with various aromatic hydrocarbons, phenols etc. These complexes usually contain the components in 1:1 ratio, and are generally coloured. Their spectra are not the same as the sum of the spectra of two individual components. Complexes of this type are called *charge-transfer complexes.* X-ray analysis of charge-transfer complex formed from 1,3,5-trinitrobenzene (acceptor) and mesitylene (donor) shows that the two rings lie in parallel planes and overlap. One molecule behaves as an electron donor (D) and another as an electron acceptor (A). (D) has a low ionisation potential and (A) has a low energy vacant orbital and a high electron affinity. Owing to their spatial arrangements, overlap occurs between the molecular orbitals, resulting in transfer of an electron from the highest occupied π orbital of (D) to the lowest unoccupied π orbital of (A). The complex may also be regarded as a non bonded molecule held together by van der Waals force where the bonding is very weak. These complexes produce a new bond to give a *charge-transfer spectrum* due to this type of electron transfer.

In the charge-transfer complex, (A) is the polynitro compound, since the ring becomes depleted of π-electron density due to –I and –R effects of $-NO_2$ groups. Thus, stability. of the complex increases with increasing number of $-NO_2$ groups in (A) and with increasing basicity of (D). 1,3,5-Trinitrobenzene does not form complex with benzene but does with mesitylene (three methyl groups have strong +R effect and thus activates the benzene ring).

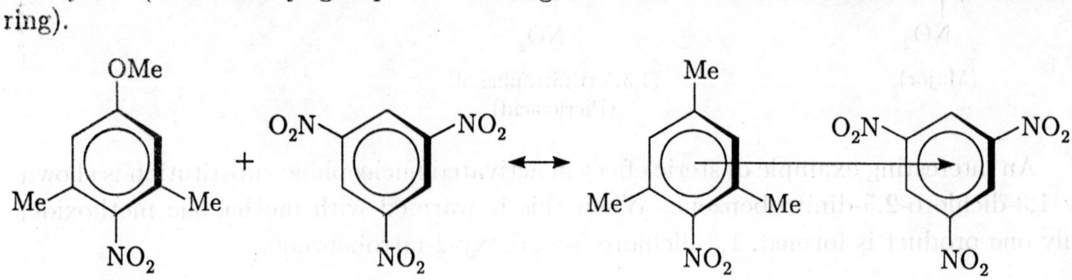

$(\overset{\oplus}{D}\overset{\ominus}{A})$

Other Nitroarenes

1.

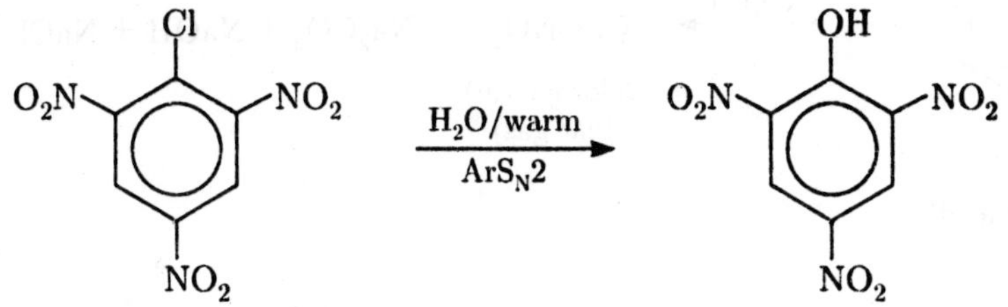

(Ring is highly activated towards aromatic nucleophilic substitution due to the presence of three $-NO_2$ groups) (*picryl chloride*)

(Picric acid)

2.

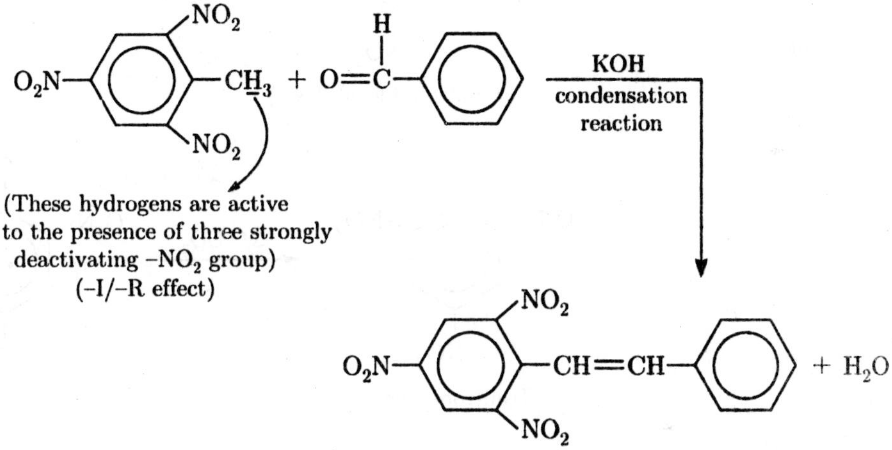

(These hydrogens are active due to the presence of three strongly deactivating $-NO_2$ group) (–I/–R effect)

(Trinitrostilbene)

The activation of methyl group may be explained in terms of stability of benzeyl anion produced.

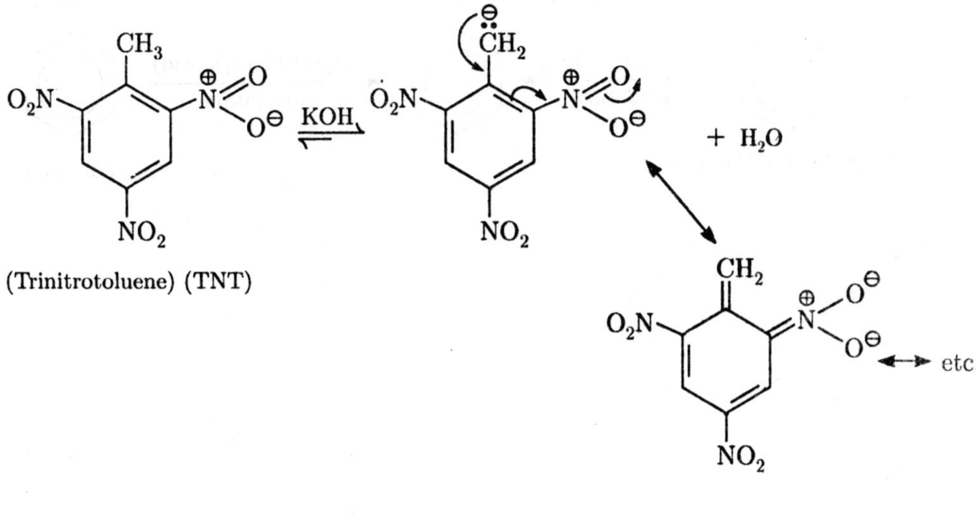

(Trinitrotoluene) (TNT)

3. 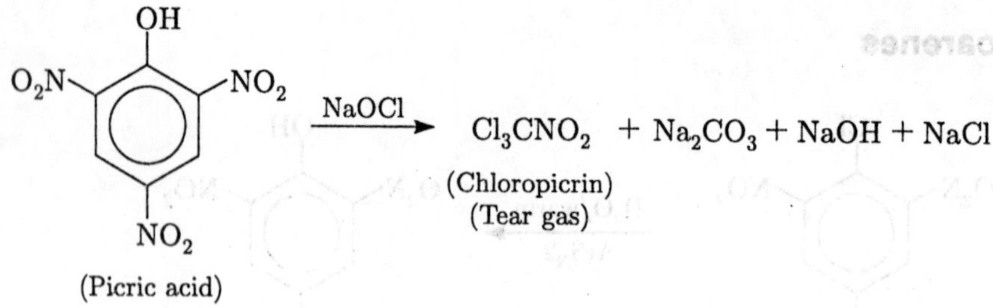

4. 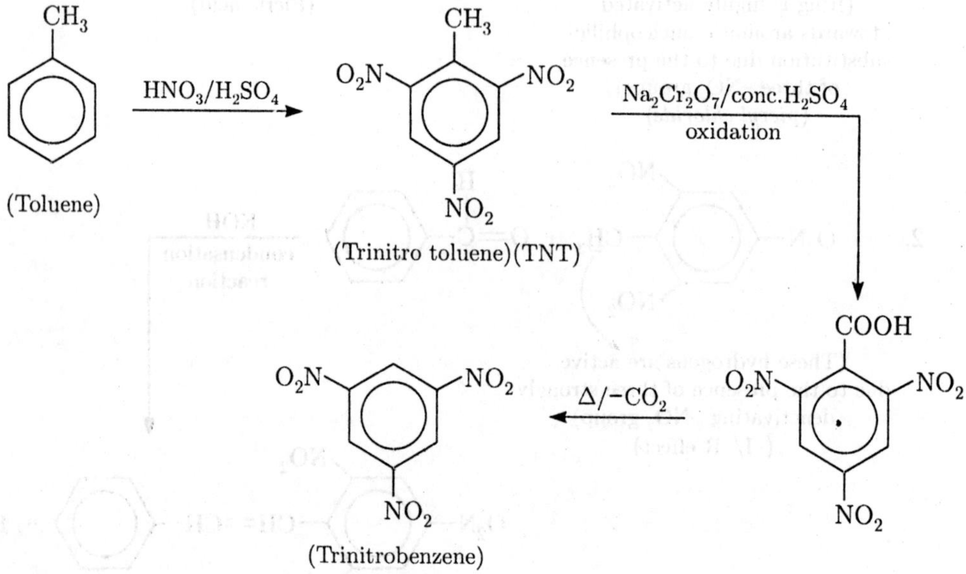

Aromatic Nitroso Compounds

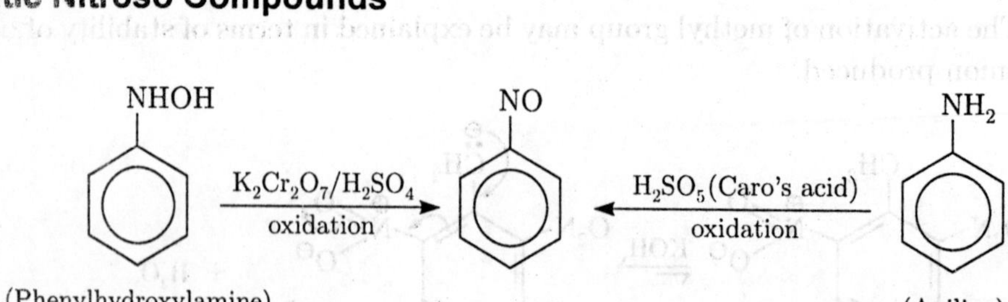

***Reduction products of nitrosobenzene* :**

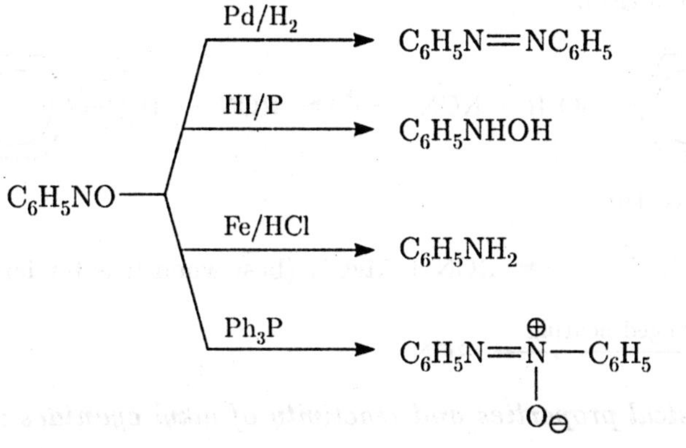

***Oxidation products of nitrosobenzene* :**

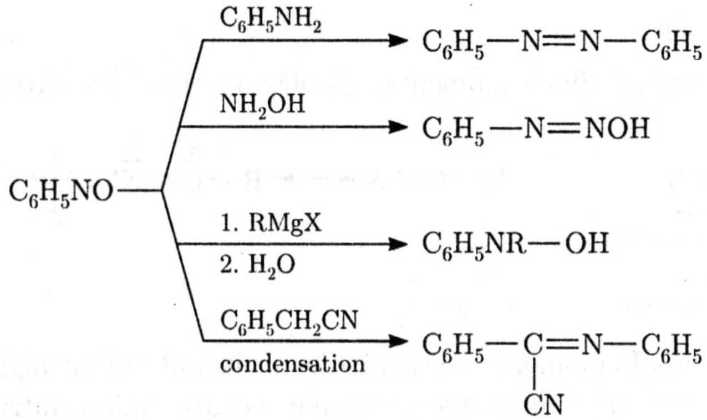

Alkyl Nitriles or Alkyl Cyanides

Cyano derivatives of alkanes are alkyl nitriles (R–CN). Alkyl nitriles are isomeric with alkyl isocyanides or isonitriles (R–NC), where R depicts an alkyl group.

***General methods of preparation of alkyl nitriles* :**

1. $RCONH_2 \xrightarrow{P_2O_5/\Delta/\text{dehydration}} RCN + H_2O$

2. $RCOOH + NH_3 \xrightarrow[\text{(Industrial method of preparation)}]{Al_2O_3/500°C} RCOONH_4 \xrightarrow{Al_2O_3} H_2O + RCONH_2 \xrightarrow{Al_2O_3/-H_2O} RCN$

3. $RCH{=}NOH \xrightarrow{P_2O_5 \text{ or } Ac_2O} RCN + H_2O$

4. $RX + KCN \xrightarrow{\text{Aqueous ethanol}/\Delta} RCN + KX$

The method is satisfactory if R is primary or secondary. Tertiary halides do not show this reaction.

5. 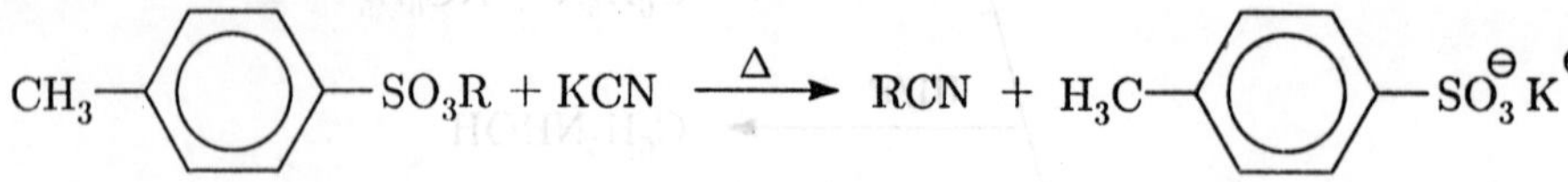

(Alkyl *p*-tosylate)

6. $RMgCl + ClCN \longrightarrow RCN + MgCl_2$ (best when R is tertiary)

7. $RNC \xrightarrow{\text{prolonged heating}} RCN$

Structure, physical properties and reactivity of alkyl cyanides :

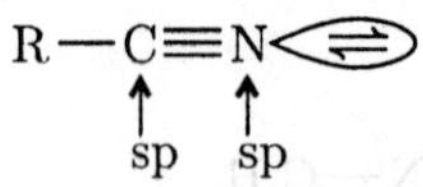 (sp) (Linear structure around the C—N bond.)

Alkyl nitriles have high dipole moment ($\mu \cong 4.0D$) and thus have strong polar character.

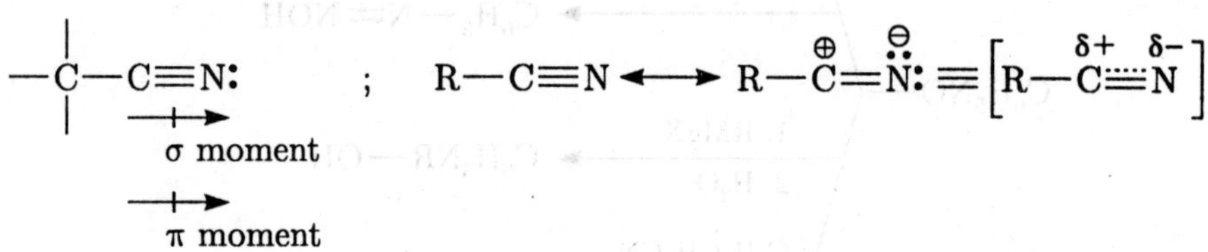

Owing to high dipole moments, alkyl nitriles melt and boil at higher temperatures than alkanes and ethers of comparable molecular weight. Again, nitriles can not form hydrogen bonding with water or protic solvents, so they are lower melting and boiling than the corresponding carboxylic acids. The lone pair of electrons on nitrogen in nitrile occupy an sp hybridised orbital which is strongly bound to the carbon nucleus and hence the donor capacity of these electrons is very poor. For this reason, nitriles are poor bases and do not dissolve appreciably in dilute acids. Cyano carbon and nitrogen have electrophilic and nucleophilic nature respectively and so they undergo addition reactions. Strong –I effect of cyano group makes the *α-hydrogen atom slightly acidic.*

Chemical Reactions Given by Alkyl Nitriles

Hydrolysis of Alkyl Nitriles to Carboxylic Acids

Alkyl nitriles can either be hydrolysed by moderately dilute acid or alkali to carboxylic acids or carboxylic acid salts.

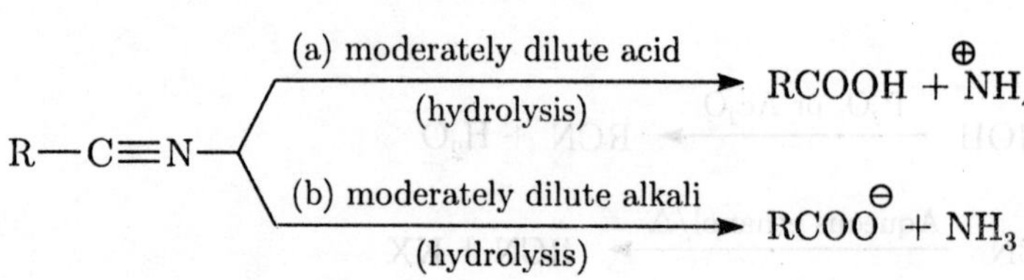

1. ***Mechanism of acid catalysed hydrolysis reaction :***

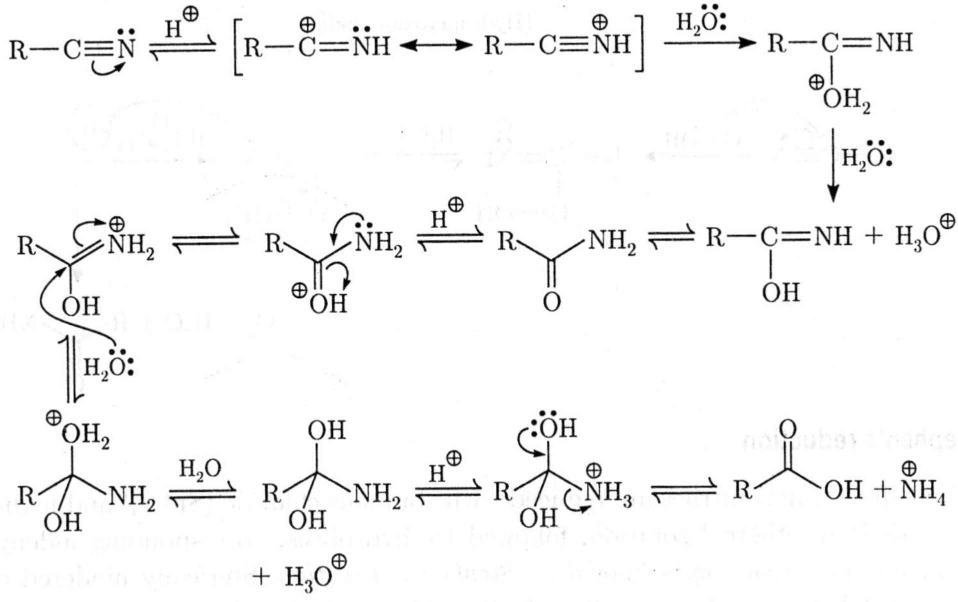

2. ***Mechanism of base-catalysed hydrolysis reaction :***

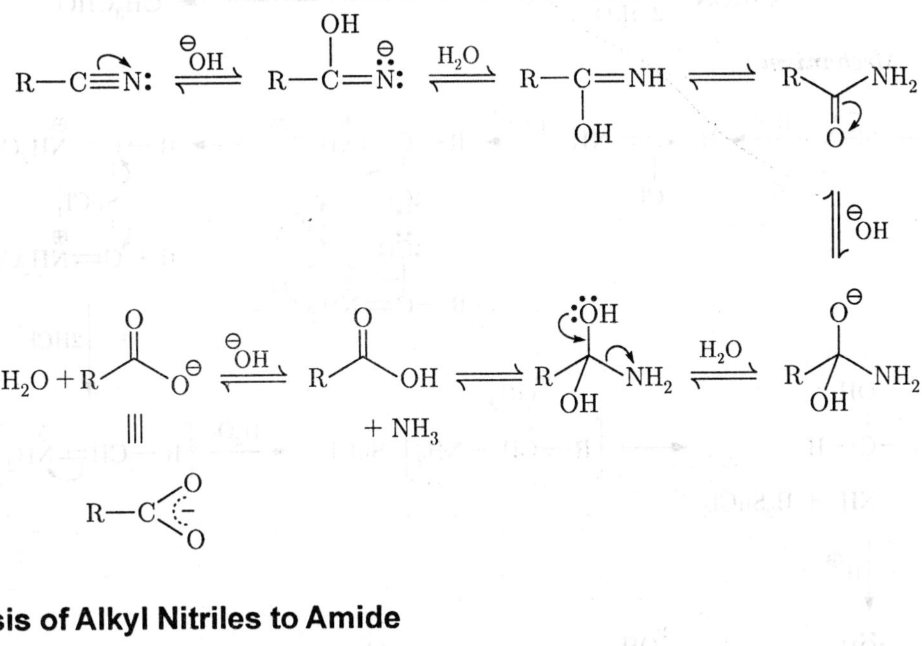

Hydrolysis of Alkyl Nitriles to Amide

An alkyl nitrile can be hydrolysed to amide by alkaline hydrogen peroxide. The rate of nucleophilic attack on the cyano carbon by hydroperoxide anion is almost ten thousand times faster than that on the amido carbon by hydroxide ion. So the formation of amide becomes much faster than it gets hydrolysed to the corresponding acid.

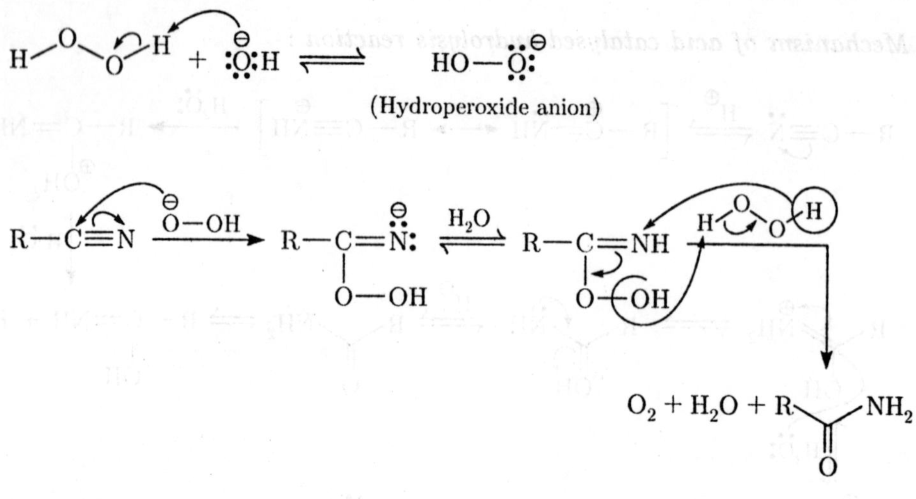

Stephen's reduction

When alkyl or aryl nitriles are reduced with stannous chloride ($SnCl_2$) and hydrochloric acid (HCl) in ethereal solution, followed by hydrolysis, corresponding aldehydes are obtained. This reaction is known as *Stephen's reduction.* Sterically hindered cyanides (*e.g.*, *o*-tolylnitriles and other *ortho* substituted benzonitriles) do not undergo this reaction.

$$CH_3CN \xrightarrow[2.\ H_2O]{1.\ SnCl_2/HCl\ \text{in ether/ethyl formate/EtOAc}} CH_3CHO$$

Mechanism :

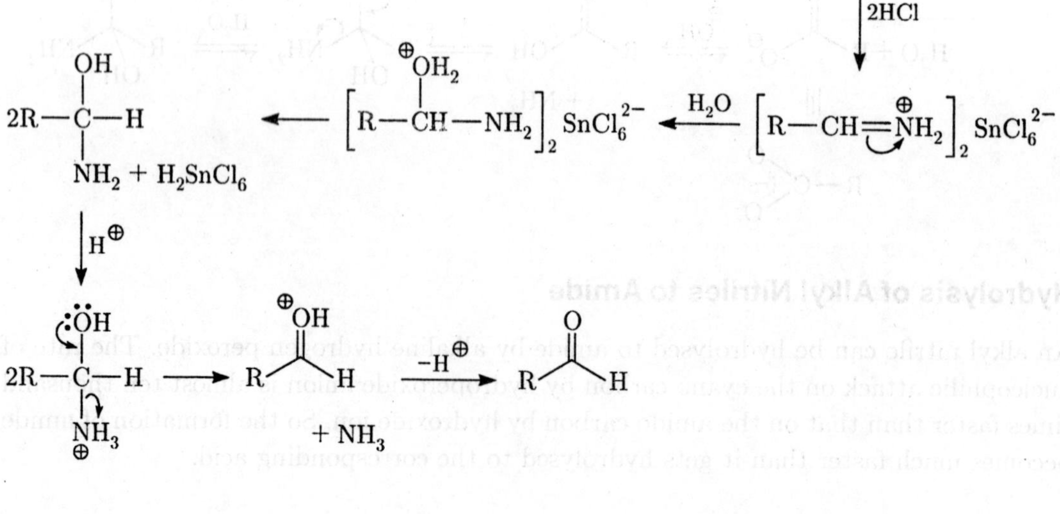

The Thorpe Nitrile Condensation

In the presence of a base (NaOEt/EtOH) or metallic sodium and ether, two molecules of a nitrile condense to form an iminonitrile in which the α–H of one molecule is involved and the reaction is known as Thorpe nitrile condensation. The condensation is analogous to aldol condensation. The iminonitrile on treatment with water gives a β-ketonitrile.

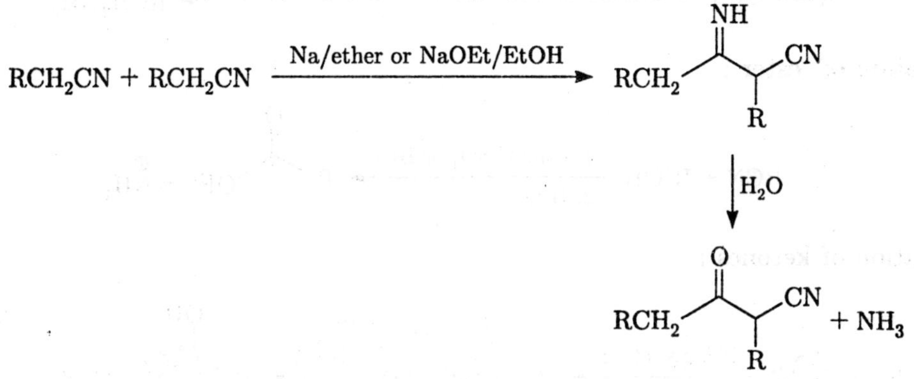

Mechanism :

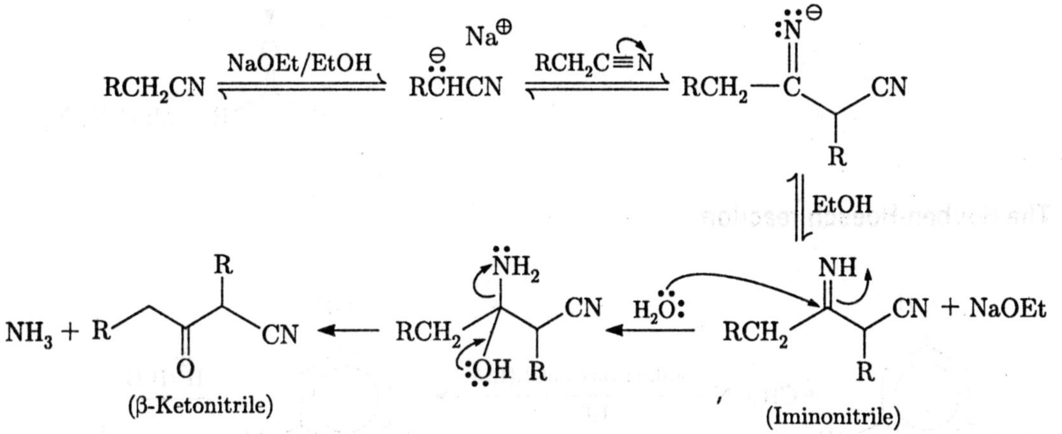

Intramolecular or Internal Thorpe condensation is also known and the reaction is called as ***Thorpe-Ziegler*** reaction. The product formed is enaminonitrile, not an iminonitrile.

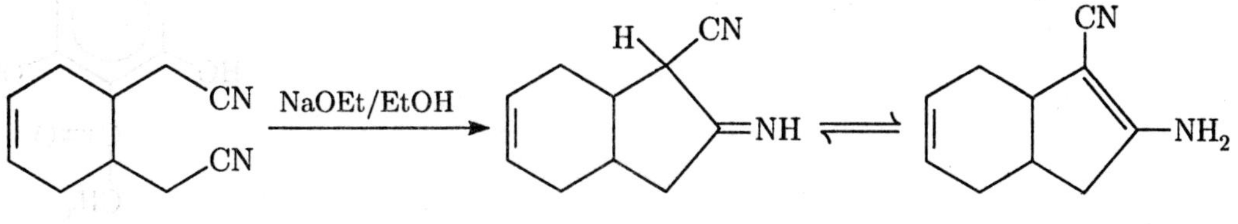

(Enaminonitrile)

The Thorpe-Zeigler reaction is a useful method for closing large rings. Five to eight membered rings and also rings containing fourteen or more carbons are prepared successfully. High yields are obtained provided high dilution techniques are used.

Reduction of cyanides :

$$R{-}C{\equiv}N \xrightarrow{\text{LiAlH}_4 \text{ or Na/ether or H}_2\text{/catalyst(Pt/Pd/Ni)}} RCH_2NH_2$$

Formation of ester :

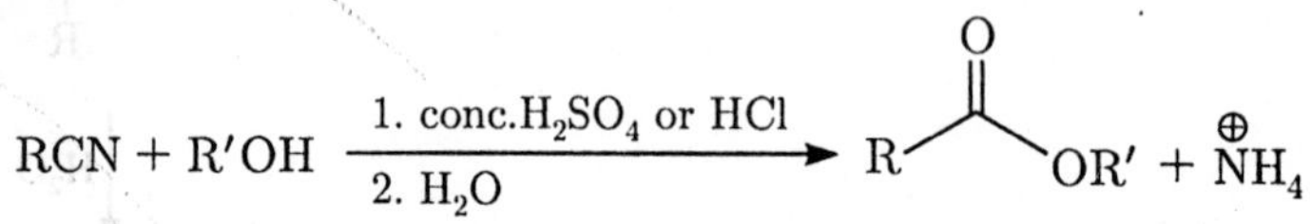

Formation of ketones :

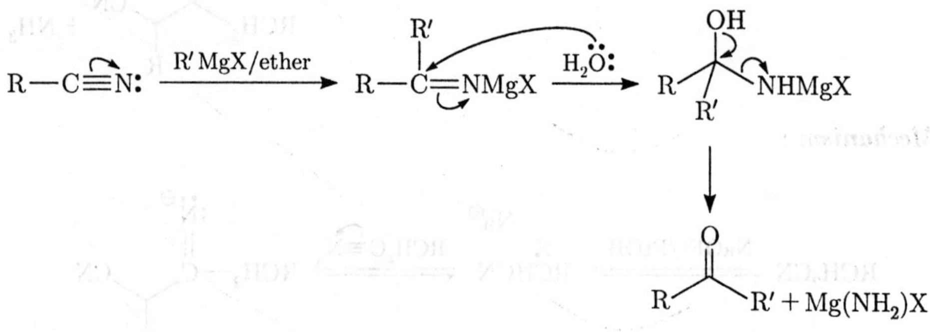

The Houben-Hoesch reaction

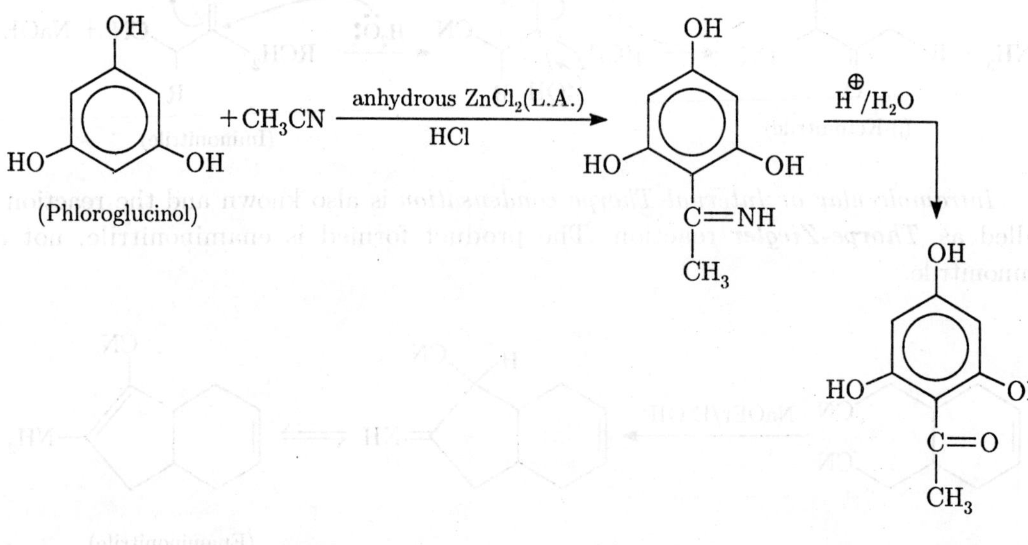

Addition of olefins :

In the presence of sulphuric acid, olefins add to nitriles to give nitrilium salts which on treatment with water gives N-tertiaryalkyl amide and the reaction is known as *Ritter reaction.*

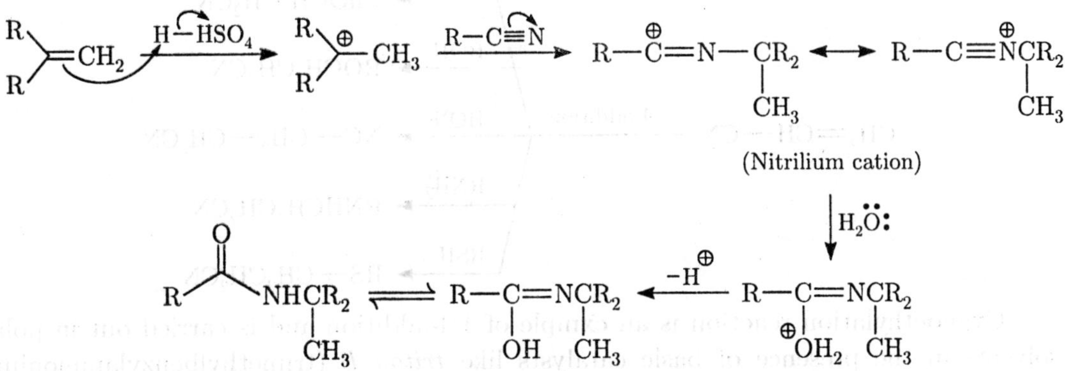

Addition of ammonia :

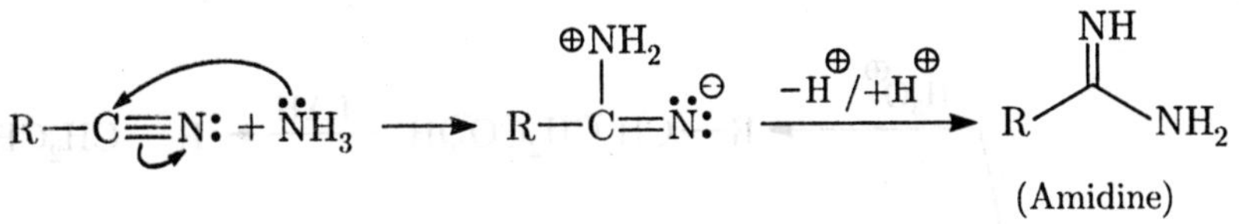

Formation of β-ketonitrile :

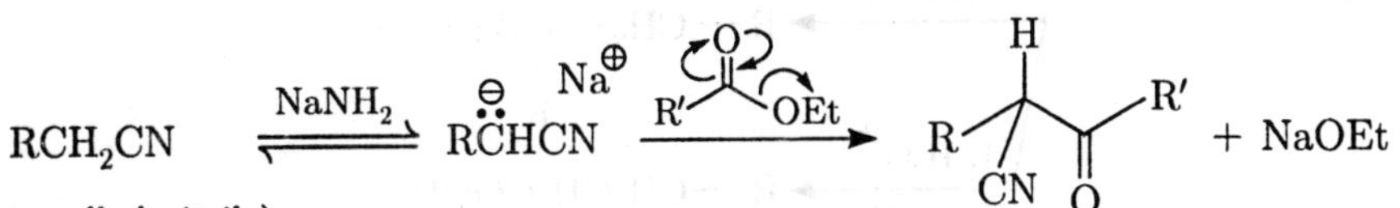

(primary alkyl nitrile) or (secondary alkyl nitrile can also be used)

Alkylation reaction :

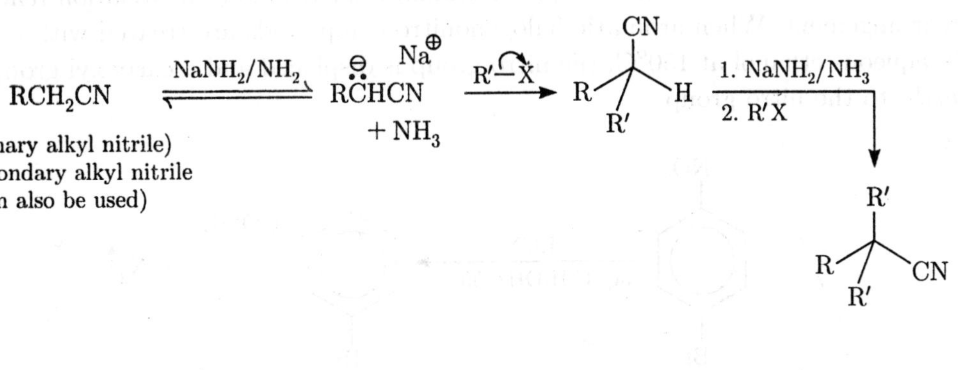

(primary alkyl nitrile) or (secondary alkyl nitrile can also be used)

Cyanoethylation reaction

The reagent for cyanoethylation is acrylonitrile ($CH_2{=}CHCN$). The substrates are compounds with active hydrogen, like phenol, alcohols, amines etc.

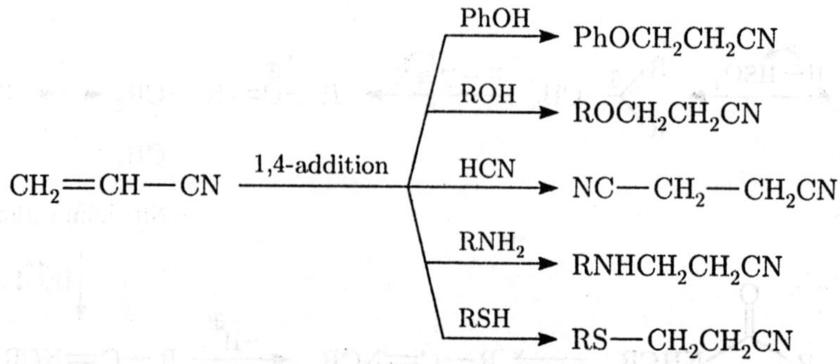

Cyanoethylation reaction is an exmple of 1,4-addition and is carried out in polar solvents in the presence of basic catalysts like *triton B* (trimethylbenzylammonium hydroxide). The reaction has immense synthetic utility where three carbon atoms are incorporated at a time. Furthermore, the cyano group can be converted to other functional groups.

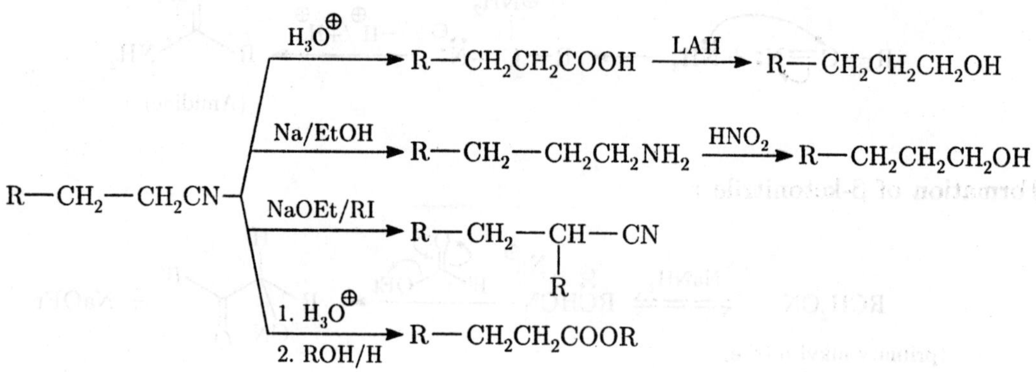

Von Richter Reaction

Von Richter reaction is an example of aromatic nucleophilic substitution reaction with rearrangement. When aromatic halogenonitro compounds are treated with cyanide ion in aqueous ethanol at 150°C, the nitro group is displaced and a carboxyl group appears *ortho* to the nitro group.

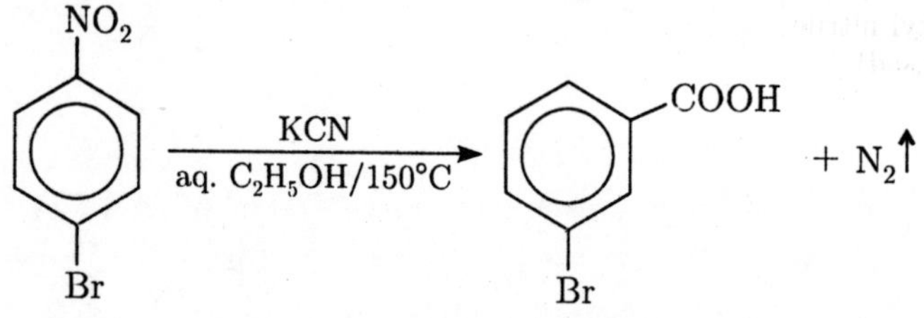

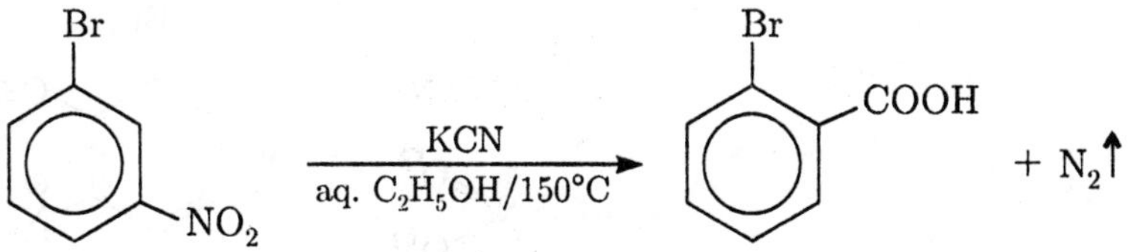

The mechanism of the reaction *does not occur via an aryne intemediate.* It is expected that the products of the reaction should be $NO_2^{\ominus}$, NH_3 and carboxylic acid as $CN^{\ominus}$ is the reagent and aryl cyanide gets hydrolysed to carboxylic acid and ammonia. But molecular nitrogen (N_2) is the major byproduct of the reaction and the following mechanism has been proposed which does not involve aryl cyanide as intermediate.

Mechanism of the reaction :

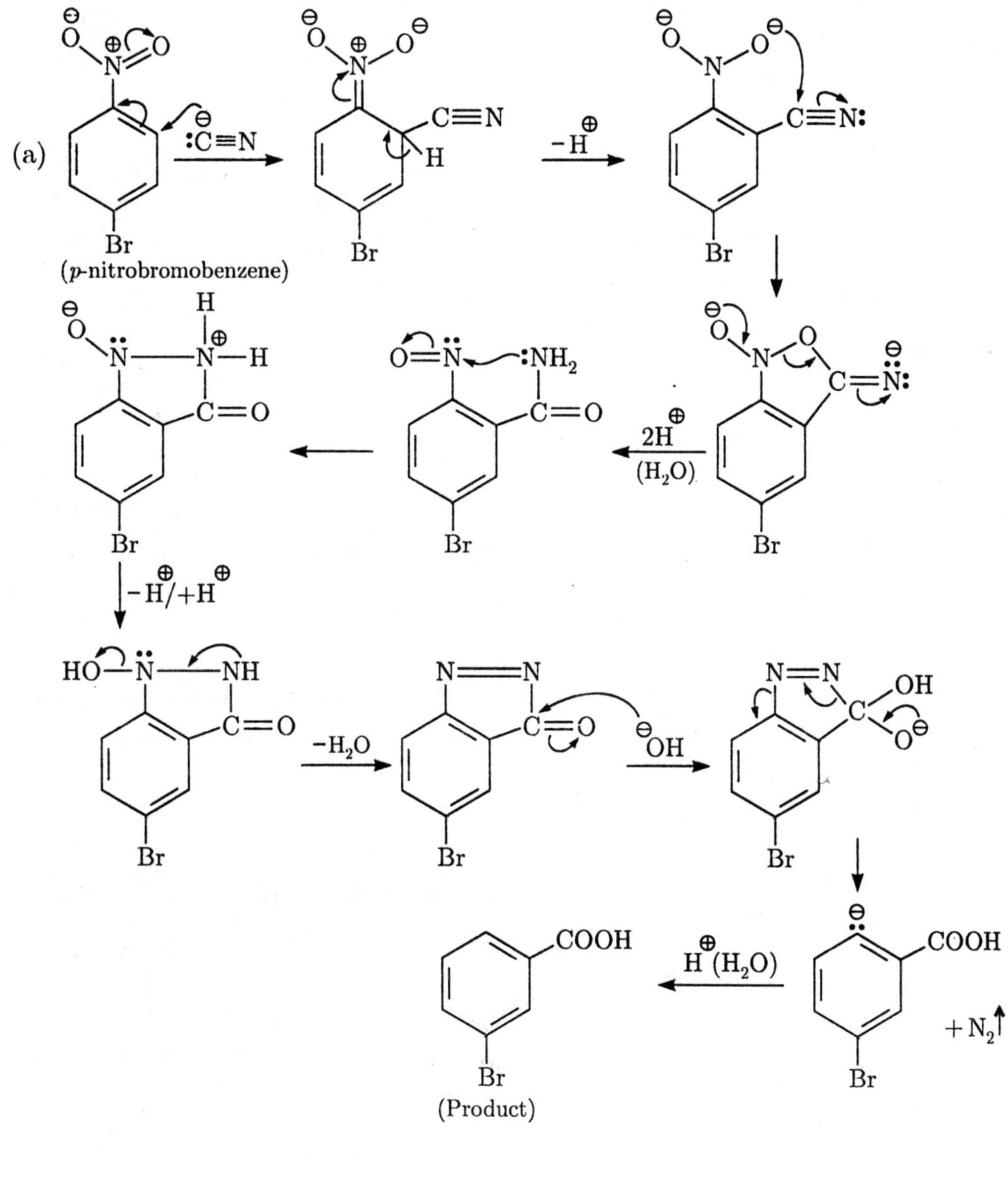

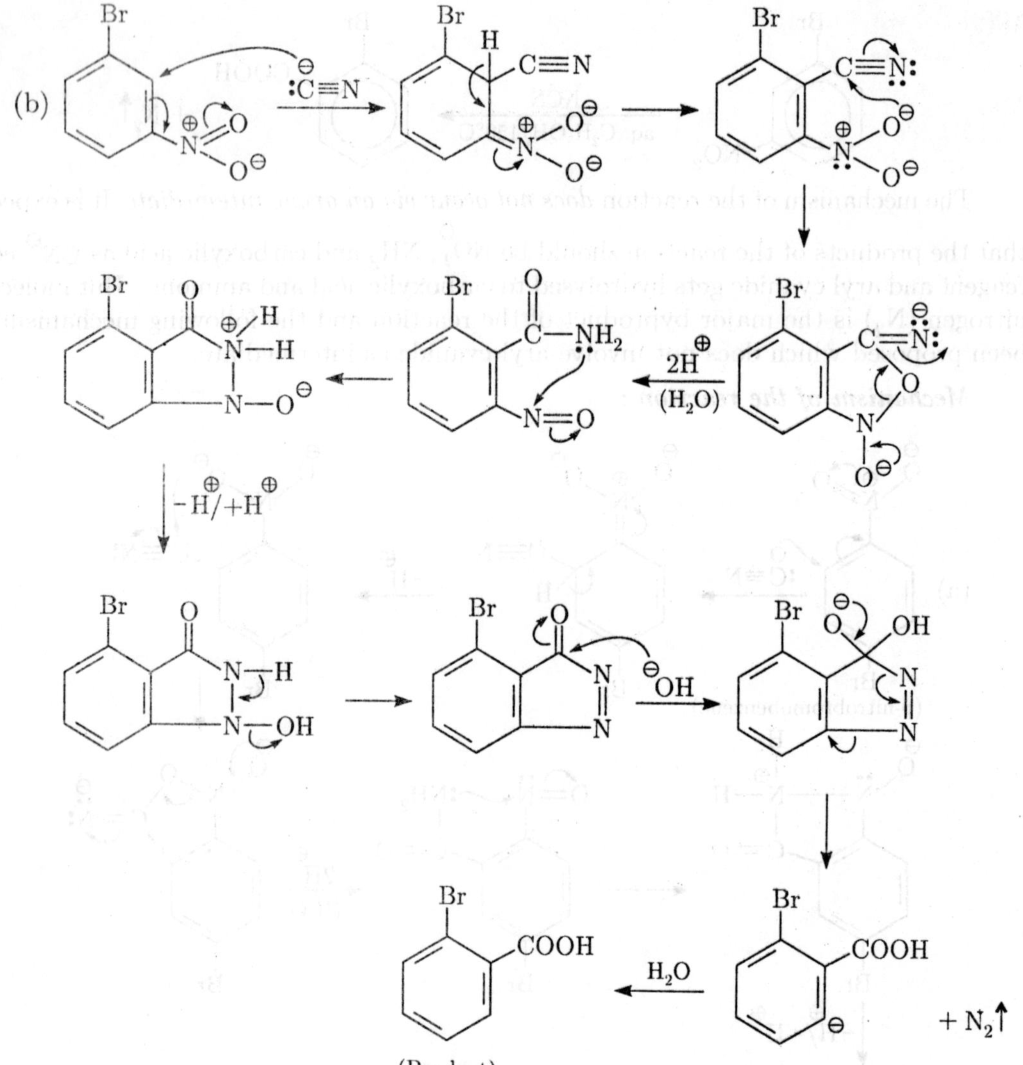

(Product)

An interesting application of Von Richter reaction is the preparation of 2-bromo-3-methylbenzoic acid, which apparently has not been prepared by other means.

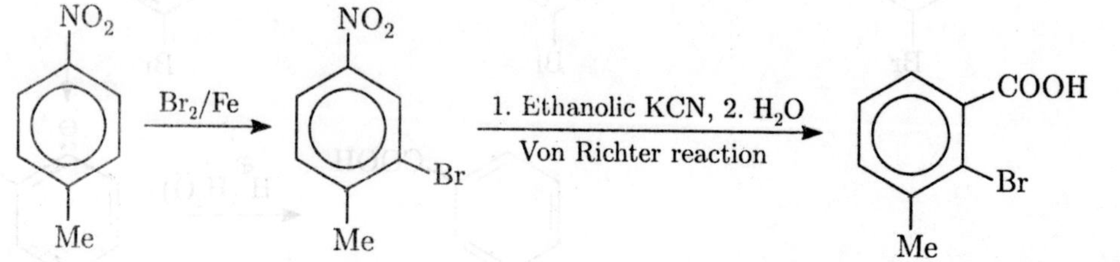

(2-Bromo-3-methylbenzoic acid)

Alkyl Isonitriles (Alkyl Isocyanides)

Alkyl isonitriles ($R-\overset{\oplus}{N}\equiv\overset{\ominus}{C}: \longleftrightarrow R-\ddot{N}=C:$) are also called alkyl isocyanides or carbylamines. They are isomeric with alkyl nitriles ($R-C\equiv N$).

General methods of preparation of alkyl isonitriles :

1. 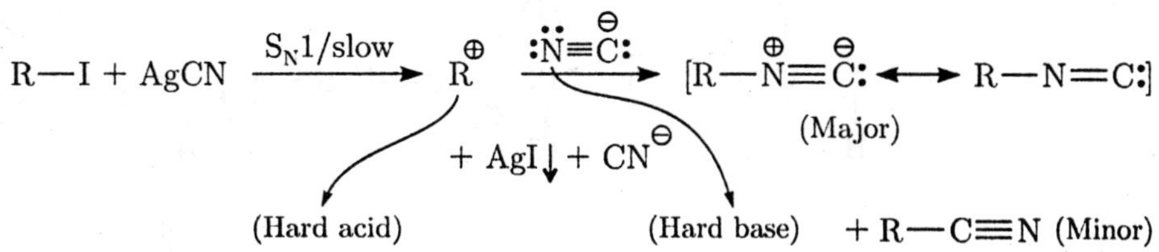

Here $\overset{\oplus}{R}$ (hard acid) prefers to combine with hard base centre nitrogen and R–NC becomes the major product. R–C≡N formed by the combination of hard acid and soft base is less favourable and so becomes minor contributory.

2. ***Carbylamine Reaction*** : When a primary amine, aliphatic or aromatic is heated wih ethanolic solution of potassium hydroxide, an isonitrile is formed and the reaction is known as *carbylamine reaction.* Isonitriles or carbylamines have unpleasant odour.

$$\underset{}{ArNH_2} + CHCl_3 + \underset{\text{(Ethanolic)}}{3KOH} \xrightarrow{\Delta} \underset{\text{(aryl isocyanide)}}{ArNC} + 3KCl + 3H_2O$$

$$R-NH_2 + CHCl_3 + \underset{\text{(Ethanolic)}}{3KOH} \xrightarrow{\Delta} \underset{\text{(alkyl isocyanide)}}{RNC} + 3KCl + 3H_2O$$

Mechanism of the reaction :

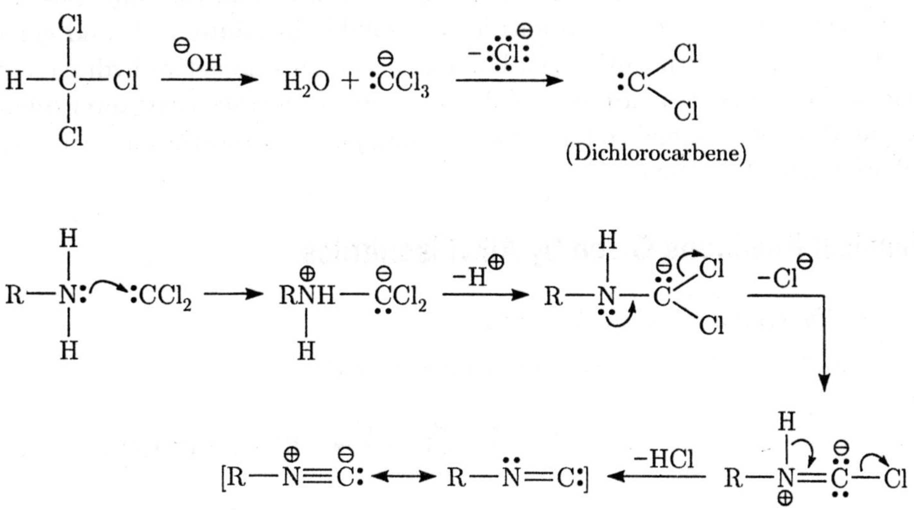

3. ***From N-alkylformamides*** :

$$RNHCHO \xrightarrow[\text{dehydration}]{POCl_3/\text{pyridine}} RNC + H_2O$$

Mechanism :

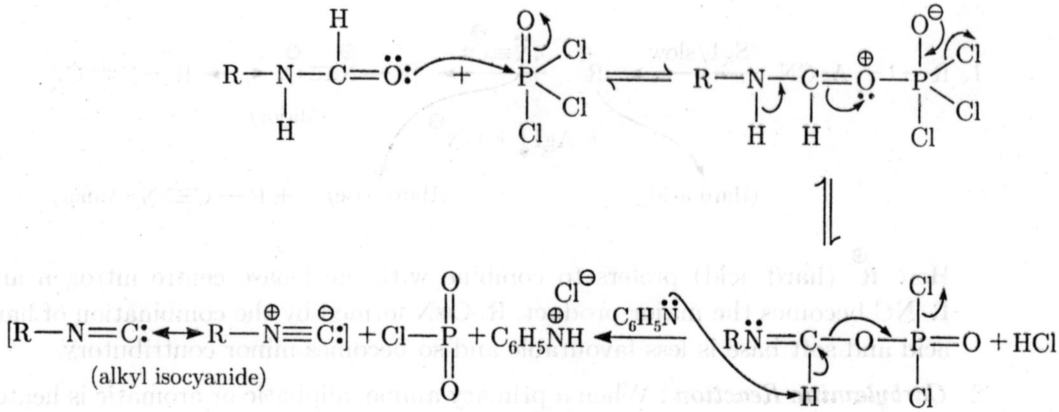

Structure, reactivity and physical properties of isonitriles :

$$R-\overset{\oplus}{N}\equiv\overset{\ominus}{C}: \longleftrightarrow R-\ddot{N}=C: \quad , \quad \mu \cong 3.0D$$

(π-Moment) (σ-Moment)

The dipole moments of isonitriles are less (μ=3.0D) than the dipole moment of nitriles (μ=4.0D) as in the former molecule, the direction of π-moment and σ-moment operate opposite to each other. Isonitriles show considerable basicity as the more electropositive carbon atom bears the negative charge and the conjugate acid becomes stable. For the same reason, isonitriles are soluble in dilute acids and get hydrolysed. Isonitriles can not form hydrogen bond as it contains no active hydrogen atom and so even the lower members are not soluble in water. Isonitriles have lower dipole moments compared to nitriles, and so have lower boiling points. Isonitriles have nauseating odour and are particularly toxic.

Chemical Reactions Given by Alkyl Isonitriles

1. ***Hydrolysis of Alkyl Isonitriles***

(a) *Hydrolysis of isonitriles by dilute acid* :

$$R-\overset{\oplus}{N}\equiv\overset{\ominus}{C}: \xrightarrow{H^{\oplus}} RNH_2 + HCOOH$$

Mechanism :

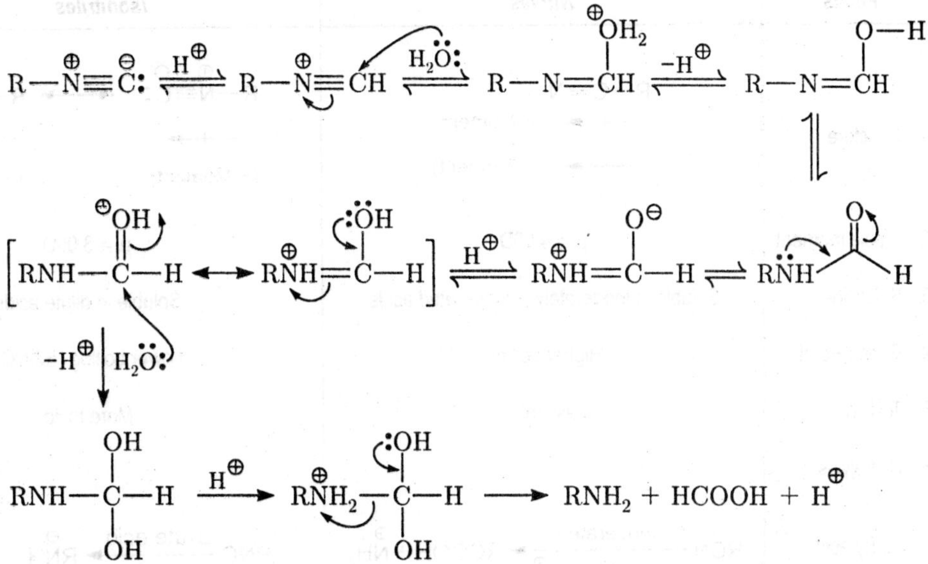

(b) *Hydrolysis of isonitriles by bases* : Isonitriles are *not hydrolysed* by alkali. Nitrogen bears a positive charge and all the valencies (four) of nitrogen are satisfied (in $R-\overset{\oplus}{N}\equiv\overset{\ominus}{C}:$, nitrogen is *tetracovalent*). So it can not accomodate an extra lone pair of electrons. Carbon bearing negative charge can not coordinate with negatively charged $\overset{\ominus}{O}H$ anion.

$$R-\overset{\oplus}{N}\equiv\overset{\ominus}{C}: \xrightarrow[\times]{\overset{\ominus}{O}H} \textbf{No alkaline hydrolysis}$$

2. ***Reduction*** :

$$R-\overset{\oplus}{N}\equiv\overset{\ominus}{C}: \xrightarrow{H_2/Pt \text{ or } Sn/conc.HCl} RNHCH_3$$

3. ***Addition of halogen*** :

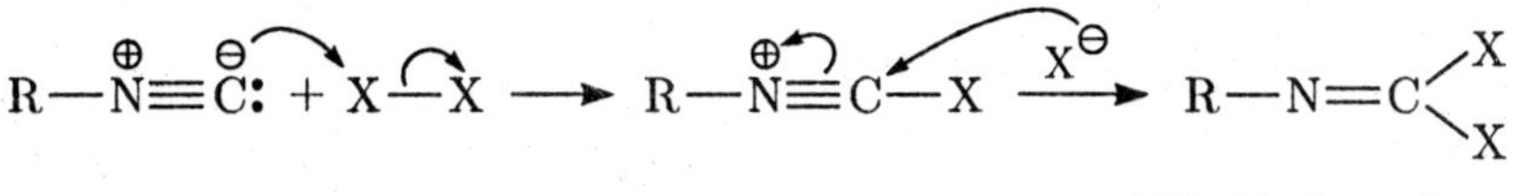

(Alkyl iminocarbonyl halide)

4. ***Addition of sulphur*** :

$$R-\overset{\oplus}{N}\equiv\overset{\ominus}{C}: + S \longrightarrow R-\ddot{N}=C=S$$

(Alkyl isothiocyanate)

Distinction between Nitriles and Isonitriles

Points	*Nitriles*	*Isonitriles*
1. Structure	$R-C\equiv N$ $\longrightarrow$ (σ-Moment) $\longrightarrow$ (π-Moment)	$R-\overset{\oplus}{N}\equiv\overset{\ominus}{C}{:} \longleftrightarrow R-\ddot{N}=C{:}$ $\longrightarrow$ (π-Moment) $\longleftarrow$ (σ-Moment)
2. Dipole moment	$\mu \cong 4.00D$	$\mu \cong 3.00D$
3. Solubility	Soluble in moderately concentrated acids	Soluble in dilute acids
4. Boiling Point	Higher boiling	Lower boiling (≅20°C)
5. Toxicity	Less toxic	More toxic
6. Hydrolysis		
(a) By acid	$RCN \xrightarrow[\text{conc. acid } (H_3\overset{\oplus}{O})]{\text{moderately}} RCOOH + \overset{\oplus}{N}H_4$	$RNC \xrightarrow[(H_3\overset{\oplus}{O})]{\text{dilute acid}} R\overset{\oplus}{N}H_3 + HCOOH$
(b) By alkali	$RCN \xrightarrow[(\overset{\ominus}{O}H/H_2O)]{\text{aq. alkali}} RCO\overset{\ominus}{O} + NH_3$	$RNC \xrightarrow{\overset{\ominus}{O}H/H_2O}$ No reaction
7. Reduction	$RCN \xrightarrow{H_2/Pt} RCH_2NH_2$ (primary amine)	$RNC \xrightarrow{H_2/Pt} RNHCH_3$ (Secondary methylamine)

4 Aromatic Polynuclear Hydrocarbons

Naphthalene

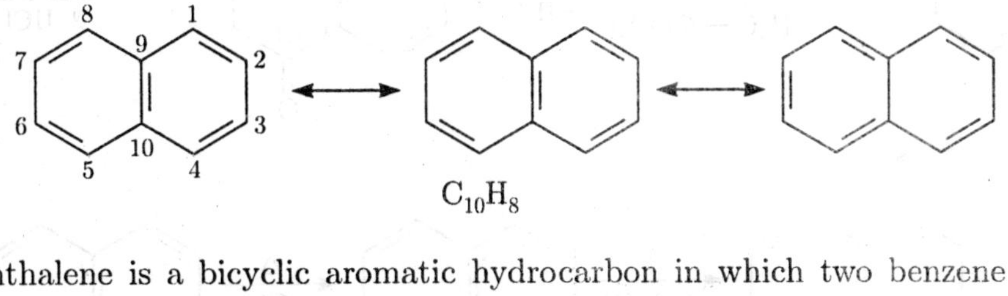

$C_{10}H_8$

Naphthalene is a bicyclic aromatic hydrocarbon in which two benzene rings are fused in *ortho* positions. Naphthalene has molecular formula $C_{10}H_8$. It is the single largest constituent of coal tar (9%), having m.p. 80°C. It is highly volatile.

Synthesis of naphthalene and alkylnaphthalene

1. 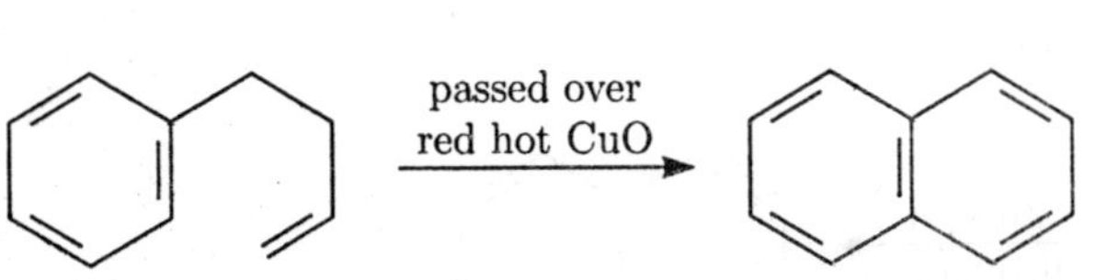

(4-Phenylbut-1-ene) (Naphthalene)

2.

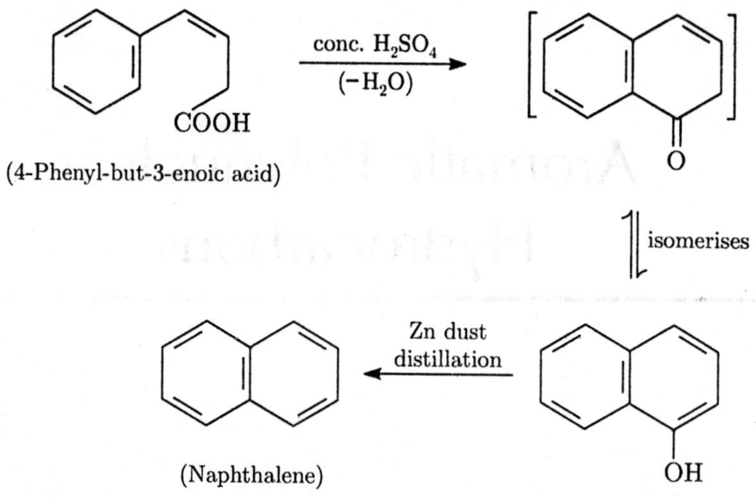

3. ***From benzaldehyde and ethyl succinate–Fitting and Erdmann Synthesis***

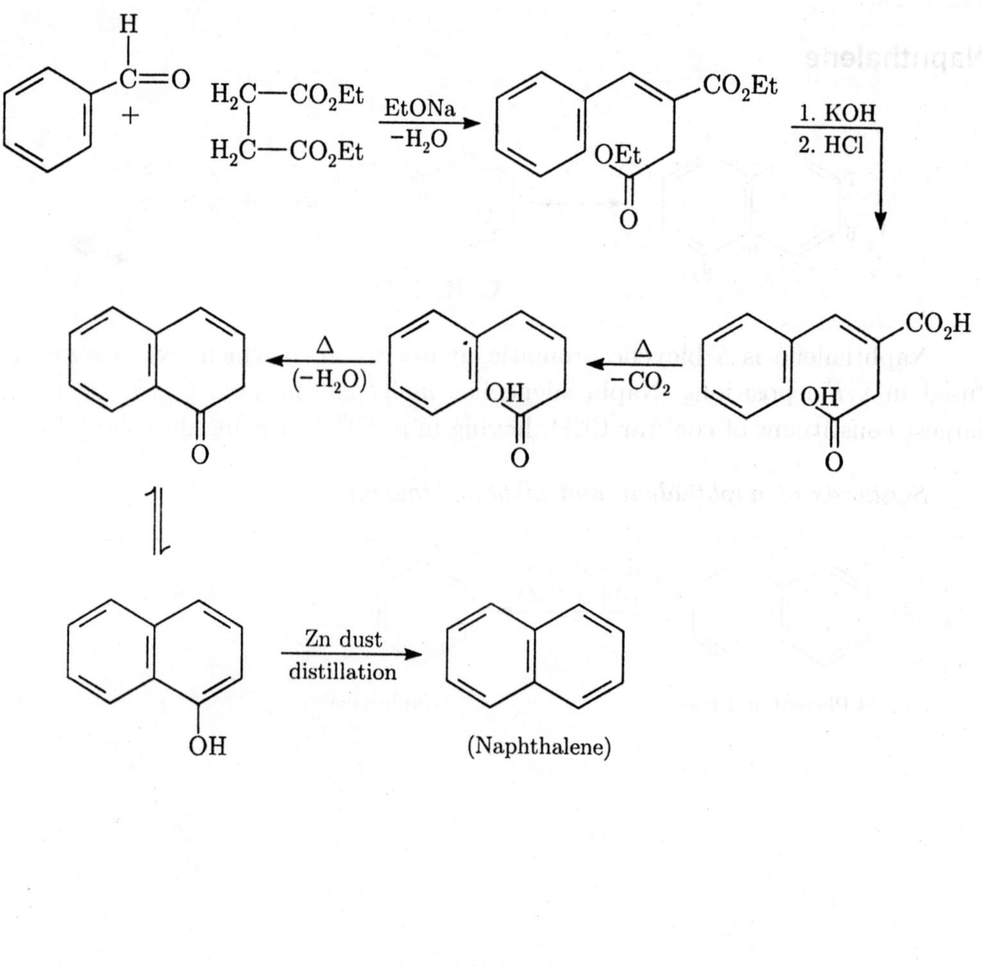

4. ***Synthesis from benzene and succinic anhydride–The Haworth Synthesis***

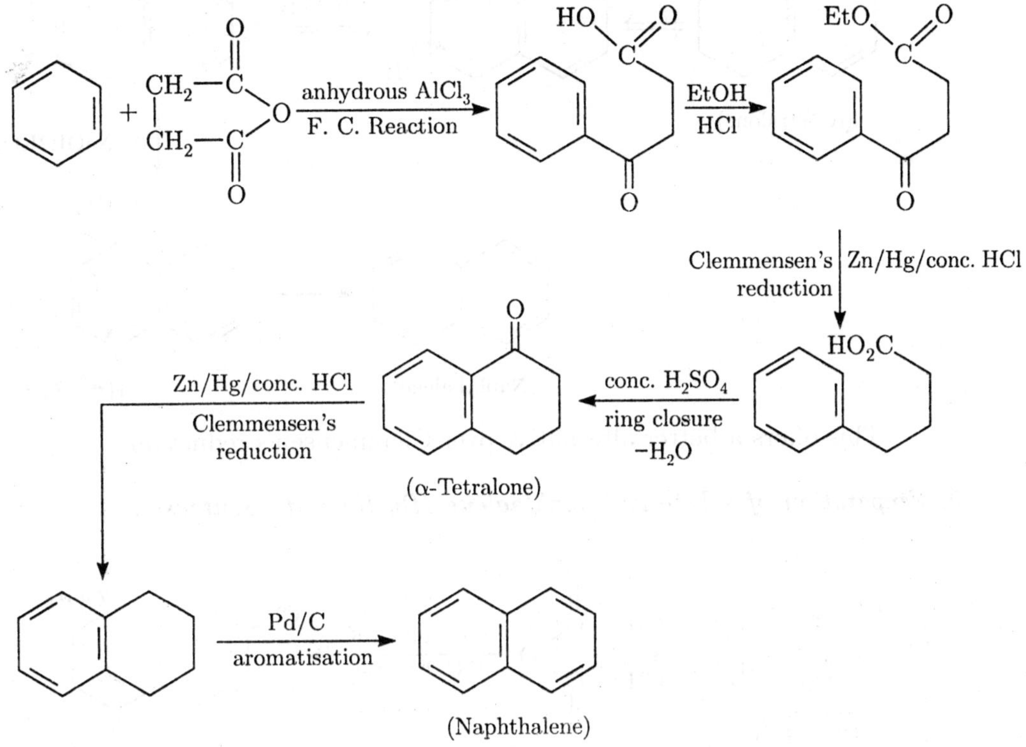

Two points are to be noted.

(a) Ring closure may be effected by Friedel-Crafts reaction also.

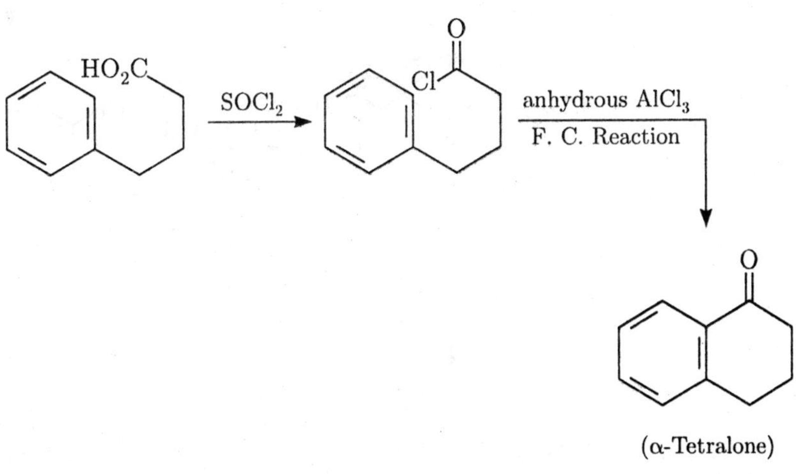

(b) Formation of cyclic ketones via *intramolecular acylation* can be effected by H_3PO_4, HF and especially by PPA (polyphosphoric acid) also. Anhydrous $SnCl_4$ can also be used in place of anhydrous, $AlCl_3$.

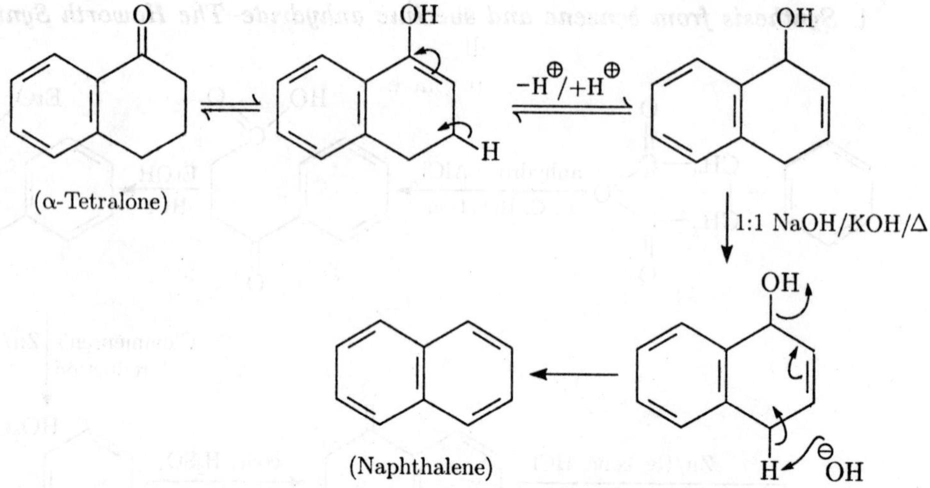

This offers a better alternative over Clemmensen's reduction.

5. ***Preparation of substituted naphthalene (By Haworth Synthesis)***

(a)

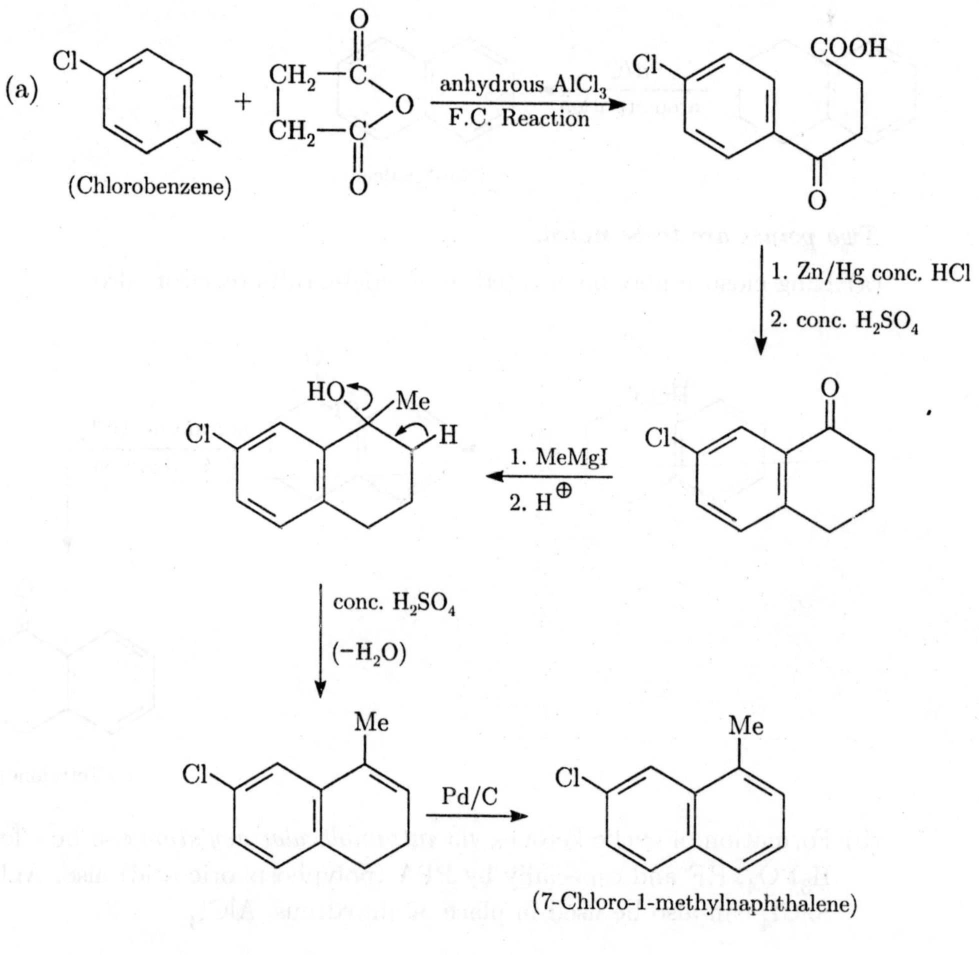

(b)

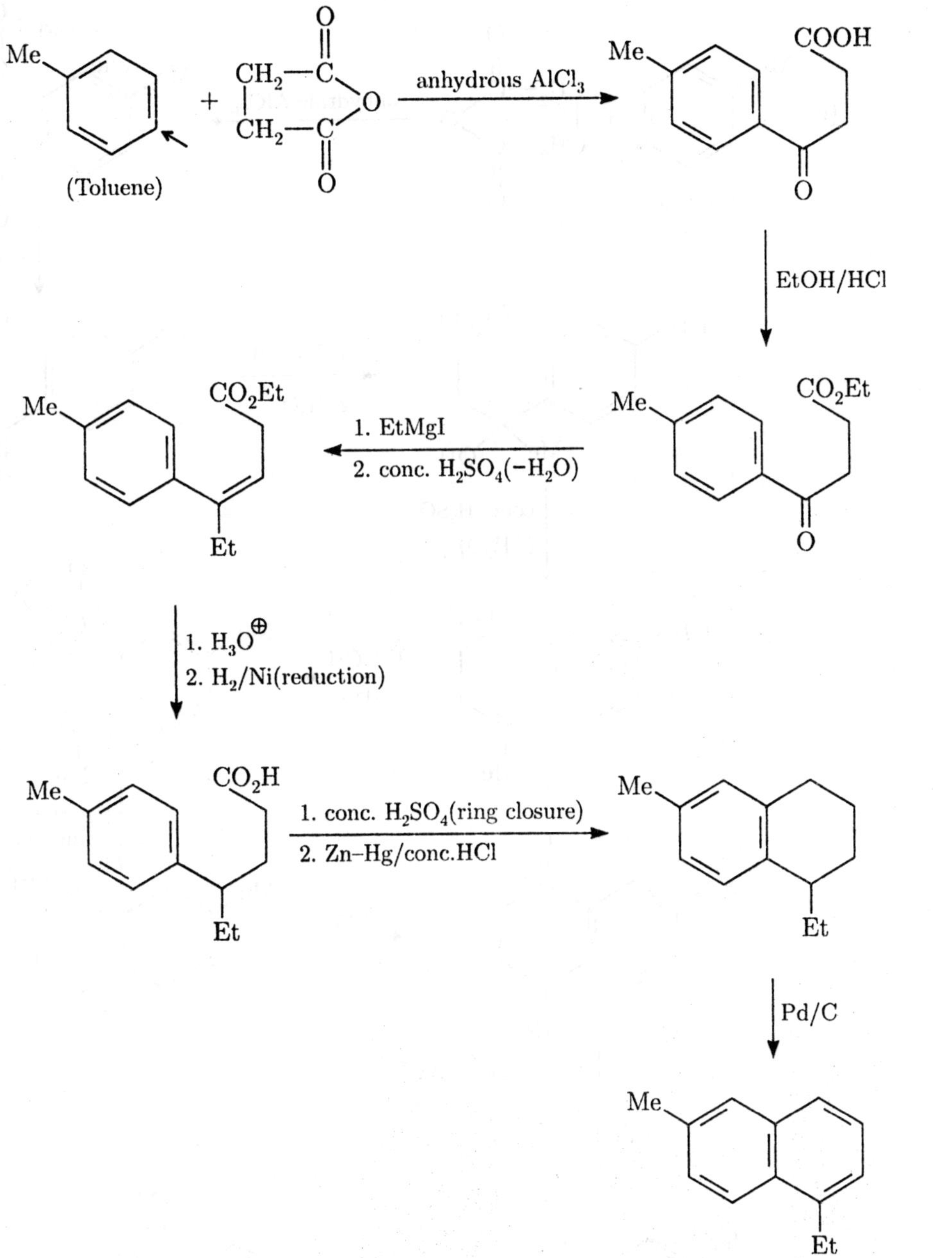

(4-Ethyl-7-methylnaphthalene)

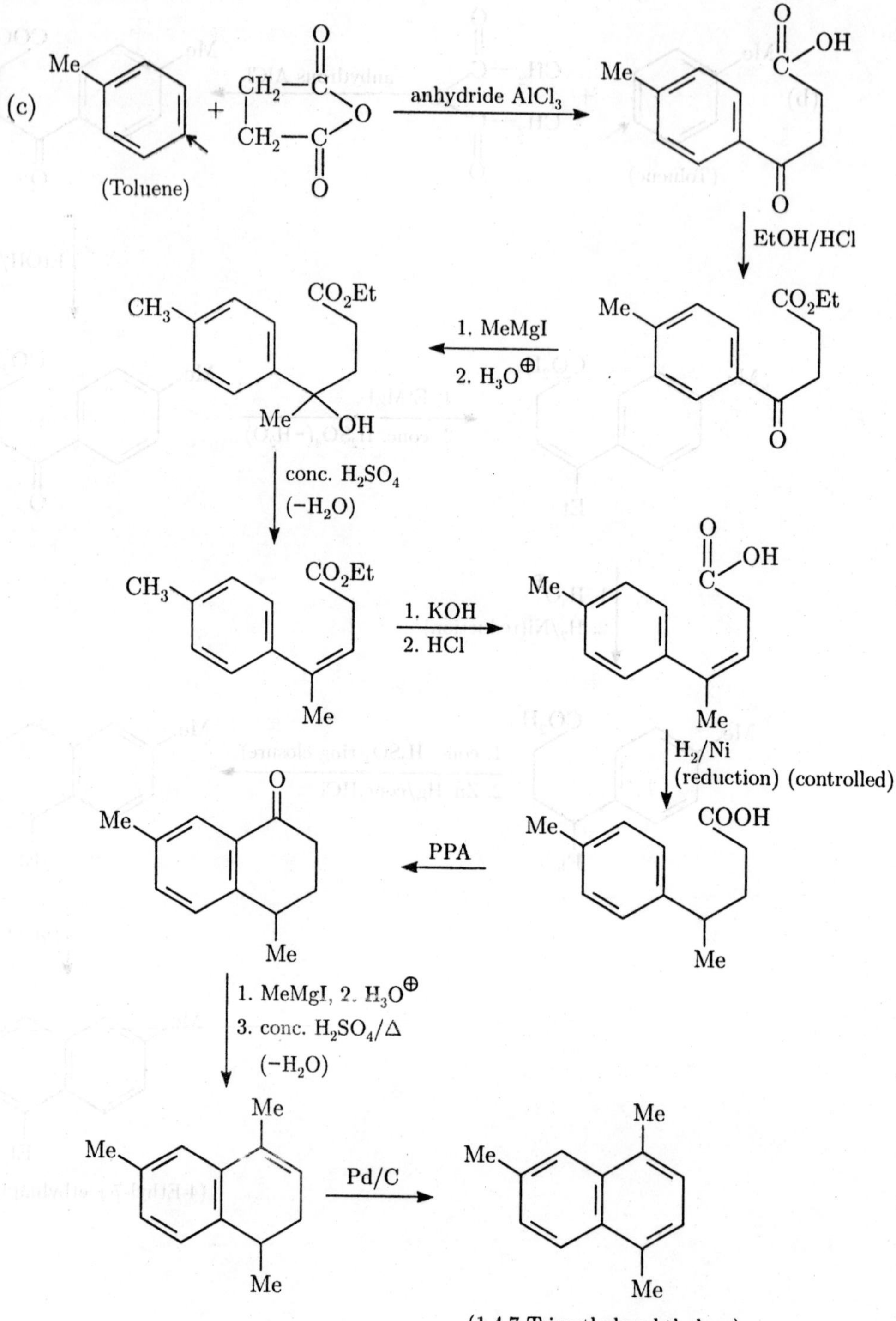

(1,4,7-Trimethylnaphthalene)

Methyl or any alkyl group may be introduced at the 1,4 and 7-positions by the proper choice of Grignard reagent and alkylbenzene.

Structure of Naphthalene

1. Analytical data and molecular weight determination suggest the molecular formula for naphthalene is $C_{10}H_8$.
2. Naphthalene resembles benzene in chemical reactions like nitration, sulphonation, halogenation etc. Its hydroxy derivatives resemble phenols. Naphthalene can not be oxidised by nitric acid or other mild oxidising agents. So Erlenmeyer proposed a symmetric structure of naphthalene as follows.

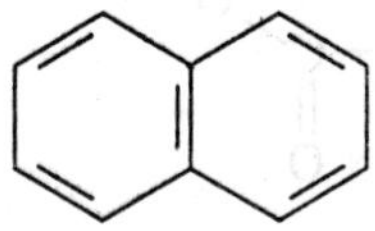

3. On oxidation, naphthalene gives *phthalic acid* which indicates naphthalene must contain

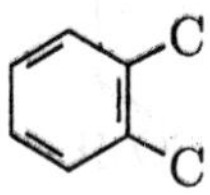
moiety, *i.e.*, a benzene ring with two side chains in *ortho* positions.

Naphthalene $\xrightarrow{\text{oxidation}}$ 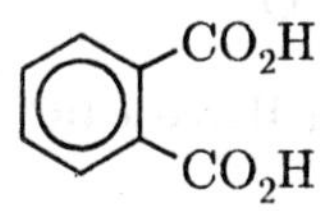 (phthalic acid), signifies that,

naphthalene is

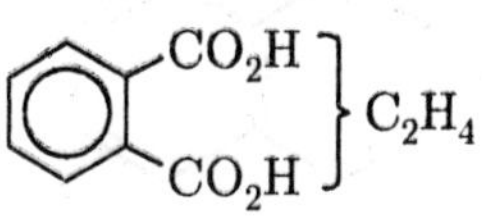

4. Next, a series of reactions are taken into consideration.

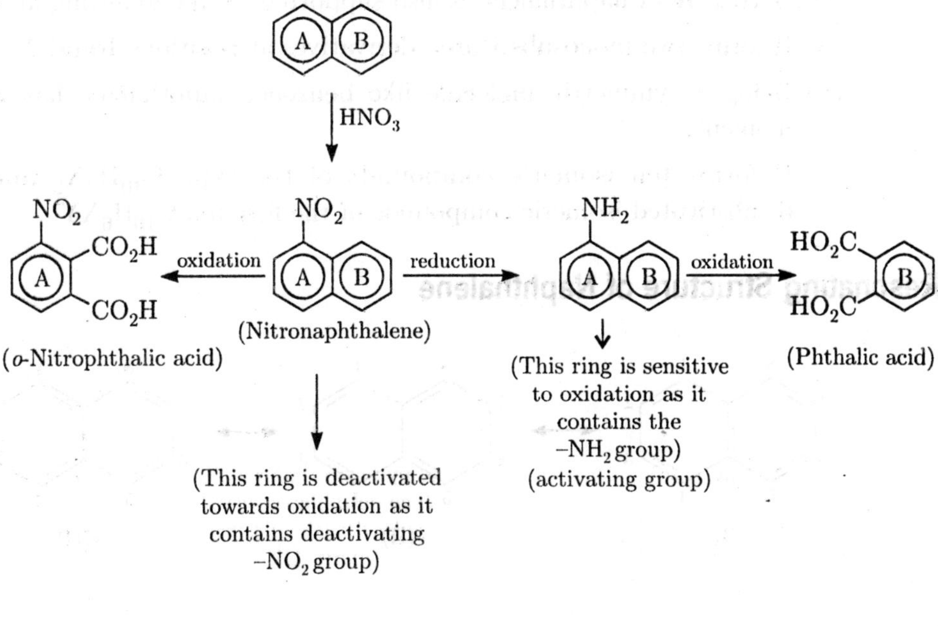

So, the inference is that, the benzene ring in phthalic acid obtained by oxidation of aminonaphthalene is not the same ring as that is obtained by oxidation of nitronaphthalene. So, naphthalene contains *two benzene rings.*

5. The bicyclic nature of naphthalene is further supported by its synthesis from benzene and succinic anhydride by Haworth's process.

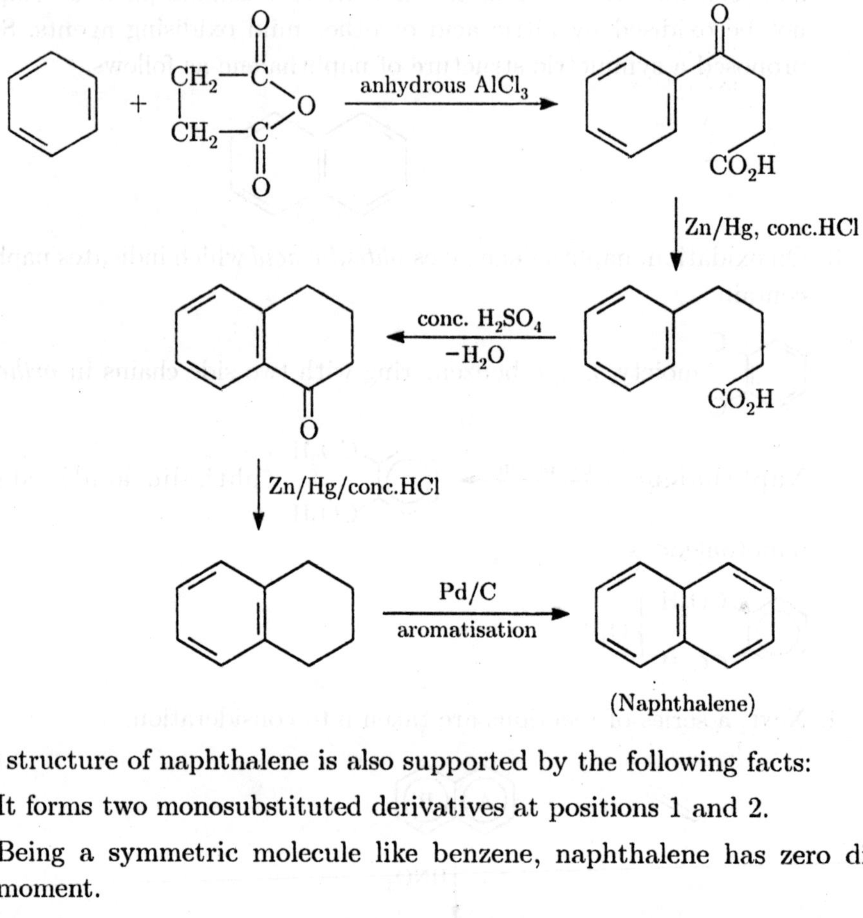

(Naphthalene)

6. The structure of naphthalene is also supported by the following facts:
   (a) It forms two monosubstituted derivatives at positions 1 and 2.
   (b) Being a symmetric molecule like benzene, naphthalene has zero dipole moment.
   (c) If forms ten isomeric compounds of the type $C_{10}H_6X_2$ and fourteen disubstituted isomeric compounds of the formula $C_{10}H_6XY$.

Resonating Structure of Naphthalene

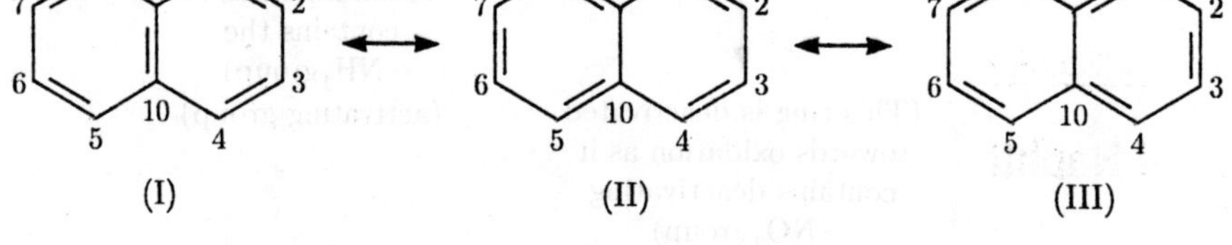

Naphthalene contains two benzene rings, so the resonance energy should be approximately equal to (2×150.6=301.2 kJ/mol), but the resonance energy of naphthalene actualy found is 255.2 kJ/mol. Hence naphthalene is *less aromatic than benzene and will be more reactive.*

From the resonating structures it is obvious that the C_1–C_2 bond length will be the average of two carbon-carbon double bond lengths and one carbon-carbon single bond length, while that of C_2–C_3 will be the average of two C–C single bond and one C–C double bond lengths. Thus, C_1–C_2 bond is shorther than C_2–C_3 bond length and thus the former has more double bond character than the latter. 2-Naphthol couples with benzenediazonium chloride at 1-position in alkaline medium where under the same condition, 1-substituted 2-naphthol fails to do so. This is due to the more double bond character of C_1–C_2 bond which makes the coupling possible.

Structure (I) is most contributory as it contains two benzenoid rings. Naphthalene is aromatic by Huckel's (4n + 2)π electron rule where n=2. All the ten bonding π electrons occuping five bonding molecular orbitals. Being aromatic, naphthalene is planar and symmetric (μ=o).

Chemical Properties of Naphthalene

1. ***Reduction*** :

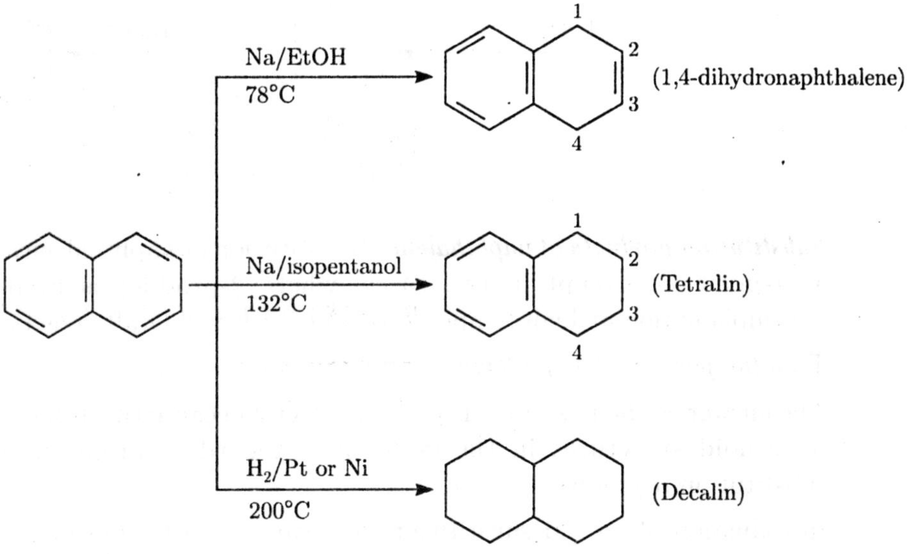

2. ***Oxidation*** :

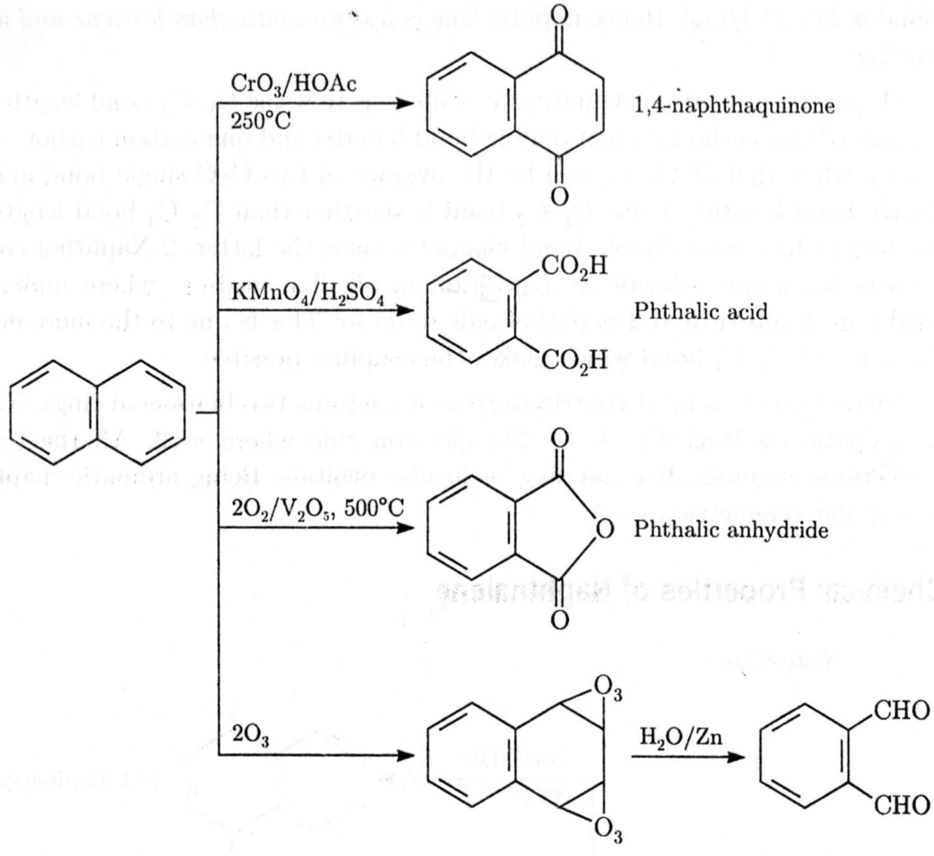

(Naphthalene diozonide) (Phthalaldehyde)

3. ***Substitution products of naphthalene*** : Substitution at naphthalene always occurs at 1-position, except in two cases, where 2-product is predominant — (a) sulphonation at high temperature and (b) Fridel-Crafts reaction.

Why the position 1 is preferred over position 2?

The answer is, the position 1 is preferred over 2 because the former retains more benzenoid structures in the σ-complex, regarding aromatic electrophilic substitution reactions.

Introduction of second substituent can give rise to homonuclear substitution (within the same ring) or heteronuclear substitution (in the other ring).

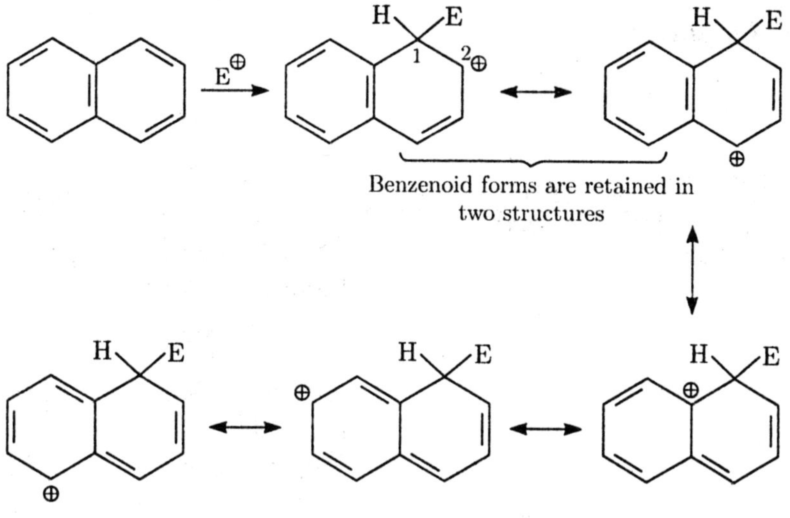

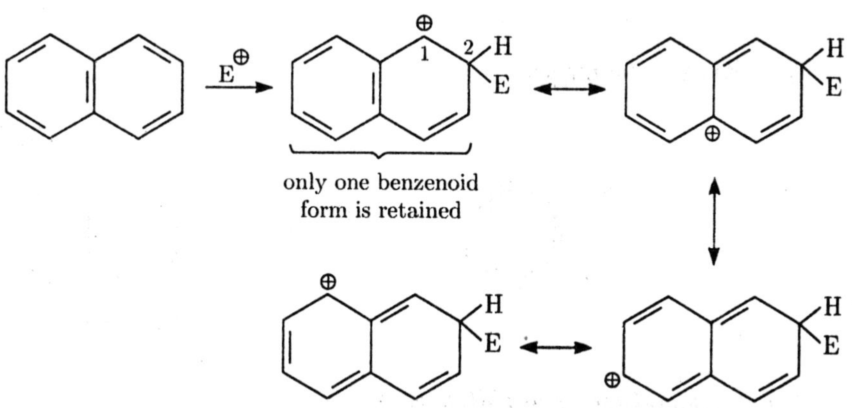

(a) When Cl, Br, OH, CH_3, NHR or $NHCOCH_3$ are present in position 1, homonuclear substitution occurs at position 4 predominantly and to a lesser extent at position 2.

(b) Presence of OH, CH_3, NHR, $NHCOCH_3$ at position 2, homonuclear substitution occurs at position 1. All these groups are *o*/*p* orientating.

(c) When $-NO_2$ or $-SO_3H$ are present at positions 1/2, heteronuclear substitution occurs at positions 5 or 8. When halogen or $-NH_2$ is present at position 2, heteronuclear substitution occurs at positions 5 or 8.

4. (a) ***Nitration*** :

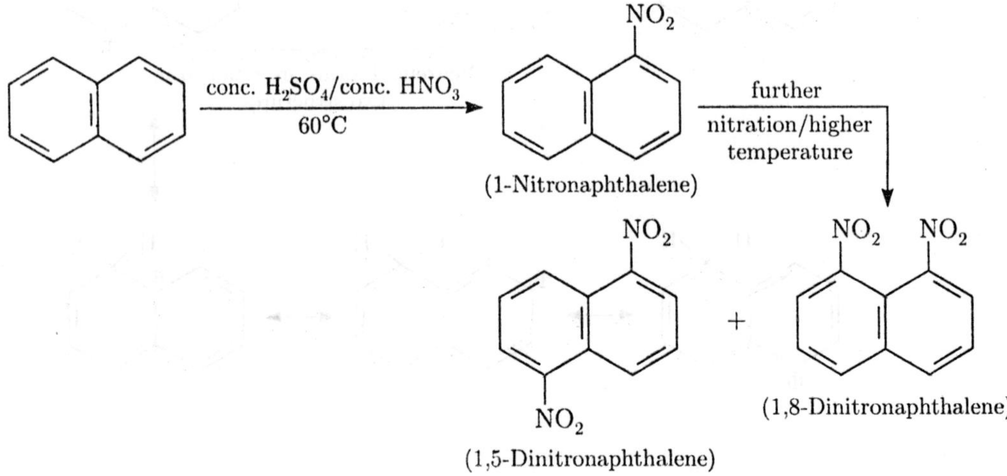

(1-Nitronaphthalene)

(1,5-Dinitronaphthalene)

(1,8-Dinitronaphthalene)

(b) ***Chloromethylation*** :

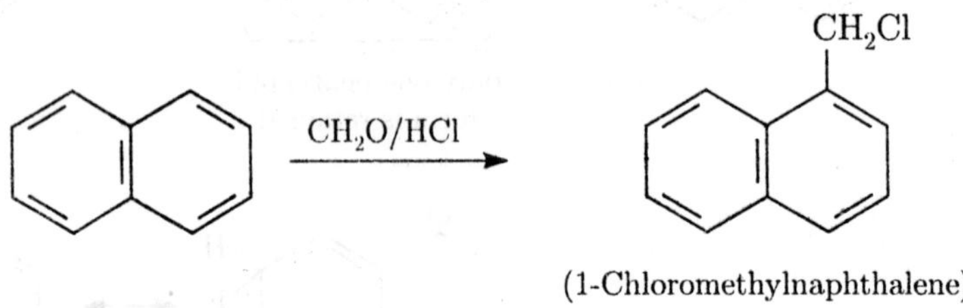

(1-Chloromethylnaphthalene)

(c) ***Sulphonation of naphthalene*** :

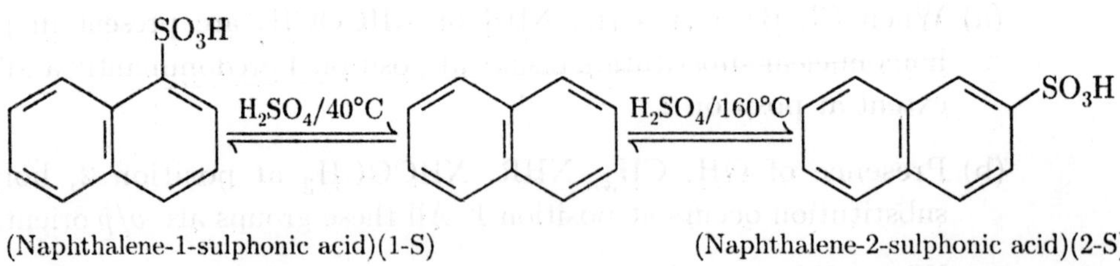

(Naphthalene-1-sulphonic acid)(1-S)

(Naphthalene-2-sulphonic acid)(2-S)

When heated with conc. H_2SO_4, 1-acid (1-S) is converted to 2-acid (2–S). Thus, 1-acid is kinetically controlled and 2-acid is thermodynamically controlled product. The reason for greater stability of 2-acid may be due to a steric repulsion between $-SO_3H$ group and hydrogen at 8 position in 1-acid.

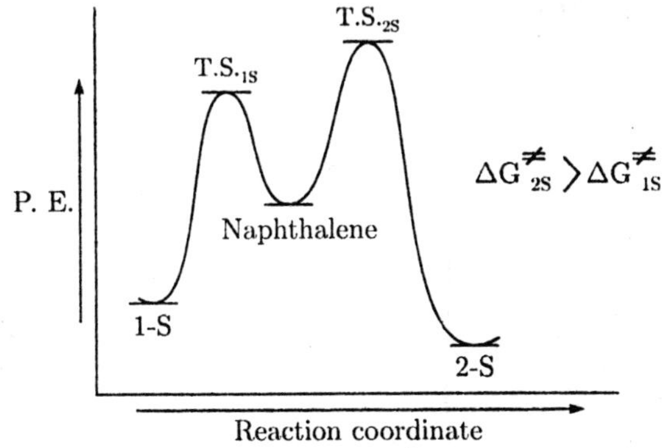

Fig. 4.1 :

(d) ***The Friedel-Craft Reaction*** :

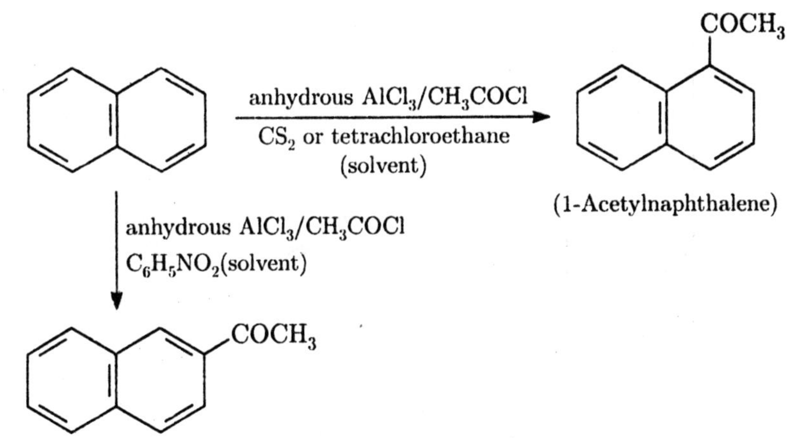

(1-Acetylnaphthalene)

(2-Acetylnaphthalene)

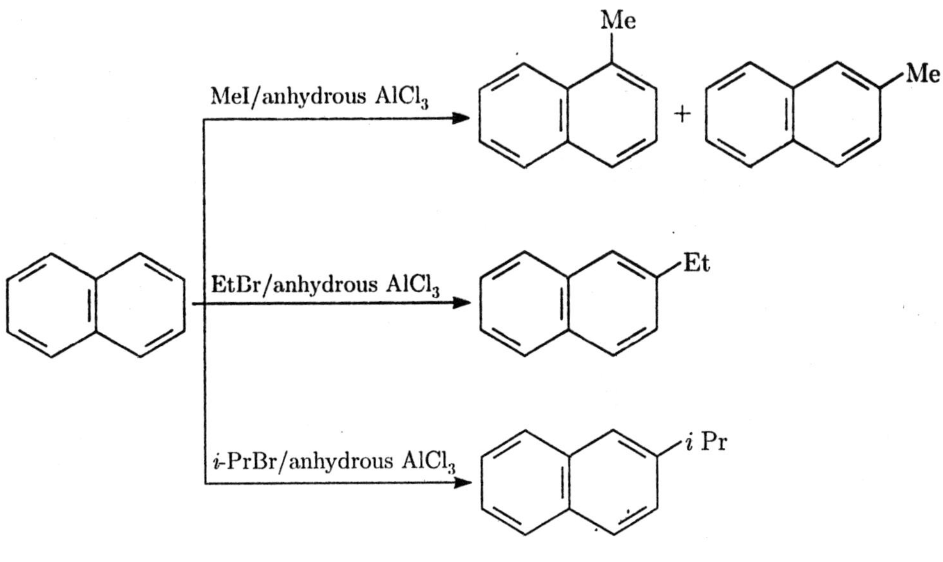

(e) ***Halogenation*** :

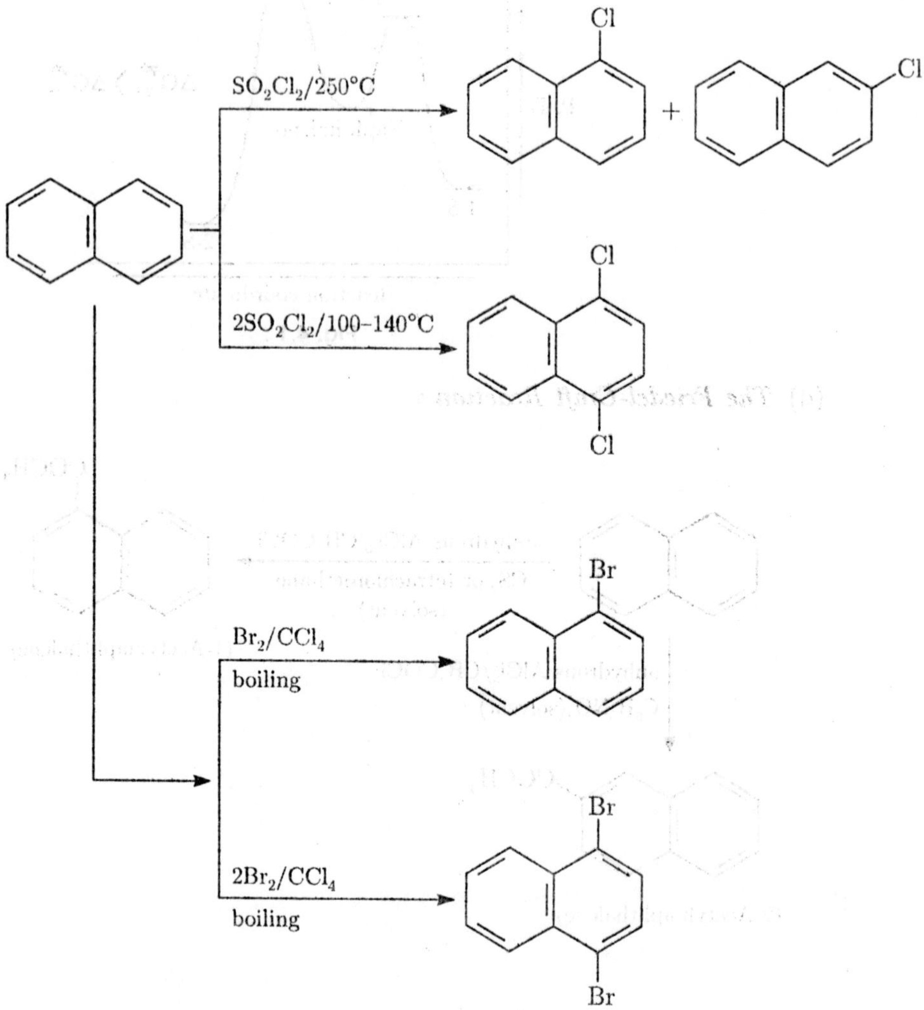

(f)

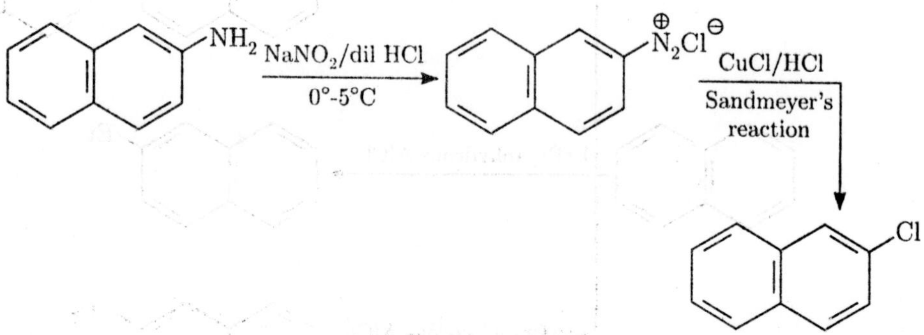

Mechanism of the reaction (Chlorination of naphthalene by SO_2Cl_2) :

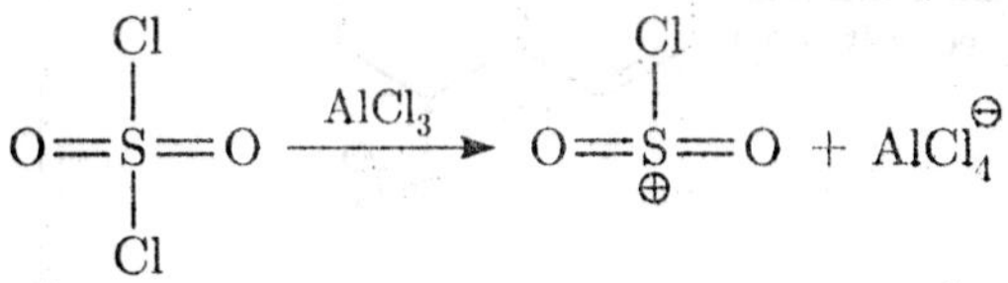

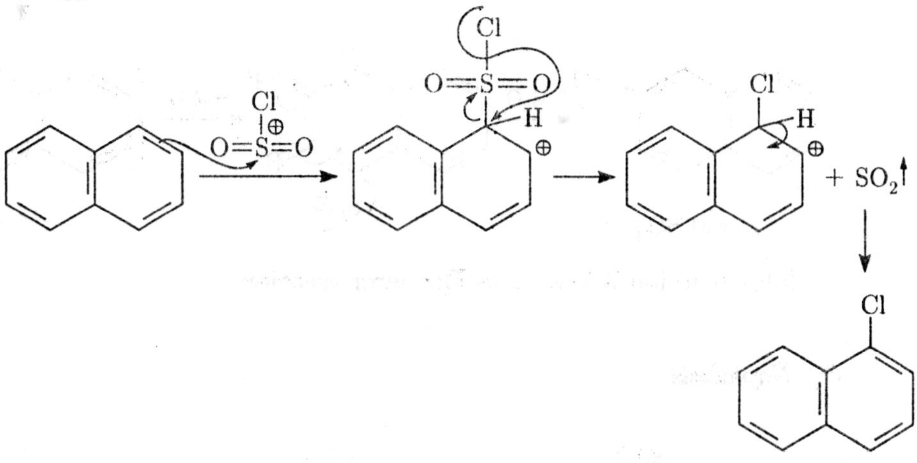

(1-chloronaphthalene)

5. ***Preparation of naphthalene derivatives***

(a) ***Naphthylamines :***

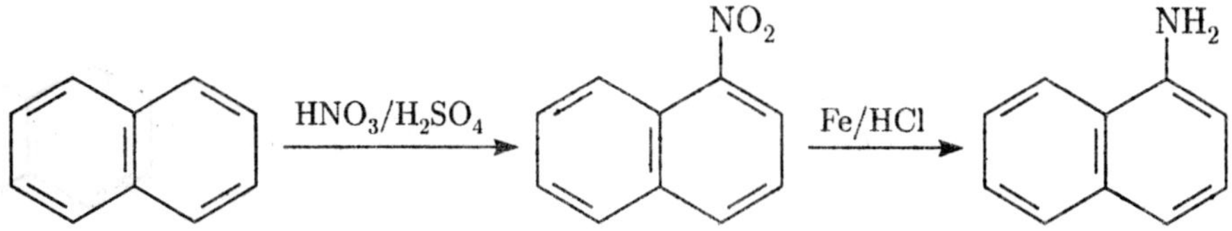

(1-Naphthylamine)

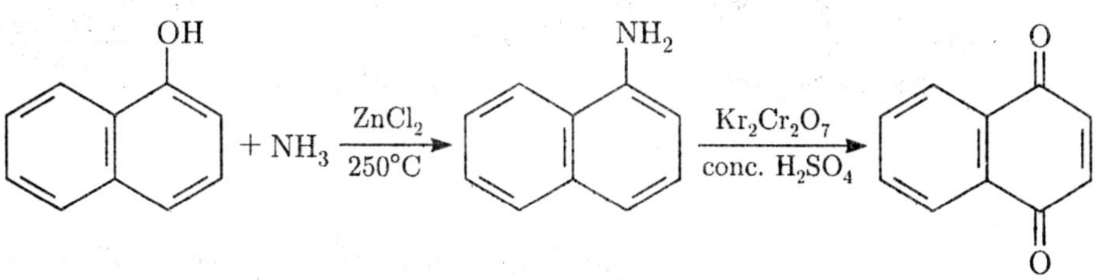

(Naphthaquinone)

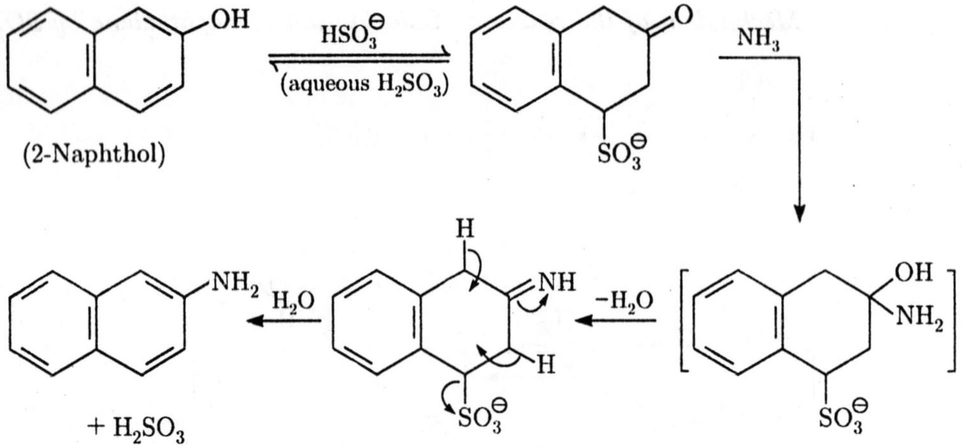

This reaction is known as **Bucherer reaction**

(b) ***Naphthols*** :

(i) 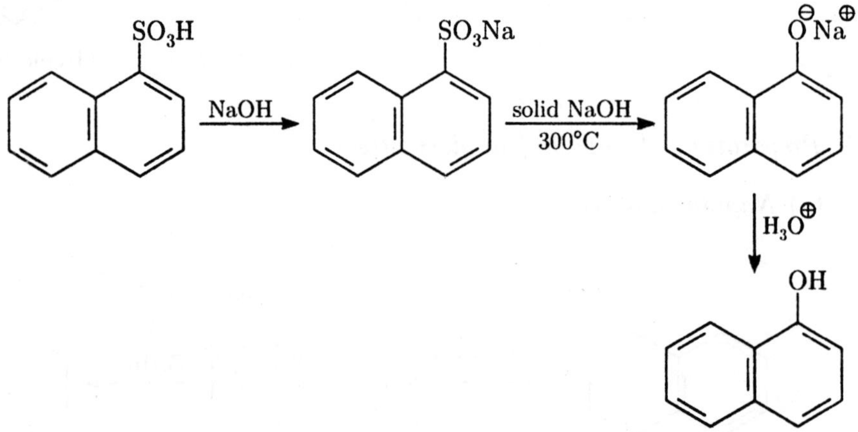

(1-Naphthol)

(ii) 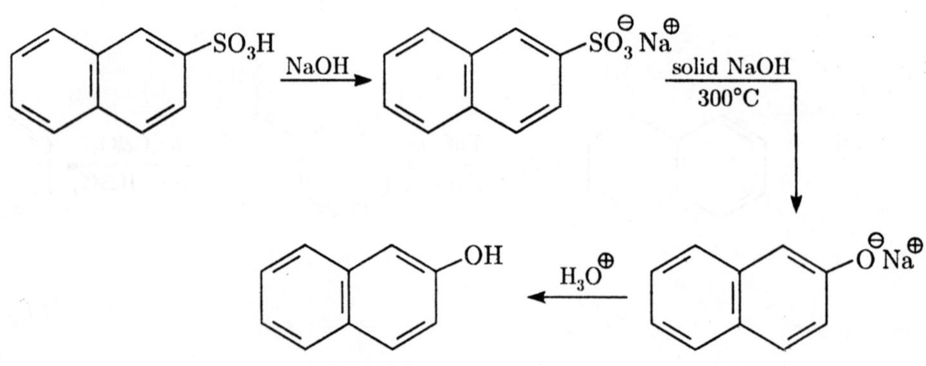

(2-Naphthol)

(iii) 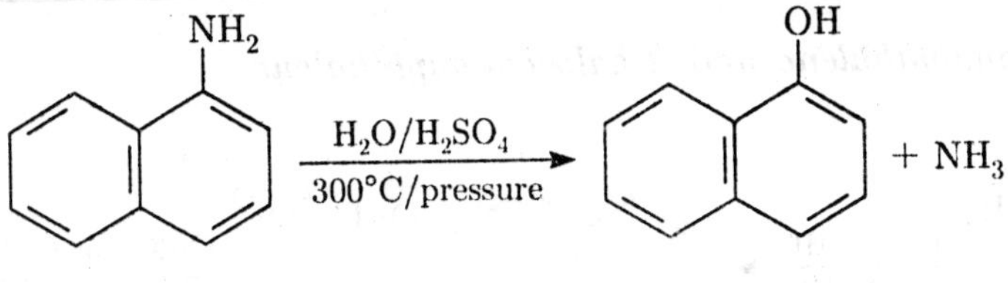

(iv) 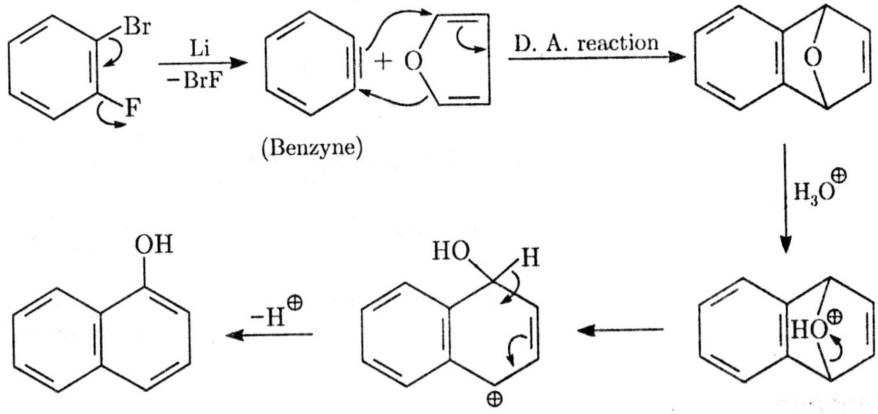

(Benzyne)

(1-Naphthol)

(c) ***Naphthoic acids*** :

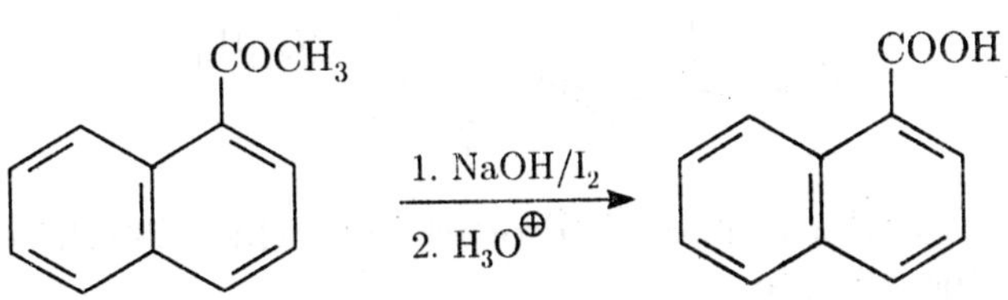

(1-Naphthoic acid)

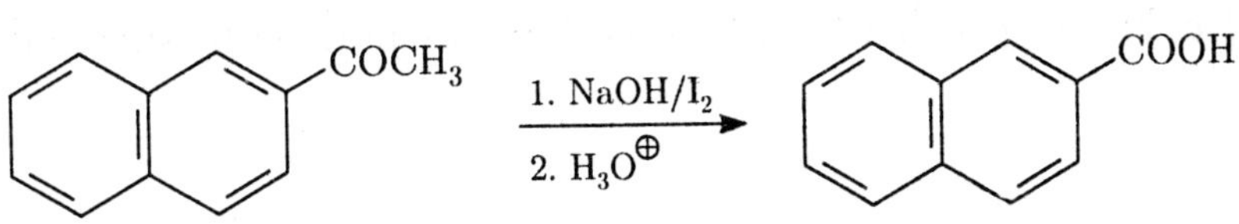

(2-Naphthoic acid)

(d) 2-*Cyanonaphthalene* and 2-*halogenonaphthalene*

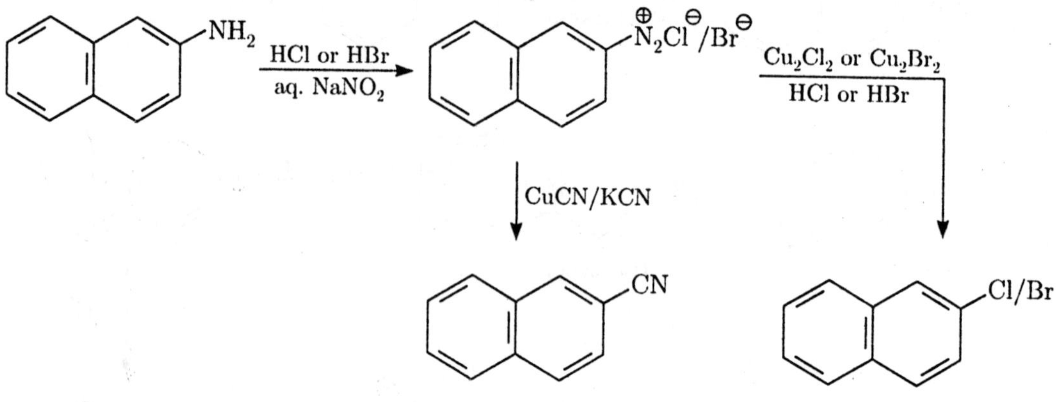

(2-Cyanonaphthalene)

(2-Chloro- or 2-bromonaphthalene)

Anthracene

The structure of anthracene is as follows:

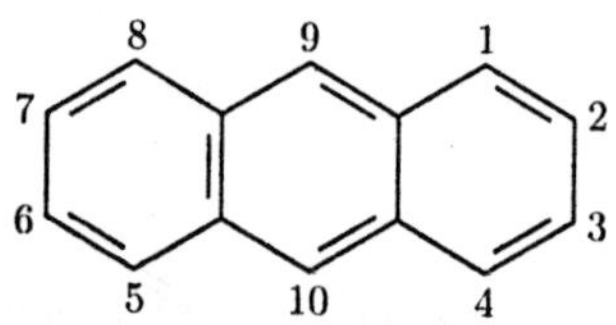

($C_{14}H_{10}$)

Anthracene is a tricyclic aromatic hydrocarbon in which the three benzene rings are fused together in a linear manner.

Anthracene is obtained from anthracene oil fraction of coal tar by cooling the latter and pressing the solid (which crystallises out) free from liquid. Crude anthracene contains phenanthrene and carbazole. This is powdered, washed with solvent naphtha which dissolves anthracene. Then anthracene is finally purified by sublimation.

Synthesis of Anthracene

1. 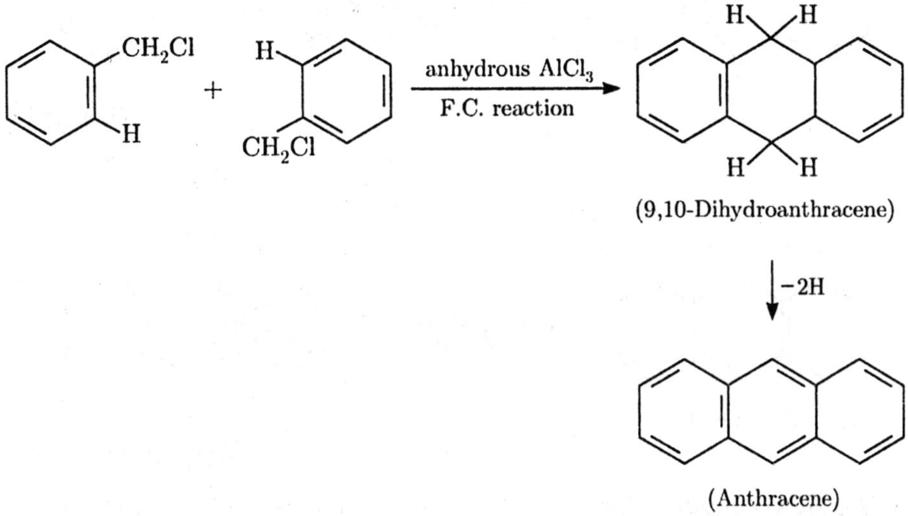

2. 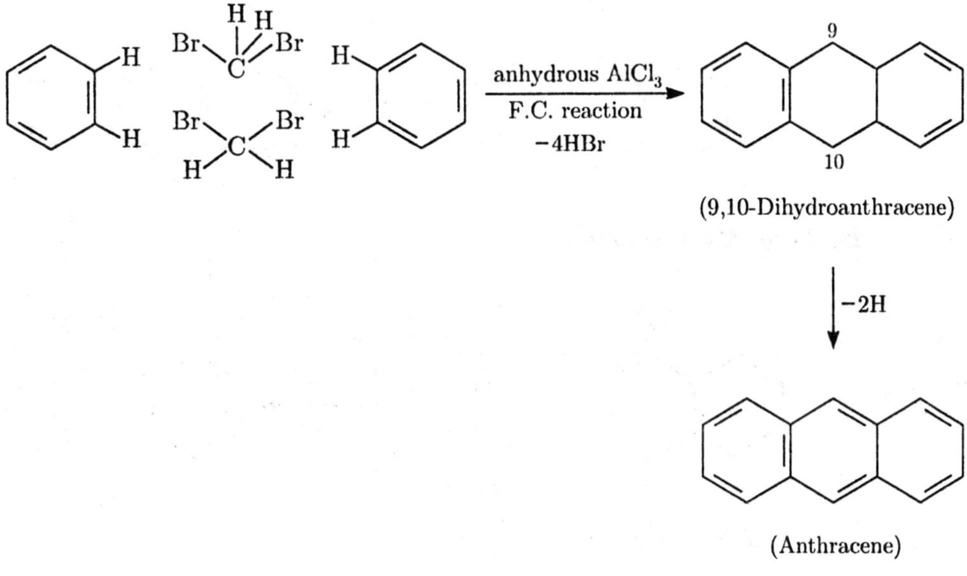

3. 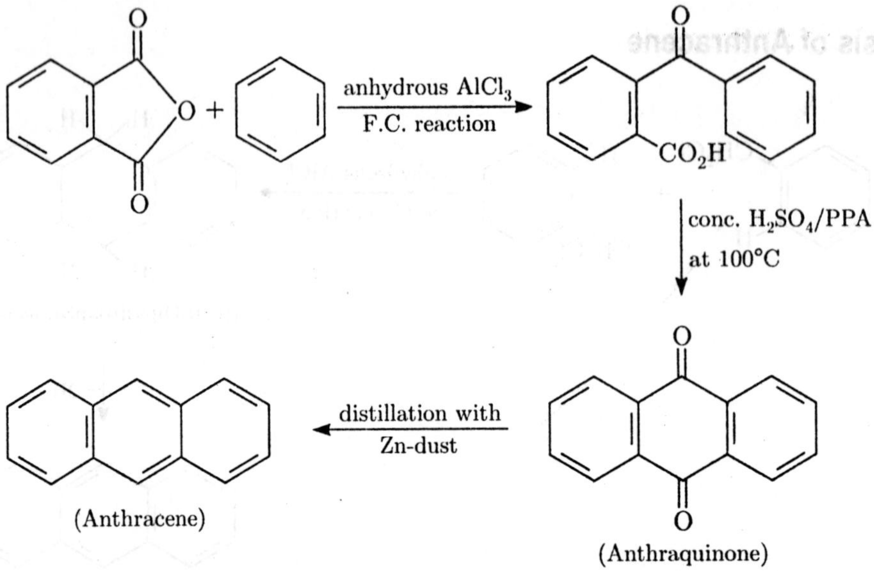

4. ***By Elbs reaction*** : Pyrolysis of a diaryl ketone containing a methyl or methylene group *ortho* to the carbonyl group.

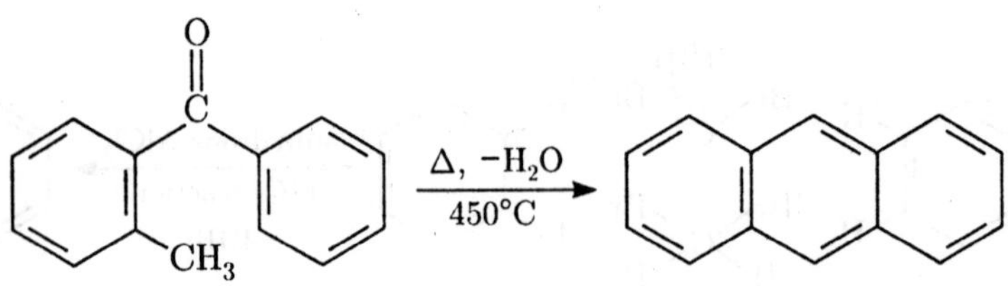

5. ***By Diels-Alder reaction*** :

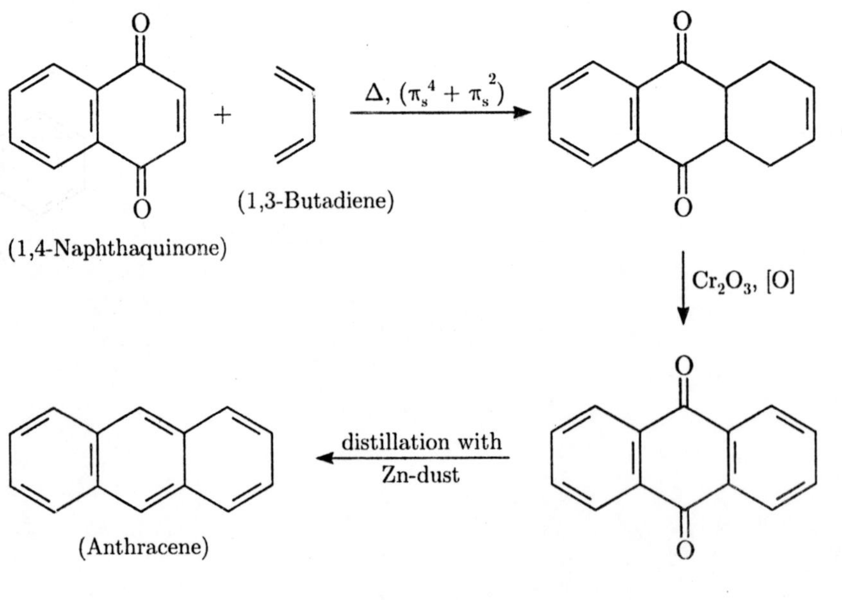

6. ***By Fittig reaction*** :

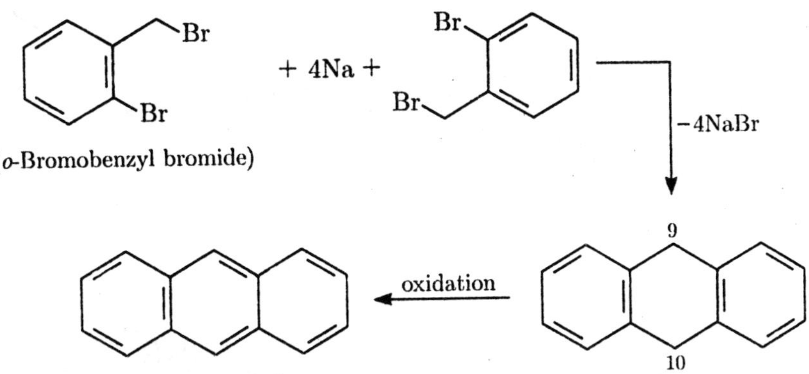

(o-Bromobenzyl bromide)

(Anthracene)

(9,10-Dihydroanthracene)

Chemical Reactions of Anthracene

Anthracene (m.p. 216°C) is very reactive at 9,10 positions. Electrophilic substitutions to form σ-complexes at 1- or 2- positions leave a "naphthalene fragment" whereas σ-complex at position 9 leaves two separate benzene rings intact, the latter being more stable. For polynuclear hydrocarbons the σ-complex that contains largest number of isolated benzene rings will be more stable. The resonance energy of two benzene rings is (150×2=300 kJ/mol), whereas the resonance energy of napthalene is 250 kJ/mol.

1. ***Reduction***

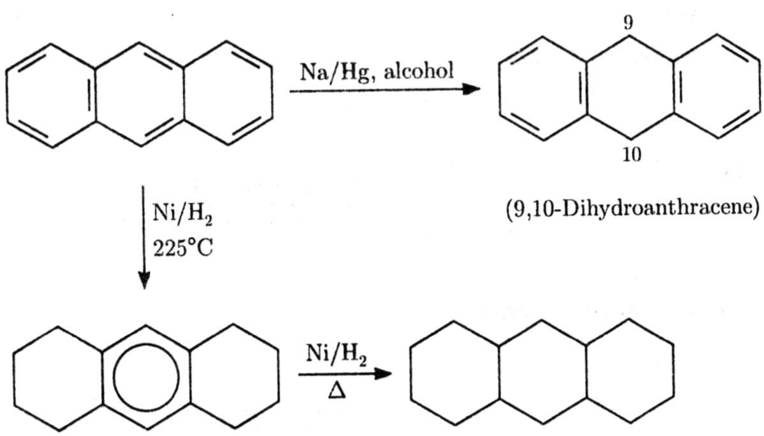

(9,10-Dihydroanthracene)

(1,2,3,4,5,6,7,8-Octahydroanthracene)

2. ***Oxidation*** :

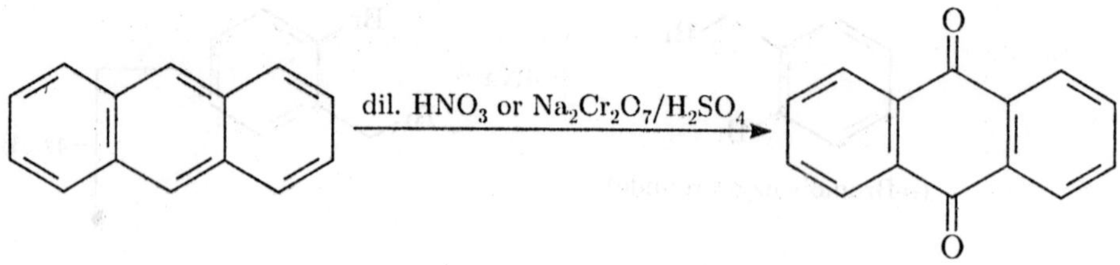

(Anthraquinone)

3. 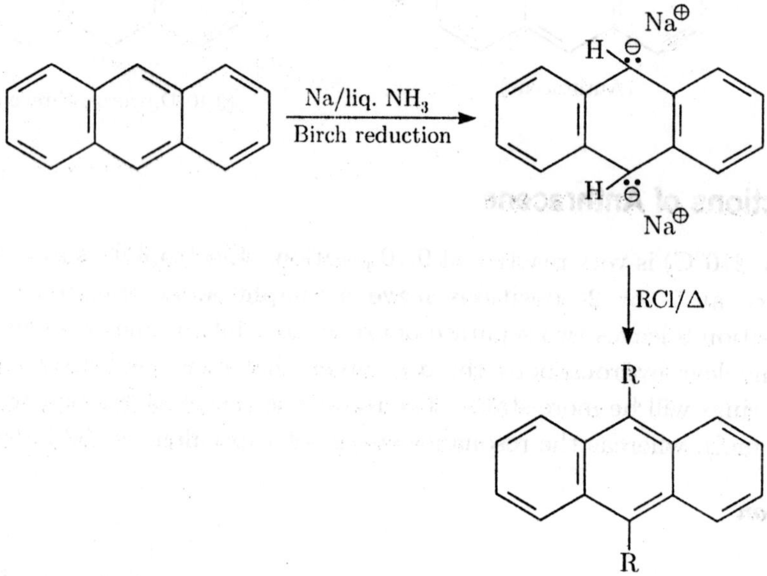

4. ***Fiedel-Crafts acylation*** :

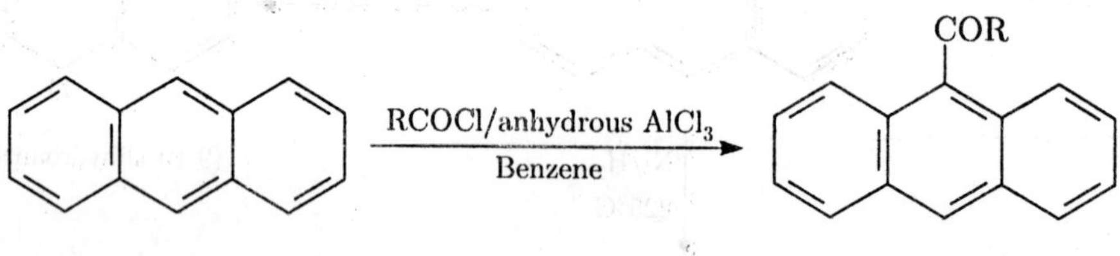

5. ***Formylation reaction*** :

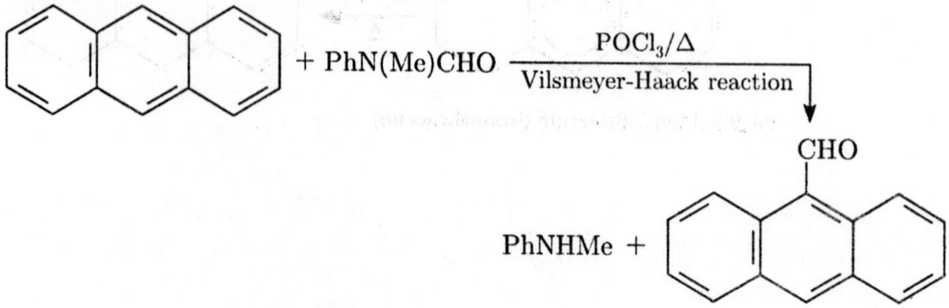

6. ***Nitration*** :

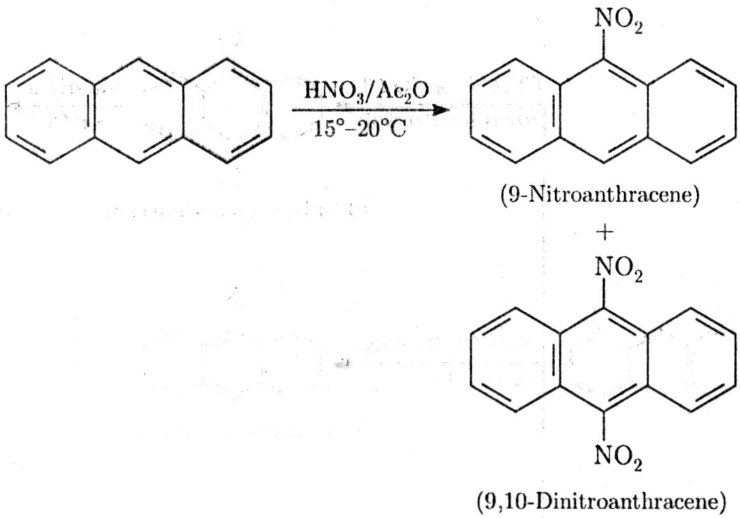

7. ***Sulphonation*** :

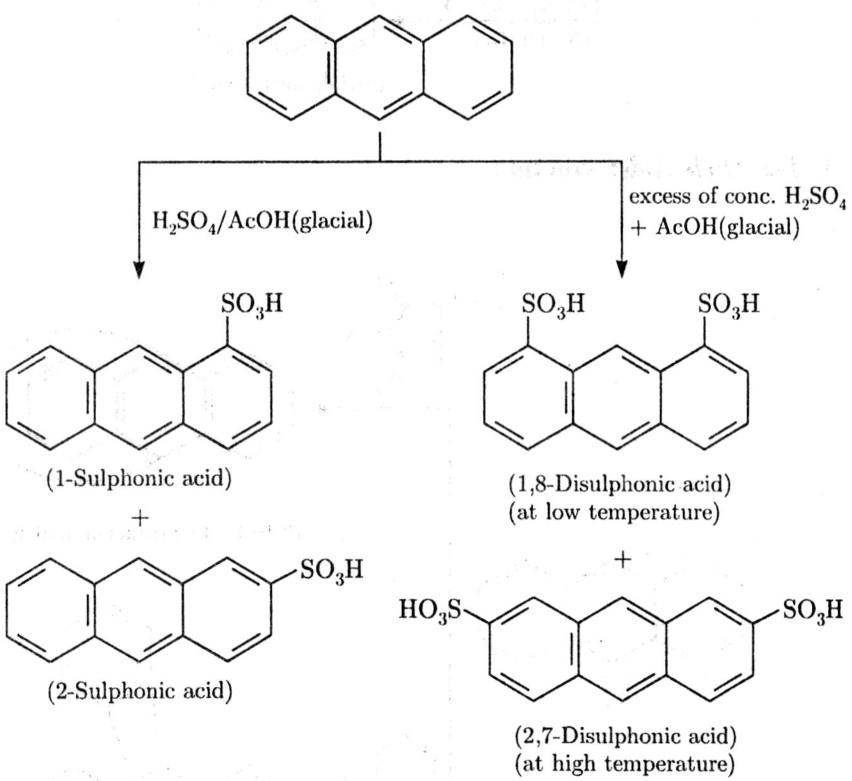

2-Sulphonic acid is favoured at high temperature, but 1-sulphonic acid shows no tendency to get rearranged to 2-sulphonic acid at high temperature in contrast to naphthalene system.

8. ***Halogenation*** :

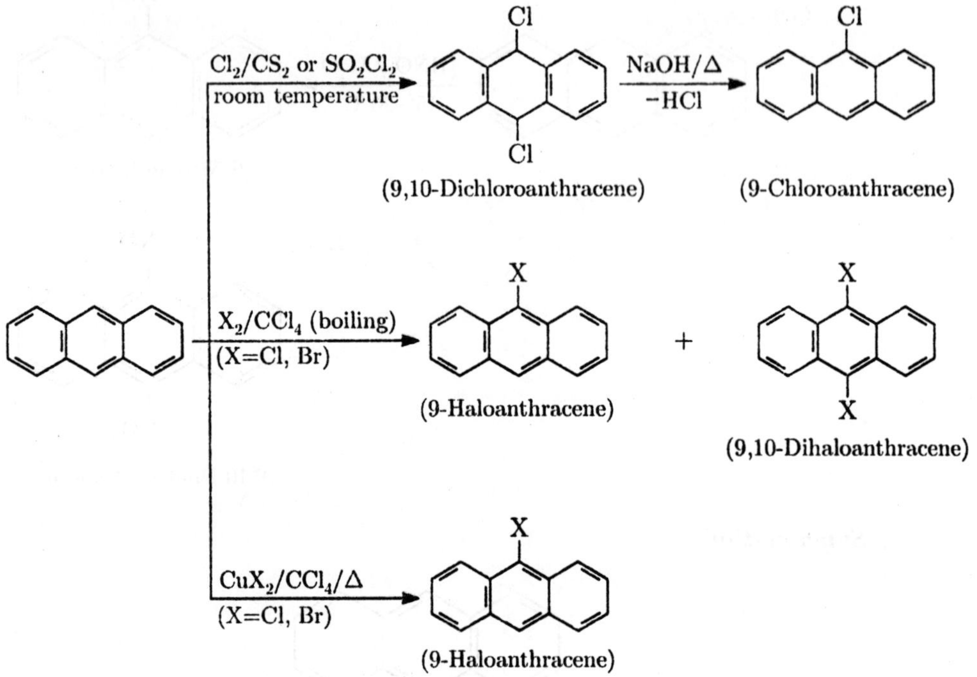

9. ***The Diels-Alder reaction*** :

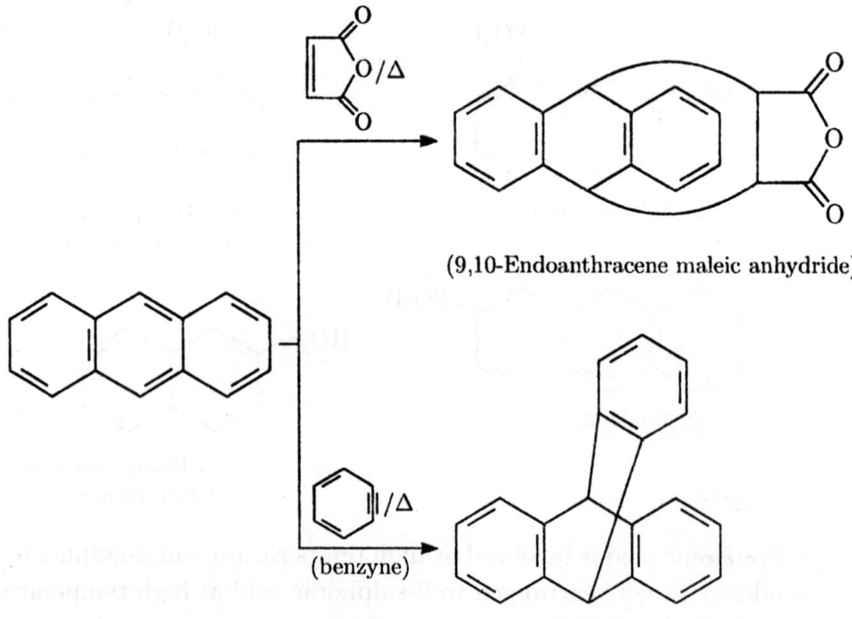

Mechanism of electrophilic substitution reactions in anthracene

1.

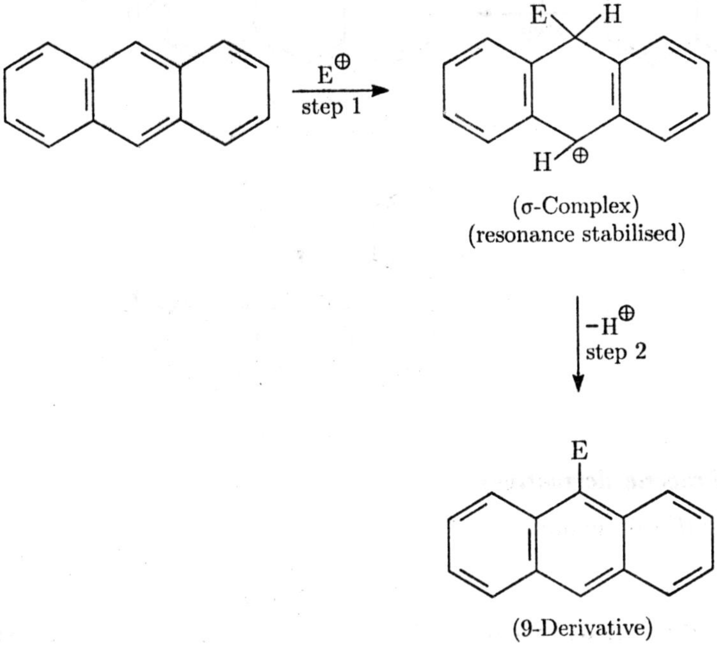

2.

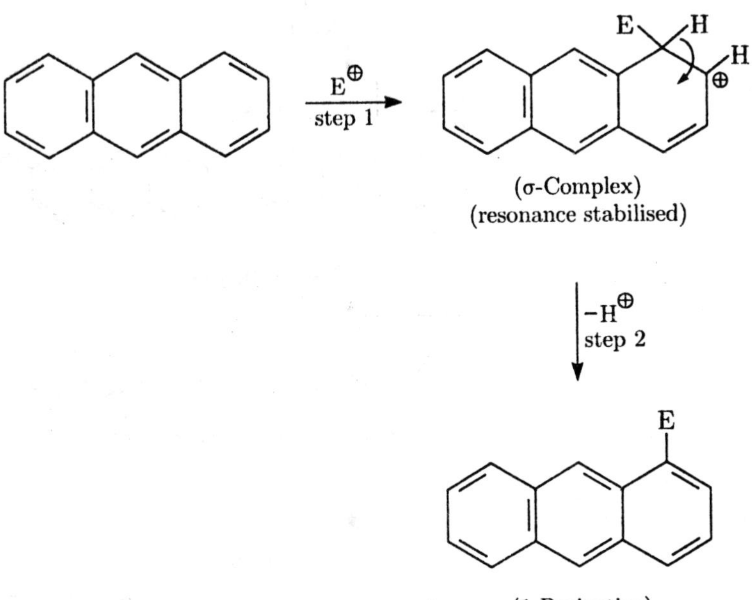

3. 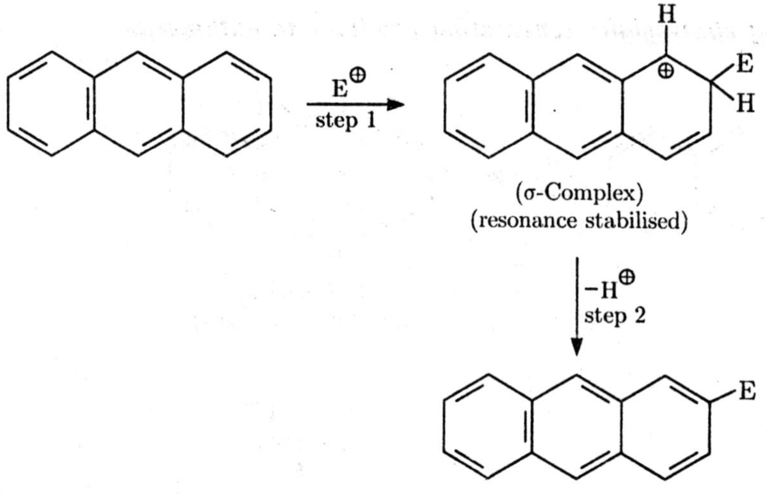

(2-Derivative)

Synthesis of anthracene derivatives

1. *Synthesis of anthroic acids*

(a) 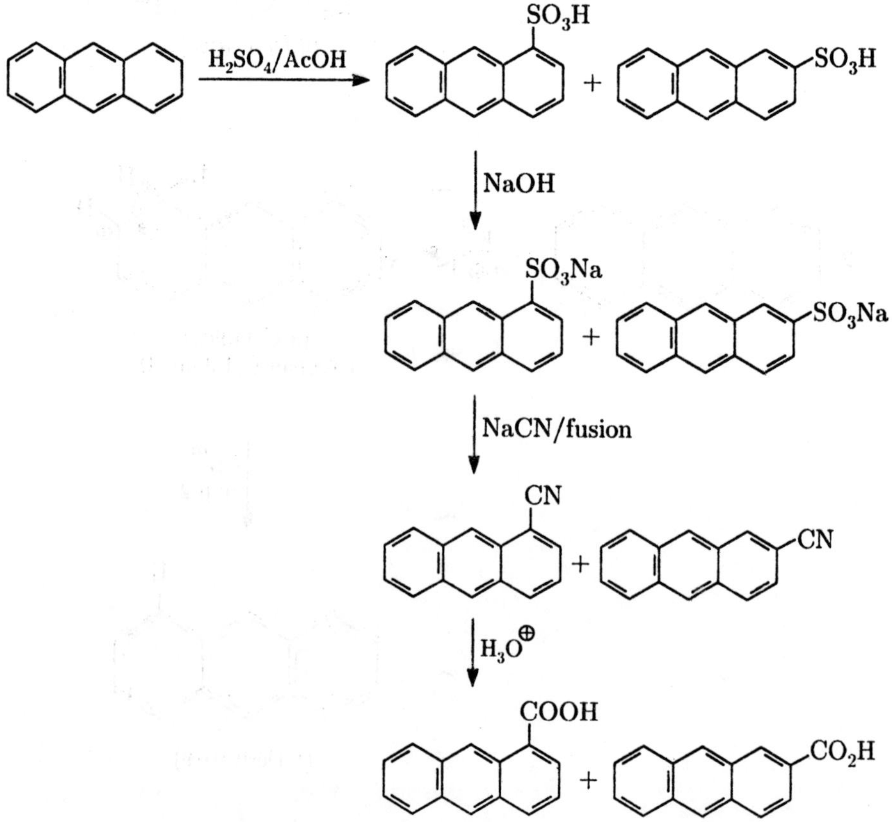

(1-Anthroic acid) (2-Anthroic acid)

(b)

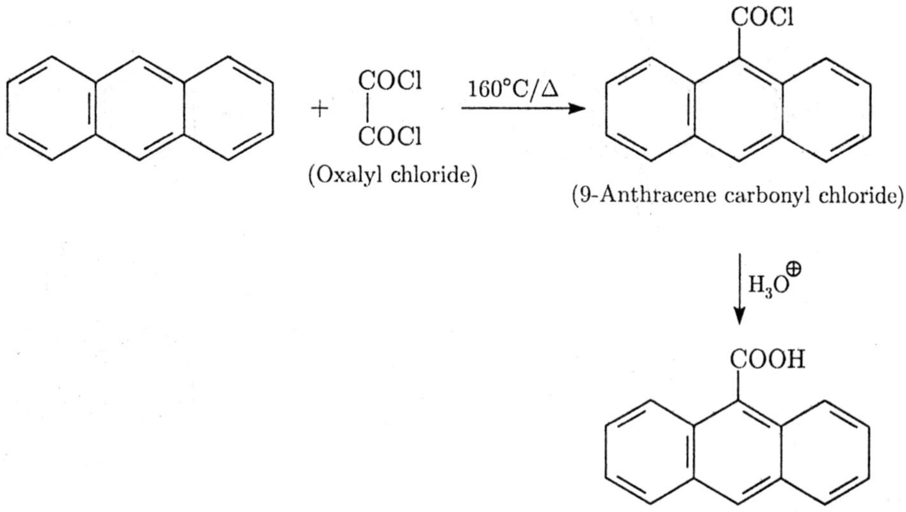

(Oxalyl chloride)

(9-Anthracene carbonyl chloride)

(9-Anthroic acid)

2. *Synthesis of hydroxyanthracenes (anthrols)*

(a)

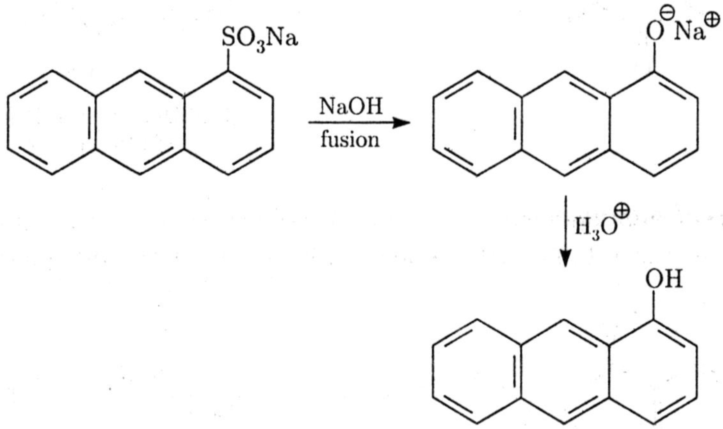

(1-Anthrol)

(b)

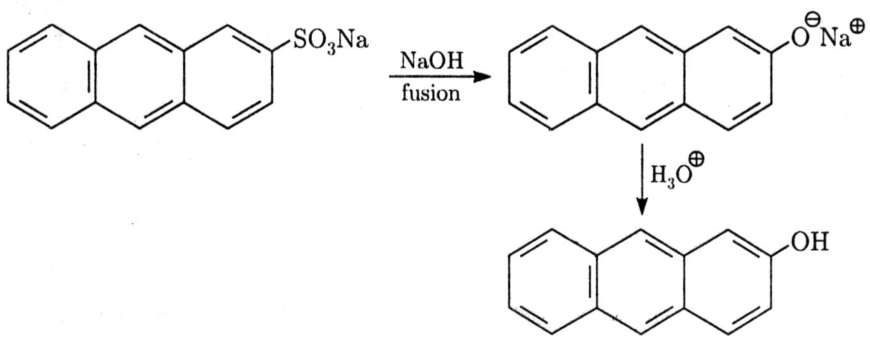

(2-Anthrol)

(c)

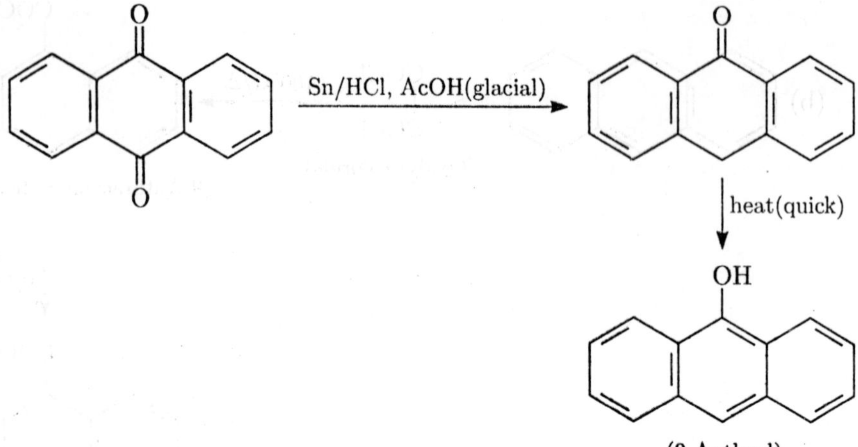

(9-Anthrol)

(d)

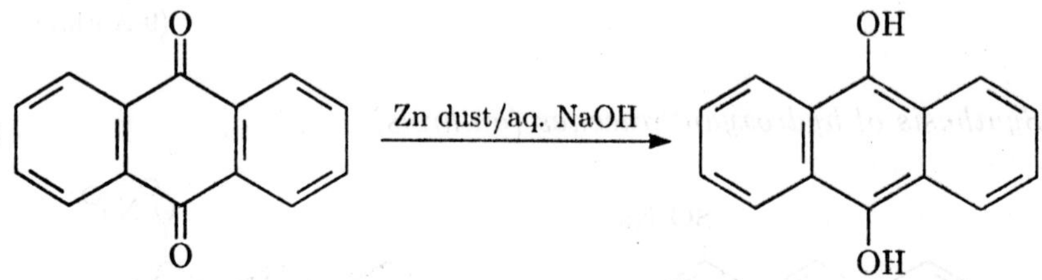

(9,10-Dihydroxyanthracene)
(Anthraquinol)

3. ***Synthesis of anthraquinone*** : Out of nine possible isomeric forms of anthraquinone, only three- 1,2; 1,4 and 9,10 are known, 9,10 being the most important.

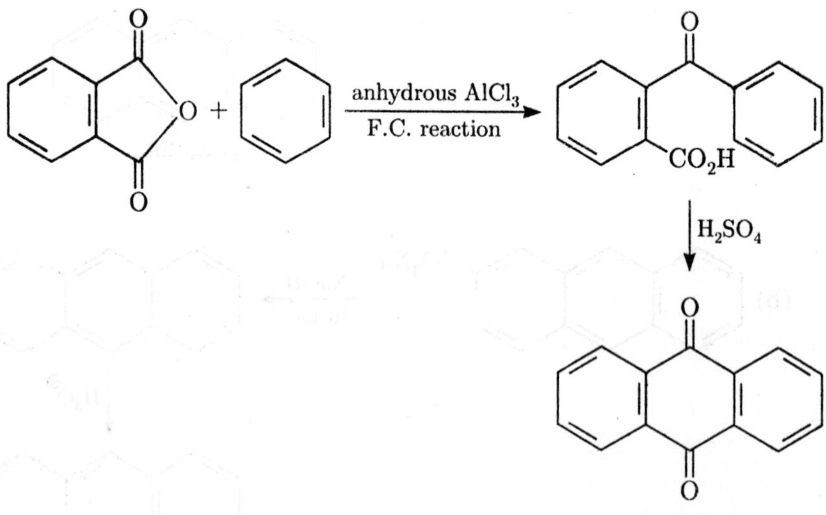

(9,10-Anthraquinone)

Anthraquinone resembles little with *p*-benzoquinone.

4. ***Preparation of Alizarin (a dye)***

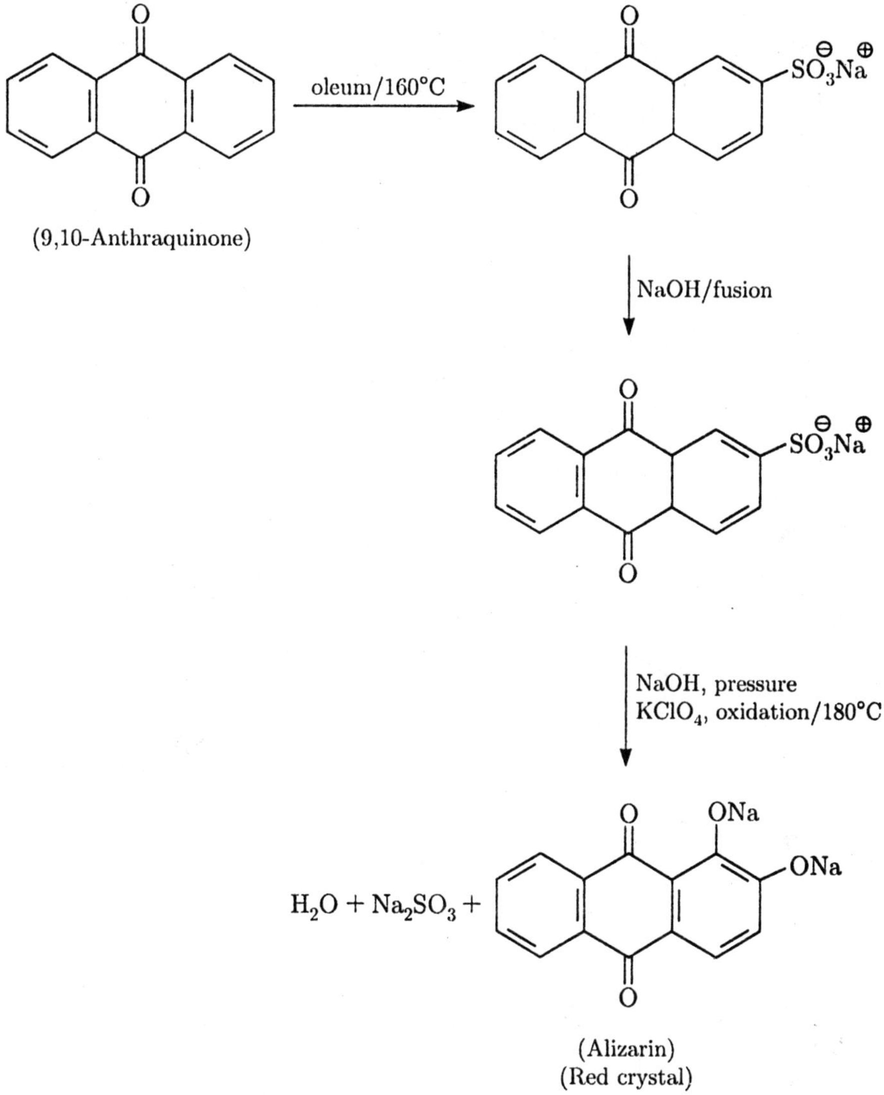

Alizarin in alkaline solution gives purple colour.

Structure of Anthracene

Analysis and molecular weight determination of anthracene show that the molecular formula of it is $C_{14}H_{10}$. Anthracene exibits the properties of both unsaturated and aromatic compounds.

Synthesis of anthracene can be done by either of the following ways.

1. 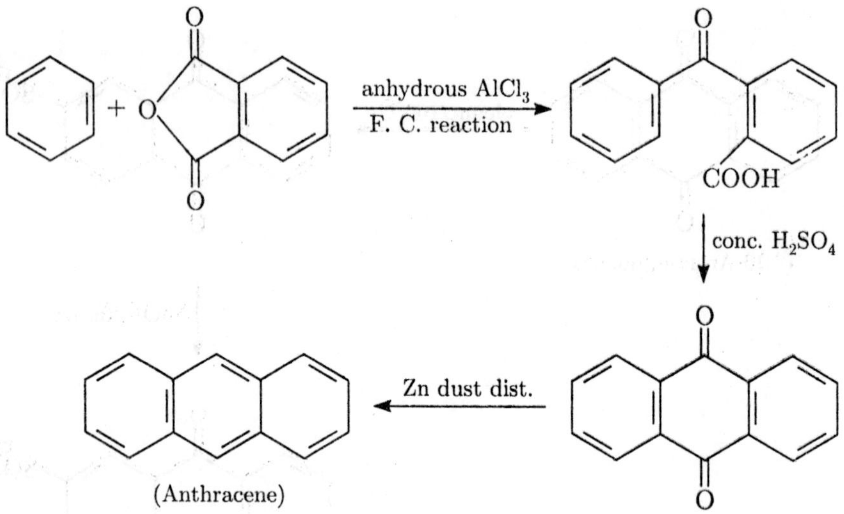

2. 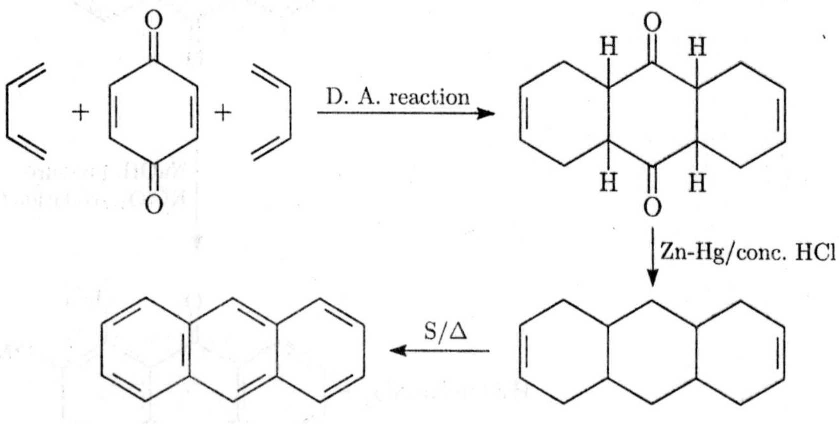

3. 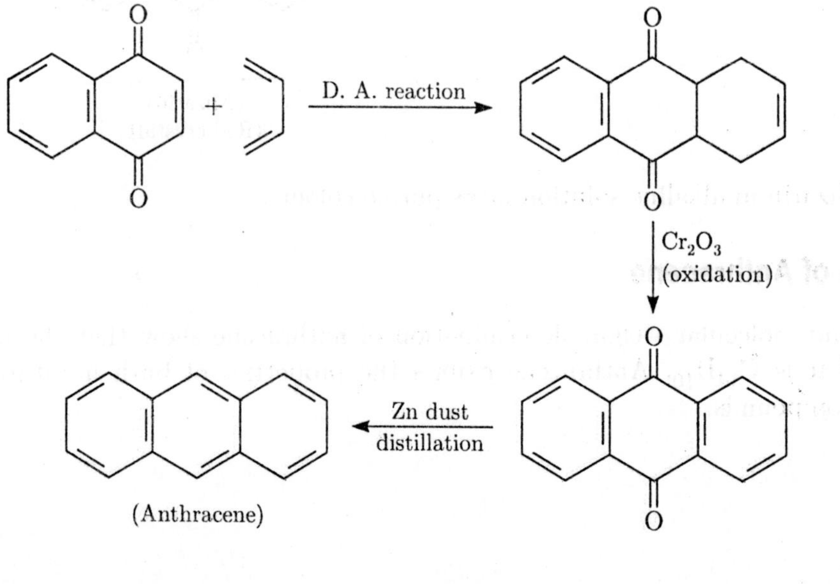

The synthetic routes leading to anthracene suggest that the molecule is a linear combination of three benzene rings in which first and the third ring are fused at the *ortho* positions of second ring as shown below.

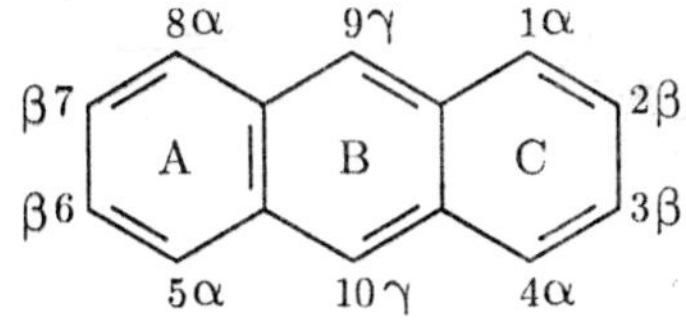

Three possible monosubstituted products (1 or α, 2 or β or 9 or γ) and 15 possible disubstituted products are possible if the substituents are identical.

The valence bond theory shows that the anthracene molecule is a resonance hybrid of the following four structures.

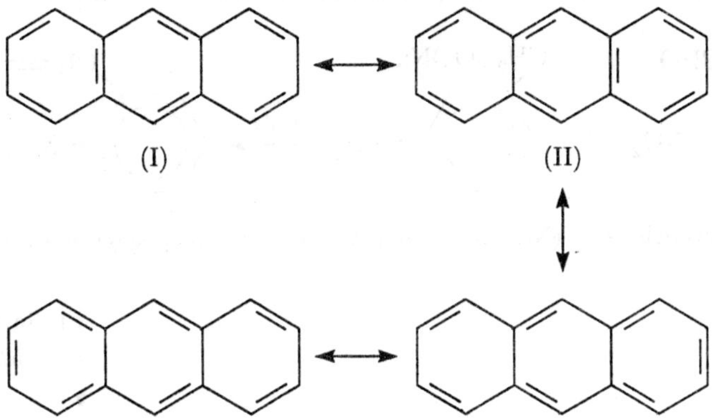

(I) (II) (IV) (III)

Since each of structures (I) and (II) contains two benzenoid rings, they contribute maximum to the hybrid. The resonance energy of anthracene is 351.5 kJ/mol.

From the stand point of molecular orbital theory anthracene is an aromatic compound containing 14 delocalised π electrons in seven bonding π orbitals in a flat (planar) structure which encompass all the three rings. Huckel's (4n+2) π electron rule, where n=3, satisfies the aromaticity of anthracene. So the structure of anthracene may be represented as,

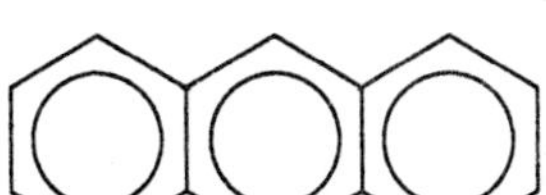

Phenanthrene

Phenanthrene (C_4H_{10}) is isomeric with anthracene and is an example of *angular polynuclear hydrocarbon*. It occurs in anthracene oil-fraction of coal tar and is separated from anthracene by means of *solution* in solvent naphtha.

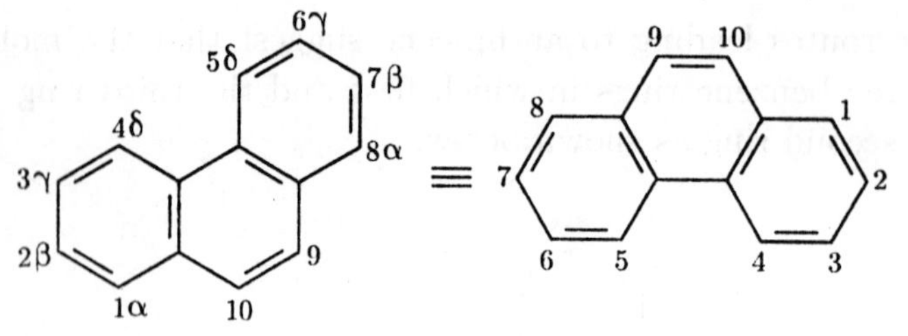

Synthesis of phenanthrene

1. *Pschorr synthesis* : It is an extension of Perkin's reaction. *o*-Nitrobenzaldehyde is heated with sodium salt of β-phenyl acetate in the presence of acetic anhydride. Reducing and diazotising the product α-phenyl-*o*-nitrocinnamic acid and treating the diazonium salt with H_2SO_4 and Cu powder, phenanthrene-9-carboxylic acid is produced and this on strong heating, forms phenanthrene.

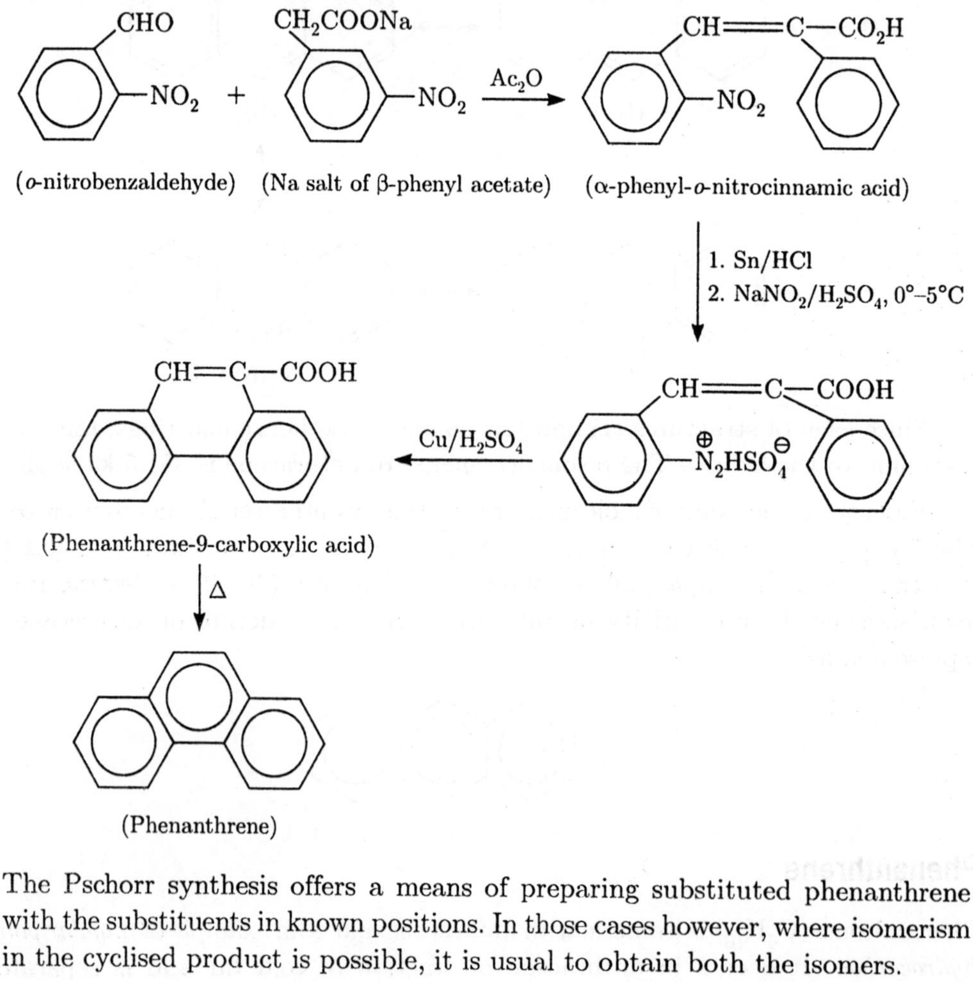

The Pschorr synthesis offers a means of preparing substituted phenanthrene with the substituents in known positions. In those cases however, where isomerism in the cyclised product is possible, it is usual to obtain both the isomers.

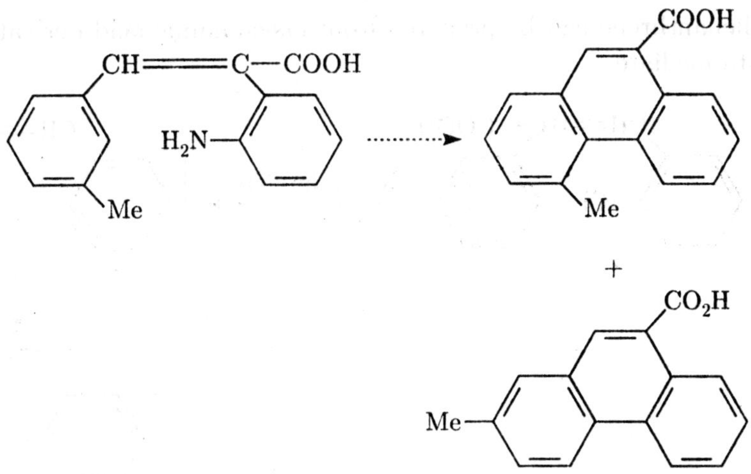

A further point to note that since ring closure is effected between two rings, these rings must be in the *cis*-position, *e.g.*, *cis*-*o*-aminostilbene gives phenanthrene, but the *trans* isomer does not.

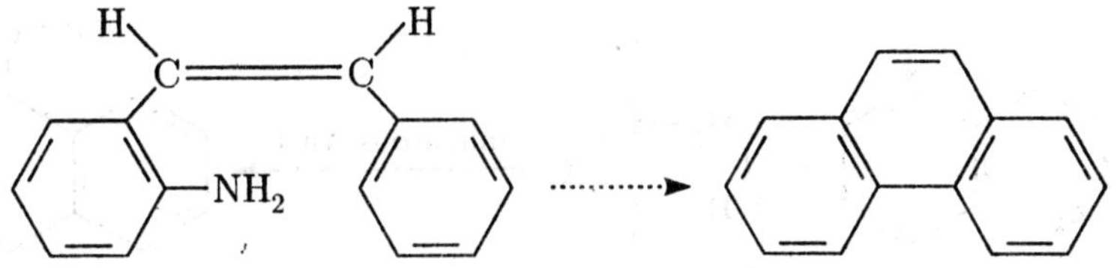

(*Cis*-isomer)

(Phenanthrene)

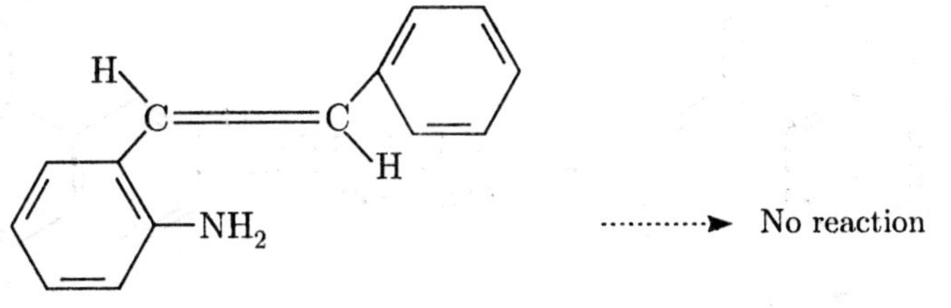

(*Trans*-isomer)

2. Phenanthrene can be prepared from *cis*-cinnamic acid derivatives *via* benzyne intermediate.

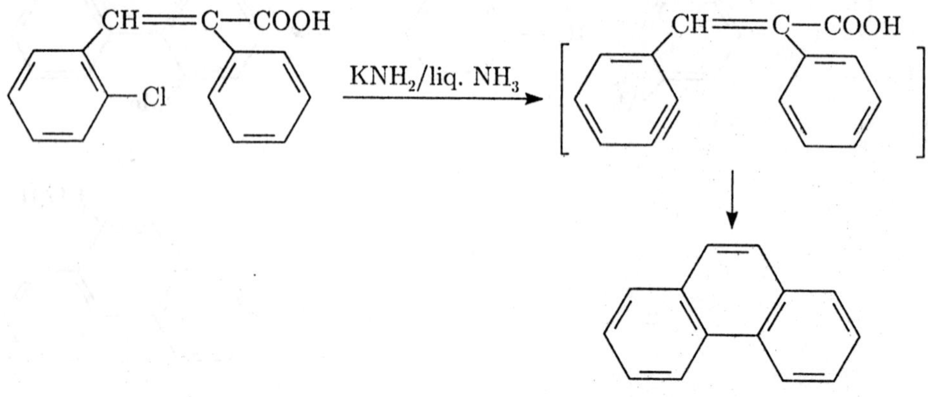

(Phenanthrene)

3. ***Haworth synthesis*** : This is an extension of Friedel-Crafts reaction.

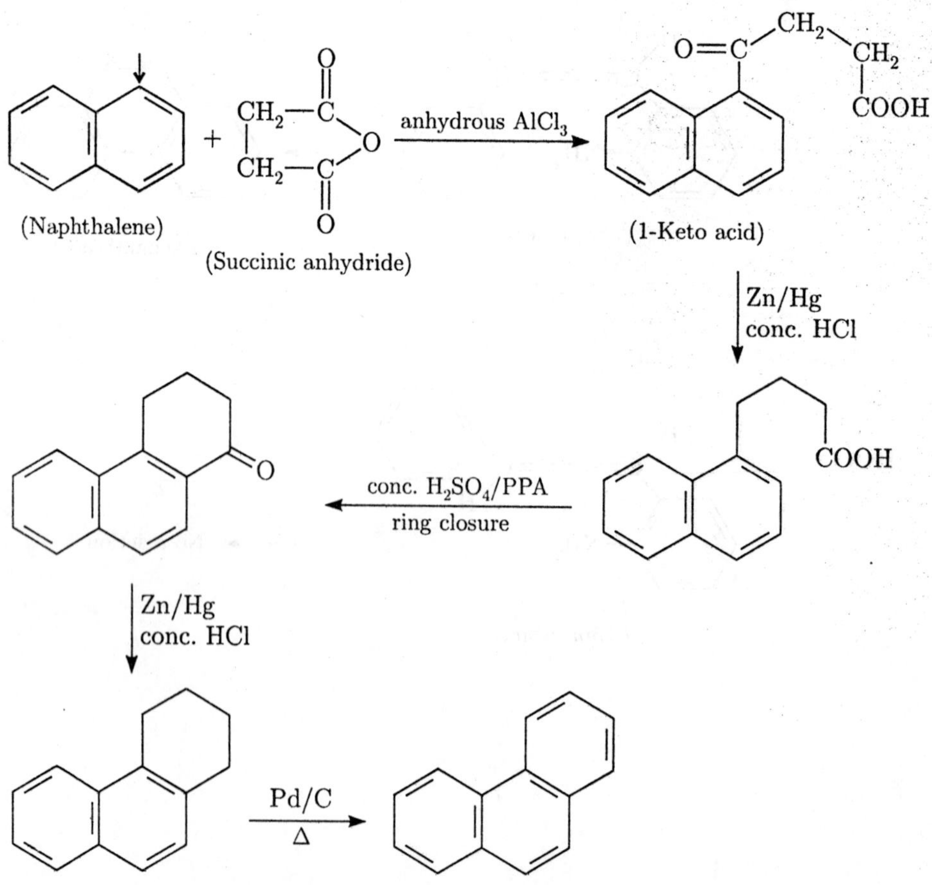

(Phenanthrene)

Succinoylation occurs in 2-position also.

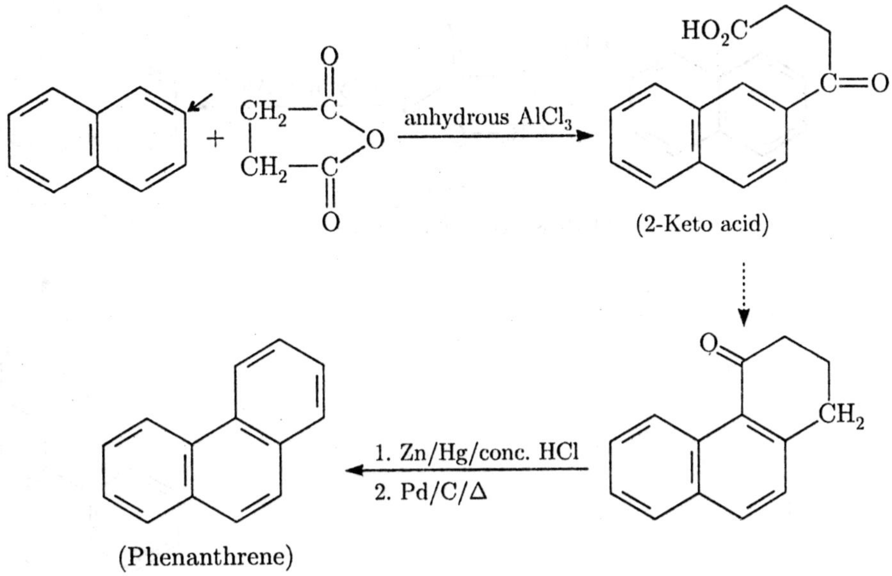

(2-Keto acid)

(Phenanthrene)

No anthracene is formed. 1-keto acid and 2-keto-acid may be readily separated. 2-keto-acid gives phenanthrene by using ring closure at 1-position, but *no anthracene* is found by ring closure at position 3. The Howarth synthesis is very useful for preparing alkylphenanthrenes with the alkyl groups in known positions, *e.g.*, after the ring closure of 1-keto acid.

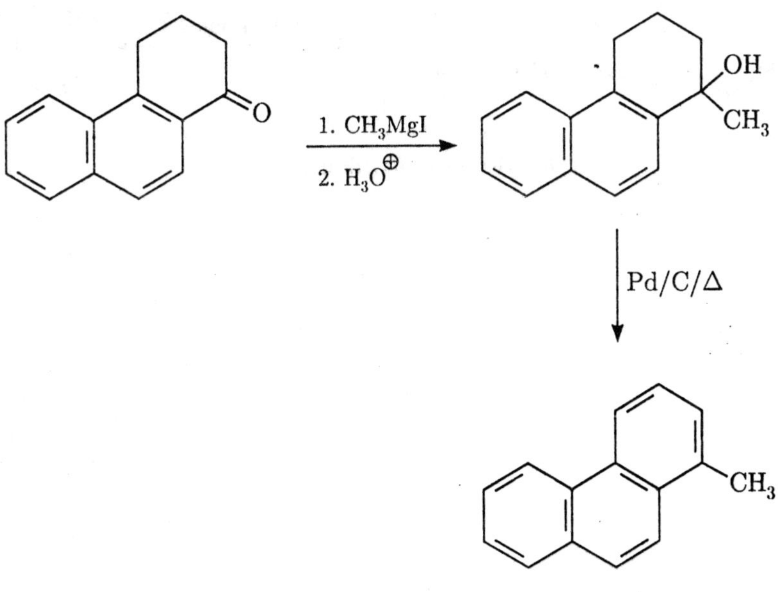

(1-methylphenanthrene)

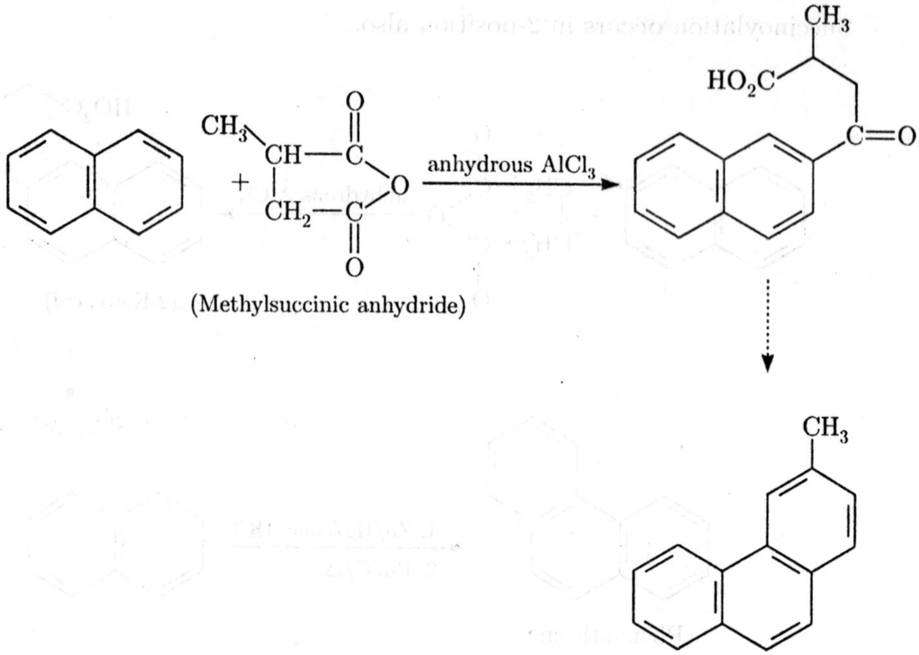

(Methylsuccinic anhydride)

(3-methylphenanthrene)

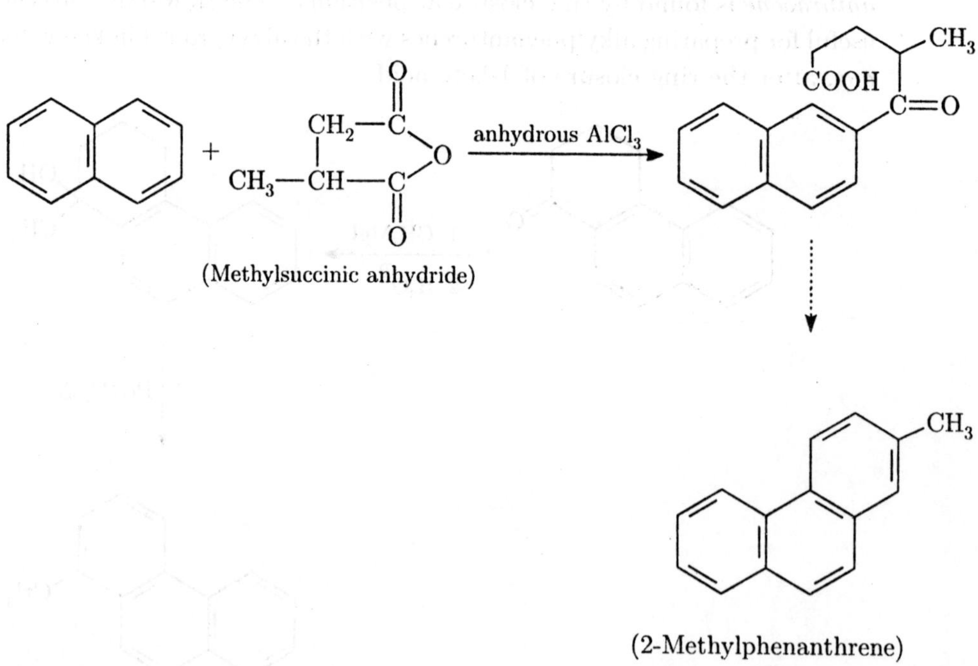

(Methylsuccinic anhydride)

(2-Methylphenanthrene)

Condensation occurs at the less hindered keto group, *i.e.*, at the one which is further removed from the methyl substituent.

4. α-Bromoketone derivatives of naphthalene may be used in the malonic ester synthesis to prepare alkylphenanthrenes.

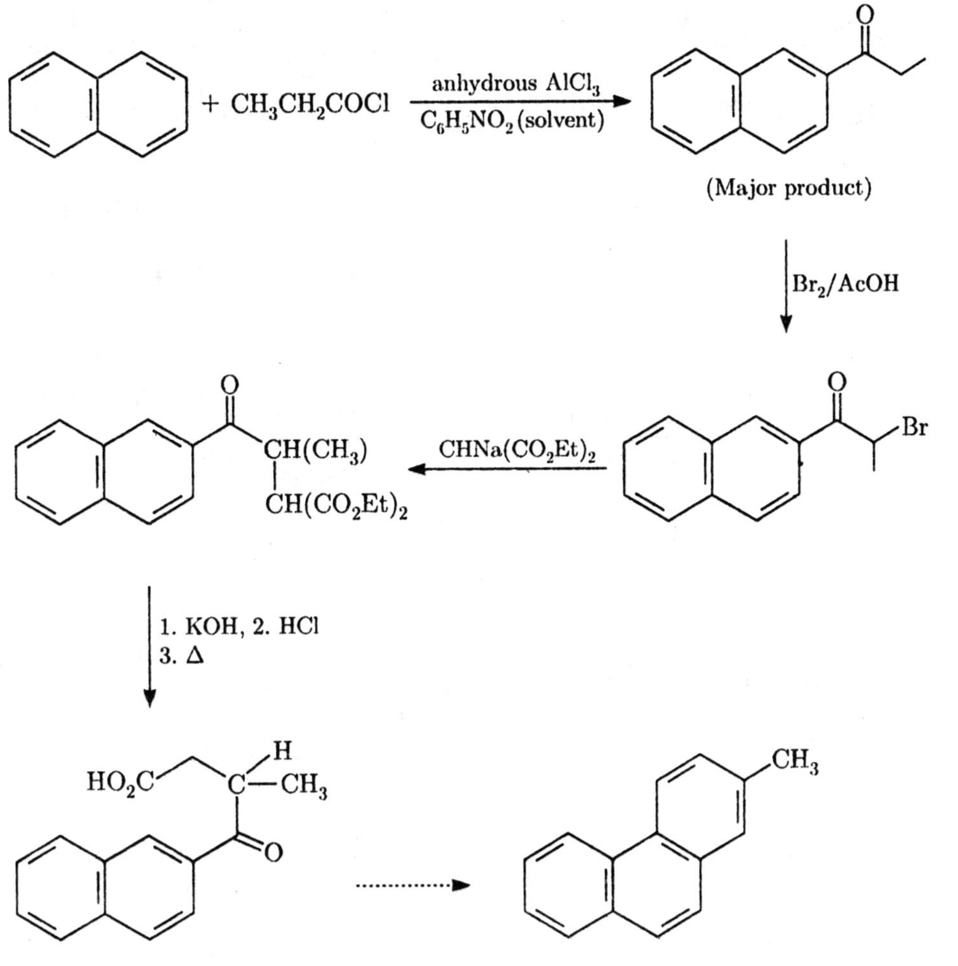

(2-Methylphenanthrene)

5. ***Stobbe condensation*** :

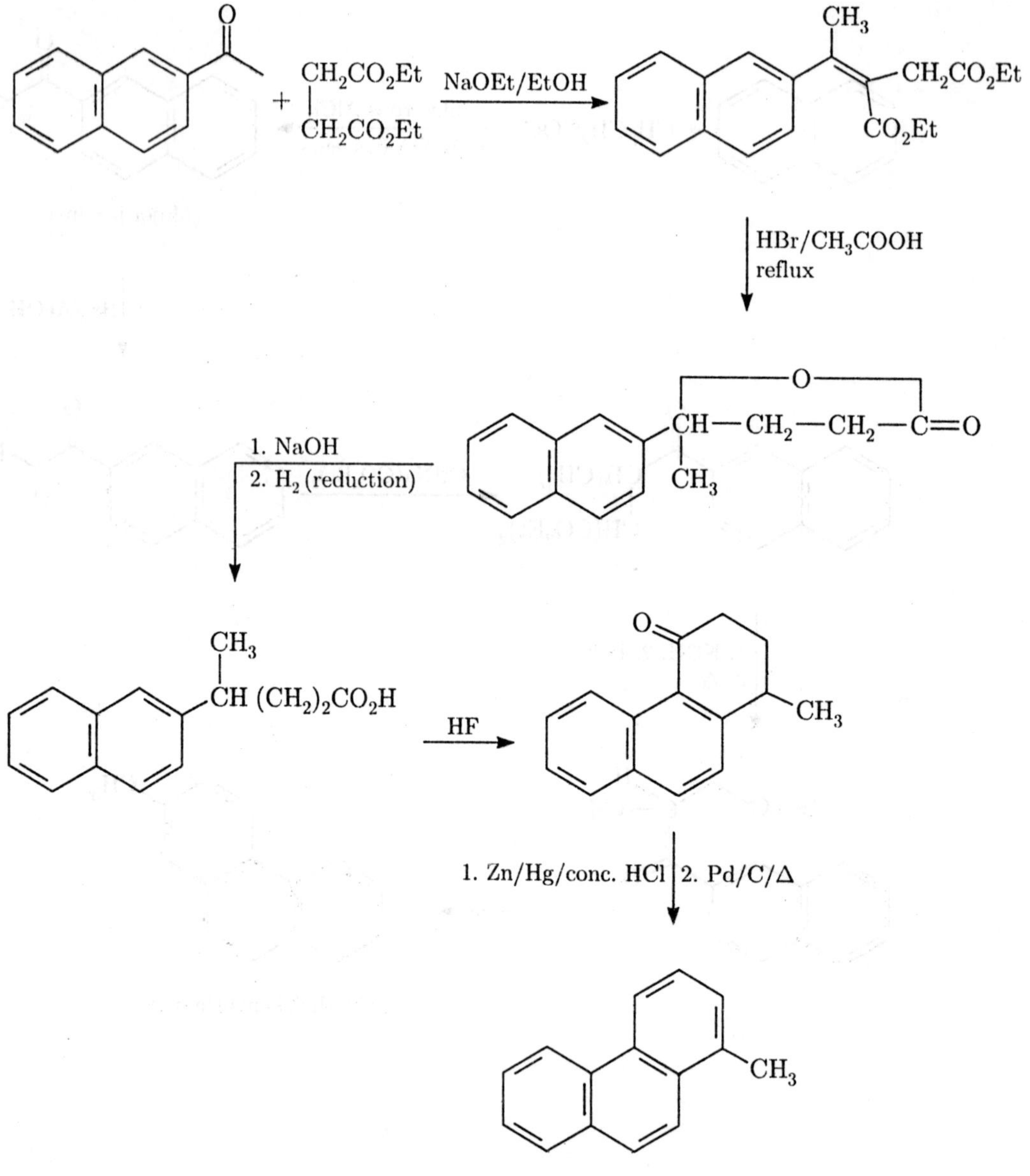

(1-Methylphenanthrene)

Mechanism of Stobbe condensation :

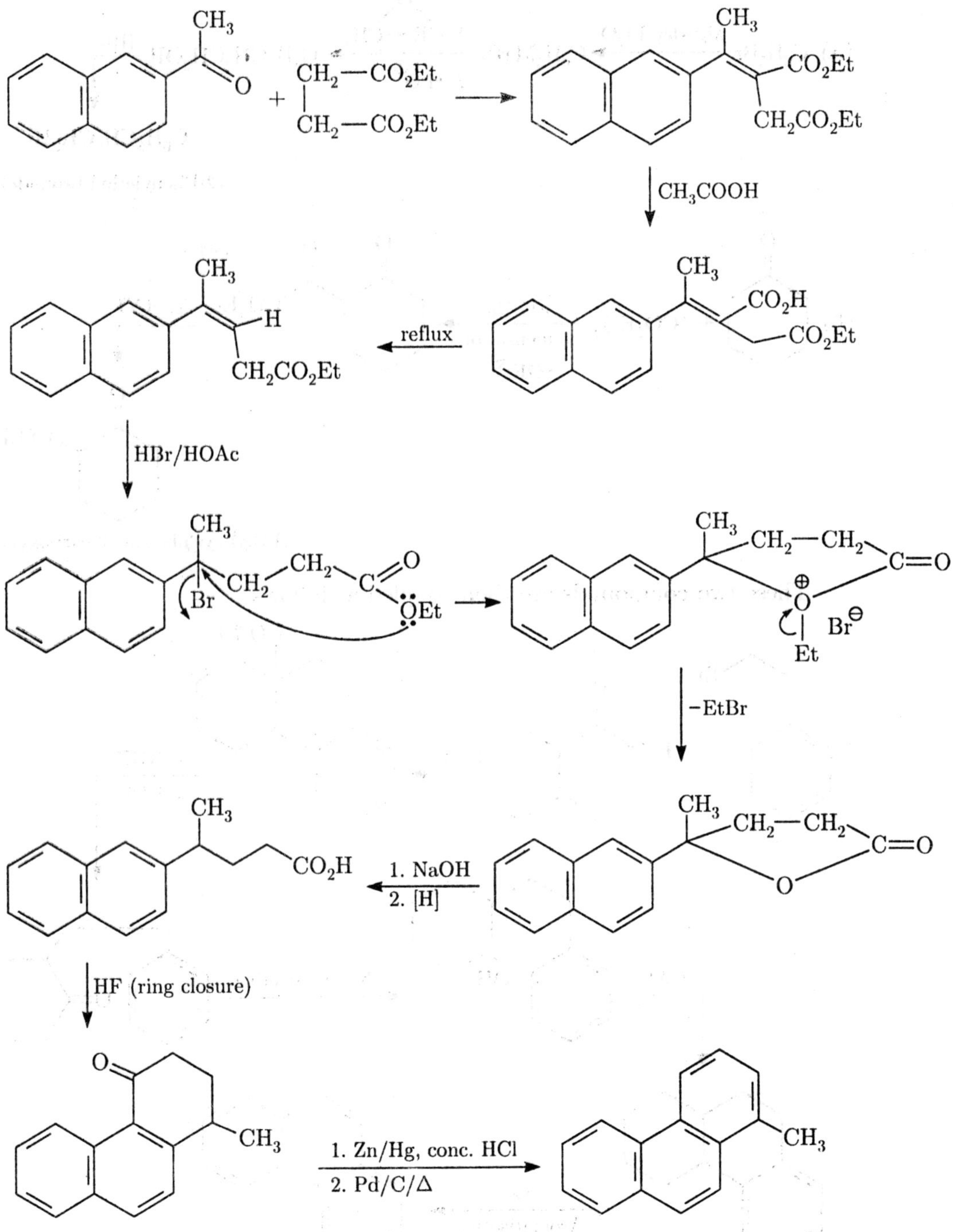

(1-Methylphenanthrene)

6. ***Bardhan-Sengupta synthesis*** : Starting materials for Bardhan-Sengupta synthesis are 2-phenylethyl bromide and ethyl cyclohexane-2-carboxylate.

(a) $$C_6H_5Br \xrightarrow{\text{Mg/dry } Et_2O} C_6H_5MgBr \xrightarrow[\text{2. } H_3O^{\oplus}]{\text{1. } \overset{\text{O}}{CH_2-CH_2}} C_6H_5CH_2CH_2OH \xrightarrow{HBr} C_6H_5CH_2CH_2Br$$

(2-Phenylethyl bromide)

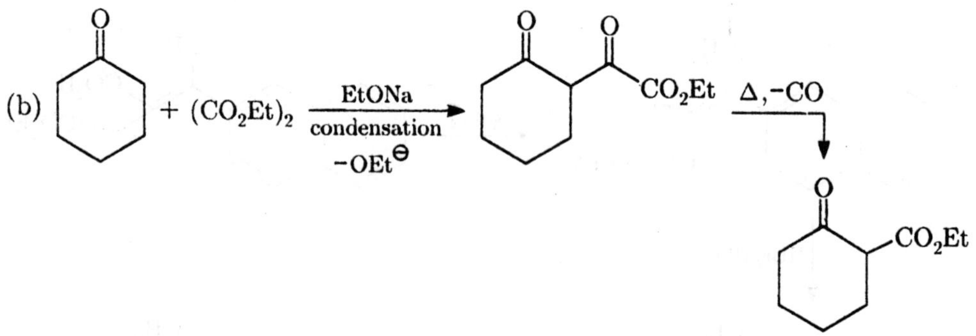

(Ethyl cyclohexane-2-carboxylate)

These two compounds are then coupled as follows.

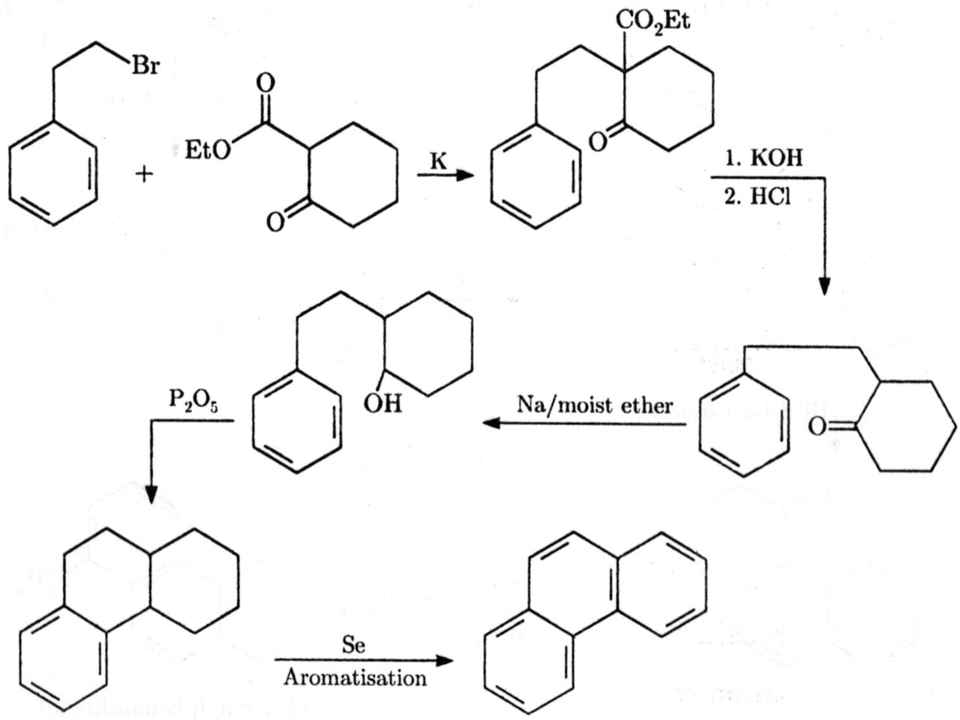

(Phenanthrene)

7. ***Bogert-Cook synthesis*** :

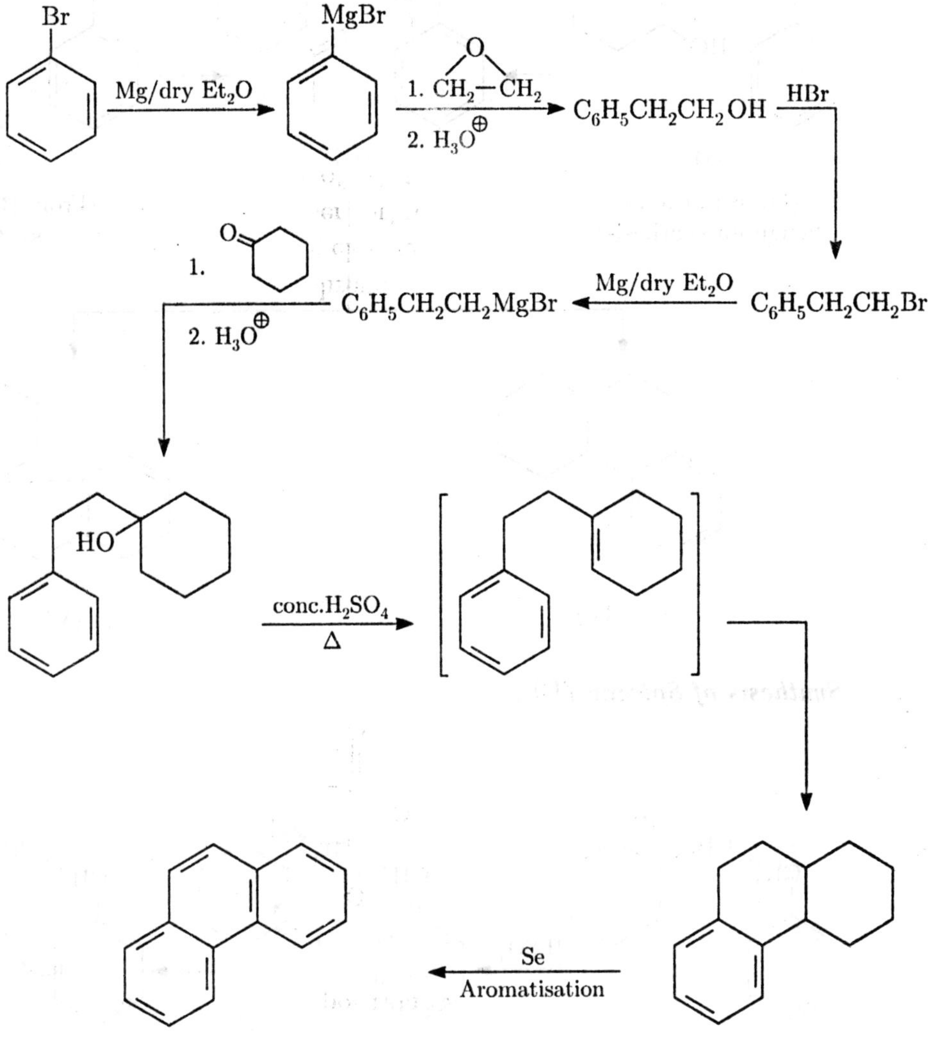

(Phenanthrene)

It might be noted that the Bardhan-Sengupta and Bogert-Cook method both proceed *via* the formation of a common intermediate (III), which then produces a mixture of octahydrophenanthrene (IV) and the spirane (V).

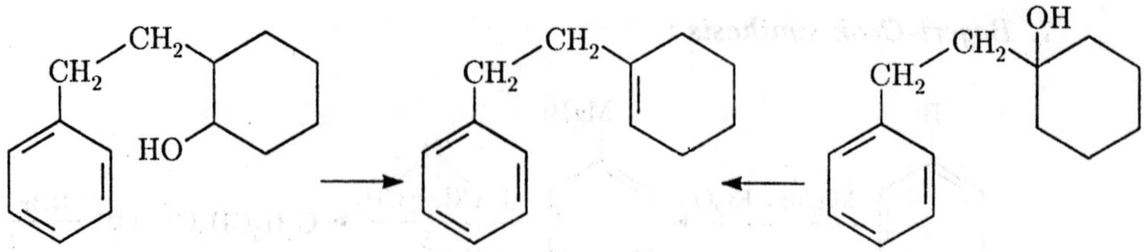

(I) (From Bardhan-Sengupta synthesis)

(III)

(II) (From Bogert-Cook synthesis)

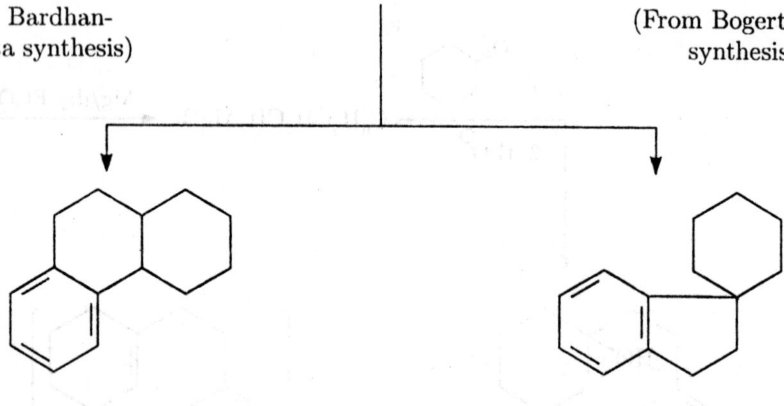

(IV)

(V)

Synthesis of Spirane (V) :

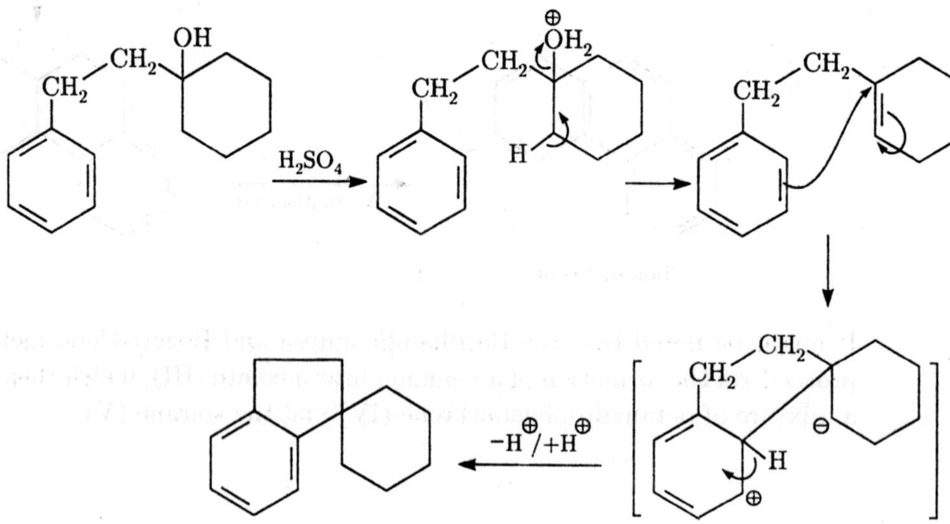

(Spirane V)

8. ***Preparation of substituted phenanthrenes (Bacon et al)*** :

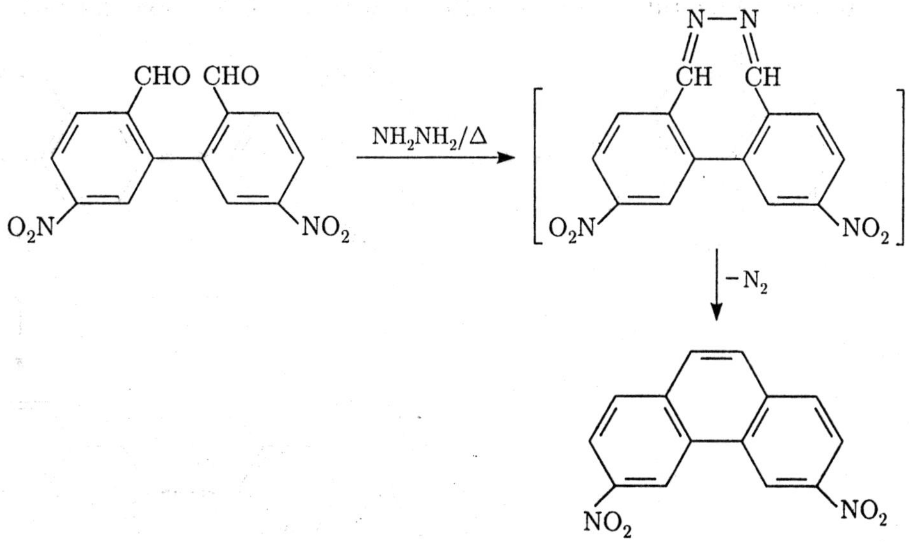

(2,7-Dinitrophenanthrene)

9.

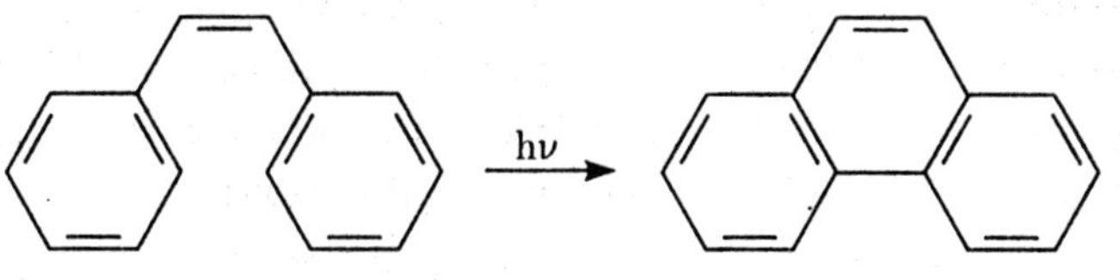

(*Cis*-stilbene) (Phenanthrene)

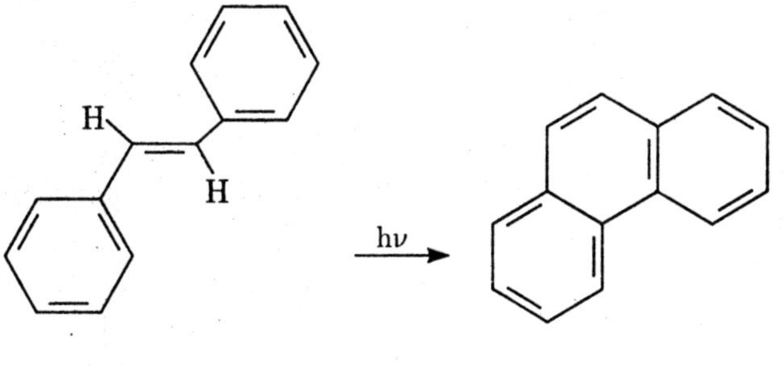

(*Trans*-stilbene) (Phenanthrene)

Resonating structures of phenanthrene : Phenanthrene is best represented as a resonance hybrid of five resonating structures (R. E. = 387 kJ/mol).

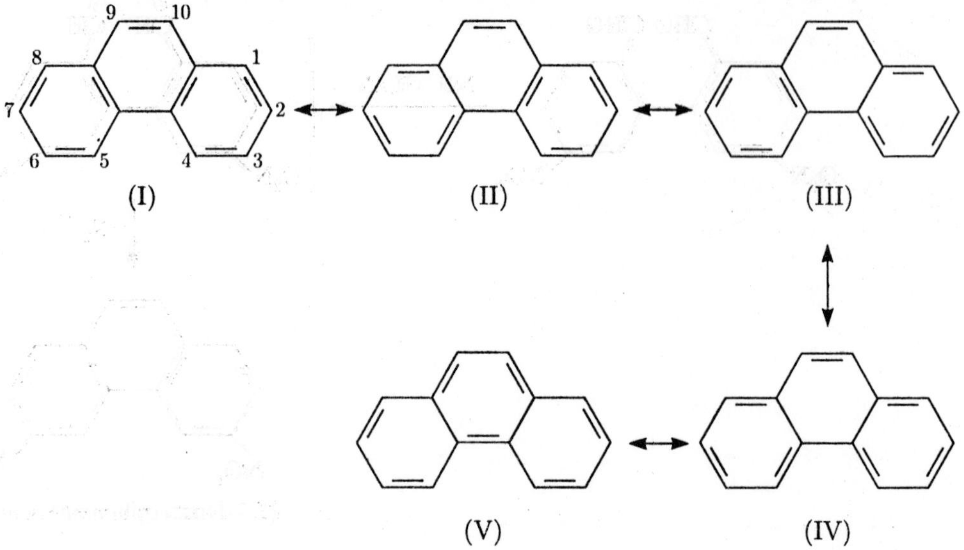

Five monosubstituted products are possible at the positions 1,2,3,4 and 9, respectively.

Properties of phenanthrene : Phenanthrene (m.p. 99°C) shows blue fluoresence and is very active at 9,10 positions. Phenanthrene is catalytically reduced to 9,10-dihydrophenanthrene (CuO/Cr_2O_3) and adds on bromine (Br_2) to form 9,10-phenanthrene dibromide. These addition reactions resemble an olefinic double bond.

1.

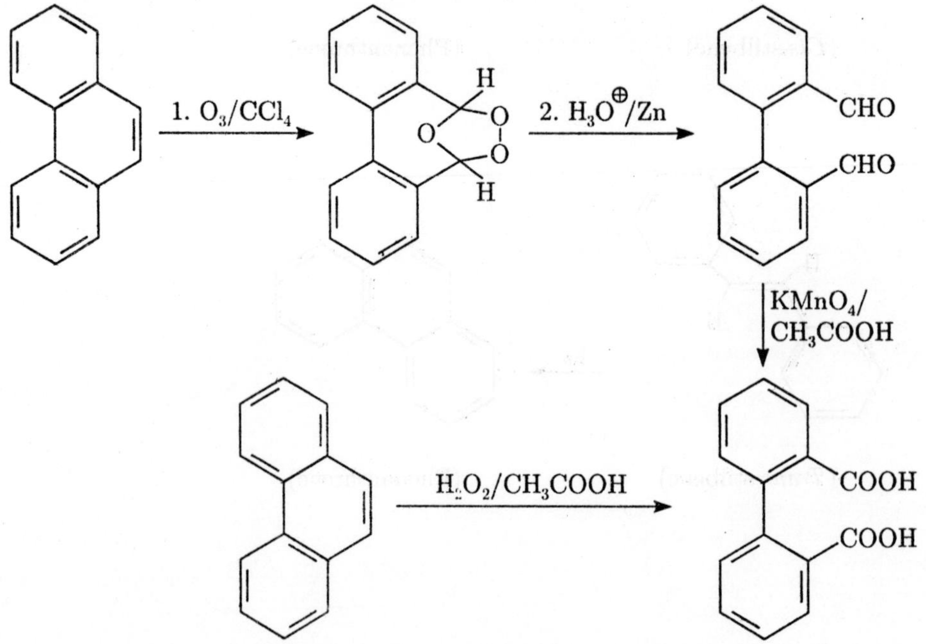

2.

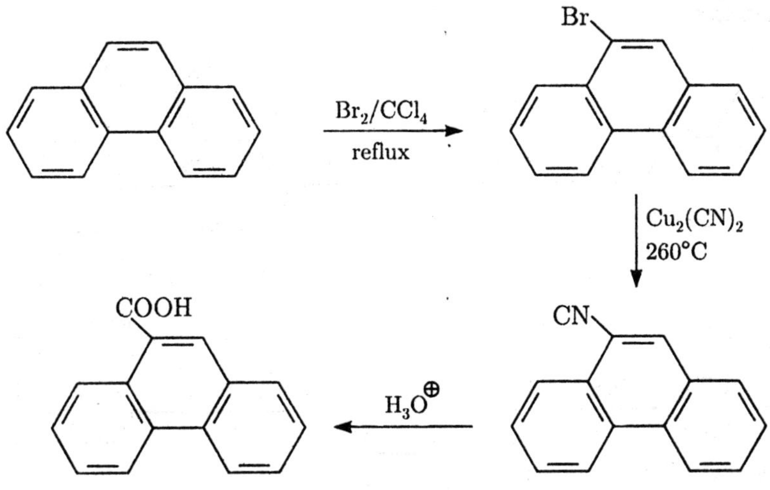

(Phenanthrene-9-carboxylic acid)

3.

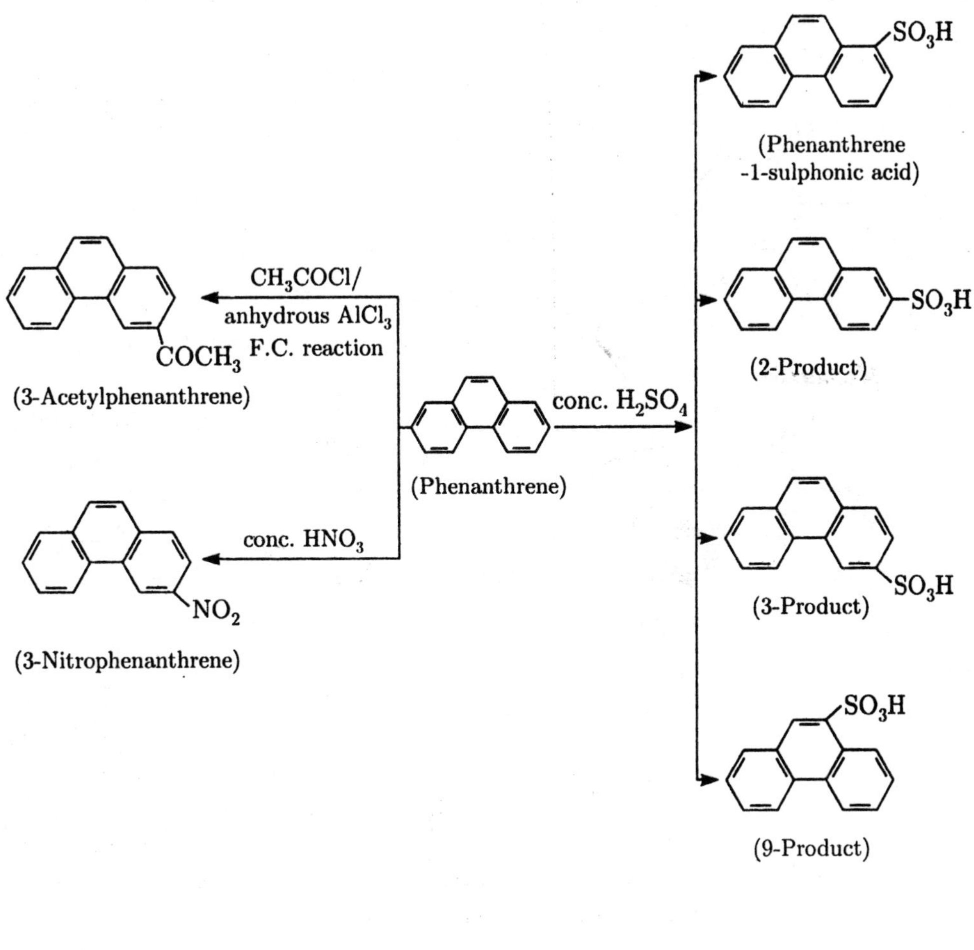

Phenanthroquinone

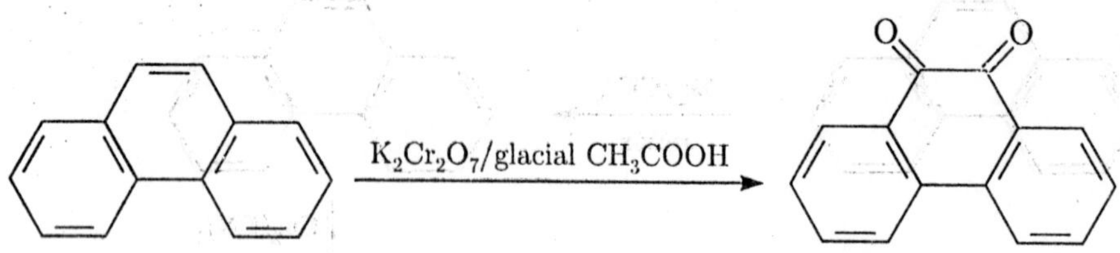

(9,10-Phenanthraquinone)

1.

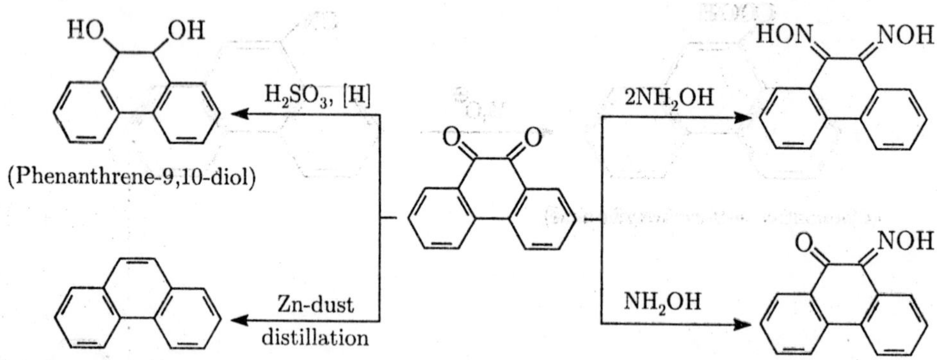

(Phenanthrene)

2.

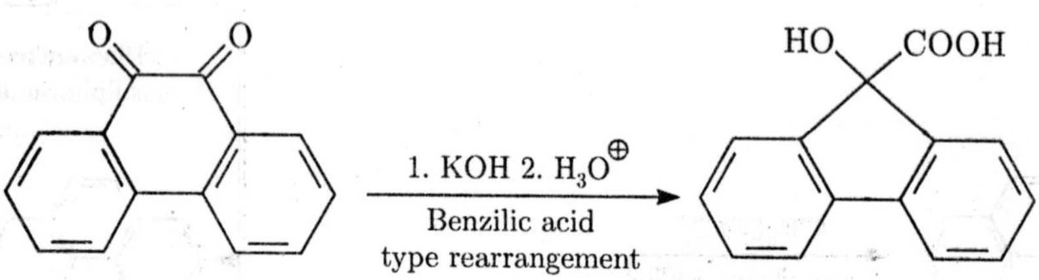

(9-Hydroxyfluorene-9-Carboxylic acid)

Mechanism :

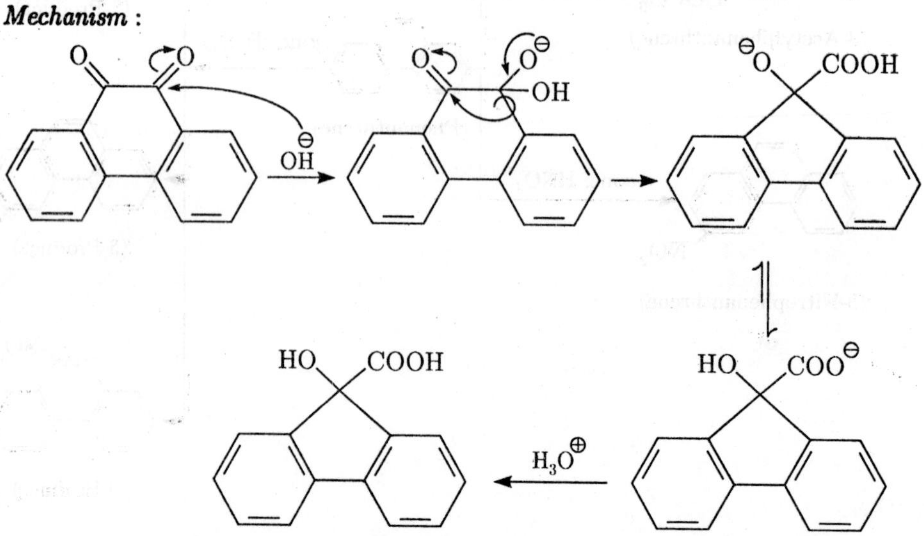

(9-Hydroxyfluorene-9-Carboxylic acid)

3. 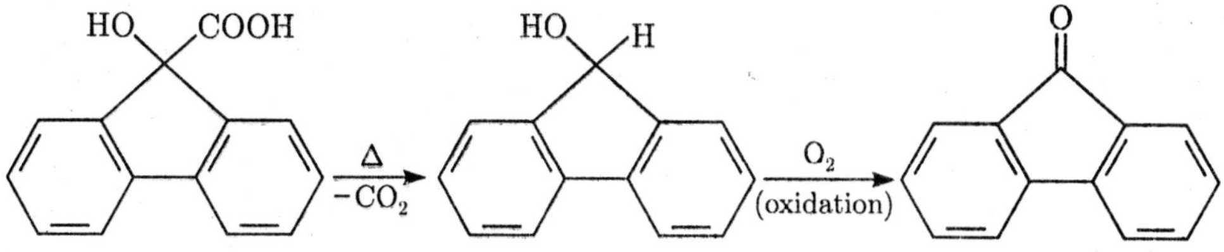

(Fluorenone)

4. 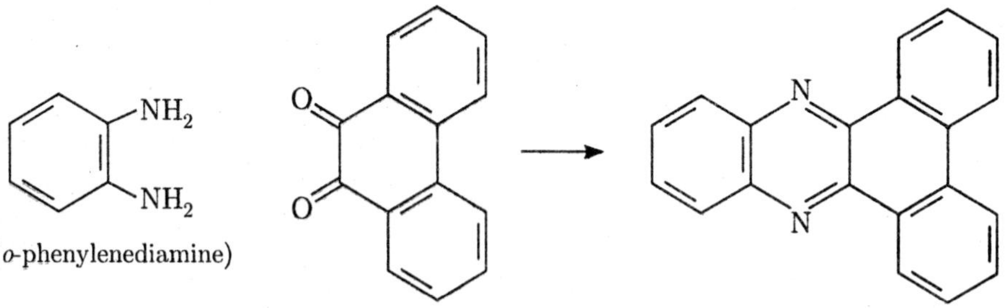

(*o*-phenylenediamine) (9,10-Phenanthraquinone) (Phenazine)

Molecular overcrowding in phenanthrene : A molecule becomes overcrowded when at least one pair of non-bonded atoms are closer to each other than the sum of their van der Waals radii. Two extremes are possible. Two atoms remain very close to each other not affecting the rest of the molecule; but it causes too much of steric repulsion. If the molecule be deformed so that the atoms get separated by their van der Waals radii, there would be a steric strain. In practice, a compromise between steric repulsion and steric strain is seen.

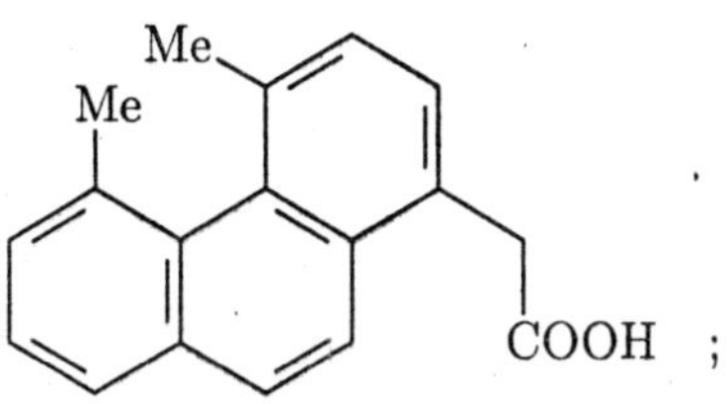

(I)

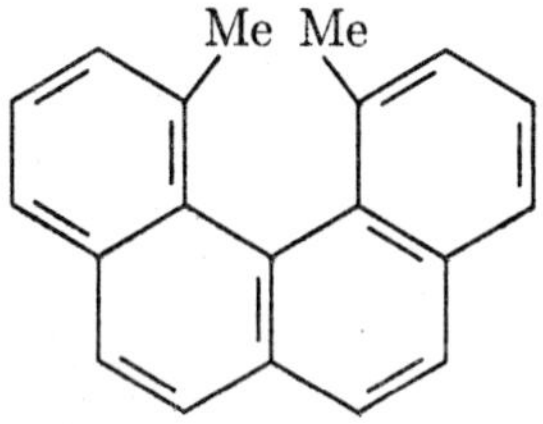

(II)

These molecule (I and II) are *not planar*, so is asymmetric and can be resolved.

Phenanthrene itself is not absolutely planar in the crystalline state and this non-planarity may be due to *molecular overcrowding.*

Index

A

$A_{AC}1$ 441, 446-449
$A_{AC}2$ 441, 444-446
$A_{AL}1$ 441, 450
$A_{AL}2$ 441, 452
Absorption spectroscopy 1, 2, 32
  absorption bands of different bonds in IR 55-61
  absorption frequency in IR 36
  absorption of IR and vibrational transition 36
  anisotropic effect 73
  anisotropic effect of
    alkenes 73
    alkynes 74
    aromatic compounds, annulenes 75
    carbonyl compouds 74
  auxochromes 4
Acyloin condensation 193, 199
Ad_N2 reaction (examples) 142
  acetal hydrolysis 157, 496-498
  acetals and cyclic acetals 151-153, 476, 487-494
Ad_N2 reaction to C=O 138, 139, 140, 199, 200, 201, 203
Ad_N-E reactions 200, 201, 202
Ad_N-S_N 203
Alcohols :
  acylation of OH group 468
  benzoylation of OH group 469
  conversion of CH(OH) to CO by dehydrogenation 459
  conversion to mesylates and tosylates 468
  dehydration of alcohols to alkenes 463-466
  dehydration of alcohols to ethers 466, 467
  D-exchange 470
  distinction between three classes of alcohols 479
  esterification 469
  methods of preparation 454-457
  oxidation of alcohols 460-463
  reaction with CS_2 478
  reaction with diazomethane 470
  reaction with epoxides 470
  reaction with hydrogen halide 472
  reaction with isocyanates 476
  reaction with metals (Na, Li) 467
  reaction with $SOCl_2$ and PBr_3 471
  structure, reactivity and physical properties 458
  sulphonates and inorganic esters 474
  trans esterification 469
  β-elimination 471
Aldol condensation :
  aldol reactions with nitriles 230
  applications of aldol reactions 234
  crossed aldol reaction 215-220
  directed aldol reactions 220, 221, 337
  lithium enolates in aldol reactions 222, 223, 224
  reaction and mechanism 210-215
  silyl-enol ethers in aldol reactions 224
  stereochemistry of 232
Alkyl isonitriles :
  distinction with nitriles 870
  methods of preparation 867
  reactions 868, 869

alkyl nitrites 837, 838
ambident nucleophiles 826
Amines :
- acetylation and benzoylation of 770
- amonolysis reactions 737
- aromatic amine-an ambident nucleophile 769
- azoxybenzene 805
- bromination of 771
- distinction between threc classes of amines 758-760
- N-alkyl or arylaldimine 775
- nitration of 772
- oxidation of amines 761-763
- preparation of amines 737-746
- reactions 763-768
- separation of three classes of amines 755-757
- structure, reactivity and physical properties 755
- sulphonation of 773
- *p*-aminoazobenzene 804

Anthracene :
- alizarine 899
- anthracene derivatives 896-899
- anthraquinone 890, 898
- anthrols 897
- chemical reactions of 891-899
- Diels-Alder reaction of 894
- electrophilic substitution of 895
- formylation of 892
- Friedel-Crafts acylation of 892
- halogenation of 894
- nitration of 893
- oxidation of 892
- reduction of 891
- structure of 899-901
- sulphonation of 893
- syntheses of 889-891

Arlenmeyer's azalactone synthesis 241
- acid chlorides 387-391
- anionotropy 347, 363

Arndt-Eistert synthesis 813
Aromatic electrophilic substitution :
- ArS_E2 589-604
- Chloromethylation reaction 641-643
- electrophiles 589
- energy profiles of ArS_E2 reactions 592, 593
- evidences of ArS_E2 mechanisms 594
- Friedel-Crafts acylation 632-641
- Friedel-Crafts alkylation 632-637, 679
- halogenation 625-632
- *ipso* substitution 643-648
- *m*- directing groups 596
- nitration 611-619,k 845-848
- *o*-, *p*- directing groups 596
- orientation in monosubstituted benzene 596
- orientations in disubstituted benzene 602-604
- *orthopara* ratio 604
- poly-electrophilic substitution in aromatic compounds 607
- radical addition to aromatic π-bonds 609
- stability of σ-complex and orientation 597-602
- sulphonation/desulphonation 619-625
- π-complex in ArS_E2 reactions 590-591
- σ-complex in ArS_E2 reactions 590, 591

Aromatic nitro compounds :
- charge transfer complexes of 854
- reduction of 848-852

Aromatic nitroso compounds 856
- addition of ammonia to 863
- addition of olefin to 863
- Alkyl nitrites or cyanides 857-866
- alkylation of 863
- formation of β-ketonitrile 863

Aromatic nucleophilic substitution 653, 853
- amino phenols 725, 726
- ArS_N1 654
- ArS_N2 655
- aryne (benzyne) intermediate 662-673
- nucleophiles 655

B

$B_{AC}1$ 441, 451
$B_{AC}2$ 441, 442-444
$B_{AL}1$ 441, 449
$B_{AL}2$ 441, 451
Bamberger reaction 852
Bardhan-Sengupta synthesis 910
Bathochromic shift/Red shift 5
Beckmann rearrangement 748-751
Benzilic acid rearrangement 279-282
benzimidazole 784
Benzoin condensation 266-270
Benzoquinones (*o*- and *p*) 322-330
benztriazole 782
Bismarck Brown 783
blue shift 5
Bogert-Cook synthesis 911
Bouveault-Blanc reduction 192
butyl lithium 565

C

18-Crown-6 586
2-cyanonaphthalene 888
Carboxylic acid derivatives :
  basicity 375, 376
  nucleophilic substitution 376
  physical properties 375
carboxylic acids:
  base-catalysed hydrolysis
    of esters 383, 388-390
  nucelophilic substitution
    at acylcarbon 418-420
  physical properties of 395
  reactions 396
  reactions of 426-253
  synthesis of 392-395
  synthesis of derivatives 420-425
catechol 720, 721
Chemistry of carbonyl compounds :
  synthesis of aldehydes and ketones 107-135
  by alkaline hydrolysis of dihaloalkanes 128
  by from esters and dimethyl
  sulphoxide (Corey *et. al*) 124
    by Grignard reagent 117
  by heating mixture of calcium salts 123
  by ketonic hydrolysis of
    ethylacetoacetate 118
  by side chain oxidation of arenes 130
  Cannizzaro reaction 177-184
  Catechol 324
  cationotropy 347
  chloranil 328
  Claisen condensation 247-255
  Clemmensen reduction 203-207
  from arene diazonium salts 132
  from carboxylic acids 129
  from esters by DIBAL-H 127
  from nitriles by DIBAL-H 127
  2-chloroquinol 326
Chloromethylation 641, 684, 685
Chromophores 3,4
Claisen rearrangement 730-736
Cope elimination 769
Cram's rule 527, 528
Cresols 718, 719
Cummene peroxide method 675
Curtius rearrangement 743, 751-753

D

2,3-dicyanoquinol 326
Darzens glycidic ester condensation 121, 247
Dakin reaction 720, 721
decarboxylation of carboxylic acids 402-418
description of spectrometers 2
Determination of pK_a by UV-spectroscopy 30
diazoacetic ester :
  physical properties and structure of 817
  preparation of 817
  reactions of 818, 819
diazoketones 819-824
diazomethane-properties and structure 809

diazonium salts :
2,3-diaminophenazine 784
diazoamino and aminoazo compounds 803
diazocoupling reactions 694, 695, 787-797
displacement of diazo group 798-806
formation of diazohydroxides 786
formation of diazophenols 786
formation of double salts and polyhalides 786
formation of hydrazines 787
preparation of 784-786
structure elucidation of 802
DIBAL-H 127, 174
Dieckmann condensation 255-258
Diels-Alder synthesis of anthracene 890
dienone-phenol rearrangement 331, 332
dihydric phenols 719-723
dinitrobenzenes 852
Doebner condensation 262

E

E2 reaction 475
effective chromophores 3, 29
Elbs persulphate oxidation 711
Elbs reaction for synthesis of anthracene 890
Electrolytic reduction of carbonyl compounds 190
electronic energy levels 10
electrophilic substition of carbonyl compounds 299
Emission spectroscopy 1
enamines 341-346
end absorption 5
enolates 332-341
Eschweiler-Clarke methylation reaction 278
esterification of carboxylic acids 383-387
Etard reaction 130
ethers :
auto oxidation 509
cleavage of ethers 506-508
epoxides 510-522
ester formation 509
formation of oxonium salts 505
reaction with halogens 508
structures physical properties of ethers 504
synthesis 499-504
extent of absorption 28
Friedel-Crafts reaction 478

F

Fermi resonance 48
field effects in IR 41
Finger print region in IR 48
Fischer-Hepp rearrangement 777-778
Fittig synthesis of anthracene 891
Fitting and Erdmann synthesis of naphthalene 872
Forbidden transition 9,11
Fries rearrangement 680-684

G

1,2-glycols 457-458, 482-486
Gabriel phthalimide synthesis 739-742
Gattermann aldehyde synthesis 131, 649
Gattermann-Koch formylation 649
Gomberg reaction 800
Grignard reagents :
abnormal behaviour of Grignard reagents 542-544
preparation 523-524
reactivity 525-526
stereoselectivity of Grignard reaction 527
structure 525
synthetic uses 528-542

H

2-halogenonaphthalene 888
9-hydroxyfluorene-9-carboxylic acid 916
haloform reaction 301-308, 478
halogenation of phenols 689-692
Haworth synthesis of naphthalene 872-875
Haworth synthesis of phenanthrene 904
Hell-Volherd-Zelinsky (H.V.Z.) reaction 397-401

hemiacetals 148-151, 486-488
Henrys reaction 230, 831
Hofmann exhaustive methylation 764-768
Hofmann rearrangement 742, 746-748
Hofmann's mustard oil reaction 761
Hofmann-Martins rearrangement 775-777
Hooke's law 35
Houben-Hoesch acylation 641, 704-708
Hunsdiecker reaction 402-403
hydration of alkynes to aldehydes
  and ketones 116
hydroboration-oxidation of alkynes 125
hydroxyquinol 723
hydroxyquinol triacetate 328
hyperchromic effect 5
hypochromic effect 5
Hypsochromic shift/Blue shift 5

I

indophenol 331
Infrared spectroscopy :
  infrared regions (near, mid and far) 32
intramolecular aldol reactions 226-230
IR absorption :
  beat bands 47
  common terminologiesin IR
  conditions of 36
  factors 37
  overtone bands 47
  problems of 62-64
isocyanic acid 477

J

Japp-klingemann reaction 797

K

Karplus equation 92
Ketals 486
Keto-enol tautomerism 350-362
Knovenagel condensation 258-262
Kolbe's electrolytic method
  for decarboxylation 404
Kolbe-Schmidt reaction 701-704

L

Lambert-Beers Law 8
lead tetracetate oxidation 483
Lederer-Manasse reaction 706-710
Leuckart reaction 743
Libermann's test 760
lithium aluminium hydride ($LiAlH_4$) 169-172
lithium dimethyl cuprate 567-570
lithium enolates 222, 336-339
Lossen rearrangement 743, 753
Lucas test 480

M

1-methylphenanthrene 905, 908, 909
2-methylphenanthrene 906, 907
Mannich base 270
Mannich reaction 270-278, 696, 775
Meerwin reaction 801
Meerwin-Pondorf-Verley reduction 185-188
Michael reaction 314-320, 833
Michler's ketone774
Modes of molecular vibration in IR 44

N

^{1}H-NMR spectroscopy :
  chemical shift in NMR 69-71
  effect of hydrogen bond in NMR 76
  equivalent and non-equivalent
    protons in NMR 79
  ^{1}HNMR spectrum of ethanol 89, 90
  integrals in ^{1}HNMR, peakarea 77
  m-dichloro- and *m*-dinitrobenzene 102
  m-nitrochlorobenzene 102
  nitrobenzene and halobenzene 100
  o-nitrochlorobenzene 101
  o-xylene 105
  p-dinitro and *p*-dichlorobenzene 103
  p-nitroanisole 105
  p-nitrochlorobenzene 104
  radiofrequency absorption in NMR 66
  relaxation process in NMR 68
  shielding and deshielding in NMR 71
  solvents used in NMR (TMS etc.) 69, 77
  spin-spin coupling and peak splitting in NMR 79-87

theory of NMR 67
toluene 100
N,N-dimethyl-N′,N-dinitrosoterepththalimide (NTA) 809
Naphthalene :
chemical properties of 879-888
chloromethylation of 882
Fiedel-Craft reaction of 883
halogenattion of 884
naphthoic acids 887
naphthols 886
naphthylamines 885
nitration of 882
structure of 877-879
sulphonation of 882
synthesis of 871-876
nitration of phenols 686-689
nitroalkanes :
acidity of α-H of 829
bromination of 831
condensation reactions of 831-833
distinction of 836, 837
hydrolysis of 833
methods of preparation of 825-828
NEF carbonyl synthesis 829-830
nitration reactions, examples 839-851
reduction of 834-836
structure and physical properties of 828
nitrosation of phenols 694
Nucleophilic addition of :
2,4-dinitrophenyl hydrazine (2,4-DNP) 202
ammonia 144
Grignard reagent 160-163
hydroxylamine 201
nitration of carbonyl compounds 299
nitrosation of carbonyl compounds 296
Nystrom and Brown reduction by LiAlH4 169
organolithium 163
organozinc 164
phenylhydrazine 202
primary amine 201
semicarbazide 202
sodium bisulphite 145
stereochemistry of nucleophilic addition 176
water 158-160
Nucleophilic addition to
carbon-oxygen double bond 136
orbitals involved 136
angle of nucleophilic attack to C=O 137

O

Oppenaur oxidation 188-190
organometallic compounds :
organocopper compounds 553-555
organolithium compounds 547-552
organomagnessium compounds 523-547
organonitrogen compounds 825
organosilicon compounds 556-564
problems on organometallics 578-587
Orton rearrangement 779, 780
oxidation of 1,2-glycols (by HIO_4 and $Pb(OAc)_4$ 114
Oxidation of alcohols to aldehydes and ketones 111, 112
oxidation of aldehydes and ketones 292
oxidation of aldehydes and ketones by selenium dioxide 293-295
ozonolysis 113

P

9,10-phenanthraquinone 783, 917
periodic acid oxidation 487
Perkin reaction 238-245
Phenanthrene :
Bacon *et al* synthesis of 913
Bardhan-Sengupta synthesis of 910
Bogert-Cook synthesis of 911
Haworth synthesis of 904
molecular overcrowding in phenanthrene 917
properties of 914
Pschorr synthesis of 902
resonating structures of 914
synthesis by Stobbe condensation 908
synthesis of 902-913

phenols :
- chloromethylation of phenols 684, 685
- condensation reactions of phenols 716-717
- C-substitution 679
- diazocoupling reaction of phenols 694-695
- Friedel-Crafts reaction of phenols 679
- Fries rearrangement 680-684
- general methods of preparation 674, 675
- halogenation of phenols 689-692
- *m*-phenylenediamine 780, 781, 782
- nitration of phenols 686-689
- nitrosation of phenols 694
- *o*-phenylenediamine 780, 782, 783, 784
- O-substitution 677
- oxidation of phenols 710-716
- phenylenediamines-distinction of 782
- phloroglucinol 723
- *p*-phenylenediamine 780, 781, 783, 784
- pyrogallol 723
- reactions (ring substitution *vs* O-substitution 676
- sulphonation of phenols 693

phenoquinone 330
Phosphorescence 1
picric acid 855
pinacol-pinacolone rearrangement 128
prototropy 347-350, 356

Q

quinhydrone 329
quinol 323, 324, 722
quinones 322

R

Red shift 5
Reduction of carbonyl compounds
- by DIBAL-H 173
- by $LiAlH_4$ 169-172
- by $NaBH_4$ 173-175

Reduction of α,β-unsaturated carbonyl compounds 321
Reformatsky reaction 164-168
Reimer-Tiemann reaction 134, 135, 652, 696-701
resorcinol 722
Ritter reaction 744
ring -chain tautomerism 362-363
ring strain effect in IR 42
Rosenmund reduction 116, 391

S

spectroscopy 1
stretching frequency :
- effects of hydrogen bonding 49-54
- examples of 50-55
- Sandmeyer reaction 800
- Schmidt rearrangement 753, 754
- Schotten-Baumann technique 388
- selenium dioxide as oxidant 292-295
- silyl enol ethers 224
- sodiumborohydride 173-175
- Sommelet's reaction 119
- spiranes 912
- Stephen's reduction 117, 860
- Stobbe condensation 263-265, 908
- Stork enamine synthesis 341
- Strecker synthesis 274
- sulphonation of phenols 693

T

m-toluidine 774
tautomerism 346-372
TBAF 339
thioacetals and cyclic thioacetals 153-155, 493-496
Thrope nitrile condensation 861
Tischenko reaction 184
TMS as solvent in NMR 69
Transition moment 29
trihydric phenols 723-724
trimethylsilyl choride 339, 570-572
trimethylsilyl cyanide 572-573
trimethylsilyl iodide 574-578
trinitrostilbene 855
trinitrotoluene (TNT) 855

U

2-chlorocyclohexanone 18
Applications of UV-spectroscopy :
benzene and derivatives 16
carbonyl compounds 13
comparison and determination of structure 27
conjugated polyynes and enynes 16
conjugated systems 13
cross conjugated systems 15
designation of UV absorption bands 12
detection of intermediate in reaction 27
determination of configuration 26
dicarbonyl compounds 19
effect of angular distortion, cross-conjugation and steric inhibition of resonance 23
effect of exocyclic double bond on UV-spectra 24
effect of pH on UV spectra 21
effect of s-*cis* and s-*trans* conformation 24
inductive effect on UV spectra 22
position of λ_{max} 20
presence of chromophore 25
steric effect on UV spectra 22
study of structural features in solvents 27
UV spectroscopy and rate of reaction 30
UV-spectra of
α,β-unsaturated carbonyl compounds 18, 19
α,β-unsaturated carbonyl compounds :
nucleophilic addition to 308-314
Ulmann biaryl ether synthesis 499

V

valence tautomerism 347, 364-366
vibrational coupling in IR 45-47, 48
Vibrational frequency factors (mass, nature of vibration, nature of bond electronic effect) 37-41
Victor Meyers reaction 480
Victor-Meyers test 836
Vilsmeyer-Haack formylation 132, 133, 651, 727-730
vinyl ethers 265
Von Pechmann method 807
Von Richter reaction 864-866

W

Williamson ether synthesis 499
Wittig reaction 283-291
Wolff rearrangement 813, 815
Wolf-Kishner reduction 208-210

Y

Ylids (definition and examples) 283
Ylids and Wittig reaction 284

Z

zeropoint energy 34